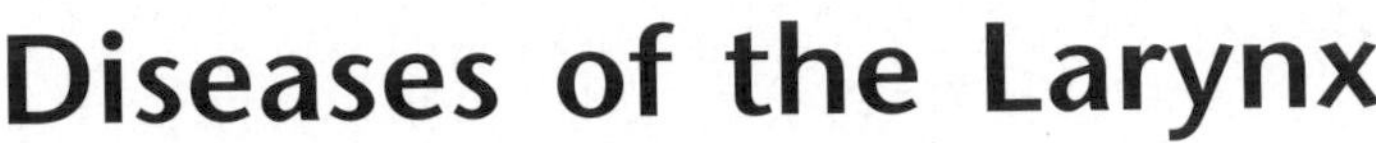

Diseases of the Larynx

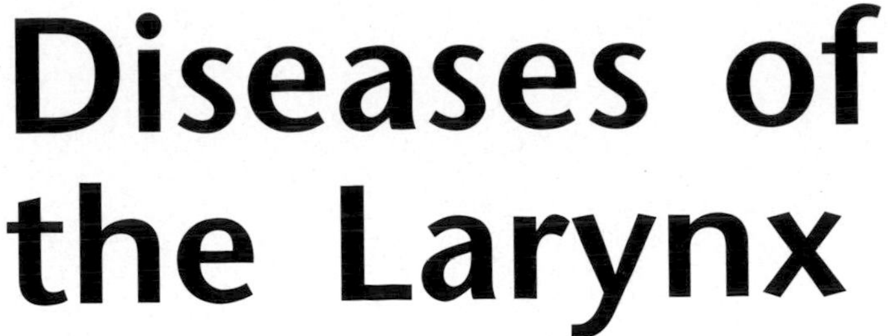

Diseases of the Larynx

Edited by

Alfio Ferlito MD

Professor and Chairman, Department of Otolaryngology – Head and Neck Surgery, Udine University School of Medicine, Udine, Italy

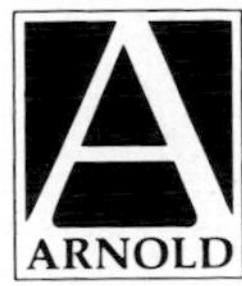

A member of the Hodder Headline Group

LONDON

Co-published in the USA by Oxford University Press Inc., New York

First published in Great Britain in 2000 by
Arnold, a member of the Hodder Headline Group,
338 Euston Road, London NW1 3BH

http://www.arnoldpublishers.com

Co-published in the United States of America by
Oxford University Press Inc.,
198 Madison Avenue, New York, NY10016
Oxford is a registered trademark of Oxford University Press

British Library Cataloguing in Publication Data
A catalogue record for this book is available from the British Library

Library of Congress Cataloging-in-Publication Data
A catalog record for this book is available from the Library of Congress

ISBN 0 340 76016 8

1 2 3 4 5 6 7 8 9 10

Publisher: Nick Dunton
Project Editor: Sarah de Souza
Production Editor: James Rabson
Production Controller: Iain McWilliams

Typeset in 9/11.5 Stone Serif by Scribe Design, Gillingham, Kent
Printed and bound in Great Britain by the University Press, Cambridge

This book is dedicated to my family

Contents

About the Editor

Alfio Ferlito is Professor and Chairman of the Department of Otolaryngology - Head and Neck Surgery at the University of Udine School of Medicine. He graduated in medicine at the University of Bologna. After 2 years at the University of Trieste, he worked at the ENT Department of Padua University from 1970 to 1997.

He has been the author or co-author of more than 300 refereed publications in medical journals. He has already edited a three-volume book entitled *Cancer of the Larynx* (CRC Press, Boca Raton, 1985) and two other books entitled *Neoplasms of the Larynx* (Churchill Livingstone, Edinburgh, 1993) and *Surgical Pathology of Laryngeal Neoplasms* (Chapman and Hall, London, 1996), and co-authored two books entitled *Granulomas and Neoplasms of the Larynx* (Churchill Livingstone, Edinburgh, 1988) and *Surgery for Cancer of the Larynx and Related Structures* (Saunders, Philadelphia, 1996). He has also edited a special issue on *Neuroendocrine Neoplasms of the Larynx* (1991) and co-edited a special issue on *Cancer of the Larynx: Current Concepts in the Treatment of the Neck* (2000), both published in the ORL Journal for Oto-Rhino-Laryngology and its Related Specialties.

He serves as editor, co-editor or reviewer for the following journals: Annals of Otology, Rhinology and Laryngology; Archives of Otolaryngology - Head and Neck Surgery; Laryngoscope; Head and Neck; Journal of Voice; American Journal of Otolaryngology; Acta Oto-Laryngologica (Stockholm); Operative Techniques in Otolaryngology-Head and Neck Surgery; European Archives of Oto-Rhino-Laryngology; Otolaryngology - Head and Neck Surgery; Journal of Laryngology and Otology; ORL Journal for Oto-Rhino-Laryngology and its Related Specialties; Journal of Otolaryngology; Current Opinion in Otolaryngology and Head and Neck Surgery; Journal of Medical Speech-Language Pathology; Auris Nasus Larynx; ORL Digest; ORL Update; American Journal of Rhinology; Otolaryngology Journal Club Journal; Oto-Rhino-Laryngologica Nova; Cancer; Indian Journal of Otology; Applied Pathology; Advances in Therapy; Ear, Nose and Throat Journal; Head and Neck Diseases; Head and Neck Pathology.

He is a member of various scientific societies, i.e. the American Laryngological Association, the Royal Society of Medicine of London, the Collegium Oto-Rhino-Laryngologicum Amicitiae Sacrum, the Japan Laryngological Association, the American Laryngological Rhinological and Otological Society, the American Society for Head and Neck Surgery, the Society of Head and Neck Surgeons, the American Broncho-Esophagological Association, the Association for Research in Otolaryngology, the American Academy of Otolaryngology - Head and Neck Surgery, the International Broncho-Esophagological Society, the Oto-Rhino-Laryngological Society of Japan, the American Association for the Advancement of Science, the Hungarian Association of Otorhinolaryngologists, the Slovenian Association of Otorhinolaryngologists, the New York Academy of Sciences, the Laryngeal Cancer Association, the International Academy of Pathology, the European Working Group on Human Auditory and Vestibular Histopathology, and the Voice Foundation.

He was visiting professor at the Departments of Otolaryngology of the Universities of Yale (1985, 1987, 1988), Pittsburgh (1988) and Amsterdam (1996), and the House Ear Institute of Los Angeles (1993). He collaborated as a member of the World Health Organization's Committee on *Histological Typing of Tumours of the Upper Respiratory Tract and Ear* (published in 1991) and is a member of the Laryngeal Cancer Association's Committee on the Classification of Laryngeal Cancer. He was consultant to Yale University.

One of his chief interests is the promotion of international cooperation in cancer research.

Contributors

Jean Abitbol, MD
Ancien Interne - Chef de Clinique à la Faculté de Médecine de Paris, Otolaryngology – Phoniatre – Laser Surgery, Paris, France

Patrick Abitbol, MD
Interne des Hopitaux de Paris, Otolaryngologist – Head and Neck Surgery, Paris, France

David Albert, FRCS
Great Ormond Street Hospital, London, UK

Peter W Alberti, MB BS PhD FRCS FRCSC
Professor of Otolaryngology, University of Toronto, Senior Staff Otolaryngologist, Toronto General Hospital, Toronto, Ontario, Canada

James C Alex, MD
Assistant Professor, Section of Otolaryngology, Head and Neck Surgery, Director, Division of Facial Plastic and Reconstructive Surgery, Yale University School of Medicine, New Haven, Connecticut, USA

Mário Andrea, MD PhD
Professor of Otolaryngology, Director of Department of Otolaryngology, Faculty of Medicine of Lisbon, University of Lisbon, Lisbon, Portugal

Abigail Arad-Cohen, MD
Instructor in Otolaryngology/Sackler Faculty of Medicine, Tel-Aviv University, Tel-Aviv, Israel

Byron J Bailey, MD FACS
Weiss Professor and Chairman, Department of Otolaryngology, University of Texas Medical Branch, Galveston, Texas, USA

Juan Bartual-Pastor, MD
Professor of Otolaryngology, Director of the ENT Clinic, University of Cadiz, Servicio de Otorrinolaringologia - Hospital Universitario de Puerto Real, Spain

Barry Kenneth Bradbury Berkovitz, BDS MSc PhD
Reader in Anatomy, Division of Anatomy, Cell and Human Biology, GKT School of Biomedical Sciences, King's College London, Guy's Campus, London, UK

Andrew Blitzer, MD DDS
Professor of Clinical Otolaryngology, Columbia University, Director, New York Center for Voice and Swallowing Disorders, New York, USA

Boudewijn J M Braakhuis, PhD
Senior Research Scientist, Section of Tumour Biology, Department of Otolaryngology/Head and Neck Surgery, University Hospital Vrije Universiteit, Amsterdam, The Netherlands

Carol R Bradford, MD
Associate Professor and Division Chief, Head and Neck Division, Department of Otolaryngology, Head and Neck Surgery, The University of Michigan Cancer Center, Ann Arbor, Michigan, USA

Mitchell F Brin, MD
Associate Professor, Bachmann/Strauss Endowed Chair in Neurology, Director, Movement Disorders Program, Mount Sinai School of Medicine, New York, USA

Allan C D Brown, MB ChB FRCA
Associate Professor of Anesthesiology and Otolaryngology, Head and Neck Surgery, Director, Difficult Airway Clinic, University of Michigan, Ann Arbor, Michigan, USA

Antonino Carbone, MD
Director, Division of Pathology, National Cancer Institute, IRCCS, Aviano, Italy

Thomas E Carey, PhD
Distinguished Research Scientist, Director, Laboratory of Head and Neck Cancer Biology, Department of Otolaryngology, Head and Neck Surgery, The University of Michigan Cancer Center, Ann Arbor, Michigan, USA

Amy Y Chen, MD
Fellow, Head and Neck Surgery, MD Anderson Cancer Center, Houston, Texas, USA

Mark C Courey, MD
Assistant Professor, Department of Otolaryngology, Vanderbilt University Medical Center, Nashville, Tennessee, USA

Agnes Czibulka, MD
Chief Resident in Otolaryngology, Instructor, Yale School of Medicine, New Haven, Connecticut, USA

Lawrence W DeSanto, MD
Professor Emeritus, Otolaryngology, Head and Neck Surgery, Department of Otolaryngology-Head & Neck Surgery, Mayo Clinic, Scottsdale, Arizona, USA

Kenneth O Devaney, MD
Associate Professor of Pathology, University of Michigan School of Medicine, Ann Arbor, Michigan, USA

Oscar Dias, MD PhD
Assistant Professor, Department of Otolaryngology, Faculty of Medicine of Lisbon, Lisbon, Portugal

Frederik G Dikkers, MD PhD
Department of Otorhinolaryngology, University Hospital Groningen, Groningen, The Netherlands

Olivier Dupuis, MD
Radiation Oncologist, Centre Jean Bernard, Le Mans, France

Adel K El-Naggar, MD PhD
Professor of Pathology and Head and Neck Surgery, The University of Texas, MD Anderson Cancer Center, Texas Medical Center, Houston, Texas, USA

François Eschwège, MD
Professor, Head of Radiotherapy Department, Institute Gustave Roussy, Villejuif, France

Alfio Ferlito, MD
Professor and Chairman, Department of Otolaryngology - Head and Neck Surgery, Udine University School of Medicine, Udine, Italy

Marvin P Fried, MD FACS
Professor and Chairman, Department of Otolaryngology, Montefiore Medical Center, Albert Einstein College of Medicine, Medical Arts Pavillion, Bronx, New York, USA

Imrich Friedmann, MD DSc FRCS DCP FRCPath
Professor Emeritus of Pathology, University of London, Emeritus Consultant Pathologist, Northwick Park/St Mark's Hospitals, Harrow, UK

C Gaelyn Garrett, MD
Assistant Professor, Vanderbilt University Medical Center, Department of Otolaryngology, Vanderbilt Voice Center, Nashville, Tennessee, USA

Javier Gavilán, MD
Professor and Chairman, Department of Otorhinolaryngology, La Paz, University Hospital, Madrid, Spain

Helmuth Goepfert, MD
Professor and Chairman, Department of Head and Neck Surgery, UTMD Anderson Cancer Center, Houston, Texas, USA

David H Henick, MD
Clinical Assistant Professor, Department of Otorhinolaryngology, Albert Einstein College of Medicine, Montefiore Medical Center, Bronx, New York, USA

Reinhardt J Heuer, PhD
Senior Speech Language Pathologist; Senior Scientist, American Institute for Voice and Ear Research; Adjunct Associate Professor, Department of Speech-Language-Hearing, Temple University, Philadelphia, Pennsylvania, USA

Simon A Hickey, MA FRCS
Consultant Otorhinolaryngologist/Head and Neck Surgeon, Department of Otorhinolaryngology/Head and Neck Surgery, Torbay Hospital, Lawesbridge, Torquay, Devon, UK

Minoru Hirano, MD PhD
President of Kurume University, Kurume, Japan

Satoshi Imaizumi, PhD
Associate Professor, Department of Speech and Cognitive Sciences, Graduate School of Medicine, University of Tokyo, Tokyo, Japan

John K Joe, MD
Resident Physician, Section of Otolaryngology, Department of Surgery, Yale University School of Medicine, New Haven, Connecticut, USA

Jonas T Johnson, MD FACS
Professor, Departments of Otolaryngology and Radiation Oncology, University of Pittsburgh School of Medicine, The Eye and Ear Institute Building, Pittsburgh, Pennsylvania, USA

Edward E Kassel, DDS MD FRCPC
Associate Professor, Department of Medical Imaging, University of Toronto, Mount Sinai Hospital, Toronto, Ontario, Canada

Thomas Keane, MB MRCPI FRCPC
Professor and Chair, Division of Radiation Oncology, University of British Columbia, British Columbia Cancer Agency, Vancouver, British Columbia, Canada

James H Kelly, MD FACS
Associate Professor, Department of Otolaryngology, Head and Neck Surgery and Department of Neurology, Johns Hopkins Medical Institutions, Chairman, Department of Otolaryngology, Head and Neck Surgery, Greater Baltimore Medical Center, Baltimore, Maryland, USA

Helen Kim, MD
Department of Head and Neck Surgery, Montefiore Medical Center, Bronx, New York, USA

John A Kirchner, MD
Professor Emeritus, Yale University School of Medicine, Department of Surgery, Section of Otolaryngology, New Haven, Connecticut, USA

Peter Kitzing, MD PhD
Department of Otolaryngology, Section of Phoniatrics, University Hospitals, Malmö, Sweden

Peter D Lacy, MB FRCSI
Fellow, Department of Otolaryngology, Washington University School of Medicine, St Louis, Missouri, USA

Arthur M Lauretano, MD FACS
Instructor in Otology and Laryngology, Harvard Medical School, Boston, Massachusetts, USA

Kelvin C Lee, MD
Associate Professor, Department of Otolaryngology, New York University, New York City, New York, USA

Dennis T H Lim, FRCS(Edin) MMeD(Surg) FRCS(Glasgow)
Department of Surgery, Singapore General Hospital, Singapore

Hans F Mahieu, MD PhD
Professor, Department of Otolaryngology/Head and Neck Surgery, University Hospital Vrije Universiteit, Amsterdam, The Netherlands

G Christoph Mahnke, MD
Department of Otorhinolaryngology, Head and Neck Surgery, University of Kiel, Kiel, Germany

Arnold G D Maran, MD FRCS
Professor of Otolaryngology, University of Edinburgh, Lauriston Building, The Royal Infirmary, Edinburgh and Royal College of Surgeons of Edinburgh, Nicolson Street, Edinburgh, UK

Trevor McGill, MD FACS FRCSI
Clinical Director of Otolaryngology, Children's Hospital, Associate Professor of Otology and Laryngology, Harvard Medical School, Boston, Massachusetts, USA

Jesus E Medina, MD
Paul and Ruth Jonas Professor and Chairman, University of Oklahoma Health Sciences Center, Department of Otorhinolaryngology, Oklahoma City, Oklahoma, USA

Neil Molony, MD BSc FRCS
Specialist Registrar, Department of Otolaryngology, Royal Infirmary of Edinburgh, Edinburgh, UK

Bernard J Moxham, BSc PhD BDS
Chairman of Anatomy, School of Molecular and Medical Biosciences, Anatomy Unit, University of Wales, Cardiff, UK

Yasushi Murakami, MD PhD
Emeritus Professor, Department of Otolaryngology, Kyoto Prefectural University of Medicine, Kawaramachi, Kamikyo-ku Kyoto, Japan

Andrew H Murr, MD
Associate Professor, Department of Otolaryngology, Head and Neck Surgery, University of California, San Francisco, California, USA

H Bryan Neel III, MD PhD
Professor and Past Chairman, Department of Otolaryngology, Head and Neck Surgery, Mayo Medical Center, Rochester, Minnesota, USA

Arnold M Noyek, MD FRCS
Professor of Otolaryngology and Radiology, University of Toronto, Mount Sinai Hospital, Toronto, Ontario, Canada

Laurie A Ohlms, MD
Assistant in Otolaryngology, Children's Hospital, Assistant Professor of Otology and Laryngology, Harvard Medical School, Boston, Massachusetts, USA

Jan Olofsson, MD PhD
Professor and Chairman, Department of Otolaryngology – Head and Neck Surgery, Haukeland University Hospital, Bergen, Norway

Robert H Ossoff, DMD MD
Guy M. Maness Professor and Chairman, Department of Otolaryngology, Vanderbilt University Medical Center, Nashville, Tennessee, USA

Jay F Piccirillo, MD FACS
Associate Professor and Director, Clinical Outcomes Research Office, Department of Otolaryngology – Head and Neck Surgery, Washington University School of Medicine and Attending Staff, Barnes-Jewish Hospital, St Louis, Missouri, USA

Lou Reinisch, PhD
Assistant Professor and Director of Laser Research, S-2100 Medical Center North, Department of Otolaryngology, Vanderbilt University Medical Center, Nashville, Tennessee, USA

William J Richtsmeier, MD PhD
Chief of Otolaryngology – Head and Neck Surgery, Bassett Health Care, Cooperstown, New York, USA

Frank L Rimell, MD
Assistant Professor, Pediatrics and Otolaryngology, University of Minnesota, Minneapolis, Minnesota, USA

Alessandra Rinaldo, MD
Clinical and Research Fellow, Department of Otolaryngology – Head and Neck Surgery, Udine University School of Medicine, Udine, Italy

Clark A Rosen, MD
Assistant Professor, Department of Otolaryngology, School of Medicine, Department of Communication Science and Disorders, School of Health and Rehabilitation Sciences, University of Pittsburgh, Pittsburgh, Pennsylvania, USA

Deborah Caputo Rosen, RN PhD
Clinical Psychologist, Bala Cynwyd, Pennsylvania, USA

Douglas A Ross, MD FACS
Chief of Otolaryngology, West Haven VA Medical Center, Associate Professor of Surgery, Section of ENT, New Haven, Connecticut, USA

Umberto Saffiotti, MD
Scientist Emeritus, National Cancer Institute, National Institutes of Health, Bethesda, Maryland, USA

Clarence T Sasaki, MD
Chief of Otolaryngology, Yale-New Haven Medical Center, Charles W Ohse Professor, Yale School of Medicine, Chief, Section of Otolaryngology, Vice-Chairman, Department of Surgery, New Haven, Connecticut, USA

Robert Thayer Sataloff, MD DMA
Professor of Otolaryngology - Head and Neck Surgery, Jefferson Medical College; Chairman, Department of Otolaryngology - Head and Neck Surgery, Graduate Hospital; Adjunct Professor, Department of Otolaryngology - Head and Neck Surgery, The University of Pennsylvania; Adjunct Professor, Department of Otolaryngology - Head and Neck Surgery, Georgetown University School of Medicine, Philadelphia, Pennsylvania, USA

Harm K Schutte, MD PhD
Professor of Physiology and Pathophysiology of Voice Production, Director of Groningen Voice Research Laboratory, Department of Biomedical Engineering, Faculty of Medical Sciences, University of Groningen, Groningen, The Netherlands

Jatin P Shah, MD FACS Hon FRCS(Edin) Hon FDSRCS(Lond)
Chief, Head and Neck Service, Professor of Surgery, EW Strong Chair in Head and Neck Oncology, Memorial Sloan-Kettering Cancer Center, New York, USA

Carl E Silver, MD
Chief, Head and Neck Surgery, Montefiore Medical Center, Bronx, New York; Professor of Surgery, Professor of Otolaryngology, Albert Einstein College of Medicine, Bronx, New York, USA

J Gershon Spector, MD FACS
Professor, Department of Otolaryngology – Head and Neck Surgery, Division of Head and Neck Oncology, Washington University School of Medicine, St Louis, Missouri, USA

Gordon B Snow, MD PhD
Professor and Chairman, Department of Otolaryngology/Head and Neck Surgery, University Hospital Vrije Universiteit, Amsterdam, The Netherlands

Marshall Strome, MD MS FACS
Professor of Otolaryngology, Chairman, Department of Otolaryngology and Communicative Disorders, The Cleveland Clinic Foundation, Cleveland, Ohio, USA

Randal S Weber, MD FACS
Professor and Vice Chair, Department of Otorhinolaryngology, Director, Center for Head and Neck Cancer, University of Pennsylvania Health System, Philadelphia, Pennsylvania, USA

Ranny van Weissenbruch, MD PhD
Department of Otorhinolaryngology, University Hospital Groningen, Groningen, The Netherlands

Charles Williams Vaughan, MD FACS
Chief, Department of Otolaryngology, Head and Neck Surgery, Associate Clinical Professor in Otolaryngology, Boston University School of Medicine, Boston, Massachusetts, USA

Mark C Witte, MD
Instructor, Department of Otorhinolaryngology, Mayo Medical School, Rochester, Minnesota, USA

Ian J Witterick, MD FRCS
Department of Otolaryngology, Mount Sinai Hospital, Toronto, Ontario, Canada

Gregory T Wolf, MD
Professor and Chair, Department of Otolaryngology, Head and Neck Surgery, University of Michigan, Ann Arbor, Michigan, USA

Thomas P U Wustrow, MD FACS
Professor Dr. med., HNO Gemeinschaftspraxis, München, Germany

Eiji Yanagisawa, MD FACS
Clinical Professor of Otolaryngology, Yale University School of Medicine; Attending Otolaryngologist, Yale-New Haven Hospital, New Haven CT; Attending Otolaryngologist, Hospital of St Raphael, New Haven, Connecticut, USA

Robert F Yellon, MD
Assistant Professor of Otolaryngology, University of Pittsburgh School of Medicine; Co-Director, Department of Pediatric Otolaryngology; Director of Clinical Services, Department of Pediatric Otolaryngology, Children's Hospital of Pittsburgh, Pittsburgh, Pennsylvania, USA

Preface

The larynx is a complex and dynamic structure and many different functions have been identified in the literature. However, three functions are the most important for the clinician: these are protective, respiratory and phonatory. As the amount of our knowledge relating to the numerous diseases continues to expand dramatically, it has become increasingly difficult to keep up-to-date on the latest issues that relate to the larynx.

The purpose of this book is to review current knowledge of laryngeal diseases in a single volume, with contributions from pediatric and adult laryngologists, voice and speech pathologists, anatomists, pathologists, radiologists, anesthesiologists, oncologists, chemotherapists, radiotherapists, and other specialists with a particular interest in the larynx.

The contributors have been selected in view of their standing, international repute and vast experience. It has been a pleasure to collaborate with these distinguished authorities and there has been a valid and continuous exchange of opinions and information during the preparation of the text.

Diseases of the Larynx is a large multi-authored compendium intended primarily for otolaryngologists and is also recommended for speech and language pathologists and for all physicians involved in the diagnostic, clinical, therapeutic and prognostic problems. It is our earnest hope that the reader will find the book useful, informative and enjoyable.

I would like to thank the editors and publishers of several medical journals for allowing me to reproduce illustrations and a few chapters.

My grateful thanks also go to Frances Coburn for her help in shaping the English of the chapters assigned to myself.

Finally, I would like to thank Nicholas J Dunton, Director of Science, Technology and Medical Publishing, and the entire production staff of Arnold for their advice, hard work and encouragement throughout the preparation of the book.

Alfio Ferlito, MD

History of laryngology

Peter W Alberti

The larynx was the first internal organ to be routinely examined; as this skill developed during the 1850s, so did the specialty of laryngology. Before that time the larynx was but one of many internal organs the function of which was known through the ages, but which only came into prominence when obstruction of the airway by croup and diphtheria led to strangulation and death.

The first written description of diphtheria is given by the Greek Aretaeus who was also famous for discovering the Eustachian tubes. Later Hippocrates also described diphtheria as it involved the throat, but beyond the epiglottis, the larynx was a mystery. On the other hand, he and the Greeks placed much emphasis on the nature of the voice in the diagnosis of disease.

Celsius, one of the master physicians and scientists of Rome, described Angine Grave but it was left to Galen, the father of Roman medicine, to bring science to the larynx. Galen was a physician from Pergamon, close to the Aegean coast of modern Turkey, who operated a private health spa before moving to Rome where he was a much sought after physician, a great scientist and medical writer. He was the first to describe the intralaryngeal muscles, noting six pairs, and was able to distinguish those that opened the vocal cords from those that closed them. He was aware of the laryngeal ventricles and their function in producing mucus to lubricate the cords, which he described as the seat of the voice. He also noted that section of the recurrent nerves in pigs leads to loss of phonation.

There matters rested for more than a millennium. The teachings of Galen remained immutable; dissections were proscribed by the Church and autopsies were not undertaken. Changes occurred slowly in the thirteenth and fourteenth centuries but gathered speed in the Renaissance. Only then was the human body studied systematically, and with it, the larynx. The great anatomist Vesalius described three cartilages of the larynx and the two arytenoids, the muscles and the intrinsic musculature of the cords. The first book about the organs of speech and hearing and perhaps the most beautiful, *De Vocis Auditusque Organis* by Casserius,[15] was published in 1600. He drew perfectly the anatomy of the larynx and the ear, in man and animals and related the two organs together as the organs of communication. Nicolas Habicot, in 1602, described the movements of the larynx and in particular how it rose during deglutition and dropped back to its normal position again when the swallow was completed. He is also remembered for turning tracheotomy into a practical operation.[64]

Many medical schools were founded in the eighteenth century as a direct result of the Enlightenment, that heady international explosion of intellectual discussion that brought with it a belief in rational thought and material explanation of many phenomena. In medicine the movement was led from Leiden and included the establishment of the medical schools in Edinburgh and Vienna. It can be argued that the search for knowledge that this engendered led directly to the nineteenth century development of specialties, including laryngology.

Andersch gave a good description of the innervation of the larynx in 1790 and Swan, the English anatomist, painstakingly elaborated this in a work published in 1830. Henle described various epithelia of the larynx in the early nineteenth century.[74] According to Weir,[74] Antoine Ferrein was the first to undertake acoustic experiments on an excised larynx and showed that air passing closed vocal cords produced a sound, and that the intensity of the sound depended upon the force of the air. He thought the vocal folds were the equivalent of violin strings, giving them the name vocal cords. It was Dutrochet in 1806 who correctly compared the vibration of the vocal folds to a passive double reed.[74]

For many centuries croup and diphtheria were the most important diseases to involve the larynx because they were common and lethal. For example, in the sixteenth and seventeenth centuries an epidemic of croup spread through Europe. This was known in Spanish as *garrotillo* after the infamous instrument of the inquisition. In the eighteenth and the nineteenth centuries also, croup and diphtheria killed in large numbers. Croup was well described by Home[30] of England in 1765, by Bard[7] of Philadelphia in 1771, and by Boerhaave,[9] who devoted one aphorism to it, 'angina aquosa, oedematosa, catarrhosa tenuis, est impedimenta, vel dolend respirandi, vel degltiendi exercitatio, cum tumore lymphatico partium, quibus illa fit, vel vicinarum'. As far as diphtheria was concerned, matters were so serious that Napoleon offered a prize for work about the management of the disease following the death of a nephew. It was finally well categorized by Bretonneau[11] in his famous book of 1826.

Understanding of the structure and function of the body, and with it the larynx, was an essential prelude to an improved understanding of what malfunctioned in disease, although management languished until the nineteenth century when the true nature of infections became known with the work of Pasteur and Koch. Whilst autopsies were gradually becoming more common in the eighteenth century, the larynx was rarely examined. Morgagni[52] in 1761 was the first to give a postmortem account of laryngeal infection. The first textbook on the pathology of the larynx was published by Albers[1] in 1829, the same year that Laennec, the founder of auscultation of the chest, described the autopsy appearance of the larynx in a case of tuberculosis. Laryngeal tuberculosis was common, frequently occurring as an end stage in those suffering from pulmonary phthisis. It was well described by Trousseau and Belloc[69] in a book that remains relevant today. In the nineteenth century, chronic infections of the larynx were common and tumors much rarer than today because people did not live so long nor smoke so much. One of the earliest clinical texts devoted entirely to the larynx, by Ryland,[57] published in 1837, devotes only 8 of a total of more than 300 pages to tumors.

In the early nineteenth century, vocal problems were common and serious. In the New World, nonconformist ministers rode long distances between towns, preached for hours and then moved on to preach some more. Their voice disorders gave rise to the generic term 'dysphonia clericorum',[50] the voice dysfunction of any professional speaker whether teacher, lawyer or preacher. Even in the pre-laryngoscopic days there were practitioners specializing in diseases of the larynx. A notable exponent, Horace Green,[22] the father of American laryngology, was deft at blindly applying the larynx sponges soaked in medication carried on whale bone probangs. There was a noisy controversy, during which he was roundly condemned as a fake because of the common belief that it was impossible to enter the larynx, disproved only when, in a patient with a tracheotomy, he was able to demonstrate that a sponge on a probang introduced through the mouth could be passed through the larynx and out through the tracheostome. He too, was one of the first to directly excise a laryngeal polyp in a child where, because the larynx is in a higher place than in an adult, it is easier to see directly through the mouth. Zeitels[76] believes he came close to being the founder of direct laryngoscopy. Nonetheless, until the discovery of mirror laryngoscopy and the development of techniques to exploit it, laryngology remained an arcane art.

It cannot be emphasized enough that the emergence of a specialty of laryngology depended not only on the ability to see the larynx, great feat though that was, but also on the development of a whole system of medical care based around this technique, illumination, instrumentation, understanding of these processes and therapeutic techniques. Let us follow these developments.

There had been many attempts to see into internal organs using specula and various sources of illumination. Up to the early nineteenth century, only sunlight was really bright enough, for artificial light consisted of candles or simple oil lamps. Nonetheless, by the early 1800s attempts were made to develop instruments to look into and illuminate such organs as the bladder, the vagina, the uterus, and the larynx. Bozzini developed a light carrier with many different specula to illuminate various organs. The light was poor, the instrument was a curiosity but he is recognized as an innovator. His travails are beautifully described by the Reuters.[56] The Englishman Babington developed a device like two spoons hinged together, one of which was used to depress the tongue and the other of which was a mirror to look at the larynx. He recognized the need to open an air space at the back of the mouth but the mechanism was inappropriate. Avery, another Englishman, built a cumbersome device which had all the features of modern indirect laryngoscopy, a head band carrying a perforated mirror with a light in front (in this case a candle) and a mirror, attached by a tube to the front of the head band, to insert into the patient's mouth.[47] Apparently he did view the larynx but did not wish to publish his findings until he could corroborate what he saw by photographs!

Another pioneer deserves mention – Pierre Segalas,[60] a urologist who realized that one tube could be used both to illuminate an organ and to see it. Previous efforts had relied on twin tubes. The simple expedient of a perforated 45° mirror placed in a tube, which allowed the observer to see straight down the tube and light to be reflected from the mirror also down the tube, made all endoscopy possible. The same concept was used by Desmoreaux[18] who became known as the father of endoscopy, leaving the pioneer Segalas unrecognized for almost a century. In other countries too, people were experimenting with endoscopy, including examination of the larynx.

It fell to a singing teacher, Manuel Garcia, to bring the matter to the fore. The time was right and the circumstances propitious. Garcia, one of a family of singing teachers, was anxious to know how the voice was produced and, seeing sunlight reflected off a window while walking through the gardens of the Tuilleries in Paris, in 1854, had a flash of inspiration. He obtained a dental mirror and a hand mirror and in the quiet of his hotel room reflected sunlight onto the dental mirror which he held in the back of his throat and saw his larynx in the same hand mirror that was bringing in the sun's rays. As a trained singer he was able to control his tongue and larynx and suppress a gag reflex. Garcia not only saw the larynx, but where he differed from others is that he made observations on its function, which he communicated to the Royal Society of London.[2]

The story moves to Vienna. Türk,[70] a neurologist, independently was experimenting with laryngeal mirrors but became aware of the work of Garcia. He could only work in the summer, because of lack of appropriate lighting in the winter, and had difficulty controlling his own larynx (it was a slow, laborious study). His mirrors were borrowed by Czermak, a physician in Vienna and physiologist in Budapest, born in Prague, who had greater facility with the laryngeal mirror and an inventive turn of mind; he produced a series of mirrors and other devices to make laryngoscopy easier. A feud developed between the two about priority, which became known as the Turkish wars and did much to popularize laryngology. Incidentally, as neither would recognize the claim of the other, this led to Garcia being labeled the father of laryngology. Vienna became the center of a new medical specialty.

It is difficult now, one and a half centuries later, to appreciate what impact this discovery made. The larynx was the first internal organ that could be reliably examined. It gave rise to a rich and beautifully illustrated literature. There were more books written about laryngology in the first decade after its discovery in 1856 than about any subject before or since until the discovery of the roentgen ray 40 years later. At first there was a profusion of texts describing what was seen, often with color illustrations produced by artists looking over the shoulders of clinicians like Türk[70] and Von Bruns;[72] the modern reader can still marvel at their artistic merit and didactic value. With these illustrations and descriptions came a better understanding of the pathology and clinical findings, which in turn led to more and improved therapy for laryngeal disease.

As so often happens when a subject becomes clinically important, basic science is found wanting and develops rapidly alongside. Johannes Muller, the great German physiologist, in the first part of the eighteenth century made many experiments using excised larynges and tracheas to produce vocalization and the correlates of human sound. He was the first to include the pharynx and mouth in his experimental setup. Details are given in Willemot's exhaustive text.[75] In 1871, Van Luschka published what is probably the best text of laryngeal anatomy ever to have been printed;[71] Semon worked hard on the functional innervation of the larynx,[61] and in 1891, Hajek gave a description of laryngeal lymphatics which would support the concept of partial and particularly horizontal, partial laryngectomy.[25]

Much was done to turn the technique of laryngeal inspection into the specialty of laryngology. The laryngeal mirror at various times was attached to the light and table, with the patient's head moved on to the mirror, which had many shapes, square and lozenge, oval and ultimately simply round. The handle was bent in many ways and at many angles until the simple straight form of today was found to be adequate. Light was shone onto the laryngeal mirror in a variety of ways, sometimes daylight in a darkened room through a hole in the blind, sometimes from a mirror fixed on a table lamp, and sometimes from a mirror attached to the examiner, at first held in the teeth and then on spectacles and later on a head band. It was soon perforated to provide parallax free illumination.

Candles were an inadequate light source, and sunshine, if present at all, was only available between the hours of 11:00 and 14:00 in the winter of northern Europe. It took the development of the argon light and the gas mantle to provide enough illumination for this specialty; the electric light invented by Swan and popularized by Edison was certainly the key to endoscopy, although it was originally shunned by most mirror laryngoscopists until well into the twentieth century.

Many instruments were devised to remove lesions of the larynx indirectly while looking through the laryngeal mirror: forceps to remove lesions, applicators to paint on medication, electrocautery to burn growths, all in the days before any anesthetic. The laryngologist held the mirror in one hand and the instrument in the other, while the patient held their own tongue. Some examiners became remarkably deft at the technique and none more so than an Englishman, Morrell MacKenzie.[47] He practiced in London, had many foreign fellows, a huge number of patients and published widely. He thus was influential in spreading knowledge of the newly fledged specialty. However, it should be noted that two Americans, Ellsworth and Solis Cohen, attended Czermak's first course and laryngology was quickly established in New York.[66]

Likewise, in Europe, in addition to Vienna,[51] early clinics were established by Merkel in Leipzig and by Voltolini in Breslau.[75] Voltolini was the inventor of an oxyhydrogen incandescent light that much aided examination both of the ear and the larynx. Clinics were rapidly established in France and Italy and the discipline was born, but as a medical subspecialty practiced by chest physicians, neurologists and general internists. If major surgery was required, a general surgeon collaborated. Indeed, Felix Semon's contract with St Thomas' Hospital in London, appointing him as laryngologist, expressly forbade him to put knife to skin and whenever a tumor needed excision, he collaborated with Sir Henry Butlin, a general surgeon.[61]

The honor of being the first surgeon laryngologist probably goes to the American, Solis Cohen. His textbook,

Diseases of the Throat,[16] remains a valuable source today and arguably has had as great an impact in English speaking countries as MacKenzie's famous text, *A Manual of Diseases of the Nose and Throat*.[49] Cohen's surgical results were excellent, the first to perform a total laryngectomy in the USA, the first to have a patient survive 20 years, the first to separate the air and food passages in total laryngectomy, the first to have a patient develop esophageal speech, a great man whose life is well summarized by Zeitels.[77]

For the first 20 years, laryngology was practiced without local anesthetic. Türk had attempted to anesthetize the larynx with a mixture of morphine and wine and failed.[70] Koeller[42] only discovered the anesthetic properties of cocaine in the 1880s and applied it widely but it was his disciple Jelinek[37] who first described its use in the larynx for this purpose. Fauvel[19] had used cocaine earlier but as a speech stimulant. This use remained in common practice for singers until the middle of the twentieth century, popularized by the opera singer Nelly Melba as an essential ingredient of Melba's mix.

The early clinicians dealt with infections, tumors and neurological disorders such as cord palsies. To begin with they did not distinguish between benign and malignant disease, between polyps, nodes and cancers and certainly they did not recognize the difference between malignancy occurring in the larynx and that in the pharynx.

Chronic infections dominated: syphilis, typhus, tuberculosis. Clinical practices before Pasteur's concepts were understood and Koch's postulates introduced actually did much to spread disease. Camel hair brushes were used on patient after patient, often without cleaning, to apply medications such as silver nitrate to the surface of the larynx, a perfect way to spread disease. And yet new knowledge was gained and the specialty grew.

Great efforts were made to photograph the larynx to demonstrate both the normal and diseased state, which were quickly successful. In Vienna stereo photographs of the larynx were taken by Czermak in the early 1860s,[45] using magnesium ribbon as the illuminating source, a device reminiscent of today's high-speed cameras to which the patient was applied; others, like the American, French, who in 1871 published a text entitled, *On a Perfected Method of Photographing the Larynx*, relied on sunlight and small plate film.[20] These techniques were not bettered until Holinger produced his brilliant photographs in the late 1940s.[29]

Laryngology was initially a medical specialty, but surgical approaches were developed in parallel, mainly to deal with malignant diseases of the area. These will be dealt with later.

The second half of the nineteenth century can be characterized as the era of indirect laryngoscopy practiced by medical laryngologists and a steady evolution of various forms of laryngectomy by general surgeons. Surgery and laryngology came together with the invention of direct endoscopic procedures, laryngoscopy and bronchoesophagoscopy. There were attempts to devise endoscopes, such as MacKenzie's esophagoscope, but they were not successful. It was Kirstein of Berlin who first described direct laryngoscopy in 1895,[40] an invention that was dependent upon adequate electric light. Three years later Killian developed bronchoscopy and also adopted direct laryngoscopy[38] and added direct suspension to laryngoscopy, a technique which is still in use today.[39] Brünings, a distinguished pupil of Killian, did much to develop the techniques of direct laryngoscopy.[14] He demonstrated the importance of posterior pressure on the thyroid cartilage and developed an attachment for the laryngoscope that did this semiautomatically; he even introduced a telescope for magnification, both ideas well ahead of their time. Initially this procedure was undertaken under local anesthetic in a sitting patient with the examiner standing behind the patient looking over the head. His book was translated into English in 1912 by Howarth[13] and greatly influenced the development of laryngology in the UK. Simultaneously in the USA, Jackson developed bronchoesophagology and laryngology.[35] He was a wonderful technical exponent of endoscopy and a great teacher.

Returning to the nineteenth century, diphtheria too, continued to be a major problem with frequent epidemics and a high mortality rate from laryngeal obstruction. Tracheostomy was practiced, but with a high perioperative mortality. This was a terrible ordeal for a child, already choking to death and then subjected to a throat cutting procedure, without anesthetic. Other methods of management were eagerly sought.[3] Intubation of the larynx was introduced by Bouchut[10] in the late 1850s but only perfected by O'Dwyer approximately 25 years later.[53] He devised intralaryngeal tubes of different sizes, together with a device to introduce them and another to effect removal, all in the awake child. These tubes saved thousands of lives and were in regular use until the 1940s.

Throughout the mid-nineteenth century there had been attempts to operate externally upon the larynx, including several isolated descriptions of laryngofissure for tumor or papilloma. This required considerable fortitude on the part of the patient, who was usually awake and not anesthetized, as well as courage and skill on the part of the surgeon.

It is difficult to overestimate the impact of anesthesia in the development of surgery. In all branches, including surgery of the larynx, it led to rapid and often dramatic advances. The great German surgeon Trendelenburg[68] described a technique of endotracheal anesthesia using chloroform that greatly facilitated surgery of the upper airways, making it possible as a controlled procedure.

The pioneering German general surgeons applied the scientific approach to this area as well as to other parts of the body. They devised the operation of laryngectomy, and Langenbeck was the first to complete experiments in dogs; however, he could not find a suitable patient, so it fell to Billroth to perform the first successful semi-total laryngectomy on New Year's Eve, 1874. Billroth left the epiglottis in place and did not separate the air and food passages. He also introduced a speech prosthesis, which effectively plugged the opening between the pharynx and the trachea. Although he believed separation of the trachea and pharynx would be necessary, he was so pleased with the success of the original operation that he felt the latter was unnecessary, delaying successful laryngectomies for years. His operation was published,[23] and was widely practiced with dismal results (although there were exceptions such as the laryngectomy of Bottini whose patient survived 15 years and that of Solis Cohen). Patients died at surgery, and postoperatively of 'schluck pneumonia' (aspiration pneumonia), so that Gluck wrote of the period 1870–1880:

> *a normal course surely was seldom seen by the old authors, erysipelas, phlegmon, secondary haemorrhage, mediastinitis, bronchitis and septic broncho-pneumonia, septicaemia, shock, particularly delirium cardis with consequent cardiac paralysis, carried off the patient.*[21]

Of the first 103 total laryngectomies, 40% died within 8 weeks of the operation and a further 20% had a short-term recurrence, only nine patients surviving 12 months.[74]

Two things were necessary to turn the tide, one surgical, the other pathological. Surgical therapy was disastrous until the pharynx and trachea were totally separated. Whilst Gluck claimed credit, the need for this was recognized in many parts of the world, almost simultaneously. I like to think that it was that giant of American laryngology, Solis Cohen, who first introduced it. The second issue was that classification of diseases and organs was virtually nonexistent. Operations were done for the wrong disease, such as tumors at the base of the tongue, in the pharynx and in the esophagus as well as in the larynx. It was only with Isambert's suggestion,[33] in 1876, later amplified by Krishaber[43] that laryngeal carcinoma be separated into intrinsic and extrinsic, that the different natural histories began to be appreciated and the indications for surgery became clearer.

In addition to total laryngectomy, two other operations were tried because of the need to preserve voice wherever possible. Laryngofissure was originally suggested by Desault, and undertaken by Pelletan in 1788 to remove a foreign body from the larynx;[75] Brauers of Louvain, Belgium in 1834 was the first to use the procedure for removal of a growth. It was undertaken from time to time during the mid-nineteenth century, but with varying success. Billroth performed eight such procedures between 1870 and 1884, but only one patient was cured. It was greeted with skepticism, but once the indications were secure, towards the end of the nineteenth century Semon, Butlin, Moure and others such as Chiari, Schmigelow, Delavan and Jackson helped to define the procedure as extremely effective for cancer confined to the middle of one vocal cord. It was still possible if disease extended to the anterior commissure, and could always be converted to a hemi- or total laryngectomy. It became the mainstay of treatment for early cancer of the vocal cords.[36] Billroth, in 1878, also introduced the operation of vertical partial laryngectomy,[58] which Semon later defined as 'an operation in which no less than an entire wing of the thyroid cartilage and possibly additionally, an arytenoid and parts of the cricoid are removed'.

At the beginning of the twentieth century, the stage was set for rapid advances in laryngology and the management of cancer, although the results for the surgical treatment of laryngeal cancer were truly dismal. Thus in 1909, at the New York Academy of Medicine, Bryson Delavan, in discussing papers by Chevalier Jackson, G Brewer and J Wright, stated:

> *after much study and observations of this subject, I am compelled to believe that operations in general for the cure of carcinoma of the larynx have, in the aggregate, materially lessened the sum total of the duration of human life.*[17]

And yet, results were already improving. The technique of total laryngectomy became standardized and the results were quite good. However, surgeons and patients were seeking means to retain or restore the voice which was, as it is now, a problem. As we have seen, the original total laryngectomy by Billroth was accompanied by the introduction of a voice prosthesis, several types of which were developed. As the original procedure maintained a fistula between the respiratory and digestive tract, they were relatively successful. However, as soon as both passages were separated, prosthesis use was a major problem, and many types were invented, some of which, like the electrolarynx, are still in use today. By the late 1920s, small tumors were treated by laryngofissure, which preserved voice, and larger ones by total laryngectomy, with its attendant loss of voice. St Clair Thomson and Colledge give an excellent revue of the status in western Europe in the 1920s.[67]

Efforts were made to retain voice in tumors of intermediate size by reintroducing vertical hemilaryngectomy which, after the deplorable results of Gluck and other early pioneers, was not really used for a quarter of a century until, in 1929, Hautant[27] revived the procedure with the important technical improvement of primary closure over a stent to maintain the lumen. Only when a better appreciation of the indications for the procedure was arrived at, was its value truly realized. Quintal of Uruguay, after 1928, was undertaking partial laryngectomies of many types: his most famous pupil was Alonso, who developed a huge practice and already in 1944, reported on the treatment of 800 personal cases of carcinoma of the larynx.[8] He credits Huet,[32] in a paper published in Paris in 1938, with removing a ventricular tumor, the middle of the hyoid, the pre-epiglottic space and the upper part of the thyroid cartilage, i.e., with developing the horizontal partial laryngectomy.

Alonso is generally regarded as the modern father of horizontal partial laryngectomy. He restated the goals of surgery for carcinoma of the larynx when he wrote, 'We feel that the two principal objectives to be striven for are, first, the preservation of the life of the patient and second, the preservation, if possible, of the function of the organ of speech'.[4] Ogura[55] made the next major contribution, in converting the operation into a one state procedure, finding it was not necessary to leave a pharyngostome.

For those with a total laryngectomy, much was tried to restore useful speech, but until recently little was uniformly successful. Esophageal voice was already recognized by Solis Cohen, but although taught up to the present day, it is a difficult technique that works well only in the minority of patients. Various artificial noise makers were tried: vibrators on the neck, reeds in external pipes from the tracheostome to the mouth, vibrating devices in oral prostheses, implanted electric vibrators and more besides; only the external electrolarynx has withstood the test of time, and it produces a monotonous sound. Surgeons attempted to develop fistulae that would allow air to pass from the trachea to the pharynx, but not food or saliva in the opposite direction. The pioneering efforts of Guttman,[24] who was the first to create a tracheohypopharyngeal fistula and of Asai,[5,6] who popularized the concept by developing various types of laryngoplasty, as he termed them, must be recognized, although their techniques were not sufficiently reliable to become generally adopted. However, the concept of a fistula that allowed air to pass into the hypopharynx which acted as a pseudolarynx by vibrating, was correct. Singer and Blom[62] and Singer *et al.*[63] developed a simpler plastic fistula which is inserted at or after laryngectomy and allows speech without aspiration. This, or similar valves have become the mainstay of post-laryngectomy speech rehabilitation.

Radiotherapy, a nonsurgical treatment of laryngeal cancer, is an ideal way of preserving voice. Its early history as a treatment for laryngeal disease is well reviewed by Lederman,[44] who lists no less than eight different clinicians who used x-ray treatment in the larynx in 1901 and 1902. Low-voltage external irradiation, and intraluminal radium both produced perichondritis of the laryngeal cartilages as well as great excoriation of the skin. The first really effective radiotherapeutic treatment for intrinsic cancer of the larynx was implantation of radium needles inside the laryngeal skeleton, developed by Finzi and Harmer,[26] which was the standby from the mid-1930s until high-voltage external beam irradiation was introduced with the cobalt bomb in the mid-1950s.

The management of benign laryngeal diseases also underwent great change. Operative endoscopic laryngology was revolutionized by the introduction of the operating microscope by Scalco *et al.*[59] Jako and Kleinsasser simultaneously but separately developed techniques of microlaryngoscopy, developing the instruments and methodology and teaching widely about them. Kleinsasser's textbook proved a landmark in this area,[41] because he not only described a technique, he also showed how it could be incorporated into practice.

It is difficult to imagine that the laser was only invented in the mid-1950s. It was adopted into medicine very early, especially in ophthalmology. There were several separate efforts made to develop a CO_2 laser, correctly considered appropriate for soft tissue surgery, but early bench models were huge. It was to the credit of Strong and Jako[65] that they introduced the first working model, attached to a microscope and used for a variety of microlaryngeal procedures, of a family of devices that have subsequently had application in many branches of otolaryngology as well as other disciplines.

The respiratory movement of the vocal cords had been well known since the discovery of the laryngeal mirror; phonatory movements waited until the adaptation of the stroboscope for laryngoscopy by Oertel in 1895.[54] The device was a mechanical one, widely distributed but difficult to use. Fletcher's high-speed photography of the vocal cords in action, produced by the Bell Laboratories, marked a further major advance. Electronic stroboscopes were introduced in the 1950s but relied upon the U-shaped stroboscopic tube, which did not produce adequate light. It took the development of the spot stroboscopic bulb, created for the American moon missions, to make the modern stroboscopes possible.

Telescopes have been used to view the larynx indirectly and directly. Proud, of Kansas City, turned a nasopharyngoscope in an infant and viewed the larynx. He demonstrated the feasibility of the technique but the lenses and illumination were inappropriate. With the development of the Hopkins rod system, and adequate illumination provided by glass fibers,[31] telescopes became practical for all endoscopic use, including laryngoscopy, and have been widely adopted.

The other great advance has been the introduction of the flexible endoscope. The principle was described by Tyndall in the nineteenth century and forgotten until it was rediscovered by Baird in 1927; he was famous as the founder of the first public television broadcasting system. However, it had no practical importance until the 1970s when new methods of making fibers were developed. Subsequently it has revolutionized the practice of all forms of aerodigestive endoscopy.

Laryngologists have been interested in the phonatory and speech-producing function of the larynx. Casserius' landmark book[15] has been referred to and there were publications in the eighteenth century such as Von Rempelen's book on the mechanisms of speech[73] and, indeed, Garcia was primarily interested in the vocal function of the larynx. MacKenzie published one of the first books on hygiene of the vocal cords.[48] Luschinger and Arnold's book of 1949[46] marks a watershed in our knowledge of speech and he and others were responsible for the development of a separate specialty, phoniatrics. At the same time, in North America, the clinical management of speech split off as a nonmedical discipline, speech and language pathology.

Preserving or improving the voice has always been a major goal, the surgical approaches to which are broadly described as phonatory surgery, whether this be careful techniques to remove lesions from the larynx or the restoration of function after paralysis of a vocal cord. Early techniques for dealing with benign laryngeal lesions were often crude, and right up to modern times frequently consisted of stripping the epithelium from the vocal cord, which often led to scarring of the regenerated epithelium to the underlying muscle, obliteration of the loose areolar layer between the two, and continuing or worsened hoarseness. The microscope provided the tool and Hirano,[28] who has made a lifelong study of how the cords vibrate in phonation, both in health and disease, the theoretical underpinning of the need to maintain the substantia propria. As a result surgeons have altered techniques for dealing with laryngeal lesions, becoming much more conservative in their surgical approaches, whether by laser or by microsurgical instruments, and thus achieving much better phonatory results.

Likewise, the weak breathy voice associated with unilateral vocal cord paralysis has been a challenge to laryngologists from early days. Successive generations have appreciated that if it were possible to medialize the affected cord, the voice might improve. Already Brünings, in the early years of the twentieth century, developed a technique for the endolaryngeal injection of hard paraffin;[12] the concept was correct but the oil gradually dispersed and produced an inflammatory reaction that led to the abandonment of the technique. It was revived by Lewy in the 1970s, who injected a much more inert material, Teflon, using Brüning's technique with great success. Nonetheless, it was not perfect and Isshiki *et al.*[34] adapted another older technique, that of buttressing the cord with a piece of cartilage. Originally undertaken through a laryngofissure, he devised a method of inserting it through a window cut in the thyroid ala which has been widely adopted.

The history of laryngology mirrors many of the developments of medicine in the past 150 years: anatomical studies giving way to physiological investigation; the emergence first of descriptive and then of experimental pathology as a guide to clinical management; ever bolder surgical techniques made safe by better anesthetic techniques and a better understanding of pathology and microbiology; and all tempered by an increasing respect for function and a wish to prevent handicap.

References

1. Albers JFH. *Die Pathologie und Therapie der Kehlkopfkrankheiten.* Leipzig, 1829. Cited by Weir.[74]
2. Alberti PW. The evolution of laryngology and laryngectomy in the mid 19th century. *Laryngoscope* 1975; **85:** 288–98.
3. Alberti PW. Tracheotomy versus intubation. A 19th century controversy. *Ann Otol Rhinol Laryngol* 1984; **93:** 333–7.
4. Alonso JM. Conservation of function in surgery of the larynx: bases, techniques and results. *Trans Am Acad Ophthalmol Otolaryngol* 1952; **56:** 722–30.
5. Asai R. Laryngoplasty. *J Jpn Broncho-Esophagol Soc* 1960; **12:** 1–3. Cited by Asai.[6]
6. Asai R. Laryngoplasty after total laryngectomy. *Arch Otolaryngol* 1972; **95:** 114–19.
7. Bard S. *An Inquiry into the Nature, Cause and Cure of Angina Suffocativa.* New York: Inslee and Car, 1771. Cited by Willemot.[75]
8. Barretto PM. The historical development of laryngectomy. IV. The South American contribution to the surgery of laryngeal cancer. *Laryngoscope* 1975; **85:** 299–321.
9. Boerhaave H. *Aphorismi de Cognoscendis et Curandis Morbis.* Lugduni Batavorum: J. Vander Linden, 1709. Cited by Willemot.[75]
10. Bouchut E. D'une nouvelle methode de traitement de croup par le tubage du larynx. *Bull Acad Natl Med* 1858; **23:** 1160–2. Cited by Willemot.[75]
11. Bretonneau PF. *Des Inflammations Speciales du Tissu Muqueux et en Particulier de la Diphtérite, ou Inflammation Pelliculaire.* Paris: Crevot, 1826. Cited by Willemot.[75]
12. Brünings W. Eine neue Behadlungsmethode einseitiger Rekurrenslahmungen. *Verh Vereins Dtsch Laryngol, Würzburg.* 1911. Cited in Brünings.[13]
13. Brünings W. *Direct Laryngoscopy, Bronchoscopy and Oesophagoscopy.* London: Baillière, Tindall and Cox, 1912.
14. Brünings W, Albrecht, W. *Direkte Laryngoskopie, Bronchoskopie und Oesophagoskopie.* Wiesbaden: Bergmann, 1910.
15. Casserius J. *De Vocis Auditusque Organis Historia Anatomica.* Ferrariae, 1600.
16. Cohen JS. *Diseases of the Throat.* New York: William Wood, 1872.
17. Delavan JB. Discussion – carcinoma of the larynx. *Proc NY Acad Med* 1909.
18. Desmoreaux AJ. 'Endoscope'. In: *Dictionnaire de Medicine et Chirurgie Practique.* Vol 13. Paris: Baillière, 1870. Cited by Willemot.[75]
19. Fauvel C-H. Cited by Jelinek.[37]
20. French TR. On a perfected method of photographing the larynx. *NY Med J* 1884; **4:** 653–6.
21. Gluck T. In: Katz, Preysing, Blumenfeld (eds). Kabitzch, Würzburg. *Handbuch der Speziellen Chirurgie.* IV band. Cited by Thomson SC, Colledge L.[67]
22. Green H. *Diseases of the Air Passages.* New York: Wiley and Putnam, 1846.
23. Gussenbauer C. Ueber die erster durch Th. Billroth am menschen ausage fuhert Kehlkopf-Extirpation und die Anwendung eines künstlichen Kehlkopfes. *Arch Klin Chir* 1874; **17:** 343–56.
24. Guttman MR. Tracheohypopharyngeal fistulization: a new procedure for speech reproduction in the laryngectomized patients. *Trans Am Laryngol Rhinol Otol Soc* 1935; **41:** 219–26.
25. Hajek J. Anatomische untersuchungen über das larynxödem. *Langenbecks Arch Klin Chir* 1891; **42:** 46–93.
26. Harmer WD. *The Relative Value of Radiotherapy in the Treatment of Cancers of the Upper Air-Passages.* London: Murray, 1932.
27. Hautant A. A propos du traitment du cancer du larynx. *Ann Mal Oreil Larynx* 1929; **48:** 671–4.
28. Hirano M. *Clinical Examination of Voice.* New York: Springer-Verlag, 1981.
29. Holinger P. Endoscopic photography in otolaryngology and broncho-esophagology. *Proceedings of the 4th*

International Congress in Otorhinolaryngology 1951; **2:** 691–711. Cited by Willemot.[75]
30. Home F. *An Inquiry into the Nature, Cause and Cure of Croup*. Edinburgh: Kincaid and Bell, 1765. Cited by Willemot.[75]
31. Hopkins HH, Kapany NS. A flexible fibrescope using static scanning. *Nature* 1954; **173:** 39–41. Cited by Weir.[74]
32. Huet PC. Présentation de malades. Cancer de l'epiglottectomie. *Ann Otolaryngol Chir Cervicofac* 1938; **57:** 1052–5. Cited by Willemot.[75]
33. Isambert E. Contribution à l'étude du cancer du laryngé. *Ann Mal Oreil Larynx* 1876; **2:** 1–23.
34. Isshiki N, Morita H, Okamura H, Hiramoto M. Thyroplasty as a new phonosurgical technique. *Acta Otolaryngol (Stockh)* 1974; **78:** 451–7.
35. Jackson C. *Peroral Endoscopy and Laryngeal Surgery*. St Louis: Laryngoscope Co., 1915.
36. Jackson C, Jackson CL. *Cancer of the Larynx*. Philadelphia: Saunders, 1939.
37. Jelinek E. Das Cocain als anästheticum und analgeticum für den pharynx und larynx. *Wien Med Wochenschr* 1884; **34:** 1334–7, 1364–7. Cited by Majer EH, Skopec M.[51]
38. Killian G. Ueber directe Bronchoskopie. *Munch Med Wochenschr* 1898; **45:** 844–7. Cited by Willemot.[75]
39. Killian G. Die Schwebelaryngoscopie. *Arch Laryngol Rhinol (Berl)* 1912; **26:** 277–317.
40. Kirstein A. Autoskopie des Larynx und der Trachea (Laryngoscopia directa, Euthyskopie, Besichtigung ohne Spiegel). *Arch Laryngol Rhinol (Berl)* 1895; **3:** 156–64.
41. Kleinsasser O. *Mikrolaryngoscopie und Endolaryngeale Mikrochirurgie*. Stuttgart: Schattauer-Verlag, 1968.
42. Koeller C. Über die Verwendung des Cocain zur Anästhesirung am Auge. *Wien Med Wochenschr* 1884; **34:** 43–4.
43. Krishaber M. Contribution à l'étude du cancer du larynx. *Gaz Hebd Med Chir* 1879; **16:** 518–23.
44. Lederman M. History of radiotherapy in the treatment of cancer of the larynx, 1896–1939. *Laryngoscope* 1975; **85:** 333–53.
45. Lesky E. *The Vienna Medical School of the 19th Century*. Baltimore: Johns Hopkins University Press, 1976.
46. Luschinger R, Arnold GE. *Lehrbuch der Stimme und Sprachheilkunde*. Wien: Springer-Verlag, 1949.
47. MacKenzie M. *The Use of the Laryngoscope in Diseases of the Throat, with an Appendix on Rhinoscopy*. London: Churchill, 1865.
48. MacKenzie M. *Essay on Growths in the Larynx*. London: Churchill, 1871.
49. MacKenzie M. *Disease of the Pharynx, Larynx and Trachea*. New York: William Wood, 1880.
50. Mackness J. *Dysphonia Clericorum*. London: Longman, 1848.
51. Majer EH, Skopec M. *Zur Geschichte der Oto-rhino-laryngologie in Osterreich*. Wien: Brandstatter Verlag, 1985.
52. Morgagni GB. *De Sedibus et Causis Morborum per Anatomen Indagatis, libri quinque*. Typog. Remondimiani Venetiis, 1761. Cited by Willemot.[75]
53. O'Dwyer J. Two cases of croup treated by tubage of the glottis. *NY Med J* 1885; **46:** 146–51.
54. Oertel M. Das Laryngo-Stroboskop und die Laryngostroboskopiche Untersuchung. *Arch Laryngol Rhinol (Berl)* 1895; **3:** 1–16.
55. Ogura JH. Supraglottic subtotal laryngectomy and radical neck dissection for carcinoma of the epiglottis. *Laryngoscope* 1958; **68:** 983–1003.
56. Reuter HJ, Reuter MA. *Philip Bozzini and Endoscopy in the 19th Century*. Stuttgart: Max Nitze Museum, 1988.
57. Ryland FA. *A Treatise on the Diseases and Injuries of the Larynx and Trachea*. London: Longman, 1837.
58. Salzer F. Larynxoperationen in der Klinik Billroth, 1870–1884. *Langenbecks Arch Klin Chir* 1885; **31:** 848–88, cited by Willemot.[75]
59. Scalco AN, Shipman WF, Tabb HG. Microscopic suspension laryngoscopy. *Ann Otol* 1960; **69:** 1134–8.
60. Segalas PS. *Traite de Retentions d'Urine et de Maladies qu'elles Produisent*. Paris: Mequingon-Marvis, 1823. Cited by Willemot.[75]
61. Semon F. *The Autobiography of Sir Felix Semon*. London: Jarrolds, 1926.
62. Singer MI, Blom ED. Tracheo-esophageal puncture: a surgical prosthetic method for post laryngectomy speech restoration. *3rd Int Plast Reconstr Surg Head Neck*. New Orleans, 1979: Abstract.
63. Singer MI, Blom ED, Hamaker RC. Further experience with voice reconstruction after total laryngectomy. *Ann Otol Rhinol Laryngol* 1981; **90:** 498–502.
64. Stevenson RS, Guthrie D. *A History of Otolaryngology*. Edinburgh: Livingstone, 1949.
65. Strong MS, Jako GJ. Laser surgery in the larynx. Early clinical experience with continuous CO_2 laser. *Ann Otol* 1972; **81:** 791–8.
66. *The American Laryngological Association, 1878–1978, Washington DC. A Centennial History*. Washington, DC: American Laryngological Association.
67. Thomson SC, Colledge L. *Cancer of the Larynx*. London: Paul, Trench, Trubner and Co., 1930.
68. Trendelenburg F. Erfahrungen über die Tamponade der Trachea. *Langenbecks Arch Klin Chir* 1873; **15:** 352–68. Cited by Willemot.[75]
69. Trousseau A, Belloc H. *Traité Pratique de la Phthisie Laryngée, de la Laryngite Chronique et des Maladies des Voix*. Paris: Baillière, 1837.
70. Türk L. *Atlas zur Klinik der Kehlkopfkrankheiten*. Wien: Braumüller, 1860.
71. Van Luschka H. *Der Kehlkopf des Menschen*. Tübingen: Laupp, 1871.
72. Von Bruns V. *Atlas zur Laryngoskopie und Laryngoskopichen Chirurgie*. Tübingen, Laupp, 1865.
73. Von Rempelen W. *Mechanismus der Menschlichen Sprache*. Wien: Degen, 1791.
74. Weir N. *Otolaryngology. An Illustrated History*. London: Butterworths, 1990.
75. Willemot J. Naissance et développement de l'oto-rhinolaryngologie dans l'histoire de la médicine. *Acta Otorhinolaryngol Belg* 1981; **35(Suppl 2,3,4):** 1–1622.
76. Zeitels SM. Premalignant epithelium and microinvasive cancer of the vocal fold: the evolution of phonomicrosurgical management. *Laryngoscope* 1995; **105(Suppl 67):** 1–51.
77. Zeitels SM. Jacob Da Silva Solis-Cohen: America's first head and neck surgeon. *Head Neck* 1997; **19:** 342–6.

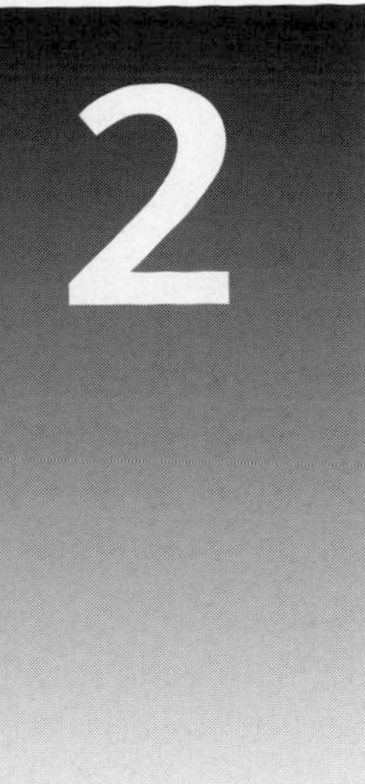

Laryngeal development

David H Henick

Over the century, conflicting concepts regarding the development of the human larynx have evolved. During the past decade, solid-model reconstructions of primate and human specimens have prompted a reexamination of existing theories. In contrast to earlier theories, more recent observations of laryngeal development adequately explain the occurrence of laryngotracheal malformations.

There have been several landmark studies on the origin and development of the larynx. Probably the most influential was the contribution of His in 1885.[7] His proposed that the respiratory primordium (RP) appeared as an outpouching from the cephalic portion of the pharynx by the third week of gestation. He described a tracheoesophageal septum, which began as a groove behind the RP and ascended to the level of the fourth pharyngeal pouch, dividing the foregut lumen into a ventral trachea and a dorsal esophagus. Zaw-Tun and Burdi rejected the concept of a tracheoesophageal septum and demonstrated that the separation of the trachea and esophagus was not the result of an ascending process, but of the descending outgrowth of the RP.[14]

A series of schematic drawings in this chapter portray the developing embryo in whole-section, coronal, axial and sagittal planes during the embryonic and fetal periods.[5] This presentation clarifies the changing anatomic relations that occur over time.

Figure 2.1 illustrates His' concept of an ascending tracheoesophageal septum, which begins at the level of the RP, dividing the foregut to form the trachea and esophagus.[7] Zaw-Tun and Burdi, however, found that the RP does not remain static, but is a descending out-growth of the foregut lumen, which ultimately gives rise to the entire respiratory system.[14]

Figure 2.2, an illustration taken from Arey, represents the classic description of laryngeal development.[1] This dorsal view of the developing laryngopharyngeal region is

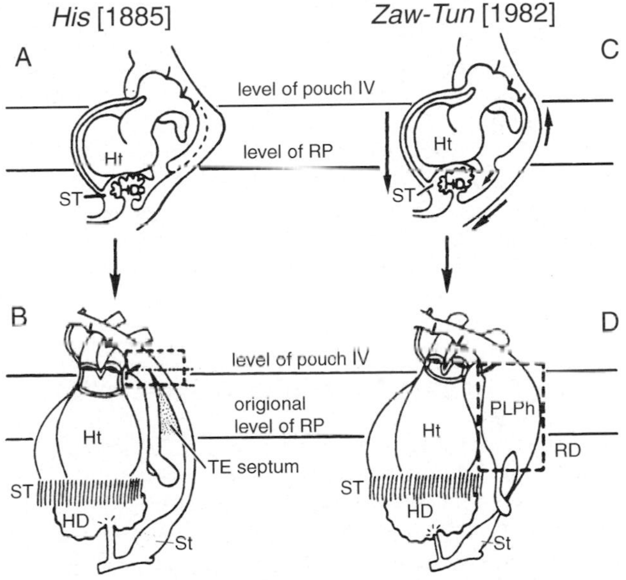

Figure 2.1 *Comparison of the His and the Zaw-Tun concepts of laryngeal development. His described an ascending tracheoesophageal septum (TES), whereas Zaw-Tun demonstrated that development results from descending outgrowth of the respiratory primordium (RP). The stippled box represents the distance between the fourth pharyngeal pouch and the tracheoesophageal separation point. According to His, this distance decreased over time; Zaw-Tun showed that the distance remained constant. HD, hepatic diverticulum; HT, heart; PLPh, primitive laryngopharynx; RD, respiratory diverticulum; RP, respiratory primordium; St, stomach.*

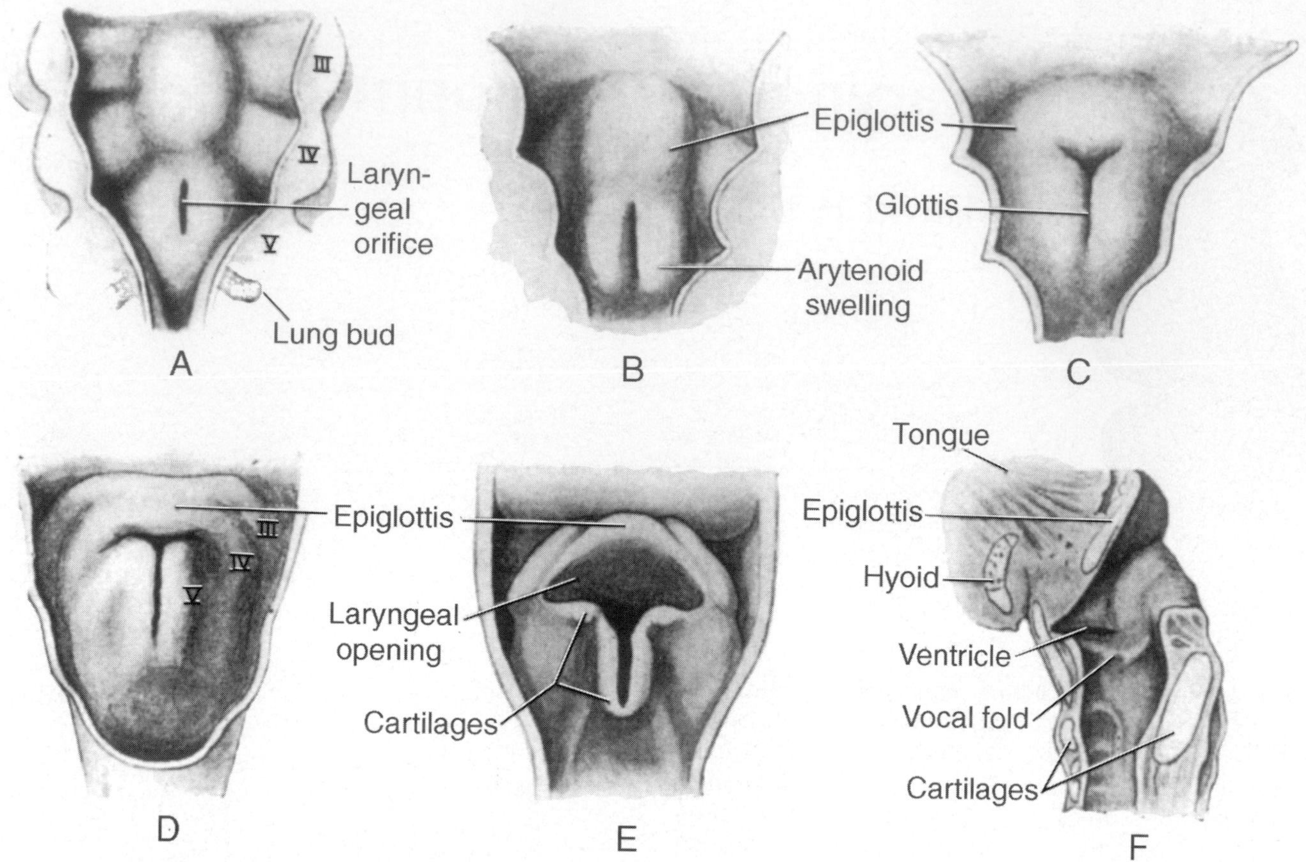

Figure 2.2 *Laryngeal development according to Arey[1]. This dorsal view of the developing laryngopharyngeal region (A–E) is similar to an endoscopic perspective. F shows a sagittal section of the adult larynx.*

similar to the endoscopic perspective. However, these illustrations provide only one perspective of laryngeal development, so the dynamic changes occurring in the axial, sagittal, and coronal planes of the developing embryonic larynx are not clearly demonstrated.

As a reference point, Figure 2.2(a) demonstrates the level of the pharyngeal floor, which is equivalent to the level of the fourth pharyngeal pouch. Because of the conflicting theories of development, the sagittal slit seen in the pharyngeal floor (labeled 'laryngeal orifice') has been interpreted by several authors to represent different anatomic sites. Frazer believed that it represented the opening to the infraglottic region,[3] Kallius, the opening to the glottic region,[8] and Zaw-Tun and Burdi, the opening to the supraglottic larynx.[14]

There is also disagreement regarding where the obliteration of the pharynx – the epithelial lamina (EL) – occurs during normal development. Kallius believed that it occurred above the level of the pharyngeal floor, giving rise to arytenoid swellings,[8] whereas Frazer believed that it occurred below the pharyngeal floor, giving rise to the infraglottis.[3] Walander, however, has demonstrated that it occurs precisely at the level of the pharyngeal floor, giving rise to the glottic region.[13]

Current concepts

The human embryologic collection available in the Carnegie Institute, located at the Armed Forces Institute of Pathology in Washington, DC, and the wax-model reconstructions of the human larynx prepared by Dr Harry Zaw-Tun from the Patton Embryologic Collection at the University of Michigan School of Medicine, were used for most the observations presented in this chapter.

Human development is divided into the embryonic period (the first 8 weeks of gestation) and the subsequent

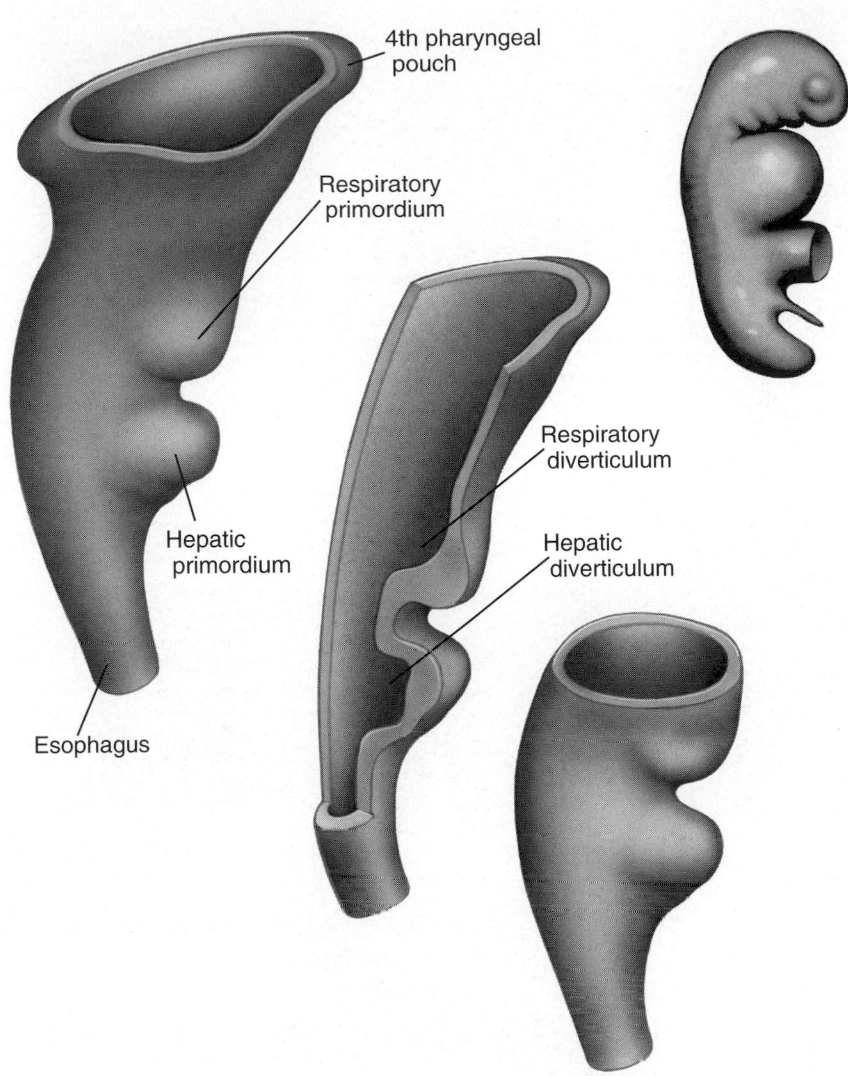

Figure 2.3 *Epithelial lining of the developing laryngopharyngeal region of phase I embryo. The respiratory primordium (RP) is first seen separated from the hepatic primordium (HP) by the septum transversum.*

fetal period (the last 32 weeks of gestation).[4] According to the Carnegie staging system, the embryonic period has 23 stages of development. Each stage has a characteristic feature not seen in a previous stage. Laryngeal development is first seen in stage 11. In this chapter, laryngeal development during the embryonic period is divided into eight phases; each is correlated with the corresponding Carnegie stages. Although development occurs as a continuum, studying these eight phases facilitates an understanding of the important developmental events. Several critical stages occur during the development of the laryngeal vestibule, and developmental arrests at these critical stages can give rise to correlational congenital anomalies.

Phase I

Figure 2.3 shows the epithelial lining of the developing laryngopharyngeal region of a phase I embryo (Carnegie stage 11). The first sign of the respiratory system is seen as an epithelial thickening along the ventral aspect of the foregut known as the RP. The RP is separated from the hepatic primordium by the septum transversum, a structure that eventually develops into the central tendon of the diaphragm. In this early stage, the foregut lumen is widely patent.

Phase II

Figure 2.4 shows the laryngopharyngeal regions of a Carnegie stage 12 embryo in comparison with a mature fetal larynx viewed in a midsagittal plane. The respiratory diverticulum (RD) is a ventral outpouching of the foregut lumen, which expands into the RP. The site of the origin of the RD is called the primitive pharyngeal floor; the primitive pharyngeal floor eventually develops into the infraglottic region of the adult larynx. The primitive

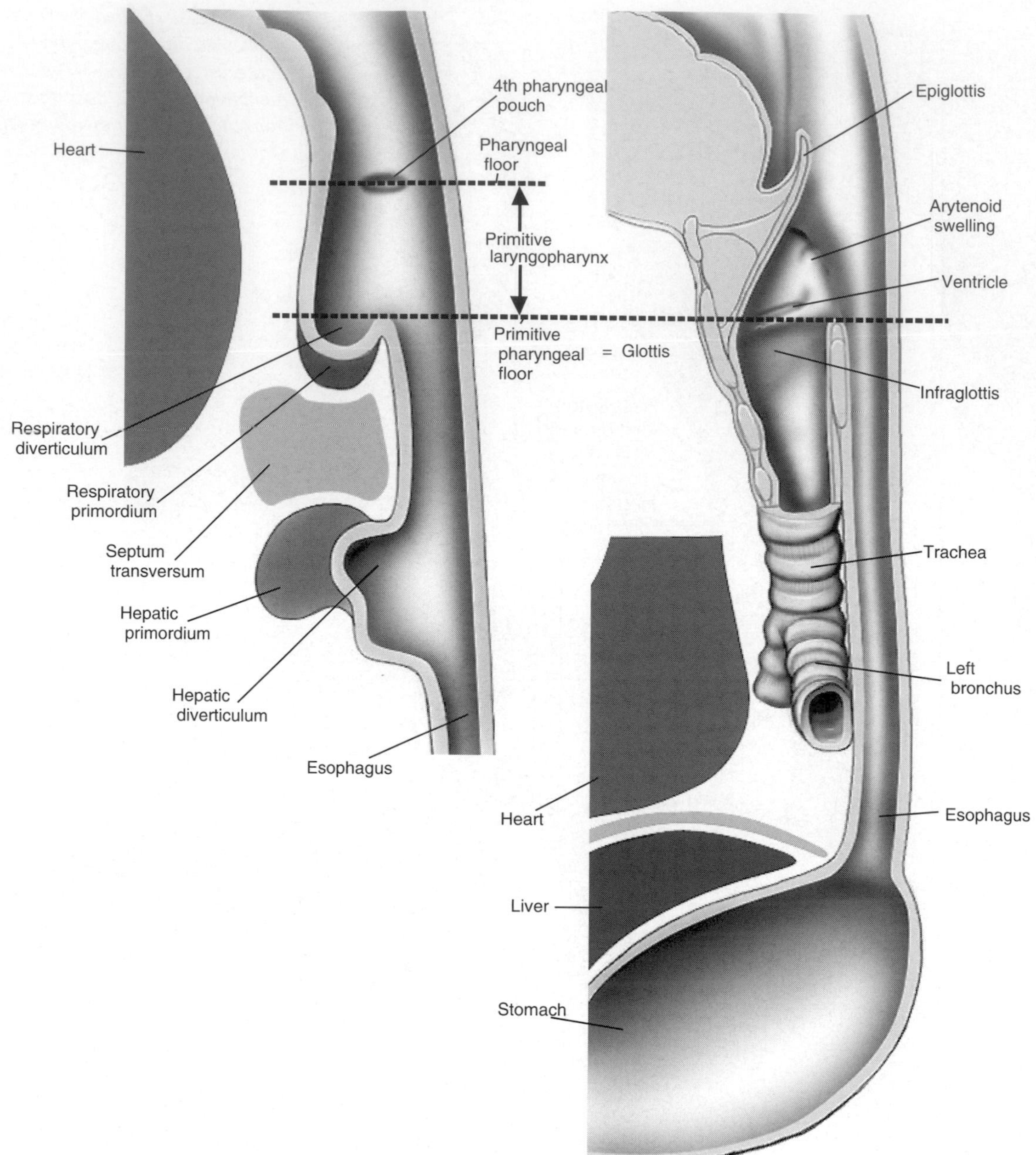

Figure 2.4 *Laryngopharyngeal regions of a phase II embryo and the mature fetal larynx. The primitive pharyngeal floor (PPhF) eventually develops into the glottic region. The cephalic portion of respiratory diverticulum (RD) develops into the infraglottic (IG) region. The primitive laryngopharynx (PLPh) develops into the supraglottic larynx.*

pharyngeal floor is separated from the pharyngeal floor – the level of the fourth pharyngeal pouch – by a segment of foregut originally classified by Zaw-Tun and Burdi as the primitive laryngopharynx; this eventually becomes the supraglottic larynx.

Figure 2.5 shows the later portion of Carnegie stage 12. The RD gives rise to bilateral projections called bronchopulmonary buds, which eventually develop into the lower respiratory tract. Removing the dorsal wall of the foregut offers a view of the pharyngeal floor, as demonstrated by Arey.[1] The vertical slit represents the entrance into the primitive laryngopharynx.

Dynamic changes to the developing foregut region occur at this and subsequent stages. For example, the heart and the hepatic primordium proliferate at a rapid rate on opposing surfaces of the septum transversum. These differential forces, exerted on the adjacent foregut region, lead to a dramatic lengthening of the foregut. The result can be seen as the distance between the RP and the hepatic primordium increases.

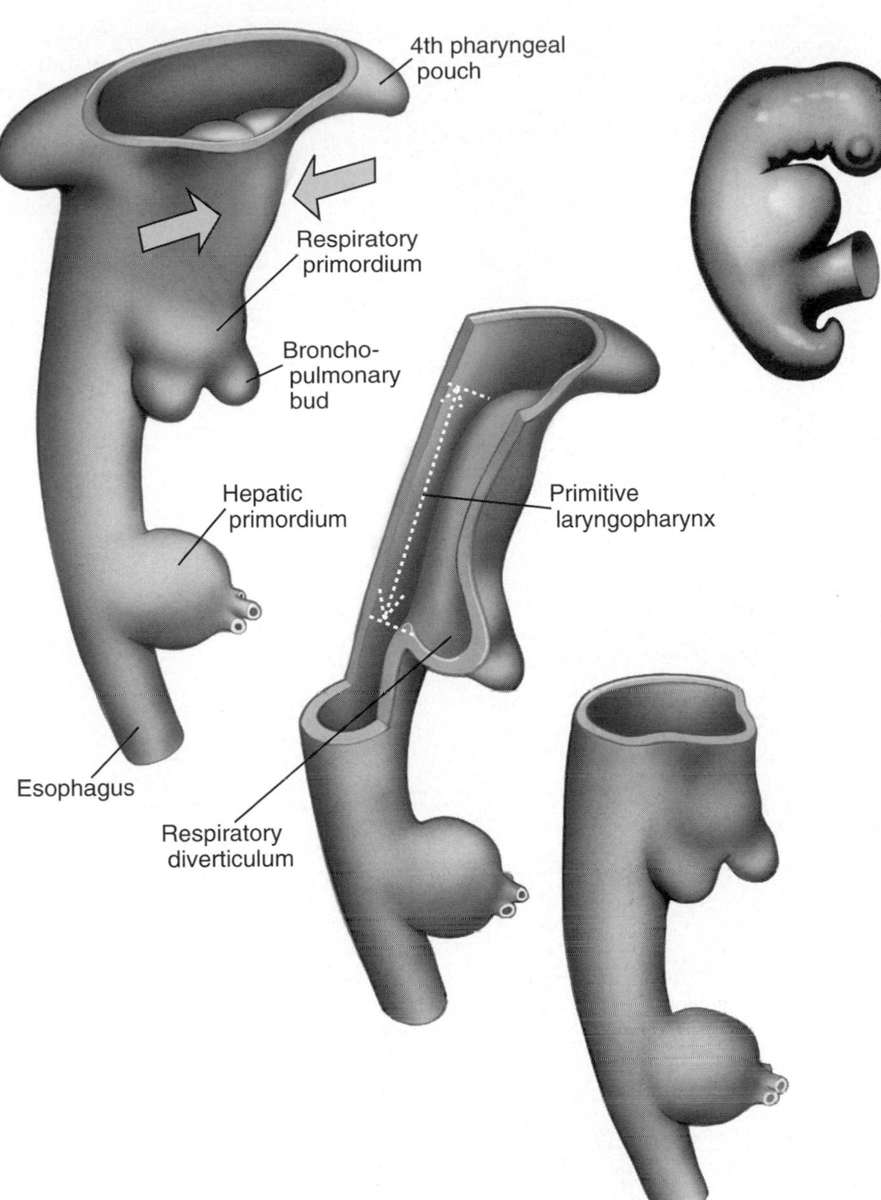

Figure 2.5 *Later portion of phase II. The respiratory diverticulum (RD) gives rise to bronchopulmonary buds (BPB). The vertical slit represents the entrance into the primitive laryngopharynx (PLPh).*

Phase III

Figure 2.6 portrays a phase III embryo (Carnegie stages 13 and 14). As the upper foregut region and the RD migrate superiorly, the bronchopulmonary buds are drawn caudally and inferiorly.[11] As a result, the two main bronchi develop; the carina develops; the infraglottis develops from the cephalic aspect of the RD, with the characteristic shape of an inverted triangle when sectioned in the sagittal plane and an upright triangle when sectioned in the coronal plane (analogous to the conus elasticus in the adult larynx); and the distance between the carina and the RD lengthens, giving rise to the trachea.

During this stage, dramatic lengthening of the trachea and esophagus occurs. Anatomically, the esophagus is close to the carina. Vascular compromise to the developing esophagus may cause esophageal atresia or tracheoesophageal fistula (Figs 2.7 and 2.8). Vascular compromise to the trachea at this phase may cause tracheal agenesis or tracheal stenosis with complete tracheal rings (Fig 2.8). These anomalies are associated with relatively normal laryngeal and pulmonary development because the insult is limited to the region of the developing trachea.

Phase IV

Figure 2.9 represents a phase IV embryo (Carnegie stage 15). The primitive laryngopharynx (PLPh) is seen as the foregut segment extending from the fourth pharyngeal pouch above to the infraglottis below. The ventral portion of this foregut region becomes compressed bilaterally by

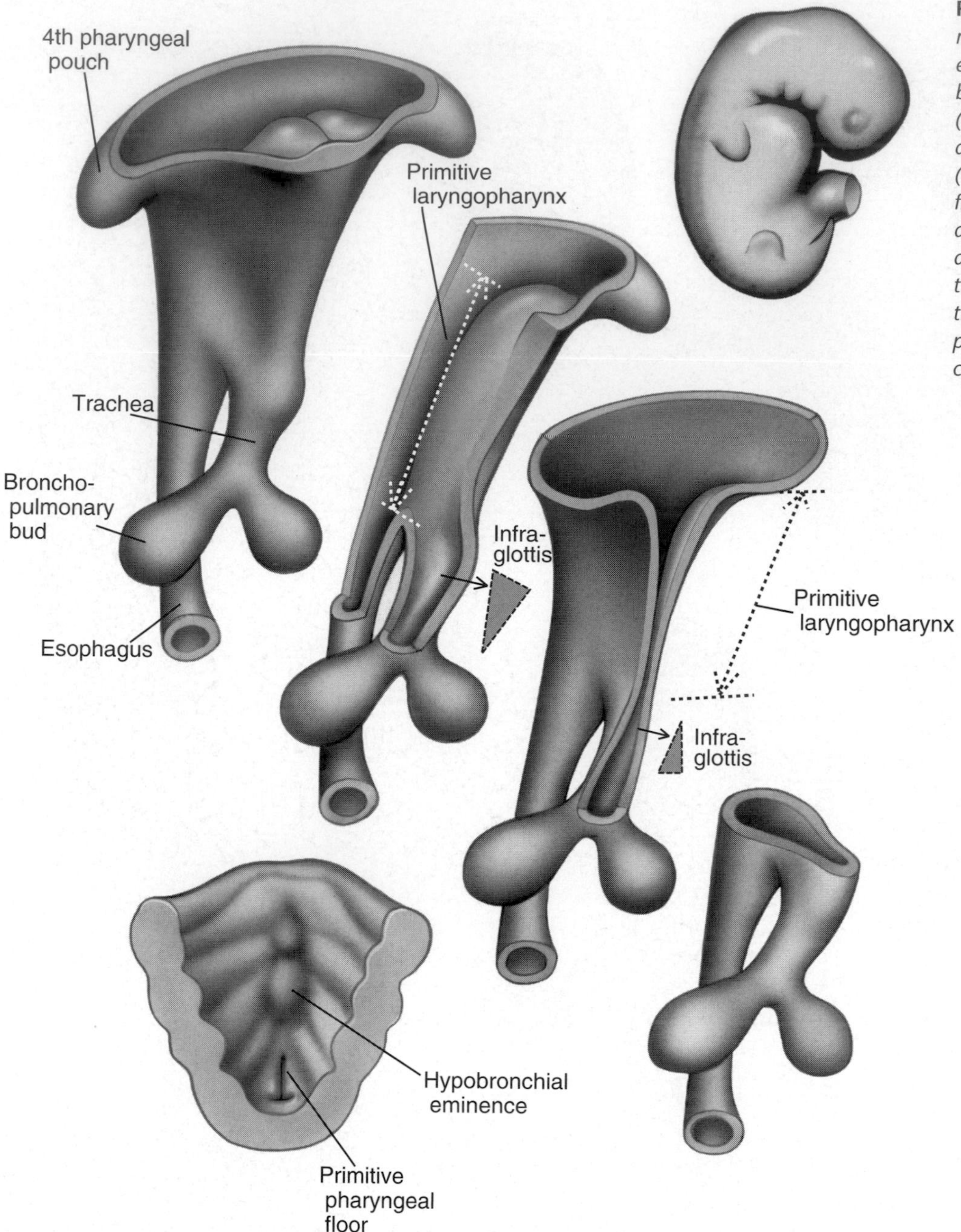

Figure 2.6 *Phase III embryo. As the respiratory diverticulum (RD) lengthens from the bronchopulmonary buds: (1) the main bronchi develop; (2) carina develops from the caudal aspect of the RD; (3) the infraglottis (IG) is a distinct region that develops from the cephalic aspect of the RD and that has a characteristic shape – an inverted triangle when sectioned in the sagittal plane, and an upright triangle when sectioned in the coronal plane; (4) the trachea develops as the carina and RD separate.*

the developing mesoderm of the laryngeal cartilages, muscles and branchial arch arteries. Eventually, obliteration of the ventral lumen of the PLPh occurs to give rise to the epithelial lamina (EL).

Bilateral elevations of the median pharyngeal floor give rise to the arytenoid swellings. This occurs at the same anatomic level as the fourth pharyngeal pouch. At this stage, the characteristic shape of the infraglottis is seen in both the sagittal and coronal planes. In addition, the infraglottis has separated from the carina with the formation of the trachea. A small elevation, which develops from the most posterior aspect of the hypobronchial eminence, is the epiglottic swelling. With removal of the dorsal wall of the foregut, the entrance to the primitive laryngopharynx now has a 'T' shape between the two arytenoid swellings and the central epiglottic swelling.

Phase V

Figure 2.10 represents phase V (Carnegie stage 16). The EL continues to obliterate the PLPh from a ventral to dorsal direction. Obliteration of the PLPh is complete, except for

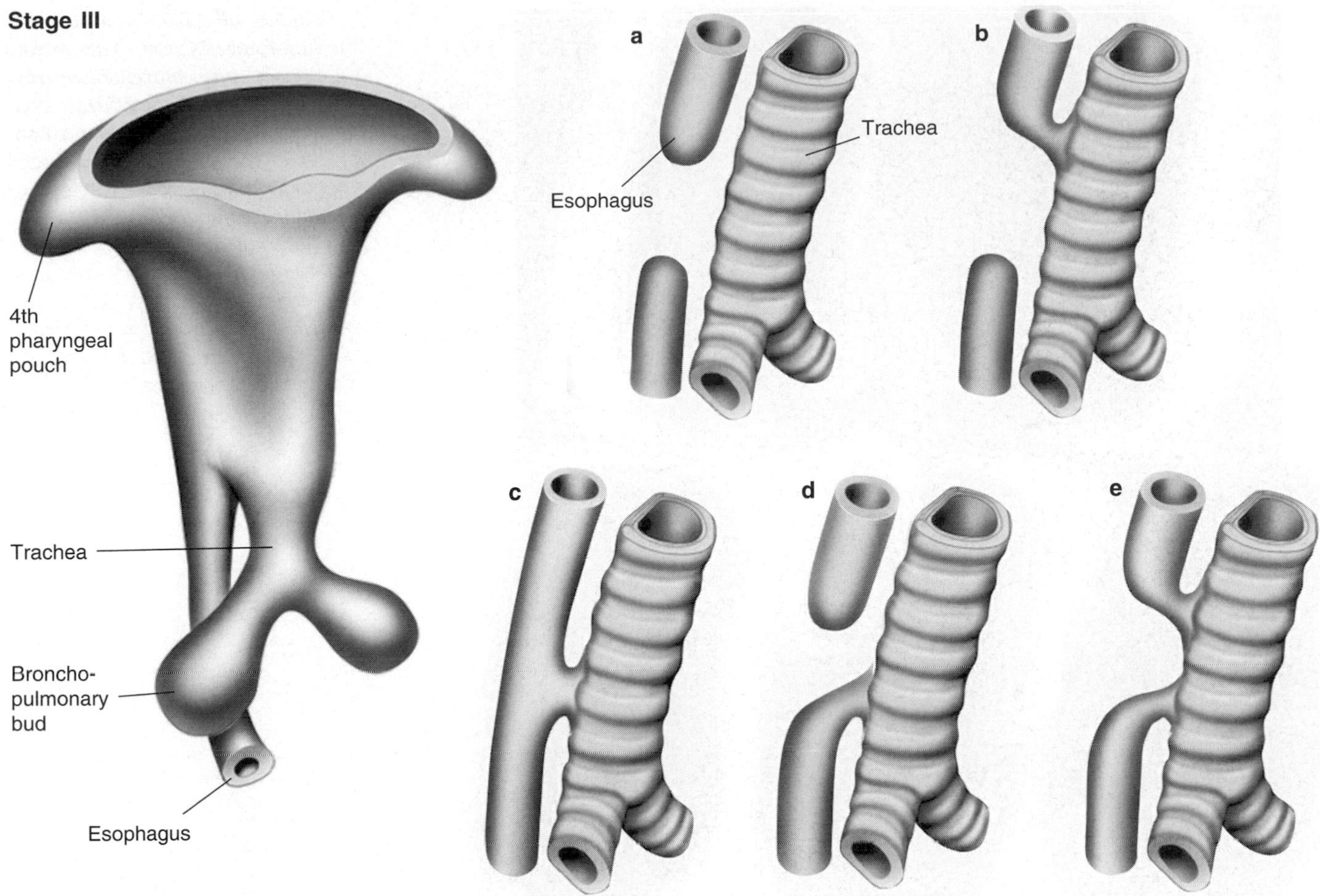

Figure 2.7 *Esophageal atresia and the spectrum of tracheoesophageal fistulae.*

a narrow communication between the hypopharynx and the infraglottis called the pharyngoglottic duct. In addition, a depression called the laryngeal cecum (LC) begins to develop between the arytenoid swellings and the epiglottis. The LC descends along the ventral aspect of the EL. From a dorsal perspective, the T-shaped entrance into the PLPh has developed more definition.

Phase VI

Figure 2.11 shows the phase VI embryo (Carnegie stages 17 and 18). The LC, which originates as a triangular lumen extending along the ventral aspect of the arytenoid swellings, continues its caudal descent until it reaches the level of the glottic region.

Phase VII

Figure 2.12 represents the phase VII embryo (Carnegie stages 19–23). The EL begins to recanalize from a dorsocephalic to ventrocaudal direction. In the process, communication is reestablished between the ventral LC and the dorsal pharyngoglottic duct. The last portion of the primitive laryngopharynx to recanalize is at the glottic level. Incomplete recanalization of the EL can give rise to the full spectrum of supraglottic and glottic webs and atresia.

Phase VIII

Figure 2.13 represents the phase VII embryo before the recanalization of the EL. Failure of the EL to recanalize completely causes a type 1 atresia, resulting in supraglottic stenosis. Recanalization of the EL, except at the glottic level, produces a glottic web. Incomplete recanalization of the EL causes a type 2 atresia. In types 1 and 2 atresia, there is likely to be an associated subglottic stenosis, because the earlier insult prevented complete expansion and development of the infraglottic region. At this stage, there still are no signs of the laryngeal ventricle, which is one of the last structures to develop.

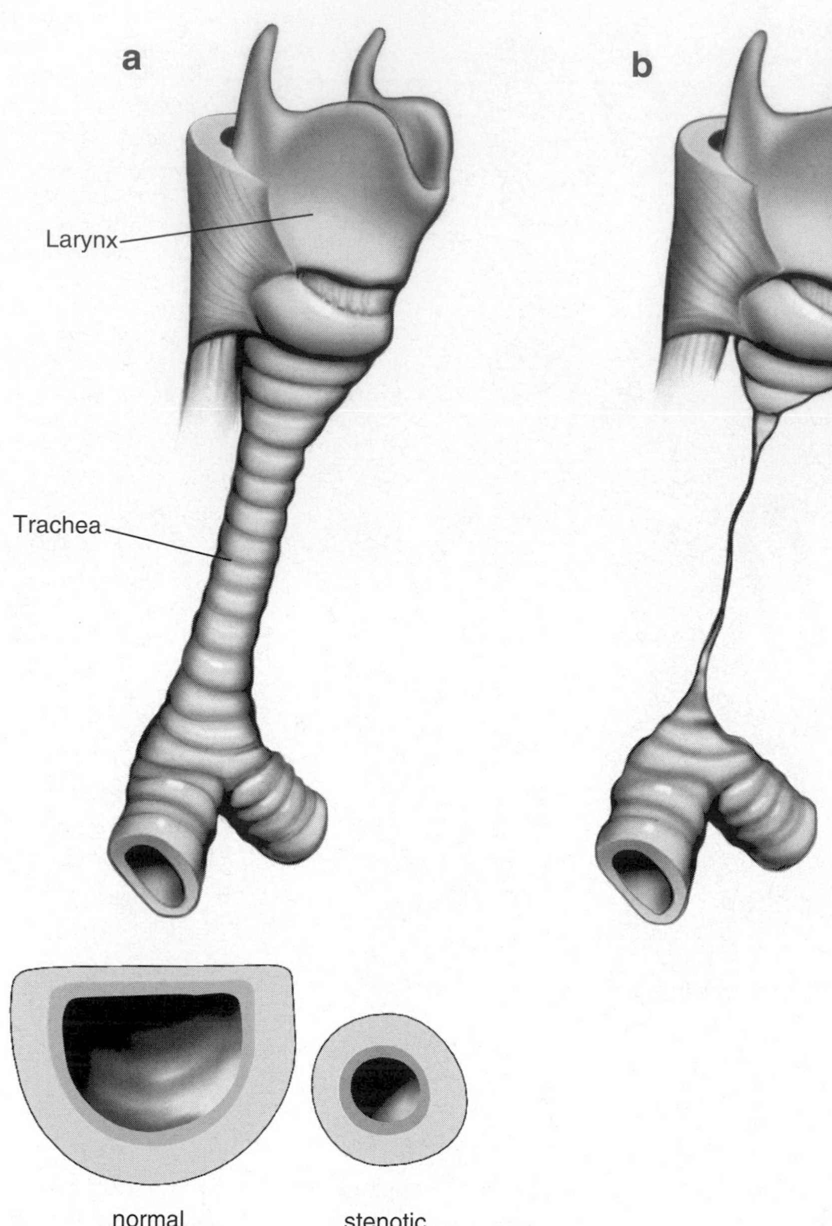

Figure 2.8 *(a) Tracheal stenosis. Axial sections demonstrate normal tracheal anatomy (left) and complete tracheal rings (right). (b) Tracheal agenesis. Relatively normal laryngeal and pulmonary development occur with both anomalies.*

Figure 2.14 represents the phase VIII embryo, which corresponds to the fetal period – the last 32 weeks of gestation that follow the 8 weeks of the embryonic period. The Carnegie staging system concludes at the end of the embryonic period and does not apply to the fetal period. No standard staging system, comparable to the Carnegie system, exists for the fetal period. Ventricular outgrowths from the lateral aspects of the LC give rise to the laryngeal ventricles. With the complete recanalization of the EL, a complete communication is established between the supraglottis and the infraglottis.

Considerations

Development of the laryngeal cartilages and muscles is first seen in a stage 14 embryo, initially as triangular-shaped condensation of mesodermal anlage appears adjacent to the primitive laryngopharynx.[14] Eventually, the laryngeal mesodermal anlage consolidates into two distinct regions, a hyoid and a thyrocricoid anlage. Fusion of the laryngeal mesodermal anlage occurs dorsally in the cricoid region by stage 18. Chondrification begins along the ventral aspect of the cricoid in stage 17 and progresses

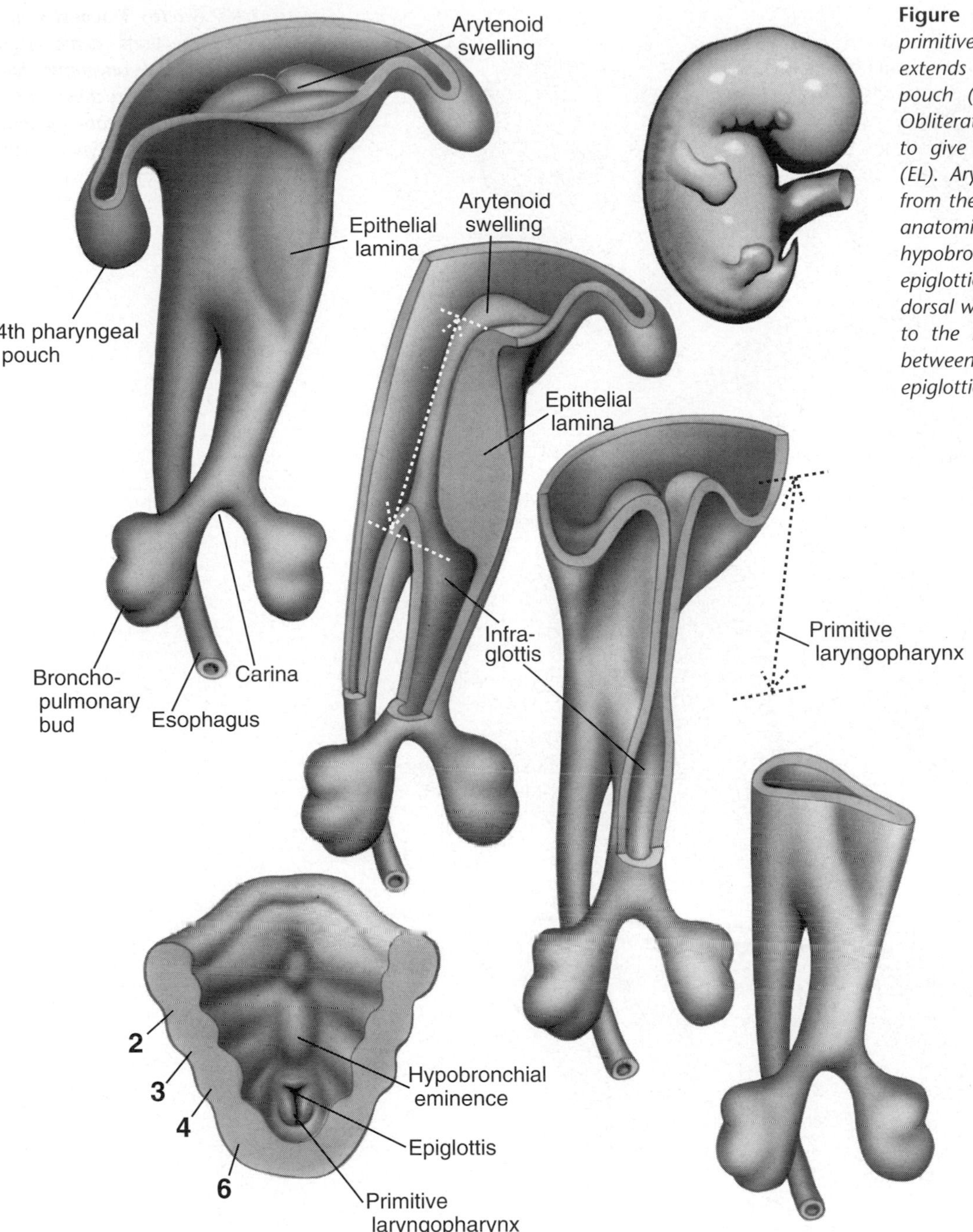

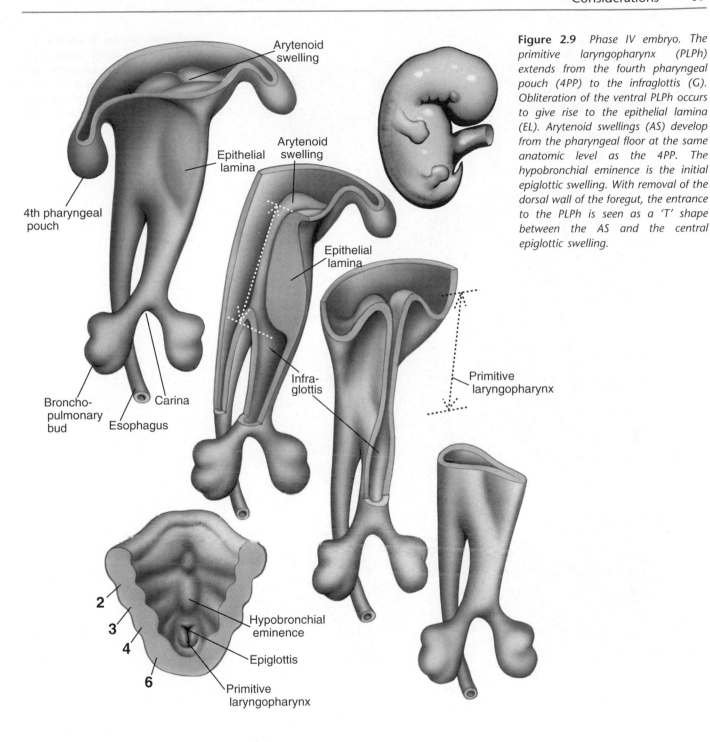

Figure 2.9 *Phase IV embryo. The primitive laryngopharynx (PLPh) extends from the fourth pharyngeal pouch (4PP) to the infraglottis (G). Obliteration of the ventral PLPh occurs to give rise to the epithelial lamina (EL). Arytenoid swellings (AS) develop from the pharyngeal floor at the same anatomic level as the 4PP. The hypobronchial eminence is the initial epiglottic swelling. With removal of the dorsal wall of the foregut, the entrance to the PLPh is seen as a 'T' shape between the AS and the central epiglottic swelling.*

dorsally until fusion occurs along the posterior cricoid lamina by stage 20. It is the incomplete fusion dorsally of the laryngeal mesodermal anlage or the chondrification process that can give rise to the full spectrum of laryngotracheal clefts seen clinically. Four types of clefts have been classified by Benjamin and Inglis:[2]

- type 1, cleft is limited to the interarytenoid area;
- type 2, partial cricoid cleft;
- type 3, total cricoid cleft which remains above the thoracic inlet; and
- type 4, laryngotrachealesophageal cleft.

The arytenoid cartilages eventually form from condensation within the laryngeal mesoderm. A precartilaginous template with vocal, muscular, and apical processes is complete by stage 21 which emulates the adult form. The vocal process is the last portion of the arytenoid to

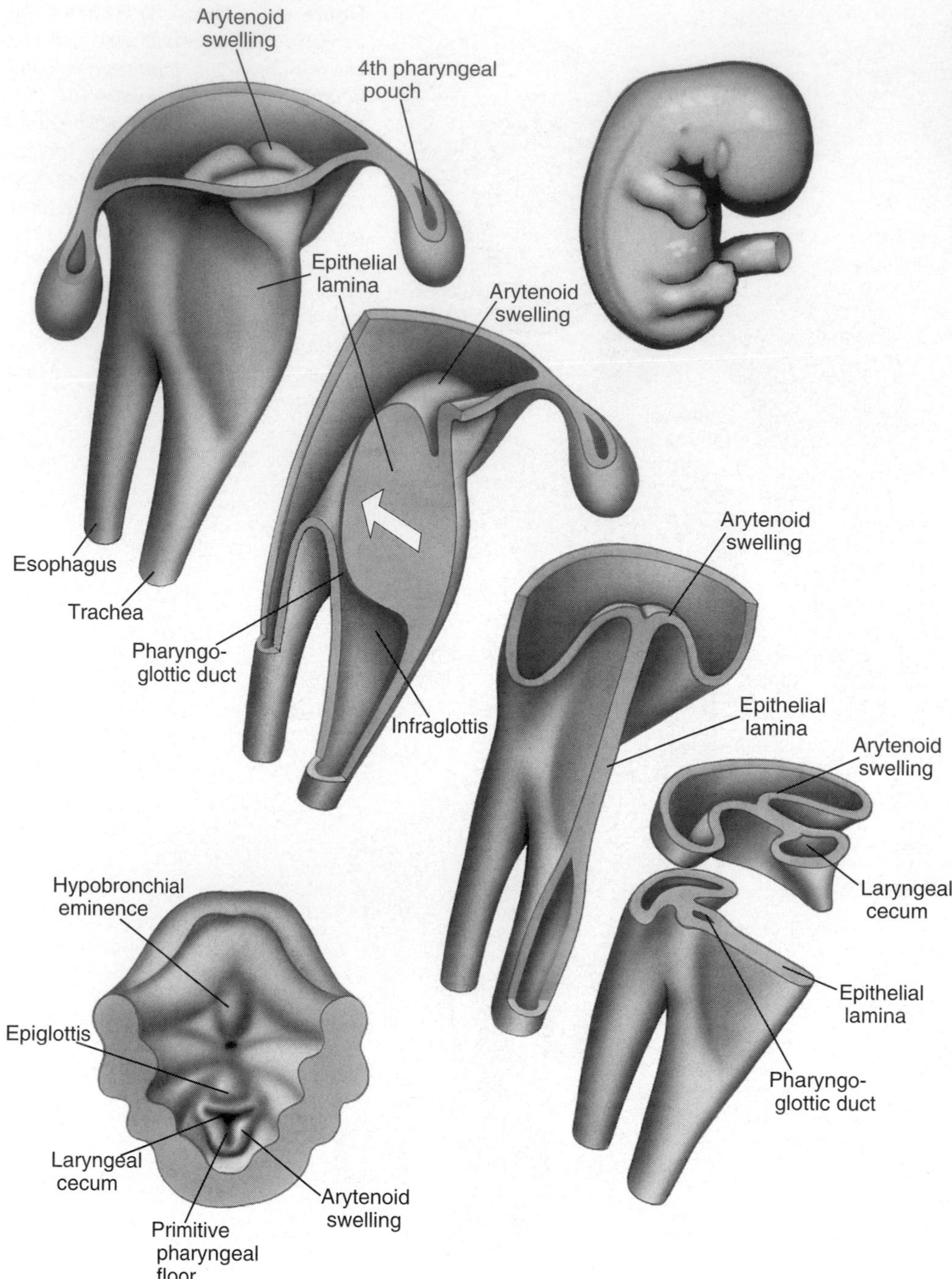

Figure 2.10 *Phase V embryo. The epithelial lamina (EL) continues to obliterate the primitive laryngopharynx (PLPh) from a ventral to dorsal direction, except for the pharyngoglottic duct (PhGD). The laryngeal cecum (LC) is a depression between the arytenoid swelling (AS) and the epiglottis.*

completely chondrify. Laryngeal hyaline cartilages develop from branchial mesoderm, whilst elastic cartilages are derived from the mesoderm on the floor of the pharynx.[9] Most of the arytenoid is composed of hyaline cartilage. However, the vocal processes develop in association with the vocal folds and consist of elastic cartilage. The arytenoid cartilages are pyramidal in shape. The base articulates with the cricoid cartilage. The apex attaches to the corniculate cartilage of Santorini and aryepiglottic fold. The vocal process projects anteriorly to connect with the vocal ligament, and the muscular process is the point of insertion of most of the muscles that move the arytenoid. The cricoarytenoid facets are well defined, smooth and symmetrical. Each arytenoid articulates with an elliptical facet on the posterior superior margin of the cricoid ring. The cricoid facet is approximately 6 mm long and has a cylindrical shape.[10] Most cricoarytenoid motion is rocking; however, along the long axis of the cricoid facet, gliding also occurs. The cricoarytenoid joint is an arthrodial joint, supported by a capsule lined with synovium and supported posteriorly by the cricoarytenoid ligament.[12] The cricoarytenoid joint controls abduction

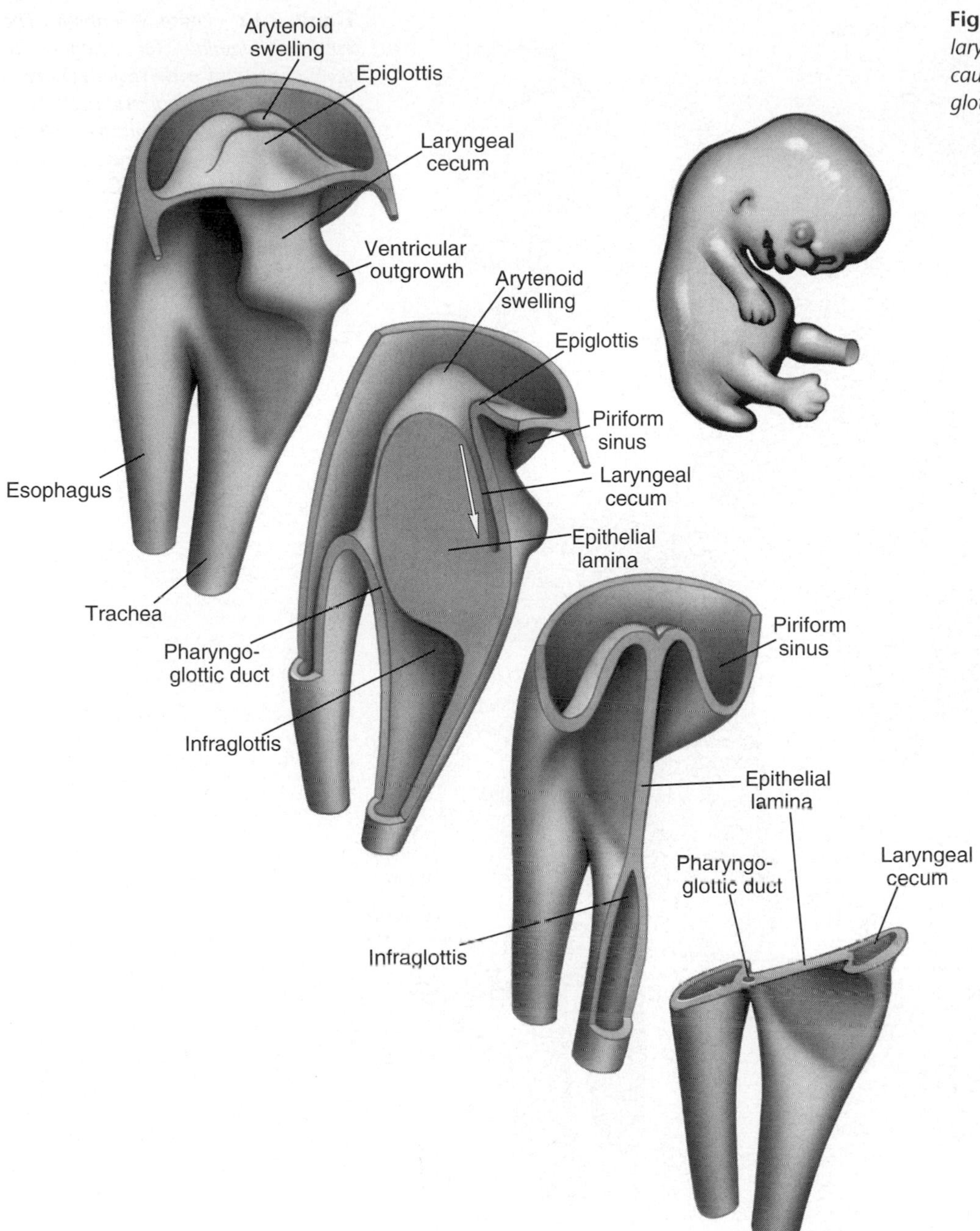

Figure 2.11 *Phase VI embryo. The laryngeal cecum (LC) continues its caudal descent to the level of the glottic region.*

and adduction of the true vocal cords, thereby facilitating respiration, phonation and protection of the airway.

The extrinsic laryngeal muscles develop from the epicardial ridge as part of the infrahyoid muscle mass. It separates into superficial and deep layers, and each layer eventually divides into two masses. The superficial layer splits longitudinally to form lateral and medial parts, resulting in the sternohyoid and omohyoid muscles. The deep layer attaches to the oblique line of the thyroid cartilage, separating into lower and upper parts to eventually form the sternothyroid muscles. Arytenoid motion is controlled by the intrinsic laryngeal muscles: posterior cricoarytenoid, lateral cricoarytenoid, arytenoideus, oblique arytenoid and thyroarytenoid. It is also affected by the cricothyroid muscle, which increases longitudinal tension of the vocal fold (which attaches to the vocal process of the arytenoid), and to a lesser degree by the thyroepiglottic muscle, which tenses the aryepiglottic fold.

In the postnatal period, the thyroid and hyoid cartilages which were formally attached, begin to separate and ossification begins. Hyoid bone ossification begins by the

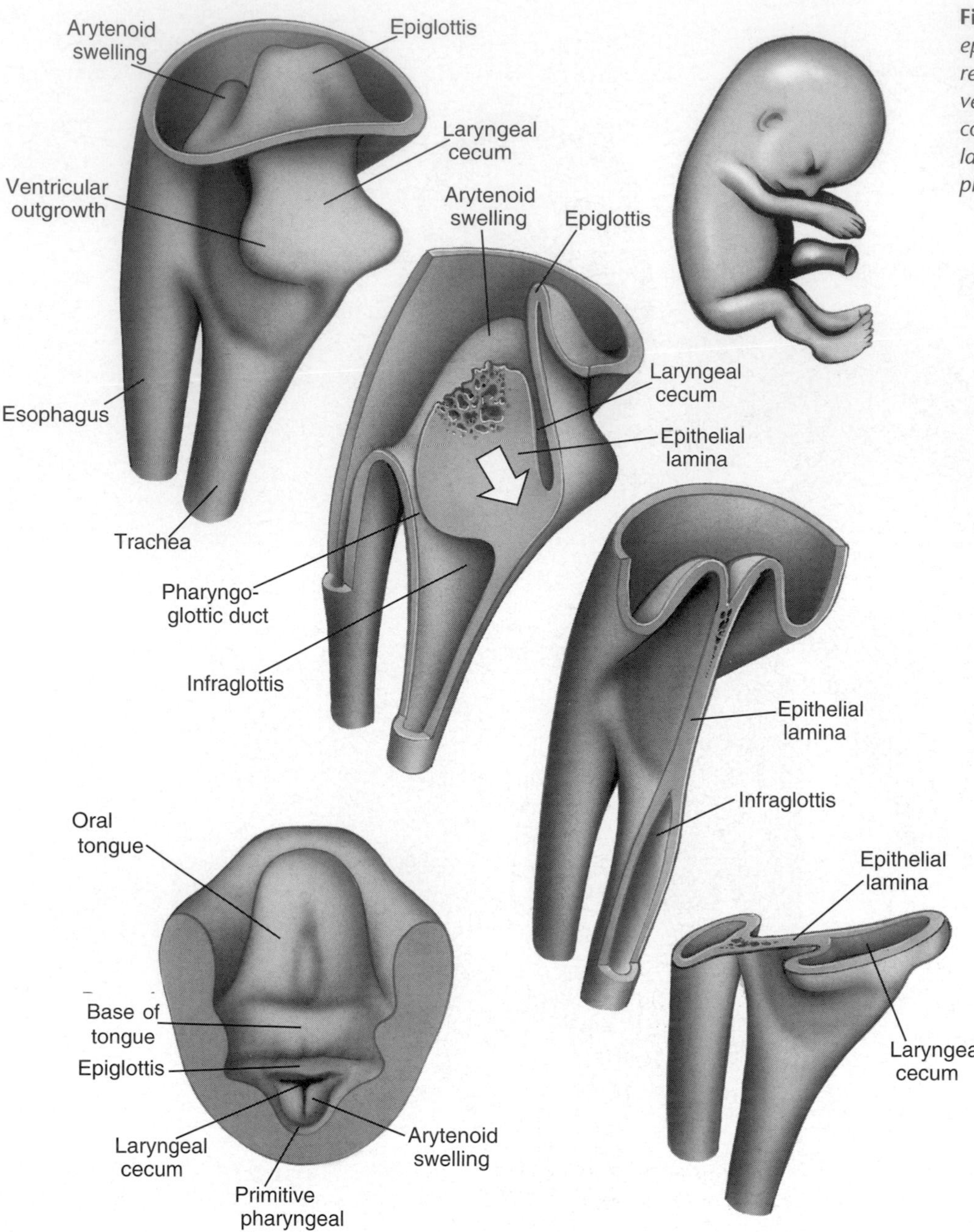

Figure 2.12 *Phase VII embryo. The epithelial lamina (EL) begins to recanalize from a dorsocephalic to a ventrocaudal direction to reestablish communication between the ventral laryngeal cecum (LC) and the dorsal pharyngoglottic duct (PhGD).*

age of 2 years. The thyroid and cricoid cartilages ossify during the early 20s, and the arytenoid cartilage ossifies in the late 30s. The superior half of the cricoid cartilage is 'V'-shaped and there is a transition in shape towards the inferior half of the cricoid, which is circular. This is the framework for the characteristic shape of the subglottic larynx identified as early as stage 3 of embryonic development. Except for the cuneiform and corniculate cartilages, the entire laryngeal skeleton is ossified by 65 years of age. At birth, the arytenoids, cuneiform cartilages and soft tissue of the posterior supraglottic larynx are proportionally larger in the infant compared to the adult larynx. In infancy, the membranous portion of the vocal cord is equal in length to the vocal process of the arytenoid. By adulthood, the membranous portion accounts for approximately two-thirds to three-quarters of vocal fold length.[6] Total vocal fold length is 6–8 mm in the infant and increases to 12–17 mm in the adult female and 17–23 mm in the adult male. The epiglottis in the infant larynx is omega-shaped, proportionally

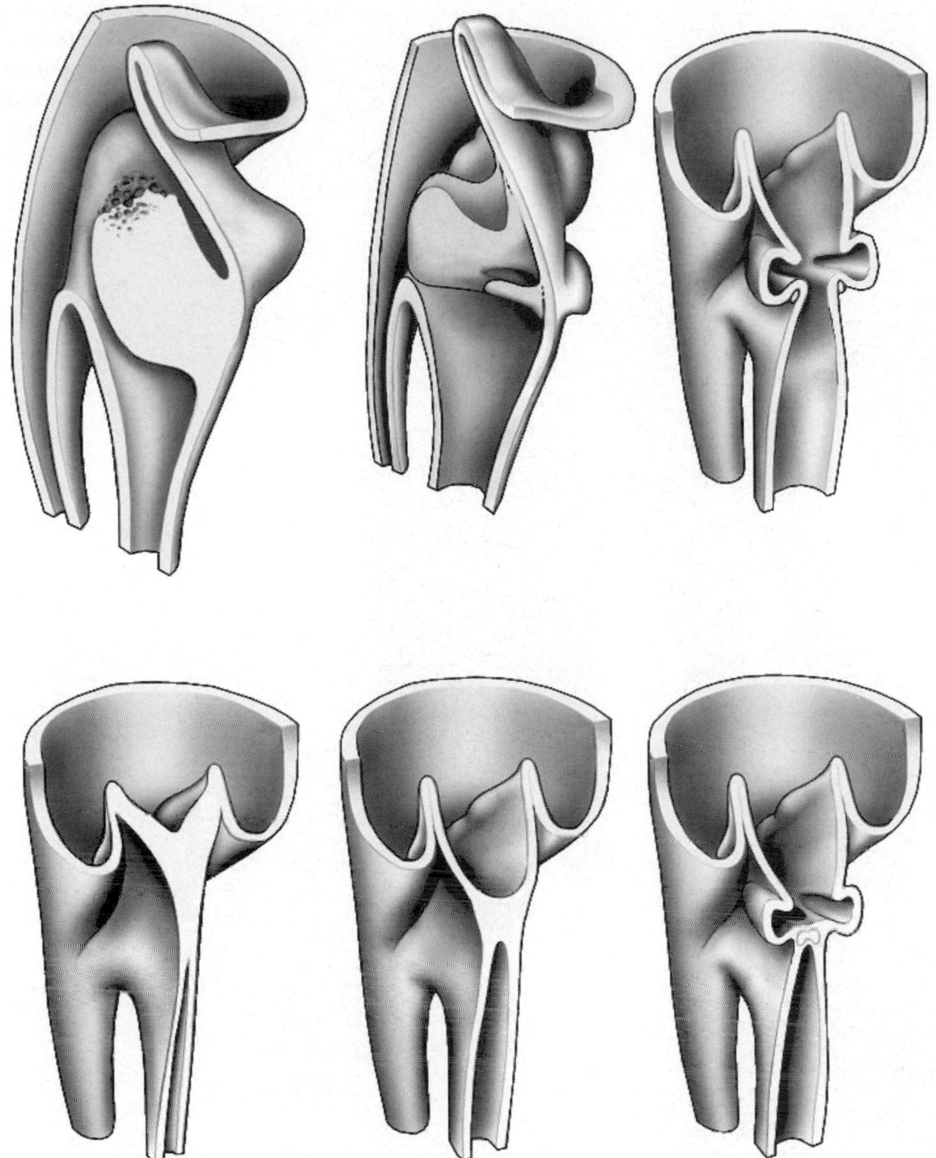

Figure 2.13 *Phase VII embryo prior to the recanalization of the epithelial lamina (EL). (a) Type 1 atresia results in a complete supraglottic stenosis. (b) Type 2 atresia causes a supraglottic stenosis. Communication between supraglottis and infraglottis is usually maintained through a patent pharyngoglottic duct. (c) Type 3 atresia produces a glottic web.*

narrower and tilted more posteriorly compared to the adult larynx.

At birth, the larynx is high in the neck, resting at about the level of the third and fourth cervical vertebrae (C3 and C4). It descends to approximately the level of C6 by age 5 years. It continues its gradual descent to the level of C7 by age 15–20 years. As a result of the caudal descent of the larynx, vocal tract length relationships change and average voice pitch tends to become lower. However, the lower anatomic position of the human larynx has made it more vulnerable to aspiration.

Conclusions

Figure 2.15 summarizes the eight phases of laryngeal development. Tracheoesophageal fistula, esophageal atresia and tracheal agenesis probably result from the early insults during embryogenesis and the rapid elongation of the foregut. Vascular compromise of these structures may play an important role in the pathogenesis of these anomalies.

The PLPh is the foregut segment that gives rise to the supraglottic larynx. It becomes obliterated ventrally by

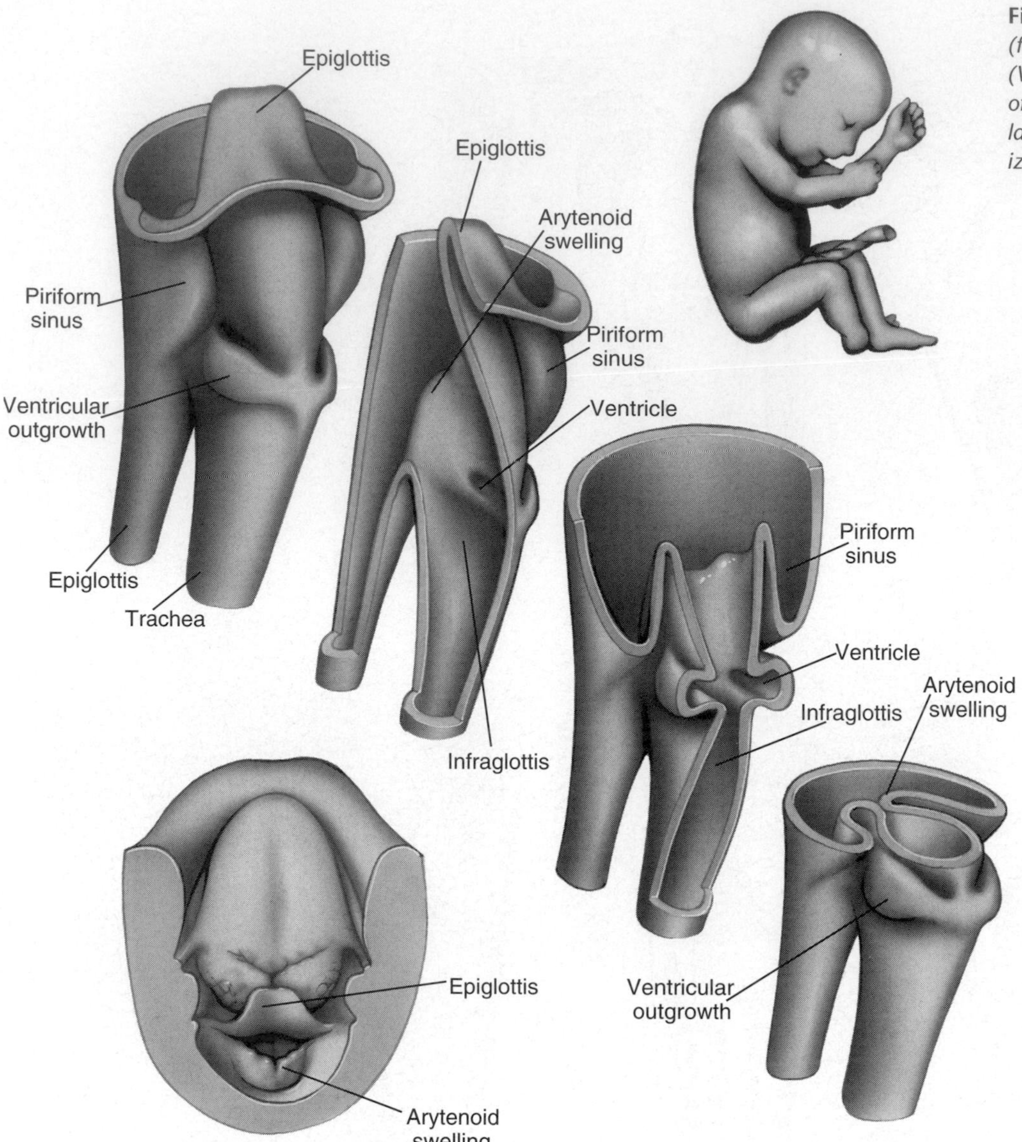

Figure 2.14 *Phase VIII embryo (fetal period). Ventricular outgrowths (VO) develop from the lateral aspects of the laryngeal cecum. The epithelial lamina (EL) has completely recanalized.*

the EL, which ultimately gives rise to the dorsal pharyngoglottic duct. The LC descends along the ventral aspect of the EL to the glottic level. Eventually, the EL recanalizes to join the dorsal pharyngoglottic duct with the ventral LC to give rise to the supraglottic vestibule. Incomplete recanalization produces a variety of supraglottic and glottic anomalies.

The infraglottis, seen early in development, has the characteristic shape of the adult conus elasticus. At no point during normal development is this lumen obliterated. If it is, congenital subglottic stenosis can occur, with a concomitant supraglottic stenosis, as seen with types 1 and 2 laryngeal atresia.

References

1. Arey LB. *Developmental Anatomy*, 7th edn. Philadelphia: Saunders, 1965: 260.
2. Benjamin B, Inglis A. Minor congenital laryngeal cleft: diagnosis and classification. *Ann Otol Rhinol Laryngol* 1989; **87:** 417–20.
3. Frazer JE. The development of the larynx. *J Anat Physiol* 1910; **44:** 156–91.
4. Henick DH. Three-dimensional analysis of murine laryngeal development. *Ann Otol Rhinol Laryngol* 1993; **102(Suppl 159):** 1–24.
5. Henick DH, Holinger LD. Laryngeal development. In:

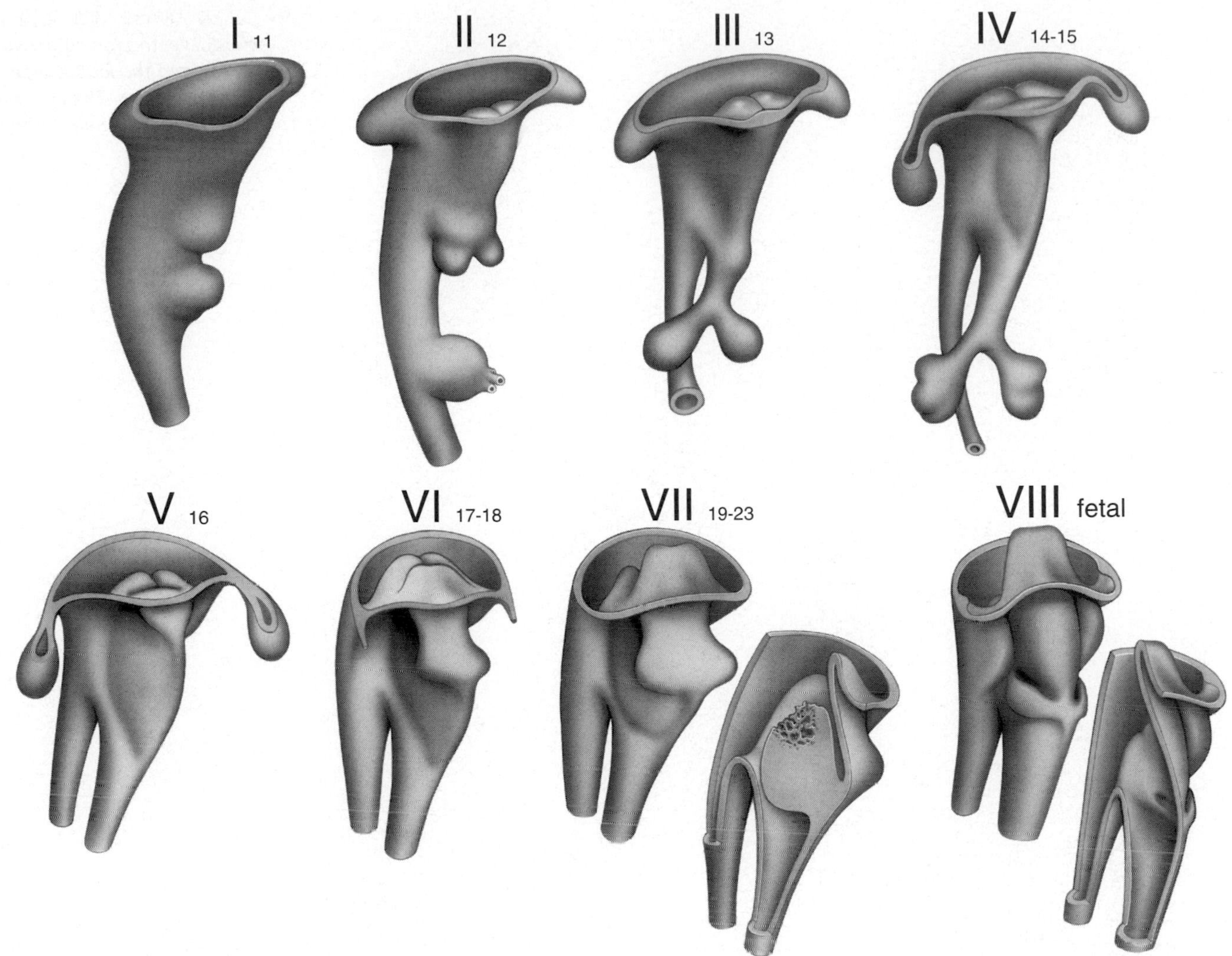

Figure 2.15 *Summary of the eight phases of laryngeal development.*

Holinger LD, Lusk RP, Green CG, eds. *Pediatric Laryngology and Bronchoesophagology.* Philadelphia: Lippincott-Raven, 1997: 1–17.

6. Hirano M, Kurita S, Kiyokawa K, Sato K. Posterior glottis. Morphological study in excised human larynges. *Ann Otol Rhinol Laryngol* 1986; **95:** 576–81.
7. His W. *Anatomic menschilicher Embryonen. III. Zur Geschichte der Organe.* Leipzig: Vogel, 1885: 12–19.
8. Kallius E. Beitraage zur entwicklungsgeschichte des kehlkopfes. *Anat Hefte Wiesbaden* 1897; **9:** 303–63.
9. Langman J. *Medical Embryology,* 3rd edn. Baltimore: Williams & Wilkins, 1975: 269–72.
10. Maue WM, Dickson DR. Cartilages and ligaments of the adult human larynx. *Arch Otolaryngol* 1971; **94:** 432–9.
11. O'Rahilly R, Muller F. Respiratory and alimentary relations in staged human embryos. New embryological data and congenital anomalies. *Ann Otol Rhinol Laryngol* 1984; **93:** 421–9.
12. Pennington CL. External trauma of the larynx and trachea. Immediate treatment and management. *Ann Otol* 1972; **81:** 546–54.
13. Walander A. Prenatal development of the epithelial primordium of the larynx in the rat. *Acta Anat (Basel)* 1950; **10(Suppl 13):** 1–140.
14. Zaw-Tun HA, Burdi AR. Re-examination of the origin and early development of the human larynx. *Acta Anat (Basel)* 1985; **122:** 163–84.

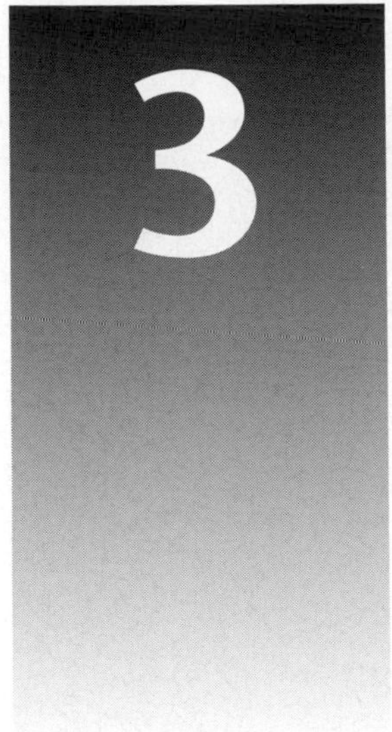

Anatomy of the larynx

Barry K B Berkovitz, Simon A Hickey and Bernard J Moxham

The adult larynx is situated in the midline of the neck, at the level of the third to the sixth cervical vertebrae. It extends from the laryngeal inlet, near the base of the tongue, to the trachea. At its inlet, the larynx communicates with the oropharynx and laryngopharynx (hypopharynx). The larynx itself is connected to the hyoid bone. The average distance from the upper edge of the hyoid bone to the lower border of the cricoid cartilage is about 63 mm in the male and 51 mm in the female.[13]

The larynx acts primarily as a sphincter,[39] preventing the entry of food or foreign material into the airway. The airway is protected by three main mechanisms:

- a sphincter-like action of the musculature at the inlet of the larynx;
- displacement of the epiglottis over the inlet; and
- elevation and anterior displacement of the larynx.

During swallowing, the vocal folds (cords) are approximated and breathing is momentarily inhibited. The rigidity of the cartilages of the larynx also helps maintain the patency of the upper airway. The larynx has become secondarily adapted for speech. During speech (and momentarily before coughing and sneezing), the vocal folds are also approximated.

Few features of the larynx are visible externally. Anteriorly, the larynx is almost completely covered by the infrahyoid (strap) muscles and by the thyroid gland, the isthmus of which lies in the midline just below the cricoid cartilage. The only feature visible is the laryngeal prominence of the thyroid cartilage. This is more prominent in the male larynx. The larynx may be brought nearer the anterior surface of the skin by extending the neck. The posterior aspect of the larynx forms the anterior wall of the laryngopharynx. Laterally is found the carotid sheath and its contents. Below, the larynx is continuous with the trachea. The reader is referred to standard anatomical textbooks for some generalized accounts of the anatomy of the larynx (e.g. references 1, 22, 56, 61, 63 and 66).

The laryngeal inlet

The laryngeal inlet (aditus) is bounded anteriorly and superiorly by the epiglottis, posteriorly and inferiorly by the mucosa of the arytenoid cartilages and the interarytenoid region, and laterally by the aryepiglottic folds. Posteriorly, the aryepiglottic folds contain the cuneiform and corniculate cartilages, producing swellings of the mucosa called the cuneiform and corniculate tubercles. The midline groove between the two arytenoid cartilages is termed the interarytenoid notch. The pharynx extends along the sides of the laryngeal inlet to form the piriform fossae. Superiorly, the epiglottis and tongue are separated by depressions called the valleculae. The valleculae are bounded by the median and lateral glossoepiglottic folds.

The internal anatomy of the larynx

The interior of the larynx (Figs 3.1–3.4) is divided into compartments by two paired folds, the vestibular cords (alternatively termed the ventricular folds or false cords) and the vocal cords (alternatively termed the vocal folds).

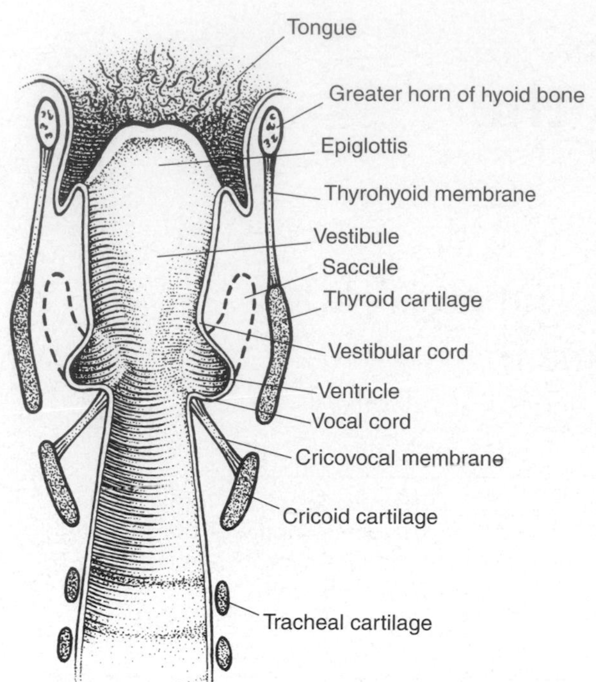

Figure 3.1 *Diagram showing the internal anatomy of the larynx as displayed in a coronal section viewed from behind.*

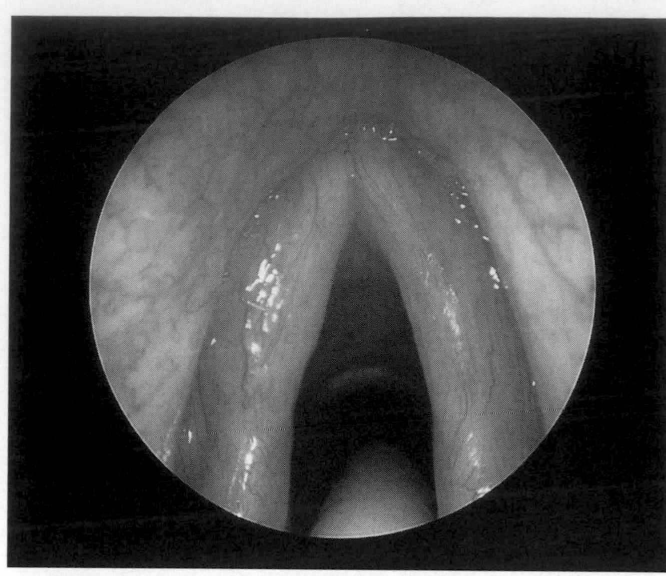

Figure 3.2 *Laryngoscopic view of the glottis.*

Between the laryngeal inlet and the vestibular cords lies the vestibule. Between the vestibular cords and the vocal cords are two slit-like spaces, the laryngeal ventricles or sinuses. The region bounded by the vocal cords is called the rima glottidis or glottis. Between the glottis and the level of the inferior margin of the cricoid cartilage lies a region which, through common usage, is known as the subglottis. The term supraglottis refers to that part of the larynx that lies above the glottis and includes the laryngeal ventricles, vestibular cords, the laryngeal surface of the epiglottis, arytenoids and the laryngeal aspects of the aryepiglottic folds. The definition of the precise margins of the glottis remains the subject of debate.

The vestibular cord

Each vestibular cord is a thick ridge of mucosa which covers a thin layer of connective tissue, the inferior free edge of the quadrangular membrane. It is attached anteriorly to the inner surface of the thyroid cartilage beneath the attachment of the petiole of the epiglottis, and attached behind to the body of the arytenoid cartilage. A variable amount of muscle (ventricularis muscle) derived from the thyroarytenoid muscle is present within the vestibular cord.[66] As the vestibular cords can move with the arytenoid cartilage, they can help close off the fissure (rima vestibuli) between them. When viewed from above, the vestibular cords partly obscure the vocal cords. Because of the presence of a loose and vascular submucosa, the vestibular cords appear pink *in vivo*.

The vocal cord

Anteriorly, the vocal cords approximate and are attached to the inner surface of the thyroid cartilage (below the attachment of the vestibular cord). Posteriorly, the vocal cords diverge to their attachment onto the vocal process of the arytenoid cartilage. The anterior three-fifths of the vocal cord is formed by the vocal ligament, the thickened free edge of the cricovocal membrane. The space between the vocal cords is termed the glottis. That portion of the glottis adjacent to the anterior three-fifths is called the intermembranous glottis. The posterior two-fifths of the glottis is bounded by the vocal processes of the arytenoid cartilage and is called the intercartilaginous glottis. The average length of the intermembranous glottis, measured from fresh autopsy material, is 14–15 mm in men and about 11 mm women.[13,29] The length of the intercartilaginous glottis is approximately 9 mm in men and about 7 mm in women.[29] As the mucosa overlying the vocal ligament is thin and lies directly on the vocal ligament, the normal vocal cord appears pearly white *in vivo*. The mucosa is loosely attached to the vocal ligament and a potential space exists which readily collects edema fluid in disease. Known as Reinke's space, it extends along the length of the free margin of the vocal ligament and, to a variable extent, onto the superior surface of the cord. The site where the vocal cords meet anteriorly is known as the anterior commissure. Fibres of the vocal ligament here pass through the thyroid cartilage to blend with the overlying perichondrium, forming Broyles' ligament.[6] Broyles' ligament contains blood vessels and lymphatics and therefore is a potential route for the spread of malignant tumors from the larynx.

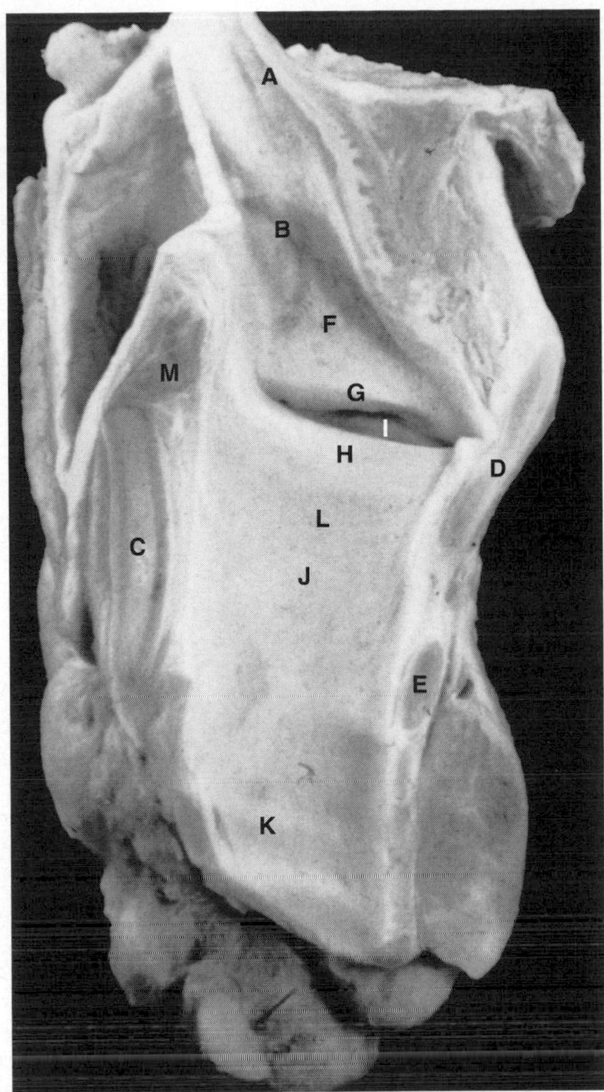

Figure 3.3 *Internal anatomy of the larynx viewed laterally: A, epiglottis; B, vestibule of supraglottis; C, lamina of cricoid cartilage; D, lamina of thyroid cartilage; E, arch of cricoid cartilage; F, mucosa covering quadrangular membrane; G, vestibular fold (false cord); H, vocal fold (true cord); I, ventricle of larynx; J, subglottic cavity; K, trachea; L, mucosa covering cricovocal membrane; M, interarytenoid muscle.*

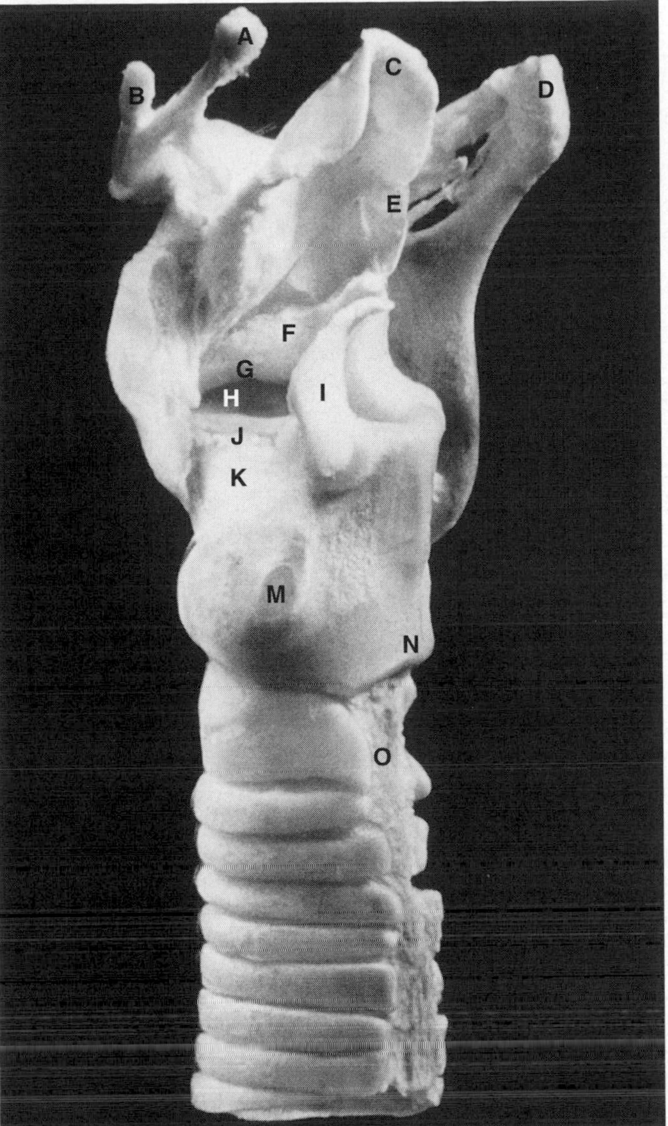

Figure 3.4 *Dissection of larynx with the left ala of the thyroid cartilage removed, showing the internal anatomy. A, greater horn of hyoid bone; B, lesser horn of hyoid bone; C, epiglottis; D, superior horn of thyroid cartilage; E, aryepiglottic fold; F, quadrangular membrane; G, vestibular cord; H, ventricle of larynx; I, arytenoid cartilage; J, vocal cord; K, cricovocal membrane; L, inferior horn of thyroid cartilage; M, facet of cricoid cartilage for articulation with inferior horn of thyroid cartilage; N, lamina of cricoid cartilage; O, first tracheal ring.*

The laryngeal ventricle and saccule

The laryngeal ventricle is the slit-like space that lies between the vestibular and vocal cords. A pouch of mucosa of varying size, the saccule extends upwards from the anterior end of each ventricle to lie between the vestibular cord and the inner surface of the alae of the thyroid cartilage (see Fig 3.12). The saccule is the site of mucous glands whose secretions help to lubricate the vocal cords which themselves lack glands. The orifice of the saccule into the ventricle is guarded by a delicate fold of mucosa, the ventriculosaccular fold.[26] The wall of the saccule contains the thyroarytenoid muscle. Pathological enlargement of the saccule, known as a laryngocele, may give symptoms of hoarseness and stridor.

The skeleton of the larynx

The skeleton of the larynx (Figs 3.4–3.7) consists of a series of single and paired cartilages united by ligaments and membranes. The larger, single cartilages are the thyroid and cricoid cartilages. The smaller, paired carti-

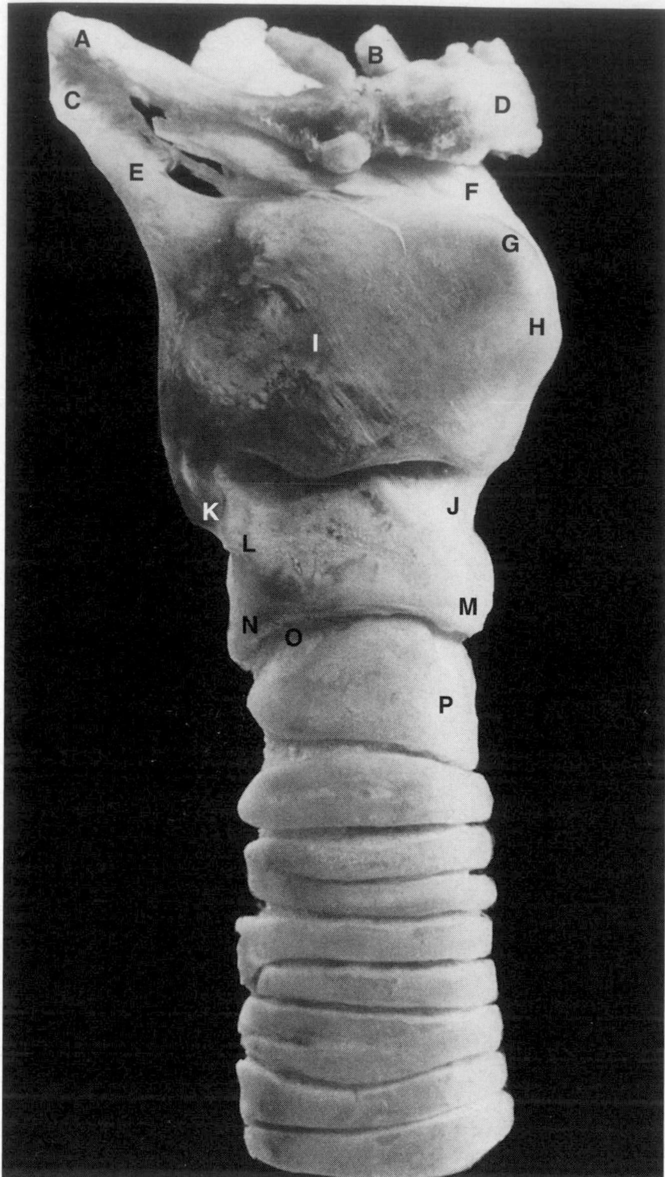

Figure 3.5 *Skeleton of larynx viewed laterally. A, greater horn of hyoid bone; B, lesser horn of hyoid bone; C, lateral thyrohyoid ligament; D, body of hyoid bone; E, superior horn of thyroid cartilage; F, thyrohyoid membrane; G, thyroid notch; H, thyroid prominence; I, lamina of thyroid cartilage with oblique line; J, anterior cricothyroid ligament; K, inferior horn of thyroid cartilage; L, capsule of cricothyroid joint; M, arch of cricoid cartilage; N, lamina of cricoid cartilage; O, cricotracheal ligament; P, first tracheal ring.*

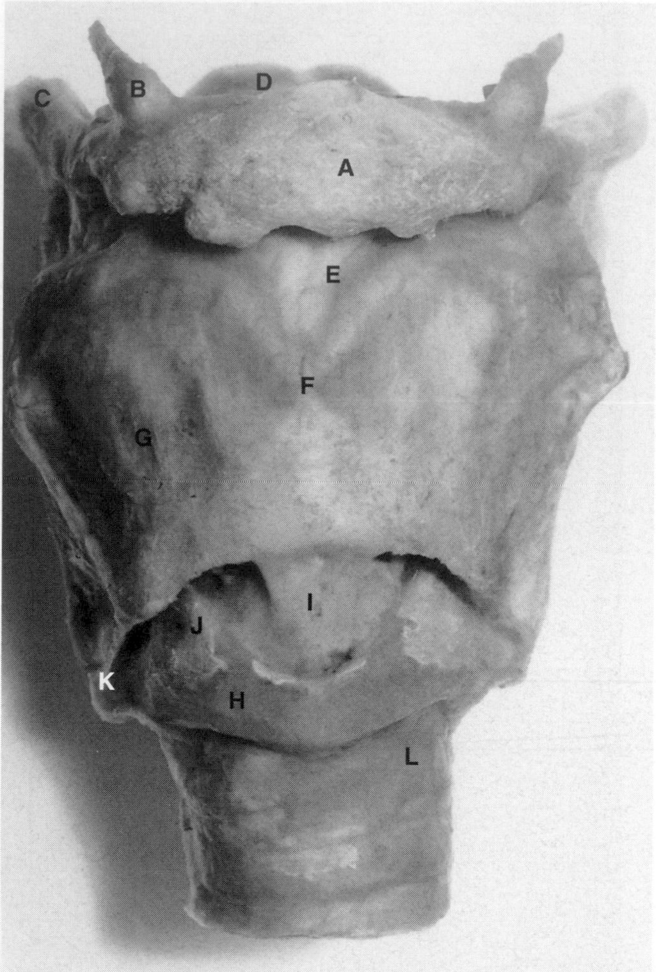

Figure 3.6 *Skeleton of larynx viewed anteriorly: A, body of hyoid bone; B, lesser horn of hyoid bone; C, greater horn of hyoid bone linking with superior horn of thyroid cartilage via a lateral thyrohyoid ligament; D, superior margin of epiglottis; E, thyrohyoid membrane; F, thyroid prominence; G, lamina of thyroid cartilage; H, arch of cricoid cartilage; I, anterior cricothyroid ligament; J, cricovocal membrane; K, cricothyroid joint; L, first tracheal ring.*

lages are the arytenoid cartilage and the rudimentary corniculate and cuneiform cartilages. Dimensions associated with the main cartilages have been reported in the literature.[13,28] The thyroid, cricoid and major part of the arytenoid cartilages are composed of hyaline cartilage, whilst the remaining laryngeal cartilages consist of elastic cartilage. This fact is of importance when considering calcification of the cartilages. Because the larynx is attached to the hyoid bone, this bone must be included in a description of the movements of the larynx. This bone will be considered briefly here, as will the epiglottis.

The hyoid bone

The hyoid bone is situated in the upper part of the front of the neck, between the third and fourth cervical vertebra. It lies at the base of the tongue, just above the laryngeal skeleton. It is horseshoe-shaped and consists of a central body, spanning the midline, with greater and lesser horns (cornua) on each side.

The body is quadrilateral and is curved so that its anterior surface appears convex when viewed from the front. A vertical median ridge is frequently present on the anterior

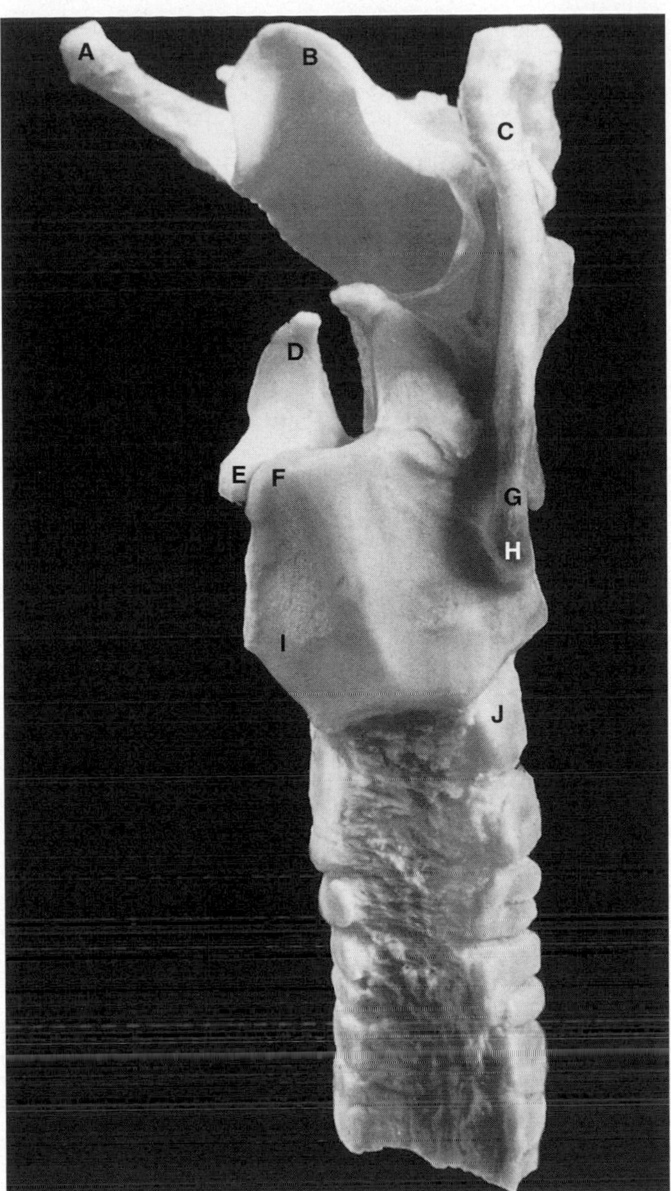

Figure 3.7 *Dissection of larynx viewed posteriorly with the left ala of the thyroid cartilage removed. A, greater horn of hyoid bone; B, epiglottis; C, superior horn of thyroid cartilage; D, apex (corniculate cartilage); E, muscular process; F, articular surfaces of crico-arytenoid joint; G, inferior horn of thyroid cartilage; H, articulation between thyroid and cricoid cartilages; I, lamina of cricoid cartilage; J, first tracheal ring.*

surface. The posterior surface is smooth and concave. The greater horns of the hyoid bone project backwards from the lateral margins of the body. At their posterior tips, they end in tubercles. The lesser horns of the hyoid bone are small and project upwards at the junction between the body and the greater horns. The union of the lesser horns with the rest of the hyoid bone may be osseous, but in most instances the lesser horns are connected by fibrous tissue (occasionally by synovial joints).

The hyoid bone is maintained in its position by the action of the numerous muscles, ligaments and membranes attached to it. It is suspended from the styloid process of the temporal bone by the stylohyoid ligament, which is attached to the lesser horn.

The thyroid cartilage

This is the largest and most prominent cartilage. It forms most of the anterior and lateral walls of the larynx. The overall shape of the thyroid cartilage takes the form of a shield. It consists of two flattened, quadrilateral laminae, which are joined anteriorly to form the laryngeal prominence. Above this prominence, posterior extensions of the laminae project upwards and downwards as the superior and inferior horns. The inferior horn articulates with the cricoid cartilage to form the cricothyroid articulation. An articular facet at the inferior horn is only well-defined in about 20% of cases.[28] On the external surface of each lamina lies the oblique ridge, which is the site for muscle attachments. The ridge runs downwards and forwards, from the superior horn towards the lower border of the cartilage, although it is only truly oblique at its inferior extremity.[68] The oblique ridge is bounded above and below by a tubercle. The thyroid cartilage shows sexual dimorphism; in the male it increases markedly in size at puberty and the thyroid prominence becomes very distinct.

The cricoid cartilage

Unlike the thyroid cartilage, the cricoid cartilage forms a complete ring. Indeed, it is the only complete cartilaginous ring within the airway. It comprises the most inferior and posterior part of the larynx and supports the entrance to the trachea. The shape of the cricoid cartilage resembles that of a signet ring, showing a narrow arch anteriorly and a flat, quadrangular lamina posteriorly. The lamina shows a midline vertical crest which gives attachment to the suspensory ligament of the esophagus[3] and which separates two concave areas associated with the origin of the posterior cricoarytenoid muscles. The height of the cricoid lamina averages nearly 25 mm in men and 21 mm in women.[13] Where the arch meets the lamina, small articular facets for the inferior horns of the thyroid cartilage may be found. However, these are often poorly developed and articular facets may only be evident in about 20% of cases.[15,28] The superior edge of the lamina has sloping shoulders and contains well-defined articular facets for the arytenoid cartilages. The cricoid cartilage may be more prominent in the female.

The arytenoid cartilage

The arytenoid cartilages lie in the posteroinferior part of the larynx, on the superior edge of the lamina of the cricoid cartilage. They contribute to the margin of the laryngeal inlet. Each cartilage is pyramidal in shape, with a base and three surfaces: medial, posterior and anterolateral. The base of the arytenoid cartilage is concave and presents a smooth articulating surface for the cricoid cartilage. The arytenoid cartilage has a process anteriorly, the vocal process (for attachment of the vocal ligament), and a process laterally, the muscular process (for the attachment of the posterior and lateral cricoarytenoid muscles).

The epiglottis

The epiglottis consists of a thin lamina of elastic cartilage covered on all sides with mucous membrane. It is leaf-shaped, the anterior surface of the stalk (or petiole) providing the means of attachment to the larynx via a thyroepiglottic ligament. A depression for this ligament lies just below the thyroid notch on the inner surface of the thyroid cartilage. The epiglottis is also anchored to the body of the hyoid bone by a hyoepiglottic ligament. The sides of the epiglottis are attached to the arytenoid cartilages by the aryepiglottic folds. Median and lateral glossoepiglottic folds pass from the root of the tongue to the anterior surface of the epiglottis. The epiglottis projects upwards and backwards over the vestibule of the larynx and gives the appearance of a lid. However, it does not seem to function as such, as its surgical removal has few adverse effects on deglutition. The posterior surface of the cartilage of the epiglottis shows numerous small indentations or perforations. In these lie mucous glands.

The minor cartilages of the larynx

The corniculate cartilages surmount the arytenoid cartilages, thus completing their pyramidal shapes.

The cuneiform cartilages lie within the aryepiglottic folds, at the laryngeal inlet, and provide some support for this thin fold.

Small triticeal cartilages are found in the ligaments joining the tips of the superior horns of the thyroid cartilage to the tips of the greater cornua of the hyoid bone.

Calcification of the laryngeal cartilages

As the thyroid, cricoid and most of the arytenoid cartilages consist of hyaline cartilage, they are capable of undergoing calcification. This normally commences at about 18 years of age. Initially, the calcification involves the lower and posterior parts of the thyroid cartilage, spreading to involve the remaining cartilages. Ossification of the arytenoid cartilage commences at the base. The degree and frequency of ossification of the thyroid and cricoid cartilages appears to be lower in females.[24] Predilection for tumor invasion may be enhanced by ossification of the laryngeal cartilages.[65]

In the arytenoid cartilage, the tip of the vocal process, as well as the upper portion from the vocal process to the apex, is comprised of noncalcifying, elastic cartilage. This may have considerable functional significance. The vocal process may bend at the elastic cartilage during adduction and abduction, whilst the two arytenoid cartilages will contact mainly at their elastic superior portions during adduction.[53]

Articulations of the laryngeal cartilages

The inferior horn of the thyroid cartilage articulates with the cricoid cartilage at a synovial joint, the cricothyroid joint. This joint has a well-developed capsule that is strengthened posteriorly by fibrous bands.[15,40] The capsule and ligaments are rich in elastin fibres, while collagen types I and III are present.[15] Both rotation and gliding movements occur at this joint.[15] The joint permits a rotary movement with activity of the cricothyroid muscle, such that the thyroid cartilage tilts forwards and downwards, with upward movement of the arch of the cricoid cartilage (see Fig 3.21d).

The joint between the base of the arytenoid cartilage and the lamina of the cricoid cartilage, the cricoarytenoid joint, is also synovial. The capsule of the joint is loose, allowing both rotatory and medial and lateral gliding movements.[63] The arytenoids can slide apart down the facet of the cricoid lamina and, at the same time, rock backwards when moving from the adducted position to the abducted one. In moving from the resting position to full adduction, the arytenoid cartilages pass up the slope of the facet on the cricoid lamina, towards each other and rock inwards.[54] The joint is strengthened by a ligament which, although traditionally called the posterior cricoarytenoid ligament, is primarily medial in position.[42,54] It has been postulated that the major determinant of the position taken up by the denervated vocal cord is not dependent on the musculature as is generally assumed, but on the resting position of this cricoarytenoid ligament.[14]

A synovial or cartilaginous joint links the corniculate cartilage to the arytenoid cartilage.

The laryngeal membranes

Considerable differences in terminology are found in different textbooks concerning the nomenclature of the laryngeal membranes (see Figs 3.4 and 3.8). In some, the cricovocal membrane and the anterior cricothyroid ligament are collectively called the cricothyroid ligament, the cricovocal membrane being designated the lateral cricothyroid ligament. Such terminology ignores the fact that the cricovocal membrane shows a thickened ligament only where it becomes the vocal ligament. Furthermore, it is attached not only to the thyroid cartilage, but also to the arytenoid cartilage. Another collective term found in the literature is conus elasticus. To add to the confusion, some anatomists restrict the term conus elasticus to the anterior cricothyroid ligament.

The larynx has thyrohyoid, quadrangular and cricovocal membranes. The single thyrohyoid membrane is external to the larynx, whereas the paired quadrangular and cricovocal membranes are internal. All the

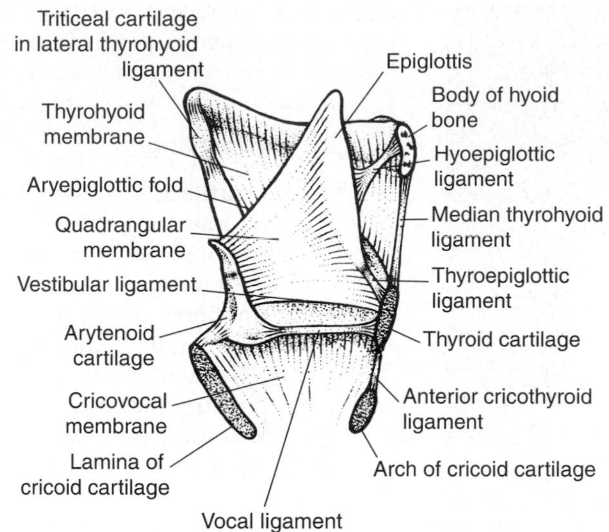

Figure 3.8 *Diagram of sagittal section of the larynx illustrating the laryngeal membranes.*

membranes are composed of fibroelastic tissue. There are also two ligaments, the anterior cricothyroid ligament and the cricotracheal ligament.

The thyrohyoid membrane

This membrane extends from the upper border of the thyroid cartilage to the upper border of the inner surface of the hyoid bone (both body and greater horns). Between the membrane and the hyoid bone lies a bursa.

The thyrohyoid membrane is thickened in three places to form ligament-like structures. In the midline is found the median thyrohyoid ligament. At the lateral margins are found the lateral thyrohyoid ligaments, connecting the tips of the superior horns of the thyroid cartilage to those of the greater horns of the hyoid bone. The lateral ligaments may contain triticeal cartilages.

The thyrohyoid membrane is pierced by the superior laryngeal vessels and the internal laryngeal nerves as they pass into the larynx.

The quadrangular membrane

Each quadrangular membrane passes from the lateral margin of the epiglottis to the arytenoid cartilage. It is often poorly defined. The membrane shows two free borders. The upper border slopes posteriorly to form the aryepiglottic ligament, which comprises the central component of the aryepiglottic fold. It is less defined in its upper portion. Posteriorly, it passes through the fascial plane of the esophageal suspensory ligament to help form a median corniculopharyngeal ligament that extends into the submucosa adjacent to the cricoid cartilage. This ligament may exert vertical traction.[3] The lower border of the quadrangular membrane is more defined and forms the vestibular cords.

The cricovocal membrane

This membrane is more pronounced than the quadrangular membrane, and arises from the side of the larynx at the upper border of the arch of the cricoid cartilage. It passes internally, deep to the lamina of the thyroid cartilage, to become attached anteriorly to the inner surface of the thyroid cartilage close to the midline, and posteriorly to the vocal process of the arytenoid cartilage. The attachment of the cricovocal membrane lies halfway between the thyroid notch and inferior border of the thyroid cartilage in the female, whilst in the male it lies one-third of this distance. The cricovocal membrane has an upper free margin that passes across the larynx. This is thickened to form the vocal ligament.

The anterior (median) cricothyroid ligament

This ligament (see Fig 3.5) is considered by some anatomists to be a superficial part of the cricovocal membrane. It is situated anteriorly in the midline, passing from the upper border of the cricoid cartilage to the lower border of the thyroid cartilage.

The cricotracheal ligament

This ligament (see Fig 3.3) joins the lower border of the cricoid cartilage to the first cartilaginous tracheal ring.

The paraluminal spaces and other relationships of the larynx

The ligaments and membranes of the larynx, together with the skeletal elements, allow for the delineation of a number of potential spaces or compartments. The three most commonly considered are the pre-epiglottic, the paraglottic and the subglottic spaces. However, these spaces are not closed compartments completely separated from each other and thus the spread of tumors is possible. Knowledge of the anatomy of these spaces and the potential pathways of spread of tumors from them have had a major influence on the surgical approach to malignant disease in this region.

The pre-epiglottic space

The pre-epiglottic space might be expected to lie anterior to the epiglottis. In reality, it also extends beyond the lateral margins of the epiglottis, giving it the form of a horseshoe.[27,43] It is primarily filled with adipose tissue and appears to contain no lymph nodes.[11] Its upper boundary is formed by the weak hyoepiglottic membrane, which is strengthened medially as the median hyoepiglottic ligament. Its anterior boundary is the thyrohyoid

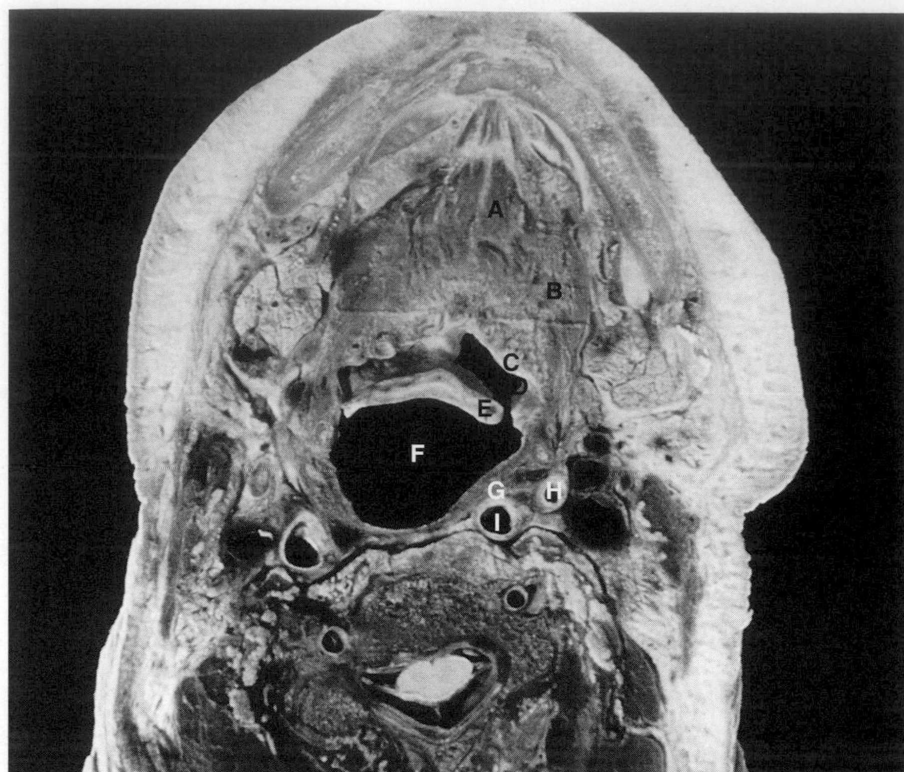

Figure 3.9 *Horizontal section of the neck at the level of the valleculae. A, genioglossus muscle; B, hyoglossus muscle; C, linguinal tonsil; D, vallecula; E, epiglottis; F, laryngopharynx; G, middle constrictor of pharynx; H, external carotid artery; I, internal carotid artery; J, internal jugular vein.*

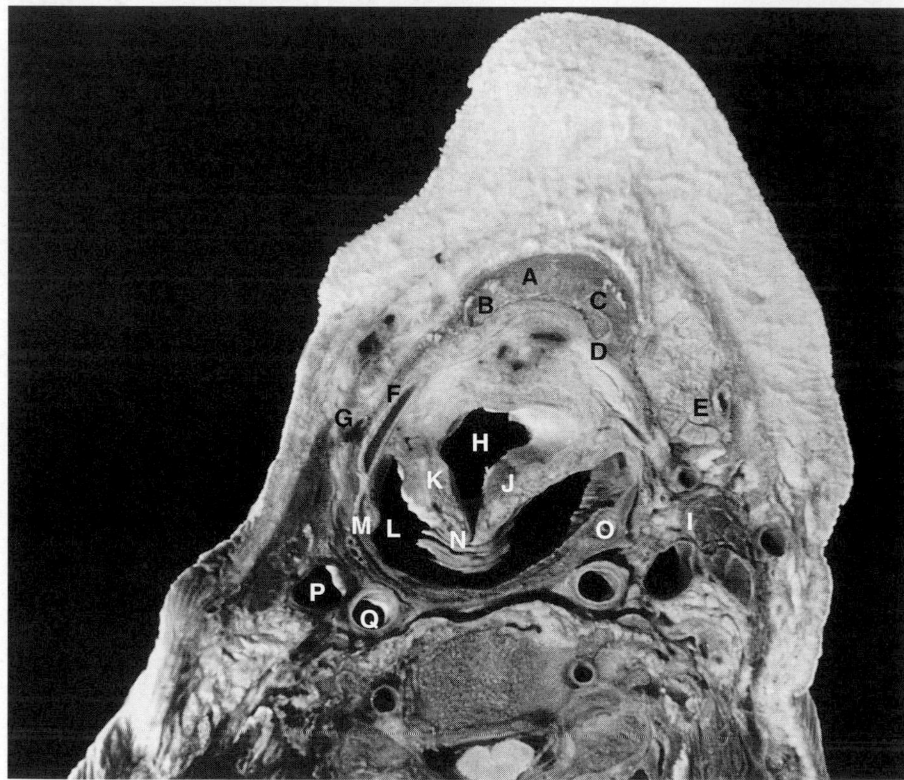

Figure 3.10 *Horizontal section of the neck at the level of the ventricle of the larynx. A, sternohyoid muscle; B, omohyoid muscle; C, body of hyoid bone; D, lesser horn of hyoid bone; E, submandibular salivary gland; F, lamina of thyroid cartilage; G, neurovascular bundle of infrahyoid muscles; H, vestibule of larynx; I, superior thyroid vessels; J, arytenoid cartilage; K, aryepiglottic fold; L, pyriform fossa; M, superior horn of thyroid cartilage; N, corniculate cartilage; O, superior horn of thyroid cartilage; P, internal jugular vein; Q, common carotid artery.*

membrane, which is strengthened medially as the median thyrohyoid ligament. Its lower boundary is the thyroepiglottic ligament, which continues laterally with the quadrangular membrane behind. Behind, it extends beyond the margins of the epiglottis. Its upper lateral border is the greater horn of the hyoid bone.[43] Inferolaterally, the pre-epiglottic space is in continuity with the paraglottic space (see below) and is often invaded from

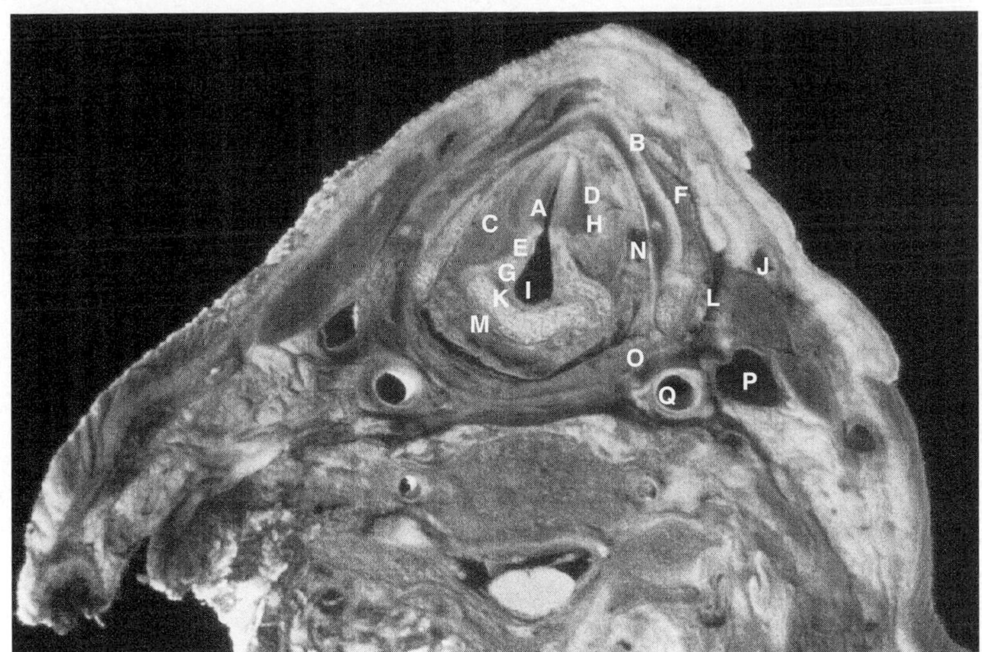

Figure 3.11 *Horizontal section of the neck at the level of the vocal cords. A, vocal cord; B, lamina of thyroid cartilage; C, lateral crico-arytenoid muscle; D, laryngeal sinus; E, vocal ligament; F, thyrohyoid muscle; G, vocal process of arytenoid cartilage; H, saccule; I, glottis; J, anterior jugular vein; K, lamina of cricoid cartilage; L, superior thyroid vessels; M, posterior crico-arytenoid muscle; N, paraglottic space; O, inferior constrictor of pharynx; P, internal jugular vein; Q, common carotid artery.*

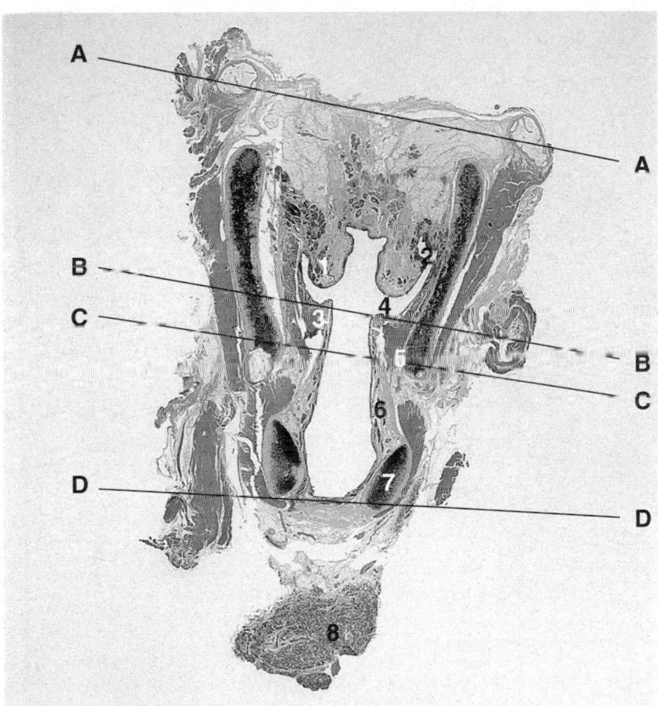

Figure 3.12 *Longitudinal section of the larynx. Hematoxylin and eosin. 1, vestibular cord; 2, saccule; 3, vocal cord; 4, ventricle; 5, thyroid cartilage; 6, cricovocal membrane; 7, cricoid cartilage; 8, thyroid gland.*

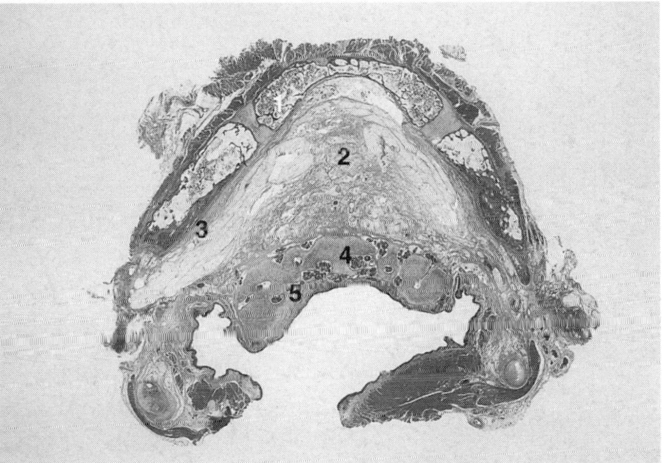

Figure 3.13 *Horizontal section of the larynx at the level of the hyoid bone (level A, Fig 3.12). Hematoxylin and eosin. 1, body of hyoid bone; 2, hyo-epiglottic ligament; 3, pre-epiglottic space; 4, epiglottis; 5, mucous glands.*

the latter by the laryngeal saccule. It is also in continuity with the mucosa of the laryngeal surface of the epiglottis via multiple perforations in the cartilage of the epiglottis. It is through these perforations that malignancies of the laryngeal surface of the epiglottis may invade the fat and areolar tissue of the pre-epiglottic space.

The paraglottic space

The paraglottic space is a region of adipose tissue that contains the internal laryngeal nerve. It is bounded laterally by the thyroid cartilage and thyrohyoid membrane. Superomedially, in most individuals it is continuous with the pre-epiglottic space. However, the two spaces may be partitioned by a fibrous septum. Inferomedially lies the cricovocal membrane. Posteriorly lies the mucosa of the

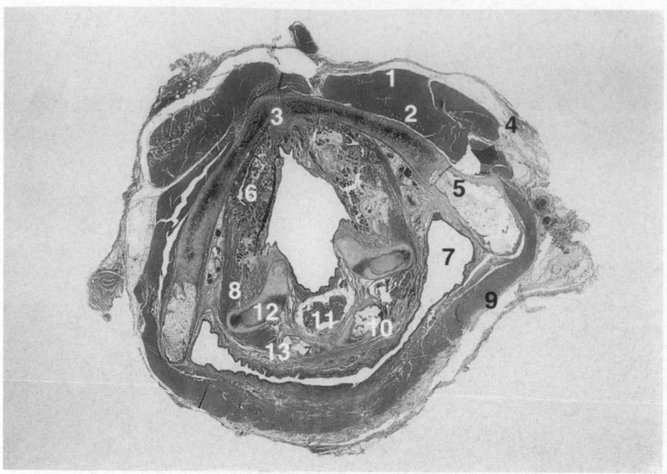

Figure 3.14 *Horizontal section of the larynx at the level of the ventricle (level B, Fig 3.12). Hematoxylin and eosin. 1, sternohyoid muscle; 2, sternothyroid muscle; 3, Broyles' ligament; 4, omohyoid muscle; 5, thyroid cartilage; 6, saccule and saccular glands; 7, pharynx (pyriform fossa); 8, lateral criso-arytenoid muscle; 9, inferior constrictor muscle; 10, cricoid cartilage; 11, interarytenoid muscle; 12, arytenoid cartilage; 13, posterior crico-arytenoid muscle.*

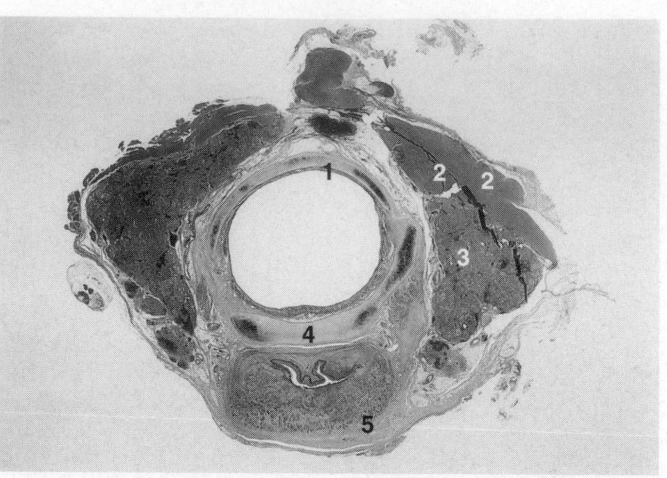

Figure 3.16 *Horizontal section of the larynx at the level of the subglottis (level D, Fig 3.12). Hematoxylin and eosin. 1, first ring of trachea; 2, strap muscles; 3, thyroid gland; 4, cricoid cartilage; 5, oesophageal lumen.*

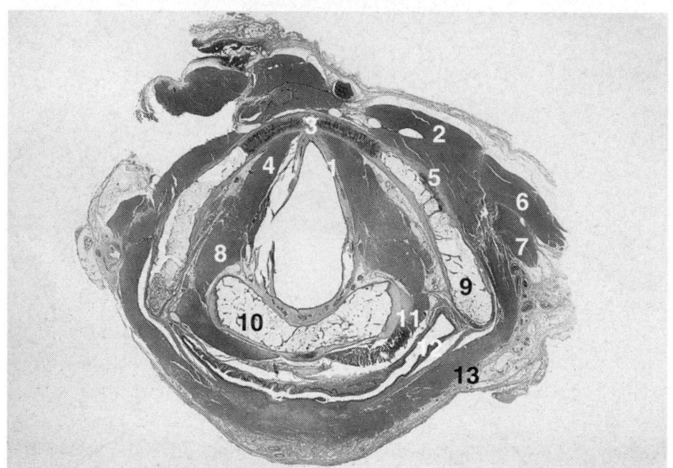

Figure 3.15 *Horizontal section of the larynx at the level of the vocal cords (level C, Fig 3.12). Hematoxylin and eosin. 1, vocal ligament; 2, sternohyoid muscle; 3, Broyles' ligament; 4, thyro-hyoid muscle; 5, sternothyroid muscle; 6, omohyoid muscle; 7, thyrohyoid muscle; 8, lateral crico-arytenoid muscle; 9, thyroid cartilage; 10, cricoid cartilage; 11, posterior crico-arytenoid muscle; 12, pharynx; 13, inferior constrictor muscle.*

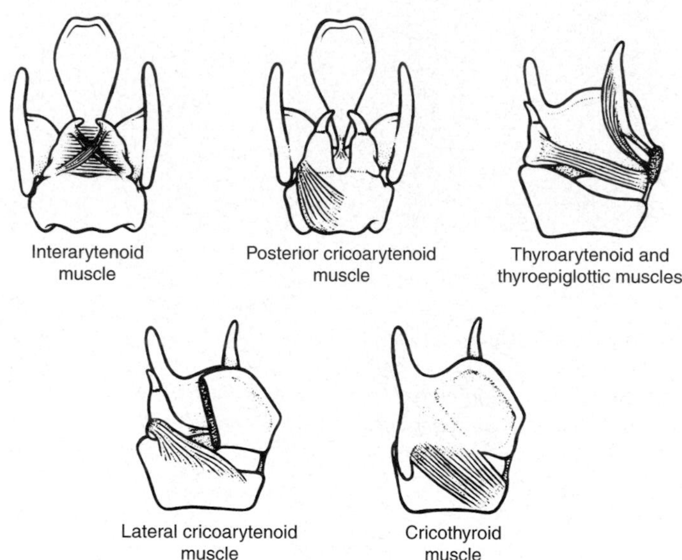

Figure 3.17 *Diagram illustrating the intrinsic muscles of the larynx.*

piriform fossa. Inferiorly is the region of the lower border of the thyroid cartilage. Anteroinferiorly, however, there are deficiencies through the paramedian gap by the side of the anterior cricothyroid ligament. Posteroinferiorly, adipose tissue extends towards the cricothyroid joint.[41,44] Some believe the thyroarytenoid muscle should be excluded as a component of the paraglottic space (see, e.g. reference 44). The paraglottic space contains the laryngeal ventricle and part, or all, of the laryngeal saccule.

The permeability and resistance of the potential laryngeal spaces have been studied by placement of dye in the loose connective tissue of postmortem larynges. A close correlation was found between the findings of these laboratory-based studies and clinical studies, although the

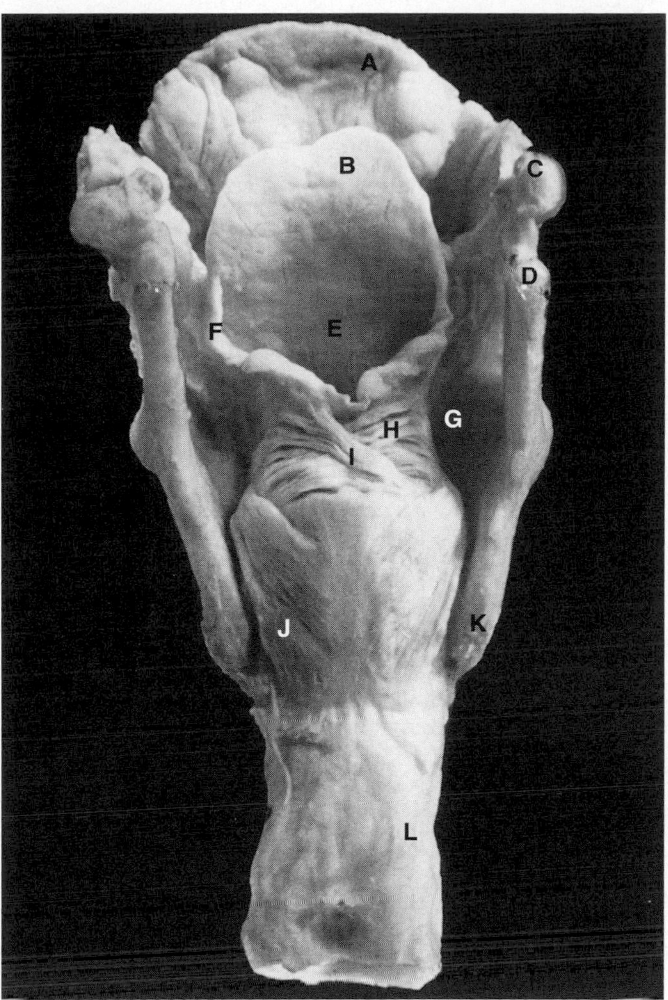

Figure 3.18 *Dissection of the posterior surface of the larynx, showing laryngeal musculature: A, posterior third of tongue; B, epiglottis; C, greater horn of hyoid bone; D, superior horn of thyroid cartilage; E, vestibule; F, aryepiglottic fold; G, pyriform fossa; H, transverse part of interarytenoid muscle; I, oblique part of interarytenoid muscle; J, posterior crico-arytenoid muscle; K, inferior horn of thyroid cartilage; L, trachea.*

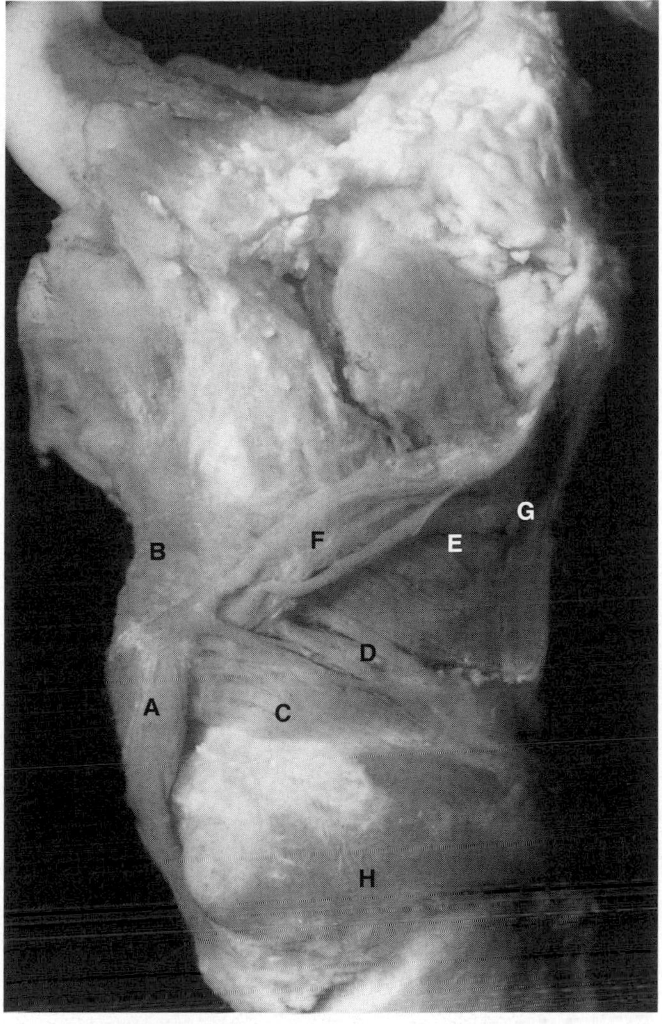

Figure 3.19 *Dissection of the larynx viewed internally and laterally, showing the laryngeal musculature: A, posterior cricoarytenoid muscle; B, interarytenoid muscle; C, lateral cricoarytenoid muscle; D, thyroarytenoid muscle (vocalis); E, thyroepiglottic muscle; F, upper fibers of thyroarytenoid muscle; G, lamina of thyroid cartilage; H, arch of cricoid cartilage.*

results tend to suggest that limitation of tumor expansion by the cricovocal membrane may be less significant than is generally considered.[64,65]

The anatomy of the paraglottic space is important in determining paths of spread to the thyroarytenoid muscles and then to the limits of the space to become transglottic, before extending out of the larynx or into the subglottis. Supraglottic tumors may also spread into the paraglottic space and reach the subglottis, or extend beyond the limits of the larynx. Ventricular tumors may obstruct mucous outflow from the saccule and cause its expansion within the paraglottic space to form a secondary laryngocele; the tumor itself may also spread transglottically, and thereby fix the vocal cord. Fixation of the vocal cord is a good indicator of a tumor within the paraglottic space. The proximity of the mucosa at the piriform fossa makes its removal in surgery mandatory for such disease.

The subglottic space

The subglottic space is bounded laterally by the cricovocal membrane, medially by the mucosa of the subglottic region, above by the undersurface of Broyles' ligament in the midline. Below, it is continuous with the inner surface of the cricoid cartilage and its mucosa.[61]

The relationships of the larynx are illustrated in Figs 3.6–3.16.

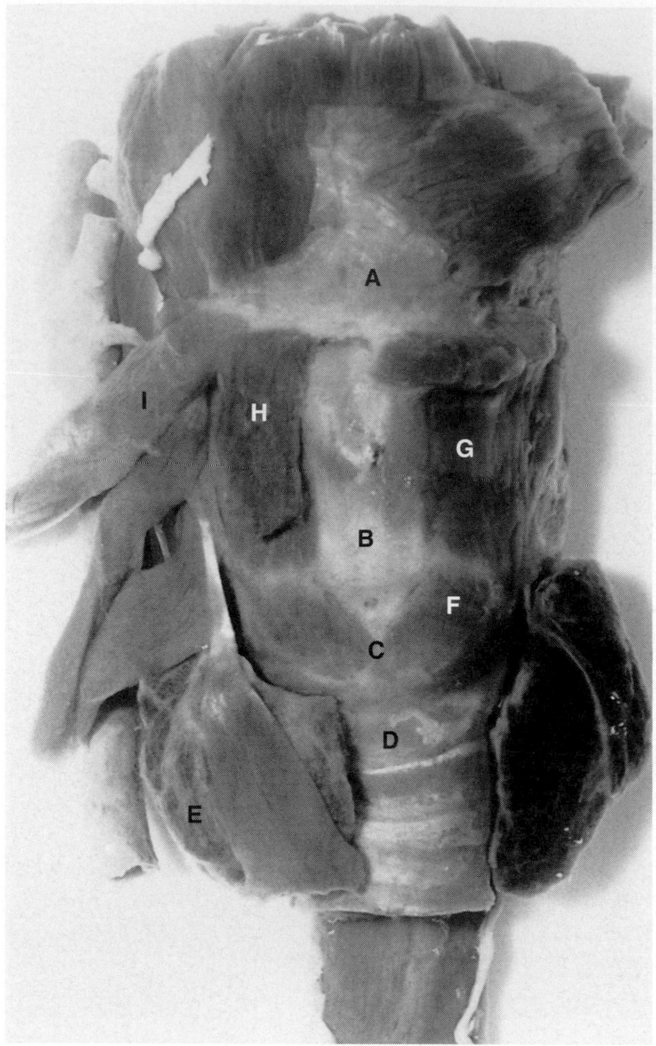

Figure 3.20 *Dissection of the larynx viewed anteriorly, showing the cricothyroid and intrahyoid strap muscles: A, body of hyoid bone; B, thyroid prominence; C, arch of cricoid cartilage; D, first tracheal ring; E, thyroid gland; F, cricothyroid muscle; G, thyrohyoid muscle; H, sternohyoid muscle; I, omohyoid muscle.*

The muscles of the larynx

The muscles can be categorized as extrinsic or intrinsic. The extrinsic muscles of the larynx have an attachment outside the larynx and include the infrahyoid (strap) muscles of the neck, and the stylopharyngeus, palatopharyngeus and inferior constrictor muscles of the pharynx. The extrinsic muscles are responsible for movements of the whole larynx (i.e. elevation and depression during swallowing, respiration and phonation). The thyrohyoid, stylopharyngeus and palatopharyngeus muscles elevate the larynx. The omohyoid, sternohyoid and sternothyroid muscles depress the larynx. Of these three latter muscles, sternothyroid is the only one that has an attachment onto the larynx and which therefore depresses the larynx by direct action. The omohyoid and sternohyoid muscles can cause depression of the larynx only indirectly by putting pressure on the larynx.

Because the larynx and the hyoid bone are connected by the thyrohyoid membrane and muscles, elevation of the larynx occurs not only by the action of the thyroarytenoid muscle, but also by the actions of the suprahyoid musculature (mylohyoid, digastric, stylohyoid and geniohyoid muscles).

The role of the extrinsic muscles during respiration appears variable. Thus, the larynx in some patients has been seen to rise during inspiration, in others it descends, whilst in some patients there is little change.[30] The extrinsic muscles can affect the tone and pitch of the voice through raising and lowering the larynx.

The intrinsic muscles of the larynx (Figs 3.17–3.20) are confined to the larynx and comprise the posterior cricoarytenoid, lateral cricoarytenoid, interarytenoid, thyroarytenoid and cricothyroid muscles. With the exception of the interarytenoid muscle, the muscles are paired.

The mass of muscle related to adduction far outweighs that related to abduction.[5] In this context, it is of interest to note that histological examination of normal larynges revealed evidence of some degenerative changes in the posterior cricoarytenoid muscle, the single muscle associated with abduction, but none in the remaining muscles.[20] The intrinsic muscles of the larynx are mainly concerned with the activities of the vocal cords. Extensions of the interarytenoid and thyroarytenoid muscles (the aryepiglottic and thyroepiglottic muscles) modify the inlet of the larynx.

Whereas most of the intrinsic muscles lie internally (under cover of the thyroid cartilage or the mucosa), the cricothyroid muscles appear on the outer and anterior aspect of the larynx.

The posterior cricoarytenoid muscle

This is the only muscle (Fig 3.18) that opens the glottis (Fig 3.21a) and it arises from a broad depression on the posterior surface of the lamina of the cricoid cartilage. Passing upwards and laterally, it is inserted into the muscular process of the arytenoid cartilage. The fibers appear to be arranged into two functional groups. The upper fibers, being almost horizontal, rotate the arytenoid cartilage and abduct the vocal cords. The lower fibers, being more vertical, pull the arytenoid cartilages down the sloping superior margin of the cricoid cartilage, thus separating them. The innervation also exhibits two main branches, one supplying the horizontal component and one supplying the more vertical fibers.[48]

The muscle is innervated by the recurrent laryngeal branch of the vagus nerve, while deriving its blood supply from the laryngeal branches of the superior and inferior thyroid arteries, especially the inferior and posterior arteries.

In about 6% of cases, an additional strip of muscle is seen in relation to the lower border of the posterior

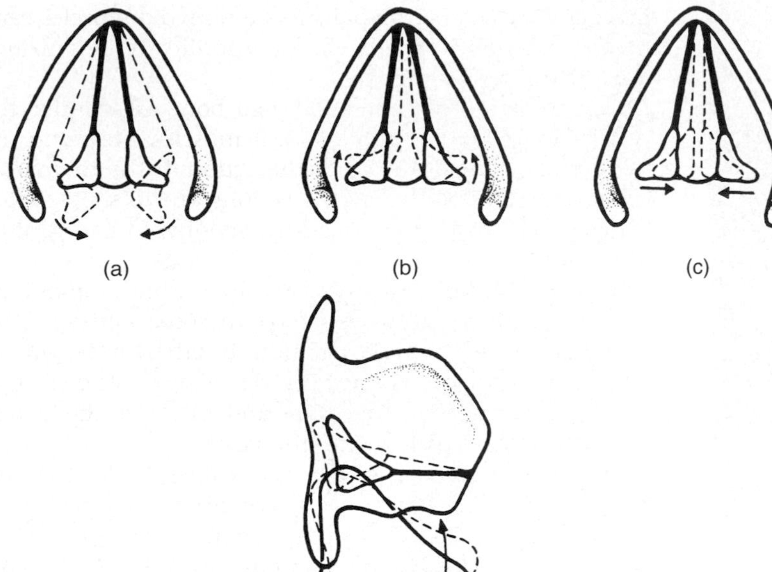

Figure 3.21 *Diagram illustrating movements of the laryngeal joints: (a, b, c) cricoarytenoid joints; (d) cricothyroid joints. (a) Movement related to posterior cricoarytenoid muscle. (b) Movement related to lateral cricoarytenoid muscle. (c) Movement related to interarytenoid muscle. (d) Movement related to cricothyroid muscle.*

cricoarytenoid muscle, arising from the cricoid cartilage and inserting onto the posterior aspect of the inferior horn of the thyroid cartilage. This has been called the ceratocricoid muscle.[55]

The lateral cricoarytenoid muscle

This muscle (Fig 3.19) originates from the lateral side of the upper border of the arch of the cricoid cartilage. It extends upwards and backwards, beneath the thyroid cartilage, to insert onto the muscular process of the arytenoid cartilage. The lateral cricoarytenoid muscle rotates the arytenoid cartilage in a direction opposite to that of the posterior cricoarytenoid muscle, thereby closing the glottis (Fig 3.21b). The recurrent laryngeal nerve supplies the lateral cricoarytenoid muscle, with a single branch that forms a homogeneous nerve plexus located in the middle of the muscle. This suggests the muscle acts as a 'single' unit, unlike the other intrinsic muscles of the larynx.[47] The muscle receives its blood supply from the laryngeal branches of the superior and inferior thyroid arteries.

The interarytenoid muscle

This muscle (see Figs 3.3 and 3.19) runs posteriorly between the muscular processes of the arytenoid cartilages. It is a single muscle in two parts. Many of its fibers run transversely, across the posterior surfaces of the arytenoids (the transverse arytenoid part), but some run obliquely from the muscular process of one arytenoid to the apex of the opposite cartilage (the oblique arytenoid part). The oblique fibers form two bands that cross to produce a distinctive 'X' shape. Some of the oblique fibers continue into the aryepiglottic folds as the aryepiglottic muscles. The transverse part of the interarytenoid muscle closes the intercartilaginous part of the glottis by approximating the arytenoid cartilages. This is accomplished by drawing the arytenoids upward along the sloping shoulders of the cricoid lamina, without rotation (Fig 3.21c). It may also cause lateral rocking of the arytenoid cartilage and its vocal process, aiding the posterior cricoarytenoid muscle in abduction.[10,32] The aryepiglottic muscles modify the inlet of the larynx. However, their poor development limits their action as sphincters of the inlet.

The interarytenoid muscle is innervated bilaterally by the recurrent laryngeal nerves. The muscle also receives branches from the internal laryngeal nerve, although it is not clear as to whether these branches contain any distinct motor input.[2,33,36,45,49] The nerves form a dense, anastomotic plexus which is highly variable.[33] The blood supply is derived from the laryngeal branches of the superior and inferior thyroid arteries.

The thyroarytenoid muscle

This muscle (see Fig 3.19) lies lateral to the vocal cord and has several different functional components. Perhaps for this reason it possesses by far the most dense anastomotic network of nerves seen in any of the intrinsic laryngeal muscles.[49] The thyroarytenoid muscle arises on the inner surface of the thyroid cartilage in the midline. It also arises from the cricovocal membrane. The thyroarytenoid muscle passes backwards, upwards and outwards to be inserted into the base and anterior surface of the arytenoid cartilage. The lower and deeper fibers form a

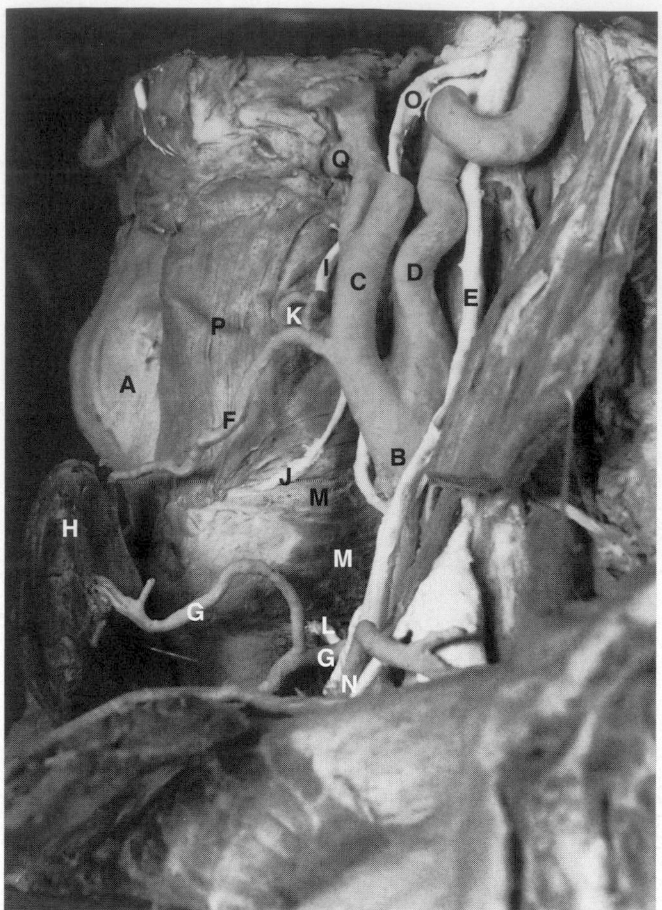

Figure 3.22 *Lateral view of larynx illustrating major arteries and nerves: A, thyroid cartilage; B, common carotid artery; C, external carotid artery; D, internal carotid artery; E, vagus nerve; F, superior thyroid artery; G, inferior thyroid artery; H, thyroid gland; I, internal laryngeal nerve; J, external laryngeal nerve; K, superior laryngeal artery; L, recurrent laryngeal nerve; M, inferior constrictor muscle; N, thyrocervical trunk; O, superior laryngeal nerve; P, thyrohyoid muscle; Q, lingual artery.*

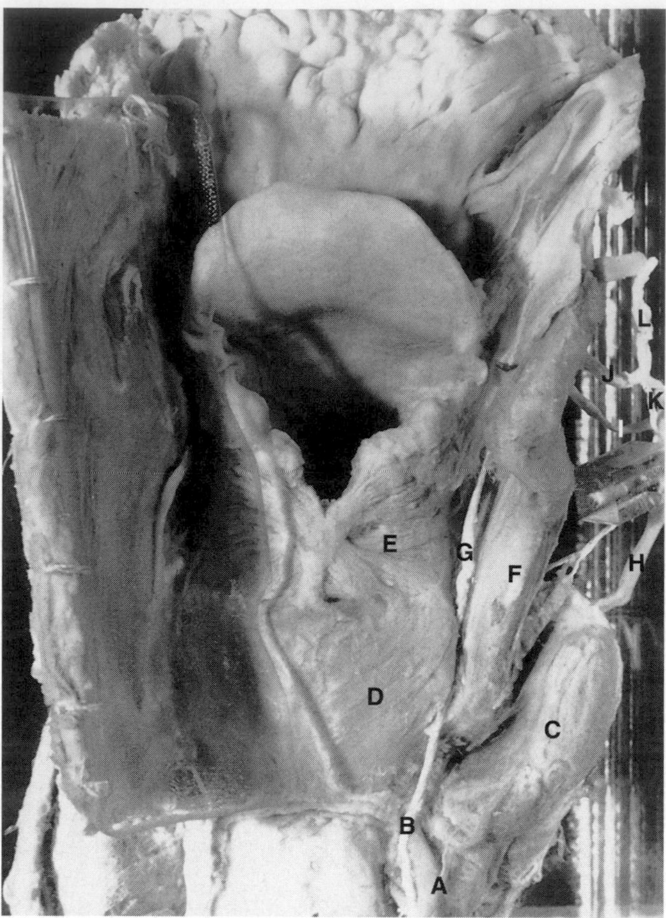

Figure 3.23 *Posterior view of larynx, illustrating major arteries and nerves: A, inferior thyroid artery; B, recurrent laryngeal nerve; C, thyroid gland; D, posterior cricoarytenoid muscle; E, interarytenoid muscle; F, posterior border thyroid cartilage; G, internal laryngeal nerve; H, superior thyroid artery; I, superior laryngeal artery; J, external laryngeal nerve; K, superior laryngeal nerve.*

distinct bundle that runs parallel with, and lateral to, the vocal ligament. This bundle is referred to as the vocalis muscle and is attached to the vocal process of the arytenoid cartilage. There is doubt as to whether the fibers of vocalis are also attached to the vocal ligament. The upper fibers of the thyroarytenoid muscle may extend into the aryepiglottic fold to form the thyroepiglottic muscle.

A distinct strip of muscle at the superolateral border of the thyroarytenoid and surrounding the ventricle occurs in about 80% of cases and has been termed the superior thyroarytenoid.[26] In addition, a variable amount of muscle fiber is found within the substance of the vestibular cord and has been called the ventricularis muscle.[26]

The primary function of the thyroarytenoid muscle is to shorten the vocal ligament and adjust the tension within it during phonation. In addition, it can rotate the arytenoid cartilage medially and so aid closure of the glottis. Increased tension of the muscle increases pitch, whilst decreased tension decreases pitch. Contraction of vocalis will alter the profile of the vocal cord and change the timbre of the voice. The thyroepiglottic muscles widen the inlet of the larynx. All parts of the thyroarytenoid muscle are supplied by the recurrent laryngeal nerve. In addition, a communicating branch is derived from the external laryngeal nerve, although it is not clear whether such branches carry motor or sensory fibers.[49]

The arterial blood supply is derived from the laryngeal branches of the superior and inferior thyroid arteries.

The cricothyroid muscle

The cricothyroid muscle (Fig 3.20) arises from the anterior and anterolateral parts of the external surface of the arch of the cricoid cartilage. Its fibers pass upwards and backwards to insert into the thyroid cartilage. Two distinct parts can be recognized. The anterior and superior fibers constitute the straight part of the cricothyroid muscle. This inserts into the lower border of the thyroid lamina. The posterior and inferior fibers constitute the oblique part of the cricothyroid muscle and insert into the inferior horn of the thyroid cartilage.

The cricothyroid muscle elongates and exerts tension on the vocal ligament. This is accomplished by elevating the arch of the cricoid cartilage and tilting back the upper border of its lamina (Fig 3.21d). As a result, the distance between the angle of the thyroid cartilage and the vocal processes of the arytenoids is increased. A similar activity results if the muscles pull the thyroid cartilage forward. Indeed, this is thought to be the principal activity during phonation, as the lamina of the cricoid cartilage is held in position against the vertebral column by the cricotracheal muscles.

Unlike the other intrinsic muscles of the larynx, the cricothyroid muscle is innervated not by the recurrent laryngeal nerve but by the external branch of the superior laryngeal nerve. The arterial supply to the muscle is provided by the cricothyroid branch of the superior thyroid artery and by the inferior laryngeal branch of the inferior thyroid artery.

The blood supply of the larynx

The blood supply of the larynx (Figs 3.22 and 3.23) is derived mainly from two pairs of arteries: the superior and inferior laryngeal arteries. The superior laryngeal artery is normally derived from the superior thyroid artery, a branch of the external carotid artery, as this artery passes down towards the upper pole of the thyroid gland. However, in about 15% of cases, it arises directly from the external carotid artery between the origins of the superior thyroid and lingual arteries.[60] The superior laryngeal artery runs down towards the larynx, with the internal branch of the superior laryngeal nerve lying above it.[12] It enters the larynx by penetrating the thyrohyoid membrane and divides into several branches that supply the larynx from the tip of the epiglottis down to the inferior margin of the thyroarytenoid muscle.[9,60] The smaller inferior laryngeal artery is a branch of the inferior thyroid artery, which itself is derived from the thyrocervical trunk of the subclavian artery. The inferior laryngeal artery runs up and into the larynx, deep to the lower border of the inferior constrictor muscle. It is accompanied in its course by the recurrent laryngeal nerve and enters the larynx just behind the cricothyroid articulation.[22]

A posterior laryngeal artery of variable size has been described as a regular feature which arises as an internal branch of the inferior thyroid artery.

The cricothyroid artery arises from the superior thyroid artery or from its anterior branch,[12] and may contribute to the supply of the larynx. It follows a variable course, either superficial or deep to the sternothyroid muscle. If superficial, it may be accompanied by branches of the ansa cervicalis. If deep, it may be related to the external laryngeal nerve.[68] It can anastomose with the artery of the opposite side and with the laryngeal arteries.

A rich anastomosis exists between the corresponding laryngeal arteries on both sides and between the laryngeal arteries of the same side.

The superior laryngeal arteries supply the greater part of the tissues of the larynx, from the epiglottis down to the level of the vocal folds, including the majority of the laryngeal musculature. The inferior laryngeal artery supplies the region of the cricothyroid muscle, whilst the posterior laryngeal artery supplies the tissue in the region of the posterior cricoarytenoid muscle.[60]

Venous return from the larynx occurs via superior and inferior laryngeal veins (see Fig 3.17). These run parallel to the laryngeal arteries. They drain into the superior and inferior thyroid veins, respectively.

The innervation of the larynx

The chief nerves (Figs 3.22 and 3.23) supplying the larynx are the superior laryngeal and recurrent laryngeal branches of the vagus, both of which contain sensory and motor fibers. The vocal cords form a dividing line for both the sensory and the secretomotor innervation of the mucosa within the larynx. Above the vocal cords, the mucosa is innervated by the internal laryngeal branch of the superior laryngeal nerve. Below the vocal cords, the mucosa is supplied by the recurrent laryngeal nerve. However, there is evidence of overlap in the region of the vocal cords.[49,67] The motor supply to the intrinsic muscles of the larynx is derived mainly from the recurrent laryngeal nerve. The cricothyroid muscle, however, is supplied by the external branch of the superior laryngeal nerve.

The superior laryngeal nerve leaves the trunk of the vagus at its inferior (nodose) ganglion. It curves downwards and forwards by the side of the pharynx, medial to the internal carotid artery. It divides into two branches, a smaller external branch and a larger internal branch, about 1.5 cm below the ganglion, although rarely both branches may arise from the ganglion.[25] The superior laryngeal nerve, or its branches, receive one or more communications from the superior cervical sympathetic ganglion: most frequently, the connection is with the external laryngeal nerve.[58]

The internal laryngeal nerve descends below the level of the greater horn of the hyoid bone to pass between the middle and inferior constrictor muscles of the pharynx. It enters the larynx by piercing the thyrohyoid membrane, with the superior laryngeal artery lying below it.[12] On entering the larynx, the nerve divides into an ascending branch (which supplies the mucosa of the piriform fossa) and a descending branch (which supplies the supraglottic mucosa). On the medial wall of the piriform fossa, descending branches give twigs to the interarytenoid muscle[36,45] and there are communicating branches with the recurrent laryngeal nerve.[33,36,46,49,59] The precise nature and function of these communicating nerves have yet to be determined.

The external branch continues downwards and forwards on the lateral surface of the inferior constrictor muscle to which it contributes some small branches. In about 30% of cases, the nerve is located within the fibers of the constrictor muscle.[8] It passes beneath the sternothyroid muscle, below its insertion into the oblique line of the thyroid cartilage and supplies the cricothyroid muscle. A communicating nerve continues from the posterior surface of the cricothyroid muscle, crosses the piriform fossa, and enters the thyroarytenoid muscle where it anastomoses with branches from the recurrent laryngeal nerve.[49,67] It is suggested that such communicating branches may provide both additional motor components to the thyroarytenoid muscle and sensory fibers to the mucosa in the region of the subglottis.[67] Of clinical importance, when considering the external laryngeal nerve, is its close relationship to the superior thyroid artery, which puts the nerve at potential risk when the artery is clamped during thyroidectomy.[8,12,25,31,68]

The external laryngeal nerve is potentially at risk where it is either particularly close to the artery (in about 20% of cases),[31] or where, instead of crossing the superior thyroid vessels about 1 cm or more above the superior pole of the gland, in about 20% of cases, it actually passes below this point.[8] The risk is likely to be exacerbated with large goiters.[7] The clinical signs of damage to the external recurrent laryngeal nerve are clearly less apparent than those associated with damage to the recurrent laryngeal nerve, as the cricothyroid muscle is the only one affected.[31]

The origins of the recurrent laryngeal nerves differ according to side. The right recurrent laryngeal nerve issues from the vagus nerve in front of the subclavian artery. It then passes below and behind the artery. The left recurrent laryngeal nerve arises in the thorax (around the arch of the aorta). Both nerves run up the neck towards the larynx in grooves between the esophagus and trachea, giving branches to each. The considerable length of the nerves makes them particularly susceptible to damage. The upper part of the recurrent laryngeal nerve has a close and variable relationship to the inferior thyroid artery, and it may pass in front of, behind, or parallel to the artery. The precise incidence of these relationships varies somewhat according to the particular study.[2,4,36,52]

The recurrent laryngeal nerve enters the larynx either by passing deep to (in two-thirds of cases) or between (in one-third of cases) the fibers of the cricopharyngeus muscle at its attachment to the lateral aspect of the cricoid cartilage,[62] supplying the muscle as it passes. At this point of entry, the nerve is in intimate proximity to the posteromedial aspect of the thyroid gland.[62] The main trunk divides into two (or more) branches, generally below the lower border of the inferior constrictor muscle. However, branching may occur higher up[35,59] to derive an anterior (mainly motor) branch sometimes called the inferior laryngeal nerve, and a posterior (mainly sensory) branch. The inferior laryngeal nerve passes posterior to the cricothyroid joint and its ligament. In this region it may (60%) or may not (40%) be covered by fibers of the posterior cricoarytenoid muscle.[40]

In following the main motor branch of the recurrent laryngeal nerve, the first branch is seen to innervate the posterior cricoarytenoid muscle. The nerve continues on to innervate the interarytenoid muscle and then the lateral cricoarytenoid muscle. The nerve subsequently terminates in the thyroarytenoid muscle.[49]

As stated previously, communications exist between the superior laryngeal nerve and its branches with the recurrent laryngeal nerve.[33,49] A communicating branch reaches the superior laryngeal nerve via the ansa Galeni.

The complexity of the distribution of motor end plates within the intrinsic muscles of the larynx appears to correlate with the functional divisions within the muscle.[16,17]

An unusual anomaly that is of relevance to laryngeal pathology and surgery, is the so-called nonrecurrent laryngeal nerve. In this condition (which has a frequency of between 0.3 and 1%), only the right side is affected and it is always associated with an abnormal origin of the right subclavian artery from the aortic arch on the left side. The right recurrent laryngeal nerve arises directly from the vagus nerve trunk high up in the neck and enters the larynx close to the inferior pole of the thyroid gland. If unrecognized, it may be susceptible to injury during surgery, as well as potentially being compressed by small tumors of the thyroid gland.[18]

Parasympathetic, secretomotor fibers run with both the superior and recurrent laryngeal nerves to glands throughout the larynx. Sympathetic fibers run to the larynx with its blood supply, having their origin in the superior and middle cervical ganglia.

The infant larynx

The infant larynx differs markedly from the adult larynx. It is relatively smaller and this has two main consequences. First, its lumen is disproportionately narrower than the adult and second, it lies higher in the neck than the adult larynx. The tip of the epiglottis is located at the level of the intervertebral disk between the first and second cervical vertebrae. This high position is associated with the ability of the infant to use its nasal airway to breathe while suckling. The epiglottis is X-shaped, with a furled petiole, and the laryngeal cartilages are soft and more pliable than the adult larynx (a fact which may predispose to airway collapse in inspiration, leading to the clinical picture of laryngomalacia). The cricothyroid ligament is relatively short, making emergency cricothyrotomy extremely difficult. The mucosa of the supraglottis is more loosely attached than the adult larynx and exhibits multiple submucosal glands. Inflammation of the supraglottis will therefore rapidly result in gross edema due to the laxity of the supraglottic soft tissues. The mucosa is also lax in the subglottis, the narrowest part of the infant larynx measuring 3.5 mm in diameter in neonates. Swelling at this point rapidly results in severe respiratory obstruction.

The saccule of the larynx is larger in children. There is also a swelling of soft tissue in the midline below the glottis on the cricoid lamina, which might help to occlude the central portion of the lumen during swallowing. There is also considerable development of glandular tissue in the region of the arytenoid cartilage.[38]

The histology of the larynx

Epithelium and associated glands

The larynx represents the junction between the upper aerodigestive tract and the lower respiratory tract. The former is predominantly lined with squamous epithelium whilst the latter is lined with pseudostratified columnar 'respiratory' epithelium. The transition from one to the other is not a smooth one and the morphology of the subepithelial glands similarly undergoes a gradual transformation from more simple structures seen submucosally in the pharynx to the typical more complex 'bronchial type' glands.

The lingual surface and upper half of the laryngeal surface of the epiglottis, together with the aryepiglottic folds have a stratified squamous epithelium. Below this a gradual transition is seen via a simple stratified columnar epithelium to pseudostratified respiratory epithelium, with stratified squamous epithelium persisting on those structures which experience regular abrasive contact with the contralateral structures during phonation, coughing and deglutition, e.g. the vocal folds and vocal processes of the arytenoids. Pathological patterns of contact will lead to pathological patterns of squamous hyperplasia, e.g. on the mucosa of the false cords, as will chronic inhalational injury, e.g. smoking.

Transmission electron microscopy (TEM) and histochemical studies of the endolaryngeal glands from the epiglottis, false cord, ventricle and true cord[37] have shown them to be complex arborized seromucinous glands confined predominantly to the lamina propria. A few glands extend more deeply, particularly over the laryngeal surface of the epiglottis and some areas, notably the free edge of the vocal folds, are devoid of glands. The serous tubules and mucous tubules drain into common collecting ducts formed principally by mitochondria-rich cells and basal cells, with intermediate cells with characteristics of goblet and respiratory glandular collector duct cells around the junction between mucus tubules and the collecting duct. The few taste buds on the laryngeal surface of the epiglottis and the gland-associated myoepithelial cells have peptidergic and cholinergic nerve endings arborizing amongst them. TEM shows the serous cells to contain a heterogeneous population of secretory granules, with seromucinous granules predominating. Histochemical studies suggest that serous cells predominantly secrete sialosulfomucins, lectins and neuraminidases, whilst mucinous cells secrete sialosulfomucins and lectins (whose nature appears to be directly related to the host's blood group).

The secretions of the laryngeal glands in particular from the laryngeal ventricle are probably important in the lubrication of apposing surfaces. However, it seems likely that most of this function tends to be served by the egress of tracheal and bronchial secretions.

The ultrastructure of the lamina propria

The ultrastructure of the laryngeal lamina propria varies between a superficial, loosely organized structure with relatively few collagen or elastic fibers, as seen in the so-called Reinke's space (above and lateral to the free edge of the vocal ligament), to deeper, much denser condensations of predominantly collagenous fibers around solid structures such as cartilages. An unusual feature is the relatively high proportion of elastic fibers seen in some regions, e.g. the epiglottic petiole and the parallel arrays in the edge of the vocal ligament (the thickened dorsal margin of the cricothyroid ligament). The density of these elastic fibers is higher on the superior surface of the vocal cord than on the inferior surface.[34]

The ultrastructure of the lamina propria of the vocal cord is of particular interest as it has a direct bearing on the process of phonation and the quality of voice produced. Light microscopy studies[21] have demonstrated the presence of a superficial 'cover' consisting of the epithelium and the superficial lamina propria and a transitional layer of intermediate and deep lamina propria lying on the muscle layer or 'body' of the vocal cord, making up a complex vibratory unit.

Electron microscopic studies have shown the fiber content of these layers to be characteristic[23] with the superficial layers containing clusters of collagen fibers (the basement membrane) and fine straight or coiled elastic fibers. It appears that these longitudinal fibers are anchored in place by looping 'anchoring fibers' which loop up through the superficial part of the lamina propria from their attachment on the lamina densa.[19]

The intermediate layers contain much thicker parallel arrays of elastic and collagen fibers running longitudinally parallel to the cord edge with finer coiled elastic and collagen fibers intertwined. The deeper layers show denser condensations of collagen fibers and coiled elastic fibers. Oxytalan microfibers have been described throughout the lamina propria with large numbers around the muscle fibers and basement membrane.

In the anterior macula flava, randomly arranged thinner elastic fibers appear to act as anchors for the thicker elastic fibers from the intermediate layer that intertwines with them. A similar arrangement is seen in the intermediate layer in the region of the posterior macula flava, just anterior to the vocal process of the arytenoid. The deep layer is connected to the intermediate layer by collagen fibers running from the adjacent cartilages.

It would appear that the elastic fibers have a role to play in restoring the cords to their resting morphology on completion of a vibratory cycle, whilst collagen fibers are important in maintaining the stratified structure of the vocal cord. In addition, the longitudinal arrangement of the elastic fibers in the intermediate layer assist the collagen and vocalis muscles to resist the considerable longitudinal forces in the vocal cord during phonation.

One might anticipate that changes in the morphology of the elastic and collagen fibers might alter the physiological function of the vocal cord as a vibrator. Age-related changes in the morphology of the elastic fibers similar to those seen in the vascular intima have been described, with the surface of the fibers becoming irregular with deposits and irregular curves.[23] Changes in the digestibility of the elastic fibers by elastase with age suggest metabolic alterations may also occur with age.[51] These changes may be associated with a change in the Young's modulus of the fibers and a resultant alteration of the voice. The macula flava, thought to be important in the synthesis of the fibrous components of the vocal cord, also shows changes in cell population and morphology with senescence. These may contribute to the changes in fiber morphology with age and an associated voice change.[50]

The laryngeal cartilages

There are three single cartilages of the larynx and six paired cartilages. All initially are made up of hyaline cartilage, but with time the epiglottis, corniculate and cuneiform cartilages and the vocal processes of the arytenoids become transformed into elastic cartilage.[57]

The spoon-shaped epiglottic cartilage is made entirely of elastic cartilage with deep pits and perforations. The fibrous networks of the elastic cartilage are curved and interlacing. The overlying epithelium is respiratory with collections of glands lining the indentations and pits in the cartilage. Relatively loosely attached in the infant epiglottis, the mucosa becomes more firmly attached as the epiglottis loses its infantile 'omega' shape and flattens into its adult shape. The mucosa of the lingual surface and upper laryngeal surface is principally squamous, whilst within the vestibule of the larynx respiratory-type epithelium is seen. The inferior portion of the anterior surface is not covered with mucosa but gives attachment to the fibers of the elastic hyoepiglottic ligament medially with adipose tissue becoming more prominent laterally.

The adult thyroid and cricoid cartilages consist of more rigid hyaline cartilage, which with age shows an increasing tendency to calcify. This tendency may start as early as the late teens. The thyroid cartilage, which has a more basophilic matrix than the cricoid, calcifies initially in the region of the inferior cornu and the process tends to spread anteriorly and superiorly. Calcification tends to occur predominantly around the margins of the cartilage with a central translucent window often persisting into old age. Occasionally a marrow cavity may form within the ossified areas.

In the infant larynx the cartilages are soft and pliable, but with age they become stiff and prone to fracture with deformation. Synovial joints are seen where the inferior cornua of the thyroid cartilage articulate with the posterolateral aspect of the lamina of the cricoid and the arytenoids articulate with the superior margin of the cricoid.

The paired arytenoid cartilages have a body of hyaline cartilage and inferior synovial joints with lax joint capsular ligaments, where they articulate with the upper part of the lamina of the cricoid cartilage. The bodies of the arytenoids may also calcify with age, as may the muscular processes. The vocal processes and apex of the arytenoid cartilages are composed of elastic fibrocartilage, which does not tend to ossify with age. The corniculate cartilages lie on the apices of the arytenoid cartilages to which they may be fused or articulate by way of a synovial joint. The cuneiform cartilages lie in the margin of the aryepiglottic folds. Both pairs of cartilages are made of elastic cartilage and show little tendency to ossify.

The laryngeal muscles

The laryngeal muscles are fine, delicate, striated muscles with small motor bundles. The fibers are fine and contain high concentrations of succinic dehydrogenase and mitochondria in the subsarcolemmal and interfibrillar areas, suggesting rapid contractility and short refractory periods. The posterior cricoarytenoid, cricothyroid and thyroarytenoid muscles have separate bellies defined by their nerve supplies whilst the vocalis muscle is innervated by a complex plexus of nerves and is composed of multiple fine motor units.

The laryngeal nerves

The nerves of the larynx derive from the superior and recurrent laryngeal nerves and histologically are seen to be made up of mixed nerves with a variety of neuronal bundles of varying degrees of myelination. Crossover between the superior and inferior nerves is seen in the anastomosis of Galen and is thought to consist purely of sensory fibers. There are significant cross-connections between the recurrent nerves and the internal laryngeal nerves in the region of the interarytenoid muscles.[49] A cross-connection between the branches of the superior laryngeal nerve and the cervical sympathetic nerve was a virtually constant feature in one cadaveric study,[58] apparently supplying the cricothyroid muscle and the thyroid gland itself. Neuroendocrine cells have been found in animal larynges and it has been suggested that similar cells may have a role to play in allergic laryngitis and spasmodic croup in the human population.[69]

Acknowledgments

We are grateful to the Museums of the Royal College of Surgeons of England for Figures 3.4, 3.5, 3.7, 3.9–3.11,

3.18, to Professor L Garey, Charing Cross and Westminster Medical School for Figures 3.5 and 3.20, to Professor C Dean, University College London for Figures 3.19 and 3.23, to Professor M Berry, United Medical and Dental Schools, London for Figure 3.3 and to Professor Sir D Harrison for Figures 3.12–3.16. We are grateful to Mr F Sambrook for photographic assistance.

References

1. Berkovitz BKB, Moxham BJ. *A Textbook of Head and Neck Anatomy*. London: Wolfe, 1988.
2. Berlin DD, Lahey FH. Dissection of the recurrent and superior laryngeal nerves. *Surg Gynecol Obstet* 1929; **49:** 102–4.
3. Bosma JF, Bartner H. Ligaments of the larynx and the adjacent pharynx and esophagus. *Dysphagia* 1993; **8:** 23–8.
4. Bowden REM. The surgical anatomy of the recurrent laryngeal nerve. *Br J Surg* 1955; **43:** 153–7.
5. Bowden REM, Sheuer JL. Weight of abductor muscles and adductor muscles of the human larynx. *J Laryngol Otol* 1960; **74:** 971–80.
6. Broyles EN. The anterior commissure tendon. *Ann Otol Rhinol Laryngol* 1943; **52:** 342–5.
7. Cernea CR, Nishio S, Hojaij FC. Identification of the external branch of the superior laryngeal nerve (EBSLN) in large goitres. *Am J Otolaryngol* 1995; **16:** 307 11.
8. Cernea CR, Ferras AR, Nishio S, Dutra A Jr, Hojaij FC, dos Santos LR. Surgical anatomy of the external branch of the superior laryngeal nerve. *Head Neck* 1992; **14:** 380–3.
9. Classen H, Klaws GR. Preparation of four-color arterial corrosion casts of the laryngeal arteries. *Surg Radiol Anat* 1992; **14:** 301–5.
10. Crumley RL. Unilateral recurrent nerve paralysis. *J Voice* 1994; **8:** 79–83.
11. Dayal VS, Bahri H, Stone PC. Preepiglottic space. An anatomical study. *Arch Otolaryngol* 1972; **95:** 130–3.
12. Durham FC, Harrison TS. The surgical anatomy of the superior laryngeal nerve. *Surg Gynecol Obstet* 1962; **118:** 33–44.
13. Eckel HE, Sittel C, Zorowka P, Jerke A. Dimensions of the laryngeal framework in adults. *Surg Radiol Anat* 1994; **16:** 31–6.
14. England RJA, Wilde AD, McIlwain JC. The posterior cricoarytenoid ligaments and their relationship to the cadaveric position of the vocal cords. *Clin Otolaryngol* 1996; **21:** 425–8.
15. Erkki A, Pitkanen R, Suominen H. Observations on the structure and the biomechanics of the cricothyroid articulation. *Acta Otolaryngol (Stockh)* 1987; **103:** 117–26.
16. Freije J, Malmgren LT, Gacek RR. Motor end-plate distribution in the human lateral cricoarytenoid muscle. *Arch Otolaryngol Head Neck Surg* 1986; **112:** 176–9.
17. Freije J, Malmgren LT, Gacek RR. Motor end-plate distribution in the human interarytenoid muscle. *Arch Otolaryngol Head Neck Surg* 1987; **113:** 63–8.
18. Friedman M, Toriumi DM, Grybauskas V, Katz A. Nonrecurrent laryngeal nerves and their clinical significance. *Laryngoscope* 1986; **96:** 87–90.
19. Gray SD, Rignatari SS, Harding P. Morphologic ultrastructure of anchoring fibres in the normal vocal fold basement membrane. *J Voice* 1994; **8:** 48–52.
20. Guindi GM, Michaels L, Bannister R, Gibson W. Pathology of intrinsic muscles of the larynx. *Clin Otolaryngol* 1981; **6:** 101–9.
21. Hirano H. Morphological structure of the vocal cord as a vibrator and its variations. *Folia Phoniat (Basel)* 1974; **26:** 89–94.
22. Hollingshead WH. *Anatomy for Surgeons. Vol. I. The Head and Neck*, 3rd edn. Philadelphia: Harper and Row, 1982.
23. Ishii K, Zhai WG, Akita M, Hirose H. Ultrastructure of the lamina propria of the human vocal fold. *Acta Otolaryngol (Stockh)* 1996; **116:** 778–82.
24. Jurik AG. Ossification and calcification of the laryngeal skeleton. *Acta Radiol Diagn* 1984; **25:** 17–22.
25. Kambic V, Zargi M, Radsel Z. Topographic anatomy of the external branch of the superior laryngeal nerve. *J Laryngol Otol* 1984; **98:** 1121–4.
26. Kotby MN, Kirchner JA, Kahane JC, Basiouny SE, el-Samaa M. Histo-anatomical structure of the human laryngeal ventricle. *Acta Otolaryngol (Stockh)* 1991; **111:** 396–402.
27. Maguire A, Dayal VS. Supraglottic anatomy; the pre- or peri-epiglottic space? *Can J Otolaryngol* 1974; **3:** 432–45.
28. Maue WM, Dickson DR. Cartilages and ligaments of the adult human larynx. *Arch Otolaryngol* 1971; **94:** 432–9.
29. McIlwain JC. The posterior glottis. *J Otolaryngol Suppl* 1991; **2:** 1–24.
30. Mitchinson AG, Yoffey JM. Respiratory displacement of larynx, hyoid bone and tongue. *J Anat* 1947; **81:** 118–20.
31. Moosman DA, DeWeese MS. The external laryngeal nerve as related to thyroidectomy. *Surg Gynecol Obstet* 1968; **127:** 1011–16.
32. Mossallam I, Nasser Kotby M, Abd-el-Rahman S, el-Samma M. Attachment of some internal laryngeal muscles at the base of the arytenoid cartilage. *Acta Otolaryngol (Stockh)* 1987; **103:** 649–56.
33. Mu L, Sanders I, Wu B-L, Biller HF. The intramuscular innervation of the human interarytenoid muscle. *Laryngoscope* 1994; **104:** 33–9.
34. Nakaaki K, Shim T. A three dimensional reconstructive study of the layer structure of the human vocal cord. *Eur Arch Otorhinolaryngol* 1993; **250:** 190–2.
35. Nguyen M, Junien-Lavillauroy C, Faure C. Anatomical intra-laryngeal anterior branch study of the recurrent (inferior) laryngeal nerve. *Surg Radiol Anat* 1989; **11:** 123–7.
36. Norland M. The larynx as related to surgery of the thyroid based on an anatomical study. *Surg Gynecol Obstet* 1930; **51:** 449–59.
37. Pastor LM, Ferran A, Calvo A, Sprekelsen C, Horn R, Marin JA. Morphological and histochemical study of human submucosal laryngeal glands. *Anat Rec* 1994; **239:** 453–67.
38. Pracy R. The infant larynx. *J Laryngol Otol* 1983; **97:** 933–47.
39. Pressman JJ. Sphincter action of the larynx. *Arch Otolaryngol* 1941; **33:** 351–77.
40. Reidenbach MM. Topographical relations between the

posterior cricothyroid ligament and inferior laryngeal nerve. *Clin Anat* 1995; **8:** 327–33.
41. Reidenbach MM. Normal topography of the conus elasticus. Anatomical bases for the spread of laryngeal cancer. *Surg Radiol Anat* 1995; **17:** 107–11.
42. Reidenbach MM. The cricoarytenoid ligament: its morphology and possible implications for vocal cord movements. *Surg Radiol Anat* 1995; **17:** 307–10.
43. Reidenbach MM. The periepiglottic space; topographic relations and histological organisation. *J Anat* 1996; **188:** 173–82.
44. Reidenbach MM. The paraglottic space and transglottic cancer: anatomic considerations. *Clin Anat* 1996; **9:** 244–51.
45. Rueger RS. The superior laryngeal nerve and the interarytenoid muscle in humans: an anatomical study. *Laryngoscope* 1972; **82:** 2008–31.
46. Sanders I, Li Y, Biller H. Axons enter the human posterior cricoarytenoid muscle from the superior direction. *Arch Otolaryngol Head Neck Surg* 1995; **121:** 754–7.
47. Sanders I, Mu L, Wu B-L, Biller HF. The intramuscular nerve supply of the human lateral cricoarytenoid muscle. *Acta Otolaryngol (Stockh)* 1993; **113:** 679–82.
48. Sanders I, Wu B-L, Mu L, Biller HF. The innervation of the human posterior cricoarytenoid muscle: evidence for at least two neuromuscular compartments. *Laryngoscope* 1994; **104:** 880–4.
49. Sanders I, Wu B-L, Mu L, Li Y, Biller HF. The innervation of the human larynx. *Arch Otolaryngol Head Neck Surg* 1993; **119:** 934–9.
50. Sato K, Hirano M. Age-related changes of the macula flava of the human vocal fold. *Ann Otol Rhinol Laryngol* 1995; **104:** 839–44.
51. Sato K, Hirano M. Age related changes of the elastic fibres in the superficial layer of the lamina propria of the vocal folds. *Ann Otol Rhinol Laryngol* 1997; **106:** 44–8.
52. Sato I, Shimada K. Arborization of the inferior laryngeal nerve and internal nerve on the posterior surface of the larynx. *Clin Anat* 1995; **8:** 379–87.
53. Sato K, Kurita S, Hirano M, Kiyokawa K. Distribution of elastic cartilage in the arytenoids and its physiologic significance. *Ann Otol Rhinol Laryngol* 1990; **99:** 363–8.
54. Sellars IE, Keen EN. The anatomy and movements of the cricoarytenoid joint. *Laryngoscope* 1978; **88:** 667–74.
55. Sharp JF. The ceratocricoid muscle. *Clin Otolaryngol* 1990; **15:** 257–61.
56. Silver CE. *Surgery for Cancer of the Larynx*. London: Churchill Livingstone, 1981.
57. Sorokin SP. The respiratory system. In: Weiss L, ed. *Histology*, 5th edn. London: Macmillan Press, 1983: 788–868.
58. Sun S-Q, Chang RWH. The superior laryngeal nerve loop and its surgical implications. *Surg Radiol Anat* 1991; **13:** 175–80.
59. Sunderland S, Swaney WE. The intraneural topography of the recurrent laryngeal nerve in man. *Anat Rec* 1952; **114:** 411–25.
60. Trotoux J, Germain MA, Bruneau X. La vascularisation du larynx. *Ann Otolaryngol Chir Cervicofac* 1986; **103:** 389–97.
61. Tucker HM. *The Larynx*. New York: Thieme, 1987.
62. Wafae N, Vieira MC, Vorobieff A. The recurrent laryngeal nerve in relation to the inferior constrictor muscle of the pharynx. *Laryngoscope* 1991; **101:** 1091–3.
63. Weir N. Anatomy of the larynx and tracheobronchial tree. In: Gleeson M, ed. *Scott-Brown's Otolaryngology. Vol. I. Basic Sciences*, 6th edn. Oxford: Butterworth Heinemann, 1997: Chapter 12.
64. Welsh LW, Welsh JJ, Rizzo TA Jr. Laryngeal spaces and lymphatics: current anatomic concepts. *Ann Otol Rhinol Laryngol Suppl* 1983; **105:** 19–31.
65. Welsh LW, Welsh JJ, Rizzo TA Jr. Internal anatomy of the larynx and the spread of cancer. *Ann Otol Rhinol Laryngol* 1989; **98:** 228–34.
66. Williams PL (ed). *Gray's Anatomy*, 38th edn. London: Churchill Livingstone, 1995.
67. Wu B-L, Sanders I, Mu L, Biller HF. The human communicating nerve. An extension of the external superior laryngeal nerve that innervates the vocal cord. *Arch Otolaryngol Head Neck Surg* 1994; **120:** 1321–8.
68. Yerzingatsian KL. Surgical anatomy of structures adjacent to the thyroid apex and post-operative voice change (a review including dissection). *J Laryngol Otol Suppl* 1987; **101:** 1–13.
69. Yu YC, Miyazaki J, Shin T. Neuroendocrine cells in the cat laryngeal epithelium. *Eur Arch Otorhinolaryngol* 1996; **253:** 287–93.

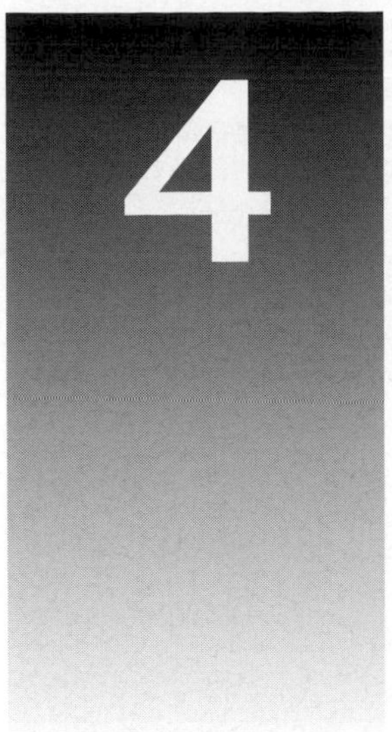

Comparative anatomy of the larynx

John A Kirchner

Anatomy

Laryngeal anatomy shows a steady progression from the primitive slit on the floor of the pharynx in the lungfish to an organ capable, in the human, of an astonishing combination of range, stability and precision unequalled in the animal kingdom. In most animals the larynx serves the simple but vital purpose of keeping everything but air out of the lung. This function has developed to a remarkable level in mammals below the primate level, but at the expense of the less vital function of vocalization.

Among the vertebrates, the larynx first appears in the lungfish, an animal that inhabits rivers that dry up at times, leaving this fish stranded in shallow pools without enough water to allow the use of gills. When the river dries up, the fish breathes air until the rains return and fill the river. During its aquatic existence the lungfish needs a mechanism for keeping water out of the lung. Its slit-like larynx, protected by a sphincter muscle, remains closed until the fish reaches the surface. During its terrestrial sojourn, the lungfish breathes by trapping air in the buccal cavity, then contracting the floor of the mouth and pharyngeal constrictor muscles to force air into the lungs. This process is an outgrowth of the buccal pump used by more primitive forms of fish for suction feeding and gill irrigation.[3] Since the larynx of the lungfish lacks a dilator muscle, the buccal pump pressure simply forces air through the membranous slit into the lung.

An evolutionary improvement over the simple slit-like larynx of the lungfish is that of the frog. It retains the sphincter muscle for airway protection, but has acquired a cricoid ring that serves as a solid base for attachment of the muscles that dilate the glottis. The combination of a complete ring and muscular dilatation serves to prevent narrowing or collapse of the lumen that might result from negative pressure during inspiration. Like the lungfish, the frog uses the buccal pump mechanism to inflate the lungs.

An animal that spends much of its time in the water, such as the crocodile, penguin or sea lion, must keep its glottis closed while opening its mouth under water to catch a fish or other prey. It reopens only when the penguin or seal has surfaced. The crocodilian larynx has an additional layer of airway protection. Its free edge, known in the crocodile as the hyoid, is rigid and functions like the mammalian epiglottis.[17] Its free edge fits snugly into a recess along the posterior edge of the soft palate. These two layers reinforce the tight seal around the top of the larynx so that the crocodile can drown its victim without drowning itself. It needs only to bring its nostrils above the surface from time to time.[2]

Among the reptiles, the snake has acquired several modifications for deglutition because it swallows objects whole, often larger than its own head, and long enough to require 15 or more minutes to pass through the mouth. It avoids suffocation during its lengthy meal by moving the larynx forward to the level of the lower teeth, below the prey. This movement is made possible by a muscle that functions like the human geniohyoid and which, in the snake, attaches to the upper trachea. With the laryngeal aditus in this forward position, the snake can take in gulps of air from time to time. The cartilaginous glottic margins resist compression as the bolus passes, as does the tracheal wall which consists of complete rings and is easily displaced laterally.[14]

In sub-primate mammals, both herbivores and carnivores, airway protection during the act of swallowing is provided by a high, intranarial epiglottis that rests against the nasopharyngeal surface of the soft palate (Fig 4.1a,b). The intranarial position is particularly important – vitally important, in fact – to the herbivores. The deer, for example, must be able to sniff the air for predators while

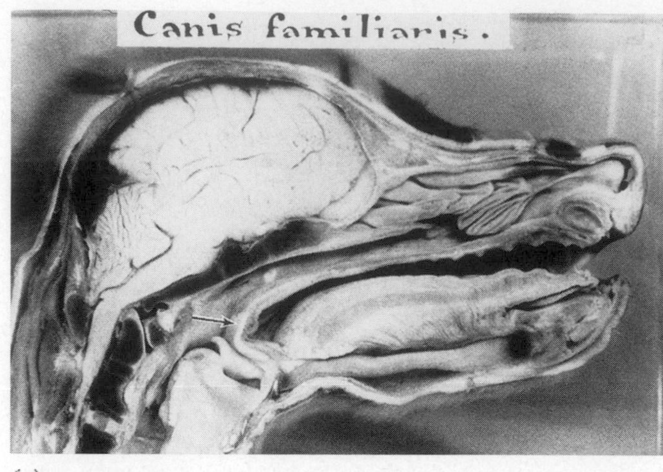

(a)

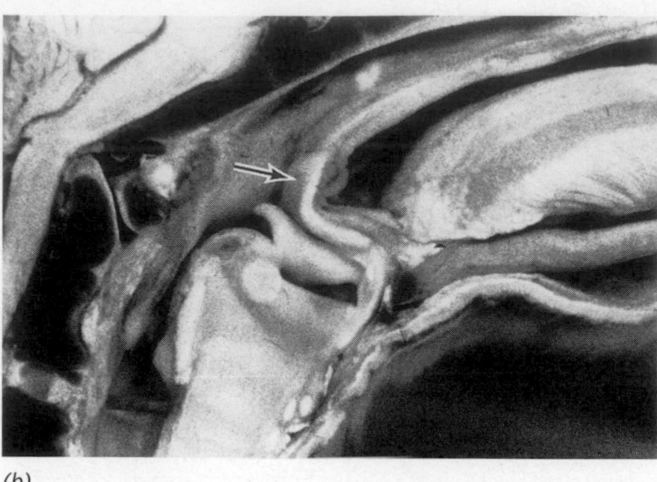
(b)

Figure 4.1 *(a) In most mammals below the level of primates, the epiglottis (arrow) lies in contact with the nasopharyngeal surface of the soft palate. This section of a dog's head is on display in the Hunterian museum, Royal College of Surgeons, London. (b) Higher power of same specimen.*

it feeds. During the act of swallowing, the side walls of the palate and upper pharynx contract around the laryngeal inlet, acting like a direct tube connecting the external air supply with the lung. According to some, this allows nasal breathing while food descends alongside the larynx through the lateral food channels. A further function of the deer's intranarial epiglottis is that the scent of an upwind predator is not masked by the aroma of food in the deer's mouth.

The newborn larynx is protected by a similar position, the epiglottis lying behind the soft palate where it rests, except when the baby cries. This position allows the infant to suckle without aspirating, and to breathe with the mouth closed. Except when the baby cries, nasal breathing is obligatory in the newborn, as demonstrated by the devastating respiratory distress caused by bilateral choanal atresia. The baby's larynx gradually descends from this intranarial position during the first few weeks, and reaches its adult level in the hypopharynx between 4 and 6 months of age.[15]

Intrapulmonary pressure

Apart from airway protection, the larynx serves an equally vital function in aquatic reptiles and amphibians, that of modulating intrapulmonary pressure. The lungs of a frog are not protected by a rib cage and would collapse like a deflated balloon in a deep dive. Not only would the lungs collapse, but so would the pulmonary capillaries as well. Such collapse is prevented by the larynx, which closes during expiration, either partially or completely, to maintain intrapulmonary pressure.

The feedback relationship between the larynx and lung has attained additional refinement in man and in those animals with well-developed, lobulated lungs. Because the larynx can alter the area of the glottic aperture from moment to moment, it can regulate the level of intrathoracic and intrapulmonary pressure by the degree of choking-off that it places on the air stream.[6] Partial closing of the glottis during inspiration lowers these pressures; partial closing during expiration raises them. As a result, intrathoracic pressure and suction influence the return flow of blood to the heart to a significant degree. A partially closed glottis during expiration squeezes some of the air back into the alveoli, accounting for the expiratory sigh and pursed lips of the emphysema victim. Similarly, the expiratory laryngeal grunt of the newborn baby with respiratory distress syndrome may represent an attempt to maintain lung inflation.

Ventilatory exchange

Ventilatory exchange under conditions of rapid respiration requires an upper airway with minimal resistance. Animals that are capable of vigorous, prolonged exercise, like the deer and the horse, need a laryngeal inlet that allows maximum entrance of air. The greatest cross-sectional area at the glottis results when the cartilaginous parts of the vocal cords make up approximately seven-tenths of the overall length. The animal that most closely approaches this optimum cross-sectional area is the horse, whose cartilaginous vocal processes occupy more than half the length of the vocal cord, about 70%.[16] Man's larynx, on the other hand, whose vocal processes make up half or less of the total length of the cord, is not suited to fast, long-distance running (Fig 4.2).[8]

Inspiratory phonation is difficult or impossible in animals possessing a laryngeal ventricle. The human vocal folds trap air in the ventricle and narrow the glottis when they approach one another close enough to produce sound during inspiration. The cat's larynx, on the other hand, having no ventricle, offers little or no obstruction

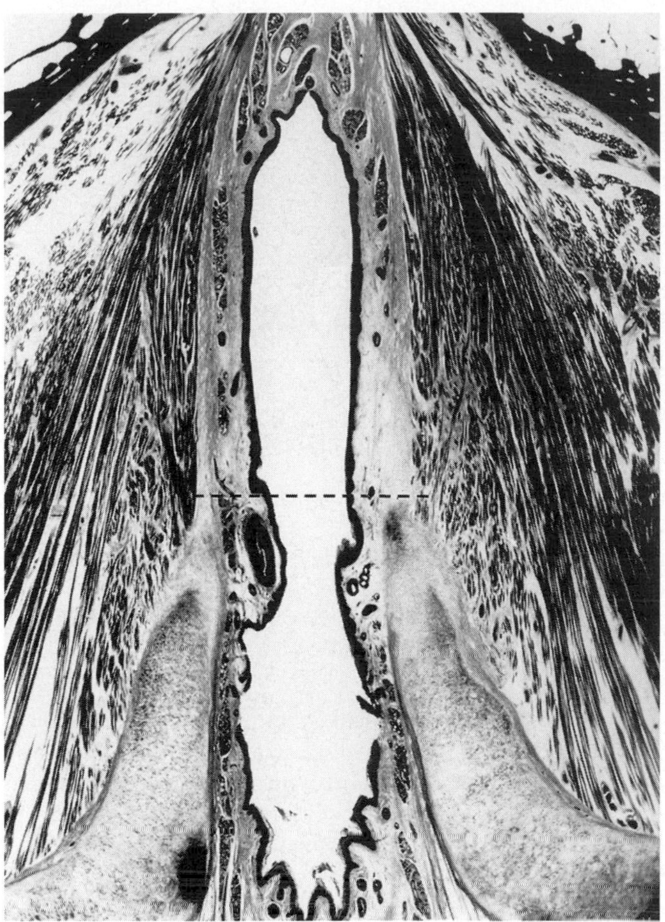

Figure 4.2 *Transverse section of adult male larynx. The vocal processes of the arytenoid cartilages usually occupy approximately 40% of the glottic length, leaving the membranous portions of the cords free to vibrate. In this specimen, the processes are unusually long, occupying some 50% of the cord's length. Dotted line indicates tips of vocal processes. In the larynx of the reptile, bird and marsupial these cartilaginous struts occupy the entire length of the cords and do not vibrate.*

to the entrance of air. The cat purrs on both inspiration and expiration. The rounded glottic apertures may also explain why the cat and cow are incapable of hiccup.

The remarkable adaptations of structure to accommodate the requirements of function develop only in animals living in the wild, where Nature takes care of their needs. With selective inbreeding of domesticated animals, desirable features such as tenacity in the bulldog or speed in the racehorse may be accompanied by crippling side effects. The English bulldog, for example, with powerful jaws that provided tenacity in the days of bull baiting, has inherited stenotic nostrils and a long, thick soft palate, both conditions obstructing its airway. The dog's nose and palate produce so much negative pressure during inspiration that the ventricular soft tissue may be sucked out of its recess and into the laryngeal lumen. This results in severe stridor, sufficient in some dogs to produce cardiopulmonary failure and death.[11]

The horse may be victimized by a disorder characterized by partial or complete paralysis of the intrinsic laryngeal muscles. The condition is the result of degeneration of the recurrent laryngeal nerve, usually the left.[5] In its advanced forms, with the left vocal fold lying weak or motionless near the midline, it causes inspiratory stridor ('roaring') and, in the Thoroughbred, can end the horse's racing career.[4] The mechanism for recurrent laryngeal neuropathy is not known, but the recurrent nerve may be vulnerable for two reasons. In addition to being the longest nerve in the horse's body, the left recurrent nerve may be subject to compression when a dilated left atrium presses against a dilated pulmonary artery during prolonged, extreme exertion. Length is probably not the major factor. In a study by Hahn and Mayhew of the larynx in 47 zebras and seven giraffes, no histologic evidence of pathology consistent with idiopathic laryngeal hemiplegia was found.[7] The disorder has been studied most intensively in the Thoroughbred, but is not limited to this breed. In a study of young mixed breed horses showing no evidence of neurogenic changes in the intrinsic laryngeal muscles, the number of myelinated fibers was found to be significantly lower in the left than in the right recurrent laryngeal nerve.[12] The discrepancy, and the fact that recurrent laryngeal neuropathy has been observed in yearlings before they started a racing career, suggest a genetic factor in the disorder. Animals living in the wild, unlike the racehorse, have not been subjected to artificial inbreeding for speed.

Sound production

Sound originating in the larynx requires glottic margins that are soft and pliable enough to be set into vibration by air from the lungs. A method of sound production analogous to the buccal pump of the lungfish is used by the male bullfrog, in which air is driven back and forth between lungs and closed mouth across membranous vocal cords. Vocal sacs alongside the floor of the mouth are inflated during this process and add resonance to the calls. Female frogs are not equipped with vocal sacs and are usually silent.[1]

In some animals a larynx is present, but is not used for the production of voice. Many herbivorous animals live in open country where they can easily be seen by their companions and have little use for voice. The larynx of the antelope, giraffe, horse and camel, although capable of sound, is rarely used for this purpose. In other animals the vocal cords may not be capable of vibration, as in the reptile, bird and marsupial whose glottic margins are cartilaginous. It requires more air pressure than a snake or a bird can generate to make cartilage vibrate, so that the larynx of most reptiles, lizards and birds can make only a hissing or blowing sound.

The cartilaginous rim of the bird's glottis probably represents the forerunner of vocal processes of the arytenoids found in higher animals. Because these cartilaginous edges cannot be used for singing, the bird has acquired a unique method of producing song: a pair of vibrating membranes at the lower end of the trachea, the so-called syrinx. By varying the tension within these membranes the bird can attain a wide range of musical tones. Its larynx serves only to bar the entrance of solids and liquids into the lung.

In those animals that need a voice for communication at a distance, an intranarial epiglottis hampers vocalization and requires adjustments even for simple phonation. The howling of a wolf or coyote, for example, requires that the epiglottis be disengaged from above the palate. The animal therefore throws up its head to bring the larynx down into the back of the mouth, so that the sound can be emitted through the oral cavity. The resonance and amplification gained through this maneuver allow the voice to reach potential mates at a distance.

Negus has suggested that when man's early ancestors took to the trees to escape enemies, the sense of vision gradually displaced olfaction as a means of protection. The degeneracy of olfaction liberated the epiglottis from its position in the nasopharynx, allowing a gap to be interposed so that laryngeal sounds escaping from the mouth can be articulated by the tongue, palate and lips.[13]

The Australopithecine larynx was probably positioned high in the pharynx, with vocal tracts much like those of today's monkeys or apes. The high position of the larynx would have made it impossible for them to produce some of the vowel sounds of modern speech.[9]

Voice quality depends largely on the shape, size and compliance of the true and false vocal cords. The cat's larynx, for example, has membranous folds but no vocal ligament that would provide tension and dependable changes in pitch. The human voice, having evolved as a mere byproduct of the laryngeal valve, has nevertheless attained a combination of range, stability and precision unequalled in the animal kingdom. Singing requires almost instantaneous changes in the mass, length, shape and tension of the vocal folds. This combination of changes requires two anatomic relationships that are present only in the human larynx. First, a cricothyroid joint, a structure shared with other mammals, and second, an attachment of the vocalis muscle to the conus elasticus, a relationship present only in the human larynx. The larynx of the reptile, bird or marsupial has no cricothyroid joint, the thyroid and cricoid being one solid cartilaginous or bony mass. Even if the vocal cords in these animals were made of membrane instead of cartilage, their length could not be changed. They could manage only a monotone.

Although the cricothyroid joint is present in other mammals, it is only in the human larynx that the thyroarytenoid muscle contains a vocalis segment, a component that can change the shape of the true cord by the adjustable traction it exerts on the conus elasticus. Even in our closest cousin, the ape, the thyroarytenoid muscle does not extend into a vocal ligament or conus elasticus.[17]

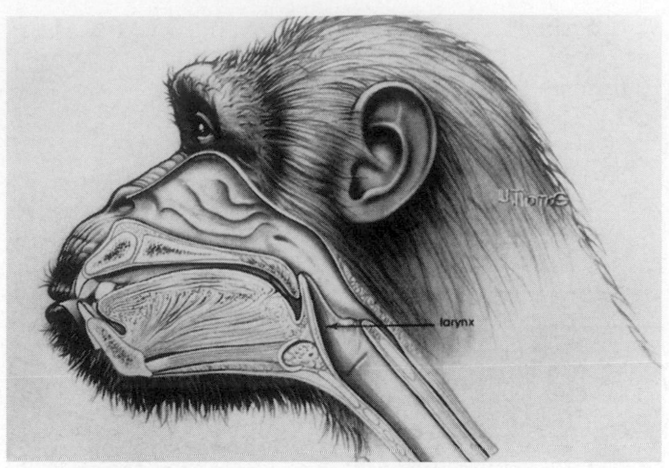

Figure 4.3 *Chimpanzee larynx during quiet respiration. During sound production the epiglottis is disengaged from its intranarial position but still remains too high in the pharyngeal cavity for effective modification of sounds produced by the vocal cords. (Reproduced with the kind permission of the author, Jeffrey Laitman, from reference 10.)*

Could a chimpanzee speak if it had the brain power? The high position of its larynx would frustrate the ape's attempts to produce certain vowel sounds of modern speech (Fig 4.3).[10] The voice would lack resonance and the fine tonal adjustments that result from changes in the shape of the human vocal folds.

Considering the range, power, versatility and stability of the human voice, it is difficult to escape the conclusion that the evolutionary development of the human larynx was directed almost as much toward communication with man's fellow creatures as toward the more vital protection of the airway.

References

1. Allen AA. Voices of the night. *National Geographic Magazine* 1950 **Apr:** 507–22.
2. Bellairs A. *The Life of Reptiles*. Vol. 1, 2. New York: Universe Books, 1970.
3. Brainerd EL, Ditelberg JS, Bramble DM. Lung ventilation in salamanders and the evolution of vertebrate air-breathing mechanisms. *Biol J Linnean Soc* 1993; **49:** 163–83.
4. Cook WR. *Specifications for Speed in the Racehorse. Airflow Factors*. Menasha: Russell Meerdink, 1989.
5. Duncan I. The pathology of equine laryngeal hemiplegia. *Acta Neuropathol (Berl)* 1974; **27:** 337–48.
6. Gautier H, Remmers JE, Bartlett D. Control of the duration of expiration. *Respir Physiol* 1973; **18:** 205–24.
7. Hahn CN, Mayhew LG. Examination of the laryngeal musculature and recurrent laryngeal nerves of zebra (*Equus burchelli*) and giraffe (*Giraffa camelopardalis*) for evidence of idiopathic laryngeal hemiplegia. In press.
8. Hirano M, Sato K. *Histological Color Atlas of the Human Larynx*. San Diego: Singular Publishing Group, 1993.

9. Laitman JT. The anatomy of human speech. *Nat Hist* 1984; **Aug:** 20–7.
10. Laitman JT. L'origine du langage articulé. *Recherche* 1986; **17:** 1164–72.
11. Leonard HC. Eversion of the lateral ventricles in dogs – 5 cases. *J Am Vet Med Assoc* 1957; **137:** 83–4.
12. Lopez-Plana C, Sautet JY, Pons I, Navarro G. Morphometric study of the recurrent laryngeal nerve in young 'normal' horses. *Res Vet Sci* 1993; **55:** 333–7.
13. Negus VE. *The Comparative Anatomy and Physiology of the Larynx*. New York: Hafner, 1962.
14. Oldham JC, Smith HM, Smith SA. *A Laboratory Prospectus of Snake Anatomy*. Champaign: Stipes Publishing, 1970.
15. Sasaki CT, Levine PA, Laitman JT, Crelin ES Jr. Postnatal descent of the epiglottis in man. *Arch Otolaryngol* 1977; **103:** 169–71.
16. Sisson S, Grossman JD. General respiratory system. In: Getty R, ed. *The Anatomy of the Domestic Animals*, 5th edn. Vol. 1. Philadelphia: Saunders, 1970.
17. Wind J. *On the Phylogeny and the Ontogeny of the Human Larynx*. Groningen: Wolters-Noordhoff, 1970.

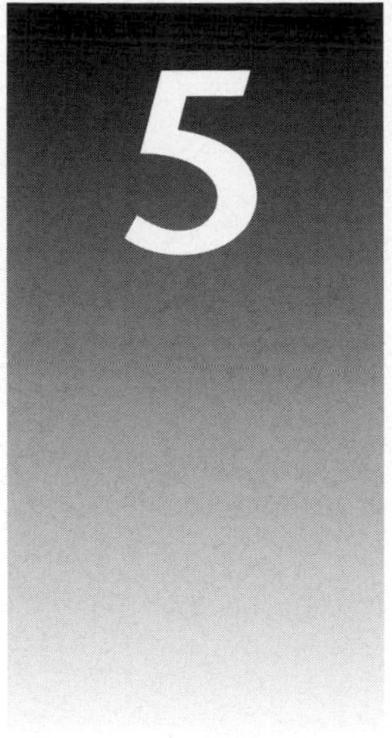

Laryngeal physiology

Agnes Czibulka, Douglas A Ross
and Clarence T Sasaki

The human larynx serves three main functions: these are protective, respiratory and phonatory. This chapter addresses the three functions in terms of structural relationships, neuromuscular reflexes and their relationship to the cardiovascular system. Also reviewed are the effects of tracheotomy and anesthesia on these reflexes.

Structural considerations

The upper airway in the adult human traverses the digestive tract in the region of the pharynx, providing sphincteric protection while complicating the respiratory function of the lower airway. Two important organic modifications developed during evolution to resolve this functional difficulty: structural adaptation and delicate coordination among the three basic laryngeal functions as dictated by precisely organized brainstem reflexes.

Many mammalian species are provided with a relatively high-riding larynx, affording its close approximation with structures of the posterior nasal cavities. The intranarial position of the larynx, which secures a continuous airway from the nose to the bronchi, decreases the risk of pulmonary contamination by swallowed matter.

The human newborn exhibits similar nasolaryngeal connection by the approximation of its epiglottis with the posterior surface of its palate, thus ensuring against aspiration.

In the adult the characteristic flat, shield-like configuration of the epiglottis serves to direct swallowed food laterally into the pyriform sinuses, away from the midline laryngeal aperture. Furthermore, in adult humans, elevation of the larynx toward the nasal cavity during the height of deglutition exaggerates this protective function. The aryepiglottic folds act as ramparts to the larynx, allowing food to pass on either side of the epiglottis along the gutter produced between each fold and the lateral pharyngeal wall. It appears that the primary function of the supraglottic larynx lies in its protection of the lower airway.

The ability of the larynx to perform as an effective valve depends on the unique shelf-like configuration of its bilateral superior and inferior folds. The ventricular folds or false cords, which are located superiorly, act as an exit valve, preventing the escape of air from the lower respiratory tract. When medialized by muscular contraction, these false cords seal even more tightly as tracheal pressure is increased below. This feature of adducted false cords is attributable to their unique shape, characterized by the down-turned direction of their free margins.

Conversely, the true cords behave as a one-way valve in the opposite direction, obstructing the ingress of air or fluid. The false cords prevent the egress of air from the lungs, and the true cords with their up-turned margins are capable of arresting its ingress.

The afferent and efferent innervation

The structural adaptation of the larynx in man aids in maintaining the functional diversity of this organ.

Sensory nerve fibers to the larynx are derived from the internal branch of the superior laryngeal nerve, which ipsilaterally innervates the superior mucosal boundary of the larynx to the level of its true vocal cords. Likewise, below the true cords, ipsilateral sensation is mediated by each recurrent laryngeal nerve. Suzuki and Kirchner, however, demonstrate a diamond-shaped area anteriorly in the midline of the subglottic space in the cat that is innervated by contributions from both external branches of the superior laryngeal nerve.[10] Afferent impulses from deep muscle receptors and the cricothyroid joints also travel cephalad in this nerve branch (Table 5.1).

Table 5.1 Sensory territories of the larynx

Nerve	*Distribution*
Superior laryngeal (internal division)	Supraglottic mucosa Thyroepiglottic joint Cricoarytenoid joint
Superior laryngeal (external division)	Anterior subglottic mucosa Cricothyroid joint
Recurrent laryngeal	Subglottic mucosa Muscle and spindles spirals
Nerve of Galen (communicating branch between superior and recurrent nerves)	Aortic arch

The density of sensory innervation appears greatest in the laryngeal inlet, an observation consistent with the concept that the aditus serves as a protective zone for the more distal respiratory system. The posterior part of the true vocal cord is more heavily innervated with touch receptors than its anterior portion.

Water chemoreceptors on the epiglottis have been experimentally implicated in the production of prolonged apnea.[3] It is generally agreed that sensory components of the superior laryngeal nerve include contributions from mucosal touch receptors, epiglottic chemoreceptors, joint receptors, aortic baroreceptors, and stretch receptors from the intrinsic laryngeal muscles.[1] Afferent impulses are delivered through the ganglion nodosum to the brainstem tractus solitarius.

The motor innervation to the intrinsic laryngeal musculature originates in the medullary nucleus ambiguus. Each recurrent laryngeal nerve ipsilaterally innervates all muscles except the cricothyroid muscle, which receives its motor impulses from the external division of its ipsilateral superior laryngeal nerve. Only the interarytenoid muscles receive bilateral motor innervation from both recurrent laryngeal nerves. The muscle that enlarges the glottic airway, as takes place on inspiration, is solely the role of the posterior cricoarytenoid muscle, which extends from the posterior aspect of the cricoid plate to the muscular process of the arytenoid (Fig 5.1a). Exerting a posterolateral force on the arytenoid body will rotate the vocal fold outward, effecting cord abduction on inspiration. Vocal cord adduction results from contraction of all other intrinsic muscles, especially by the thyroarytenoid and lateral cricoarytenoid muscles (Fig 5.1b,c). The interarytenoid muscles serve to close the posterior gap in the glottis (Fig 5.1d), whilst the cricothyroid muscle adducts and tenses the vocal cord, passively lengthening it by 30% (Fig 5.1e).

When one cricothyroid muscle is denervated by sectioning the superior laryngeal nerve, the unopposed contraction of the contralateral cricothyroid muscle results in rotation of the posterior commissure toward the inactive side, with foreshortening of the cord on the side of denervation. Unilateral recurrent laryngeal nerve injury results in paramedian positioning of the denervated cord since the unopposed action of the ipsilateral cricothyroid muscle, innervated by an intact superior laryngeal nerve, produces cord adduction on the side of the damaged recurrent laryngeal nerve.

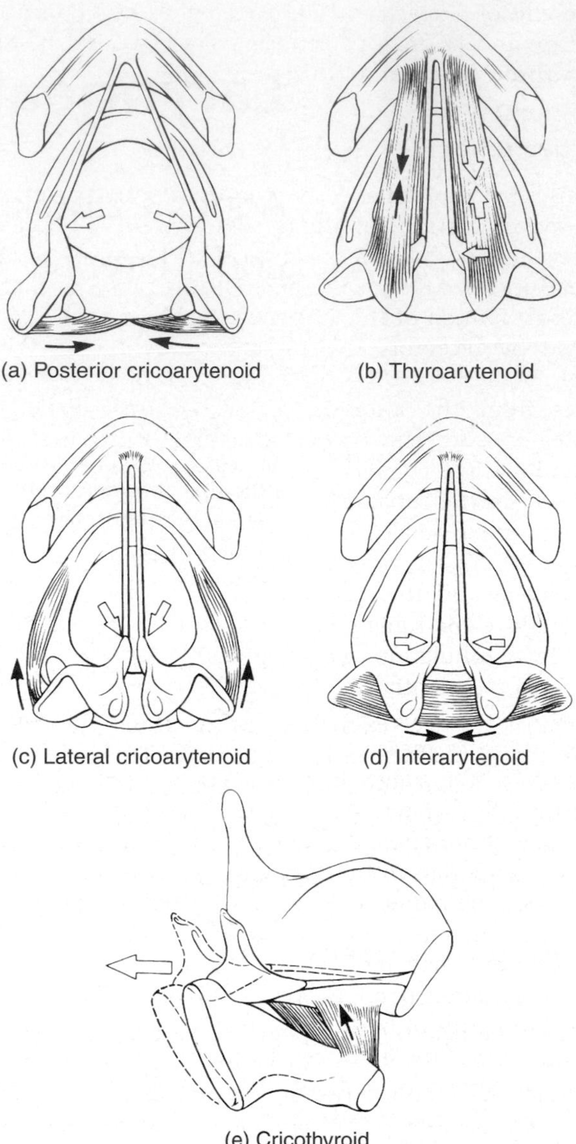

Figure 5.1 *Laryngoscopic view of the intrinsic muscles responsible for activating vocal cord position.*

Laryngeal reflexes

Basic functions of the larynx (protective, respiratory and phonatory) are derived from a complicated interrelationship of diverse polysynaptic brainstem reflexes. Protective function is entirely reflexive and involuntary, constituting one end of a spectrum that is balanced by voluntary respiratory and phonatory performances regulated involuntarily through an array of feedback reflexes.

Protective reflex

Stimulation of the upper respiratory tract, especially the larynx, evokes a strong glottic closure reflex. The afferent input reaches the brainstem via the superior and inferior laryngeal nerves. Most of the afferent impulses travel via the internal branch of the superior laryngeal nerve (SLN), generated by receptors in the supraglottic larynx. The external branch of the SLN also conducts afferent impulses from the anterior portion of the subglottic mucosa and from the deeper structures, including the cricothyroid joint. The recurrent laryngeal nerve conducts impulses from the subglottic region.

The functional analog of this reflex is reproduced as protective laryngeal closure during deglutition. Touch, and chemical and thermal stimulation of the laryngeal aditus produce the same response as seen experimentally when electrostimulation of SLN produces a low threshold-evoked action potential in the adductor branches of the recurrent laryngeal nerve. In man, the threshold of the adductor reflex is measured to be 0.5 V and possesses a latency of 25 ms, suggesting that this is a polysynaptic brainstem reflex (Fig 5.2). In commonly used animal models, the stimulation of one SLN produces simultaneous action potentials in the contralateral adductor musculature, hence the name crossed adductor reflex. Man does not possess this reflex; it is therefore possible that unilateral SLN injury may result in failure of ipsilateral cord closure, a condition predisposing to aspiration despite the anatomic integrity of both recurrent laryngeal nerves.

Bilateral SLN stimulation results in sphincteric closure of the upper airway of its three muscular tiers within the laryngeal framework. The highest occurs at the level of the aryepiglottic folds, which contain the superior-most divisions of the thyroarytenoid muscle. The contraction of these fibers approximates the aryepiglottic folds to cover the superior inlet of the larynx, and with the arytenoid cartilages in the posterior gap, completes the first of three sphincteric tiers of protection.

The second tier of protection occurs at the level of the false cords, consisting of bilateral folds forming the roof of each laryngeal ventricle.

The third tier of protection occurs at the level of the true vocal cords, which in man are shelf-like with a slightly upturned free border. The inferior division of the thyroarytenoid muscle forms the bulk of this shelf, and with the passive valvular effect of the upturned border of the true cord margin, the true vocal cord perhaps is the most significant of the three barriers to aspiration.

Mechanical stimulation applied to the upper respiratory tract, which is innervated by the trigeminal and glossopharyngeal nerves, or the electrical stimulation of all major cranial afferent nerves, produces strong laryngeal adductor responses. In the cat, reflex action potentials in the adductor branch of recurrent laryngeal nerve can be elicited by electrostimulation of the optic, acoustic, chorda tympani, trigeminal, splanchnic, vagus, radial and intercostal nerves.[12] The susceptibility of this reflex response to such diverse sensory stimulation is unique and emphasizes its primitive role in respiratory protection of the organism from a wide variety of potentially noxious influences.

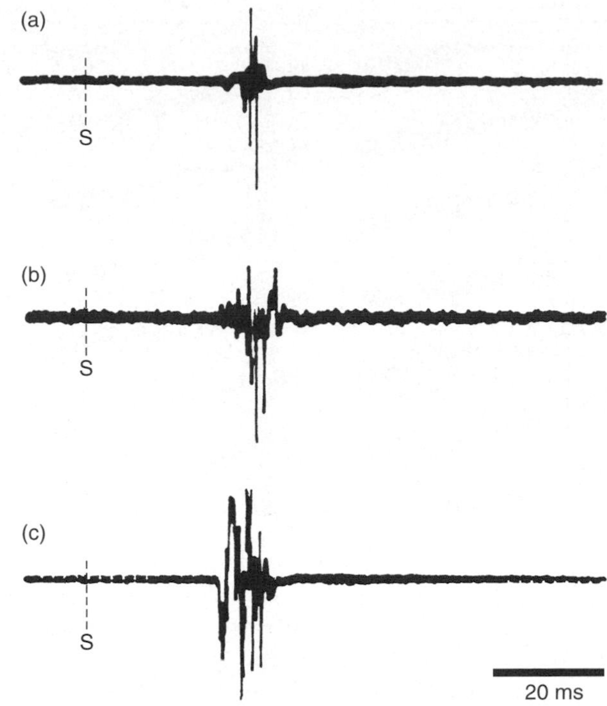

Figure 5.2 *Ipsilateral adductor responses evoked by single-shock stimulation of superior laryngeal nerve in three separate patients, (a), (b) and (c). Stimulus is represented as S. In man, no contralateral adductor reflex can be demonstrated.*

Physiologic exaggeration of the glottic closure reflex is called laryngospasm, clinically observed as a strong prolonged closure of the glottis when the adductor muscle is tonically contracted and maintained well beyond the cessation of mucosal irritation. From neurophysiologic analysis, laryngeal spasm consists of prolonged tonic adductor spike activity in the recurrent laryngeal nerve that bears no precisely reproducible temporal relationship or latency, to its initiating stimulus (Fig 5.3).[13] This observation is based on the fact that laryngeal spasm is solely mediated by stimulation of the SLN. In fact, high-frequency stimulation of other afferent nerves, capable of eliciting simple glottic closure, produces little adductor afterdischarge activity that is characteristic of laryngospasm.

Adductor motor depression caused by hypoventilation is supported by other experimental data indicating preferential abolition of postsynaptic potentials by hypoxia.[2] This experimental evidence further indicates that in

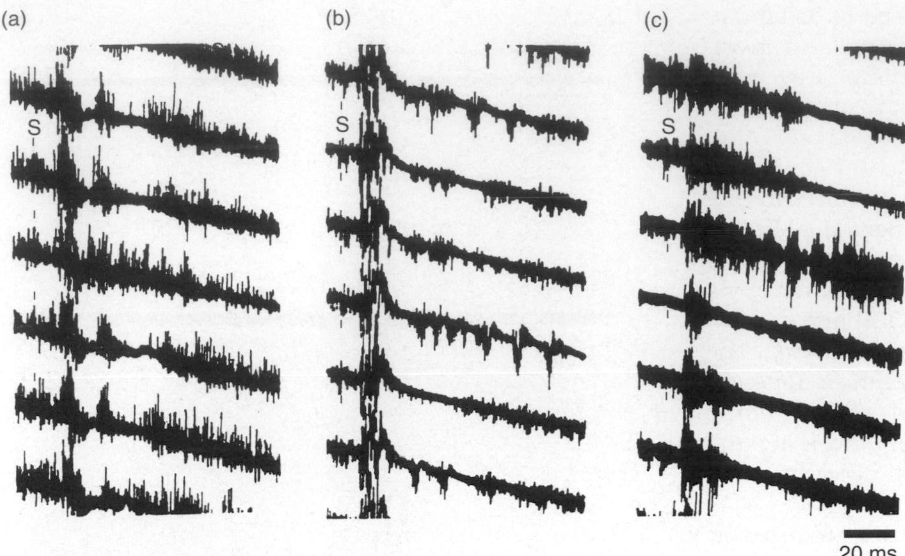

Figure 5.3 *Primary evoked responses and random high-frequency afterdischarge activity. (a) Recurrent laryngeal nerve. (b) Thyroarytenoid muscle. (c) Lateral cricoarytenoid muscle produced by repetitive stimulation of ipsilateral superior laryngeal nerve in dog (0.3 V/0.1 ms at 8 Hz).*

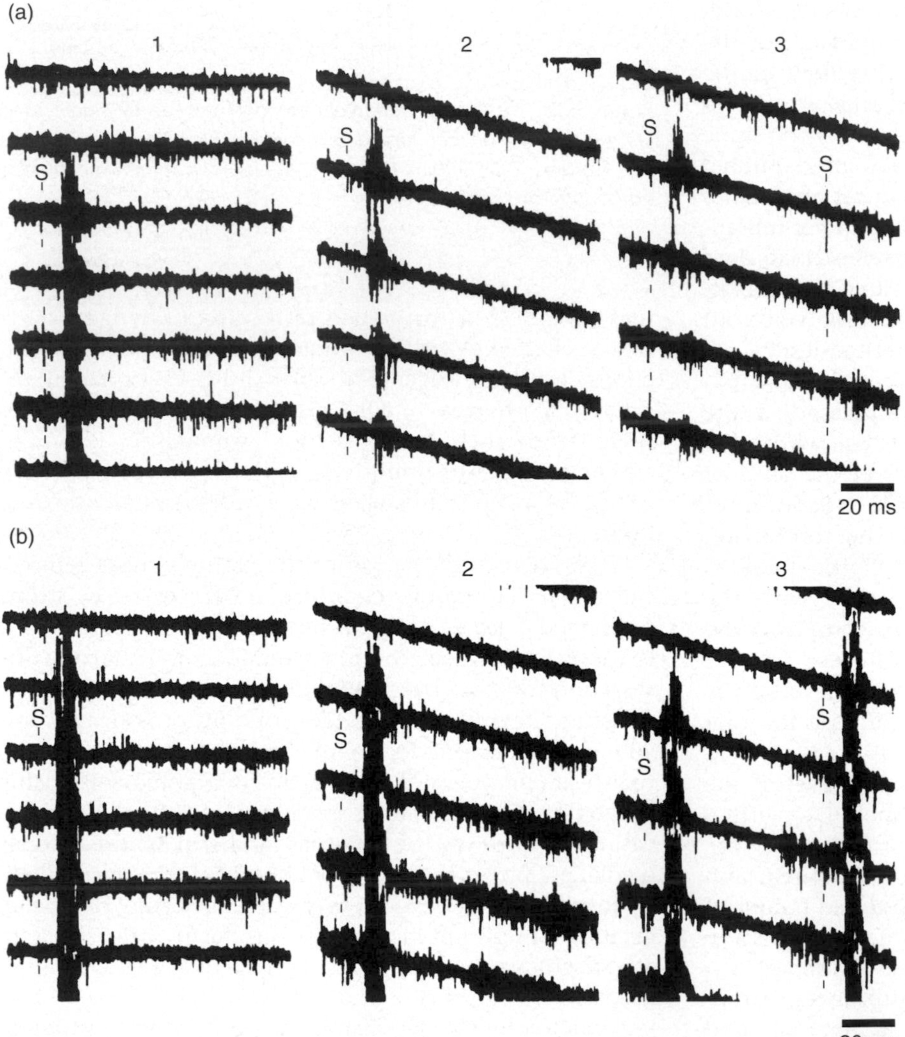

Figure 5.4 *Thyroarytenoid responses produced by repetitive superior laryngeal stimulation (0.3 V/0.1 ms). (a) Hyperventilation. (b) Hypoventilation. Column 1, 1 Hz; column 2, 8 Hz; column 3, 16 Hz. Note reduced afterdischarge activity in the hypoventilated state.*

hypoxic states, postsynaptic recovery lags behind the presynaptic recovery, producing a net depressive effect on all reflex neural activity. Hypoventilation, therefore, understandably impairs the output capability of the brainstem adductor motor aggregate to repetitive SLN stimulation (Fig 5.4). Such experimental data seem to support the clinical observation that laryngeal spasm occurs more often in well-ventilated, rather than cyanotic, patients. Superior laryngeal nerve stimulation, aside from the variety of excitatory adductor responses it produces, also exerts an inhibitory effect on the medullary inspiratory motor neurons. Not only does laryngeal abductor activity cease but phrenic activity is also inhibited, resulting in various degrees of reflex apnea.

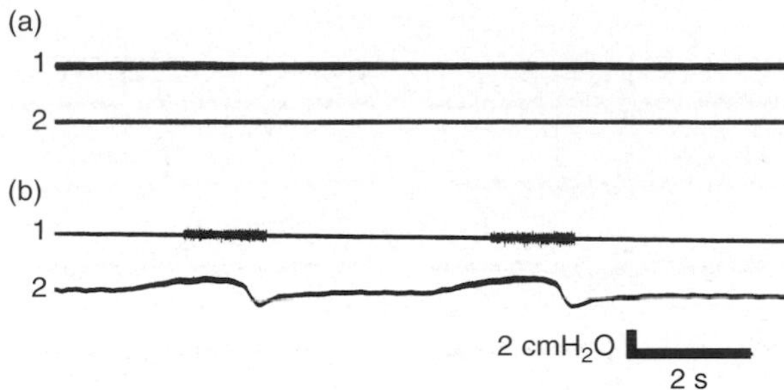

Figure 5.5 *Laryngeal abductor activity. (a) Immediately after tracheostomy. (b) With tracheostome partially closed. 1, Posterior cricoarytenoid EMG; 2, intratracheal pressure. Note disappearance of phasic abduction in tracheostomized breathing.*

Respiratory reflex

Negus in 1949 noted that the glottis opened a fraction of a second before the air was drawn in by the descent of the diaphragm.[7] In 1969, Suzuki and Kirchner established this activity as a direct effect of the medullary respiratory center.[11] Widening of the glottis occurred with rhythmic bursts of activity in the laryngeal nerve. Like phrenic activity, this rhythmicity was accentuated by hypercapnia and ventilatory obstruction and depressed by hyperventilation and hypocapnia.

Because the true vocal cords passively act to obstruct the ingress of air to the lungs, active inspiratory abduction by muscular contraction of the posterior cricoarytenoid appears mandatory to successful ventilation. The degree of inspiratory abductor activity appears to vary directly with ventilatory resistance, disappearing entirely when inspiratory resistance is removed, only to return when resistance to ventilation is reestablished (Fig 5.5).[9] Because vagotomy abolishes this response, it is felt that the afferent limb for the reflex regulation of phasic inspiratory abduction lies within the ascending vagus nerve.

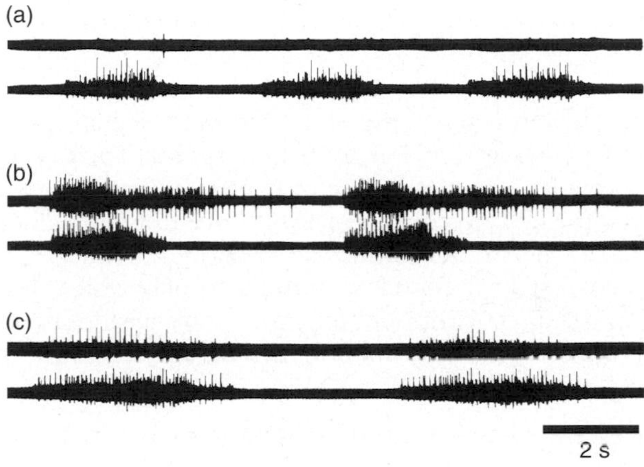

Figure 5.6 *Cricothyroid EMG (upper tracing) and phrenic EMG (lower tracing). (a) Quiet breathing. (b) Expiratory dyspnea. (c) Inspiratory dyspnea. Cricothyroid, like posterior cricoarytenoid, appears to be an inspiratory muscle.*

The cricothyroid muscle is known to be a vocal cord adductor and isotonic tensor. Neurophysiologic investigation, however, demonstrates that this muscle contracts phasically with inspiration (Fig 5.6).[14] Although its adductor function would appear counterproductive to inspiration, its role in cord lengthening actually enhances the cross-sectional diameter of the glottis by increasing its anteroposterior dimension. Posterior cricoarytenoid contraction increases the horizontal diameter of the glottic chink while its anteroposterior diameter is increased by phasic inspiratory contraction of cricothyroid muscle.

Although the cricothyroid serves as an inspiratory muscle, it also provides an important influence during expiration. In eupneic states, expiratory flow and duration are principal determinants of respiratory frequency. Variations in respiratory rate result primarily from changing the duration of the expiratory phase rather than the inspiratory phase of the respiratory cycle.[8]

In this regard, the larynx exerts a major valvular effect on ventilatory resistance, significantly influencing the expiratory phases of respiration through cricothyroid contraction.

Under normocapnic conditions, the rate of positive intratracheal pressure change appears critical to cricothyroid muscle participation. A rapid rise in tracheal pressure is more likely to initiate cricothyroid activity than a gradual rise in pressure regardless of the absolute pressure amplitude obtained.

The valvular mechanism of laryngeal constriction during expiration is based on the following understanding: during expiration, the cross-sectional area of the laryngeal aperture is reduced by virtue of elastic recoil assuming a cadaveric configuration in mid-expiration. On the one hand, Remmers and Bartlett[8] have indicated that expiratory laryngeal resistance is regulated by continued posterior cricoarytenoid activity well into the expiratory phase of respiration. Such abductor activity in early expiration retards elastic collapse of the glottis, acting in turn to retard the braking mechanism of the larynx. Cricothyroid action in conjunction with this posterior

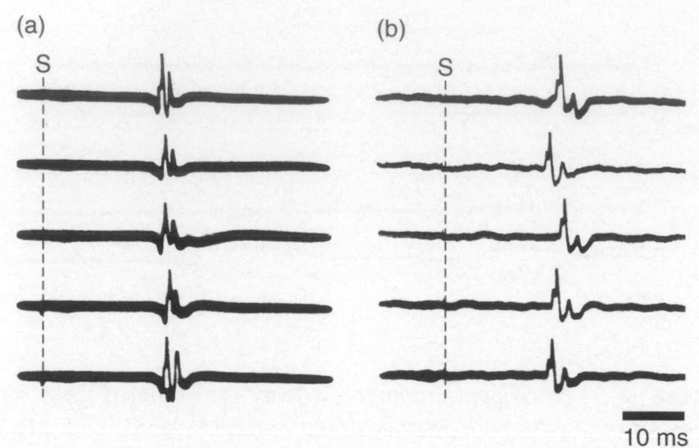

Figure 5.7 *Thyroarytenoid action potentials elicited by single-shock stimuli applied to the ipsilateral superior laryngeal nerve. (a) Control dogs. (b) Chronically tracheotomized dogs (aged 6–8 months). Note latency shift in dogs chronically tracheotomized.*

cricoarytenoid activity therefore not only maximizes the effective cross-sectional area of the laryngeal aperture but also provides a greater degree of regulatory potential with respect to the fine control of expiratory resistance. Based upon the neural regulation of cricothyroid muscle, its expiratory activity therefore appears to play a significant role in the direct control of expiratory laryngeal resistance and indirectly in the overall control of respiration itself.

The effect of tracheotomy on laryngeal function

Tracheotomy may be complicated by serious deficiencies in laryngeal function even when no prior laryngeal pathology exists.

The threshold of the adductor reflex produced by superior laryngeal nerve stimulation nearly doubles after prolonged tracheotomy, while evoked adductor reflexes undergo wide shifts in their latency. Repetitive superior laryngeal nerve stimulation produces marked attenuation of the adductor reflex, reflected in a weakened closure response after long-term tracheotomy (Figs 5.7–5.10). These changes may help to explain the onset of aspiration due to a weakened, uncoordinated closure response resulting from tracheotomy when no laryngotracheal surgical injury can be found.

Respiratory function of the larynx is even more susceptible to central alterations when the upper airway is bypassed by tracheotomy. Tracheotomy, by reducing respiratory resistance, gradually abolishes the phasic inspiratory contraction of the posterior cricoarytenoid muscle. Experimental studies in dogs showed no abductor activity with an open tracheostoma, and repeated partial closure of the tracheostoma produced no return in posterior cricothyroid muscle activity at 4 weeks after the tracheotomy. This observation helps to explain the difficulty of decannulation when laryngeal abductor activity is temporarily lost.

Phonatory reflex system

The phonatory function of the larynx is probably the least well understood of its three basic functions. With advances in investigative technique, many established hypotheses based on animal models have been challenged, a result in large measure due to the advent of more sophisticated technology based on human study. High-speed cinematography, electro- and photoglottography, improved endoscopic techniques using the video

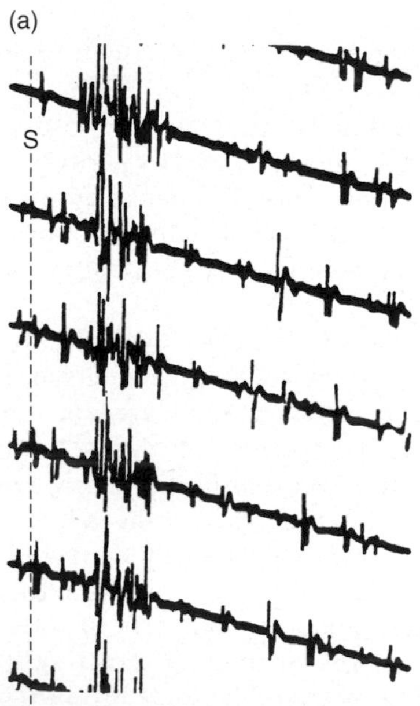

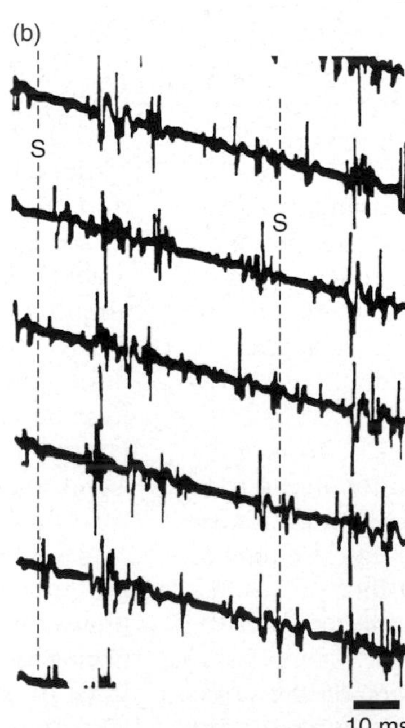

Figure 5.8 *Thyroarytenoid action potentials elicited by repetitive stimulation of ipsilateral superior laryngeal nerve control in dogs: (a) 8 Hz, (b) 16 Hz. Note numerous afterdischarges following the primary evoked response.*

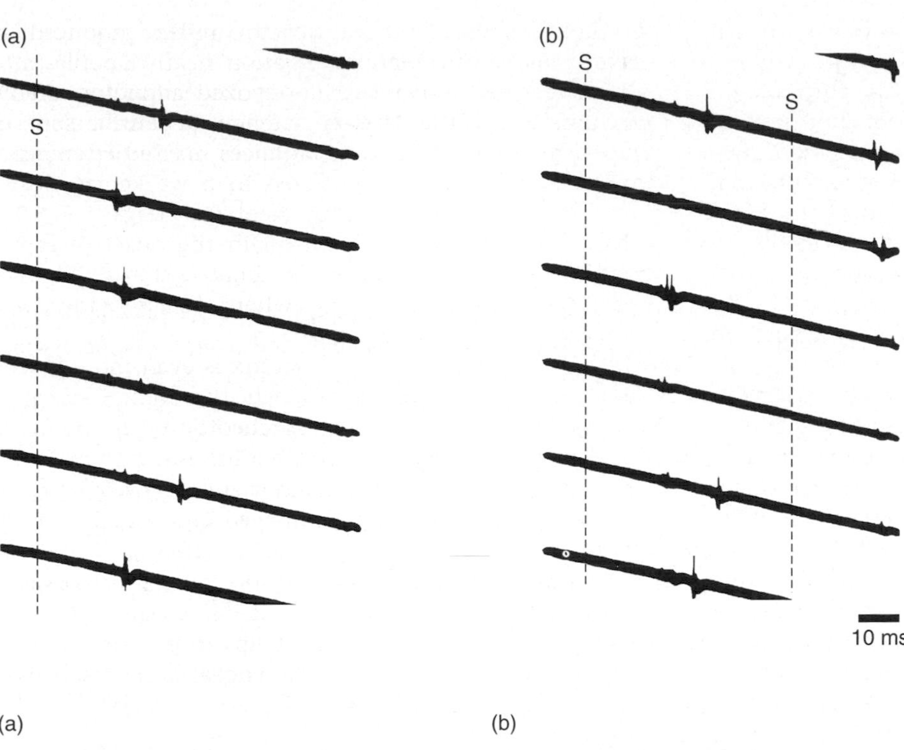

Figure 5.9 *Thyroarytenoid action potentials elicited by superior laryngeal stimulation in tracheotomized dogs: (a) 8 Hz, (b) 16 Hz. Note latency shifts. No afterdischarge activity observed.*

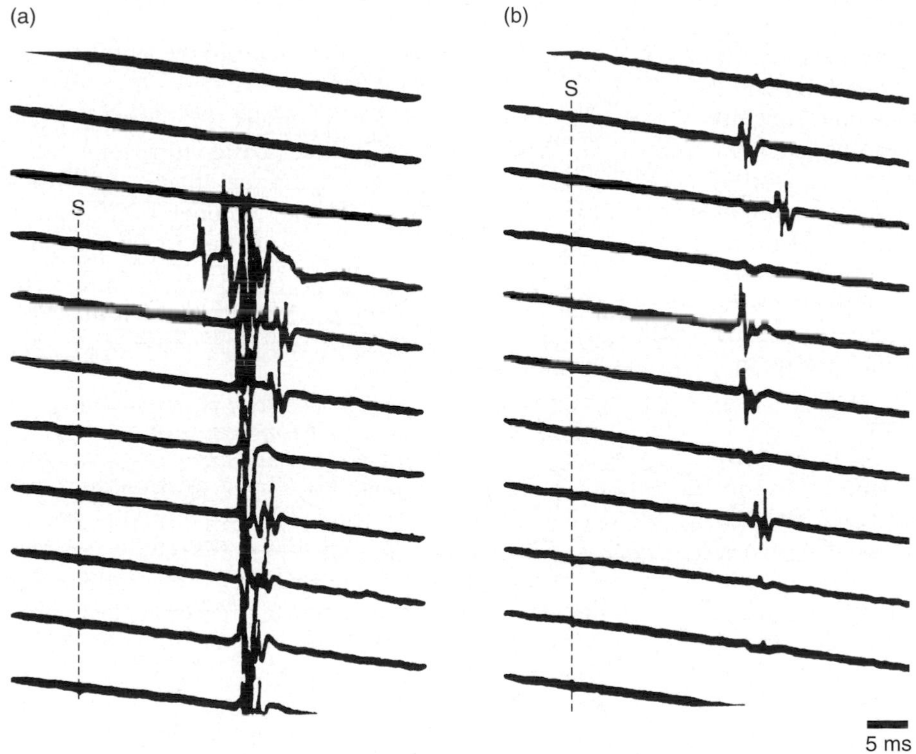

Figure 5.10 *Thyroarytenoid action potentials produced by 16 Hz superior laryngeal stimulation in chronically tracheotomized dogs. Primary evoked response attenuates within seconds of stimulus onset: (a) onset of stimulus train; (b) 1–2 seconds after onset of stimulus train.*

stroboscope, and direct human electromyographic measurements made possible by hook-wire electrodes combined with advanced aerodynamic measurements are largely responsible for these newer additions.

It is generally agreed that speech results from the production of a fundamental tone produced at the larynx and is modified by resonating chambers of the upper aerodigestive tract. Intelligible speech, therefore, represents the combined effect of the larynx, tongue, palate and related structures of the oral vestibule. The fundamental tone is produced by vibration of the vocal folds against each other, powered by the passage of air between them. The passive nature of vocal cord vibration forms the basis of the aerodynamic theory of sound generation. Such a theory is supported by the observation that the completely paralyzed larynx is capable of producing sound, as is the cadaver larynx when air is blown through it. Furthermore, vocal cord vibration ceases when a tracheostomy is performed for diversionary purposes.

The aerodynamic theory of sound production replaces the neurochronaxic theory proposed by Husson, who postulated that the central generation of recurrent laryngeal nerve impulses produces cord vibrations by active contraction of the thyroarytenoid muscles.[5] According to theory, each vibration represented the result of beat-by-beat impulses through the recurrent laryngeal nerve. This concept is no longer accepted as tenable on acoustic or neurophysiologic grounds.

Although sound production may be considered a passive function, the regulation of its acoustic quality is not. Rather, vocal cord shaping and positioning are under active neurophysiologic regulation. During phonation the vocal folds are positioned near the midline by isotonic tensing provided by the cricothyroid muscles. Additionally, the thyroarytenoid muscles provide finer shaping of the vocal folds. The effect of shaping may be appreciated when the vocal folds are viewed in the frontal plane during phonation. During the production of high-pitched notes, the folds seen on cross-section appear thin, but during low pitches the folds appear thickened considerably. Thus, the frequency of vibration depends on the vibratory mass of both cords, their anteroposterior tension, functional damping at high pitches, and subglottic pressure. As pitch increases, the true cords lengthen and tense isotonically through the action of the cricothyroid muscles. Although cord lengthening alone might serve to lower pitch, this effect is offset by cord thinning, produced by thyroarytenoid action that increases the internal tension of the true cord. It must also be recognized that the activity of the extrinsic laryngeal muscles affects pitch altering the spatial relationship between the cricoid and the thyroid cartilages. The sternothyroid muscle is felt to influence pitch in this way.

A variety of feedback mechanisms aid in the fine tuning of the voice. The contribution of auditory input is demonstrated by observing a non-professional singer's inability to hit a desired note when hearing is masked by white noise. Mucosal receptors in the pharynx and larynx also supply important information, the transmission of which can be blocked by topical anesthetics. Finally, stretch receptors in the laryngeal joint capsules give critical proprioceptive information.[1,4,6]

Despite recent advances in our understanding of the mechanisms of the larynx, the precise mechanism of voice regulation remains a matter of continued fascination.

References

1. Bowden REM. Innervation of intrinsic laryngeal muscles. In: Wyke B, ed. *Ventilatory and Phonatory Control Systems*. London: Oxford University Press, 1974: 370–91.
2. Chang H. Activation of internuncial neurons through collaterals of pyramid fibers at cortical level. *J Neurophysiol* 1955; **18:** 452–71.
3. Downing SE, Lee JC. Laryngeal chemosensitivity: a possible mechanism for sudden infant death. *Pediatrics* 1975; **55:** 640–9.
4. Gracheva MS. Sensory innervation of locomotor apparatus of the larynx. *Arkh Anat Gistol Embriol* 1963; **44:** 77–80.
5. Husson, R. Etude des phénomènes physiologiques et acoustiques fondamentaux de la voix chantée. *These Fac Sc*, Paris, June 17, 1950.
6. Koizumi H. On sensory innervation of the larynx in dog. *J Exp Med* 1953; **58:** 199–210.
7. Negus VE. *The Comparative Anatomy and Physiology of the Larynx*. London: Heinemann, 1949.
8. Remmers JE, Bartlett D Jr. Reflex control of expiratory airflow and duration. *J Appl Physiol* 1977; **42:** 80–7.
9. Sasaki CT, Fukuda H, Kirchner JA. Laryngeal abductor activity in response to varying ventilatory resistance. *Trans Am Acad Ophthalmol Otolaryngol* 1973; **77:** 403–10.
10. Suzuki M, Kirchner JA. Afferent nerve fibers in the external branch of the superior laryngeal nerve in cat. *Ann Otol* 1968; **77:** 1059–70.
11. Suzuki M, Kirchner JA. The posterior cricoarytenoid as an inspiratory muscle. *Ann Otol* 1969; **78:** 849–65.
12. Suzuki M, Sasaki CT. The effect of various sensory stimuli on reflex laryngeal adduction. *Ann Otol* 1977; **86:** 30–6.
13. Suzuki M, Sasaki CT. Laryngeal spasm: a neurophysiologic redefinition. *Ann Otol* 1977; **86:** 150–7.
14. Suzuki M, Kirchner JA, Murakami Y. The cricothyroid as a respiratory muscle. Its characteristics in bilateral recurrent laryngeal nerve paralysis. *Ann Otol* 1970; **79:** 976–83.

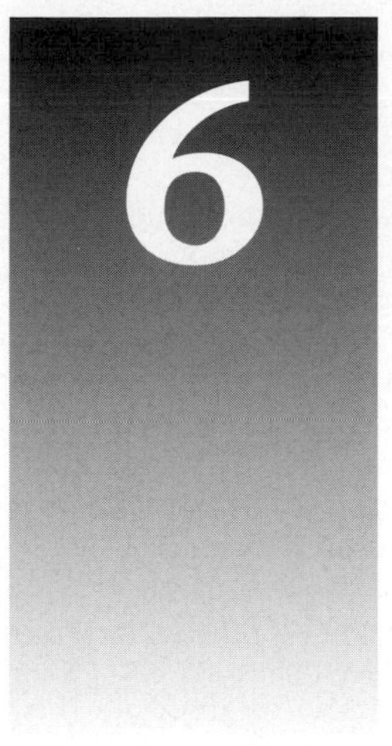

History and physical examination in patients with voice disorders*

Robert T Sataloff

Effective history taking and physical examination depend upon a practical understanding of the anatomy and physiology of voice production.[48,52–54,62] Because dysfunction in virtually any body system may affect phonation, medical inquiry must be comprehensive. The current standard of care for all voice patients evolved from advances inspired by voice professionals such as singers and actors. Even minor problems may be particularly apparent in singers and actors because of the extreme demands they place upon their voices. However, a great many other patients are voice professionals. They include teachers, sales people, attorneys, clergy, physicians, politicians, telephone receptionists, and anyone else whose ability to earn a living is impaired in the presence of voice dysfunction. Because good voice quality is so important in our society, the majority of our patients are voice professionals, and all patients should be treated as such.

The scope of inquiry and examination for most patients is similar to that required for singers and actors, except that performing voice professionals have unique needs which require additional history and examination. Questions must be added regarding performance commitments, professional status and voice goals, the amount and nature of voice training, performance environment, rehearsal practices, abusive habits during speech and singing, and many other matters. Such supplementary information is essential to proper treatment selection and patient counseling in singers and actors. However, analogous factors must also be taken into account for stockbrokers, factory shop foremen, elementary school teachers, homemakers with several noisy children, and many others. Consequently, in order to provide the broadest perspective and greatest amount of practical information, this chapter includes a discussion of history taking and physical examination in professional voice users. Physicians familiar with the requirements for these challenging patients are well equipped to evaluate all patients with voice complaints. It should be recognized that this chapter, while comprehensive, is certainly not complete. Readers interested in additional information, particularly regarding professional voice performers, are encouraged to consult other sources, including those from which this chapter is derived.[48,53,54]

Patient history

Extensive historical background is necessary for thorough evaluation of the voice, and the otolaryngologist who sees voice patients (especially singers) only occasionally cannot reasonably be expected to remember all the pertinent questions. Although some laryngologists consider a lengthy inquisition helpful in establishing rapport, many of us who see a substantial number of voice patients each day within a busy practice need a thorough but less time-consuming alternative. A history questionnaire can be extremely helpful in documenting all the necessary information, in helping the patient sort out and articulate his or her problems, and in saving the clinician time recording information. The author has developed a questionnaire[45,49,54] that has proven helpful (see Appendix, p. 76). The patient is asked to complete the relevant portions of the form in the waiting room before seeing the doctor. A similar form has been developed for voice patients who are not singers.[54]

No history questionnaire is a substitute for direct, penetrating questioning by the physician. However, the direction of most useful inquiry can be determined from a glance at the questionnaire. Obviating the need for extensive writing permits the physician greater eye contact with the patient and facilitates rapid establishment of the close rapport and confidence that are so

*Adapted in part from Sataloff RT. *Professional Voice: Science and Art of Clinical care*, 2nd edn. San Diego, Calif; Singular Publishing Group, Inc., 1997, with permission.

important in treating voice patients. The physician is also able to supplement initial impressions and historical information from the questionnaire with seemingly leisurely conversation during the physical examination. The use of the history questionnaire has added substantially to the efficiency, consistent thoroughness, and ease of managing these delightful, but often complex patients. A similar set of questions is also used by the speech-language pathologist, and many enlightened singing teachers when assessing new students.

How old are you?

Serious vocal endeavor may start in childhood and continue throughout a lifetime. As the vocal mechanism undergoes normal maturation, the voice changes. The optimal time to begin serious vocal training is controversial. For many years, most people advocated delay of vocal training and serious singing until near puberty in the female and after puberty and voice stabilization in the male. However, in a child with earnest vocal aspirations and potential, starting specialized training early in childhood is reasonable. Initial instruction should teach the child to vocalize without strain and avoid all forms of voice abuse. It should not permit premature indulgence in operatic bravado. Most experts agree that taxing voice use and singing during puberty should be minimized or avoided altogether, particularly by the male. Voice maturation (attainment of stable adult vocal quality) may occur at any age from the early teenage period to the fourth decade of life. The dangerous tendency for young singers to attempt to sound older than their vocal years frequently causes vocal dysfunction.

All components of voice production are subject to normal aging. Abdominal and general muscular tone frequently decreases, lungs lose elasticity, the thorax loses its distensibility, the mucosa of the vocal tract atrophies, mucous secretions change character, nerve endings are reduced in number, and psychoneurologic functions change. Moreover, the larynx itself loses muscle tone and bulk and may show depletion of submucosal ground substance in the vocal folds. The laryngeal cartilages ossify and the joints may become arthritic and stiff. Hormonal influence is altered. Vocal range, intensity and quality all may be modified. Vocal fold atrophy may be the most striking alteration. The clinical effects of aging seem more pronounced in female singers, although vocal fold histologic changes may be more prominent in males. Excellent male singers occasionally extend their careers into their seventies or beyond.[1,66] However, some degree of breathiness, decreased range, and other evidence of aging should be expected in elderly voices. Nevertheless, many of the changes we typically associate with elderly singers (wobble, flat pitch) are due to lack of conditioning, rather than inevitable changes of biological aging. These aesthetically undesirable concomitants of aging can often be reversed.[54]

What is your voice problem?

Careful questioning as to the onset of vocal problems is needed to separate acute from chronic dysfunction. Often an upper respiratory tract infection will send a patient to the physician's office, but penetrating inquiry may reveal a chronic vocal problem that is the patient's real concern, especially in singers and actors. Identifying acute and chronic problems before beginning therapy is important so that both patient and physician may have realistic expectations and optimal therapeutic selection.

The specific nature of the vocal complaint can provide a great deal of information. Just as dizzy patients rarely walk into the physician's office complaining of 'rotary vertigo', voice patients may be unable to articulate their symptoms without guidance. They may use the term hoarseness to describe a variety of conditions that the physician must separate. Hoarseness is a coarse or scratchy sound most often associated with abnormalities of the leading edge of the vocal folds such as laryngitis or mass lesions. Breathiness is a vocal quality characterized by excessive loss of air during vocalization. In some cases, it is due to improper technique. However, any condition that prevents full approximation of the vocal folds can be responsible. Such causes include vocal fold paralysis, a mass lesion separating the leading edges of the vocal folds, arthritis of the cricoarytenoid joint, arytenoid dislocation, unilateral scarring of the vibratory margin, senile vocal fold atrophy, psychogenic dysphonia, malingering and other conditions.

Fatigue of the voice is inability to continue to speak or sing for extended periods without change in vocal quality and/or control. The voice may show fatigue by becoming hoarse, losing range, changing timbre, breaking into different registers, or exhibiting other uncontrolled aberrations. A well-trained singer should be able to sing for several hours without vocal fatigue. Fatigue is often caused by misuse of abdominal and neck musculature or 'oversinging', singing too loudly, or too long. Vocal fatigue may also be a sign of general tiredness or serious illnesses such as myasthenia gravis.

Volume disturbance may manifest itself as inability to sing loudly or inability to sing softly. Each voice has its own dynamic range. Within the course of training, singers learn to sing more loudly by singing more efficiently. They also learn to sing softly, a more difficult task, through years of laborious practice. Actors and other trained speakers go through similar training. Most volume problems are secondary to intrinsic limitations of the voice or technical errors in voice use, although hormonal changes, aging, and neurologic disease are other causes. Superior laryngeal nerve paralysis impairs the ability to speak or sing loudly. This is a frequently unrecognized consequence of herpes infection ('cold sores') and may be precipitated by an upper respiratory tract infection.

Most highly trained singers require only about 10 minutes to half an hour to 'warm up the voice'. Prolonged warm-up time, especially in the morning, is most often caused by reflux laryngitis. Tickling or choking during singing is most often a symptom of abnormality of the vocal fold's leading edge. The symptom of tickling or choking should contraindicate singing until the vocal folds have been examined. Pain while singing can indicate vocal fold lesions, laryngeal joint arthritis, infection, or gastric acid irritation of the arytenoid region. However, pain is much more commonly caused by voice abuse with excessive muscular activity in the neck rather than an acute abnormality on the leading edge of a vocal fold. In the absence of other symptoms, these patients do not generally require immediate cessation of singing pending medical examination.

Do you have any pressing voice commitments?

If a singer or professional speaker (e.g. actor, politician) seeks treatment at the end of a busy season and has no pressing engagements, management of the voice problem should be relatively conservative and designed to assure long-term protection of the larynx, the most delicate part of the vocal mechanism. However, the physician and patient rarely have this luxury. Most often, the voice professional needs treatment within a week of an important engagement, and sometimes within less than a day. Younger singers fall ill shortly before performances, not because of hypochondria or coincidence, but rather because of the immense physical and emotional stress of the pre-performance period. The singer is frequently working harder and singing longer hours than usual. Moreover, he or she may be under particular pressure to learn new material and to perform well for a new audience. The singer may also be sleeping less than usual because of additional time rehearsing or because of the discomforts of a strange city. Seasoned professionals make their living by performing regularly, sometimes several times a week. Consequently, any time they get sick is likely to precede a performance. Caring for voice complaints in these situations requires highly skilled judgment and bold management.

Tell me about your vocal career, long-term goals, and the importance of your voice quality and upcoming commitments

To choose a treatment program, the physician must understand the importance of the patient's voice in his or her long-term career plans, the importance of the upcoming commitment, and the consequences of canceling the engagement. Injudicious prescription of voice rest can be almost as damaging to a vocal career as injudicious performance. For example, although a singer's voice is usually his or her most important commodity, other factors distinguish the few successful artists from the multitude of less successful singers with equally good voices. These include musicianship, reliability, and 'professionalism'. Canceling a concert at the last minute may seriously damage a performer's reputation. Reliability is especially critical early in a singer's career. Moreover, an expert singer often can modify a performance to decrease the strain on his or her voice. No singer should be allowed to perform in a manner that will permit serious injury to the vocal folds, but in the frequent borderline cases, the condition of the larynx must be weighed against other factors affecting the singer as an artist.

How much voice training have you had?

Establishing how long a singer or actor has been performing seriously is important, especially if his or her active performance career predates the beginning of vocal training. Active untrained singers and actors frequently develop undesirable techniques that are difficult to modify. Extensive voice use without training or premature training with inappropriate repertoire may underlie persistent vocal difficulties later in life. The number of years a performer has been training his or her voice may be a fair index of vocal proficiency. A person who has studied voice for one or two years is somewhat more likely to have gross technical difficulties than is someone who has been studying for 20 years. However, if training has been intermittent or discontinued, technical problems are common, especially among singers. In addition, methods vary among voice teachers. Hence, a student who has had many teachers in a relatively brief period of time commonly has numerous technical insecurities or deficiencies that may be responsible for vocal dysfunction. This is especially true if the singer has changed to a new teacher within the preceding year. The physician must be careful not to criticize the patient's current voice teacher in such circumstances. It often takes years of expert instruction to correct bad habits.

All people speak more often than they sing, yet most singers report little speech training. Even if a singer uses the voice flawlessly while practicing and performing, voice abuse at other times can cause damage that affects singing.

Under what kinds of conditions do you use your voice?

The Lombard effect is the tendency to increase vocal intensity in response to increased background noise. A well-trained singer learns to compensate for this tendency and to avoid singing at unsafe volumes. Singers of classical music usually have such training and frequently perform with only a piano, a situation in which the balance can be controlled well. However, singers performing in large halls, with orchestras, or in operas early in their careers tend to 'oversing' and strain their voices. Similar problems occur during outdoor concerts because of the lack of auditory feedback. This phenomenon is seen even more among 'pop' singers. Pop singers are in a uniquely difficult position; often, despite little vocal training, they enjoy great artistic and financial success and endure extremely stressful demands on their time and voices. They are required to sing in large halls not designed for musical performance, amid smoke and other environmental irritants, accompanied by extremely loud background music. One frequently neglected key to survival for these singers is the proper use of monitor speakers. These direct the sound of the singer's voice toward the singer on the stage and provide auditory feedback. Determining whether the pop singer uses monitor speakers and whether they are loud enough for the singer to hear is important.

Amateur singers are often no less serious about their music than are professionals, but generally they have less ability to compensate technically for illness or other physical impairment. Rarely does an amateur suffer a great loss from postponing a performance or permitting someone to sing in his or her place. In most cases, the amateur singer's best interest is served through conservative management directed at long-term maintenance of good vocal health.

A great many singers who seek physicians' advice are primarily choral singers. They often are enthusiastic amateurs, untrained but dedicated to their musical recreation. They should be handled as amateur solo singers, educated specifically about the Lombard effect, and cautioned to avoid the excessive volume so common in a choral environment. One good way for a singer to monitor loudness is to cup a hand to his or her ear. This adds about 6 dB[60] to the singer's perception of his or her own voice and can be a very helpful guide in noisy surroundings. Young professional singers are often hired to augment amateur choruses. Feeling that the professional quartet has been hired to 'lead' the rest of the choir, they often make the mistake of trying to accomplish that goal by singing louder than others in their sections. Such singers should be advised to lead their section by singing each line as if they were soloists giving a voice lesson to the two people standing beside them, and as if there were a microphone in front of them recording their choral performance for their voice teacher. This approach usually not only preserves the voice but also produces a better choral sound.

How much do you practice and exercise your voice?

Vocal exercise is as essential to the vocalist as exercise of other muscle systems is to the athlete. Proper vocal practice incorporates scales and specific exercises designed to maintain and develop the vocal apparatus. Simply acting or singing songs and giving performances without routine studious concentration on vocal technique is not adequate for the vocal performer. The physician should know whether the vocalist practices daily, whether he or she practices at the same time daily, and how long the practice lasts. Actors generally practice and warm up their voices for 10–30 minutes daily, although more time is recommended. Most serious singers practice for at least 1–2 hours per day. If a singer routinely practices in the late afternoon or evening but frequently performs in the morning (religious services, school classes, teaching voice, choir rehearsals, etc.), one should inquire into the warm-up procedures preceding such performances as well as cool-down procedures after voice use. Singing 'cold', especially early in the morning, may result in the use of minor muscular alterations to compensate for vocal insecurity produced by inadequate preparation. Such crutches can result in voice dysfunction. Similar problems may result from instances of voice use other than formal singing. School teachers, telephone receptionists, sales people, and others who speak extensively also often derive great benefit from 5 or 10 minutes of vocalization of scales first thing in the morning. Although singers rarely practice their scales too long, they frequently perform or rehearse excessively. This is especially true immediately before a major concert or audition, when physicians are most likely to see acute problems. When a singer has hoarseness and vocal fatigue and has been practicing a new role for 14 hours a day for the last 3 weeks, no simple prescription will solve the problem. However, a treatment regimen can usually be designed to carry the performer safely through his or her musical obligations.

Are you aware of misusing or abusing your voice during singing?

A detailed discussion of vocal technique in singing is beyond the scope of this chapter. The reader is referred to other sources.[54] However, the most common technical errors involve excessive muscle tension in the tongue, neck and larynx; inadequate abdominal support; and excessive volume. Inadequate preparation can be a devastating source of voice abuse and may result from limited practice, limited rehearsal of a difficult piece, or limited vocal training for a given role. The latter error is tragically common. In some situations, voice teachers are at fault, especially in competitive academic environments. Both singer and teacher must resist the impulse to show off the voice in works that are either too difficult for the singer's level of training or simply not suited to the singer's voice. Singers are habitually unhappy with the limitations of their voices. At some time or another, most baritones wish they were tenors and walk around proving they can sing high C in '*Vesti la giubba*'. Singers with other vocal ranges have similar fantasies. Attempts to make the voice something that it is not, or at least that it is not yet, are frequently harmful.

Are you aware of misusing or abusing your voice during speaking?

Common patterns of voice abuse and misuse will not be discussed in detail in this chapter. They are covered elsewhere in this book and in other literature.[54] Voice abuse and/or misuse should be suspected particularly in patients who complain of voice fatigue associated with voice use, whose voices are worse at the end of a working day or week, and in any patient who is chronically hoarse. Technical errors in voice use may be the primary etiology of a voice complaint, or it may develop secondarily due to a patient's effort to compensate for voice disturbance from another cause.

Dissociation of one's speaking and singing voices is probably the most common cause of voice abuse problems in excellent singers. Too frequently, all the expert training in support, muscle control and projection is not applied to a singer's speaking voice. Unfortunately, the resultant voice strain affects the singing voice as well as the speaking voice. Such damage is especially likely to occur in noisy rooms and in cars, where the background noise is louder than it seems. Backstage greetings after a lengthy performance can be particularly devastating. The singer usually is exhausted and distracted; the environment is often dusty and dry, and generally a noisy crowd is present. Similar conditions prevail at post-performance parties, where smoking and alcohol worsen matters. These situations should be avoided by any singer with vocal problems and should be controlled through awareness at other times.

Three particularly destructive vocal activities are worthy of note. Cheerleading requires extensive screaming under the worst possible physical and environmental circumstances. It is a highly undesirable activity for anyone considering serious vocal endeavor. This is a common conflict in younger singers because the teenager who is the high school choir soloist often is also student council president, yearbook editor, captain of the cheerleaders, and so on. Conducting, particularly choral conducting, can also be deleterious. An enthusiastic conductor, especially of an amateur group, frequently sings all four parts intermittently, at volumes louder than the entire choir, during lengthy rehearsals. Conducting is a common avocation among singers but must be done with expert technique and special precautions to prevent voice injury. Hoarseness or loss of soft voice control after conducting a rehearsal or concert suggests voice abuse during conducting. The patient should be instructed to record his or her voice throughout the vocal range, singing long notes at dynamics from soft to loud to soft. Recordings should be made prior to rehearsal and following rehearsal. If the voice has lost range, control, or quality during the rehearsal, voice abuse has occurred. A similar test can be used for patients who sing in choirs, teach voice or perform other potentially abusive vocal activities. Such problems in conductors can generally be managed by additional training in conducting techniques and by voice training, warm-up and cool-down exercises. Teaching singing may also be hazardous to vocal health. It can be done safely but requires skill and thought. Most teachers teach while seated at the piano. Late in a long, hard day, this posture is not conducive to maintenance of optimal abdominal and back support. Usually, teachers work with students continually positioned to the right or left of the keyboard. This may require the teacher to turn his or her neck at a particularly sharp angle, especially when teaching at an upright piano. Teachers also often demonstrate vocal works in their students' vocal ranges rather than their own, illustrating bad as well as good technique. If a singing teacher is hoarse or has neck discomfort, or his or her soft singing control deteriorates at the end of a teaching day (assuming that the teacher warms up before beginning to teach voice lessons), voice abuse should be suspected. Helpful modifications include teaching with a grand piano, sitting slightly sideways on the piano bench, or alternating student position to the right and left of the piano to facilitate better neck alignment. Retaining an accompanist so that the teacher can stand rather than teach from behind a piano, and many other helpful modifications, are possible.

What kind of physical condition are you in?

Speaking and singing are athletic activities that require good conditioning and coordinated interaction of numerous physical functions. Maladies of any part of the body may be reflected in the voice. Failure to exercise to maintain good abdominal muscle tone and respiratory endurance is particularly harmful in that deficiencies in these areas undermine the power source of the voice. Patients generally attempt to compensate for such weaknesses by using inappropriate muscle groups, particularly in the neck, causing vocal dysfunction. Similar problems may occur in the well-conditioned vocalist in states of fatigue. These are compounded by mucosal changes that accompany excessively long hours of hard work. Such problems may be seen even in the best singers shortly before important performances in the height of the concert season.

A popular but untrue myth holds that great opera singers must be obese. However, the vivacious, gregarious personality that often distinguishes the great performer seems to be accompanied frequently by a propensity for excess, especially culinary excess. This excess is as undesirable in the vocalist as it is in most other athletic artists, and it should be prevented from the start of one's vocal career. Appropriate and attractive body weight has always been valued in the pop music world and is becoming particularly important in the opera world as this formerly theater-based art form moves to television and film media. However, attempts to effect weight reduction in an established speaker or singer are a different matter. The vocal mechanism is a finely tuned, complex instrument and is exquisitely sensitive to minor changes. Substantial fluctuations in weight frequently cause deleterious alterations of the voice, although these are usually temporary. Weight reduction programs for people concerned about their voices must be monitored carefully and designed to reduce weight in small increments over long periods. A history of sudden recent weight change may be responsible for almost any vocal complaint.

Do you have allergy or cold symptoms?

Voice patients usually volunteer information about upper respiratory tract infections and 'postnasal drip', but the relevance of other maladies may not be obvious to them. Consequently the physician must seek out pertinent history. Acute upper respiratory tract infection causes inflammation of the mucosa, alters mucosal secretions, and makes the mucosa more vulnerable to injury. Coughing and throat clearing are particularly traumatic vocal activities and may worsen or provoke hoarseness associated with a cold. Postnasal drip and allergy may produce the same response. Infectious sinusitis is associated with discharge and diffuse mucosal inflammation, resulting in similar problems, and may actually alter the sound of a voice, especially the patient's own perception of his or her voice. Futile attempts to compensate for disease of the supraglottic vocal tract in an effort to return the sound to normal frequently result in laryngeal strain. The expert singer or speaker should compensate by monitoring technique by tactile rather than by auditory feedback, or by singing 'by feel' rather than 'by ear'.

Do you have breathing problems, especially after exercise?

Respiratory problems are especially important in voice patients. Even mild respiratory dysfunction may adversely affect the power source of the voice.[51,61] Occult asthma may be particularly troublesome.[10] A complete respiratory history should be obtained in most patients with voice complaints, and pulmonary function testing is often advisable.

Do you have jaw joint or other dental problems?

Dental disease, especially temporomandibular joint (TMJ) dysfunction, introduces muscle tension in the head and neck, which is transmitted to the larynx directly through the muscular attachments between the mandible and the hyoid bone, and indirectly as generalized increased muscle tension. These problems often result in decreased range, vocal fatigue, and change in the quality or placement of a voice. Such tension often is accompanied by excess tongue muscle activity, especially pulling of the tongue posteriorly. This hyperfunctional behavior acts through hyoid attachments to disrupt the balance between the intrinsic and extrinsic laryngeal musculature. TMJ problems are also problematic for wind instrumentalists, and some string players, including violinists. In some cases, the problems may actually be caused by instrumental technique. The history should always include information about musical activities including instruments other than the voice.

Have you suffered whiplash or other bodily injury?

Various bodily injuries outside the confines of the vocal tract may have profound effects on the voice. Whiplash, for example, commonly causes changes in technique, with consequent voice fatigue, loss of range, difficulty singing softly and other problems. Lumbar, abdominal and extremity injuries may also affect voice technique and be responsible for the dysphonia that prompted the voice patient to seek medical attention.

Do you have morning hoarseness, bad breath, excessive phlegm, a lump in your throat, or heartburn?

Reflux laryngitis is especially common among singers and trained speakers because of the high intraabdominal pressure associated with proper support, and because of lifestyle. Singers frequently perform at night. Many vocalists refrain from eating before performances because a full stomach can compromise effective abdominal support. They typically compensate by eating heartily at post-performance gatherings late at night and then go to bed with a full stomach. Chronic arytenoid mucosa and vocal fold irritation by reflux of gastric secretions may occasionally be associated with dyspepsia or pyrosis. However, the key features of this malady are bitter taste and halitosis on awakening in the morning, a dry or 'coated' mouth, often a scratchy sore throat or a feeling of a 'lump in the throat', hoarseness, and the need for prolonged vocal warm-up. The physician must be alert to these symptoms and ask about them routinely, otherwise the diagnosis will often be overlooked because people who have had this problem for many years or a lifetime do not even realize it is abnormal.

Do you have trouble with your bowels or belly?

Any condition that alters abdominal function, such as muscle spasm, constipation, or diarrhea, interferes with support and may result in a voice complaint. These symptoms may accompany infection, anxiety, various gastroenterological diseases and other maladies.

Do you or your blood relatives have hearing loss?

Hearing loss is often overlooked as a source of vocal problems. Auditory feedback is fundamental to speaking and singing. Interference with this control mechanism may result in altered vocal production, particularly if the person is unaware of the hearing loss. Distortion, particularly pitch distortion (diplacusis) may also pose serious problems for the singer. This appears to be due not only to aesthetic difficulties in matching pitch, but also to vocal strain which accompanies pitch shifts.[63]

Are you under particular stress or in therapy?

The human voice is an exquisitely sensitive messenger of emotion. Highly trained voice professionals learn to control the effects of anxiety and other emotional stress on their voices under ordinary circumstances. However, in some instances this training may break down or a performer may be inadequately prepared to control the voice under specific stressful conditions. Pre-performance anxiety is the most common example, but insecurity, depression, and other emotional disturbances are also generally reflected in the voice. Anxiety reactions are mediated in part through the autonomic nervous system and result in a dry mouth, cold clammy skin and thick secretions. These reactions are normal, and good vocal training coupled with assurance that no abnormality or disease is present generally overcomes them. However, long-term, poorly compensated emotional stress and exogenous stress (from agents, producers, teachers, parents, etc.) may cause substantial vocal dysfunction and may result in permanent limitations of the vocal apparatus. These conditions must be diagnosed and treated expertly. Hypochondriasis is uncommon among professional singers, despite popular opinion to the contrary.

Recent publications have highlighted the complexity and importance of psychological factors associated with voice disorders.[41,42] A more comprehensive discussion of this subject is presented elsewhere in this book. It is important for the physician to recognize that psychological problems may not only cause voice disorders, but they may also delay recovery from voice disorders that were entirely organic in etiology. Professional voice users, especially singers, have enormous psychological investment and personality identifications associated with their voices. A condition that causes voice loss or permanent injury often evokes the same powerful psychological responses seen following death of a loved one. This process may be initiated even when physical recovery is complete, following an incident (injury or surgery) that makes the vocalist realize that voice loss is possible, a 'brush with death'. It is essential for laryngologists to be aware of these powerful factors and manage them properly if optimal therapeutic results are to be achieved expeditiously.

Do you have problems controlling your weight? Are you excessively tired? Are you cold when other people are warm?

Endocrine problems warrant special attention. The human voice is extremely sensitive to endocrinological changes. Many of these are reflected in alterations of fluid content of the lamina propria just beneath the laryngeal mucosa. This causes alterations in the bulk and shape of the vocal folds and results in voice change. Hypothyroidism[22,33,35,39,40] is a well-recognized cause of such voice disorders, although the mechanism is not fully understood. Hoarseness, vocal fatigue, muffling of the voice, loss of range, and a sensation of a lump in the throat may be present even with mild hypothyroidism. Even when thyroid function test results are within the low-normal range, this diagnosis should be entertained, especially if thyroid stimulating hormone levels are in the high-normal range or are elevated. Thyrotoxicosis may result in similar voice disturbances.[33]

Do you have menstrual irregularity, cyclical voice changes associated with menses, recent menopause, or other hormonal changes or problems?

Voice changes associated with sex hormones are encountered commonly in clinical practice and have been investigated more thoroughly than have other hormonal changes.[34,58] Although a correlation appears to exist between sex hormone levels and depth of male voices (higher testosterone and lower estradiol levels in basses than in tenors),[22] the most important hormonal considerations in males occur during puberty.

When castrato singers were in vogue, castration at about age 7 or 8 years resulted in failure of laryngeal growth during puberty, and voices that stayed in the soprano or alto range and boasted a unique quality of sound.[7] Failure of a male voice to change at puberty is uncommon today and is often psychogenic in etiology.[6] However, hormonal deficiencies such as those seen in cryptorchidism, delayed sexual development, Klinefelter's syndrome, or Fröhlich's syndrome may be responsible. In these cases, the persistently high voice may be the complaint that causes the patient to seek medical attention.

Voice problems related to sex hormones are more common in female singers. Although vocal changes associated with the normal menstrual cycle may be difficult to quantify with current experimental techniques, unquestionably they occur[9,54,65] Most of the ill effects are seen in the immediate premenstrual period and are known as laryngopathia premenstrualis. This common condition is caused by physiological, anatomical and psychological alterations secondary to endocrine changes. The vocal dysfunction is characterized by decreased vocal efficiency, loss of the highest notes in the voice, vocal fatigue, slight hoarseness, and some muffling of the voice. It is often more apparent to the singer than to the listener, and these symptoms tend to be more troublesome for singers than for speakers. Submucosal hemorrhages in the larynx are common in the premenstrual period.[30] In many European opera houses, singers used to be excused from singing during the premenstrual and early menstrual days ('grace days'). This practice is not followed in the USA and is no longer in vogue in most European countries. Premenstrual changes cause significant vocal symptoms in approximately one-third of singers. Although ovulation inhibitors have been shown to mitigate some of these symptoms in some women (about 5%),[9,69] birth control pills may deleteriously alter voice range and character even after only a few months of therapy.[8,17,37,59] When oral contraceptives are used, the voice should be monitored closely. Under crucial performance circumstances, oral contraceptives may be used to alter the time of menstruation, but this practice is justified only in unusual situations. Symptoms very similar to laryngopathia premenstrualis occur in some women at the time of ovulation.

Pregnancy frequently results in voice alterations known as laryngopathia gravidarum. The changes may be similar to premenstrual symptoms or may be perceived as desirable changes. In some cases, alterations produced by pregnancy are permanent.[16,19] Although hormonally induced changes in the larynx and respiratory mucosa secondary to menstruation and pregnancy are discussed widely in the literature, there are few references to the important alterations in abdominal support. Uterine muscle cramping associated with menstruation causes pain and compromises abdominal support. Abdominal distension during pregnancy also interferes with abdominal muscle function. Any high performance voice user whose abdominal support is compromised substantially should be discouraged from performing until the abdominal impairment is resolved.

Estrogens are helpful in postmenopausal speakers and singers but generally should not be given alone. Sequential replacement therapy is the most physiologic regimen and should generally be used under the supervision of a gynecologist. Under no circumstances should androgens be given to female singers even in small amounts if any reasonable therapeutic alternative exists. Clinically, these drugs are most commonly used to treat endometriosis. Androgens cause unsteadiness of the voice, rapid changes of timbre, and lowering of the fundamental frequency (masculinization).[2,5,12,13,46,67] These changes are usually permanent.

Recently, we have seen increasing abuse of anabolic steroids. In addition to their many other hazards, these medications may alter the voice. They are (or are closely related to) male hormones and are thus capable of producing masculinization of the voice. Lowering of the fundamental frequency and coarsening of the voice produced in this fashion are generally irreversible.

Other hormonal disturbances may also produce vocal dysfunction. In addition to the thyroid gland and the gonads, the parathyroid, adrenal, pineal and pituitary glands are included in this system. Also, other endocrine disturbances may alter voice as well; for example, pancreatic dysfunction may cause xerophonia (dry voice), as in diabetes mellitus. Thymic abnormalities can lead to feminization of the voice.[27]

Have you been exposed to environmental irritants?

Any mucosal irritant can disrupt the delicate vocal mechanism. Allergies to dust and mold are aggravated commonly during rehearsals and performances in concert halls, especially older theaters and concert halls, because of numerous curtains, backstage trappings and dressing room facilities that are rarely cleaned thoroughly. Nasal obstruction and erythematous conjunctivae suggest generalized mucosal irritation. The drying effects of cold air and dry heat may also affect mucosal secretions, leading to decreased lubrication, a 'scratchy' voice and tickling cough. These symptoms may be minimized by nasal breathing, which allows inspired air to be filtered, warmed, and humidified. Nasal breathing, whenever possible, rather than mouth breathing is proper vocal technique. While the performer is backstage between appearances or during rehearsals, aspiration of dust and other irritants may be controlled by wearing a protective mask such as those used by carpenters, or a surgical mask that does not contain fiberglass. This is especially helpful when sets are being constructed in the rehearsal area.

A history of recent travel suggests other sources of mucosal irritation. The air in airplanes is extremely dry, and airplanes are noisy.[18] One must be careful to avoid talking loudly and to maintain good hydration and nasal breathing during air travel. Environmental changes can also be disruptive. Las Vegas is infamous for the mucosal irritation caused by its dry atmosphere and smoke-filled rooms. In fact, the resultant complex of hoarseness, vocal 'tickle', and fatigue is referred to as 'Las Vegas voice'. A history of recent travel should also suggest jet lag and generalized fatigue, which may be potent detriments to good vocal function.

Environmental pollution is responsible for the presence of toxic substances and conditions encountered daily. Inhalation of toxic pollutants may affect the voice adversely by direct laryngeal injury, by causing pulmonary dysfunction that results in voice maladies, or through impairments elsewhere in the vocal tract. Ingested substances, especially those that have neurolaryngologic effects, may also adversely affect the voice. Non-chemical environmental pollutants such as noise can cause voice abnormalities, as well. Laryngologists should be familiar with the laryngologic effects of the numerous potentially irritating substances and conditions found in the environment.[53] Laryngologists must also be familiar with special pollution problems encountered by performers. Numerous materials used by artists to create sculptures, drawings and theatrical sets are toxic and have adverse voice effects. In addition, performers are routinely exposed to chemicals encountered through stage smoke, and pyrotechnic effects.[23,36,44] Although it is clear that some of the 'special effects' result in serious laryngologic consequences, much additional study is needed to clarify the nature and scope of these occupational problems.

Do you smoke, live with a smoker, or work around smoke?

The deleterious effects of tobacco smoke on mucosa are indisputable. Anyone concerned about the health of his or her voice should not smoke. Smoking causes erythema, mild edema and generalized inflammation throughout the vocal tract. Both smoke itself and the heat of the cigarette appear to be important. Marijuana produces a particularly irritating, unfiltered smoke that is inhaled directly, causing considerable mucosal response. Voice patients who refuse to stop smoking marijuana should at least be advised to use a water pipe to cool and partially filter the smoke. Some vocalists are required to perform in smoke-filled environments and may suffer the same effects as the smokers themselves. In some theaters, it is possible to place fans upstage or direct the ventilation system so as to create a gentle draft toward the audience, clearing the smoke away from the stage. 'Smoke eaters' installed in some theaters are also helpful.

Have you noted voice or bodily weakness, tremor, fatigue, or loss of control?

Even minor neurologic disorders may be extremely disruptive to vocal function. Specific questions should be asked to rule out neuromuscular and neurologic diseases such as myasthenia gravis, Parkinson's disease, tremors, other movement disorders, spasmodic dysphonia, multiple sclerosis, central nervous system neoplasm, and other serious maladies that may be present with voice complaints.[3,51]

What medications and other substances do you use?

A history of alcohol abuse suggests the probability of poor vocal technique. Intoxication results in incoordination and decreased awareness, which undermine vocal discipline designed to optimize and protect the voice. The effect of small amounts of alcohol is controversial. Although many experts oppose its use because of its vasodilatory effect and consequent mucosal alteration, many people do not seem to be adversely affected by small amounts of alcohol, such as a glass of wine with a meal. However, some people have mild sensitivities to certain wines or beers. Patients who develop nasal congestion and rhinorrhea after drinking beer, for example, should be made aware that they probably have a mild allergy to that particular beverage and should avoid it before voice commitments.

Patients frequently acquire antihistamines to help control 'postnasal drip' or other symptoms. The drying effect of antihistamines may result in decreased vocal fold lubrication, increased throat clearing, and irritability leading to frequent coughing. Antihistamines may be helpful to some voice patients, but they must be used with caution.

When a voice patient seeking the attention of a physician is already taking antibiotics, it is important to find out the dose and the prescribing physician, if any, as well as whether the patient frequently treats him/herself with inadequate courses of antibiotics often supplied by colleagues. Singers, actors, and other speakers sometimes have a 'sore throat' shortly before important vocal presentations and start themselves on inappropriate antibiotic therapy, which they generally discontinue after their performance.

Diuretics are also popular among some performers. They are often prescribed by gynecologists, at the vocalist's request, to help deplete excess water in the premenstrual period. They are not effective in this scenario because they can not diurese the protein-bound water in the laryngeal ground substance. Unsupervised use of these drugs may cause dehydration and consequent mucosal dryness.

Hormone use, especially use of oral contraceptives, must be mentioned specifically during the physician's inquiry. Women frequently do not mention them routinely when asked whether they are taking any medication. Vitamins are also frequently not mentioned. Most vitamin therapy seems to have little effect on the voice. However, high-dose vitamin C (5–6 g/day), which some people use to prevent upper respiratory tract infections, seems to act as a mild diuretic and may lead to dehydration and xerophonia.[31]

Cocaine use is common, especially among pop musicians. This drug can be extremely irritating to the nasal mucosa, causes marked vasoconstriction, and may alter the sensorium, resulting in decreased voice control and a tendency toward vocal abuse.

Many pain medications (including aspirin and ibuprofen), psychotropic medications and many others may be responsible for voice complaint. Laryngologists must be familiar with the laryngologic effects of the many substances ingested medically and recreationally.[55]

Do any foods seem to affect your voice?

Various foods are said to affect the voice. Traditionally, singers avoid milk and ice cream before performances. In many people, these foods seem to increase the amount and viscosity of mucosal secretions. Allergy and casein have been implicated, but no satisfactory explanation has been established. Restriction of these foods from the diet before a voice performance may be helpful in some cases. Chocolate may have the same effect and should be viewed similarly. Chocolate also contains caffeine, which may aggravate reflux or cause tremor. Voice patients should be asked about eating nuts. This is important not only because some people experience effects similar to those produced by milk products and chocolate, but also because they are extremely irritating if aspirated. The irritation produced by aspiration of even a small organic foreign body may be severe and impossible to correct rapidly enough to permit performance. Highly spiced foods may also cause mucosal irritation. In addition, they seem to aggravate reflux laryngitis. Coffee and other beverages containing caffeine also aggravate gastric reflux and may alter secretions and necessitate frequent throat clearing in some people. Fad diets, especially rapid weight-reducing diets, are notorious for causing voice problems. Lemon juice and herbal teas are considered beneficial to the voice. Both may act as demulcents, thinning secretions, and may very well be helpful. Eating a full meal before a speaking or singing engagement may interfere with abdominal support or may aggravate upright reflux of gastric juice during abdominal muscle contraction.

Did you undergo any surgery prior to the onset of your voice problems?

A history of laryngeal surgery in a voice patient is a matter of great concern. It is important to establish exactly why the surgery was done, by whom it was done, whether intubation was necessary, and whether voice therapy was instituted pre- or postoperatively if the lesion was associated with voice abuse (vocal nodules). If the vocal dysfunction that sent the patient to the physician's office dates from the immediate postoperative period, surgical trauma must be suspected.

Otolaryngologists frequently are asked about the effects of tonsillectomy on the voice. Singers especially may consult the physician after tonsillectomy and complain of vocal dysfunction. Certainly removal of tonsils can alter the voice.[21,68] Tonsillectomy changes the configuration of the supraglottic vocal tract. In addition, scarring alters pharyngeal muscle function, which is trained meticulously in the professional singer. Singers must be warned that they may have permanent voice changes after tonsillectomy; however, these can be minimized by dissecting in the proper plane to lessen scarring. The singer's voice generally requires 3–6 months to stabilize or return to normal after surgery. As with any procedure for which general anesthesia may be needed, the anesthesiologist should be advised preoperatively that the patient is a professional singer. Intubation and extubation should be performed with great care and the use of nonirritating plastic rather than rubber endotracheal tubes is ideal.

Surgery of the neck, such as thyroidectomy, may result in permanent alterations in the vocal mechanism through scarring of the extrinsic laryngeal musculature. The cervical (strap) muscles are important in maintaining laryngeal position and stability of the laryngeal skeleton; they should be retracted rather than divided whenever possible. A history of recurrent or superior laryngeal nerve injury may explain a hoarse, breathy, or weak voice. However, in rare cases even a singer can compensate for recurrent laryngeal nerve paralysis and have a nearly normal voice.

Thoracic and abdominal surgery interfere with respiratory and abdominal support. After these procedures, singing and projected speaking should be prohibited until pain has subsided and healing has occurred sufficiently to allow normal support. Abdominal exercises should be instituted before resumption of vocalizing. Singing and speaking without proper support are often worse for the voice than not using the voice for performance at all.

Other surgical procedures may be important factors if they necessitate intubation or if they affect the musculoskeletal system so that the person has to change stance or balance. For example, balancing on one foot after leg surgery may decrease the effectiveness of the support mechanism.

Physical examination

A comprehensive history frequently reveals the cause of a voice problem even before a physical examination is performed. However, a specialized physical examination, often including objective assessment of voice function, is essential.[48,50,54] This includes a complete ear, nose and throat examination; examination of the singer during the act of singing, or a professional speaker during mock performance; slow motion evaluation of the vocal folds using strobovideolaryngoscopy; and quantitative measures of voice function. A physical examination outside the head and neck is also often indicated, particularly neurological and pulmonary examination. Generally, only laryngologists subspecializing in voice care have all the necessary equipment and team collaborators for optimal comprehensive assessment. Interestingly, many of the new technologic devices used in the voice laboratory have also proven extremely helpful adjuncts to traditional voice teaching.

Complete ear, nose and throat examination

Examination of the ears must include assessment of hearing acuity. Even a relatively slight hearing loss may result in voice strain as a singer tries to balance his or her vocal intensity with that of associate performers. Similar effects are encountered among speakers, but they are less prominent in the early stages of hearing loss. This is especially true of hearing losses acquired after vocal training has been completed. The effect is most pronounced with sensorineural hearing loss. Diplacusis makes vocal strain even worse. With conductive hearing loss, singers tend to sing more softly than appropriate rather than too loudly, and this is less harmful.

During an ear, nose, and throat examination the conjunctivae and sclerae should be observed routinely for erythema that suggests allergy or irritation, for pallor that suggests anemia, and for other abnormalities such as jaundice. These observations may reveal the problem reflected in the vocal tract even before the larynx is visualized.

The nose should be assessed for patency of the nasal airway, character of the nasal mucosa, and nature of secretions, if any. A patient who is unable to breathe through the nose because of anatomic obstruction is forced to breathe unfiltered, unhumidified air through the mouth. Pale gray allergic mucosa or swollen infected mucosa in the nose suggests abnormal mucosa elsewhere in the respiratory tract.

Examination of the oral cavity should include careful attention to the tonsils and lymphoid tissue in the posterior pharyngeal wall, as well as to the mucosa. Diffuse lymphoid hypertrophy associated with a complaint of 'scratchy' voice and irritative cough may indicate infection. The amount and viscosity of mucosal and salivary secretions should also be noted. Xerostomia is particularly important. Dental examination should focus not only on oral hygiene but also on the presence of wear facets suggestive of bruxism. Bruxism is a clue to excessive tension and may be associated with dysfunction of the temporomandibular joints, which should also be assessed routinely. Thinning of the enamel of the central incisors in a normal or underweight patient may be a clue to bulimia. However, it may also result from excessive ingestion of lemons, which some singers eat to help thin their secretions.

The neck should be examined for masses, restriction of movement, excess muscle tension and scars from prior neck surgery or trauma. Laryngeal vertical mobility is also important. For example, tilting of the larynx produced by partial fixation of cervical muscles cut during previous surgery may produce voice dysfunction, as may fixation of the trachea to overlying neck skin. Particular attention should be paid to the thyroid gland. Examination of posterior neck muscles and range of motion should not be neglected. The cranial nerves should also be examined. Diminished fifth nerve sensation, diminished gag reflex, palatal deviation, or other mild cranial nerve deficits may indicate cranial polyneuropathy. Postviral, infectious neuropathies may involve the superior laryngeal nerve and cause weakness, fatigability and loss of range and projection in the voice. The recurrent laryngeal nerve is also affected in some cases. More serious neurologic disease may also be associated with such symptoms and signs.

Laryngeal examination

Examination of the larynx begins when the patient enters the physician's office. The range, ease, volume and quality of the speaking voice should be noted. Technical voice classification is beyond the scope of most physicians. However, the physician should at least be able to discriminate substantial differences in range and timbre such as between bass and tenor, or alto and soprano. More detailed definitions of voice classification may be found elsewhere.[54] Although the correlation between speaking and singing voices is not perfect, a speaker with a low comfortable bass voice who reports that he is a tenor may be misclassified and singing inappropriate roles with consequent voice strain. This judgment should be deferred to an expert, but the observation should lead the physician to make the appropriate referral. Excessive volume or obvious strain during speaking clearly indicates that voice abuse or misuse is present and may be contributing to the patient's voice complaint.

Any patient with a voice problem should be examined by indirect laryngoscopy at least. Judging voice range, quality, or other vocal attributes by inspection of the vocal folds is not possible. However, the presence or absence of nodules, mass lesions, contact ulcers, hemorrhage, erythema, paralysis, arytenoid erythema (reflux), and other anatomic abnormalities must be established. Erythema of the laryngeal surface of the epiglottis is often associated with frequent coughing or clearing of the throat or with muscular tension dysphonia and is caused by direct trauma from the arytenoids during these maneuvers. A mirror or laryngeal telescope may provide a better view of the posterior portion of the vocal folds than is obtained with flexible endoscopy.

Fiberoptic laryngoscopy can be performed as an office procedure and allows inspection of the vocal folds in patients whose vocal folds are difficult to visualize indirectly. In addition, it permits observation of the vocal mechanism in a more natural posture than does indirect laryngoscopy. In the hands of an experienced endoscopist, this method may provide a great deal of information about both speaking and singing techniques. The combination of a fiberoptic laryngoscope with a laryngeal stroboscope may be especially useful. This system permits magnification, photography and detailed inspection of vocal fold motion. Sophisticated systems that permit fiberoptic strobovideolaryngoscopy are currently available commercially and are an invaluable asset for routine clinical use. The video system also provides a permanent record, permitting reassessment, comparison over time, and easy consultation. A refinement not currently available commercially is stereoscopic fiberoptic laryngoscopy, accomplished by placing a laryngoscope through each nostril, fastening the two together in the pharynx, and observing the larynx through the eyepieces.[20] This method allows visualization of laryngeal motion in three dimensions. However, it is practical primarily in a research setting.

Rigid endoscopy with anesthesia may be reserved for the rare patient whose vocal folds cannot be assessed adequately by other means or for patients who need surgical procedures to remove or biopsy laryngeal lesions. In many cases this may be done with local anesthesia, avoiding the need for intubation and the traumatic coughing and vomiting that may occur even after general anesthesia administered by mask. Coughing after general anesthesia may be minimized by using topical anesthesia in the larynx and trachea. However, topical anesthetics may act as severe mucosal irritants in a small number of patients. They may also predispose the patient to aspiration in the postoperative period. If a patient has had difficulty with a topical anesthetic administered in the office, it should not be used in the operating room. When used in general anesthesia cases, topical anesthetics should be applied at the end of the procedure. Thus, if inflammation occurs, it will not interfere with microsurgery. Postoperative duration of anesthesia is also optimized. The author has had the least difficulty with 4% Xylocaine.

Objective tests

Reliable, valid, objective analysis of the voice is extremely important and is an essential part of a comprehensive physical examination. It is as invaluable to the laryngologist as audiometry is to the otologist.[54,56] Familiarity with some of the measures currently available is helpful.

Strobovideolaryngoscopy

Strobovideolaryngoscopy is the single most important technologic advance in diagnostic laryngology with the possible exception of fiberoptic laryngoscopy.

Stroboscopic light allows routine slow-motion evaluation of the mucosal cover layer of the leading edge of the vocal fold. This state-of-the-art physical examination permits detection of vibratory asymmetries, structural abnormalities, small masses, submucosal scars, and other conditions that are invisible under ordinary light.[54,57] For example, in a patient who has a poor voice after laryngeal surgery and a 'normal looking larynx', stroboscopic light often reveals adynamic segments that explain the problem even to an untrained observer (such as the patient). The stroboscope is also extremely sensitive in detecting changes caused by fixation from small laryngeal neoplasms in patients who are being followed for leukoplakia or after laryngeal irradiation. Documentation of the procedure by coupling stroboscopic light with the video camera allows later reevaluation by the laryngologist or other health care providers.

A relatively standardized method of subjective assessment of videostroboscopic pictures is in wide clinical use,[4,24] allowing comparison of results among various physicians and investigators. Characteristics assessed include fundamental frequency, symmetry of bilateral movements, periodicity, glottal closure, amplitude, mucosal wave, presence of nonvibrating portions, and other unusual findings (such as a tiny polyp).

Other techniques to examine vocal fold vibration

Other techniques to examine vocal fold vibration include ultrahigh-speed photography, electroglottography (EGG), photoelectroglottography and ultrasound glottography, and most recently videokymography.[64] Ultrahigh-speed photography provides images similar to those provided by strobovideolaryngoscopy but requires expensive, cumbersome equipment and delayed data processing. Electroglottography (EGG) uses two electrodes on the skin of the neck above the thyroid laminae. A weak, high-frequency voltage is passed through the larynx from one electrode to the other. Opening and closing of the vocal folds varies the transverse electrical impedance, producing variation of the electrical current in phase with vocal fold vibration. The resultant tracing is called an electroglottogram. It traces the opening and closing of the glottis and can be compared with stroboscopic images.[32] Electroglottography allows objective determination of the presence or absence of glottal vibrations and easy determination of the fundamental period of vibration and is reproducible. It reflects the glottal condition more accurately during its closed phase. Photoelectroglottography and ultrasound glottography are less useful clinically.[25]

Measures of phonatory ability

Objective measures of phonatory ability are among the easiest and most readily available to the laryngologist, helpful in the treatment of professional vocalists with specific voice disorders, and are quite useful in assessing the results of surgical therapies. Maximum phonation time is measured with a stopwatch. The patient is instructed to sustain the vowel /a/ for as long as possible after deep inspiration, vocalizing at a comfortable frequency and intensity. The frequency and intensity may be determined and controlled by an inexpensive frequency analyzer and sound level meter. The test is repeated three times, and the greatest value is recorded. Normal values have been determined.[25] Frequency range of phonation is recorded in semitones and documents the vocal range from the lowest note in the modal register (excluding vocal fry) to the highest falsetto note. This is the physiologic frequency range of phonation and disregards quality. The musical frequency range of phonation measures lowest to highest notes of musically acceptable quality. Tests for maximum phonation time, frequency ranges, and many of the other parameters discussed later (including spectrographic analysis) may be preserved on a tape recorder for analysis at a convenient future time and used for pre-treatment and post-treatment comparisons. Recordings should be made in a standardized, consistent fashion.

Frequency limits of vocal register may also be measured. The registers are (from low to high) vocal fry, chest, mid, head and falsetto. However, classification of registers is controversial, and many other classifications are used. Although the classification listed above is common among musicians, at present, most voice scientists prefer a scheme that classifies registers as pulse, modal and loft. Overlap of frequency among registers occurs routinely. Testing the speaking fundamental frequency often reveals excessively low pitch, an abnormality associated with chronic voice abuse and development of vocal nodules. This parameter may be followed objectively throughout a course of voice therapy. Intensity range of phonation (IRP) has proven a less useful measure than frequency range. It varies with fundamental frequency (which should be recorded) and is greatest in the middle frequency range. It is recorded in sound pressure level (SPL) re: 0.0002 microbar. For normal adults who are not professional vocalists, measuring at a single fundamental frequency, IRP averages 54.8 dB for males and 51 dB for females.[11] Alterations of intensity are common in voice disorders, although IRP is not the most sensitive test to detect them. Information from these tests may be combined in a fundamental frequency-intensity profile,[25] also called a phonetogram.

Glottal efficiency (ratio of the acoustic power at the level of the glottis to subglottal power) provides useful information but is not clinically practical because measuring acoustic power at the level of the glottis is difficult. Subglottic power is the product of subglottal pressure and airflow rate. These can be determined clinically. Various alternative measures of glottic efficiency have been proposed, including the ratio of radiated acoustic power to subglottal power,[28] airflow intensity profile,[47] and ratio of the root mean square value of the AC component to the mean volume velocity (DC component).[29] Although glottal efficiency is of great interest, none of these tests is particularly helpful under routine clinical circumstances.

Aerodynamic measures

Traditional pulmonary function testing provides the most readily accessible measure of respiratory function. The most common parameters measured include:

- tidal volume, the volume of air that enters the lungs during inspiration and leaves during expiration in normal breathing;
- functional residual capacity, the volume of air remaining in the lungs at the end of inspiration during normal breathing. It may be divided into expiratory reserve volume (maximal additional volume that can be exhaled) and residual volume (the volume of air remaining in the lungs at the end of maximal exhalation);
- inspiratory capacity, the maximal volume of air that can be inhaled starting at the functional residual capacity;
- total lung capacity, the volume of air in the lungs following maximal inspiration;
- vital capacity, the maximal volume of air that can be exhaled from the lungs following maximal inspiration;
- forced vital capacity, the rate of air flow with rapid, forceful expiration from total lung capacity to residual volume;
- FEV_1, the forced expiratory volume in 1 second;
- FEV_3, the forced expiratory volume in 3 seconds;
- maximal mid-expiratory flow, the mean rate of air flow over the middle half of the forced vital capacity (between 25% and 75% of the forced vital capacity).

For singers and professional speakers with an abnormality caused by voice abuse, abnormal pulmonary function tests may confirm deficiencies in aerobic conditioning or reveal previously unrecognized asthma.[10] Flow glottography with computer inverse filtering is also a practical and valuable diagnostic for assessing flow at the vocal fold level, evaluating the voice source, and imaging the results of the balance between adductory forces and subglottal pressure.[53,62] It also has therapeutic value.

The spirometer, readily available for pulmonary function testing, can be used for measuring airflow during phonation. However, it does not allow simultaneous display of acoustic signals, and its frequency response is poor. A pneumotachograph consists of a laminar air resistor, a differential pressure transducer, and an amplifying and recording system. It allows measurement of airflow and simultaneous recording of other signals when coupled with a polygraph. A hot-wire anemometer allows determination of airflow velocity by measuring the electrical drop across the hot wire. Modern hot-wire anemometers containing electrical feedback circuitry that maintains the temperature of the hot wire provide a flat frequency response up to 1 kHz and are useful clinically.[29]

The four parameters traditionally measured in analyzing the aerodynamic performance of a voice are: subglottal pressure (Psub), supraglottal pressure (Psup), glottal impedance and volume velocity of airflow at the glottis. These parameters and their rapid variations can be measured under laboratory circumstances. However, clinically their mean value is usually determined as follows:

$$P_{sub}\ P_{sup} = MFR \times GR$$

where MFR is the mean (root mean square) flow rate and GR is the mean (root mean square) glottal resistance. When vocalizing the open vowel /a/, the supraglottic pressure equals the atmospheric pressure reducing the equation to:

$$P_{sub} = MFR \times GR$$

The mean flow rate is a useful clinical measure. While the patient vocalizes the vowel /a/, the mean flow rate is calculated by dividing the total volume of air used during phonation by the duration of phonation. The subject phonates at a comfortable pitch and loudness either over a determined period of time or for a maximum sustained period of phonation.

Air volume is measured by the use of a mask fitted tightly over the face or by phonating into a mouthpiece while wearing a nose clamp. Measurements may be made using a spirometer, pneumotachograph or hot-wire anemometer. The normal values for mean flow rate under habitual phonation, with changes in intensity or register, and under various pathologic circumstances, have been determined.[25] Normal values are available for both adults and children. Mean flow rate is a clinically useful parameter to follow during treatment for vocal nodules, recurrent laryngeal nerve paralysis, spasmodic dysphonia and other conditions.

Glottal resistance cannot be measured directly, but it may be calculated from the mean flow rate and mean subglottal pressure. Normal glottal resistance is 20–100 dynes/cm^5 at low and medium pitches and 150 dynes/cm^5 at high pitches.[28] Subglottal pressure is less useful clinically because it requires an invasive procedure for accurate measurement. It may be determined by tracheal puncture, transglottal catheter, or measurement through a tracheostoma using a transducer. Subglottal pressure may be approximated using an esophageal balloon. Intratracheal pressure, which is roughly equal to subglottal pressure, is transmitted to the balloon through the trachea. However, measured changes in the esophageal balloon are affected by intraesophageal pressure, which is dependent upon lung volume. Therefore, estimates of subglottal pressure using this technique are valid only under specific, controlled circumstances. The normal values for subglottal pressure under various healthy and pathologic voice conditions have also been determined by numerous investigators.[25]

The phonation quotient is the vital capacity divided by the maximum phonation time. It has been shown to correlate closely with maximum flow rate[26] and is a more convenient measure. Normative data determined by various authors have been published.[25] The phonation quotient provides an objective measure of the effects of treatment and is particularly useful in cases of recurrent laryngeal nerve paralysis and mass lesions of the vocal folds, including nodules.

Acoustic analysis

Acoustic analysis of voice signals is both promising and disappointing. The skilled laryngologist, speech-language therapist, pathologist, musician, or other trained listener frequently infers a great deal of valid information from the sound of a voice. However, clinically useful technology for analyzing and quantifying subtle acoustic differences is still not ideal. In many ways, the tape recorder is still the laryngologist's most valuable tool for acoustic analysis. Recording a patient's voice under controlled, repeatable circumstances before, during, and at the conclusion of treatment allows both the physician and the patient to make a qualitative, subjective acoustic analysis. Objective analysis with instruments may also be made from recorded voice samples.

Care must be taken to use a standardized protocol, and utilizing sophisticated instrumentation available[54] may be valuable for both medical diagnosis and studio feedback. Acoustic analysis equipment can determine frequency, intensity, harmonic spectrum, cycle-to-cycle perturbations in frequency (jitter), cycle-to-cycle perturbations in amplitude (shimmer), harmonics/noise ratios, breathiness index and many other parameters. The DSP SONA-GRAPH Model 5500 (Kay Elemetrics, Pine Brook, New Jersey) is an integrated voice analysis system. It is equipped for sound spectrography capabilities. Spectrography provides a visual record of the voice. The acoustic signal is depicted using time (x axis), frequency (y axis) and intensity (z axis), shading of light vs dark. Using the band pass filters, generalizations about quality, pitch and loudness can be made. These observations are used in formulating the voice therapy treatment plan. Formant structure and strength can be determined using the narrow-band filters, of which a variety of configurations are possible. In those clinical settings where singers and other professional voice users are routinely evaluated and treated, this feature is extremely valuable. A sophisticated voice analysis program (an optional program) may be combined with the Sona-Graph and is an especially valuable addition to the clinical laboratory. The voice analysis program (CSL, Kay Elemetrics) measures speaking fundamental frequency, frequency perturbation (jitter), amplitude perturbation (shimmer), harmonics-to-noise ratio, and provides a great number of other useful values. An electroglottograph (EGG) may be used in conjunction with the Sona-Graph to provide some of these voicing parameters. Examining the EGG waveform alone is possible with this setup, but its clinical usefulness has not yet been established. An important feature of the Sona-graph is the long-term average (LTA) spectral capability, which allows for analyzing longer voice samples (30–90 seconds). The LTA analyzes only voiced speech segments, and may be useful in screening for hoarse or breathy voices. In addition, computer interface capabilities (also an optional program) have solved many data storage and file maintenance problems.

In analyzing acoustic signals, the microphone may be placed at the level of the mouth or may be positioned in or over the trachea. Position should be standardized in each office or laboratory.[38] Various techniques are being developed to improve the usefulness of acoustic analysis. Because of the enormous amount of information carried in the acoustic signal, further refinements in objective acoustic analysis should prove particularly valuable to the clinician.

Laryngeal electromyography

Electromyography requires an electrode system, an amplifier, an oscilloscope, a loudspeaker, and a recording system. Electrodes are placed transcutaneously into laryngeal muscles. It may be extremely valuable in confirming cases of vocal fold paresis, in differentiating paralysis from arytenoid dislocation, in distinguishing recurrent laryngeal nerve paralysis from combined recurrent and superior nerve paralysis, diagnosing other more subtle neurolaryngologic pathology, and in documenting functional voice disorders and malingering. It is also recommended for needle localization when using botulinum toxin for the treatment of spasmodic dysphonia and other conditions.

Psychoacoustic evaluation

Because the human ear and brain are the most sensitive and complex analyzers of sound currently available, many researchers have tried to standardize and quantify psychoacoustic evaluation. Unfortunately, even definitions of basic terms such as hoarseness and breathiness are still controversial. Psychoacoustic evaluation protocols and interpretations are not standardized. Consequently, although subjective psychoacoustic analysis of voice is of great value to the individual skilled clinician, it remains generally unsatisfactory for comparing research among laboratories or for reporting clinical results.

Evaluation of the singing voice

The physician must be careful not to exceed the limits of his or her expertise especially in caring for singers. However, if voice abuse or technical error is suspected, or if a difficult judgment must be reached on whether to allow a sick singer to perform, a brief observation of the patient's singing may provide invaluable information. This is accomplished best by asking the singer to stand and sing scales either in the examining room or in the soundproof audiology booth. Similar maneuvers may be used for professional speakers including actors (who can vocalize and recite lines), clergy and politicians (who can deliver sermons and speeches), and virtually all other voice patients. The singer's stance should be balanced, with the weight slightly forward. The knees should be bent slightly and the shoulders, torso, and neck should be relaxed. The singer should inhale through the nose whenever possible allowing filtration, warming and humidification of inspired air. In general, the chest should be expanded, but most of the active breathing is abdominal. The chest should not rise substantially with each inspiration, and the supraclavicular musculature should not be involved obviously in inspiration. Shoulders and neck muscles should not be tensed even with deep inspiration. Abdominal musculature should be contracted shortly before the initiation of the tone. This may be evaluated visually or by palpation. Muscles of the neck and face should be relaxed. Economy is a basic principle of all art forms. Wasted energy and motion and muscle tension are incorrect and usually deleterious.

The singer should be instructed to sing a scale (a five-note scale is usually sufficient) on the vowel /a/, beginning on any comfortable note. Technical errors are usually most obvious as contraction of muscles in the neck and chin, retraction of the lower lip, retraction of the tongue, or tightening of the muscles of mastication. The singer's mouth should be open widely but comfortably. When singing /a/, the singer's tongue should rest in a neutral position with the tip of the tongue lying against the back of the singer's mandibular incisors. If the tongue pulls back or demonstrates obvious muscular activity as the singer performs the scales, improper voice use can be confirmed on the basis of positive evidence. The position of the larynx should not vary substantially with pitch changes. Rising of the larynx with ascending pitch is also evidence of technical dysfunction. This examination also gives the physician an opportunity to observe any dramatic differences between the qualities and ranges of the speaking voice and the singing voice.

Remembering the admonition not to exceed his or her expertise, the physician who examines many singers can often glean valuable information from a brief attempt to modify an obvious technical error. For example, deciding whether to allow a singer with mild or moderate laryngitis to perform is often difficult. On the one hand, an expert singer has technical skills that allow him or her to compensate safely. On the other hand, if a singer does not sing with correct technique and does not have the discipline to modify volume, technique, and repertoire as necessary, the risk of vocal injury may be increased substantially even by mild inflammation of the vocal folds. In borderline circumstances, observation of the singer's technique may greatly help the physician in making a judgment.

If the technique appears flawless, we may feel somewhat more secure in allowing the singer to proceed with performance commitments. More commonly, even good singers demonstrate technical errors when experiencing voice difficulties. In a vain effort to compensate for dysfunction at the vocal fold level, singers often modify their technique in the neck and supraglottic vocal tract. In the good singer, this usually means going from good technique to bad technique. The most common error involves pulling back the tongue and tightening the cervical muscles. Although this increased muscular activity gives the singer the illusion of making the voice more secure, this technical maladjustment undermines vocal efficiency and increases vocal strain. The physician may ask the singer to hold the top note of a five-note scale; while the note is being held, the singer may simply be told, 'Relax your tongue'. At the same time the physician points to the singer's abdominal musculature. Most good singers immediately correct to good technique. If they do, and if upcoming performances are particularly important, the singer may be able to perform with a reminder that meticulous technique is essential. The singer should be advised to 'sing by feel rather than by ear', to consult his or her voice teacher, and conserve the voice except when it is absolutely necessary to use it. If a singer is unable to correct from bad technique to good technique promptly, especially if he or she uses excessive muscle tension in the neck and ineffective abdominal support, it is generally safer not to perform with even a mild vocal fold abnormality. With increased experience and training, the laryngologist may make other observations that aid in providing appropriate treatment recommendations for singer patients. Once these skills have been mastered for the care of singers, applying them to other patients is relatively easy, so long as the laryngologist takes the time to understand the demands of the individual's professional, avocational and recreational vocal activities.

If treatment is to be instituted, at least a tape recording of the voice is advisable in most cases and essential before any surgical intervention. The author routinely uses strobovideolaryngoscopy for diagnosis and documentation in virtually all cases as well as many of the objective measures discussed. Such testing is extremely helpful clinically and medicolegally.

Additional examinations

A general physical examination should be performed whenever the patient's systemic health is questionable. Debilitating conditions such as mononucleosis may be noticed first by the singer as vocal fatigue. A neurologic assessment may be particularly revealing. The physician must be careful not to overlook dysarthrias and dysphonias characteristic of movement disorders and of serious neurologic disease. Dysarthria is a defect in rhythm, enunciation and articulation that usually results from neuromuscular impairment or weakness such as may occur after a stroke. It may also be seen with oral deformities or illness. Dysphonia is an abnormality of vocalization usually originating from problems at the laryngeal level.

Physicians should be familiar with the six types of dysarthria, their symptoms, and their importance.[14,15]

Flaccid dysarthria occurs in lower motor neuron or primary muscle disorders such as myasthenia gravis and tumors or strokes involving the brainstem nuclei. Spastic dysarthria occurs in upper motor neuron disorders (pseudobulbar palsy) such as multiple strokes and cerebral palsy. Ataxic dysarthria is seen with cerebellar disease, alcohol intoxication and multiple sclerosis. Hypokinetic dysarthria accompanies Parkinson's disease. Hyperkinetic dysarthria may be spasmodic, as in Gilles de la Tourette's disease, or dystonic, as in chorea and cerebral palsy. Mixed dysarthria occurs in amyotrophic lateral sclerosis. The preceding classification actually combines dysphonic and dysarthric characteristics, but is very useful clinically. The value of a comprehensive neurolaryngologic evaluation cannot be overstated.[43] More specific details of voice changes associated with neurological dysfunction and their localizing value are available elsewhere.[3,54]

It is extremely valuable for the laryngologist to assemble an arts medicine team that includes not only a speech-language pathologist, singing voice specialist, acting voice specialist, and voice scientist, but also medical colleagues in other disciplines. Collaboration with an expert neurologist, pulmonologist, endocrinologist, psychologist, psychiatrist, internist, physiatrist, and others with special knowledge of, and interest in, voice disorders is invaluable in caring for patients with voice disorders. Such interdisciplinary teams have not only changed the standard of care in voice evaluation and treatment, but are also largely responsible for the rapid and productive growth of Voice as a subspecialty.

References

1. Ackerman R, Pfan W. Gerotologische Untersuchungen zur Storunepanfalligkeit der Sprechstimme bei Berufssprechern. *Folia Phoniatr (Basel)* 1974; **25:** 95–909.
2. Arndt HJ. Stimmstorungen nach Behandlung mit Androgenen und anabolen Hormonen. *Munch Med Wochenschr* 1974; **116:** 1715–20.
3. Aronson AE. *Clinical Voice Disorders*, 3rd edn. New York: Thieme, 1990: 70–193.
4. Bless D, Hirano M, Feder RJ. Video stroboscopic evaluation of the larynx. *Ear Nose Throat J* 1987; **66:** 289–96.
5. Bourdial J. Les troubles de la voix provoqués par la thérapeutique hormonale androgène. *Ann Otolaryngol Chir Cervicofac* 1970; **87:** 725–34.
6. Brodnitz F. Hormones and the human voice. *Bull NY Acad Med* 1971; **47:** 183–91.
7. Brodnitz F. The age of the castrato voice. *J Speech Hear Disord* 1975; **40:** 291–5.
8. Brodnitz F. Medical care preventive therapy (panel). In: Lawrence VL, ed. *Transcripts of the Seventh Annual Symposium. Care of the Professional Voice.* New York: The Voice Foundation, 1978; **3:** 86.
9. Carroll C. Arizona State University at Tempe: personal communication with Dr Hans von Leden. September, 1992.
10. Cohn JR, Sataloff RT, Spiegel JR, Fish JE, Kennedy K. Airway reactivity-induced asthma in singers (ARIAS). *J Voice* 1991; **5:** 332–7.
11. Coleman RJ, Mabis JH, Hinson JK. Fundamental frequency sound pressure level profiles of adult male and female voices. *J Speech Hear Res* 1977; **20:** 197–204.
12. Damste PH. Virilization of the voice due to anabolic steroids. *Folia Phoniatr (Basel)* 1964; **16:** 10–18.
13. Damste PH. Voice changes in adult women caused by virilizing agents. *J Speech Hear Disord* 1967; **32:** 126–32.
14. Darley F, Aronson AE, Brown JR. Differential diagnosis of patterns of dysarthria. *J Speech Hear Res* 1969; **12:** 246–9.
15. Darley F, Aronson AE, Brown JR. Clusters of deviant speech dimensions in the dysarthrias. *J Speech Hear Res* 1969; **12:** 462–96.
16. Deuster CV. Irreversible Stimmstorung in der Schwangerscheft. *HNO* 1977; **25:** 430–2.
17. Dordain M. Etude statistique de l'influence des contraceptifs hormonaux sur la voix. *Folia Phoniatr (Basel)* 1972; **24:** 86–96.
18. Feder RL. The professional voice and airline flight. *Otolaryngol Head Neck Surg* 1984; **92:** 251–4.
19. Flach M, Schwickardi H, Simen R. Welchen Einfluss haben Menstruation and Schwangerschaft auf die augsgebildete Gesangsstimme? *Folia Phoniatr (Basel)* 1968; **21:** 199–210.
20. Fujimura O. Stero-fiberoptic laryngeal observation. *J Acoust Soc Am* 1979; **65:** 70–2.
21. Gould WJ, Alberti PW, Brodnitz F, Hirano M. Medical care preventive therapy (panel). In: Lawrence VL, ed. *Transcripts of the Seventh Annual Symposium. Care of the Professional Voice.* New York: The Voice Foundation, 1978; **3:** 74–6.
22. Gupta OP, Bhatia PL, Agarwal MK, Mehrotra ML, Mishr SK. Nasal pharyngeal and laryngeal manifestations of hypothyroidism. *Ear Nose Throat J* 1977; **56:** 10–21.
23. Herman H, Rossol M. Artificial fogs and smokes. In: Sataloff RT, ed. *Professional Voice: the Science and Art of Clinical Care*, 2nd edn. San Diego: Singular Publishing Group, 1997: 413–27.
24. Hirano M. Phonosurgery: basic and clinical investigations. *Otologia (Fukuoka)* 1975; **21:** 239–442.
25. Hirano M. *Clinical Examination of the Voice.* New York: Springer-Verlag, 1981: 1–98.
26. Hirano M, Koike Y, von Leden H. Maximum phonation time and air usage during phonation. *Folia Phoniatr (Basel)* 1968; **20:** 185–201.
27. Imre V. Hormonell bedingte Stimmstorungen. *Folia Phoniatr (Basel)* 1968; **20:** 394–404.
28. Isshiki N. Regulatory mechanism of voice intensity variation. *J Speech Hear Res* 1964; **7:** 17–29.
29. Isshiki N. Functional surgery of the larynx. *Report of the 78th Annual Convention of the Oto-Rhino-Laryngological Society of Japan, Kyoto University, Fukuoka,* 1977.
30. Lacina V. Der Einfluss der Menstruation auf die Stimme der Sangerinnen. *Folia Phoniatr (Basel)* 1968; **20:** 13–24.
31. Lawrence VL. Medical care for professional voice (panel). In: Lawrence VL, ed. *Transcripts from the Annual Symposium. Care of the Professional Voice.* New York: The Voice Foundation, 1978; **3:** 17–18.
32. Leclure FLE, Brocaar ME, Verscheeure J. Electroglottography and its relation to glottal activity. *Folia Phoniatr (Basel)* 1975; **27:** 215–24.

33. Malinsky M, Chevrie-Muller, Cerceau N. Etude clinique et electrophysiologique des alterations de la voix au cours des thyrotoxioses. *Ann Endocrinol (Paris)* 1977; **38**: 171–2.
34. Meuser W, Nieschlag E. Sexualhormone und Stimmlage des Mannes. *Dtsch Med Wochenschr* 1977; **102**: 261–4.
35. Michelsson K, Sirvio P. Cry analysis in congenital hypothyroidism. *Folia Phoniatr (Basel)* 1976; **28**: 40–7.
36. Opperman DA. Pyrotechnics in the entertainment industry: an overview. In: Sataloff RT, ed. *Professional Voice: the Science and Art of Clinical Care*, 2nd edn. San Diego: Singular Publishing Group, 1997: 393–402.
37. Pahn V, Goretzlehner G. Stimmstorungen durch hormonale Kontrazeptiva. *Zentralbl Gynakol* 1978; **100**: 341–6.
38. Price DB, Sataloff RT. A simple technique for consistent microphone placement in voice recording. *J Voice* 1988; **2**: 206–7.
39. Ritter FN. The effect of hypothyroidism on the larynx of the rat. *Ann Otol Rhinol Laryngol* 1964; **67**: 404–16.
40. Ritter FN. In: Paparella M, Shumrick D, eds. *Endocrinology in Otolaryngology*. Vol. I. Philadelphia: Saunders, 1973: 727–34.
41. Rosen DC, Sataloff RT. Psychological aspects of voice disorders. In: Rubin J, Korovin G, Sataloff RT, Gould WJ, eds. *Diagnosis and Treatment of Voice Disorders*. New York: Igaku-Shoin Medical Publishers, 1995: 491–501.
42. Rosen DC, Sataloff RT. *Psychology of Voice Disorders*. San Diego: Singular Publishing Group, 1997: 1–261.
43. Rosenfield DB. Neurolaryngology. *Ear Nose Throat J* 1987; **66**: 323–6.
44. Rossol M. Pyrotechnics: health effects. In: Sataloff RT, ed. *Professional Voice: the Science and Art of Clinical Care*, 2nd edn. San Diego: Singular Publishing Group, 1997: 407–11.
45. Rubin JS, Sataloff RT, Korovin G, Gould WJ. *Diagnosis and Treatment of Voice Disorders*. New York: Igaku-Shoin, 1995: 1–525.
46. Saez S, Francoise S. Récepteurs d'androgènes: mise en evidence dans la fraction cytosolique de muqueuse normale et d'epitheliomas phryngolarynges humains. *C R Acad Sci III* 1975; **280**: 935–8.
47. Saito S. Phonosurgery, basic study on the mechanism of phonation and endolaryngeal microsurgery. *Otologia (Fukuoka)* 1977; **23**: 171–384.
48. Sataloff RT. Professional singers: the science and art of clinical care. *Am J Otolaryngol* 1981; **2**: 251–66.
49. Sataloff RT. Efficient history taking in professional singers. *Laryngoscope* 1984; **94**: 1111–14.
50. Sataloff RT. The professional voice: part II, physical examination. *J Voice* 1987; **1**: 191–201.
51. Sataloff RT. *Professional Singers: the Science and Art of Clinical Care*. New York: Raven Press, 1991: 77–9, 159–78.
52. Sataloff RT. The human voice. *Sci Am* 1992; **267**: 108–15.
53. Sataloff RT. The impact of pollution on the voice. *Otolaryngol Head Neck Surg* 1992; **106**: 701–5.
54. Sataloff RT. *Professional Voice: the Science and Art of Clinical Care*, 2nd edn. San Diego: Singular Publishing Group, 1997: 1–1069.
55. Sataloff RT, Rosen DC, Hawkshaw M. Medications: effects and side-effects in professional voice users. In: Sataloff RT, ed. *Professional Voice: the Science and Art of Clinical Care*, 2nd edn. San Diego: Singular Publishing Group, 1997: 453–65.
56. Sataloff RT, Spiegel JR, Carroll LM, Darby KS, Hawkshaw MJ, Rulnick RK. The clinical voice laboratory: practical design and clinical application. *J Voice* 1990; **4**: 264–79.
57. Sataloff RT, Spiegel JR, Carroll LM, Schiebel BR, Darby KS, Rulnick RK. Strobovideolaryngoscopy in professional voice users: results and clinical value. *J Voice* 1988; **1**: 359–64.
58. Schiff M. The influence of estrogens on connective tissue. In: Asboe-Hansen G, ed. *Hormones and Connective Tissue*. Munksgaard Press, 1967: 282–341.
59. Schiff M. 'The pill' in otolaryngology. *Trans Am Acad Ophthalmol Otolaryngol* 1968; **72**: 76–84.
60. Schiff M. Comment at the *Seventh Symposium on Care of the Professional Voice, The Juilliard School, New York*, June 15 and 16, 1978.
61. Spiegel JR, Cohn JR, Sataloff RT, Fish JE, Kennedy K. Respiratory function in singers: medical assessment, diagnoses, treatments. *J Voice* 1988; **2**: 40–50.
62. Sundberg J. *The Science of the Singing Voice*. DeKalb: Northern Illinois University Press, 1987: 1–194.
63. Sundberg J, Prame E, Iwarsson J. Replicability and accuracy of pitch patterns in professional singers. In: Davis PJ, Fletcher NJ, eds. *Vocal Fold Physiology: Controlling Chaos and Complexity*. San Diego: Singular Publishing Group, 1995: 291–306.
64. Svec J, Shutte H. Videokymography: high-speed line scanning of vocal fold vibration. *J Voice* 1996; **10**: 201–5.
65. von Gelder L. Psychosomatic aspects of endocrine disorders of the voice. *J Commun Disord* 1974; **7**: 257–62.
66. von Leden H. Speech and hearing problems in the geriatric patient. *J Am Geriatr Soc* 1977; **25**: 422–6.
67. Vuorenkoski V, Lenko HL, Tjernlund P, Vuorenkoski L, Perheentupa J. Fundamental voice frequency during normal and abnormal growth, and after androgen treatment. *Arch Dis Child* 1978; **53**: 201–9.
68. Wallner LJ, Hill BJ, Waldrop W. Voice changes following adenotonsillectomy. *Laryngoscope* 1968; **78**: 1410–18.
69. Wendler J. Zyklusabhangige Leistungsschwankungen der Stimme und ihre Beeinflussung durch Ovulationshemmer. *Folia Phoniatr (Basel)* 1972; **24**: 259–77.

Appendix

Patient history form for professional voice users

Name——————————————— Age———— Sex———— Race————————

Height——————————————— Weight——————— Date———————

1. How long have you had your present voice problem?
   Who noticed it?
   Do you know what caused it? Yes No
   If so, what?
   Did it come on slowly or suddenly? Slowly Suddenly
   Is it getting: Worse Better Same ?

2. Which symptoms do you have? (Please check all that apply)
   - Hoarseness (coarse or scratchy sound)
   - Fatigue (voice tires or changes quality after speaking for a short period of time)
   - Volume disturbance: (trouble speaking) softly, loudly
   - Loss of range: high, low
   - Prolonged warm-up time (over 30 min to warm up voice)
   - Breathiness
   - Tickling or choking sensation while speaking
   - Pain in throat while speaking
   - Other (please specify):

3. Have you ever had training for your singing voice?
   Yes No

4. Have there been periods of months or years without lessons in that time?
   Yes No

5. How long have you studied with your present teacher?
   Teacher's name:

   Teacher's address:

   Teacher's telephone number:

6. Please list previous teachers and years during which you studied with them:

7. Have you ever had training for your singing voice?
   Yes No
   If so, list teachers and years of study:

8. In what capacity do you use your voice professionally?
   - Actor
   - Announcer (television/radio/sports arena)
   - Attorney
   - Clergy
   - Politician
   - Salesperson
   - Teacher
   - Telephone operator or receptionist
   - Other (please specify):

9. Do you have an important performance soon?
   Yes No
   Date(s):

10. Do you do regular voice exercises?
    Yes No
    If yes, describe:

11. Do you play a musical instrument?
    Yes No
    (a) If yes, please check all that apply:
    - Keyboard (piano, organ, harpsichord, other ___________)
    - Violin, viola, cello
    - Bass
    - Plucked strings (guitar, harp, other ___________)
    - Brass
    - Wind with single reed
    - Wind with double reed
    - Flute, piccolo
    - Percussion
    - Bagpipes
    - Accordion
    - Other (please specify):

12. Do you warm up your voice before practice or performance?
    Yes No

13. Do you warm down after using it?
    Yes No

14. How much are you speaking at present (average hours per day)?
    Rehearsal Performance Other

15. Please check all that apply to you:
    - Voice worse in the morning
    - Voice worse later in the day, after it has been used
    - Sing performances or rehearsals in the morning
    - Speak extensively (teacher, clergy, attorney, telephone, work, etc.)
    - Cheerleader
    - Speak extensively backstage or at post-performance parties
    - Choral conductor
    - Frequently clear your throat
    - Frequent sore throat
    - Jaw joint problems
    - Bitter or acid taste; bad breath or hoarseness first thing in the morning
    - Frequent 'heartburn' or hiatal hernia
    - Frequent yelling or loud talking
    - Frequent whispering
    - Chronic fatigue (insomnia)
    - Work around extreme dryness
    - Frequent exercise (weight lifting, aerobics, etc.)
    - Frequently thirsty, dehydrated
    - Hoarseness first thing in the morning
    - Chest cough
    - Eat late at night
    - Ever used antacids
    - Under particular stress at present (personal or professional)
    - Frequent bad breath

- Live, work, or perform around smoke or fumes
- Traveled recently: When:
  Where:

16. Your family doctor's name, address and telephone number:

17. Your laryngologist's name, address and telephone number:

18. Recent cold?
    Yes No

19. Current cold?
    Yes No

20. Have you been evaluated by an allergist?
    Yes No
    If yes what allergies do you have:
    [none, dust, mold, trees, cats, dog, foods, other]
    (Medication allergies are covered elsewhere in this history form)
    If yes, give name and address of allergist:

21. How many packs of cigarettes do you smoke per day?
    - Smoking history
    - Never
    - Quit. When?
    - Smoked about _____ packs per day for _____ years
    - Smoked _____ packs per day. Have smoked for _____ years

22. Do you work in a smoky environment?
    Yes No

23. How much alcohol do you drink?
    none, rarely, a few times per week, daily
    If daily, or few times per week, on average, how much do you consume?
    1, 2, 3, 4, 5, 6, 7, 8, 9, 10, more glasses per day, week of beer, wine, liquor
    Did you used to drink more heavily?
    Yes No

24. How many cups of coffee, tea, cola, or other caffeine-containing drinks do you drink per day?

25. List other recreational drugs you use:
    marijuana, cocaine, amphetamines, barbiturates, heroin, other __________________

26. Have you noticed any of the following? (Check all that apply)
    - Hypersensitivity to heat or cold
    - Excessive sweating
    - Change in weight: gained/lost _____ lb. In _____ weeks/ _____ months
    - Change in your voice
    - Change in skin or hair
    - Palpitation (fluttering) of the heart
    - Emotional lability (swings of mood)
    - Double vision
    - Numbness of the face or extremities
    - Tingling around the mouth or face
    - Blurred vision or blindness
    - Weakness or paralysis of the face
    - Clumsiness in arms or legs
    - Confusion or loss of consciousness

- Difficulty with speech
- Difficulty with swallowing
- Seizure (epileptic fit)
- Pain in the neck or shoulder
- Shaking or tremors
- Memory change
- Personality change
- For females:
- Are you pregnant? Yes No
- Are your menstrual periods regular? Yes No
- Have you undergone hysterectomy? Yes No
- Were your ovaries removed? Yes No
- At what age did you reach puberty?
- Have you gone through menopause? Yes No

27. Have you ever consulted a psychologist or psychiatrist?
    Yes No

28. Are you currently under treatment?
    Yes No

29. Have you injured your head or neck (whiplash, etc.)?
    Yes No

30. Describe any serious accidents related to this visit:

31. Are you involved in legal action involving problems with your voice?
    Yes No

32. List names of spouse and children:

33. Brief summary of ENT problems, some of which may not be related to your present complaint.
    - Hearing loss
    - Ear pain
    - Ear noises
    - Facial pain
    - Lump in face or head
    - Lump in neck
    - Dizziness
    - Stiff neck
    - Facial paralysis
    - Nasal obstruction
    - Nasal deformity
    - Nose bleeds
    - Mouth sores
    - Trouble swallowing
    - Trouble breathing
    - Eye problem
    - Excess eye skin
    - Excess facial skin
    - Jaw joint problem
    - Other (please specify):

34. Do you have or have you ever had:
    - Diabetes
    - Seizures
    - Hypoglycemia
    - Psychological therapy or counseling

- Thyroid problems
- Frequent bad headaches
- Syphilis
- Ulcers
- Gonorrhea
- Kidney disease
- Herpes
- Urinary problems
- Cold sores (fever blisters)
- Arthritis or skeletal problems
- High blood pressure problems
- Severe low blood pressure
- Cleft palate
- Intravenous antibiotics or diuretics
- Asthma, lung or breathing problems
- Heart attack
- Angina
- Irregular heartbeat
- Rheumatic fever
- Other heart problems
- Unexplained weight loss
- Cancer of ________________
- Other tumor ______________
- Blood transfusions
- Hepatitis
- Tuberculosis
- AIDS
- Glaucoma
- Meningitis
- Multiple sclerosis
- Other illnesses (please specify):

35. Do any blood relatives have:
    - Diabetes
    - Hypoglycemia
    - Cancer
    - Heart disease

36. Other major medical problems such as those above. Please specify:

37. Describe serious accidents unless directly related to your doctor's visit here.
    - None
    - Occurred with head injury, loss of consciousness, or whiplash
    - Occurred without head injury, loss of consciousness, or whiplash
    - Describe:

38. List all current medications and doses (include birth control pills and vitamins).
    - None
    - Codeine
    - Medication allergies
    - Novocaine
    - Penicillin
    - Tetracycline
    - Erythromycin
    - Keflex/Ceclor/Ceftin
    - Iodine
    - x-Ray dyes
    - Adhesive tape

- Other (please specify):

39. List operations:
    - Tonsillectomy (age ______)
    - Adenoidectomy (age ______)
    - Appendectomy (age ______)
    - Heart surgery (age ______)
    - Other (please specify):

40. List toxic drugs or chemicals to which you have been exposed:
    - Streptomycin, neomycin, kanamycin
    - Lead
    - Mercury
    - Other (please list):

41. Have you had x-ray treatments to your head or neck (including treatments for acne or ear problems as a child), treatments for cancer, etc.?
    Yes No

42. Describe serious health problems of your spouse or children.

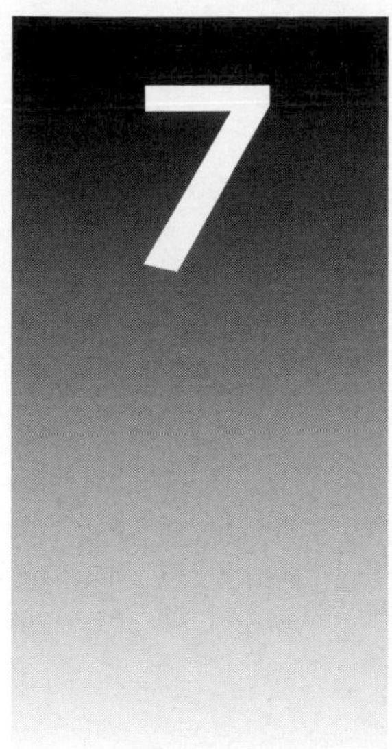

Videolaryngoscopy and laryngeal photography

Eiji Yanagisawa

Since Thomas French of New York published a paper entitled 'On a perfected method of photographing the larynx'[13] with a laryngeal mirror and a primitive camera, many different methods of laryngeal documentation have been proposed. They include:

indirect laryngoscopic photography[12,30]
direct laryngoscopic photography[12,16–18,31]
fiberscopic photography[10,11,19,32–34,42–45,47,48,51,52,60]
telescopic photography[1,4–9,14,22,27,28,35,37,39,40,43–52,54–58,60]
microscopic photography.[20,21,24–26,29,30,36,38,50,53,55,56,58]

Laryngeal documentation can be accomplished by different modalities: still photography, videography, cinematography and digital imaging. Although still photography of the larynx is a valuable method of laryngeal documentation today, videography is increasingly gaining favor. Cinematography was a popular effective means of documentation and presentation. However, because of the cost of films, time-consuming film development and editing, and the availability of newer generation video projectors for large screens, cinematography was practically replaced by videography. With the continuing advances in computer technology, digital imaging will undoubtedly play a significant role in laryngeal documentation.

In this chapter, various techniques of videolaryngoscopy (videography of the larynx) and laryngeal still photography as well as newer digital imaging will be described.

Videolaryngoscopy (videography of the larynx)

Videolaryngoscopy is an examination and documentation of the anatomy, physiology and pathology of the larynx using a video camera. It also allows simultaneous voice recording and digital imaging. Videolaryngoscopy can be accomplished by using a flexible fiberscope, a rigid telescope and/or a microscope. Videolaryngoscopy can be performed either in the office or in the operating room.[53,55–57,60]

The equipment required for videographic documentation of the larynx includes endoscopes (fiberscopes and telescopes), video cameras, video adapters, light sources, video recorders, video monitors, and video printers (Figs 7.1, 7.2).

Endoscopes

For fiberscopic videolaryngoscopy, the author uses the 3.4 mm and 4.4 mm flexible fiberscopes (Olympus ENF-P3 and L3, respectively) (Fig 7.1a). The smaller scope is used for routine laryngeal fiberscopic examinations whilst the larger scope is used for fiberscopic strobovideolaryngoscopy because it provides a much larger, clearer fiberscopic image. There are other excellent fiberscopes such as Machida 4L (4.0 mm), 3L (3.3 mm) and Pentax FNL 10S (3.5 mm).

Various 90° and 70° laryngeal telescopes are available. Standard 90° telescopes include:

- 5.8 mm 20 cm long 90° telescope (Karl Storz 8700D);
- Berci–Ward 14 cm long 90° laryngopharyngoscope (Karl Storz 8702D);
- 15 cm long 90° telelaryngo-pharyngoscope with 4× magnification (Karl Storz 8704D); and
- 90° Wolf telescope (Wolf 4447.57).

The author prefers 70° telescopes (Fig 7.1b):

- Nagashima SFT-1;

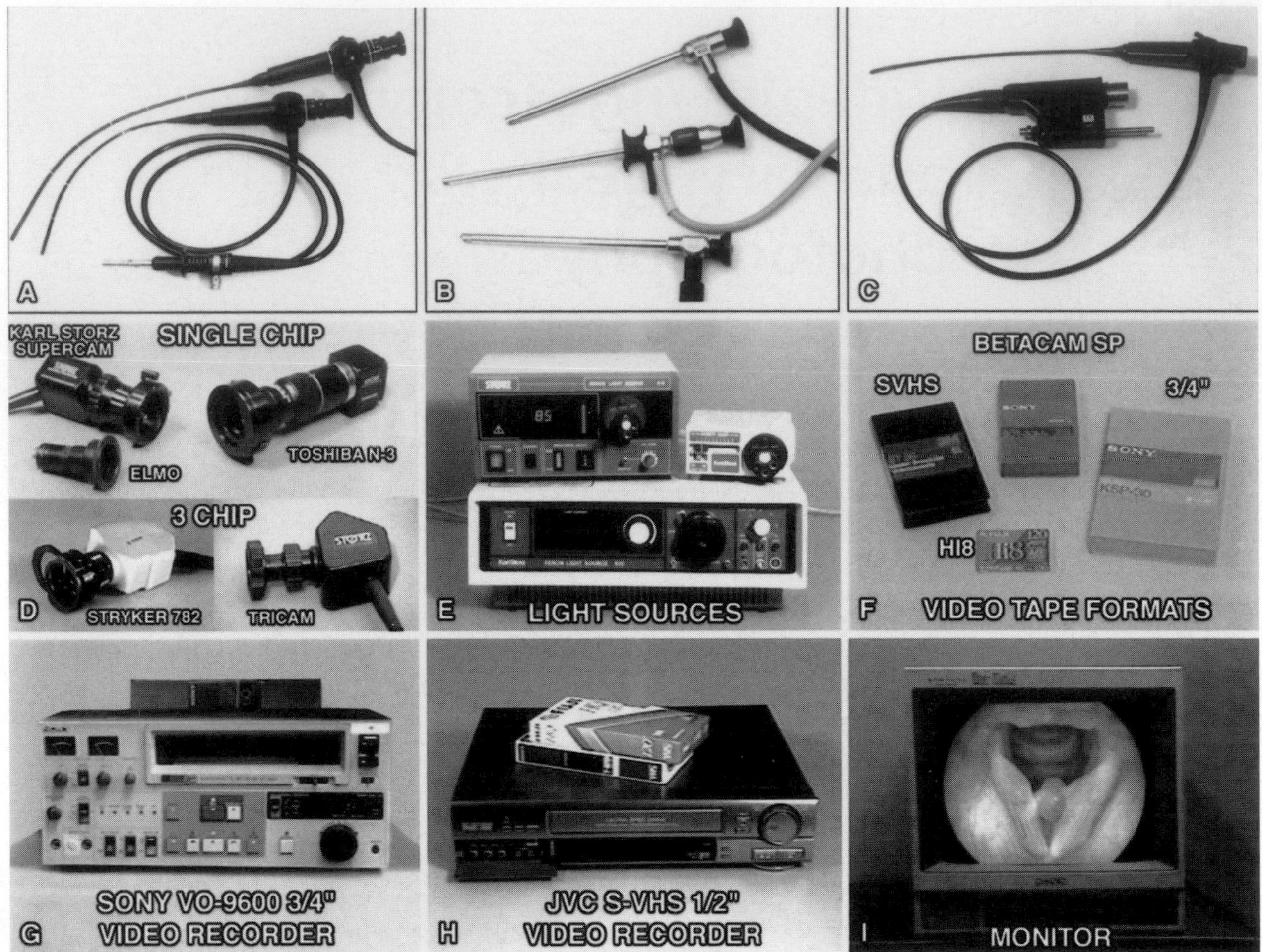

Figure 7.1 *Equipment. (a) Flexible fiberscopes: top, Olympus ENF-L3; bottom, Olympus ENF-P3. (b) 70° Rigid telescopes: top, Nagashima SFT-1; middle, Karl Storz 8706CJ; bottom, Kay 9105. (c) Pentax videoendoscope. (d) Video cameras: top left, Karl Storz supercam; middle left, Elmo EC102; top right, Toshiba N3 single chip CCD; bottom left, Stryker 782 three-chip CCD; bottom right, Karl Storz Tricam. (e) Light sources: top left, Karl Storz xenon 615; top right, Karl Storz 481C; bottom, Karl Storz xenon 610. (f) Videotape formats: SVHS, Betacam SP, 3/4 inch U-matic and Hi-8. (g) Sony VO-9600 3/4 inch video recorder. (h) JVC S-VHS ½ inch video recorder. (i) Monitor: Sony Trinitron 1343 MD.*

- Karl Storz 8706CJ; and
- Kay 9105.

The 70° telescope produces a larger, closer view of the larynx whilst the 90° telescope provides a panoramic view.

Video cameras

There are many compact single chip CCD video cameras currently available. The author has used:

- Elmo EC-102;
- Elmo EC-202; and
- Karl Storz Telecam (Fig 7.1d).

The newer three-chip CCD cameras are expensive but represent the gold standard for video cameras. They are compact and durable, and produce the brightest and clearest images. Popular models include:

- Stryker 782 (Fig 7.1d); and
- Karl Storz Tricam (Fig 7.1d).

Digital cameras represent the newest video imaging technology. Digital imaging has the advantages of:

- safe, long-term storage;
- easy computer manipulation (adjusting color, editing, enlarging, labeling, making composites, etc.);
- no image degrading with time;
- easy retrieval of images; and
- no need of a film or a tape.

This technology is not yet practical, since still high quality digital cameras or digital image capture devices are prohibitively expensive.

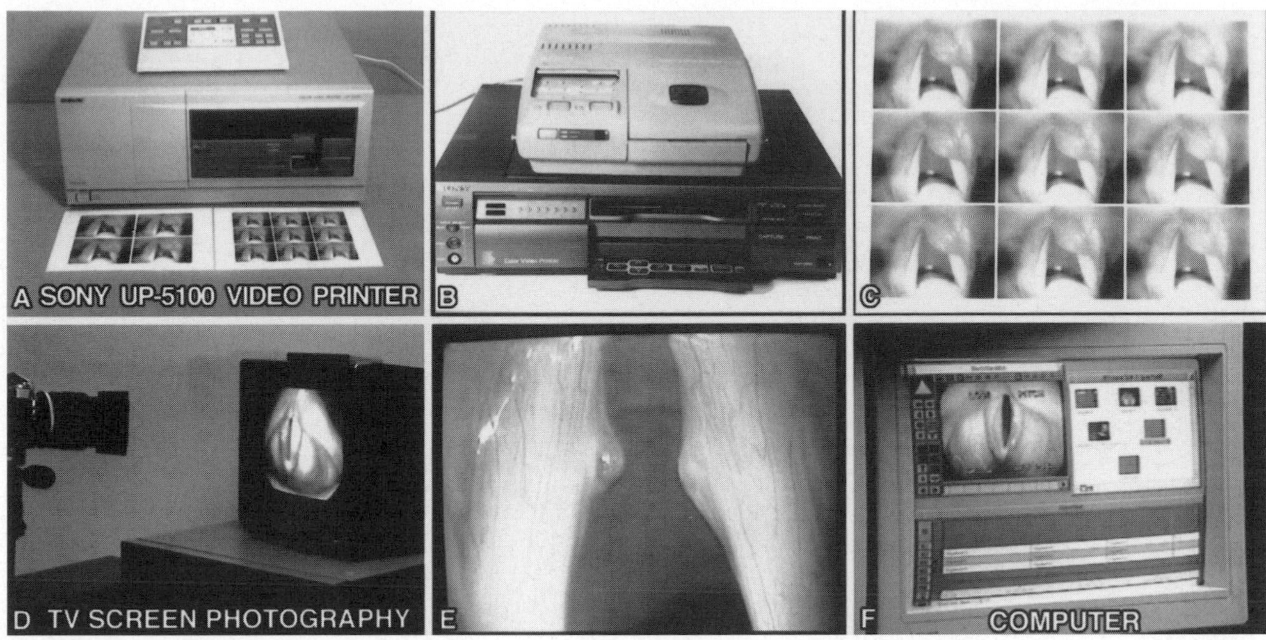

Figure 7.2 *Equipment. (a) Sony UP-5100 video color printer. (b) Top, Sony CVP M3; bottom, Sony CVP-G 700 color video printer. (c) Multiple image video prints made by Sony UP-5100. (d) TV monitor screen photography setup. (e) Slide image of laryngeal nodules by TV screen photography. (f) Computer used for digital imaging.*

Video adapters

Most modern endoscopic cameras have built-in video adapters, so that endoscopes can be connected directly. Examples of such cameras include the single-chip Supercam (Karl Storz), Telecam (Karl Storz) (Fig 7.1d), DX-cam (Karl Storz) and Wolf Endocam as well as the three-chip CCD Stryker 782 (Fig 7.1d) and Karl Storz Tricam (Fig 7.1d). The miniature CCD cameras such as Elmo MN401 and Panasonic GP KS152 may require a C-mount adapter to connect to the endoscope. Certain zoom lens adapters (Karl Storz and Nagashima) or brand specific fixed focus adapters may be used. The Karl Storz quick-connect video adapter is used to connect home video cameras to endoscopes.[47,60,61]

Light sources

The xenon cold light source is recommended for both fiberscopic and telescopic videolaryngoscopy. Popular xenon light sources include Karl Storz 610 and 615 (Fig 7.1e). The newer endoscopic cameras are very light sensitive so that excellent images can be obtained even with standard halogen light sources for telescopic videolaryngoscopy (Fig 7.1e). Fiberscopic videolaryngoscopy, however, often requires the xenon light source. Standard illuminators include the Pilling 2X Luminator, Olympus ILK-3, Machida LH-150 and Karl Storz 481C.

Video recorders

There are several video recording formats available: 3/4 inch (U-matic) (Fig 7.1g), 1/2 inch (VHS, SVHS, Betacam SP), 8 mm (Hi-8) and digital (Fig 7.1f). The 3/4 inch format records excellent images but is bulky for storage. The Betacam SP system produces high quality images but is costly. The 1/2 inch Super VHS (S-VHS) (Fig 7.1h) or the 8 mm Hi-8 formats, high-performance versions of the standard formats (i.e. VHS and 8 mm, respectively) may be more practical for people setting up new systems. These newer formats produce excellent images, and are compact and affordable. Although the standard tapes (VHS or 8 mm) can be played on the high performance players (S-VHS or Hi-8, respectively), the high performance tapes do not play well on the standard players. Digital video systems are impractical at this time due to their high cost. The author uses the 3/4 inch Sony VO-5600 and VO-9600 video recorders (Fig 7.1g).

There are also analog recorders often used by orthopedic colleagues that record still video images directly to a floppy disk. These images can be printed with a video printer. They do not record motion. Examples of these digital still video image recorders include the Panasonic Video Floppy Recorder AG810 and the Sony Still Video Recorder MVR5300.

Video monitors

There are many brands of excellent color video monitors available. High-resolution monitors are recommended, such as Sony Trinitron PVM 1343 MD (Fig 7.1i).

Video printers

High-quality pictures can be obtained from video images instantaneously using a color video printer.

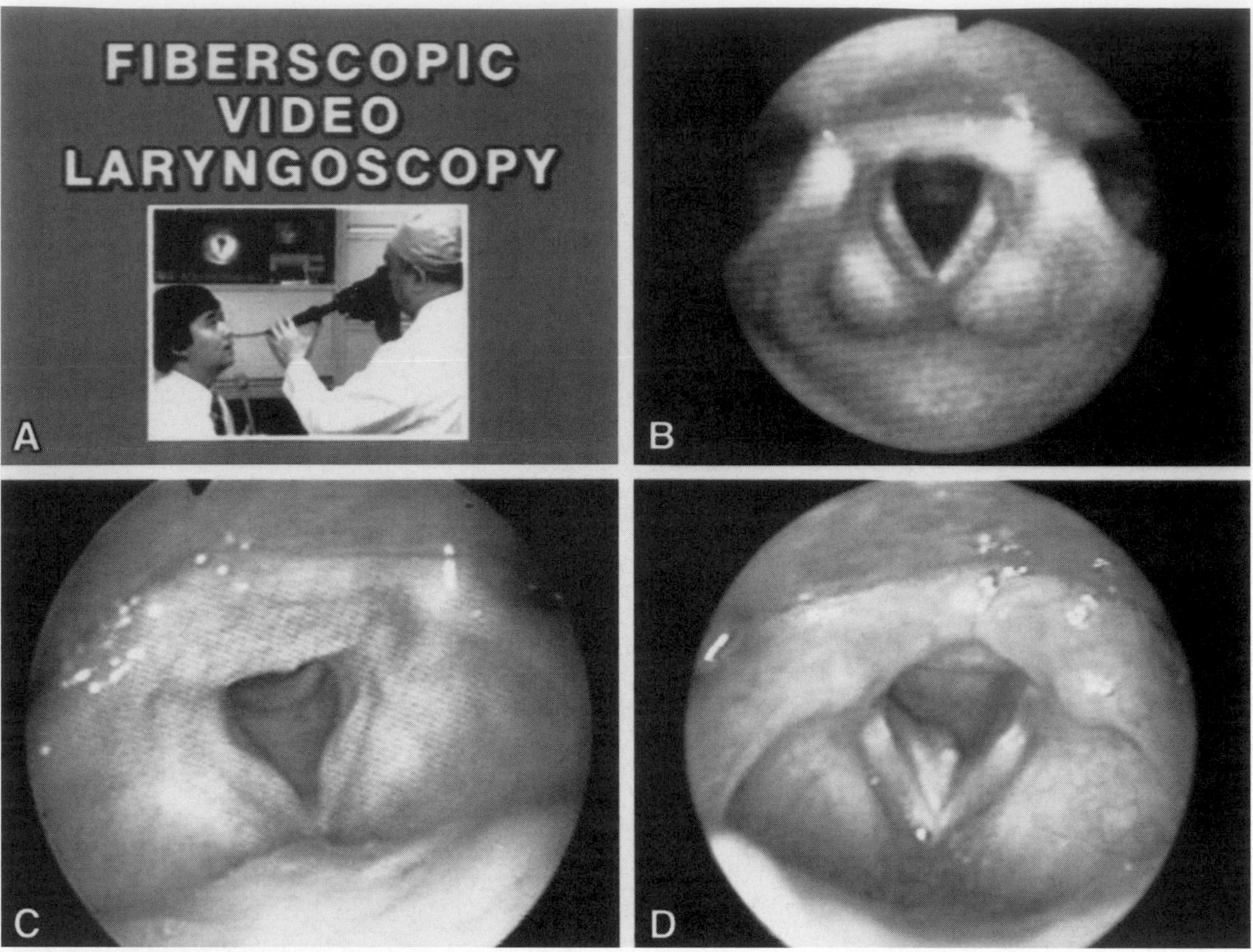

Figure 7.3 *Fiberscopic videolaryngoscopy. (a) Technique. (b) Fiberscopic image of normal larynx. (c) Fiberscopic image of polypoid vocal fold. (d) Fiberscopic image of subglottic lesion.*

Most of these printers allow for color and contrast adjustment before the print is made, and they provide the option of single or multiple images on one print (Fig 7.2a–c). Prints can be made at the time of the examination for medical records, for referring physicians, or for students and patients. Prints can also be made during review of the videotape. The author has used the Sony UP-5000, -5100 and -5600 (Fig 7.2a) and the more affordable Sony CVP-G700 and CVP M3 color video printers (Fig 7.2b).

Videolaryngoscopy in the office

Flexible fiberscopic videolaryngoscopy

Fiberscopic videolaryngoscopy is the most popular technique for video documentation of the larynx because it is the easiest and best tolerated technique and because it allows a full endoscopic examination of the upper aerodigestive tract with one pass (Fig 7.3a,b). It is of great value in evaluating and documenting the functions and pathology of the larynx, permitting simultaneous recording of natural undistorted speech.

The author currently uses the Olympus ENF-P3 (3.4 mm) and ENF-L3 (4.4 mm) fiberscopes attached to a lightweight three-chip CCD camera with a xenon light source for optimal images. Topical anesthetic (4% lidocaine) and decongestant (3% ephedrine) are applied to the wider nasal cavity. With the patient in an upright sitting position, the fiberscope is passed along the nasal floor, through the velopharyngeal port, down to the oropharynx. When the desired image is seen on the monitor, illumination and focus are optimized and recording begins. A panoramic view of the larynx is obtained. The scope is advanced to the vallecula, then over the epiglottis into the laryngeal vestibule (Fig 7.3b). Close-up views of the glottis, true vocal folds, and vestibule and sometimes even subglottis can be obtained as well as views of any lesions (Fig 7.3c,d). If the moiré effect (unwanted color strips) is noted on the monitor, turn the camera relative to the endoscope. Video prints may be captured at any point and instantly printed or else captured from video replay.[61]

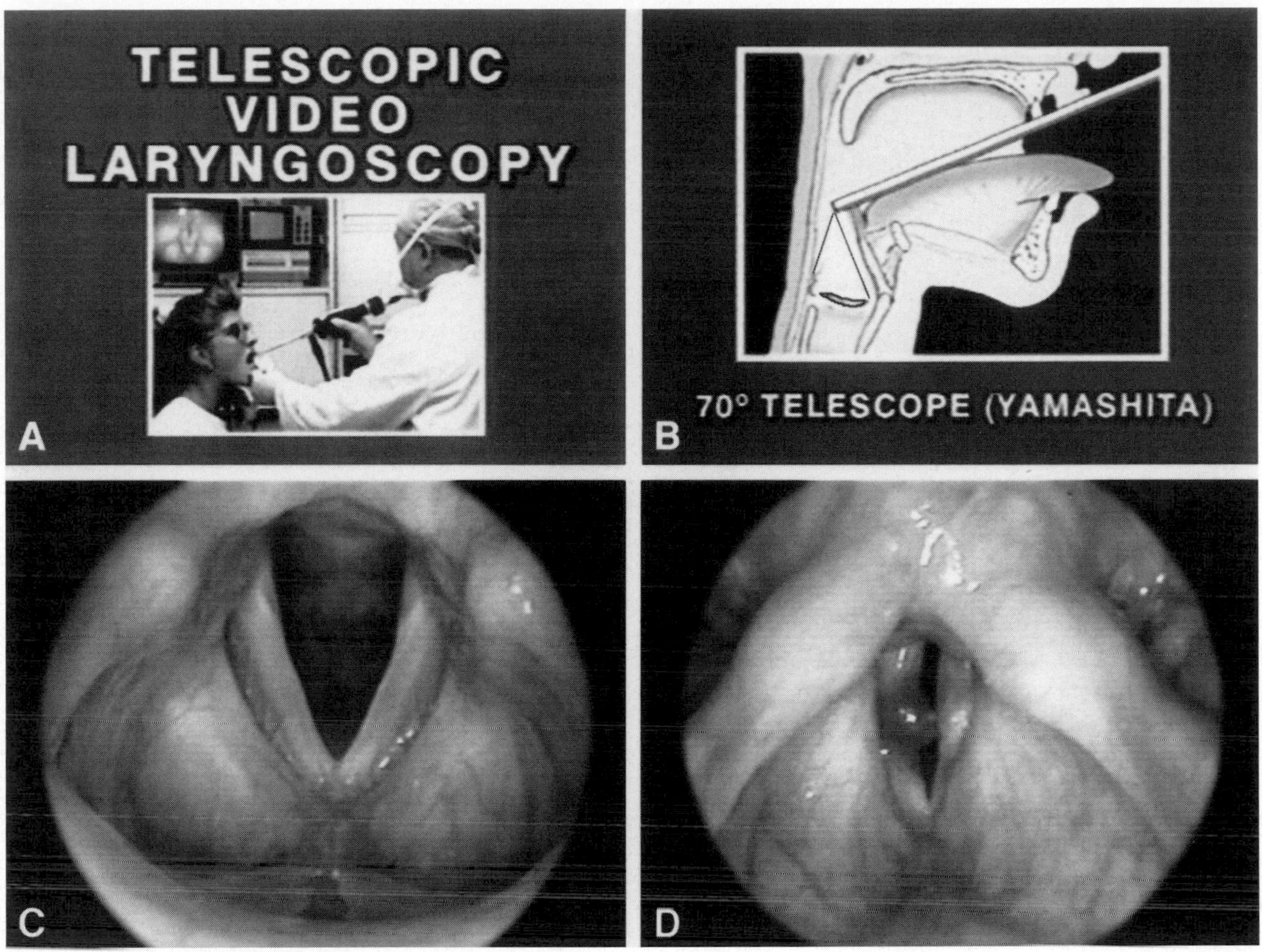

Figure 7.4 *Telescopic videolaryngoscopy. (a) Technique. (b) 70° Telescope. (c) Telescopic image of normal larynx taken by a 70° telescope. (d) Telescopic image of laryngeal polyp taken by a 70° telescope.*

Rigid telescopic videolaryngoscopy

Telescopic videolaryngoscopy with a rigid telescope is an effective method of documenting the normal physiology and pathology of the larynx, although normal undisturbed voice cannot be recorded simultaneously (Fig 7.4a–d). This is the best technique for obtaining the clearest, largest, brightest video images of the larynx. The serious laryngeal endoscopist favors this technique.

Patient preparation is important: sitting upright, good oropharyngeal topical anesthesia, and a monitor in the examiner's and patient's views. The 70° or 90° telescope is attached to a lightweight three-chip CCD camera with a xenon light source for optimal images. The telescope is dipped in hot water to prevent fogging. While the tongue is retracted with a gauze in the left hand, the telescope is carefully placed in the oropharynx and directed to the larynx (Fig 7.4a). When the desired image is seen, the illumination and focus are optimized and recording begins.

The 90° telescope provides a panoramic view of the larynx from the oropharynx; however, it tends to place the larynx more posteriorly, showing more of the base of the tongue. The 70° telescope, on the other hand, provides a closer view of the larynx as it can be angled downward to bring the lens closer to the larynx, to enlarge the image and to display both the anterior and posterior commissures (Fig 7.4a–d). The 70° scope (Fig 7.1b) is particularly useful for stroboscopic videolaryngoscopy, where the largest, clearest image is necessary. It also provides the best images of pathologic lesions. The 70° telescopes are the author's choice. Just as with fiberscopic videolaryngoscopy, video prints may be captured during the examination or later during review.[61]

Microscopic videolaryngoscopy

Microscopic videolaryngoscopy can be accomplished by using a laryngeal mirror and an operating microscope (Zeiss) to which a lightweight, miniature CCD video camera is attached. To obtain satisfactory video images of the larynx in the office is difficult and time consuming. The author has abandoned this technique in favor of fiberscopic and telescopic videolaryngoscopy.[61]

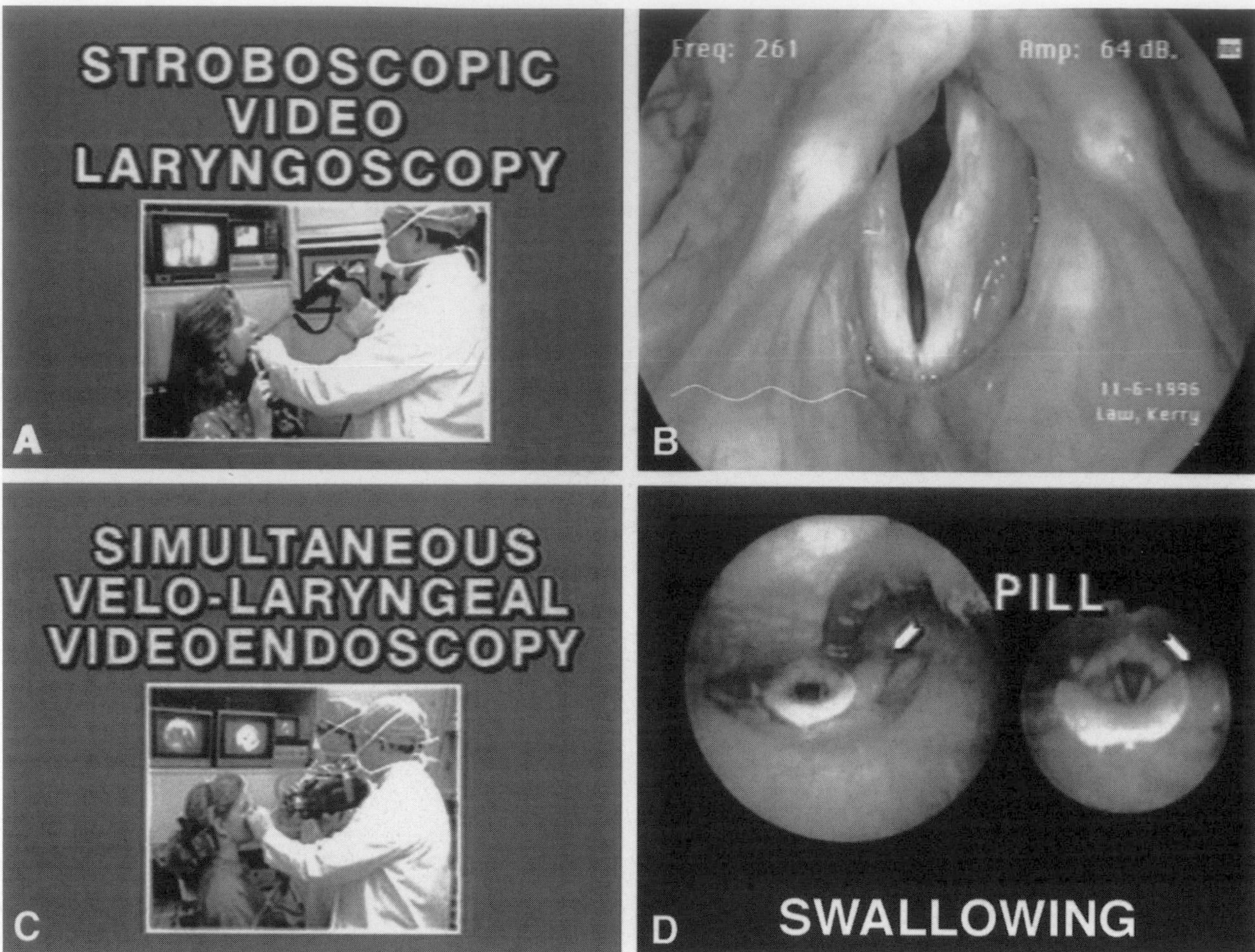

Figure 7.5 *Stroboscopic videolaryngoscopy and simultaneous velolaryngeal videoendoscopy. (a) Technique of stroboscopic telescopic videolaryngoscopy. (b) Stroboscopic view of laryngeal cyst by 70° telescope. (c) Technique of simultaneous velolaryngeal videoendoscopy. (d) Simultaneous transnasal telescopic and transnasal fiberscopic views of swallowing of a pill.*

Stroboscopic videolaryngoscopy

Stroboscopic videolaryngoscopy uses a strobe light source, timed with the true vocal fold (TVF) modal frequency, to provide a composite motion image of the TVF mucosal wave (Fig 7.5a,b).[15,23,41,50,55] This technique provides the most detailed information about TVF physiology and pathology (Fig 7.5b). As with regular videolaryngoscopy, this technique can be performed with a flexible fiberscope or a rigid 70° telescope. The fiberscope allows for very close-up views of the TVFs, but suffers from optical distortion due to the wide-angle lens and from the disruptive moiré effect. The best images are produced with the 70° telescope that allows large, bright, clear close-up images of the TVFs. The Nagashima SFT-1, Karl Storz 8706CJ and Kay 9105 are all excellent 70° rigid strobotelescopes (Fig 7.1b). Popular stroboscopy units in the USA are the Kay Elemetrics Rhino-Laryngeal Stroboscope 9100 and the Nagashima Laryngostroboscope LS-3A.[61]

Detailed discussion on stroboscopic videolaryngoscopy is found elsewhere in this book.

Simultaneous velolaryngeal videoendoscopy

Simultaneous velolaryngeal videoendoscopy is the simultaneous examination of the velum palatine (soft palate) via rigid transnasal videonasopharyngoscopy and the larynx via transnasal fiberscopic videolaryngoscopy (Fig 7.5c,d).[59] Both examinations are video- and audio-recorded in order to study the coordinated movements and positioning of the larynx and soft palate during respiration, phonation, swallowing (Fig 7.5d), coughing, straining, singing, and during other routine laryngeal functions.

The equipment used for this dual endoscopic examination include:

- flexible fiberscope (Olympus ENF-P3);
- Hopkins 4.0 mm 18 cm long, 70° rigid nasal telescope (Karl Storz 7200C);
- xenon light source;
- two video cameras;
- two video monitors;
- two video recorders;

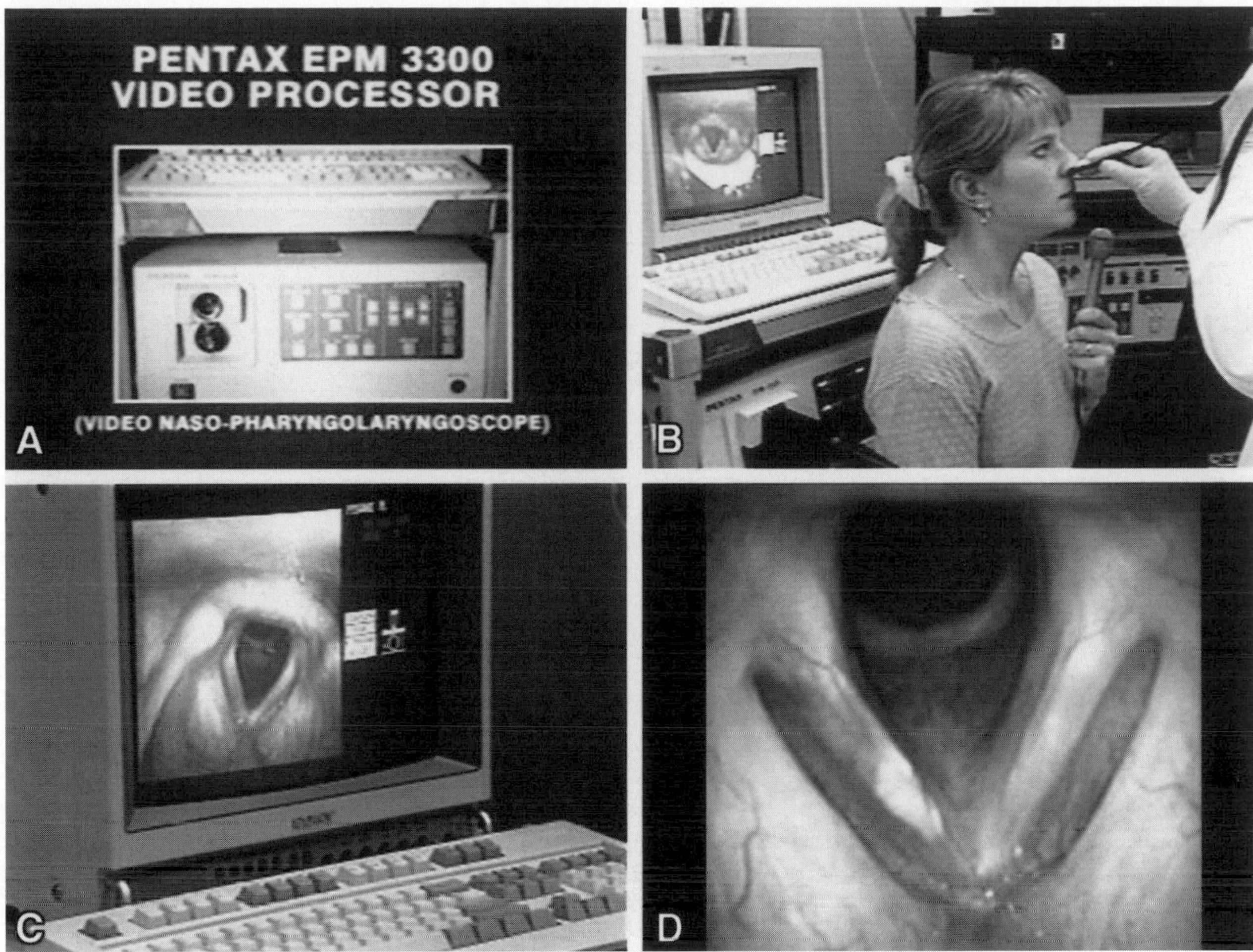

Figure 7.6 *Pentax videoendoscopic laryngoscopy. (a) Pentax EPM 3300 video processor. (b) Technique of videoendoscopic laryngoscopy using Pentax EPM 3300 videoendoscope. (c) Normal larynx shown on a monitor by digital imaging. (d) Close-up view of larynx with leukoplakia taken with Pentax system.*

- microphone;
- video printer; and
- nasal topical anesthetic and decongestant.

These examinations are best appreciated on motion video with real-time audio. Still videoprints, however, do demonstrate many of the important findings during these examinations.[61]

Pentax videoendoscopic digital imaging

Pentax videoendoscopic digital imaging system consists of:

- Pentax EPM 3300 video processor (Fig 7.6a);
- Pentax flexible video endoscope (Fig 7.1b);
- PC computer; and
- display monitor (Fig 7.6c).

This highly integrated system was primarily developed for the evaluation and documentation of gastrointestinal disorders. More recently it has been used for evaluation of the larynx (Fig 7.6d), utilizing a specifically designed shorter flexible video-naso-pharyngo-laryngoscope (VNL 1330 or 1530) (Fig 7.1c). The insertion tube diameter is 4.9 mm for VNL 1530 and 4.1 mm for VNL 1330. The examining technique is almost the same as for fiberscopic videolaryngoscopy (Fig 7.6b). Advantages include: no capture delay time, high telescopic quality pictures (Fig 7.6c), quick boot-up, ease of use, and images can be annotated and manipulated. The main disadvantages are high cost and physical size.[61]

Videolaryngoscopy in the operating room

Rigid telescopic videolaryngoscopy

Equipment required for telescopic videolaryngoscopy include:

- direct laryngoscope (Dedo/Ossoff);
- rigid Hopkins 5.0 mm, 24 cm long, 0°, 30°, 70° and

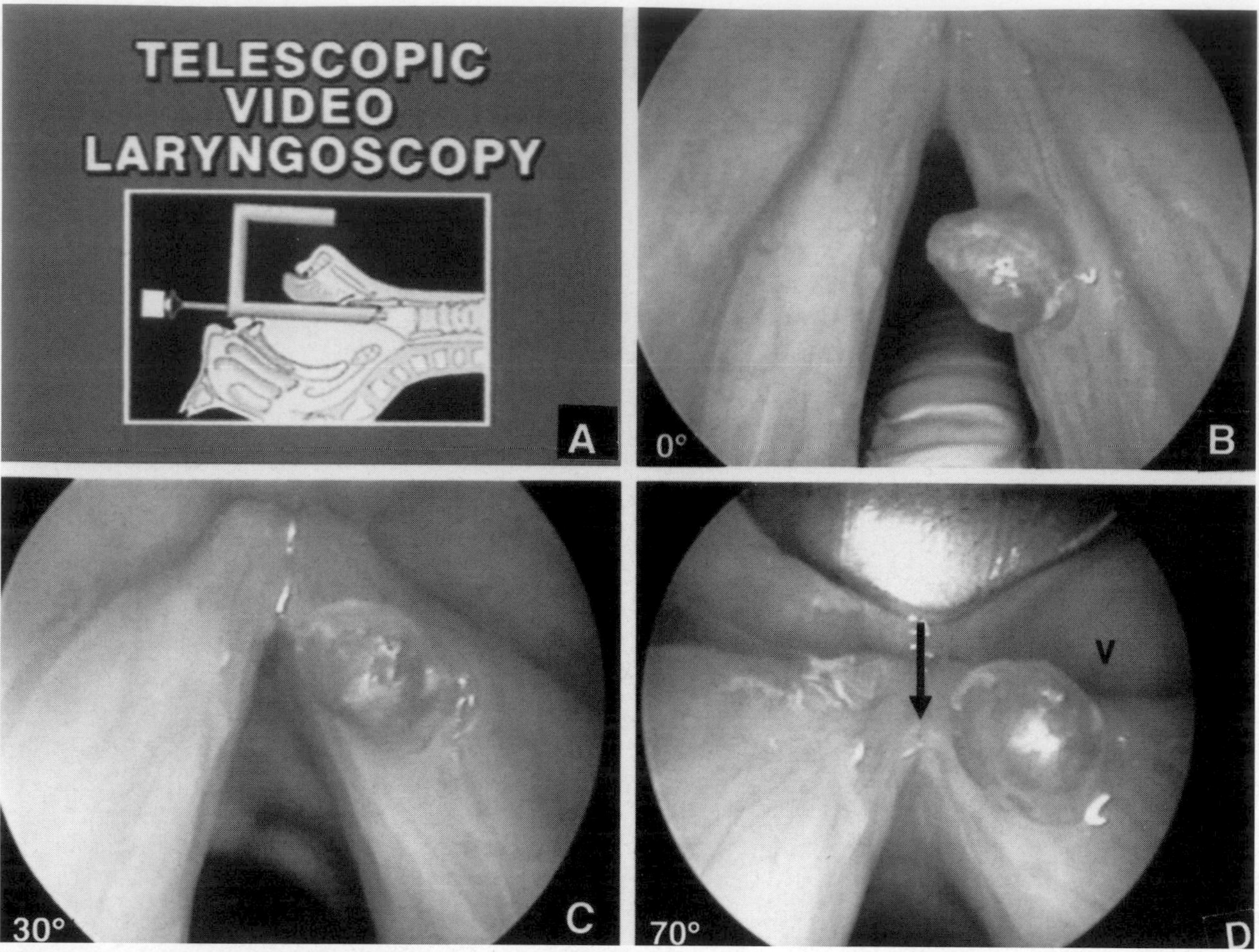

Figure 7.7 *Telescopic videolaryngoscopy. (a) Technique. (b) 0° View of a laryngeal polyp in the anterior portion of the left vocal fold. (c) The same polyp with a 30° telescope. (d) The same polyp with a 70° telescope. Note well visualized anterior commissure (arrow) and ventricle (V).*

120° endoscopes (Karl Storz 8712AA, BA, CA and DA, respectively);
- xenon light source; and
- laryngoscope suspension system.

The patient is placed under general anesthesia and intubated. Then the larynx and hypopharynx are examined as the direct laryngoscope is passed to just above the true vocal folds and suspended. A rigid telescope is passed through the laryngoscope to view and videorecord the anatomic structures and pathologic conditions of the larynx (Fig 7.7a–d).[4,50,55,56] The author primarily uses the 0° telescope for all patients undergoing microlaryngoscopy but in selected patients with laryngeal pathology of documentation value, uses 30°, 70°, 120° telescopes as recommended by Andrea and Dias.[2] The findings are videoprinted and videotaped for later review. Telescopic videolaryngoscopy while the patient is undergoing microlaryngeal surgery under general anesthesia is an excellent method of examining and documenting laryngeal anatomy and pathology. Telescopy with angled telescopes are of particular value in documenting lesions of anterior commissure, ventricles and undersurface of the vocal fold (Fig 7.7b–d).[3,50]

Kantor–Berci telescopic videomicrolaryngoscopy

Kantor, Berci *et al.*[22] introduced a new approach to microlaryngeal surgery and its documentation. Their method is akin to performing endoscopic sinus surgery using a video camera and a video monitor. Using a specially designed microlaryngoscope that houses a rigid telescope with attached camera (Fig 7.8a–c), they are able to both videorecord and perform the operation while viewing a high-resolution screen (Fig 7.8a). The required equipment includes:

- a Kantor–Berci videomicrolaryngoscope (Karl Storz 8590VJ) (Fig 7.8b) and laryngoscope suspension holder;
- a Karl Storz Supercam micro CCD video camera;
- a xenon light source (Karl Storz 615);
- a large, high-resolution TV monitor and recorder; and
- a color video printer (Sony UP-5000).

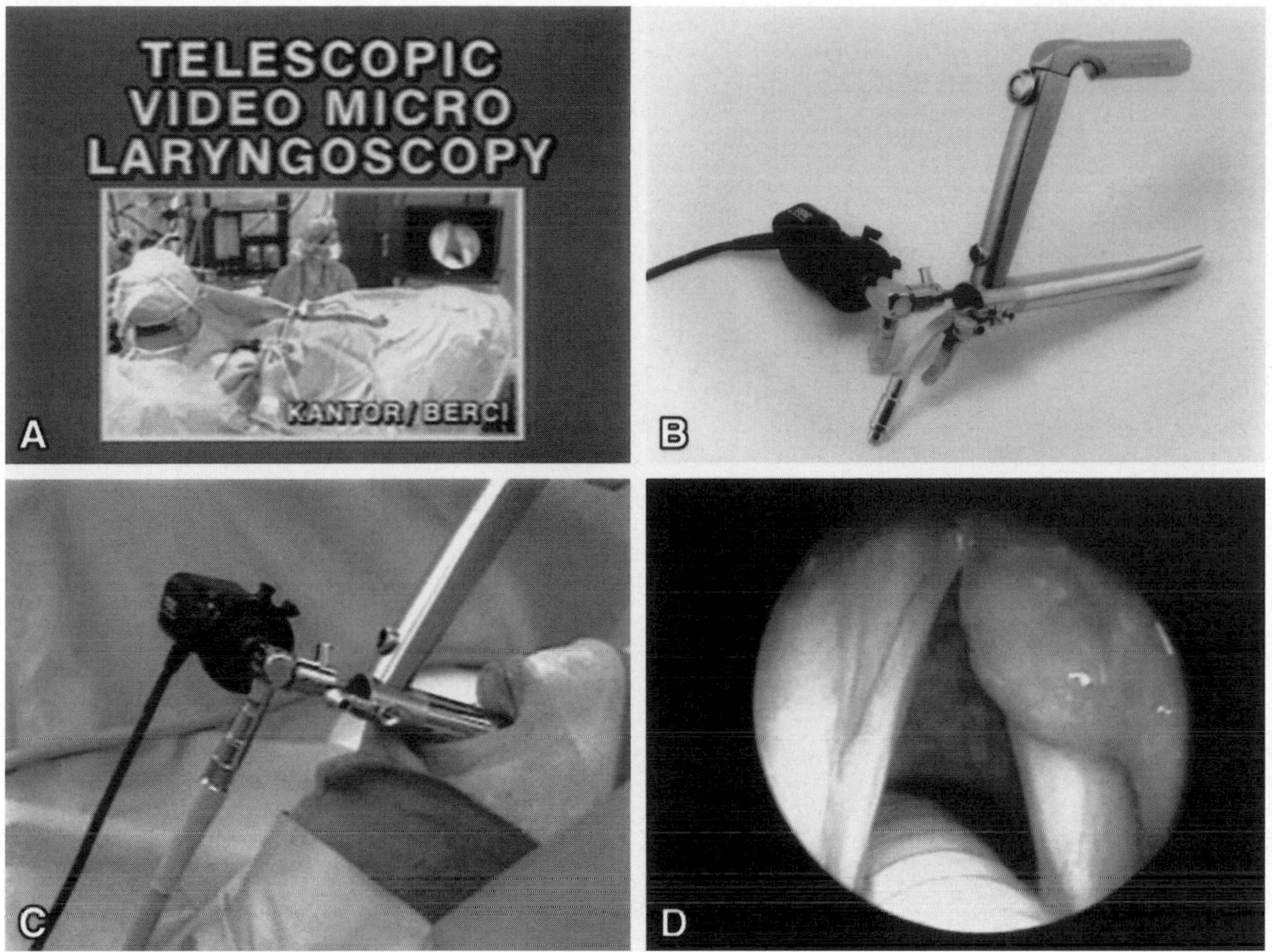

Figure 7.8 *(a) Telescopic videomicrolaryngoscopy (Kantor–Berci technique). (b) The original Kantor–Berci videomicrolaryngoscope to which a miniature CCD camera is attached. The telescope is housed in the left side of the laryngoscope. (c) The same scope positioned in the patient's larynx. (d) A large polyp arising from the anterior portion of the right false fold using this system.*

Some of the advantages of the Kantor–Berci system include the following:

- it gives a clear, sharp image with excellent depth of field (Fig 7.8d);
- it facilitates instrumentation of the larynx since the microscope is not between the surgeon and patient; and
- it provides superior documentation.

Some disadvantages are that:

- the equipment is costly;
- specialized equipment, such as the angled forceps, is needed;
- it requires a dedicated video camera;
- there is some image distortion; and
- at present no pediatric laryngoscope is available.

A newer improved Kantor–Berci microvideolaryngoscope is now available which eliminates some of the above-mentioned disadvantages.

Microscopic videolaryngoscopy

Microscopic videolaryngoscopy with the operating microscope and a color video camera remains the single most convenient and effective method to teach and document microsurgery of the larynx (Fig 7.9a–d). This is the author's preferred method of operative documentation.[61] Equipment needed includes:

- a photographic laryngoscope such as the Dedo or Ossoff (these laryngoscopes have two channels that house large-bore fiberoptic cables);
- a light source, such as the Pilling 2X;
- the Zeiss operating microscope with a straight eyepiece and 400 mm objective lens;
- a beam splitter;
- a photoadapter, such as the Zeiss or Telestill photoadapter;
- a miniature camera or pickup tube camera (Figs 7.9a, 7.13c);
- a videorecorder; and
- a color TV monitor.

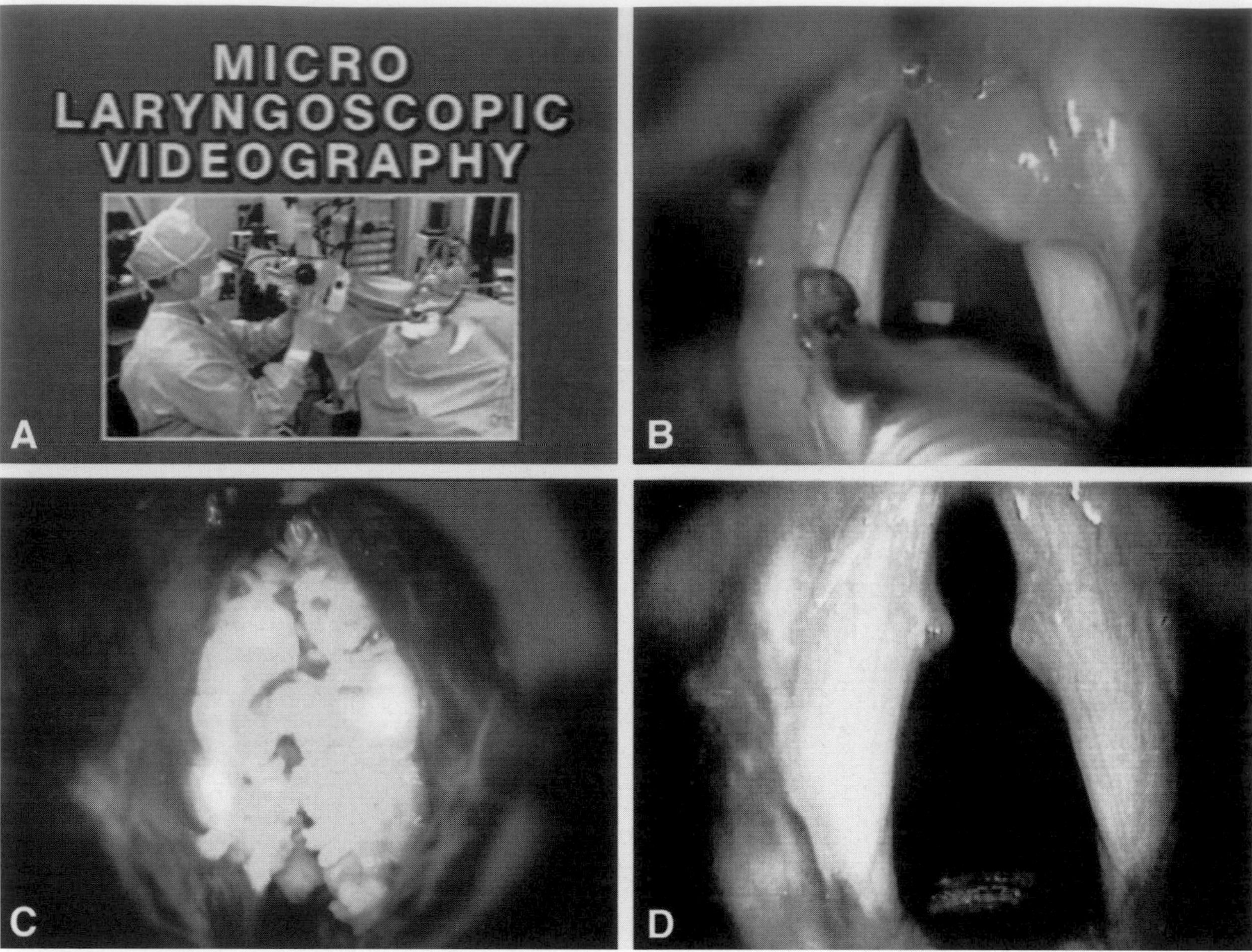

Figure 7.9 *Microscopic videolaryngoscopy. (a) Technique. (b) Microlaryngoscopic images of a large polyp arising from the anterior portion of the right false fold. (c) Microlaryngoscopic view of extensive verrucous carcinoma arising from both vocal folds. (d) Microlaryngoscopic view of vocal fold laryngeal nodules.*

With the small size and weight, the miniature single chip CCD cameras interfere minimally with the operative procedure. For those who seek the highest quality images, the three-chip CCD cameras, such as Sony DXC 960MD or Stryker 782, are recommended.

Some advantages of this system are:

- minimal interference with the operative procedure;
- live viewing by an unlimited audience;
- equipment that is readily available in most medical centers;
- variability of magnification, facilitating precise documentation of small lesions;
- video documentation for teaching surgical techniques; and
- the capability of producing instant color prints with a color video printer.

Among the disadvantages are:

- the depth of field is shallower;
- instrumentation may be difficult;
- at times surgery must be carried out through one eyepiece because of the small proximal opening of the laryngoscope; and
- refocusing at various magnifications may be necessary.

Contact videolaryngoscopy

Andrea *et al.*[3] described an innovative technique in which a microcolpohysteroscope was placed in contact with the vocal fold which had been stained with 1% methylene blue dye (Fig 7.10a,b). Video images permit endoscopic visualization of normal and pathologic vocal fold epithelium *in vivo*. The cell structures normally only seen under the microscope – epithelial layer, nucleus, nucleolus, mitoses, cytoplasmic inclusions, nucleus–cytoplasm ratio, etc. – can be seen through the endoscope. Submucosal microvasculatures and circulating red blood cells can also be seen (Fig 7.10b). Different and specific cellular epithelial patterns can be identified in different disorders of the vocal fold such as chronic laryngitis, keratosis, dysplasia,

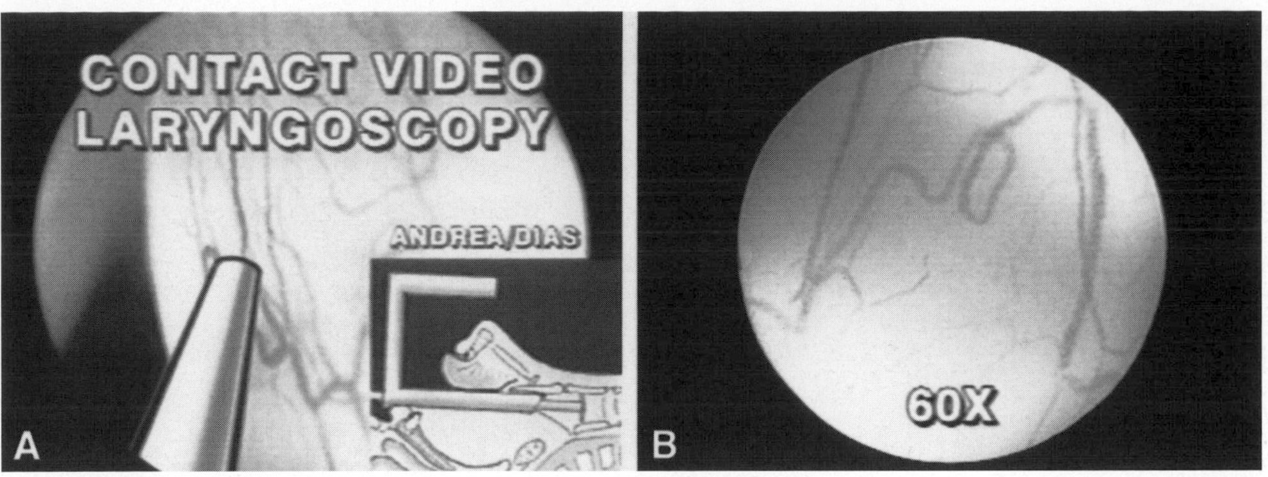

Figure 7.10 *Contact videolaryngoscopy. (a) Technique. (b) Submucosal microvasculature seen with this technique.*

papilloma and malignant tumor. More accurate determinations of cancer margins may be possible with this technique, and would allow for more precise ablation of these lesions.

Detailed discussion of contact videolaryngoscopy is found elsewhere in this book.

Laryngeal photography

Laryngeal still photography in the office

Still photography has been the traditional method of documentation of laryngeal photography. There are numerous methods of still photography of the larynx. Many of these methods will provide high-quality color slides for publication or presentation. The basic equipment is a 35 mm SLR camera (Fig 7.11) combined with a light source and a means of visualizing the larynx, such as the laryngeal mirror, laryngoscope, flexible fiberscope, rigid telescope or the operating microscope (Fig 7.12). Laryngeal photography has recently been made even easier with the use of the newer 35 mm SLR cameras with built-in autowinder combined with the TTL (through the lens) electronic flash system.

Fiberscopic still photography

Although this technique produces a grainy image that is inferior in resolution to that of the telescope, there are distinct advantages to its use. Full functional examination of the larynx can be accomplished with one insertion, even in difficult patients in whom other techniques of laryngeal examination would be difficult or impossible, for example, small children, immobilized adults, and

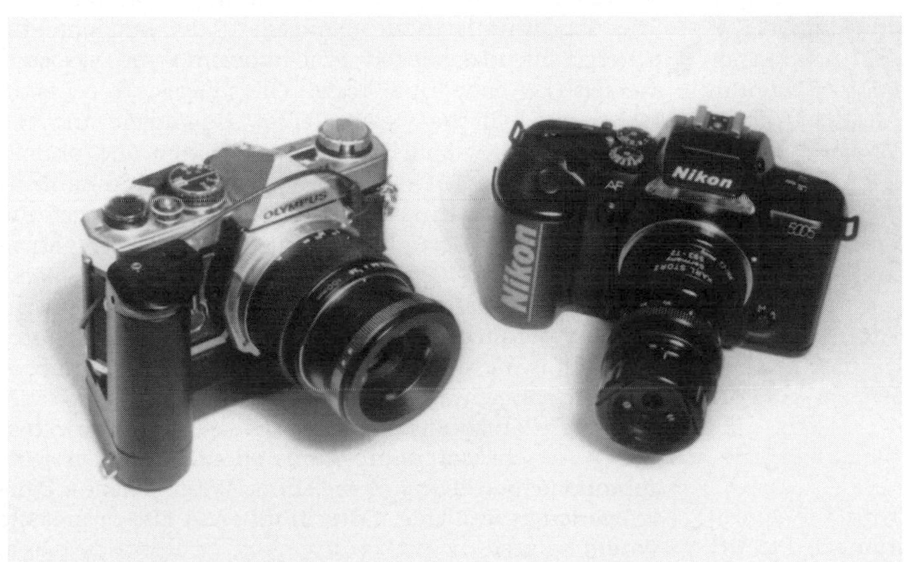

Figure 7.11 *Single lens reflex camera: left, Olympus OM2 camera with 50 mm macrolens and automatic film winder; right, Nikon N5005 camera with Karl Storz 35–140 mm zoom lens adapter, a built-in film advance system.*

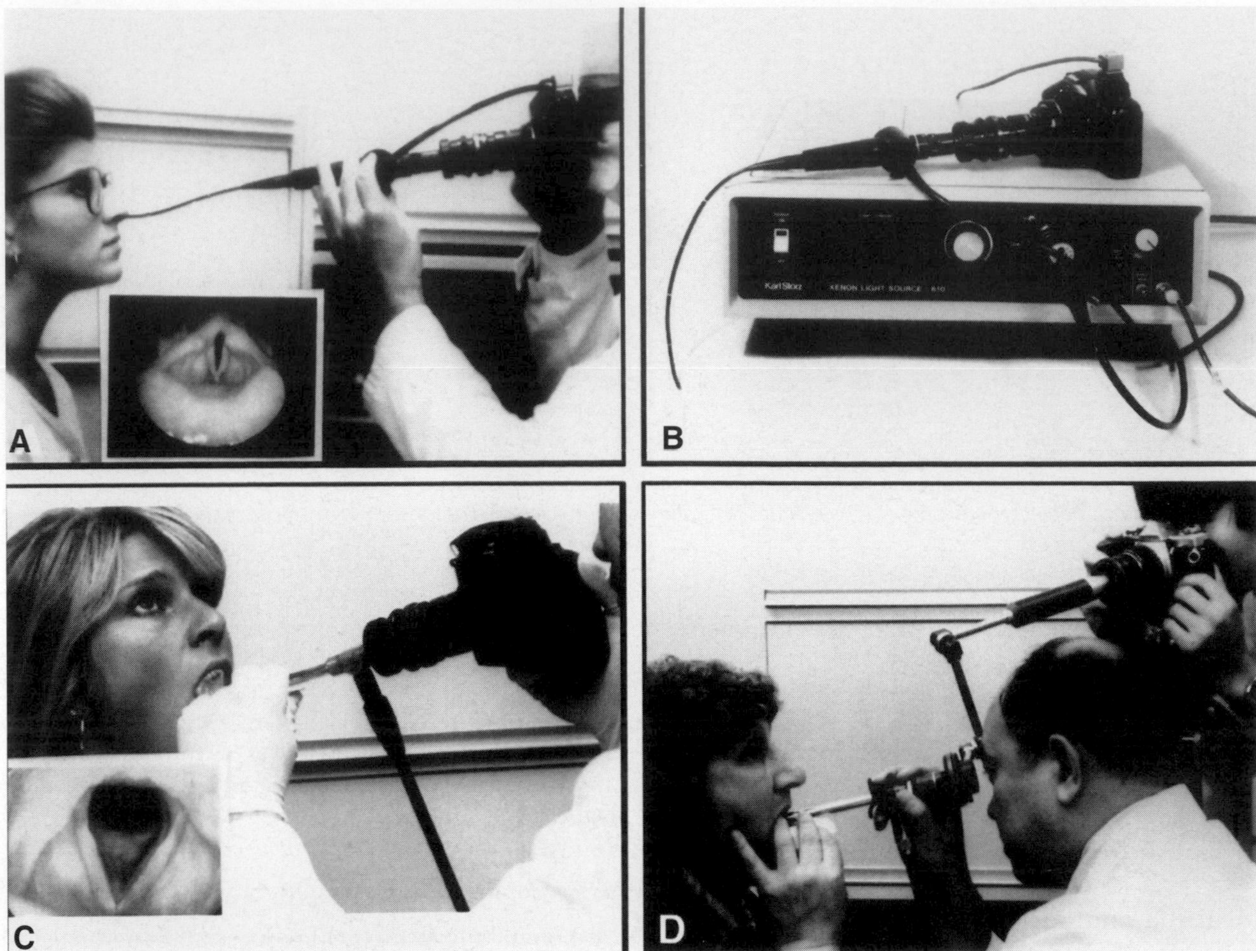

Figure 7.12 *Laryngeal still photography in the office. (a) Fiberscopic still photography. (b) Equipment for fiberscopic electronic flash still photography with Karl Storz 610 light source. (c) Telescopic still photography. (d) Telescopic still photography using Wittmoser articulated optical arm attached to the SLR camera.*

those with a hypersensitive gag or unusual supraglottic anatomy that makes visualization of the anterior larynx difficult with the telescope.[60]

This technique can be accomplished with a number of flexible scopes such as the Olympus ENF-P2 (3.4 mm) or P3 (3.6 mm). Machida 4L (4.0 mm) or 3L (3.3 mm), Pentax FNL l0S (3.5 mm), or Olympus ENF L (4.4 mm).

Equipment for photodocumentation of the author's technique consists of:

- the Olympus OM2 35 mm SLR camera with an autowinder, clear-glass focusing screen 1–9, and 2X teleconverter;
- Olympus ENF P3 or L3 fiberscope;
- Olympus SMR endoscopic coupler;
- Karl Storz xenon cold light source 610, or 615 (Fig 7.1e); and
- Ektachrome ASA 400 or 800 daylight film.

The camera is set on automatic mode with the appropriate ASA setting. The flexible scope is connected to the 2X teleconverter, which is attached to the SLR camera using either the SMR endoscopic coupler or the 100 mm macrolens with the Karl Storz quick-connect adapter. The fiberscope is then advanced to the hypopharynx through an anesthetized (4% lidocaine) and vasoconstricted (3% ephedrine) nose. The images are centered and focused in the viewfinder of the camera and the larynx is photographed during inspiration and phonation (Fig 7.12a). The clearest pictures are taken immediately after phonating 'ee'. It should be noted that the laryngeal image occupies a small portion of the photographic field and much of what the camera sees is blackened out. This situation will cause the metering system in most automatic cameras to overexpose the photograph, thus washing out the laryngeal image. To prevent this, the compensation dial of the camera should be set at –1 or –2 to underexpose the image by one or two *f*-stops. A series of photographs should be taken with appropriate bracketing of the shots. When a xenon light source is not available, faster films (ASA 800 or greater) should be used.

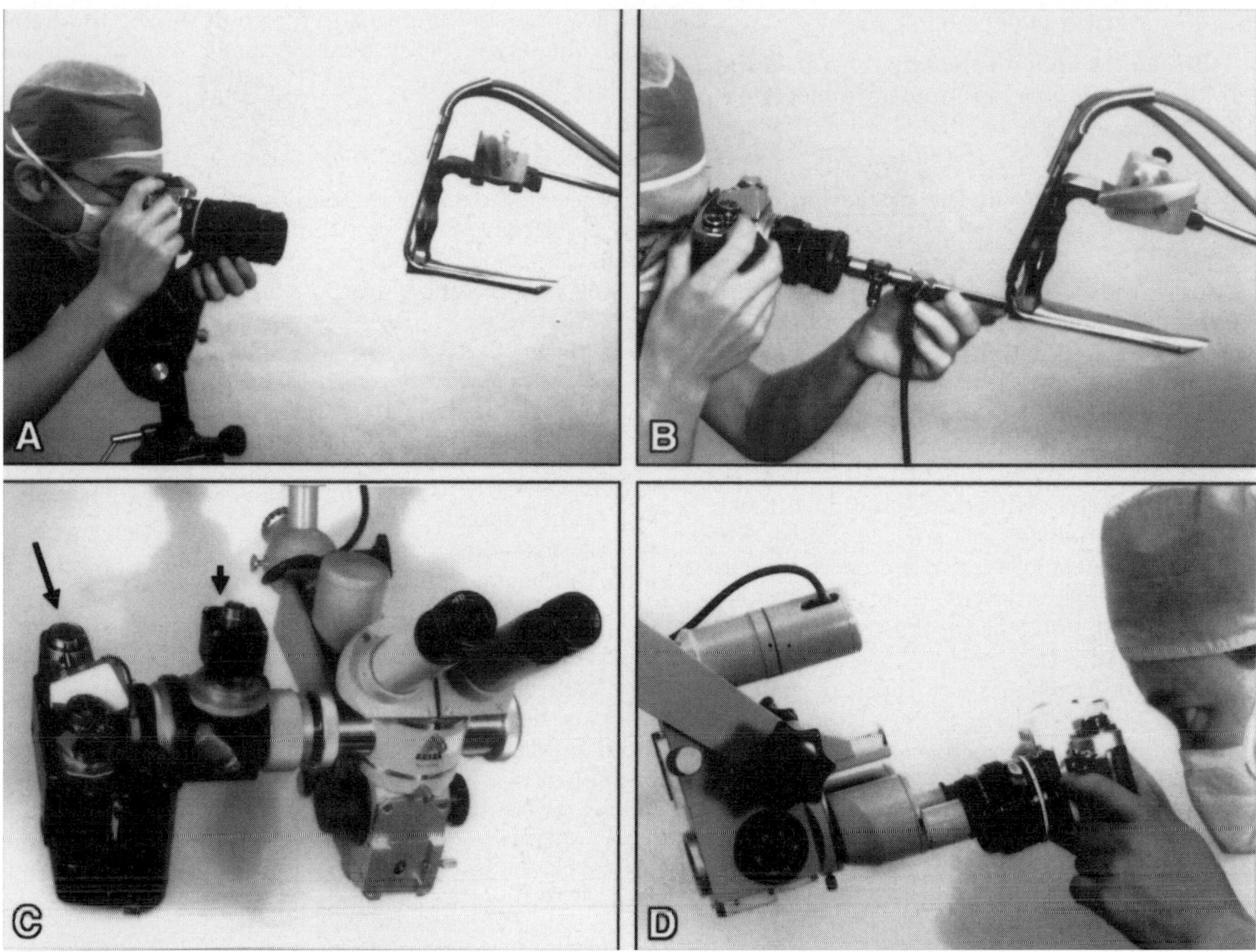

Figure 7.13 *Laryngeal still photography in the operating room. (a) Direct laryngeal still photography. (b) Telescopic still photography. (c) Microscopic still photography with SLR camera (long arrow). Note also a miniature CCD video camera on the photoadapter. (d) Microscopic still photography using a SLR camera with the macrolens placed on an eye piece of the microscope.*

More recently, the author has employed the TTL endoscopic flash photography technique as recommended by Karl Storz (Fig 7.12b). This technique uses the Nikon 5005 camera which is set to manual at a shutter speed of 1/30 second, and any aperture setting except aperture setting 'S'. The Karl Storz 610 light source is set at auto TTL and attached to the camera with a 570MN connection cord. The fiberscope is connected to the camera by the Karl Storz 593 T2 lens and the focal length can be set from 30 mm to 140 mm. The author routinely uses 140 mm since it produces a larger image. Using the TTL system obviates the need to underexpose the image or bracket the photographs.

Telescopic still photography

This method provides the clearest laryngeal images available in the office. The equipment used includes:

- the Olympus 35 mm SLR OM2 camera system described for fiberscopic laryngoscopy;
- a 70° telescope, such as KAY 9105, Nagashima SFT-1, Karl Storz 8706CJ;
- a xenon light source (Karl Storz 610, 615C) (Fig 7.1e); and
- ASA 400 or 800 Ektachrome daylight film.

With the soft palate and posterior tongue anesthetized, the patient's tongue is grasped and protruded. The telescope is advanced into the mouth, being careful not to induce gagging by touching the posterior tongue or pharynx (Fig 7.12c). Having the patient vocalize a high-pitched 'ee' will raise and fully expose the larynx in most cases. Pictures can be taken during respiration and phonation. The exposures should be bracketed using the automatic compensation dial. The Wittmoser articulated optical arm can also be used, allowing the examiner to view the larynx while an assistant takes pictures with the SLR camera positioned on a tripod (Fig 7.12d). The success rate with this method is 70–80%. The Karl Storz TTL system as described for the fiberscope can also be used in this setting.

Microscopic still laryngeal photography

Microscopic still photography of the larynx in the office is difficult and results are poor and unpredictable. Hence, the author abandoned the use of this technique.

Laryngeal still photography in the operating room

Direct laryngoscopic still photography

There are two methods of photographing the larynx directly through the laryngoscope. The first utilizes a 100 mm or 200 mm telephoto lens attached to a 35 mm SLR camera on a tripod (Fig 7.13a). Ektachrome Tungsten ASA 160 is used and pushed to 320 during processing. If the Dedo or Ossoff photographic laryngoscope with two large fiberoptic cables is used, no additional light sources are needed. The major difficulty with this technique is that it is cumbersome. Interruption of the operation and readjustment of the camera and tripod are necessary with each new photograph of the larynx. The success rate is about 70–80%. The image obtained with this method may be small but quite satisfactory.

The second method requires an aperture-preferred automatic 35 mm SLR camera such as the Nikon FE or the Olympus OM2 with a 50 mm macrolens attached. If the newer autofocus cameras such as the Nikon 6006 or 8008 are used, manual focusing should be used. This will prevent the camera from focusing on the edge of the laryngoscope. Ektachrome Tungsten ASA 160 film is used and pushed to 320 (or use ASA 320 film from the beginning). For this technique the camera is hand-held, the larynx is focused through the laryngoscope and photographed. The resulting image, although small, is quite recognizable. The photograph may be cropped and enlarged (Fig 7.14a). This is the simplest method of laryngeal photography and is recommended for the occasional laryngeal photographer.

Fiberscopic still photography

This method of still photography is rarely used in the operating room. The technique is the same as that used in the office.

Telescopic still photography

In the operating room, telescopic laryngeal photography is accomplished by passing a telescope, attached to a 35 mm SLR camera and light source, through the laryngoscope and then photographing the larynx (Fig 7.13b).

The setup the author uses includes the Hopkins 0° straightforward telescope 8700A with the Karl Storz 615 xenon light source. The telescope is attached to the Olympus OM2 camera with a 100 mm macrolens, a Karl Storz quick-connect adapter, a 1–9 focusing screen and an autowinder. ASA 400 Ektachrome daylight film is used. This method is highly successful (greater than 90%) and produces excellent pictures of the larynx (Fig 7.14b). The major drawbacks are the expense of the special telescope and adapters, and the need to interrupt surgery to photograph the larynx. The Nikon automatic camera can also be used with the Karl Storz TTL flash system.

Microscopic still photography

Laryngeal photography through the operating microscope can be accomplished with or without the use of a photoadapter (Fig 7.13c,d).[50,55,56,58] High-quality images or varying magnification are possible with this technique (Fig 7.14c,d).

Microscopic photography with the use of a photoadapter
Microscopic photography with the use of a photoadapter requires the following equipment:

- Zeiss operating microscope
- a beam splitter
- a photoadapter
- an automatic 35 mm SLR camera; and
- a ring adapter for the camera.

High-speed Ektachrome Tungsten ASA 160 film is used and pushed to 320 when processed. After the laryngoscope is suspended, the microscope with the attached beam splitter, photoadapter and 35 mm SLR camera are positioned for microlaryngoscopy (Fig 7.13c). Photographs can now be taken at any time. Two major advantages of this technique are that the surgeon is the photographer and that there is minimal disruption of the operation. Other advantages include:

- the ability to photograph at varying magnifications (63, 103, 253 and 403);
- full field image of the larynx at higher magnifications obviates the need for copying and enlarging the slides for presentation; and
- with the use of a Telestill or dual photoadapter, TV and movie documentation is possible.

The disadvantages are:

- the expense of the beam splitter and photoadapter;
- shallow depth of field, especially at high magnification; and
- the need for brilliant illumination, such as that provided by the Dedo or Ossoff (Pilling) photographic laryngoscope.

The success rate is approximately 70%.

Microscopic photography without the use of a photoadapter
This simple, inexpensive means of laryngeal photography known as the 'microscopic macrolens technique'[58] requires only:

- the Zeiss operating microscope;
- an 'aperture-preferred' automatic 35 mm SLR camera, such as the Nikon FE, Pentax ME, Olympus OM2, etc.
- a 50 mm macrolens; and
- the Dedo or Ossoff photographic laryngoscope.

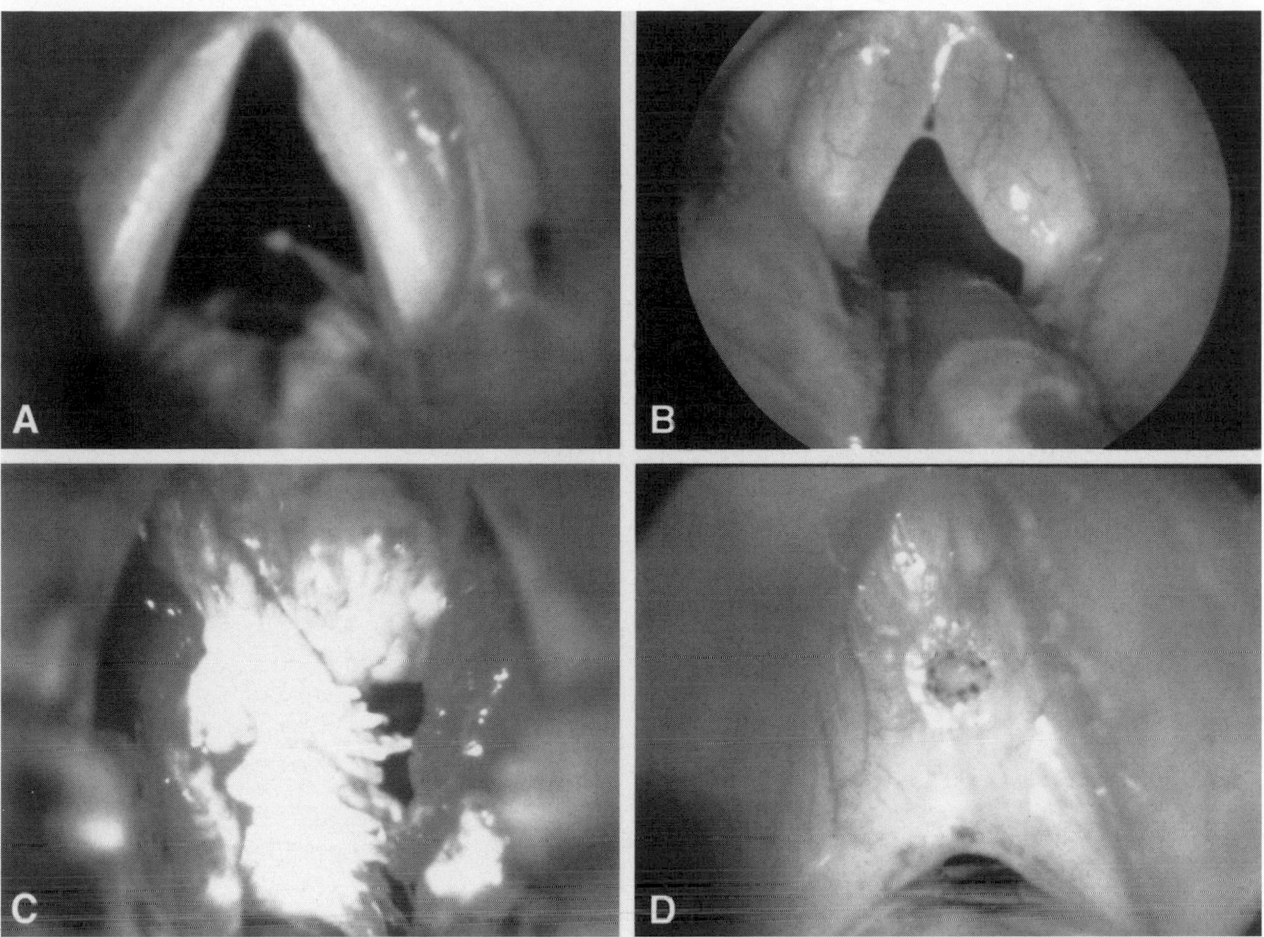

Figure 7.14 *Still photographs taken with different techniques. (a) Picture of laryngeal polyps taken by direct laryngoscopic photography. (b) Marked Reinke's edema taken by telescopic still photography. (c) Verrucous carcinoma taken by microscopic photography using a still camera and a photoadapter. (d) Fusion of both vocal folds taken by microscopic photography using a macrolens on the SLR camera (macrolens technique).*

Ektachrome Tungsten ASA 160 film is used and pushed to 320 (Figs 7.13d, 7.14d).

During microscopic laryngoscopy the larynx is focused through the microscope with the eyepiece set at 0. The microscope is then locked in place. With the camera focused at infinity and the aperture wide open (usually f3.5), the camera is placed on the microscope eyepiece and the laryngeal image centered and brought into sharp focus through the camera (Fig 7.13a). The picture is then taken. Surprisingly good-quality photographs, with a success rate of 70–80%, can be taken with this simple technique (Fig 7.13b). Some disadvantages are that occasionally it may be difficult to hold the camera still on the eyepiece, and it requires interruption of surgery. The ultimate success of this technique depends on illumination, critical focusing, and the stability of the patient, microscope and camera.

Transfer of video images to prints and slides

Video images can be transferred to prints and slides in several ways.

TV monitor photography

This technique is to photograph the desired image on the video monitor using daylight Ektachrome ASA 400 color print or slide film in a standard 35 mm SLR camera equipped with a 50 mm macrolens and an orange-colored filter (Kodak CC40R or Tiffen CC40) (see Fig 7.2d). The camera is placed on the tripod and focused on the video monitor (see Fig 7.2e). The room is darkened to avoid reflection on the monitor. The shutter speed is set at 1/2 second or slower or else there will be streaks across the picture. The exposure is bracketed using the *f*-stop.

Video printer photography

The second technique to transfer video images to print and slides uses a videoprinter (see Fig 7.2a,b). High performance video printers produce excellent pictures, quickly, from video images, The color and contrast can be adjusted before the print is made, and the printer gives the option of single or multiple images on one print. The

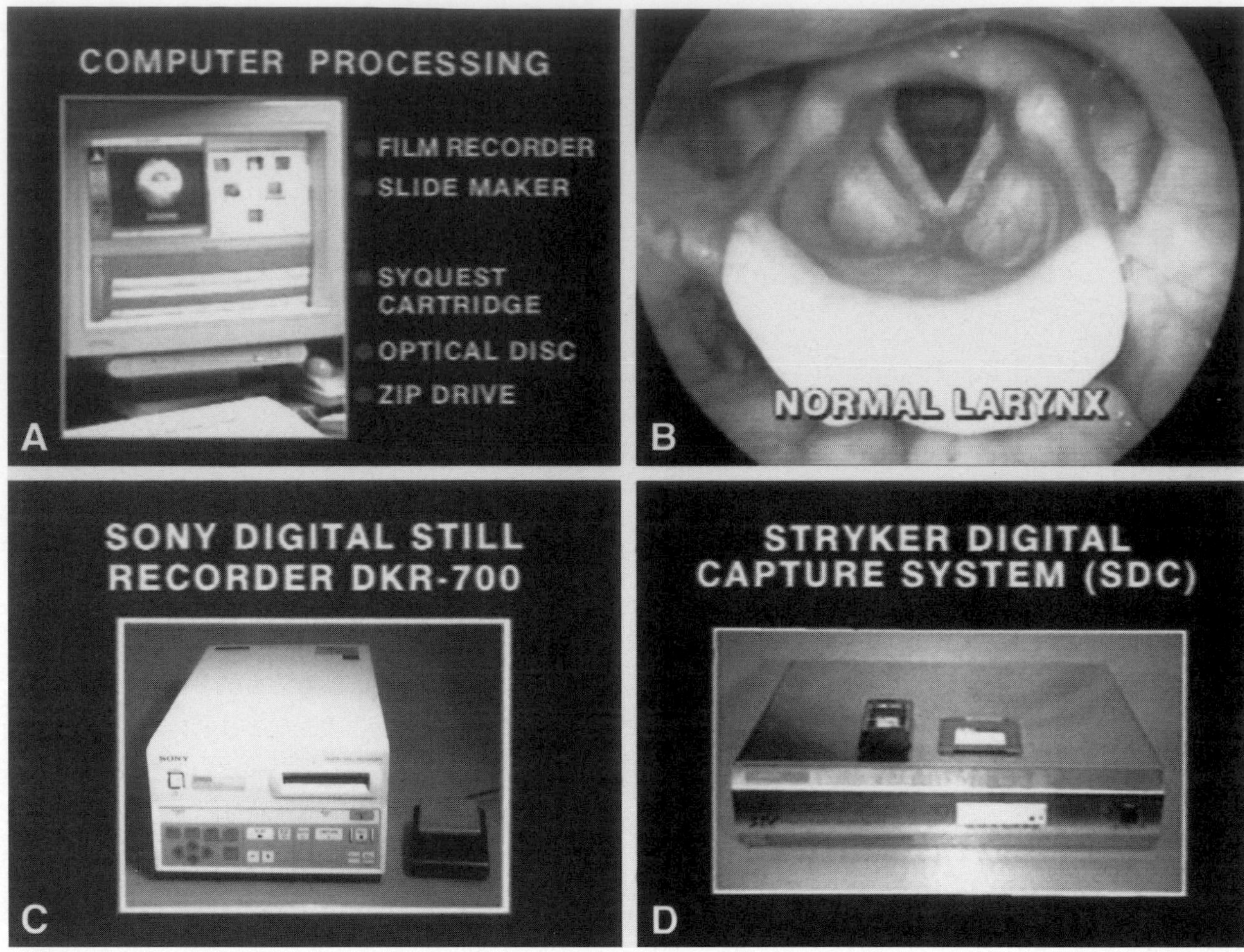

Figure 7.15 *Digital imaging. (a) Computer processing and digital imaging. (b) Laryngeal image produced from prerecorded videotape. (c) Sony digital still recorder DKR-700. (d) Stryker digital capture system (SDC).*

photographs in this chapter were all produced by the Sony UP-5100 color video printer (Fig 7.2a). Slides can be made simply by photographing the color videoprints using color slide film such as Ektachrome Tungsten ASA 160. A more affordable color video printer such as Sony CVP M3 is now available.

Computer and digital imaging

The third technique of video-to-print/slide transfer is to use a computer to digitize images from the videotape (see Fig 7.2f, 7.15a–d). Software is available that can capture video images either as still frames or as full-motion video. These digitized images may be made into composite pictures and labeled and saved as a computer file. The image may be printed with a computer printer. Dye sublimation prints produce high-quality photo-realistic prints, but these printers are prohibitively expensive. Lesser quality images can be made on most computer printers. As described above, slide photographs may be shot from these computer prints. Alternatively, the computer file may be transferred to photo prints or 35 mm slides by a computer service bureau (usually via high-capacity removable storage devices such as Syquest, optical drives or zip drive).

Digital imaging is the newest technology for permanently recording images without a film or a videotape. An image obtained via a video camera can now be converted to an electronic signal that a computer can read, record and store in a digital fashion.

More recently, digital image capture devices, such as Sony DKR-700 Digital Still Recorder (Fig 7.15c) and Stryker Digital Capture System (SDC) (Fig 7.15d), have been introduced. These newer image capture devices allow the digital images to be transferred from a video camera to a computer disk. No videotape is needed. The image obtained can be displayed on a computer monitor, annotated and stored. These devices are very useful but costly.

Stryker Surgislide Slidemaker

The Stryker Surgislide Slidemaker is a relatively new analog image capture device for the production of 35 mm

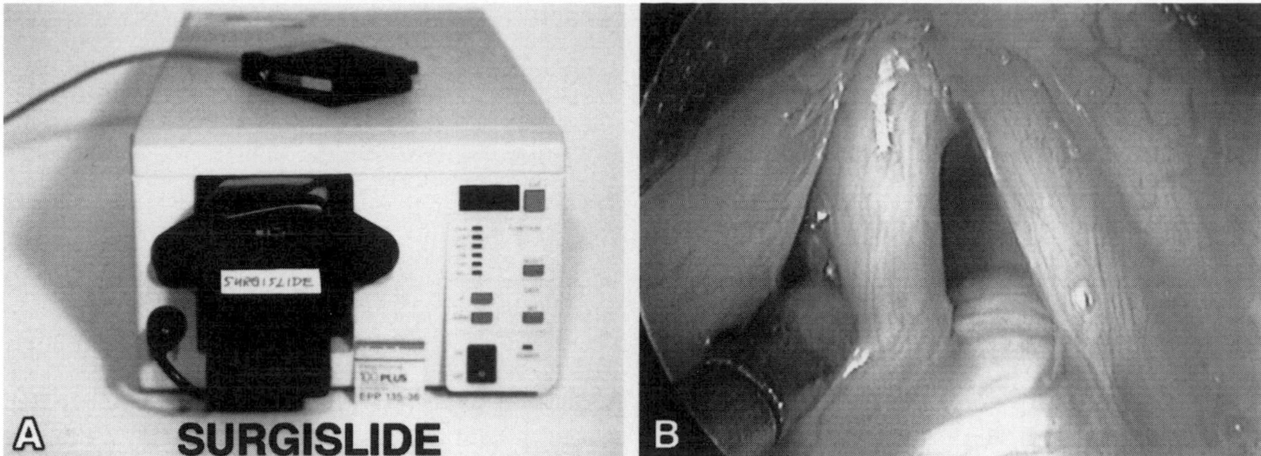

Figure 7.16 *Surgislide photography. (a) Stryker Surgislide Slidemaker. (b) Still photography (35 mm) from video image using the Surgislide Slidemaker.*

slides from either a video camera or a prerecorded video image. The recommended film is ASA 100 Professional Ektachrome. A 35 mm automatic SLR camera is attached to the front of the image capture device (Fig 7.16a). This system produces excellent color slides (Fig 7.16b). The advantage of the Stryker Surgislide Slidemaker is the ability to capture images directly onto 35 mm slide film without the need for additional hardware or software. However, the disadvantage is its high cost.

Conclusions

Laryngeal documentation can be achieved either in the office or in the operating room, utilizing still photographic, videographic and digital imaging techniques. Although still photography still remains as a valuable method of laryngeal documentation, videography has become a widely accepted method of laryngeal documentation today, because it allows documentation of anatomy, pathology, motion and simultaneous voice recording.

In this chapter various methods of videography and still photography of the larynx are described. Telescopic documentation both in the office and in the operating room produces superior structural images with higher resolution. Although fiberscopic documentation generally produces inferior quality images at present, it is of great value for documenting laryngeal function and voice recording. Microscopic video documentation is the preferred practical method of laryngeal documentation and teaching of microlaryngeal surgery in the operating room.

More recently, digital imaging technique has been introduced to laryngeal documentation. The advantages of digital imaging include safe, long-term storage, easy computer manipulation, easy retrieval and no image degrading with time. The main disadvantage is its high cost. However, as this technology improves and the cost decreases, the use of digital imaging will likely become widespread.

References

1. Alberti PW. Still photography of the larynx – an overview. *Can J Otolaryngol* 1975; **4:** 759–65.
2. Andrea M, Dias O. *Atlas of Rigid and Contact Endoscopy in Microlaryngeal Surgery.* Philadelphia: Lippincott-Raven, 1995.
3. Andrea M, Dias O, Santos A. Contact endoscopy during microlaryngeal surgery – a new technique for endoscopic examination of the larynx. *Ann Otol Rhinol Laryngol* 1995; **104:** 333–5.
4. Benjamin B. Technique of laryngeal photography. *Ann Otol Rhinol Laryngol* 1984; **93(Suppl 109):** 1–11.
5. Benjamin B. *Diagnostic Laryngology – Adults and Children.* Philadelphia: Saunders, 1990.
6. Benjamin B. Art and science of laryngeal photography. *Ann Otol Rhinol Laryngol* 1993; **102:** 271–82.
7. Berci G. *Endoscopy.* New York: Appleton-Century-Crofts, 1976.
8. Berci G, Caldwell FH. A device to facilitate photography during indirect laryngoscopy. *Med Biol Illus* 1963; **13:** 169–76.
9. Berci G, Calcaterra T, Ward PH. Advances in endoscopic techniques for examination of the larynx and nasopharynx. *Can J Otolaryngol* 1975; **4:** 786–92.
10. Brewer DW, McCall G. Visible laryngeal changes during voice study. *Ann Otol Rhinol Laryngol* 1974; **83:** 423–7.
11. Davidson TM, Bone RC, Nahum AM. Flexible fiberoptic laryngo-bronchoscopy. *Laryngoscope* 1974; **84:** 1876–82.
12. Ferguson GB, Crowder WJ. A simple method of laryngeal and other cavity photography. *Arch Otolaryngol* 1970; **92:** 201–3.
13. French TR. On a perfected method of photographing the larynx. *NY Med J* 1884; **4:** 655–6.
14. Hahn C, Kitzing P. Indirect endoscopic photography of the larynx – a comparison between two newly constructed laryngoscopes. *J Audiov Media Med* 1978; **1:** 121–30.
15. Hirano M. *Clinical Evaluation of Voice.* Wien: Springer-Verlag, 1981.
16. Holinger PH. Photography of the larynx, trachea, bronchi and esophagus. *Trans Am Acad Ophthalmol Otolaryngol* 1942; **46:** 153–6.

17. Holinger PH, Tardy ME. Photography in otorhinolaryngology and bronchoesophagology. In: English GM, ed. *Otolaryngology*. Philadelphia: Lippincott, 1986; Vol. 5, 1–21.
18. Holinger PH, Brubaker JD, Brubaker JE. Open tube, proximal illumination, mirror and direct laryngeal photography. *Can J Otolaryngol* 1975; **4:** 781–5.
19. Inouye T. Examination of child larynx by flexible fiberoptic laryngoscope. *Int J Pediatr Otorhinolaryngol* 1983; **5:** 317–23.
20. Jako GJ. Laryngoscope for microscopic observations, surgery and photography. *Arch Otolaryngol* 1970; **91:** 196–9.
21. Jako GJ, Strong S. Laryngeal photography. *Arch Otolaryngol* 1972; **96:** 268–71.
22. Kantor E, Berci G, Partlow E, Paz-Partlow M. A completely new approach to microlaryngeal surgery. *Laryngoscope* 1991; **101:** 678–9.
23. Kitzing P. Stroboscopy – a pertinent laryngological examination. *J Otolaryngol* 1985; **14:** 151–7.
24. Kleinsasser O. Entwicklung und Methoden der Kehlkopffotografie (Mit Beschreibung eines neuen einfachen Fotolaryngoskopes). *HNO* 1963; **1:** 171–6.
25. Kleinsasser O. *Microlaryngoscopy and Endolaryngeal Microsurgery*. Philadelphia: Saunders, 1968.
26. Kleinsasser O. *Tumors of the Larynx and Hypopharynx*. New York: Thieme, 1988: 124–30.
27. Mambrino L, Yanagisawa E, Yanagisawa K, Gallo O. Endoscopic ENT photography – a comparison of pictures by standard color films and newer color video printers. *Laryngoscope* 1991; **101:** 1229–32.
28. Muller-Hermann F, Pedersen P. Modern endoscopic and microscopic photography in otolaryngology. *Ann Otol Rhinol Laryngol* 1984; **93:** 399–402.
29. Olofsson J, Ohlsson T. Techniques in microlaryngoscopic photography. *Can J Otolaryngol* 1975; **4:** 770–80.
30. Padovan IF, Christman NT, Hamilton LH, Darling RJ. Indirect micro-laryngoscopy. *Laryngoscope* 1973; **83:** 2035–41.
31. Rosnagle R, Smith HW. Hand-held fundus camera for endoscopic photography. *Trans Am Acad Ophthalmol Otolaryngol* 1972; **76:** 1024–5.
32. Sawashima M, Hirose H. New laryngoscopic technique by use of fiberoptics. *J Acoust Soc Am* 1968; **43:** 168–9.
33. Selkin SG. The otolaryngologist and flexible fiberoptics – photographic considerations. *J Otolaryngol* 1983; **12:** 223–7.
34. Silberman HD, Wilf H, Tucker JA. Flexible fiberoptic naso-pharyngolaryngoscope. *Ann Otol Rhinol Laryngol* 1976; **85:** 640–5.
35. Steiner W, Jaumann MP. Moderne otorhinolaryngologische Endoskopie beim Kind. *Padiatr Prax* 1978; **20:** 429–35.
36. Strong MS. Laryngeal photography. *Can J Otolaryngol* 1975; **4:** 766–9.
37. Stuckrad H, Lakatos I. Uber ein neues Lupenlaryngoskop (Epipharyngoskop). *Laryngorhinootologie* 1975; **54:** 336–40.
38. Tardy ME, Tenta LT. Laryngeal photography and television. *Otolaryngol Clin North Am* 1970; **3:** 483–92.
39. Tsuiki Y. *Laryngeal Examination*. Tokyo: Kanehara Shuppan, 1956.
40. Ward PH, Berci G, Calcaterra TC. Advances in endoscopic examination of the respiratory system. *Ann Otol Rhinol Laryngol* 1974; **83:** 754–60.
41. Wendler J. Stroboscopy. *J Voice* 1992; **6:** 149–54.
42. Yamashita K. Endonasal flexible fiberoptic endoscopy. *Rhinology* 1983; **21:** 233–7.
43. Yamashita K. *Diagnostic and Therapeutic ENT Endoscopy*. Tokyo: Medical View, 1988.
44. Yamashita K, Mertens J, Rudert H. Die flexible Fiberendoskopie in der HNO-Heildunde. *HNO* 1984; **32:** 378–84.
45. Yamashita K, Oku T, Tanaka H, Sato K. VTR endoscopy. *J Otolaryngol Jpn* 1977; **80:** 1208–9.
46. Yanagisawa E. Office telescopic photography of the larynx. *Ann Otol Rhinol Laryngol* 1982; **91:** 354–8.
47. Yanagisawa E. Videolaryngoscopy using a low cost home video system color camera. *J Biol Photogr* 1984; **52:** 9–14.
48. Yanagisawa E. Videolaryngoscopy. In: Lee KJ, Stewart CH, eds. *Ambulatory Surgery and Office Procedures in Head and Neck Surgery*. Orlando: Grune & Stratton, 1986: 63-71.
49. Yanagisawa E. Documentation. In: Ferlito A, ed. *Neoplasms of the Larynx*. Edinburgh: Churchill Livingstone, 1993: 369–400.
50. Yanagisawa E. *Color Atlas of Diagnostic Endoscopy in Otorhinolaryngology*. New York: Igaku Shoin, 1997.
51. Yanagisawa E, Carlson RD. Videolaryngoscopy and laryngeal photography. In: Cummings CW, ed. *Otolaryngology and Head and Neck Surgery*. Philadelphia: Mosby, 1986: 1752–60.
52. Yanagisawa E, Carlson, RD. Physical diagnosis of the hypopharynx and the larynx with and without imaging. In: Lee KJ, ed. *Textbook of Otolaryngology and Head and Neck Surgery*. New York: Elsevier, 1989: 578–98.
53. Yanagisawa E, Driscoll BP. Laryngeal photography and videography. In: Rubin JS, Sataloff RT, Korovin GS, Gould WJ, eds. *Diagnosis and Treatment of Voice Disorders*. New York: Igaku Shoin, 1995: 269–89.
54. Yanagisawa E, Yamashita K. Fiberoptic nasopharyngolaryngoscopy. In: Lee KJ, Stewart CH, eds. *Ambulatory Surgery and Office Procedures in Head and Neck Surgery*. Orlando: Grune & Stratton, 1986: 31–40.
55. Yanagisawa E, Yanagisawa K. Stroboscopic videolaryngoscopy – a comparison of fiberscopic and telescopic documentation. *Ann Otol Rhinol Laryngol* 1993; **102:** 255–65.
56. Yanagisawa E, Yanagisawa R. Laryngeal photography. *Otolaryngol Clin North Am* 1991; **24:** 999–1022.
57. Yanagisawa E, Casuccio JR, Suzuki M. Videolaryngoscopy using a rigid telescope and video home system color camera – a useful office procedure. *Ann Otol Rhinol Laryngol* 1981; **90:** 346–50.
58. Yanagisawa E, Eibling DE, Suzuki M. A simple method of laryngeal photography through the operating microscope – 'macrolens technique'. *Ann Otol Rhinol Laryngol* 1980; **89:** 547–50.
59. Yanagisawa E, Kmucha ST, Estill J. Role of the soft palate in laryngeal functions and selected voice qualities: simultaneous velolaryngeal videoendoscopy. *Ann Otol Rhinol Laryngol* 1990; **99:** 18–28.
60. Yanagisawa E, Owens TW, Strothers G, Honda K. Videolaryngoscopy – a comparison of fiberscopic and telescopic documentation. *Ann Otol Rhinol Laryngol* 1983; **92:** 430–6.
61. Yanagisawa K, Yanagisawa E. Current diagnostic and office practice – techniques of endoscopic imaging of the larynx. *Curr Opin Otolaryngol Head Neck Surg* 1996; **4:** 147–53.

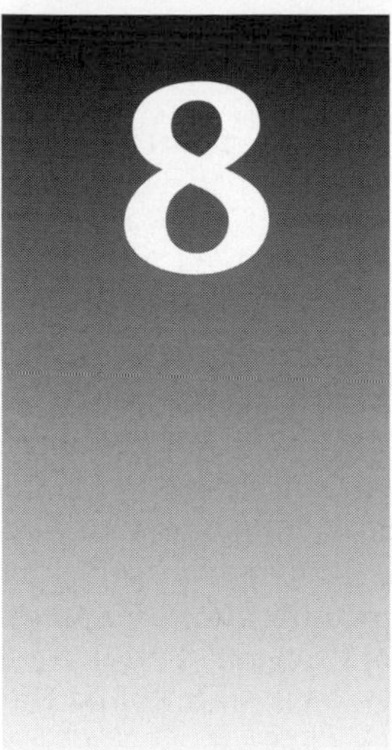

Rigid and contact endoscopy of the larynx

Mário Andrea and Oscar Dias

The use of rigid and contact endoscopy during microlaryngoscopy improves the assessment of the laryngeal pathology. It is advantageous to observe in detail the whole of the endolarynx in a routine and systematic way using rigid endoscopes with several angles of vision. This enhanced evaluation has consequences in therapeutic management, also affecting the physiopathologic understanding of laryngeal diseases.

Contact endoscopy has brought a new dimension to the evaluation of the laryngeal pathology, offering the possibility of visualizing '*in vivo*' and '*in situ*' the cells of the superficial layers of the epithelium.

In this chapter the current role of these techniques and its consequences in clinical practice are described.

Rigid endoscopy associated with microlaryngeal surgery

Currently, endoscopic evaluation of the larynx is based on rigid endoscopy, fibroscopy, stroboscopy and microlaryngoscopy, in most cases benefiting from video recording.

The complex morphology of the endolarynx justifies the existence of regions of the larynx that are difficult or even impossible to visualize, such as the anterior commissure or the Morgagni ventricle. At the anterior part, the inclination of the epiglottis, its shape and its insertion at the thyroid cartilage, close to the anterior insertion of the vocal cords, make observation of the anterior commissure difficult most times. The same happens to the floor of the Morgagni ventricle, hidden below the false cord.

When the larynx is evaluated in the office with the rigid endoscopes (70°, 90°), the images are very clear and magnified but still limited by the vertical axis of vision. Inspection of the endolarynx is more complete with the fiberscope but the quality of the image is not so sharp. In the operating room, the fact that the axis of vision of the microscope is superimposed on the laryngeal axis also limits the visualization of the vocal cords to its superior surface and border.

Previous research work on laryngeal microanatomy[1,2,9,13,20] has underlined the importance of considering the vocal cord as a topographic unit with a superior and an inferior surface in continuity with the subglottis. The orientation of the inferior surface and its relationships varies according to the site, being distinct, anteriorly, close to the anterior commissure, and posteriorly, near the vocal process.

The physiology of phonation highlights the importance of the inferior surface of the vocal cord and its free border. According to stroboscopy, the free border of the vocal cord should be considered a dynamic anatomic area, corresponding to the most superior part of the inferior surface.

With these concepts in mind, we began, some years ago, routinely using rigid endoscopes during microlaryngoscopies. The combination of rigid endoscopy with the microscope, as developed in the nose and in the ear, improved laryngeal assessment significantly and led us to propose and systematize rigid endoscopy associated with microlaryngeal surgery (REMS).[3–8,10–12,14]

The use of endoscopes intraoperatively is common, for particular cases, namely in cancer, to evaluate areas or regions that can influence or determine the choice of an operative technique.[15,24–26] However, our proposal was different, in concept and in method.

Conceptually we assume it is advantageous to observe in detail the whole of the endolarynx, in a routine and systematic way, using rigid endoscopes with several angles of vision, during microlaryngoscopy. This combination contributes to the performance of a systematized endoscopic examination of the larynx as it happens currently with CT and NMR imaging.

The increase in time taken is not significant and is largely compensated for by the information and possibility of further analysis and sharing of the video documentation.

REMS is a natural combination of the microscope and endoscopes, taking advantage of general anesthesia. The use of the endoscopes does not require the modification of routine anesthetic techniques, all patients being under regular endotracheal intubation. To perform the REMS technique, a set of four endoscopes is used, 24 cm long, 5 mm in diameter, with 0°, 30°, 70° and 120° angles of vision (KS 8712AA, 8712BA, 8712CA, 8712DA). Endoscopes of smaller diameter (4 mm) are preferred in children or in particular cases.

Rigid endoscopy offers distinct angles, better illumination, magnification, associated with a wider field of vision and a superior depth of field, allowing improved definition of the lesion's characteristics. Beyond the full assessment of the endolarynx the endoscopes permit the visualization of each site or area from different perspectives, allowing a multiperspective reconstruction of the pathology and the neighboring areas.

The type and placement of the laryngoscope is important in obtaining the best exposure of the different regions of the larynx. The 0° endoscope offers an overall vision of the aditus laryngis, vestibule, the upper part of the hypopharynx and of the superior surface of the vocal cords. Passing through the cordal level, the subglottis and trachea are reached. However, the 0° endoscope misses important regions such as the free border and the inferior surface of the vocal cord.

The 30° endoscope allows the visualization of the laryngeal surface of the epiglottis until the anterior commissure. Laterally it allows the assessment of the orifice and floor of the ventricle. By rotating the endoscope and with the endotracheal tube displaced, the posterior commissure is observed.

The 70° endoscope improves the assessment of laryngeal pathology in traditionally difficult areas. By rotating the 70° endoscope laterally and progressing from the superior margin of the vestibule to the trachea, complete evaluation of both hemilarynges is possible, including the entire Morgagni ventricle, the floor, the anterior and posterior limits and also the external and superior limit. The superior surface of the vocal cord and the anterior commissure are analyzed in detail as are the border and inferior surface of the vocal cord.

Below the ventricle, the 70° endoscope, positioned at the angle between the anesthesia tube and the vocal process of the arytenoid, offers a superb view of the glottic margins in the horizontal and vertical planes. Visualization of the height of the 'free border', the relationship of the pathology on the opposite vocal cord, the inferior surface of the vocal cords, the mucosal characteristics and shape of the inferior part of the paraglottic space, and tracheal walls is an important advantage using a 70° telescope.

In the anterior midline, the 30° and 70° endoscopes give access to the laryngeal surface of the epiglottis, the epiglottic stem and the small region that separates it from the vocal cords. The anterior commissure, the small slit between the vocal cords at the thyroid cartilage, the slim area of the free border of the vocal cords at the most anterior part, the subcommissural region, and the area corresponding internally to the cricothyroid ligament and the anterior part of the trachea are clearly observed.

The 120° endoscope permits backwards visualization of the superior limit of the ventricular orifice (false cord) and visualization of part of the vertical component of the Morgagni ventricle. Rotation of the 120° endoscope below the vocal cord allows the view of the glottosubglottic dome, including the subcommissural region, the inferior surface of the vocal cords and the small area below the base of the arytenoid cartilage.

By placing the 70° and 120° endoscopes at the anterior part of the larynx and displacing the endotracheal tube, the posterior larynx can be observed: namely, the height of the arytenoid cartilages, the cricoarytenoid junction, the internal surface of the vocal process, the subarytenoid region, and the posterior part of the subglottis.

Each endoscope allows a specific perspective. The use of one or several endoscopes is determined by the anatomy and the characteristics of the pathology.

Intraoperative telescopic images are of high quality. Rigid endoscopes can focus from a position very close to the lesion and the magnification is higher than that obtained with the microscope, improving the definition of the lesion's characteristics (shape, dimensions, limits, extension, color, surface alterations and vascular changes).

Benign pathology

When a polyp is observed with the surgical microscope, only its superior surface and the superior surface of the vocal cord can be assessed. Rigid endoscopy allows a more complete view of the polyp – its dimensions, localization, surface characteristics and color, as well as the vasculature of the polyp and nearby zones (Fig 8.1). The inferior surface of the polyp and the dimensions of its base of implantation are clearly defined.

The multiperspective view of the base of implantation – horizontal and vertical axis – allows the planning and performance of a meticulous surgical technique. The definition of the anterior and posterior limits of a polyp that are not always evident when observed through the microscope are well established with the telescopes, allowing the identification of the transition between the polyp and the normal mucosa.

Assessment of the glottis with 70° and 120° endoscopes identifies significant features of the mucosa of the inferior surface and the free border of the vocal cord, and of its vasculature, in phonation disorders.

REMS also permits a much better view of the opposite vocal cord. Areas of edema, hyperplasia, keratosis and depressions of the free border can be observed when examining the primary lesion; these areas are usually poorly visualized or possibly missed by single microscopic evaluation.

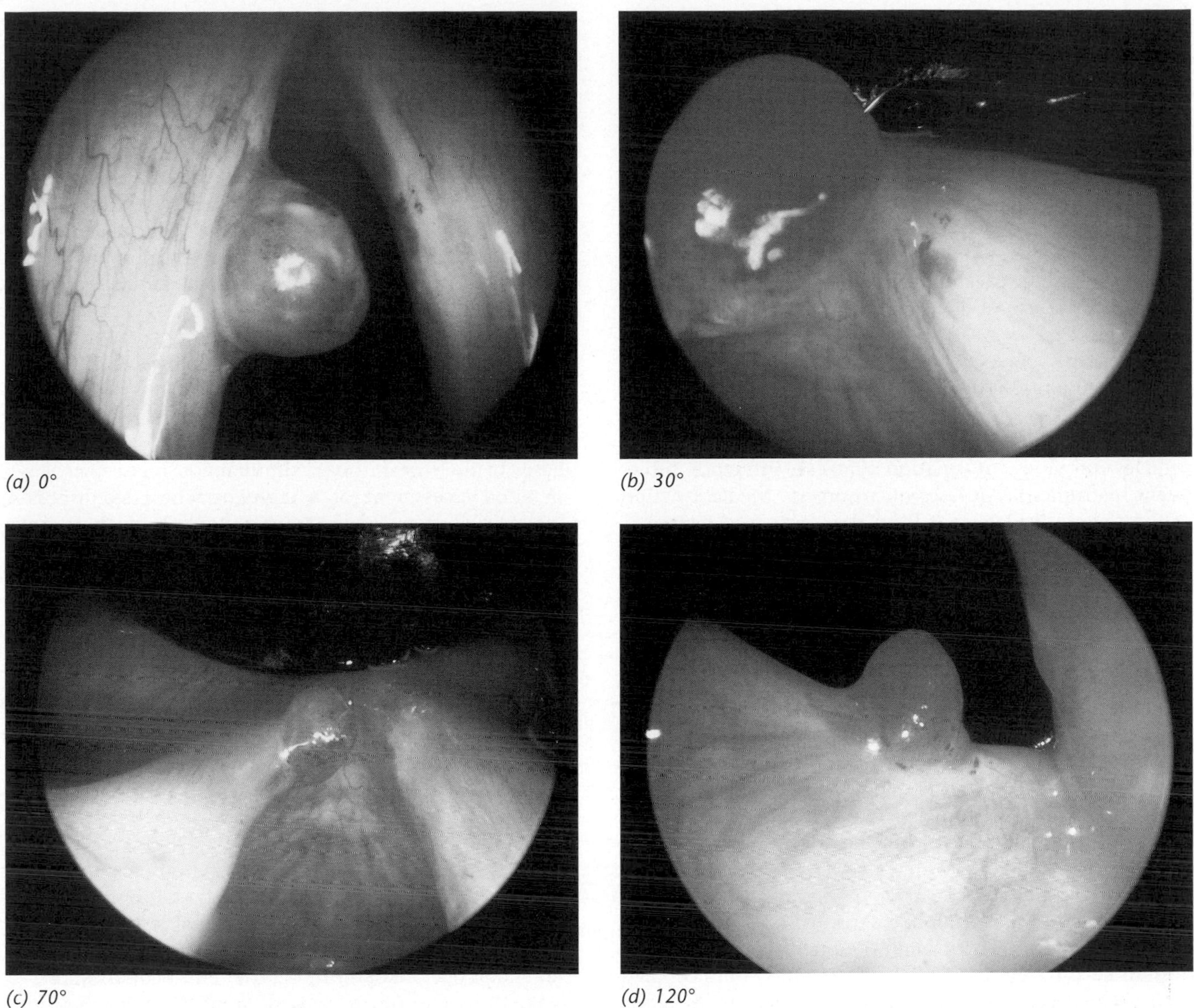

(a) 0° (b) 30°

(c) 70° (d) 120°

Figure 8.1 *Vocal cord polyp visualized with the different endoscopes (a, 0°; b, 30°; c, 70°; and d, 120°).*

The use of endoscopes also provides a much more detailed evaluation of nodules. Besides form, relief and surface characteristics, it is possible to observe the inferior surface of the vocal cord and the nodule. By looking at the nodule from below and from behind and observing all the alterations of the mucosa, the understanding of its physiopathology and its developmental stage is improved.

The notion of trauma is perceived by the symmetric keratotic and edematous areas at the inferior surface of both vocal cords. This precise assessment provides a better therapeutic approach and rigid endoscopic video images can be shared between surgeons and speech pathologists.

Cysts that have already benefited from stroboscopy become more evident with REMS. Oblique illumination increases the perception of relief. Definition of site, dimensions and vasculature of the vocal cord mucosa are assessed in great detail and the surgical approach is well established. The differential diagnosis of early stages of polyps, nodules and cysts can also be improved with the detailed evaluation through the endoscopes.

When a sulcus glottidis is diagnosed with an office procedure, the 30° and 70° endoscopes allow a more complete and detailed assessment of this entity. The elastic structure at the level of the glottis conditions the etiopathogeny of the sulcus glottidis. When performing microdissection of the glottosubglottic region, the easy dissociation of the vocal ligament from the rest of the conus elasticus is noted. This creates a 'weak' point or area at the vocal cord border that, faced with the elastic and muscular tensions and dynamic alterations occurring at the glottosubglottic region, may justify the invagination of the vocal cord epithelium.

Discrepancies among different authors can be explained by the different conditions of observation. When the patient is observed in the office, the larynx is vertical and with a permanent muscular tone. In the operating room, the larynx is horizontal, stretched by the laryngoscope, and the elastic tension is not opposed by the vocal muscles.

The coexistence of additional pathology other than that viewed by microlaryngoscopy is quite frequent, as happens with small leukoplakias, present in cases of nodules and polyps.

Phonosurgery techniques are influenced by the assessment of benign lesions. In polyps, the improved observation allowed by REMS, including the base of the lesion, the inferior surface of the vocal cord and the vascular pedicles, provides information that can influence subsequent instrumental or laser microsurgery. Medial traction of the polyp, displacing it from the vocal cord ligament, may cause unnecessary sacrifice of the mucosa of the inferior surface of the vocal cord, compromising phonation.

In microlaryngeal surgery of vocal polyps, concern is usually focused on the superior surface of the vocal cords although polyps originate from the mucosa of the inferior surface of the vocal cords. With REMS the characteristics of the base of implantation of the polyp (shape, dimensions, blood vessels) are determined with precision. The multiperspective and highly detailed assessment of benign lesions will certainly contribute to the refinement of the surgical technique and to the creation of new instruments.

Surgery through the microscope has the advantage of the simultaneous use of both hands. In some cases, surgical gestures performed through the microscope have been monitored through one of the angled endoscopes coupled with a video camera. Microlaryngeal surgery will evolve, as it has in endoscopic nasal surgery in which microscope and endoscopes are used in articulation, complementing each other.

The Kantor–Berci video laryngoscope[22,28] combines the classic laryngoscope with the benefits of rigid endoscopy imaging, substituting the conventional operating microscope. It offers excellent conditions for documentation; however, it has the limitation of only observing the vocal cords from the vertical axis.

In Reinke's edema, the endoscopes have allowed its limits to be established – anteriorly, posteriorly, laterally and also inferiorly. If the relationships between the floor of the ventricle, the anterior commissure, and the vocal process are important to define the surgical technique, REMS has permitted observation from the subglottis to the inferior surface of the vocal cord and the inferior limit of Reinke's edema. REMS also contributes to understanding the evolution of Reinke's edema and its development stage. In some cases, the vasculature of the mucosa is one of the main features; in other cases, keratosis will inhibit the observation of the blood vessels. In one case, we were able to diagnose an infiltrating tumor below Reinke's edema that extended into the subglottis. This would not have been detected at this phase if observation had been limited to the superior surface of the vocal cord.

In chronic laryngitis, the difference between microscopic observation and that allowed by the rigid endoscope is significant, as subtle color alterations, relief changes, areas of keratosis, vascular abnormalities, and edema are more objectively defined. Information about these features can be used to guide microsurgical excisions and biopsies.

Studying video endoscopic images obtained in both vocal cords and in the rest of the endolarynx contributes to the understanding of the dynamic process of disease of the laryngeal mucosa. REMS images associated with contact endoscopy evaluation demonstrate that different phases of the disease occur simultaneously.

A good assessment of a laryngotracheal stenosis is a fundamental step for its management. In fact, stenosis must be evaluated not only in a horizontal plane but the disease must be considered three-dimensionally at different levels of the larynx. The endoscopic multiperspective view in conjunction with CT and MRI provides a better assessment of stenosis.

If, in the office, the progression allowed by the fiberscope gives more complete information of the lesion than using a rigid endoscope placed in the oropharynx, the systematic use of angled optics in the operating room is extremely useful as the progression of the endoscopes allows a precise evaluation of each level of the larynx and trachea.

The site, size and thickness of a stenotic lesion can be determined in detail using the telescopes. On the other hand, the frequent association of several lesions in different levels of the airway is better assessed by combining the endoscopes. Rotation of the endoscopes allows a detailed observation in cases of stenosis of the posterior glottis and the height of the arytenoid, which is important in the assessment of granulomas. The surgical technique should be assisted at each stage through the endoscopes, choosing the optics according to the stenosed area.

The advantages offered by the REMS evaluation and peroperative control are increased even more when lasers conducted by angled fibers (KTP) are used under the control of the endoscopes. One of the main difficulties of CO_2 laser arytenoidectomy is to guarantee a complete exeresis of the arytenoid.

The height of the arytenoid and the relationship of its base, lying over the conus elasticus, are well observed with the angled endoscopes during surgery.

For several years, our preference has been to use the posterior cordotomy proposed by Kashima.[23] Microdissection of the arytenoid, vocal ligament and conus elasticus, has allowed us to recognize that the deep sectioning of the conus elasticus at the base of the arytenoid is as important as the lateral incision. Due to

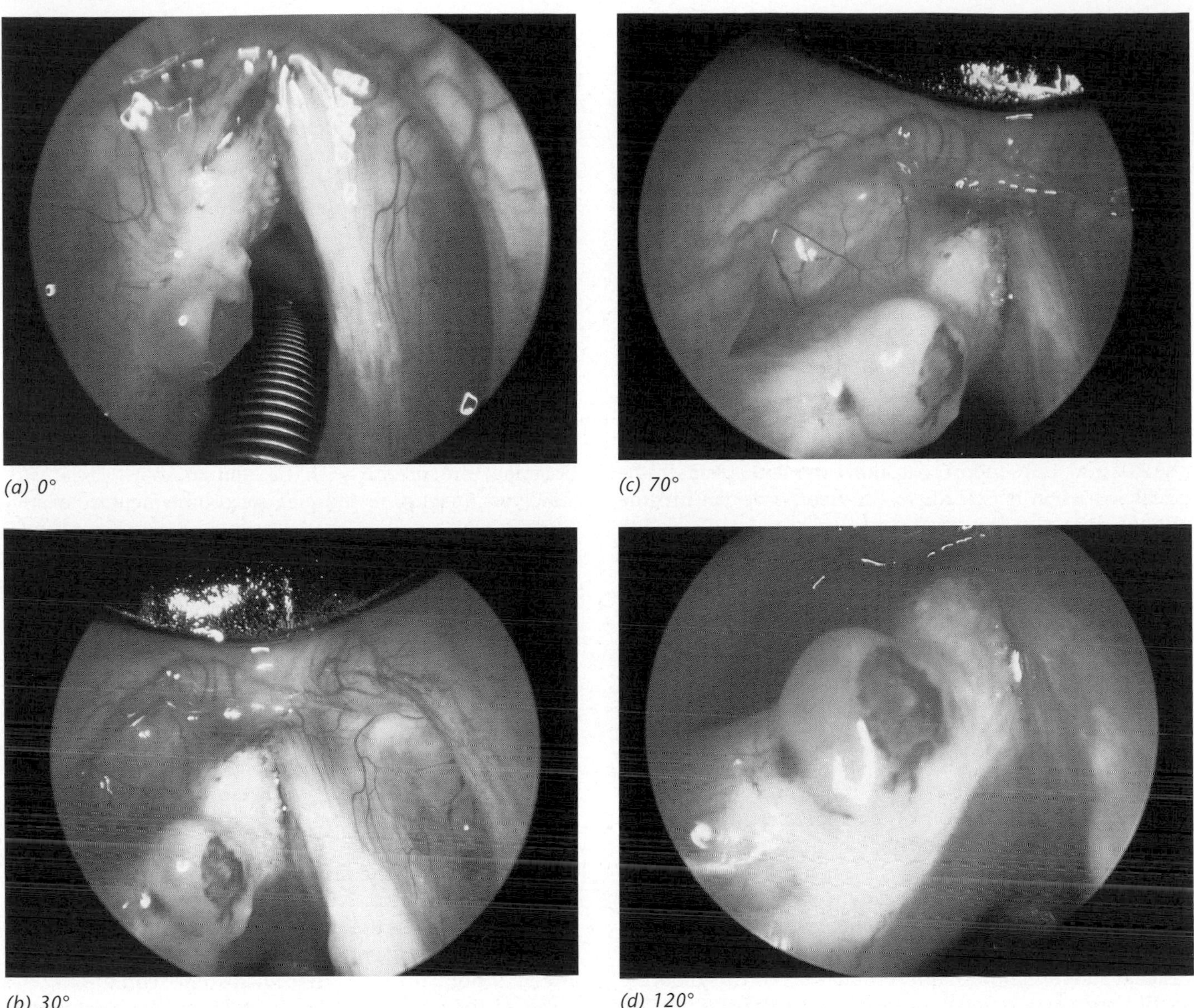

Figure 8.2 *Vocal cord tumor. The combination of the distinct endoscopes (0°, 30°, 70° and 120°) during microlaryngoscopy improves topographic assessment, definition of the lesion's characteristics and allows a multiperspective reconstruction.*

these facts, posterior cordotomy should be systematically assisted by angled endoscopes (30°, 70°). If the section of the vocal ligament is well visualized through the microscope, the depth of the cut and the interruption of the fibers of the conus elasticus are better controlled with angled optics.

Laryngeal papillomatosis and papillomas also benefit with the REMS evaluation, reducing the possibility of residual lesions. As surgery progresses, the control of the lesion, and of its anatomic relationships, are clearly evaluated with different optics. The magnifications and different angles of the endoscopes allow more precise limits of the diseased and the normal mucosa to be established. Contact endoscopy also permits the identification of very early phases of the disease.

If the introduction of the CO_2 laser has improved papillomatosis surgery, the use of endoscopes (rigid and contact) and fiber-transmitted lasers contribute to obtain even better results. The aim of treating the pathology as early as possible and preserving the anatomy of the organ can, in this way, be accomplished in better conditions.

Premalignant pathology

Office endoscopic techniques allow the observation of premalignant pathology at the superior surface of the vocal cord. Microlaryngoscopy makes it possible to have good visualization and to perform a biopsy or a microsurgical excision. In premalignant pathology, REMS allows an overall analysis not only of the lesion that justified the surgical procedure, but also a very detailed observation of the entire larynx.

Frequently, the existence of more than one lesion is noticed in areas of the vocal cord that are difficult or even impossible to visualize with conventional techniques. Beyond the main lesions, subtle abnormalities at the surface indicate different stages of pathology.

The detailed observation with the endoscopes reinforces the physiopathologic notion of a 'disease', influencing the therapeutic approach and the pathological control. Besides the inventory of the distinct lesions, REMS offers the possibility of analyzing dimensions, limits, transition areas to normal mucosa, edemas, surface characteristics, and definition of the vascular pattern. Relief perception is improved with the 30°, 70° and 120° endoscopes and provides a better definition of the site and the distance that separates lesions from distinct laryngeal landmarks. The 70° and 120° endoscopes allow the leukoplakia to be visualized when it extends to the free border and to the inferior surface of the vocal cord.

Image processing has important potential applications in this area. Attempts at using computer systems to enhance the analysis of endoscopic images are very promising, allowing the quantification of parameters such as dimensions, contours and the mapping of the lesions in the endolarynx.

Malignant pathology

Given that rigid endoscopes are useful in non-malignant pathology, their importance is even greater in oncology.

Systematic combination of rigid endoscopy with microlaryngoscopy and microlaryngeal surgery allows enhanced diagnostic precision in the early phases of malignant tumors and a precise topographic assessment for the therapeutic approach. Dimensions, shape, boundaries, vascular abnormalities and evaluation of neighboring regions may be accurately assessed with the 0°, 30°, 70° and 120° endoscopes (Fig 8.2).

Assessment with angled endoscopes is fundamental in order to plan the approach. This is justified by the ability to explore, namely, the anterior commissure, the thyroepiglottic ligament, the Morgagni ventricle, the free border and the inferior surface of the vocal cord, the arytenoid region and the subglottis. Endoscopes offer access to regions formerly difficult or impossible to explore clinically and also allow the evaluation of a particular tumor or region from different angles, enabling a multiperspective and three-dimensional reconstruction of the lesion.

Dimensions, site, surface characteristics, color alterations, boundaries, vascular abnormalities and edema in neighboring regions are also assessed with the various endoscopes. All these facts improve biopsy performance.

Angled endoscopes make it possible to perform biopsies in areas not accessible to the microscope, as happens in some anatomic regions or in cases in which the tumoral volume does not allow, or limits, the assessment and the biopsy. The macroscopic characteristics of the tumor – infiltrating, ulcerative, etc. – is another parameter that can be explored by the surgeon using endoscopes. This is particularly evident in tumors of the laryngeal surface of the epiglottis. In these tumors, microscopic observation is always limited and can even be impaired by the placement of the laryngoscope. The 70° endoscope (in some cases it is preferable to use 4 mm endoscopes) can provide an excellent view of tumors spreading to the preepiglottic space. The same happens in the case of tumors of the false cord and of the Morgagni ventricle.

Full exploration of the subglottic mucosa became possible with rigid endoscopy. If it is possible to determine the inferior limit of a vocal cord tumor on the surface, deep subglottic invasion can also be explored as the conus elasticus is pushed by the tumor.

The staging of the majority of the laryngeal tumors became more precise with CT and in some cases MRI. However, imaging techniques are complementary examinations, whilst endoscopy, even under general anesthesia, is an observation technique, which allows the detection of early stages of tumor spread. REMS will contribute to make laryngeal endoscopy more systematized according to angles and planes, as currently occurs with CT and MRI.

The higher magnification permitted by the endoscopes has also allowed the identification of other pathologic alterations beyond the lesion that determined microlaryngeal evaluation. In some cases subtle abnormalities, such as localized edema, keratosis, scattered along the surface, indicate different stages of the pathology in distinct areas. The same is true in the opposite vocal cord and in the rest of the larynx.

The performance of different types of (endoscopic/external) partial surgery is also improved with the assistance of video endoscopic peroperative control. The classic vision through the microscope conditions the access to the vocal cord. This fact has some repercussions in that, in some cases, exeresis can be over-necessary and sometimes limited. Endoscopes allow a detailed evaluation of a vocal cord tumor even in the early stages. The next step is to benefit from this three-dimensional visualization in laryngeal endoscopic surgery.

It is our conviction that the systematic use of rigid endoscopes through the laryngoscope during microlaryngeal surgery will stimulate the design of new instruments and tools to improve access and exeresis, even in areas traditionally considered difficult to visualize. KTP laser angled fibers in conjunction with angled telescopes during microlaryngeal surgery improve the access and control of exeresis. Nowadays it is possible to perform a laser incision, under the control of angled endoscopes, at the floor of the ventricle without the need to sacrifice part of the false cord. The same happens when performing incisions at the anterior, posterior and also the inferior limit of the lesion under the control of rigid endoscopes.

The visualization of the endolarynx with angled endoscopes after partial surgery allowed a better under-

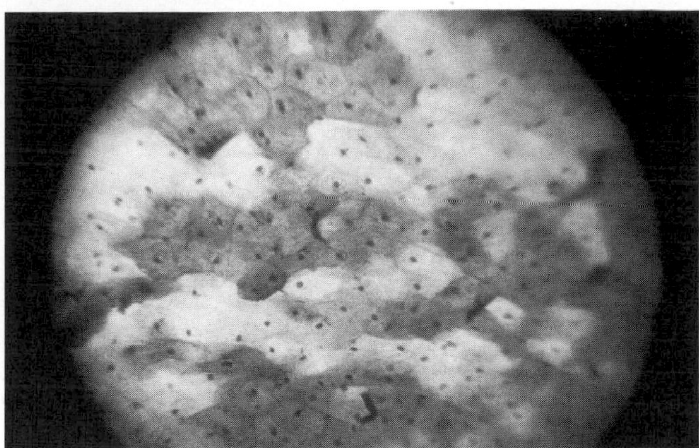

Figure 8.3 *Contact endoscopy (603). Squamous epithelium of the vocal cord visualized with the contact laryngoscope (KS 8715A) after staining of the mucosa with methylene blue (1%). There is a homogeneous cellular pattern – nucleus (dark blue) and cytoplasm (light blue) – with regular characteristics of staining, shape and dimensions.*

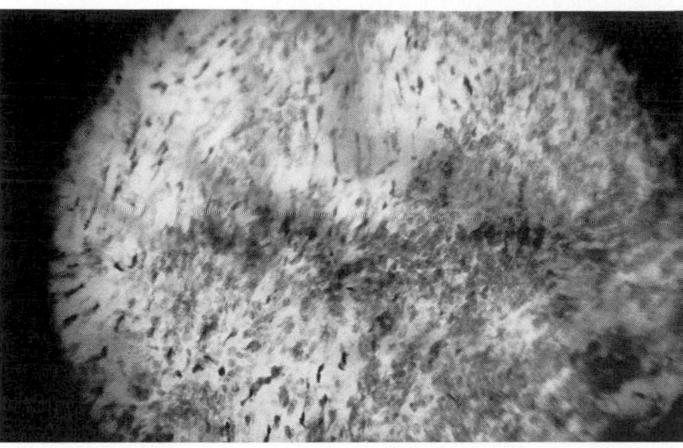

Figure 8.4 *Contact endoscopy (603). Ciliated epithelium visualized with the contact laryngoscope after staining with methylene blue (1%). The dark blue nuclei are round but the cytoplasmic limits of the cells are not so well defined as in the squamous epithelium. The filamentous structures are bundles of cilia.*

standing of the changes that occur inside the larynx. In fact it has been demonstrated that following a cordectomy, the new fold of mucosa that functions as a 'new vocal cord' is situated at a much lower plane than the opposite vocal cord. The glottic gap in phonation is not only in the horizontal plane but also in the vertical plane. When required, the exploration of the endolarynx after radiotherapy and chemotherapy also benefits with the REMS technique.

Contact endoscopy performed during microlaryngeal surgery

Contact endoscopy of the larynx is a new endoscopic technique that offers the possibility of visualizing the cells of the vocal cord epithelium '*in vivo*' and '*in situ*'. Contact endoscopy of the larynx was introduced in 1991 using the Hamou microcolpohysteroscope.[21] A contact microlaryngoscope has been developed (Karl Storz 8715A) according to our specifications, offering significant advantages in the observation of the superficial layers of the laryngeal epithelium. With the magnifications offered by this technique (603, 1503) and after staining the tissues with methylene blue, there is direct access to the cells and their characteristics. Methylene blue was chosen as a vital staining agent because of its easy accessibility and widespread clinical use. In our experience other colorants such as Lugol's iodine, Waterman's blue ink, toluidine blue, did not stain the cytoplasm and nucleus so well.

To perform the technique, the superior surface of the vocal cord is first cleaned with saline solution. Afterwards the area is carefully suctioned, followed by staining of the vocal cords with 1% methylene blue. The mucosa is gently touched with the tip of the contact endoscope, and the stained cells of the superficial layers of the epithelium become visible. Staining lasts for approximately 4–5 minutes, gradually disappearing. Methylene blue is applied again if needed. Video recording allows ongoing study and discussion of the images obtained by this *in vivo* and *in situ* study method of the tissues.

The vocal cords are covered by two types of epithelium – squamous and ciliated. When observed through contact endoscopy the squamous cells have a polyhedric shape, being in continuity with each other. The nuclei are round, darkly stained and the cytoplasm has a light blue tone. The nucleus/cytoplasm ratio is regular and the overall morphologic pattern is homogeneous (Fig 8.3).

The ciliated epithelium can also be identified by contact endoscopy. The dark blue nuclei are round, but the cytoplasmic limits of the cells are not as well defined as in the squamous epithelium. The filamentous structures displaced by the extremity of the contact endoscope are formed by bundles of cilia (Fig 8.4).

The concept of normality will probably be influenced by the introduction of contact endoscopy. The distribution of ciliated epithelium and squamous epithelium can now be assessed '*in vivo*'. How age and exogenous factors affect the distribution of the epithelium on the larynx are questions that are raised when observing contact endoscopy images. The transition zone and the relationship between ciliated and squamous tissues is not always regular and islands of metaplastic squamous epithelium can be observed among ciliated cells.

In the squamous epithelium, contact endoscopy allows the evaluation of the regularity of the cells, dimensions and color of the nucleus, nucleus/cytoplasm ratio, nuclear and cytoplasmic contours, presence of nucleoli, mitosis, cytoplasmic inclusions, keratosis and koilocytes. Contact endoscopy allows the documentation of normal squamous epithelium to patterns specific for pathology,

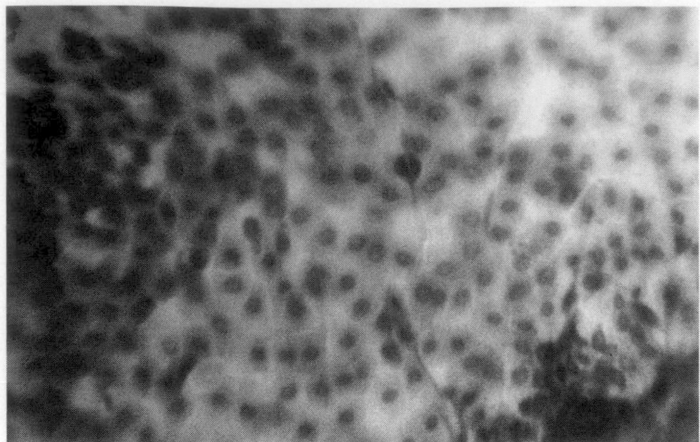

Figure 8.5 *Chronic laryngitis evaluated by contact endoscopy (150×). The squamous epithelium is homogeneous but the nuclei are larger with an increase of the nucleus/cytoplasm ratio.*

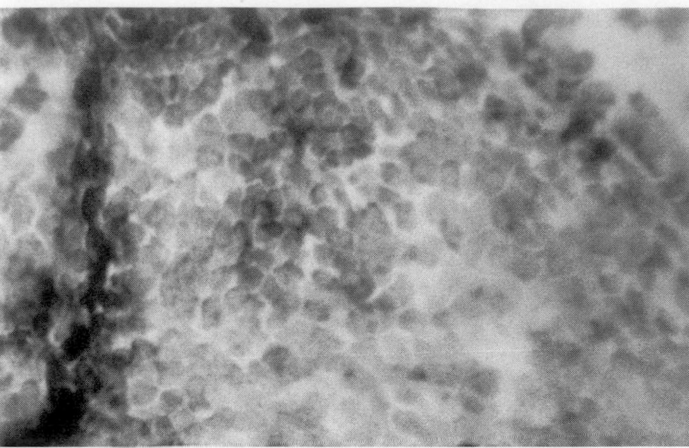

Figure 8.6 *Keratosis shown by contact endoscopy (150×). Cell squamae without nuclei due to keratinization of superficial cells.*

such as chronic laryngitis, keratosis, dysplasia, papilloma and malignant tumors. Furthermore, this technique also permits the observation of the microvascular network of the mucosa.

The present contact laryngoscope allows magnifications of 603 and 1503 to be obtained. However, with the zoom of the camera and digital image enhancement it has been possible to reach higher magnifications (4003 and 6003) in the operating room.

The dynamic migration of the cells toward the surface indicates that most of the pathology of the epithelium has an expression at the superficial layers, being accessible to observation with contact endoscopy. In chronic laryngitis studied by this method, the epithelial pattern is homogeneous, but the nuclei are of larger size, with an increase of the nucleus/cytoplasm ratio. As the cellular turnover is accelerated in the inflammatory reaction, it is possible to visualize immature cells at the surface, similar to those usually present at the intermediate layers of the normal epithelium (Fig 8.5).

Keratosis is easily documented with contact endoscopy because it occurs at the surface of the epithelium, showing distinct stages of keratinization, which can occur simultaneously in the same patient. In the initial stages of keratinization, isolated cells without nuclei are observed. More advanced stages show groups of cells without nuclei but identification of distinct cells still occurs. Furthermore, it is not possible to distinguish limits, and only large areas of amorphous or laminar structure are visible (Fig 8.6).

In some cases of leukoplakia, apart from keratosis, other types and degrees of abnormalities can be identified, such as heterogeneity of cell population with nuclei of different color, size and shape. The variety of images obtained is consistent with the macroscopic concept of leukoplakia, integrating different pathologic alterations such as hyperkeratosis, dysplasia or neoplasia.

Pathologic and cytopathologic correlation has shown that superficial assessment of dysplasia with contact endoscopy may not detect stage I dysplasia. However, those stages of dysplasia that involve the superficial layers are accessible to the contact endoscope. Thus, the more cell abnormalities that are detectable with contact videoendoscopy, the more severe the dysplasia.

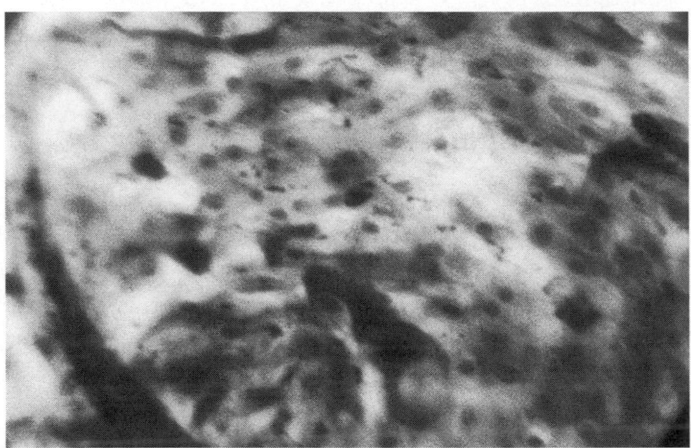

Figure 8.7 *Contact endoscopy (150×). Vocal cord carcinoma. Some nuclear abnormalities are observed: irregular dimensions and staining, irregular shape and prominent nucleolus.*

Most of the histologic and cytologic alterations, required for the diagnosis of dysplasia[16–19,27] can be documented by contact endoscopy, including the presence of severe nuclear abnormalities (size, color and shape), alterations of the nucleus/cytoplasm ratio, dyskaryosis, dyschromasia, and the presence of mitosis and anisokaryosis).

In cancer, contact videoendoscopy shows the irregularity of cell distribution and the extreme heterogeneity of cells (Fig 8.7). The nuclei have different staining properties, size and shape. The nucleus/cytoplasm ratio is very irregular. Nuclear inclusion bodies, prominent nucleoli

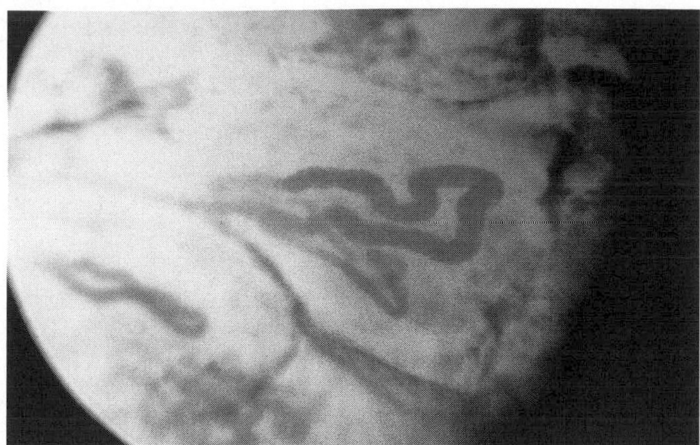

Figure 8.8 *Contact endoscopy (60×). Papilloma of the larynx in which the typical papillar arrangement with newly formed vascular axis is visualized.*

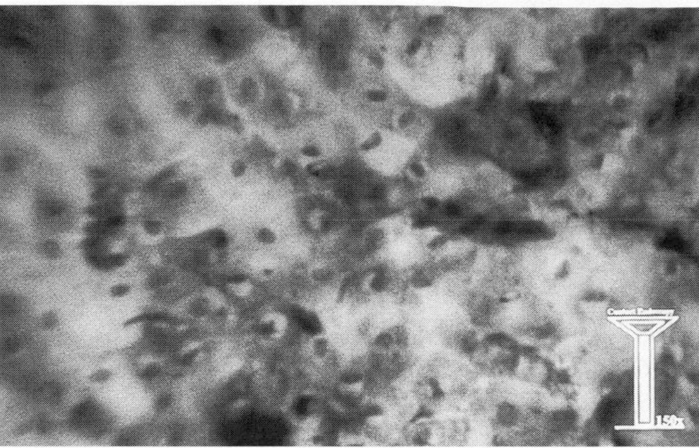

Figure 8.9 *Contact endoscopy (150×). Laryngeal papilloma in which koilocytes (balloon-shaped cells) can be identified.*

and mitosis are sometimes observed. Atypical capillaries with a very irregular pattern are also demonstrated by contact endoscopy.

If the direct demonstration of a tumoral pattern by contact endoscopy in the operating room is already a reality, a much more critical application would be to improve the assessment of transition zones, namely in the early stages, to guide biopsies and to establish safety margins.

In papillomatosis, contact endoscopy allows the visualization of papillae covered by squamous epithelium with a vascular axis (Fig 8.8). The degree of visualization of the vascular structures is determined by the degree of keratosis. In papillomas, koilocytes (balloon-shaped cells) can also be identified (Fig 8.9).

Contact endoscopy reinforces the need to approach the examination of the larynx with a different concept, being not only limited to a lesion but also looking for different stages of a disease. It allows the identification of different aspects of a disease in distinct zones and the transition to the normal epithelium. Contact video endoscopy also permits the *in vivo* observation of the vocal cord vessels, making possible video documentation of their distribution pattern and the microcirculatory dynamics at the laryngeal mucosa.

The goal of contact endoscopy is not to try to observe at the surface what should be seen with classic histologic sections. Neither should it be seen as a substitute for biopsies, but as a clinical method that adds *in vivo* and *in situ* information to the traditional pathologic and/or cytopathologic examinations.

Pathology usually evaluates tissue and cellular alterations at the basal layers of the epithelium whilst cytopathologists analyze abnormal characteristics of individual cells removed from the body. Contact endoscopy offers, on the one hand, a global type of information about the disease, along the superficial layers of the entire mucosa, enabling a mapping of the disease in different sites and stages. On the other hand, it also allows the evaluation of abnormalities at the individual cellular level (*'in vivo'* and *'in situ'* cytology).

Contact endoscopy is still in its first steps of development. Technology, clinical experience and basic science research will all contribute to improve its accuracy. The articulation of clinical observation and pathologic examination will be enhanced, requiring a closer collaboration of the specialists. Both the laryngologist and the pathologist, the cytopathologist and even the molecular biologist will need to be familiar with contact endoscopy. Improvements of the optical systems, new cell dyes and markers, fluorescent products, better techniques of illumination, including lasers of different wavelengths, recording and image processing will certainly occur in the next few years and will contribute to the development of contact endoscopy.

Rigid and contact video endoscopy correspond to a new phase of development in laryngeal endoscopy. Future developments will only be possible with the experience of different specialists and institutions. Clinical application of contact video endoscopy will progress when other territories and specialties adopt the principles of this technique.

Conclusions

Rigid and contact endoscopy of the larynx improve the evaluation of pathology, namely of the early mucosal alterations observed in the endolarynx. Endoscopic procedures in general, including office techniques and microlaryngoscopy, only allow the observation of the larynx along a vertical axis. This has limitations concerning diagnosis, physiopathologic interpretation of diseases, treatment and follow-up.

Rigid endoscopy associated with microlaryngeal surgery (REMS) improves the assessment of the entire endolarynx, including regions considered difficult or even impossible to visualize. The various endoscopes (0°, 30°, 70°, 120°) also allow a multiperspective reconstruction of the lesion and the neighboring regions.

Parameters considered to be important in the evaluation of premalignant and malignant lesions are analyzed in great detail. REMS is also of benefit with benign pathology as present phonosurgery techniques can be modified with a more accurate assessment of the lesion and subsequent excision.

The quality and detail of the information allowed by the REMS technique justify its routine use during microlaryngoscopy or microlaryngeal surgery. Apart from the endoscopes, it does not require any equipment that is not currently available in most institutions.

Contact video endoscopy performed during microlaryngoscopy allows '*in vivo*' and '*in situ*' assessment of the superficial layers of the epithelium, previously stained with methylene blue. With the magnifications permitted with this technique (603, 1503) there is direct access to the cells and their characteristics. Several parameters are evaluated – regularity of the epithelium, dimensions and color of the nucleus, nucleus/cytoplasm ratio, nucleus and cytoplasm contours, presence of nucleolus, mitosis, cytoplasmic inclusions, keratosis, koilocytes, inflammatory infiltrates.

Specific cellular epithelial patterns have already been defined in contact endoscopy: chronic laryngitis, keratosis, dysplasia, papilloma and malignant tumor. Studies have to be continued to establish the normal characteristics and distribution of the epithelium in the face of several factors and to define its clinical role in combination with pathologic and cytopathologic examinations.

Contact endoscopy offers a global type of information about disease along the superficial layers of the entire mucosa, mapping the disease in different sites and in different stages. On the other hand, it also permits the evaluation *in situ* of abnormalities at the individual cellular level.

The accuracy of contact endoscopy will certainly be enhanced with improvements in the optical system, new cell dyes and markers, fluorescent products, distinct lighting and better imaging techniques.

Rigid and contact endoscopy represent a new phase in the development of laryngeal endoscopy. With experience from different centers and technologic progress, new ideas, concepts and instruments will occur. If all this progress facilitates a more thorough examination of the larynx, it will also require a more profound knowledge and understanding of the larynx, and an intense interdisciplinary work.

References

1. Andrea M. *Vascularização arterial da laringe, distribuição macro e micro vascular.* PhD thesis, University of Lisbon, Lisbon, Portugal, 1975.
2. Andrea M. Vasculature of the anterior commissure. *Ann Otol* 1981; **90:** 18–20.
3. Andrea M, Dias O. La endoscopia rigida y de contacto asociada a la microcirugia laringea. In: Alvarez Vicente J, Sacristan Alonso T, eds. *Ponência de la Sociedad Española de ORL y Patologia Cervico-Facial.* Barcelona: Farma Cusi, 1995: 140–8.
4. Andrea M, Dias O. *Atlas of Rigid and Contact Endoscopy in Microlaryngeal Surgery.* Philadelphia: Lippincott-Raven, 1995.
5. Andrea M, Dias O. Rigid and contact endoscopy associated to microlaryngeal surgery. In: Fried M, ed. *The Larynx: a Multidisciplinary Approach,* 2nd edn. St Louis: Mosby, 1996: 75–9.
6. Andrea M, Dias O. Endoscopic assessment of early vocal cord cancer. In: Shah JP, Johnson JT, eds. *Proceedings of the 4th International Conference on Head and Neck Cancer.* Toronto, 1996: 268–73.
7. Andrea M, Dias O. Rigid and contact endoscopy during microsurgery. In: Yanagisawa E, ed. *Color Atlas of Diagnostic Endoscopy in Otorhinolaryngology.* New York: Igaku Shoin, 1997: 168–73.
8. Andrea M, Dias O. Newer techniques of laryngeal assessment. In: Cummings CW, Fredrickson JM, Harker LA, Krause CJ, Schuller DE, eds. *Otolaryngology – Head and Neck Surgery,* 3rd edn. St Louis: Mosby, 1998: 1967–78.
9. Andrea M, Guerrier Y. The anterior commissure of the larynx. *Clin Otolaryngol* 1981; **6:** 259–64.
10. Andrea M, Dias O, Paço J. Endoscopic anatomy of the larynx. *Curr Opin Otolaryngol Head Neck Surg* 1994; **2:** 271–5.
11. Andrea M, Dias O, Santos A. Contact endoscopy during microlaryngeal surgery. A new technique for endoscopic examination of the larynx. *Ann Otol Rhinol Laryngol* 1995; **104:** 333–9.
12. Andrea M, Dias O, Santos A. Contact endoscopy of the vocal cord. Normal and pathological patterns. *Acta Otolaryngol (Stockh)* 1995; **115:** 314–16.
13. Andrea M, Paço J, Guerrier Y. L'Epiglotte et ses amarrages. *Cahiers ORL* 1979; **14:** 793–803.
14. Andrea M, Dias O, Paço J, Santos A. Vocal cord assessment. Rigid and contact endoscopy associated to microlaryngeal surgery. In: Smee R, Bridger G, eds. *Laryngeal Cancer. Proceedings of 2nd World Congress on Laryngeal Cancer, Sydney.* Amsterdam: Elsevier, 1994: 233–5.
15. Benjamin B. *Diagnostic Laryngology – Adults and Children.* Philadelphia: Saunders, 1990.
16. Crissman JD. Pathology of the upper aerodigestive tract mucosa. In: Paparella M, Shumrick D, Gluckman J, Meyerhoff W, eds. *Otolaryngology. Vol. 3. Head and Neck,* 3rd edn. Philadelphia: Saunders, 1991: 495–508.
17. DeMay R. *The Art and Science of Cytopathology – Aspiration Cytology.* Chicago: ASCP Press, 1996.
18. DeMay R. *The Art and Science of Cytopathology – Exfoliative Cytology.* Chicago: ASCP Press, 1996.
19. Ferlito A. *Neoplasms of the Larynx.* Edinburgh: Churchill Livingstone, 1993.
20. Guerrier Y, Andrea M. Microvascularization de la muqueuse laryngée et trachéale – introduction à la physiopathologie des lésions sténosantes. *Ann Oto-laryngol Chir Cervicofac* 1980; **97:** 409–21.
21. Hamou JE. *Hysteroscopy and Microcolpohysteroscopy. Text and Atlas.* Norwalk: Appleton & Lange, 1991.

22. Kantor E, Berci G, Partlow E, Paz-Partlow M. A completely new approach in microlaryngeal surgery. *Laryngoscope* 1991; **101**: 676–9.
23. Kashima HK. Bilateral vocal fold motion impairment: pathophysiology and management by transverse cordotomy. *Ann Otol Rhinol Laryngol* 1991; **100**: 717–21.
24. Kleinsasser O. *Tumors of the Larynx and Hypopharynx*. Stuttgart: Thieme, 1988.
25. Kleinsasser O. *Microlaryngoscopy and Endolaryngeal Microsurgery*, 3rd edn. Philadelphia: Hanley & Belfus, 1991.
26. Lehmann W, Pidoux J, Widmann J. *Larynx Microlaryngoscopie et Histopathologie*. Cadempino: Inpharzam Medical Publications, 1981.
27. McGee J. *Oxford Textbook of Pathology*. New York: Oxford University Press, 1992.
28. Yanagisawa E, Horowitz JB, Yanagisawa K, Mambrino LJ. Comparison of new telescopic video microlaryngoscopic and standard microlaryngoscopic techniques. *Ann Otol Rhinol Laryngol* 1992; **101**: 51–60.

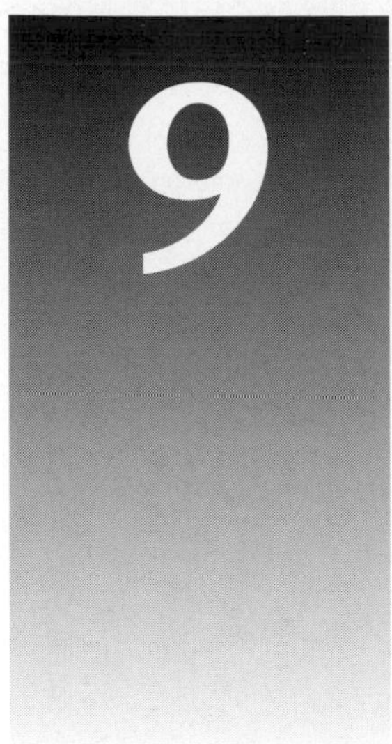

Videostroboscopy

Minoru Hirano

To modern laryngological practice, videostroboscopic examination of the larynx should be one of the essential procedures.[1,2] The key event in phonation is vibration of the vocal folds. The vibratory pattern of the vocal folds is one of the most important and crucial determinants of the voice signal. Abnormal voices are always accompanied by abnormal vibratory patterns of the vocal folds. Examination of the vibratory behavior of the vocal folds, therefore, is necessary and essential to determine the cause and mechanism of abnormal voices. Videostroboscopy is the only existing technique to examine vocal fold vibration routinely in a clinical setup.

It is strongly advised that the videostroboscopic unit is placed in the otolaryngological office so that the examination can be performed routinely as an office procedure for patients with laryngeal pathologies and/or voice problems. Videostroboscopy in laryngological practice is equivalent to microscopy in otological practice.

Principle

Stroboscopic light sources emit intermittent flashes of light synchronously with successive cycles of vocal fold vibrations. The waveform of the examinee's voice signal picked up with a microphone triggers the stroboscopic light source. When the frequency of the light flashes is the same as that of the vocal fold vibration, one can observe a clear still image of the vocal folds at a given phase point, provided that the vibrations are periodical (Fig 9.1a). When the frequency of the flashes is slightly less than that of the vocal fold vibration, causing a systematic phase delay of the consecutive light flashes, a slow motion effect is obtained (Fig 9.1b). Stroboscopy does not demonstrate fine details of each individual vibratory cycle, but it shows a vibratory behavior averaged over many successive vibratory cycles. If successive vocal fold vibrations take place periodically and the vibratory mode is entirely uniform, the stroboscopic images demonstrate exactly the slow motion images of each vibratory cycle like images of ultra-high-speed photography. However, even in normal human beings, vocal fold vibrations are aperiodical to a greater or lesser extent. There are minor cycle-to-cycle perturbations in period, amplitude and mode of vibration. In this sense, stroboscopy is a crude evaluation. Nevertheless, it is extremely useful for clinical purposes.

(a)

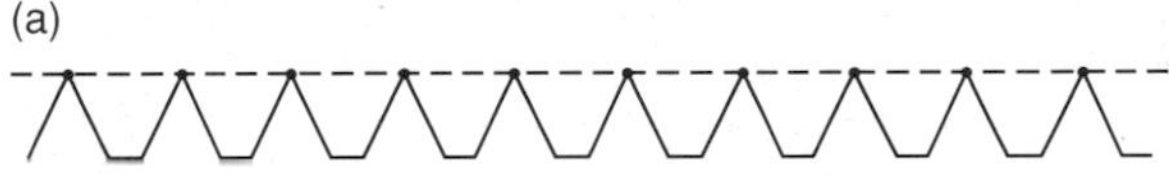

(b)

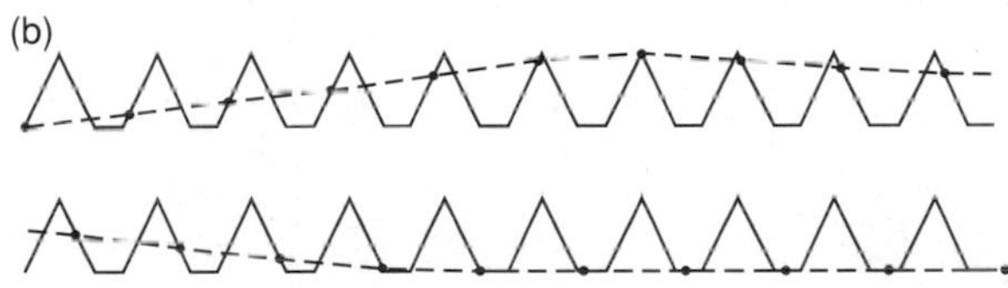

Figure 9.1 *Schematic presentation of the principle of stroboscopy. (Reproduced with permission from reference 1)*

Instrumentation

A videostroboscopic instrument basically consists of a stroboscopic unit, an endoscope, a video camera and a

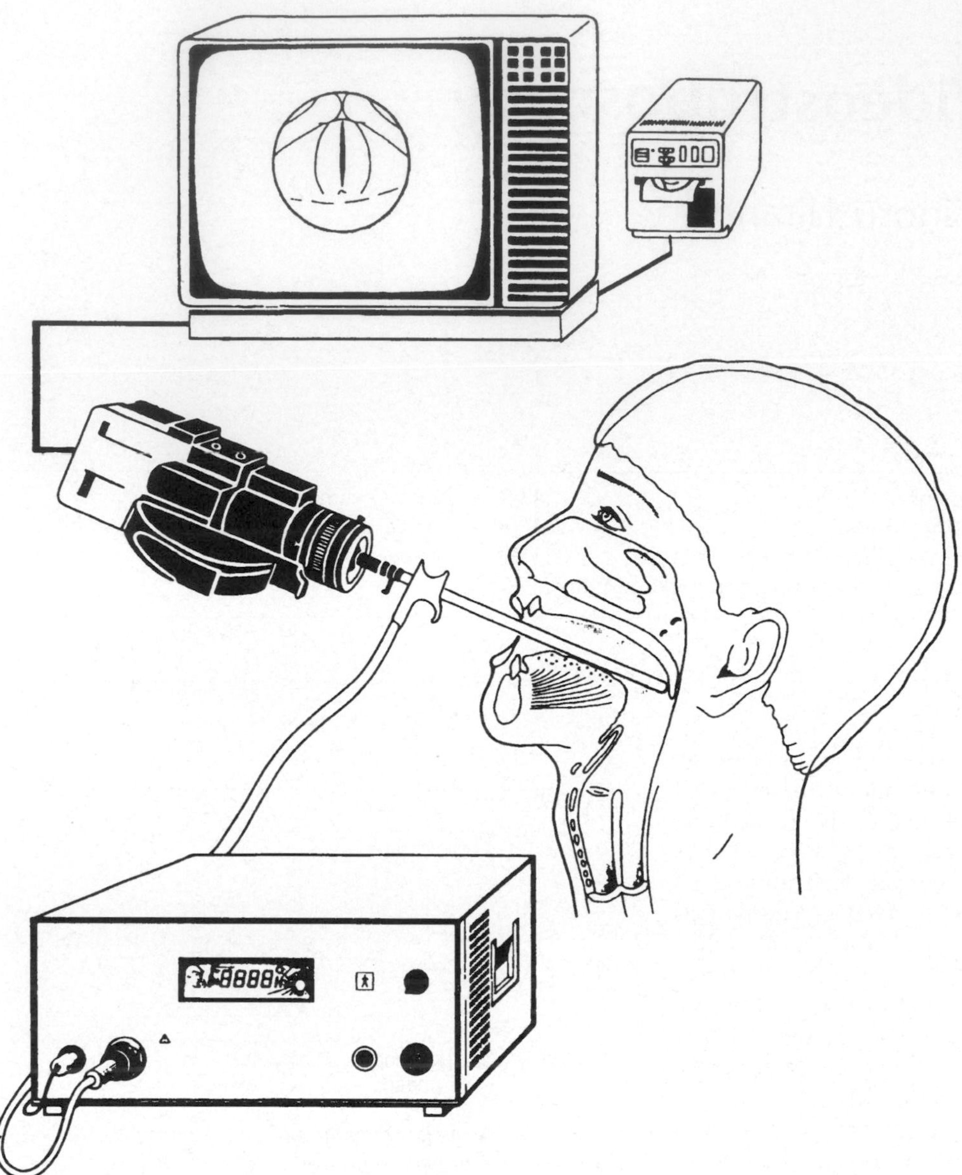

Figure 9.2 *An example of videostroboscopic system. (Reproduced with permission by Singular Publishing Group, Inc. from reference 2).*

video recorder (Fig 9.2). They are all commercially available. Two types of endoscopes, i.e. rigid telescopes and flexible fiberscopes, can be used. The use of flexible fiberscopes, however, can produce good video images only when a very bright video camera, for example the Hitachi DK-5050 three-tube camera, is employed. Rigid telescopes yield good images even with many types of chip camera or single tube camera. For those patients with a narrow supraglottis, the use of a fiberscope is required to examine the vocal folds in detail.

Normal vibratory movements

Figure 9.3 schematically demonstrates normal movements of the vocal fold during one vibratory cycle in modal register. The vibratory cycle normally consists of three phases as shown in Fig 9.4:

- the opening phase in which the vocal fold edges move laterally;
- the closing phase in which the vocal fold edges move medially; and
- the closed phase in which the bilateral vocal folds are in contact with each other.

Typically, two wave peaks emerge on the vocal folds during vibration. They are called the upper and lower lips. The two lips are not structures that are placed at consistent locations of the vocal fold but they are the peaks of traveling waves on the vocal fold mucosa. The occurrence of traveling waves is a very important phenomenon for normal vocal fold vibrations.

At the very end of the closed phase, the vocal folds are in contact with each other at the upper lip (Fig 9.3a). During the early stage of the opening phase, the entire

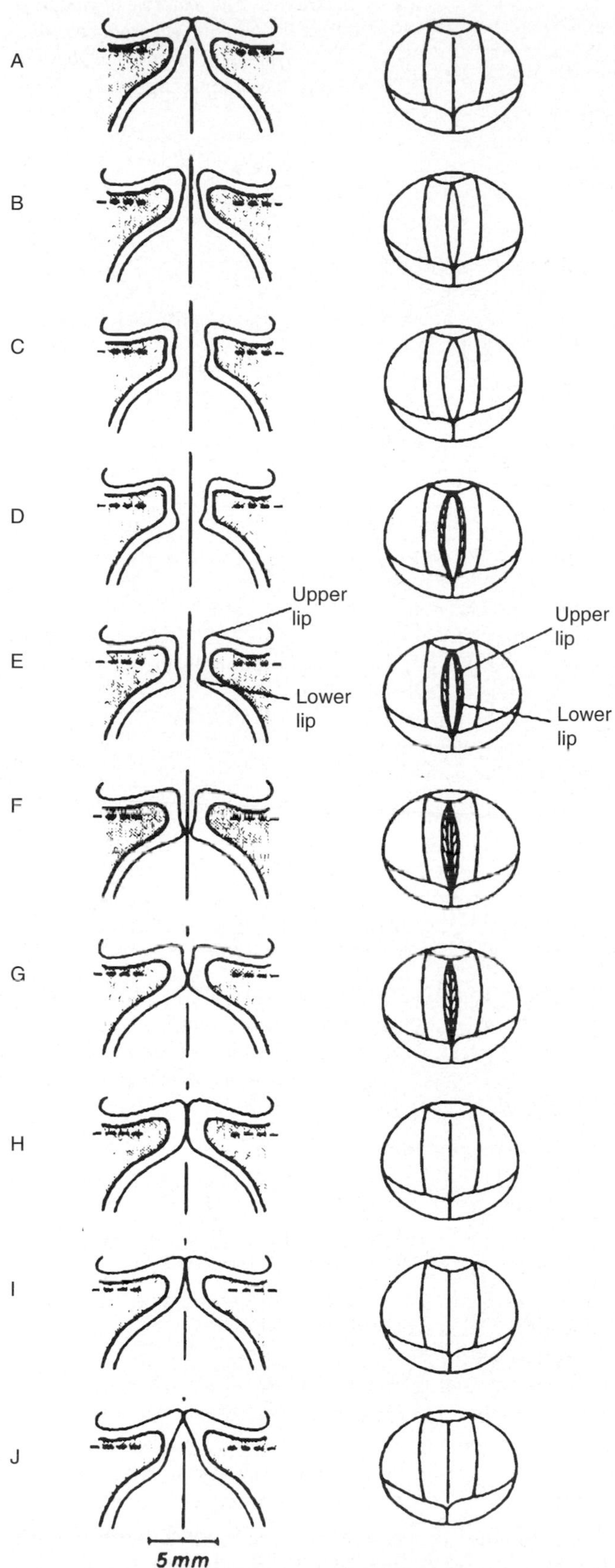

Figure 9.3 *Schematic presentation of normal vocal fold vibration. (Reproduced with permission from reference 1).*

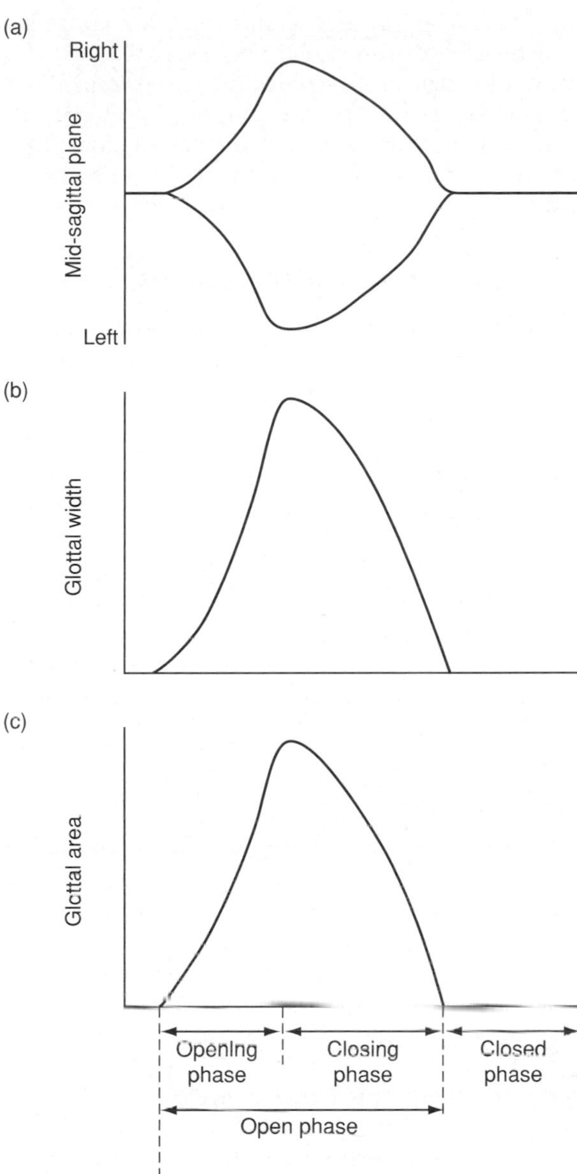

Figure 9.4 *Phases in one vibratory cycle: (a) horizontal excursion; (b) glottal width; (c) glottal area. (Reproduced with permission from reference 1).*

vocal fold moves laterally (Fig 9.3b). At the maximum opening the upper and lower lips are lined up on the same sagittal plane (Fig 9.3c). In the beginning stage of the closing phase, the lower lips start moving medially while the upper lips still keep moving laterally (Fig 9.3d). During the later stage of the closing phase, both lips move medially (Figs 9.3e,f). The lower lips usually meet earlier than the upper lips at the beginning of the closed phase (Fig 9.3g). In the early stage of the closed phase, the contact area of the two vocal folds increases (Fig 9.3h). Following the maximum contact, the vocal folds start separating from each other from the bottom portion

(Fig. 9.3i). The top portion separates from the contralateral side at the end of the closed phase (Fig 9.3j).

The vocal fold edge stroboscopically viewed from above varies. Usually, it is the tip of the upper lip at the late stage of the closed phase and during the opening phase whereas it is the tip of the lower lip during the closing phase and at the beginning of the closed phase.

Parameters for stroboscopic examination

The parameters evaluated during stroboscopic examinations are as follows:

Fundamental frequency (F0)

F0 is shown on the F0 indicator embedded in stroboscopes.

Symmetry of vibratory movements of the vocal folds

It should be checked whether or not the vibratory movements of the bilateral vocal folds are symmetrical. Normally they move symmetrically. When movements of bilateral vocal folds are asymmetrical, the asymmetry should be described in terms of amplitude and phase.

Regularity or periodicity of successive vibrations

The regularity or periodicity implies how uniform the successive vibratory movements are. Normally they look uniform under stroboscopy and are labeled as regular or periodic. When the vibratory behavior differs from cycle to cycle, the vibrations are labeled irregular or aperiodic.

Glottic closure

Whether or not the glottis closes completely during the vibratory cycle should be checked. Normally it closes at the intermembranous portion. At the intercartilaginous portion, the glottis closes completely in many normal subjects but it does not always close completely in some normal people.

Amplitude

The maximum amplitude of the lateral excursion of the edges of the vocal folds is evaluated subjectively and qualitatively. Typically, the amplitude is approximately one-third of the width of the vocal fold for the normal modal voice. The amplitude evaluated should be described as 'greater than normal', 'normal', 'smaller than normal', or 'zero'. Differences in the amplitude of the two vocal folds are also checked and described.

Table 9.1 A form for videostroboscopic findings

Fundamental frequency (Hz)

Symmetry
1. Symmetrical
2. Asymmetrical
   (a) in amplitude (+,–)
   (b) in phase (+,–)

Regularity (periodicity)
1. Regular (periodic)
2. Inconsistent (sometimes regular, sometimes irregular)
3. Irregular (aperiodic)

Glottic closure
1. Complete
2. Inconsistent (sometimes complete, sometimes incomplete)
3. Incomplete
   (a) along entire length
   (b) spindle shape
   (c) sandglass shape
   (d) irregular shape
   (e) anterior portion
   (f) posterior portion of intermembranous glottis
   (g) intercartilaginous portion
   (h) (f) and (g)
   (i) others; specify

Amplitude
1. Right: (1) great, (2) normal, (3) small, (4) zero
   Lesion: (1) great, (2) normal, (3) small, (4) zero
2. Left: (1) great, (2) normal, (3) small, (4) zero
   Lesion: (1) great, (2) normal, (3) small, (4) zero

(1) RightLeft, (2) RightLeft, (3) RightLeft

Mucosal wave
1. Right: (1) great, (2) normal, (3) small, (4) zero
   Lesion: (1) great, (2) normal, (3) small, (4) zero
2. Left: (1) great, (2) normal, (3) small, (4) zero
   Lesion: (1) great, (2) normal, (3) small, (4) zero

(1) RightLeft, (2) RightLeft, (3) RightLeft

Nonvibrating portion
1. Right: (1) none, (2) occasionally partially, (3) always partially, (4) occasionally entirely, (5) always entirely
2. Left: (1) none, (2) occasionally partially, (3) always partially, (4) occasionally entirely, (5) always entirely

Other findings
1. None
2. Noted; specify:

Mucosal wave

The wave that travels on the vocal fold mucosa during vibration is called mucosal wave. The occurrence of mucosal wave is a very important sign of the existence of normal pliable mucosa. The size and extent of the mucosal wave are evaluated subjectively and qualitatively and described as 'greater than normal', 'normal', 'smaller than normal', or 'absent'. Differences in the mucosal wave between the two vocal folds are also described.

Nonvibrating portion

Whether or not there is any portion of the vocal fold that does not move should be checked, in other words, that remains still during phonation. The absence of vibratory movement can occur either occasionally or always, and either partially or entirely.

Other findings

If there are any other findings, they should be described. Table 9.1 shows an example of a form for videostroboscopic findings.

Normal variations

The vibratory pattern of normal vocal fold varies significantly depending on the F0 and sound pressure level (SPL) of phonation, vocal register and mode of phonation. There are the following general tendencies:

- As the F0 increases, the amplitude of vibration, mucosal wave and the ratio of the closed phase to the entire cycle decrease.
- As the SPL increases, the amplitude, mucosal wave and relative duration of the closed phase against the entire cycle increase.
- In the falsetto or light register, the amplitude is small, mucosal wave is absent, and the intermembranous portion of the glottis does not completely close.
- Strained or hyperfunctional phonation results in a long closed phase whereas asthenic or hypofunctional phonation causes a short or no closed phase.

Typical vibratory pattern in varying diseases

Any specific disease or pathology of the phonatory organ does not always result in a given vibratory pattern. The vibratory behavior is determined not only by the disease itself, but also by the location, size, degree, extent and histopathologic characteristics of the disease and the phonatory mode including compensatory efforts. There are, however, general tendencies of vibratory behavior deviations caused by a given disease. Typical vibratory patterns for varying diseases are described here.

Acute catarrhal laryngitis

When an edematous lesion is dominant, aperiodic vibrations result. When cell infiltration and capillary dilatation are the dominant features, the amplitude of vibration and mucosal wave are small.

Chronic catarrhal laryngitis

Abnormality in vibratory behavior is frequently minimum. The vibratory amplitude and mucosal wave tend to be decreased.

Subepithelial bleeding of the vocal fold

The lesion is often unilateral. The vibratory amplitude and mucosal wave of the affected portion are small or absent. Consequently, the vibratory movements of the two vocal folds are asymmetrical.

Vocal fold nodules

Vocal fold nodules usually occur bilaterally in a roughly symmetrical fashion. The glottic closure during vibration is incomplete, presenting with an hourglass-shape glottic chink at the maximum closure. The amplitude of vibration is usually decreased. The mucosal wave on the nodule varies: when the nodule is edematous the mucosal wave is normal or slightly small at the nodule, but it is markedly reduced or absent when the nodule is histologically fibrous.

Vocal fold polyps

Vocal fold polyps are developed unilaterally or bilaterally. Unilateral lesions are more frequent than bilateral lesions. Bilateral lesions are usually asymmetrical in size and shape. The glottic closure is incomplete, presenting with gaps anterior and posterior to the polyp during maximum closure. The vocal folds show asymmetrical vibratory movements. Successive vibrations are often irregular or aperiodic. The amplitude of vibration is small or zero at the polyp and it is more or less reduced at the unaffected portion of the vocal fold. The mucosal wave on the polyp varies. It is usually absent when the polyp is histologically fibrous or hemorrhagic whereas, when the polyp is edematous and pliable, mucosal wave emerges to varying extents.

Reinke's edema

Reinke's edema is usually developed bilaterally but the lesions are often asymmetrical. A complete glottic closure takes place during vibration. The vibratory movements of the two vocal folds are frequently asymmetrical and successive vibrations are often aperiodic. The amplitude of vibration is usually small. The mucosal wave is great when the tissue is edematous, whereas it is small when the tissue is gelatinous.

Vocal fold cysts

The majority of vocal fold cysts are unilateral but some are bilateral. Glottic closure is usually incomplete during vibration. Small glottic gaps are noted anterior and posterior to the cyst during maximum glottic closure unless the cyst is very small. The vibratory movements of the two vocal folds are asymmetrical and successive vibrations are occasionally irregular. The amplitude of vibration is small on the affected side. No mucosal wave takes place on the cyst. The lack of mucosal wave is an important videostroboscopic sign to differentiate a cyst from a nodule and a small whitish polyp. A very small cyst is often overlooked without videostroboscopy. In such a case, a diagnosis of 'functional dysphonia' tends to be given.

Sulcus vocalis

Sulcus vocalis is defined as a condition in which a furrow along the vocal fold edge causes voice disorders. Bilateral lesions are more frequent than a unilateral lesion. Glottic closure is incomplete, presenting with a narrow spindle-shaped gap at the maximum closure. Cases with bilateral sulci usually display symmetrical vibratory movements. The vibratory amplitude is small. The mucosal wave is interrupted at the sulcus.

Vocal fold scar

Scar tissue is much stiffer than the normal vocal fold mucosa. The vibratory behavior varies greatly depending upon the extent of scarring. In general, the amplitude of vibration is small or zero and the mucosal wave is absent at the affected portion. A small scar can be clinically detected only with the videostroboscopic examination.

Epithelial hyperplasia/dysplasia of the vocal fold

Epithelial hyperplasia/dysplasia is developed unilaterally or bilaterally. It originates from the epithelium and enters the superficial layer of the lamina propria or Reinke's space but never involves the vocal ligament. The glottic closure is incomplete in many cases, especially when the vocal fold edge is involved. Vibratory movements of the bilateral vocal folds are often asymmetrical and successive vibrations are frequently irregular. The amplitude of vibration is reduced and the mucosal wave is absent at the affected site. The neighboring normal mucosa, however, presents with mucosal wave. The affected portion moves like a wooden board floating on waves.

Glottic carcinoma

Carcinomatous tissue is much stiffer than the normal vocal fold mucosa. This fact is reflected in the vibratory behavior clearly and facilitates early diagnosis of carcinoma, early detection of recurrence following radiotherapy and determination of the extension of subepithelial invasion.

The vibratory amplitude is small or zero and no mucosal wave takes place at the lesion. The lack of mucosal wave is a very important sign to suspect very early carcinoma. The mucosal wave should be carefully checked not only at the site of the lesion but also at the neighboring areas where the surface of the mucosa looks normal under regular light. In general, the neighboring area shows mucosal wave when there is no subepithelial carcinomatous invasion but it lacks mucosal wave when subepithelial involvement is present. Videostroboscopy is, therefore, useful to estimate the extent of subepithelial invasion. This may not be clinically very valuable when radiotherapy is employed because the entire vocal fold is usually irradiated. However, the estimation of the extent of subepithelial invasion is very important when microscopic laser surgery is chosen, in order to have a sufficient but minimum removal.

The glottic closure during vibrations is often incomplete, the bilateral vocal folds usually show asymmetrical vibrations, and successive vibrations are irregular.

Papilloma of the vocal fold

The papillomatous tissue is also much stiffer than the tissue of normal vocal fold mucosa. The vibratory behavior of a vocal fold with papilloma is basically the same as that with carcinoma.

Vocal fold paralysis

Unilateral paralysis is more frequent than bilateral paralysis.

In most cases with unilateral paralysis, the glottic closure is incomplete along the entire length, the two vocal folds show asymmetrical vibratory movements, and successive vibrations are irregular. The vibratory amplitude of the affected vocal fold varies. The mucosal wave is often reduced or absent. The lack of mucosal wave is attributed partly to the incomplete glottic closure, which interferes with a buildup of effective air pressure, and partly to the lack of the tonus of the vocalis muscle. The size of the mucosal wave, therefore, reflects the degree of muscular tonus to a certain extent.

Functional dysphonia

Videostroboscopy does not give any evidence to specify functional dysphonia. However, it is necessary in order to exclude very minor organic lesions before a diagnosis of functional dysphonia is given. Especially, small cyst, sulcus, localized minor scarring, localized small epithelial hyperplasia/dysplasia, and very early carcinoma have to be excluded with the use of videostroboscopy whenever one makes a diagnosis of functional dysphonia. They are apt to be overlooked under the routine laryngeal inspection with regular light.

References

1. Hirano M. *Clinical Examination of Voice.* Wien: Springer-Verlag, 1981.
2. Hirano M, Bless DM. *Videostroboscopic Examination of the Larynx.* San Diego: Singular Publishing Group, 1993.

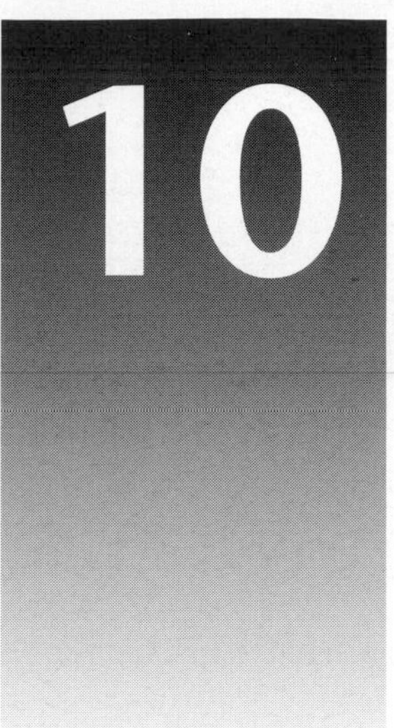

Laryngeal electromyography

Andrew Blitzer

Electromyography (EMG) is a technique to evaluate the electrical activity (micropotentials) of the neuromuscular junction. The motor unit potential (MUP) is the basic electrophysiological component of striated muscle and represents the summation of all the single muscle fiber potentials that make up the single motor unit. This represents individual motor axons within the nerve innervating the muscle in which the electrode is placed. The electromyogram can help decipher a disorder's central signal, faulty axonal transmission, abnormal neurotransmitter release or aberrant muscle response which produces a discoordinated, weak or absent muscle contraction.[22]

Laryngeal EMG was first established by Faaborg-Andersen,[10] Faaborg-Andersen and Buchthal[11] and Buchthal[7] as a useful diagnostic test. They used indirect insertion techniques of concentric electrodes and described MUPs for the laryngeal muscles ranging in amplitude from 224 to 358 µV. They found a mean duration of MUPs of 3.5–5.3 ms. These recordings were made during respiration and speaking. The maximal activity was measured during loud phonation, high potential glide, effort closure and cough. These are smaller values than is seen with monopolar electrodes.

It is often difficult to measure spontaneous activity in the laryngeal muscles because complete silence is difficult to achieve since the muscles are active during respiration. Spontaneous activity is much more clearly identified in limb muscles, where complete relaxation and electrical silence may be achieved. The spontaneous activity (fibrillation and fasciculation potentials) is characteristic of denervation and there is usually an associated decreased amplitude and number of MUPs. Fibrillation potentials are biphasic waves with an initial positive sharp deflection of 50–150 µV and a short duration of 0.5–2 ms. A positive sharp wave is also biphasic with an initial positive deflection, a variable amplitude, and a long, low, negative phase of 1–10 ms (Figs 10.1, 10.2).[21,22]

Figure 10.1 *A laryngeal EMG recording of the thyroarytenoid muscle in a patient with vocal fold paralysis, showing a fibrillation potential (spontaneous activity) suggestive of denervation.*

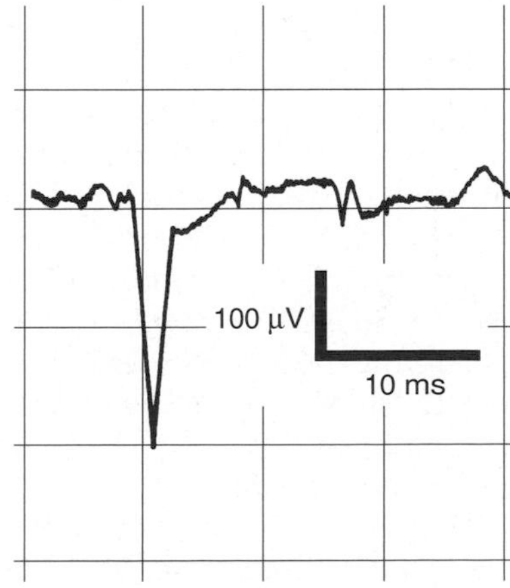

Figure 10.2 *A laryngeal EMG recording of the thyroarytenoid muscle in a patient with vocal fold paralysis, showing a positive sharp wave (spontaneous activity) suggestive of denervation.*

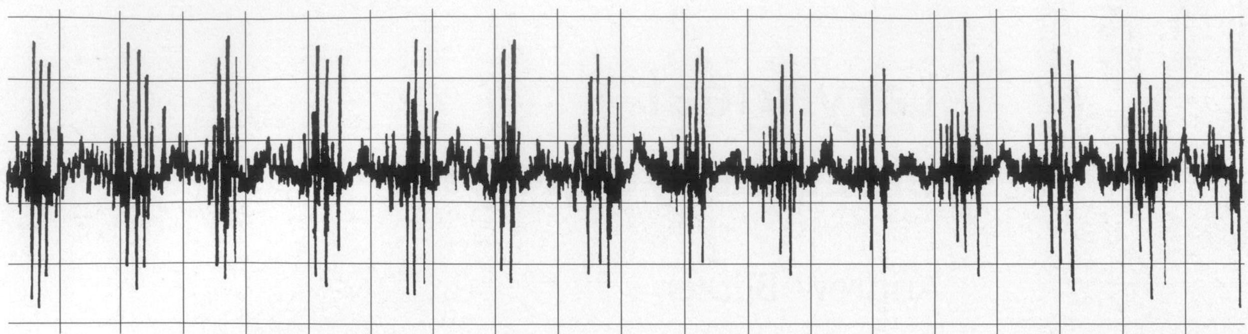

Figure 10.3 *A laryngeal EMG recording of the thyroarytenoid muscle showing complex and repetitive, time-locked discharges in a patient with essential tremor (scale 500 μV and 200 ms).*

Complex and repetitive discharges may be time-locked to similar discharges in other muscles which is characteristic of myoclonus. These tend to be slow, regular, and repetitive at 4–5 Hz. In other cases there may be MUPs which have periodic changes in amplitude and intensity which is characteristic of tremor. In contrast, myopathic conditions usually have small and fragmented MUPs of short duration, and low amplitude. Complex polyphasic potentials of long duration and large amplitude are suggestive of reinnervation, whereas potentials with normal form but an abnormal firing pattern are usually associated with central disease (Fig 10.3).[21,22,25]

A number of different techniques have been described to measure the electromyographic patterns of the larynx. The least sensitive is the use of surface electrodes which measure a large number of MUPs due to the distance from the motor end plates, and the recordings lack specificity.[16,22,28] Fujita *et al.*[12] and Rea[27] described a technique of utilizing bipolar surface electrodes in a feeding tube to measure the electrical activity of the posterior cricoarytenoid muscles. The feeding tube is inserted nasally and passed to the level of the cricopharyngeus muscle. The surface electrodes are held against the mucosa overlying the posterior cricoarytenoid (PCA) muscles. The tube can be moved to different positions to sample different areas of the PCA muscle. This technique is well tolerated and is non-invasive. Because it is a surface electrode sample, it is not accurate for assessing parameters such as individual motor unit potentials. A multiple surface electrode recording technique has been described by Boemke *et al.*;[6] however, a great variation in motor unit morphology recording may be found in the same patient. This technique is therefore not very useful for electromyographic diagnostic studies, but could be valuable for follow-up examinations of patients who are recovering from a laryngeal muscle paresis.

To increase the accuracy of the recordings of motor unit potentials, more invasive techniques are necessary. Either monopolar or concentric needles can be used to impale the muscle and allow recordings of the MUPs adjacent to the needle. The concentric needles offer the narrowest recording area with the greatest specificity. This allows for single unit potential waveform analysis. Monopolar or bipolar hooked-wire electrodes can also be used to allow multiple recordings from the same area, to sample multiple muscles, or do quantitative electromyography. The limitation is that the sampling is always from the same small area within the muscle. The needles can be placed perorally either by direct laryngoscopy or through an indirect technique. A direct percutaneous technique is most frequently used to place either monopolar, concentric or hooked-wire electrodes.[1,2,13,17,22]

We perform the percutaneous technique with the patient in the recumbent position, with the neck slightly extended. The thyroid and cricoid cartilages are palpated and used as landmarks. Local anesthesia is not used, since the procedure is relatively painless and the local anesthetic may produce an artifact in the recordings by decreasing the numbers and amplitude of the MUPs. A ground electrode is generally placed over the sternum, and a reference lead is placed over the cheek.[2,22]

Generally, anesthesia is not used in needle placement, since it may alter the recording parameters. However, topical anesthesia may be necessary in some patients who have an active gag or cough reflex, which also may interfere with proper recordings.

There are a number of factors that may alter the size, number and morphology of the MUPs found on EMG, including the muscle size, the age of the patient, and the prior activity of the muscle. Elevation of muscle temperature may also lead to change, often with numbers of polyphasic potentials.[2,22]

Since the EMG recording is state-dependent, spontaneous rest potentials are recorded as well as those produced during phonation. The normative data has been published using percutaneous needle insertion. The phase of the MUP is related to the potential recording crossing the baseline. The rise time of acceptable MUPs with this technique is shorter than 100 μs from the main spike, and selection is by a sharp or crisp sound on the audio system. The amplitude is measured only from consistently repeating MUPs and is measured from peak to peak. The maximum amplitude is measured on maximum phonation. Rest is difficult to achieve in the larynx because of

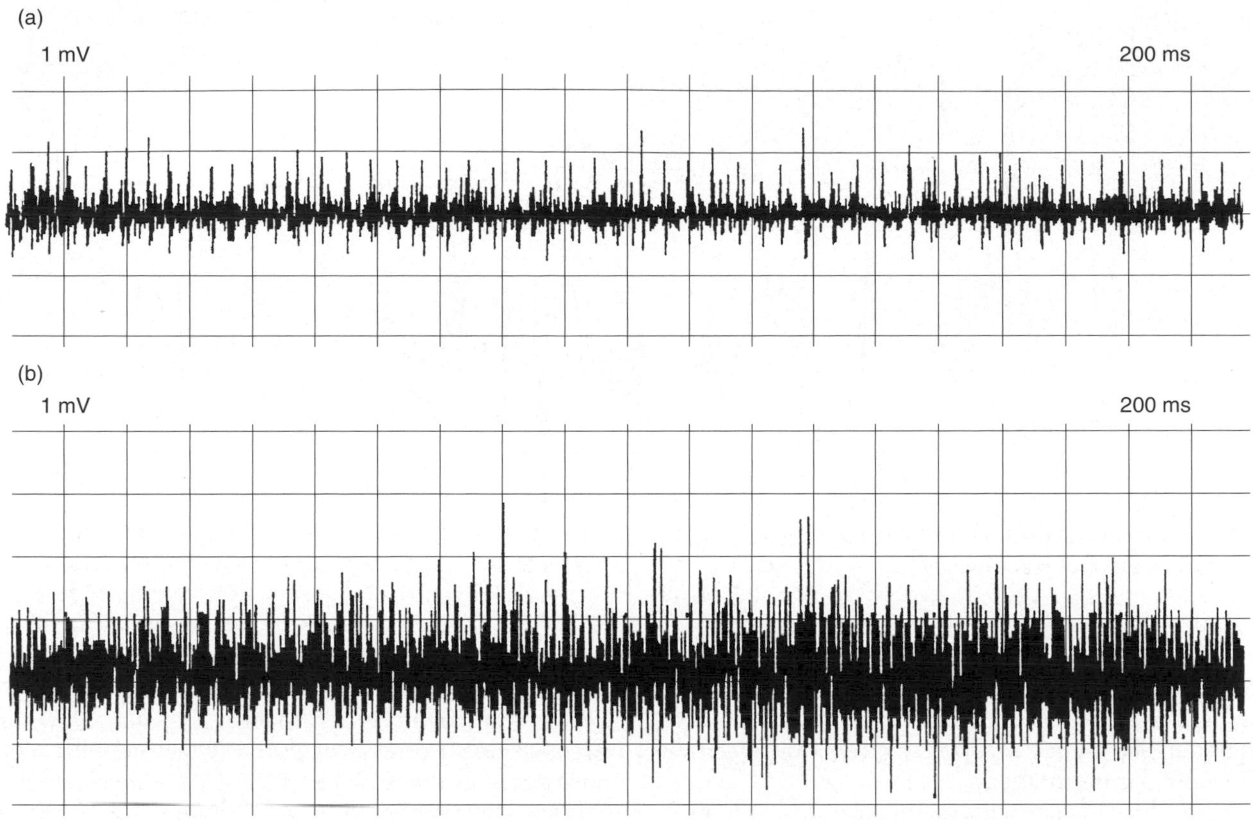

Figure 10.4 *(a) A laryngeal EMG recording of the thyroarytenoid muscle showing a normal interference pattern. (b) A laryngeal EMG recording of the thyroarytenoid muscle in a patient with vocal fold immobility showing a reduced, 'picket-fence' interference pattern (paresis).*

respiratory activity, but in relatively quiet periods abnormal spontaneous activity (fibrillations and positive sharp waves) can be identified.[7,10–12,22]

In order to study both components of the vagal innervation, both cricothyroid (CT) and both thyroarytenoid (TA) muscles are tested and compared. The PCA muscles may also be tested for an analysis of abductor signal. The EMG study is performed by passing a monopolar or concentric needle electrode through the skin overlying the CT membrane. The needle electrode is passed along the cricoid cartilage superiorly and laterally until electrical activity is identified on the EMG tracing. The patient is asked to turn and raise the head to assure that the needle is not in the strap muscles. The patient is asked to say /i/ in a high pitch to tense the CT muscle, and a burst of electrical activity will be seen.[2]

The thyroarytenoid–vocalis muscle complex, innervated by the recurrent laryngeal nerve, is tested utilizing a midline, percutaneous technique. The needle is then passed through the cricothyroid membrane and advanced superiorly and laterally until it impales the muscle. On muscle insertion, sharp sounding potentials are identified on the EMG tracing. The TA muscle complex usually has continuous motor activity during phonation. Simple manipulation of the needle allows sampling in multiple sites within the muscle.[2,22]

The potentials seen immediately after needle insertion should not be thought of as characteristic of the normal motor unit potentials, since muscle injury from the needle insertion may produce bursts of potentials. The duration of these insertional bursts is usually brief, and if they persist or if there are unusual waveforms such as myotonic or pseudomyotonic discharges, it may be from a primary myopathic process. If the muscle being tested is denervated, the needle insertion may provoke positive sharp waves or fibrillation potentials.[22]

The other portion of the recurrent nerve innervation is to the PCA muscle, the only abductor of the larynx. If there are questions about the abductive ability of the vocal fold, the PCA muscles should be tested as well. A Teflon-coated monopolar or concentric needle or hooked-wire electrode is inserted into the PCA for recordings. In the technique I have described,[2,5] the larynx is rotated away from the investigator, and the posterior edge of the thyroid lamina is lifted with the investigator's thumb. The needle electrode is then inserted along the lower half, traversing the inferior constrictor muscle and advanced until the cricoid. The needle is then pulled back slightly and the patient is asked to sniff, maximally stimulating the PCA muscle. The PCA muscle should be silent during phonation and swallowing, but very active during inspiration.[19] Utilizing surface EMG of the diaphragm and

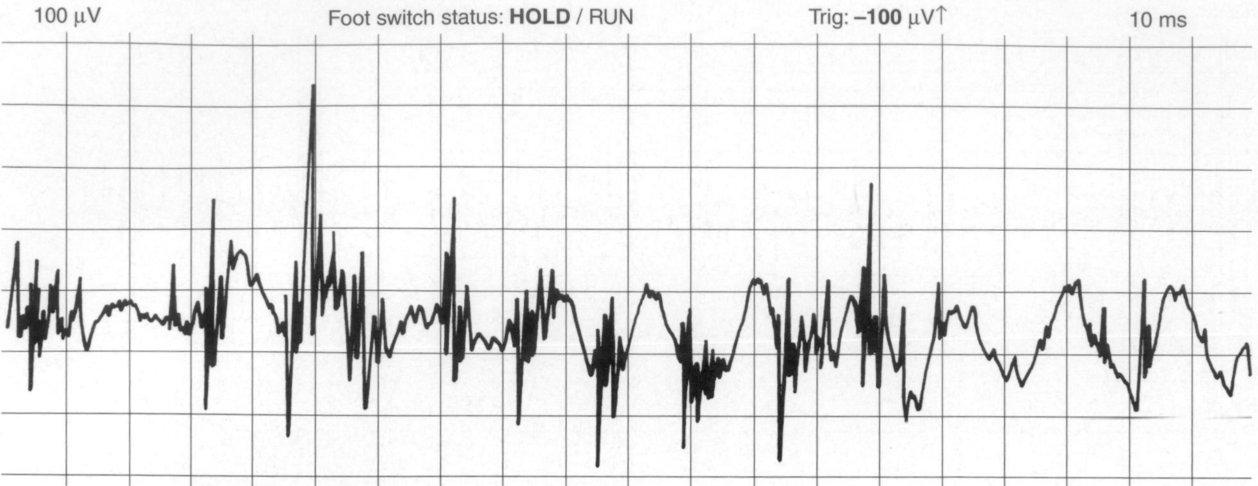

Figure 10.5 *A laryngeal EMG recording of the thyroarytenoid muscle in a patient with vocal fold immobility showing complex polyphasic potentials suggestive of reinnervation.*

needles in the PCA serves as a good predictor of respiratory drive, tidal volume, and ventilation as Scott *et al.*[30] have shown in animal studies. The PCA recordings have been found to be useful in assessing respiratory central control in premature infants.[20]

Laryngeal EMG is particularly helpful in separating mechanical from neurogenic causes of vocal fold immobility. Patients with a mechanical etiology to their vocal fold immobility, such as cricoarytenoid arthritis, cricoarytenoid joint dislocation, or posterior commissure scarring, have a normal EMG pattern. Patients with a neurogenic etiology to their vocal fold immobility often show a wide variety of abnormal activity. In cases where there is denervation, fibrillation potentials and positive sharp waves can be found. Other cases of immobility may be due to vocal fold paresis in which there is a reduced interference pattern, a decreased amplitude of potentials, and often some giant waves or polyphasic potentials suggestive of reinnervation (Figs 10.4–10.7). A denervation pattern may be found in cases of brainstem trauma; recurrent laryngeal nerve (RLN) trauma after thyroid, esophageal or mediastinal surgery; or cases of laryngeal trauma. Laryngeal EMGs may be prognostic when performed sequentially, since recovery of electrical activity will precede visualization of vocal fold motion. Lack of movement with a relatively normal EMG pattern may suggest a synkinetic pattern of recovery and may be confirmed with simultaneous PCA recording. Nahn *et al.* have found laryngeal EMG to be useful in studying the degree of recovery and synkinesis after neuropathy. Laryngeal EMG has also been used intraoperatively to identify the RLN and avoid neural injury during surgery.[20]

Palmer *et al.*[26] have found that, in some cases, other muscles should also be tested electrically (such as tongue, sternocleidomastoid, facial mimetic muscle, or pharynx) to help make the diagnosis of a denervating central process. With multiple muscle samples, the diagnosis of bulbar palsy (anterior horn cell disease), primary lateral sclerosis, Arnold–Chiari malformation, or syringomyelia can be entertained. When there is a regular, slow, repetitive abnormal firing of MUPs in the larynx, with synchronous firing in the muscles of the palate and pharynx, the diagnosis of myoclonus is easily made. Tremor disorders may also be characterized with testing of the laryngeal muscles and other muscles of the head and neck, which will show a 4–8 Hz repetitive signal. In patients where the numbers and amplitude of the MUPs decrease with repetitive function, the diagnosis of myasthenia gravis should be considered. This can be confirmed with the use of Tensilon while the patient is still connected to the EMG recorder. The patient's electrical activity should return to a normal pattern (Fig 10.8).[22]

Laryngeal electromyography has also been found useful in clarifying the diagnosis of patients who have motion disorders with dysphonia. Patients who have spasmodic dysphonia (laryngeal dystonia) have been studied extensively. When an EMG time-locked pattern is measured with a voice spectrogram, there is a delay of onset from the start of the electrical activity to the beginning of audible sound. The delay may be 0.5–1 s with a normal of 0–200 ms (Fig 10.9). Laryngeal electromyography has also helped to localize the most active places in the laryngeal muscles.[3,4,17,24,29]

Quantitative laryngeal EMG can also be performed with recordings over time in multiple muscles with multiple tasks. These are usually performed with multiple hooked-wire electrodes. The quantified data collection is then obtained by digitizing the signals at 5000 Hz, allowing motor units to be automatically detected and analyzed. The amplitude, duration, number of potentials, and rate of firing can be measured and averaged. Abnormal units may also be identified, counted and defined. Fibrillations, polyphasics, and giant potentials can be quantified and measured in a number of muscles simultaneously.[16]

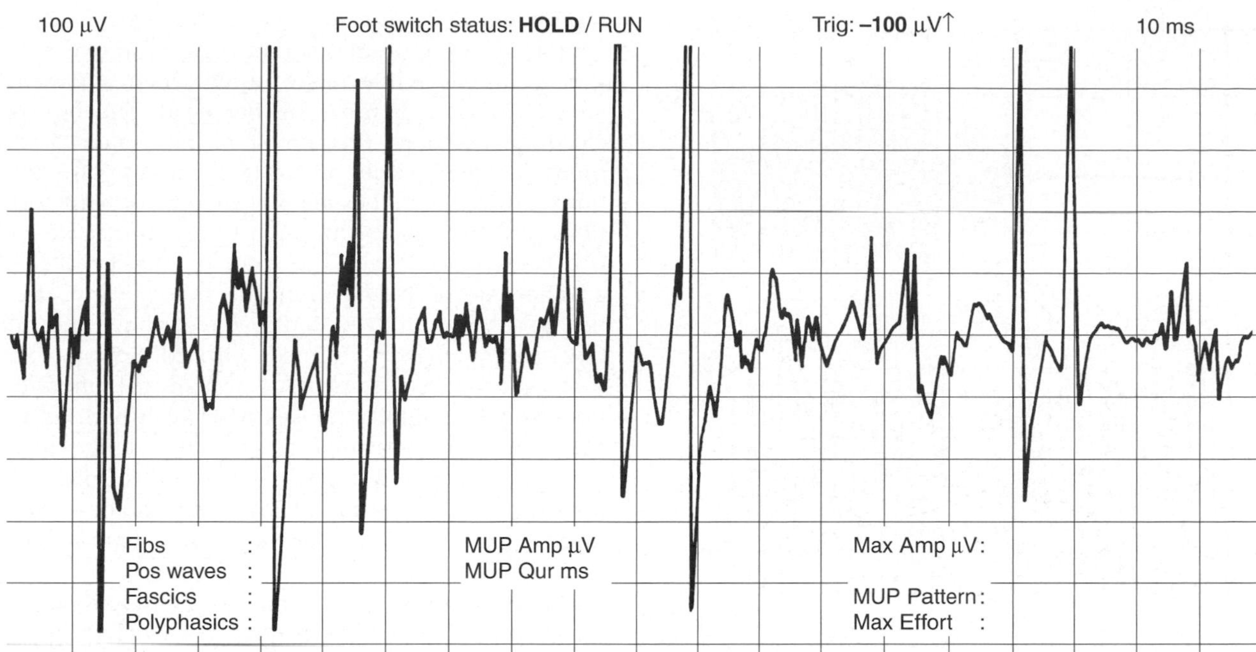

Figure 10.6 *A laryngeal EMG recording of the thyroarytenoid muscle in a patient with vocal fold immobility showing giant waves suggestive of reinnervation.*

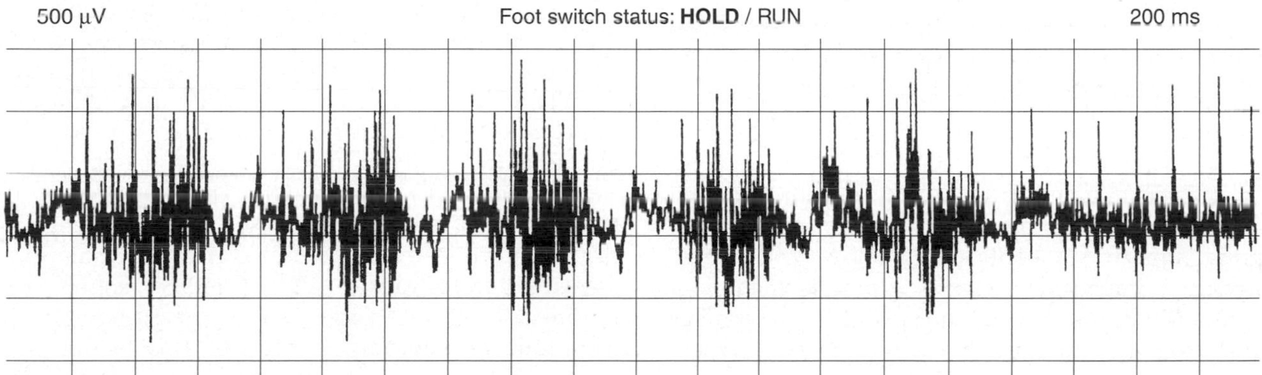

Figure 10.7 *A laryngeal EMG recording of the thyroarytenoid muscle in a patient with vocal fold immobility showing repetitive bursts of electrical activity on sniffing. This was synchronous with bursts of activity in the posterior cricoarytenoid muscle suggestive of synkinesis as the basis for the vocal fold immobility.*

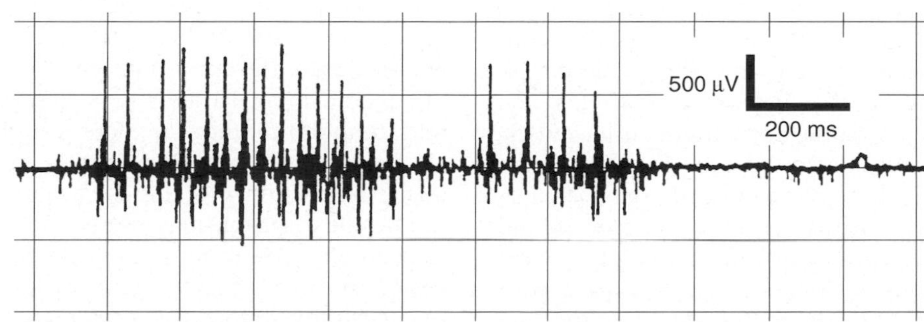

Figure 10.8 *A laryngeal EMG recording of the thyroarytenoid muscle showing decreasing amplitude and numbers of potentials with continued function. The electrical activity normalized with intravenous Tensilon consistent with the diagnosis of myasthenia gravis.*

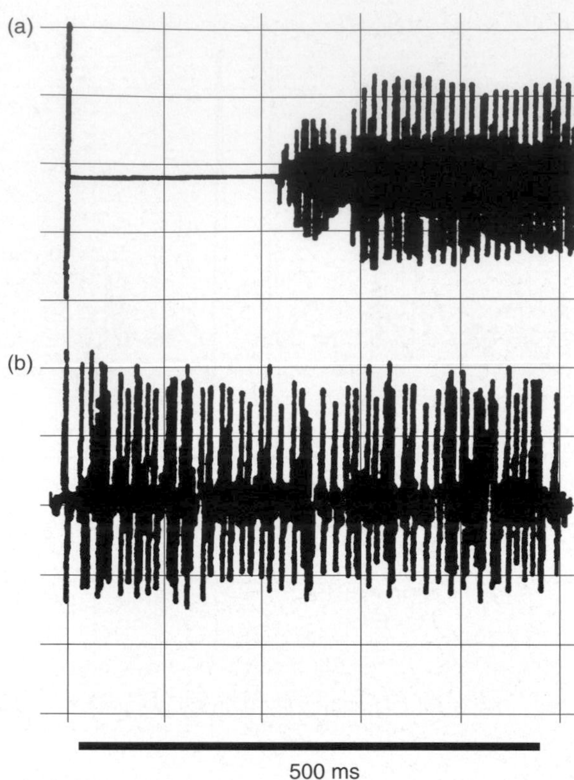

Figure 10.9 *(a) Voice spectrogram. (b) EMG of a patient with spasmodic dysphonia showing greater than 1 second delay between the onset of electrical activity and the onset of voicing.*

The characteristics of the quantitative recordings will vary depending upon the type of sensor (surface, monopolar, bipolar, concentric). To allow for accurate comparisons, impedance noise, measurement of maximum and minimum amplitudes, and the percentage maximum over the minimum must be subtracted. These measurements are most easily made using a digital computer with a signal-processing algorithm. After the signal is digitized, it is converted into microvolts using calibration signals. Filters are used to remove noise and electrode impedance signals. Quantification of maximum activities of the adductor muscles is best achieved with phonation at the top of the vocal range. The maximum abductor activity (PCA muscle) is best achieved with sniffing. Digitization of signals in real time allows the precise identification of muscle activation onset and offset. When a number of muscles are studied simultaneously, muscle activation onsets and offsets can be used to evaluate the coordination between the muscles and the patient's control of the muscles. Multiple simultaneous recordings also allow comparison of the activation of various muscle groups between different individuals. These comparisons can only be performed after the data from recordings has been normalized and quantified.[14,18,23]

The ease of moving the electrodes to many sites within the muscle being tested is the main advantage of the monopolar and concentric needle electrodes. The disadvantage of these needles is that they can move out of the site or muscle while being tested when a patient may cough, swallow or move his/her head. The hooked-wire electrodes obviate this problem, but make testing of multiple sites within the same muscle difficult. The hooked-wire electrodes are 30-gauge wires bent to form a hook and then placed through the shaft of a needle that has been placed into the muscle. The hooked-wire is advanced until it is within the muscle, and the outer needle is then removed. Multiple recordings and multiple tasks can then be performed, with continuous sampling from exactly the same area within the muscle. Two hooked-wires (bipolar hooked-wires) can be used to limit the field being measured, to give data similar to that of concentric electrodes. These hooked-wire electrodes are important for the study of MUP morphology over time, during different activities, and in different positions within the muscle.[2,9]

Thumfart[31] and Gay *et al.*[13] have described another technique of EMG recording in which there is an indirect needle insertion into the laryngeal muscles. This technique utilizes a transoral endoscopic placement of needle electrodes. Specially designed forceps have been produced to grasp the electrodes, while a zoom-telescope is used in the other hand to allow visualization of the larynx and accurate placement of the electrodes. Either mono- or bipolar hooked-wire electrodes are used. This technique has been found effective for single, multiple, simultaneous, or successive EMG recordings. This indirect technique has been found to be very effective in measuring MUPs from the TA and PCA muscles, but cannot be used for the CT. Thumfart *et al.*[32] and Haghighi and Estrem[15] have also used this technique in combination with magnetic cortical stimulation, to identify prolongation of stimulus signal ratios. Dejonckere *et al.*[8] used EMG measurements in a technique of neuromyography. In this technique, the electrodes are placed, the superior laryngeal nerve is stimulated, and the response is measured.

The relative contraindications for laryngeal electromyography are few, and include patients with bleeding disorders or coagulopathies, due to the potential to have airway or vocal fold bleeding. Patients who are immunocompromised or those patients with cardiac valvular disease or prosthetic heart valves may need prophylactic antibiotics to prevent a transient bacteremia from becoming an infection. Patients who suffer from bilateral vocal fold immobility may be poor candidates for laryngeal electromyography if their airway is relatively compromised before the procedure. The trauma associated with the needle insertion may cause swelling of the vocal folds with further compromise of the airway. The airway may need to first be secured with an intubation or tracheostomy before the needle insertion can safely be accomplished. Serum chemistry tests should be performed before the EMG since artifacts may occur from the muscle damage related to needle insertion.[2,22]

References

1. Blair RL, Berry H, Briant TDR. Laryngeal electromyography techniques and application. *Otolaryngol Clin North Am* 1978; **11:** 325–31.
2. Blitzer A. Laryngeal electromyography. In: Gould WJ, Rubin JR, Korovin G, Sataloff R, eds. *Diagnosis and Treatment of Voice Disorders.* New York: Igaku-Shoin, 1995: 316–26.
3. Blitzer A, Brin MF. Laryngeal dystonia: a series with botulinum toxin therapy. *Ann Otol Rhinol Laryngol* 1991; **100:** 85–90.
4. Blitzer A, Lovelace RE, Brin MF. Electromyographic findings in focal laryngeal dystonia (spasmodic dysphonia). *Ann Otol Rhinol Laryngol* 1985; **94:** 591–4.
5. Blitzer A, Brin MF, Stewart C, Aviv JE, Fahn S. Abductor laryngeal dystonia: a series treated with botulinum toxin. *Laryngoscope* 1992; **102:** 163–7.
6. Boemke W, Gerull G, Hippel K. Electromyography of the larynx with skin surface electrodes. *Folia Phoniatr (Basel)* 1992; **44:** 220–30.
7. Buchthal F. Electromyography of intrinsic laryngeal muscles. *J Exp Physiol* 1959; **44:** 137–48.
8. Dejonckere PH, Knoops P, Lebacq J. Evoked muscular potentials in laryngeal muscles. *Acta Otolaryngol Belg* 1988; **42:** 494–501.
9. Eichenwald EC, Howell RG, Kosch PC, Ungarelli RA, Lindsey J, Stark R. Developmental changes in sequential activation of laryngeal abductor muscle and diaphragm in infants. *J Appl Physiol* 1992; **73:** 1425–31.
10. Faaborg-Andersen K. Electromyographic investigation of intrinsic laryngeal muscles in human. *Acta Physiol Scand* 1957; **41(Suppl 140):** 1–149.
11. Faaborg Andersen KC, Buchthal F. Action potentials from internal laryngeal muscles during phonation. *Nature* 1956; **177:** 340–1.
12. Fujita M, Ludlow CL, Woodson GE, Naunton RF. A new surface electrode for recording from the posterior cricoarytenoid muscle. *Laryngoscope* 1989; **99:** 316–20.
13. Gay T, Hirose H, Strome M, Sawashima M. Electromyography of the intrinsic laryngeal muscles during phonation. *Ann Otol Rhinol Laryngol* 1972; **81:** 401–9.
14. Goodgold J, Eberstein, A. *Electrodiagnosis of Neuromuscular Disease.* Baltimore: Williams & Wilkins, 1972: 41–59.
15. Haghighi SS, Estrem SA. Comparison of evoked electromyography of the larynx to electrical and magnetic stimulation of the motor cortex of the dog. *Laryngoscope* 1991; **101:** 68–70.
16. Hallet M. Analysis of abnormal voluntary and involuntary movements with surface electromyography. In: Desmedt JE, ed. *Motor Control Mechanisms in Health and Disease.* New York: Raven, 1983: 907–15.
17. Hirano M, Ohala J. Use of hooked-wire electrodes for electromyography of the intrinsic laryngeal muscles. *J Speech Hear Res* 1961; **12:** 362–73.
18. Kimura J. *Electrodiagnosis in Disease of Nerve and Muscle.* Philadelphia: Davis, 1983.
19. Kuna ST, Smickley JS, Insalco G. Posterior cricoarytenoid muscle activity during wakefulness and sleep in normal adults. *J Appl Physiol* 1990; **68:** 1746–54.
20. Lipton RJ, McCaffrey TV, Litchy WJ. Intraoperative electrophysiologic monitoring of laryngeal muscle during thyroid surgery. *Laryngoscope* 1988; **98:** 1292–6.
21. Lovelace RE. Clinical neurophysiology of neuromuscular disease. In: Mohr JP, ed. *Manual of Clinical Problems in Neurology.* Boston: Little Brown, 1989: 326–8.
22. Lovelace RE, Blitzer A, Ludlow C. Clinical electromyography. In: Blitzer A, Brin MF, Sasaki CT, Fahn S, eds. *Neurological Disorders of the Larynx.* New York: Thieme, 1992: 66–82.
23. Ludlow CA, Baker M, Naunton RF. Intrinsic laryngeal muscle activation in spasmodic dysphonia. In: Benecke R, Conrad B, Marsden CD, eds. *Motor Disturbances I.* New York: Academic Press, 1987: 119–30.
24. Ludlow CL, Naunton RF, Bassich CJ. Procedures for the selection of spasmodic dysphonia patients for recurrent laryngeal nerve section. *Otolaryngol Head Neck Surg* 1984; **92:** 24–31.
25. Myers SJ, Lovelace RE. The motor unit and muscle action potentials. In: Downey JA, Darling RC, eds. *Physiological Basis of Rehabilitation Medicine.* Philadelphia: Saunders, 1971: 107–34.
26. Palmer JB, Holloway AM, Tanaka E. Detecting lower motor neuron dysfunction of the pharynx and larynx with electromyography. *Arch Phys Med Rehabil* 1991; **72:** 214–18.
27. Rea JL. Postcricoid surface laryngeal electrode. *Ear Nose Throat J* 1992; **71:** 267–9.
28. Redenbaugh MA, Reich AR. Surface electromyographic (EMG) and related measures in normal and vocally hyperfunctional speakers. *J Speech Hear Disord* 1989; **54:** 68–73.
29. Schaefer SD. Laryngeal electromyography. *Otolaryngol Clin North Am* 1991; **24:** 1053–7.
30. Scott SC, Inman JD, Butsch RW, Moss IR. Respiratory electromyographic estimates of ventilatory functions in piglets. *Respir Physiol* 1993; **92:** 39–51.
31. Thumfart WF. Electrodiagnosis of laryngeal nerve disorders. *Ear Nose Throat J* 1988; **67:** 380–93.
32. Thumfart WF, Pototschnig C, Zorowka P, Eckel HE. Electrophysiological investigation of lower cranial nerve diseases by means of magnetically stimulated neuromyography of the larynx. *Ann Otol Rhinol Laryngol* 1992; **101:** 629–34.

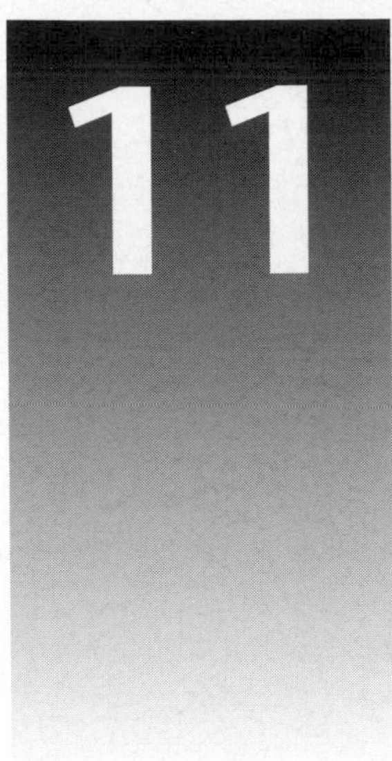

Electroglottography

Peter Kitzing

Electroglottography is a method to monitor vocal fold movements by studying their effect on a weak electrical current through the soft tissues of the neck. As it is easy to handle and entirely non-invasive, the method has attracted increasing interest and is now in common use in voice clinics as well as in phonetic laboratories.

Based on earlier studies of the effects of pulsatile variations of the bloodstream on the impedance of body tissues, so called impedance plethysmography, it was Fabre who in 1957 was the first to report on percutaneously measurable electric phenomena depending on the vibratory movements of the vocal folds during phonation. He called his new method high frequency glottography.[27] Nowadays the term glottography denotes all physiological – as opposed to optic, acoustic, or auditively perceptual – methods to study vocal fold vibrations. In addition to electroglottography, photoglottography, ultrasonoglottography and inverse-filtered flow glottography can be mentioned.[51]

In *photoglottography*, the varying amounts of light from an outside source shining through the glottis during phonation are detected by a photosensitive device.[5,55,87] The photoglottogram corresponds on the whole to the variable area of the glottis (projected area function), but artifacts, like light shining through thin parts of the mucosa even if the glottis is closed and the difficulty to calibrate the curve amplitudes, diminish the reliability of the results. Besides, the method is rather invasive, as it is necessary to place either the light source or the light sensor in the throat immediately above the glottis, so photoglottography has not become generally accepted.

Ultrasonoglottography[38,44] is another method which, though promising initially, has almost entirely been abandoned. The method is completely non-invasive. It is the only type of glottography to sense the movements of each vocal fold and thereby well suited to diagnose one-sided lesions, but the complicated and varying configurations of the vocal fold medial edges during phonation scatter the ultrasonic echoes too much to yield consistent results. In addition, progressing calcification of the thyroid cartilages prevents their penetration by ultrasound.

In inverse-filtered *flow glottography*,[42,75] the airflow through the mouth is measured by a pneumotachograph placed in a mask. The signal is inverse-filtered to eliminate the influence of the vocal tract resonators. Even if not entirely identical, the resulting flow glottogram (FLOGG) is very similar to the glottal area function and it is possible to calibrate and measure essential parts of single curves, such as the baseline and the amplitude. The mask may be somewhat cumbersome but it is not an obstacle to prevent simultaneous registrations of, e.g. oral pressure or a microphone signal. Furthermore, it has been possible to correlate special features of the FLOGG curve to spectral analysis of the voice signal,[28,32,33] thereby bridging the gap between physiologic and acoustic aspects of voice.

Electroglottography makes use of the electrical conductivity of the body tissues. Two metal electrodes, the size of about 1 cm^2, are placed on the skin on each side of the neck in the thyroid region at the level of the glottis. With the neck tissues functioning as a mass conductor with a certain impedance, an electric current can pass between the electrodes and, depending on the construction of the instrument used (constant voltage or constant current), the amount of current or the impedance through the tissues is measured. Obviously, the current has to be weak so as not to cause tissue damage or to provoke muscle contractions or nerve impulses. Typically, electroglottographs use currents of 20 mA or less, yielding a voltage across the neck of about 0.5 V. Actually, the current is not perceptible to the subject as it is high frequency (0.3–5 MHz) alternating, which also reduces signal loss at the electrode skin boundary.

The impedance of the tissues depends on their chemical quality. Adipose tissue as in obese persons, for instance, has a rather high impedance, whereas the impedance of muscle tissue and body fluids such as blood, mucus and saliva is low. Other factors that may influence the amount of current between the electrodes are the position and shape of intrinsic organs in the neck, and the moisture of the skin. The electrical signal may therefore be influenced by muscle contractions when swallowing or by respiratory and articulatory movements of the larynx, but also by changes in electrode placement. As these signal changes usually are of little interest, glottographs are equipped with high pass filters and often also with an automatic gain control (AGC) to stabilize the amplitude of the most interesting part of the signal.[6] This is the impedance variation caused by the vibratory movements of the vocal folds. As the impedance of air is almost infinitely high, even the small variations in the glottal air gap during phonation will to some extent influence the total neck impedance. By demodulation and amplification, these impedance variations can be isolated as a separate signal, the electroglottogram. However, it should always be clear that the electroglottogram only represents a small fragment (about 1%) of the entire tissue impedance between the electrodes, the necessary high amplification causing a risk for spurious signals and artifacts.

As the electric current cannot be focused directly to the vocal folds, most of it will pass through the tissues around the airway whether the glottis is open or closed. This is the reason why a number of researchers refrain from naming the signal an electro*glottogram*. Fourcin[29] has instead suggested the term electro*laryngogram*, as it represents the status of the entire larynx as a unit. Unfortunately, this terminology may be ambiguous, as laryngography also means radiologic examination of the larynx by the aid of a contrast medium.[8,57]

Those in favour of 'laryngography' usually let the upper part of the resulting curve represent the part of the cycle when the amount of current passing through the tissues is at its largest, consistent with the engineering usage to let the duty cycle be portrayed by an upwards deflection. This means that the upper parts of the curve indicate a closure of the glottis. On the other hand, many voice physiologists, used to graphs from high-speed films or photo- and flow-glottographic curves, where the upwards deflection indicates an open glottis, prefer to have the glottogram oriented in the same way with the maximum current during glottal closure being shown as a downwards deflection. Practically, this is a minor problem, as many instruments have a switch for inversion of curves, but when studying electroglottograms, their orientation should always first be made clear.

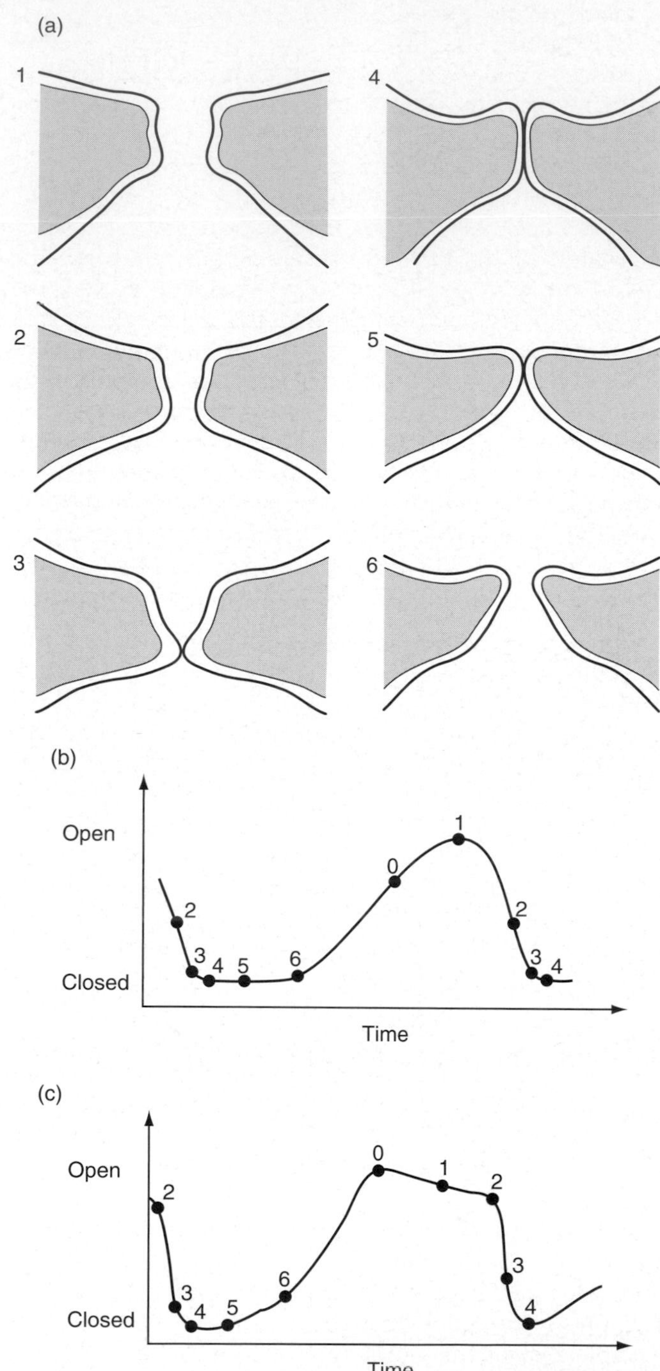

Figure 11.1 *(a) Schema of frontal sections through the glottis illustrating different moments of a vibratory cycle: 0, point of largest impedance (only shown in Fig 1b and 1c); 1, maximal open (point of largest amplitude); 2, closing; 3, closed; 4, maximum contact; 5, closed (but different from 3); 6, opening. (b) Location of these moments in the glottal area function represented by a flow glottographic (FLOGG) curve. (c) The same moments in the contact area function represented by an electroglottographic (EGG) curve.*

The electroglottographic curve

Electroglottograms are often described in terms of open and closed phases of the wave or opening and closing segments of the open phase, relating to the varying area of the glottis as depicted by high-speed movies, stroboscopy and also by photo- and inverse-filtered flow glottography. This strive is understandable as theoretical models of phonation often imply the phonatory area function of the glottis and its influence on the acoustic signal and thereby on voice quality. It is acceptable, however, only as a very coarse approximation, as the impedance of the laryngeal tissues is not related to the area of the glottis. As is nowadays generally agreed, the impedance variations detected in the electroglottogram are rather caused by variations of the contact area between the two vocal folds. In fact, during the part of the vibratory cycle, when there is no contact between the vocal folds (positions 0–2 in Fig 11.1), the electroglottogram is not sensitive to variations of the glottal area. Impedance is at a maximum, whether the air gap between the vocal folds is large or small, and it is not possible to define the acoustically important moment of the greatest glottal opening (point 1 in Fig 11.1) from an electroglottogram. Changes of the wave shape during the period when presumably there is no contact between the vocal folds can be explained as caused by electrical filters in the electroglottograph. Furthermore, it is notoriously difficult to make out the moment when the glottal opening starts (point 6 in Fig 11.1), which makes attempts to calculate the open time related to the entire period (the so-called open quotient) problematic.

Because of the risk of confounding the contact-area-depending impedance with variations of the glottal area, Fourcin[30] has avoided the qualification 'glottal' and coined the term Lx for the EGG wave. Orlikoff,[69] too, recommends a clear terminological distinction between the *vibratory* cycle, defined by contact phenomena, and the *glottal* cycle, representing the changes of the glottal area. In accordance with this, a 'contact phase' and a 'minimal contact phase' should be distinguished in the electroglottogram, and it should be acknowledged that these are not synonymous with the traditional closed and open phases of the glottal area function. The incorrect terminology is so common, however, that it will be impossible to avoid altogether in the discussion below.

When comparing the glottal area function with that of the contact area (Fig 11.1b vs 11.1c), it can be seen that the former shows the changes in greatest detail while the glottis is open, whereas the latter shows the greatest resolution of changes while the glottis is closed. The moments of opening and closing of the glottis as well as the instant of maximum opening and the glottal amplitude have been shown to correlate well with the resulting acoustic signal and thereby to voice quality.[32,33] This information can be obtained directly from the glottal area function but not from a curve representing the varying contact area between the vocal folds. Despite considerable research, the immediate relevance of the vocal fold contact ('depth of closure'[5]) to phonation remains to be shown. On the other hand, as the electroglottogram is so easily obtained it has become very popular and a great number of reports show that useful information about normal as well as pathologic phonation can be inferred from it.[6,7,15,16,18,20,30,53,69,71,78]

Qualitative appraisal of the EGG waveform

Though the exact physiological relevance of the electroglottogram remains to be shown, the shape of the EGG waves in many ways parallels different modes of phonation so well that a common application is to use the electroglottogram just qualitatively as a graphical illustration of different aspects of phonation.[64] This is shown in Figs 11.2–11.6, the interpretation of which is eased by combining the electroglottograms with inverse-filtered flow glottograms.

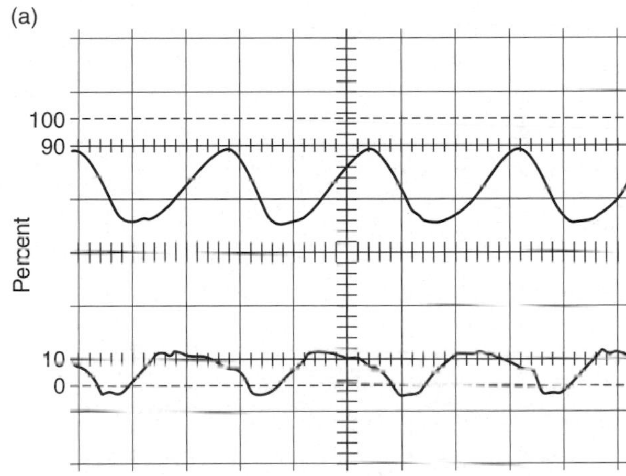

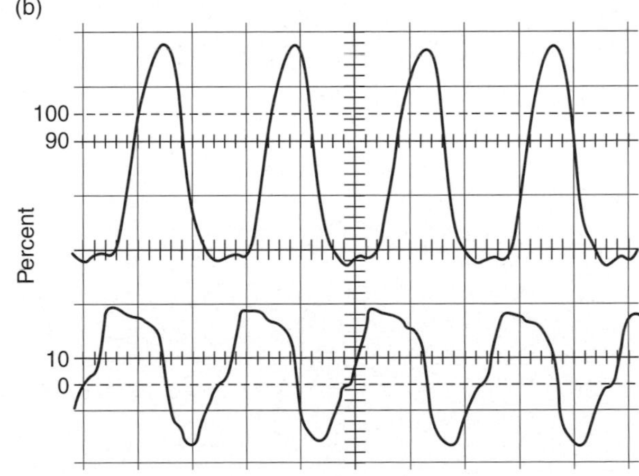

Figure 11.2 *Simultaneous flow glottogram and electroglottogram of a normal male voice at (a) low intensity, 139 Hz, and (b) high intensity, 156 Hz. Upper trace: FLOGG. Signal delayed because of distance between glottis and mouth opening. Lower trace: EGG with maximum impedance (glottal opening) shown upwards. Note the small hump in the rising part of the EGG at high intensity (see text).*

Intensity (Fig 11.2)

The registrations of increased intensity certainly show an increased EGG amplitude, as might be expected and which is common,[88] but one should keep in mind that there is no clear relationship between the amplitude of the acoustic wave and that of the EGG. Furthermore, the EGG amplitude may be influenced by the position of the larynx relative to the electrodes, e.g. by vertical movements of the larynx when singing an upwards glissando or by changes of posture. What might be less conspicuous when just looking at the curves is the increased time of vocal fold contact ('closed phase') relative to the entire period when intensity is increased. Quantitative studies have shown that this effect is consistent.[26,37,67] The small hump in the rising ('opening') part of the curve at high intensity is incidental and could be caused by a small strand of mucus forming an additional electrical path beside the contacting vocal fold edges.

(a)

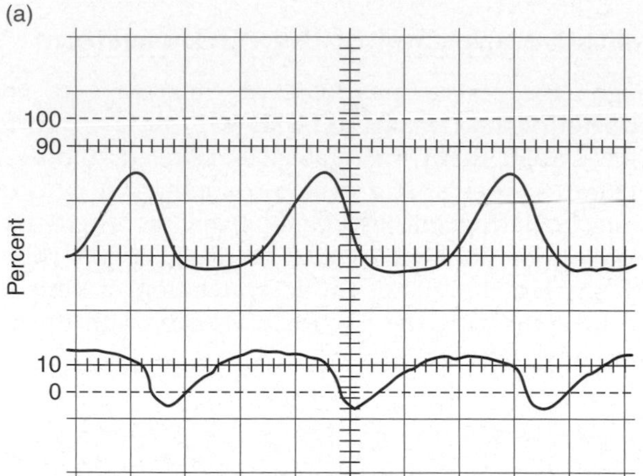

(b)

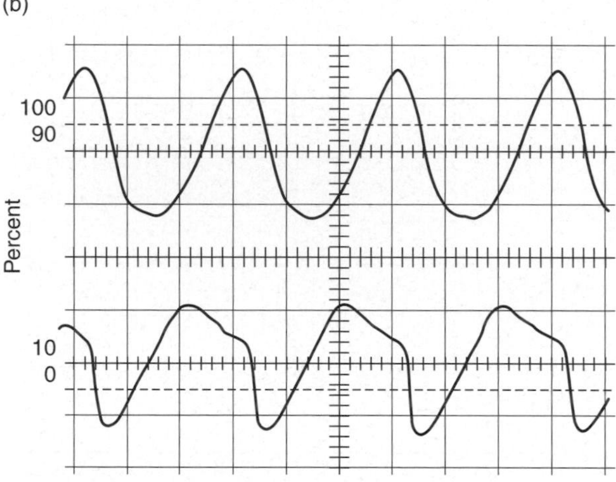

(c)

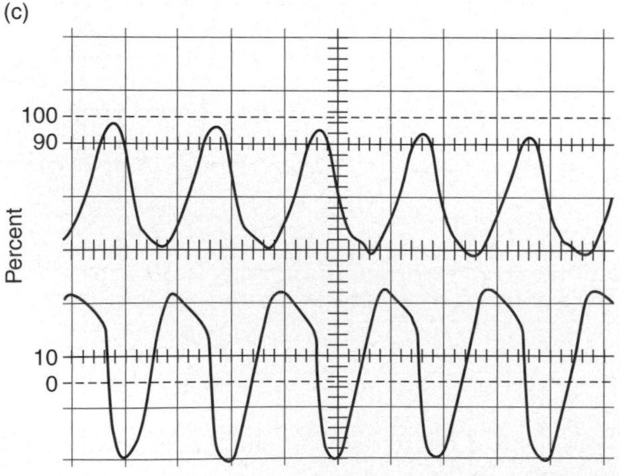

Figure 11.3 *Simultaneous flow glottogram and electroglottogram of a normal male voice at different fundamental frequencies: (a) 100 Hz, (b) 128 Hz, (c) 200 Hz.*

Fundamental frequency (Fig 11.3)

The fundamental frequency of the acoustic signal matches exactly the vibratory period of the electroglottogram.[93] As the EGG wave shape with its just one maximum per period is far less complicated than the acoustic wave, pitch extraction from the electroglottogram is more straightforward than that from the acoustic signal. Actually, simple and accurate measurements of the voice fundamental frequency is one of the most important applications of the electroglottographic method (see below).

Quality (Fig 11.4)

One important aspect of voice quality is described by the continuum leaky–flow–strained. This is well reflected in the electroglottogram by the increasing contact time ('closed phase') relative to the entire period. However, especially in the example from the strained voice, it becomes evident that the time of contact by no means agrees with the closure time of the flow glottogram; nor can one be sure that the dip of minimum contact in the electroglottogram represents a complete closure of the glottis. As was shown by Orlikoff,[69] it is actually perfectly possible to produce an entirely normal electroglottogram even if – because of a laryngeal paresis – a large part of the glottis remains continuously open during the entire vibratory cycle.

Registers and perturbations (Figs 11.5, 11.6)

Vocal register relates to both fundamental frequency and voice quality. Apart from the obvious differences in period length, the shape of the electroglottogram varies in a characteristic manner. In chest or modal register, it typically shows a somewhat rounded contact ('closed') phase, whereas in falsetto or loft register, this part of the wave is usually more pointed, due to the thinning of the vocal folds and the very short closure of the glottis. By aid of glottography, it is possible to differentiate between falsetto and operatic head register.[49,82,94] Furthermore, the ability of professional singers to equalize the transition between different registers without voice breaks can be

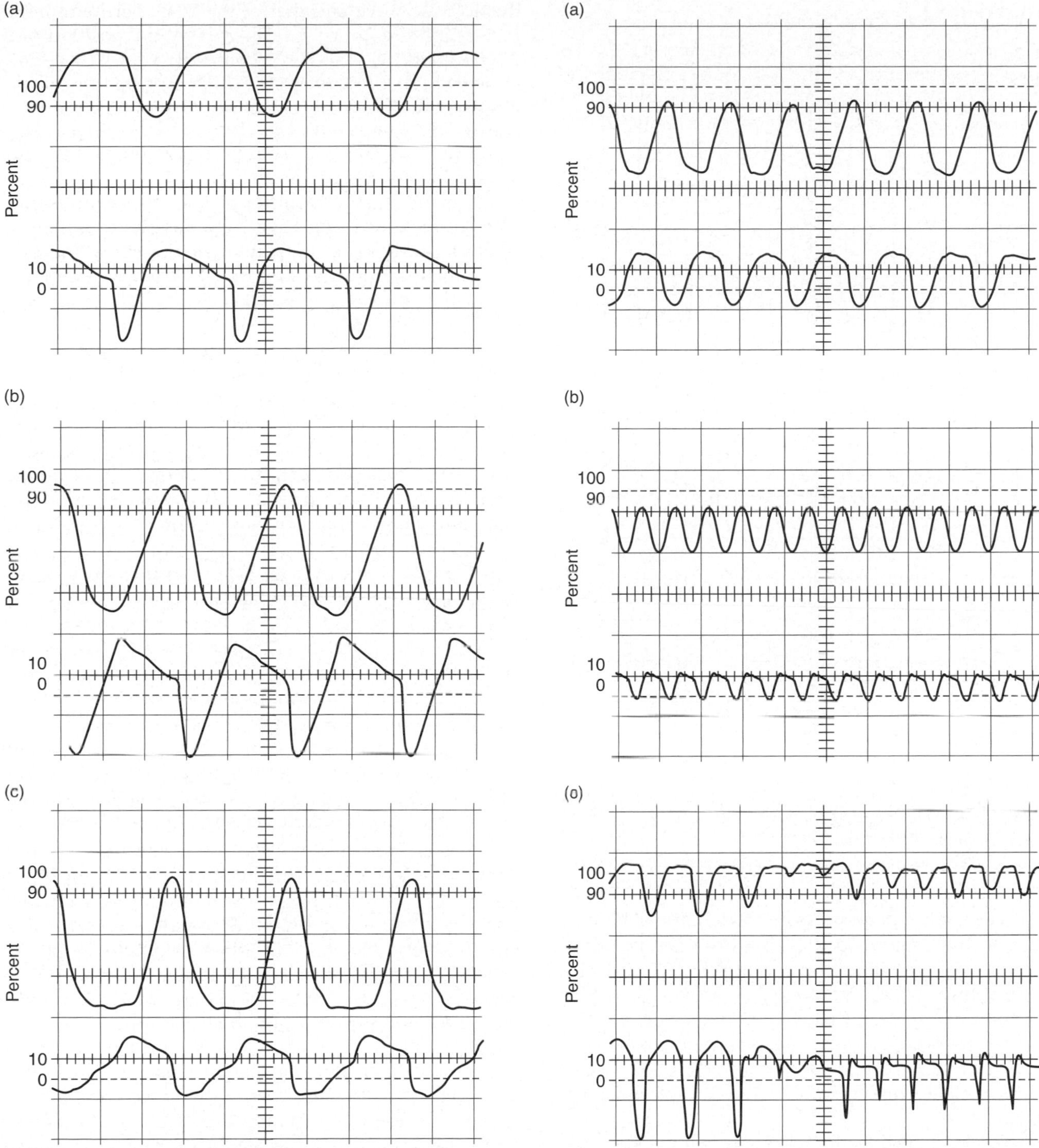

Figure 11.4 *Simultaneous flow glottogram and electroglottogram of a normal male voice at (a) leaky, (b) flow, and (c) strained voice quality.*

Figure 11.5 *Simultaneous flow glottogram and electroglottogram of a normal male voice at different registers: (a) chest register, (b) head register, and (c) voice break from chest to head register.*

easily shown.[79] It is also possible to document regular cyclic variations of phonation due to vibrato and trillo.[25]

Irregularities of vibration stand out especially well in the electroglottogram. This is illustrated by the example of a voice break (Fig 11.5c), where the wave shape in the very moment of register shift is similar to glottograms of creaky voices (pulse register, not illustrated here as such).

Vibratory irregularities (perturbations) are common at the start of phonation. This is illustrated in the examples of soft and hard glottal attack (Fig 11.6). At the hard

(a)

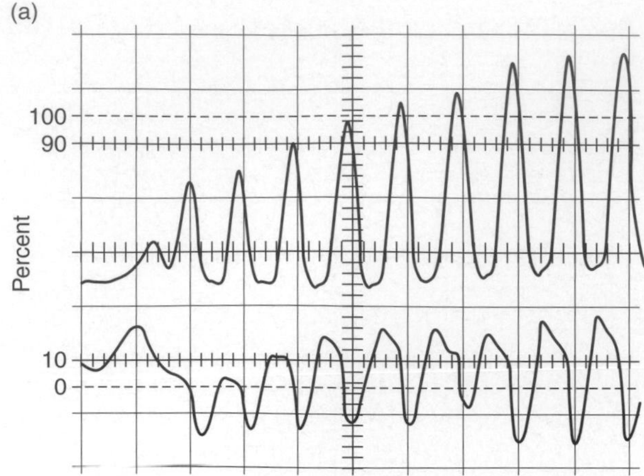

(b)

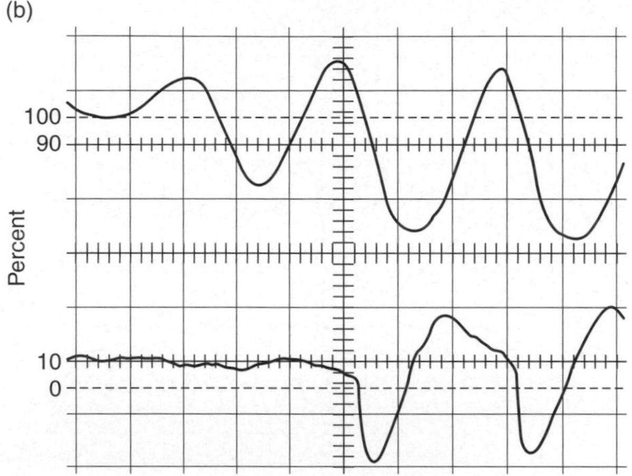

Figure 11.6 *Simultaneous flow glottogram and electroglottogram of a normal male voice at (a) hard vocal attack, and (b) at soft attack. For explanation see text.*

attack, it takes seven periods before the vibrations become regular, and they appear in the EGG from the very start of phonation. In the example of soft attack (recorded with a different time scale), by comparison with the flow glottogram it can be seen that the electroglottogram does not register the first two waves. Even if there are (acoustically relevant) vibrations of the vocal folds, these cannot be seen in the electroglottogram if the folds do not make contact.

Irregularities of the electroglottogram should be interpreted cautiously. Even if conspicuous, their cause may be very trivial, like a strand of mucus between the vocal folds. On the other hand, there may occur sequences of largely normal electroglottograms even in cases of full-blown vocal fold cancer.[53]

Quantifying EGG findings

Period-to-period irregularities or so-called perturbations of the period time and amplitude of the acoustic voice signal have been generally regarded as an important correlate to rough or harsh voice quality and hence as a sign of laryngeal pathology. They are called jitter and shimmer, respectively. A very simple way of quantifying the occurrence of waveform irregularities is by just counting their number and relating it to the total of inspected waves. Electroglottograms have been treated in this way and even with this crude method it has been possible to distinguish dysphonic voices from normal ones.[74]

Automatic measurements of period perturbations (jitter) have been shown to have 76% discriminating power between pathologic and normal voices whereas the discriminating power dropped to chance level (50%) when the same analysis was applied on microphone signals of sampled speech instead of electroglottograms.[86] To get a more secure period detection, some researchers transform the electroglottogram to its first derivative.[17,39,85] However, small irregularities and artifacts in the original signal may cause spurious spikes in the differentiated glottogram, so the derivation hardly means any advantage.[16] One way to control for common measurement errors in jitter extraction is to compare pitch period information obtained simultaneously from the acoustic and the EGG signal.[80]

It is possible to carry out EGG measurements even on children down to an age of about 7 years.[61,97] In children with velopharyngeal incompetence due to (surgically treated) cleft palate or after earlier adenotonsillectomy, EGG-based measurements of jitter were found to be positively correlated with ratings of perceived nasality, whereas shimmer was correlated to hoarseness.[97]

Besides measuring of jitter, EGG period perturbations may be depicted by the scattering of data points in EGG-based intonation contours. A somewhat similar method is to plot successive periods against each other in scatter-plots, which have been called 'digrams' or 'bihistograms'.[29,35] In such displays, most perturbations can be seen to occur in the lower frequency range, where the voice may sound creaky or harsh. Another measure of hoarseness is to analyze frequency distributions for the occurrence of low-frequency periods, and a reduction of the number of such low-frequency vibrations has been reported to signal perceived vocal improvement after therapy.[3,21,66,96]

EGG- and microphone-based measurements of frequency and jitter are comparable as both depend on the period length. The same does not hold for amplitude and shimmer, as there is no simple relation between the vocal fold contact area and the amplitude of the lip-radiated voice signal. However, there is some evidence that EGG amplitude perturbations may be a more sensitive gauge of perceived vocal disorder than acoustic measures of shimmer.[45,70] For normal phonation, EGG amplitude perturbation of about 0.2 dB appears typical, which is roughly half the normal acoustic amplitude perturbation (shimmer).[45,61]

A frequently used method of quantifying EGG findings is by computing quotients between various time segments of the wave or between such segments and the entire period, thus creating parameters to be correlated with different qualities of the voice. EGG data compare with photoglottographic measurements, indicating that the relative closure time tends to decrease with rising pitch, i.e. decreased time of vocal fold contact relative to the entire period (closed quotient) or increased open quotient, and to increase with growing intensity.[26,37,55,58,67] From this later correlation it can be inferred that the closed quotient also correlates with subglottal pressure, a fact that does not always seem to be recognized by researchers who uncritically use this quotient as a measure of vocal hyperfunction (pressed phonation).[91] An increase of the open quotient has been shown to distinguish pathologic from normal phonation but not to be useful for separating different lesions. However, when measuring pathologic voices, the described EGG parameters often become less dependable because of decreased signal-to-noise ratio. The magnitude of the method error has been shown to be approximately 15–18 % in such cases.[18,50]

Errors when metrically measuring single-period segments can be avoided by mathematical treatment of the entire curve, which has become feasible with increased computer capacity. The resulting global quotients, which thus represent an average across a number of periods, are obviously not directly related to individual glottal vibratory events, and their relevance has to be shown by statistical matching with various types of phonation. One such quotient is the so-called surface quotient. The EGG wave is divided by a line at equal distance from its maximum and minimum, and the S-quotient is computed by dividing the area of the resulting 'closed' part of the cycle with the area of the 'open part'. The S-quotient has been shown to increase with raised vocal intensity and to be decreased in pathologic voices.[23,24]

Another 'global' quotient is the quasi-open quotient, QOQ, also called β (beta) by some researchers. It is computed by dividing the EGG cycle by a zero line, so that the area of the part above the line (corresponding to high impedance) equals that under the line. The time corresponding to the part with the highest impedance ('open' part) is divided by the entire period. With this method a tendency has also been shown towards increased relative glottal closure when intensity was raised[36,37] as well as in hyperfunctional, strained voice quality, whereas the contrary was true for hypofunctional, 'loose' quality voices.[31]

Methods as described above to 'globally' define certain parts of the EGG curve to be used for computing quotients have been called criterion-level methods by Rothenberg and Mahshie.[78] With these methods, quotients can be defined by determining either the area or the amplitude of the waveform above or below a certain criterion level. The above-mentioned methods used 50% levels of distance or area, respectively. Using a 25% distance criterion for the EGG duty cycle, a 'contact quotient' ('closed quotient') was found to vary directly with vocal SPL.[67] A similar criterion level dependent variable is the EGG 30% open quotient. In a study comprising also stroboscopy and flow glottography, this quotient was shown to differ between various states of adduction (voice strain), though the variable seemed to be dependent also on F_0.[42]

EGG and measurements of fundamental frequency

Vocal pitch is one of the most important criteria when describing voice quality. It is a psychological entity, and its physical equivalent is fundamental frequency, F_0. The fundamental frequency of speech or speaking fundamental frequency, SFF, is of great interest in the voice clinic and also in phonetic research. Unfortunately, analysis of the SFF from the acoustic (microphone) signal is all but trivial, one reason for this being the fact that the acoustic voice spectrum may be entirely void of energy in the frequency region of the fundamental, and another that the signal may be so rich in strong overtones that these are wrongly taken for the fundamental by the analyzing device, so-called octave error.[43] These difficulties may be overcome by complex circuitry or computer algorithms, but many researchers prefer to use electroglottography for F_0 tracking because of its obvious advantages: it is almost as non-invasive as a microphone, it is not sensible to ambient noise and the EGG waveshape is so uncomplicated that it takes only simple zero-crossing to extract the period time or – by its inversion – the vocal vibratory frequency.

By definition, this is identical to the fundamental frequency of the acoustic signal. However, the EGG frequency at least of pathologic voices cannot without qualification be directly taken as a measure of SFF or rather the speaking voice pitch. When estimating the pitch level of speech, listeners tend in fact to neglect aperiodic and low frequency parts of the signal. These are perceived rather as signals of a certain quality, such as creakiness or harshness, and as pointed out above, they may as such be used as an objective measure of hoarseness.[1] Automated calculations of the EGG vibratory frequency consequently give lower results than estimations of mean pitch by auditory perception. For the measurements to correspond correctly to the perceived pitch, low-frequency period measurements of creaky phonation have to be eliminated. This has been accomplished in different ways, e.g. by discarding all measurements differing from the mean of the original distribution by more than an octave.[14] Another method is to introduce a periodicity criterion by accepting measurements only when two or three consecutive EGG periods, respectively, correspond to the same class range, forming so-called histograms of second or third order.[29]

The Glottal Frequency Analyzer (GFA) is a special device for measuring the mean speaking fundamental frequency, and its range and distribution in classes of semitones. Here frequency measurements at the extremes of the main distribution are discarded, once the distribution has dropped below a certain level (Fig 11.7). The results have been shown to correlate well (r = 0.98) with the pitch

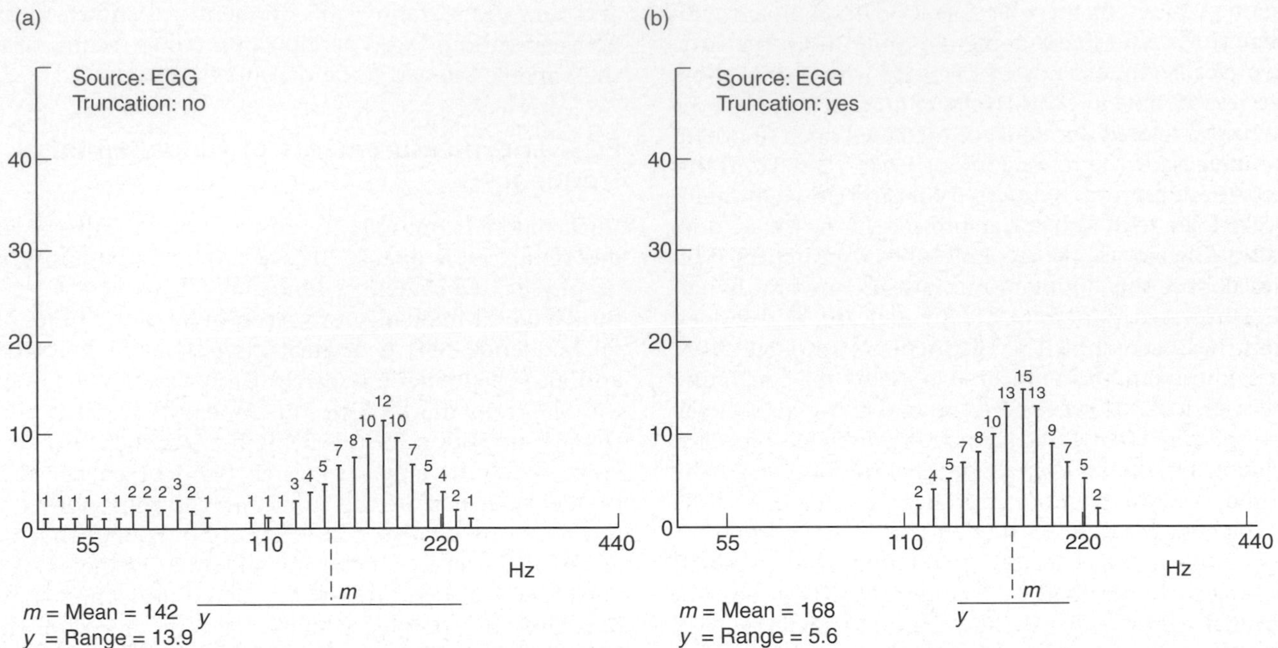

Figure 11.7 *(a) EGG-based measurement of 1000 glottal vibratory periods by aid of the Glottal Frequency Analyzer (GFA). Distribution by classes of semitones is shown as percentage of entire sample. Female subject, Reinke's edema. Mean 142 Hz, mode 175 Hz, range 13.9 semitones. Note occurrence of low-pitched vibrations below 100 Hz. (b) Same analysis as in (a) after discarding the low-frequency measurements. Mean 168 Hz, range 5.6 semitones. Estimated speaking pitch by trained listeners: 170 Hz.*

estimates of expert listeners, even if the analysis was made on pathologic voices. The pitch was on an average estimated to be only slightly (2.5%) higher than the GFA measurements, while SFF measurements by sonograms have been shown to give almost 4% lower results than those of the GFA.[21,47]

The mode of the distribution does not seem to be ideally suited as a central tendency measure of SFF because even normal voices often show asymmetric or bimodal distributions. In these cases as well as in pathologic voices in general, estimation of pitch by just listening (and comparing to a given pitch from a tuning fork, or the like) is rather difficult. Therefore, the access to a dependable method of measuring voice pitch is especially helpful in the voice clinic. Average SFF for female voices reported in the literature is 211 Hz, and the range (± 1 SD) is 5.4 semitones on average. The correspondent values for male voices are 124 Hz and 5.8 semitones. However, these values are not generally applicable as they are clearly language dependent. Swedish speakers, for instance, use much lower SFF (180 Hz and 113 Hz, respectively), while a group of French female speakers, studied by the aid of the same GFA method, speak at even higher average pitch (222 Hz).[21,47,56]

In studies of puberty, EGG-based measurements of the SFF have shown to be useful as quantifiable secondary male sex characteristics, highly correlating with serum levels of the sex hormones.[72,73] Besides depending on age and sex, the SFF is also dependent on the emotional character of the speech and the general situation, where the speech takes place. Provided such factors are kept under control when obtaining the speech sample, the mean SFF is strikingly stable and has been found to vary between successive observations of the same subjects at a time interval of about 2 months by only 2%.[47]

Considering such a high reproducibility, EGG-based measurements of SFF changes become highly relevant for the work in a voice clinic. The most conspicuous findings are the lowered SFF in female subjects either by virilizing hormones or by smoking, and the elevated pitch in males due to puberphonia (mutational falsetto).[12] As to organic voice disorders, GFA has proven especially useful as a means of monitoring the treatment of Reinke's edema, as the changes from pathologically lowered SFF to normal after surgery and voice therapy can be distinctly documented.[52]

Clinical applications of electroglottography

Electroglottography has found numerous clinical applications even if no single anatomic or physiologic condition can be diagnosed by EGG only.[95] It has been used especially for the assessment of laryngeal function in connection with interventions such as thyroplasties,[85] endotracheal intubation[59,60] and cricothyroidotomy,[34] as well as to study the effect of anti-inflammatory drugs after such interventions.[63] Computerized electroglottography in combination with sonography has been used for voice evaluation of myomucosal shunts after total laryngectomy.[10] Another application is to monitor laryngeal function in different types of neuromuscular impairments[92] and in laryngeal paralysis,[40] when the acoustic analysis alone cannot tell if compensatory contact between the vocal folds is made and where the very inability to obtain an EGG signal may be a pertinent clinical finding.[69] Spasmodic dysphonia and stuttering have been studied with the findings of altered EGG waveforms and perturbations.[9,13,22] Intonation contours based on electroglottograms have been used to analyze dysphonia due to hearing impairment as well as for a pattern matching biofeedback therapy of these patients.[1] EGG feedback has also proven to be useful in clinical voice therapy.[11]

By not using the high pass filter of the glottograph, slow changes of tissue impedance in the neck may be assessed. In this way it is possible to monitor the movements of the soft palate, for example before uvulo-palatoplasty for severe snoring[19] or the vertical movements of the larynx, e.g. when swallowing.[62,81,90] Swallowing movements can be monitored particularly well by the aid of a special multichannel electroglottograph including two electrodes on each side of the neck. This arrangement also simplifies optimal electrode placement.[77]

For clinical applications many authors prefer to use electroglottography in combination with other methods to investigate vocal function like videostroboscopy,[2,46,83,84,88,89] where the EGG signal also can be used to trigger the stroboscope. Other such combinations are with photoglottography,[40,41,48,54,65] and inverse-filtered flow glottography.[42,76]

Conclusions

Because electroglottograms are so very easy to come by, the risk is great that they are used incautiously. It should always be remembered, that 'the EGG is not the voice',[69] and that it represents changes of contact between the vocal folds and not of the varying area of the glottis.

Among the drawbacks of electroglottography may be mentioned technical difficulties to get a signal if the neck impedance is increased by subcutaneous adipose tissue or by scarring, e.g. after thyroid surgery. Similar difficulties occur when the vibration-induced impedance variations are reduced either due to diminished vibratory amplitudes (laryngeal paresis) or to small dimensions of the vocal folds as in small female subjects, in whom the obtuse angle between the thyroid plates may cause additional difficulties by impeding optimal electrode placement.

Correct electrode placement, both vertically and horizontally, is in any case critical to obtain a good EGG signal, and the best position should be tried out by monitoring the signal amplitude on an oscilloscope. The subject should not wear a metal necklace as this may function as an electric conductor interfering with the impedance between the electrodes. The same effect may be caused by moist and greasy skin, which may have to be dried with alcohol to get an acceptable signal. At small EGG amplitudes, the content of overtones in the acoustic signal tends to be reduced. This is an ideal situation to track the period time with just a contact microphone, which can be used in these cases as a complementary signal source.[4]

Automatic gain control and electric filters cause distortions of the EGG wave shape. The user should be aware of these effects, and especially seek information as to the cutoff frequency of the high pass filter in her/his instrument.

It should also be acknowledged that apart from the exact and dependable measure of the glottal period, no single feature of the EGG curve can be unequivocally correlated to the dimensions or movements of the vibrating glottis, which makes the computation of different suggested quotients as parameters of vocal function rather questionable. Not even glottal closure can be inferred from the electroglottogram with certainty, as a negative excursion of the curve signals just a minimum of impedance which may occur even when the glottis stays partly open during the entire vibratory cycle. Finally, small irregularities of the wave, like 'knees' and 'bumps', may be caused simply by unimportant mucous strands whereas the wave may show normal configuration even in serious conditions, such as cancer (see also reference 20).

As to the advantages of electroglottography, the fact that the signal is so easy to access is without doubt one of the best reasons for the vast popularity this method enjoys. It is almost as non-invasive as a microphone, but contrary to the acoustic signal it is entirely immune to ambient noise and to interference from the varying resonances of the vocal tract and articulation.[68] Contrary to the acoustic signal, it represents a perfect base for vibratory period measurements,[93] thereby easing fundamental frequency tracking, to be used as intonation curves or as objective measures of the mean pitch of speech. Again contrary to the microphone signal, the configuration of the EGG wave varies in accordance with different qualities of phonation, such as the increased relative contact time in loud and pressed phonation, the vibratory irregularities in rough voice, and the typical differences in wave shape relating to chest and falsetto register. Though exact correspondence between the EGG wave shape and the glottal area function and thereby the acoustic qualities of the voice remains to be established, the described changes of the EGG wave are evident enough to serve as a general illustration of what is going on in the larynx at different modes of phonation, and in this way the method may serve as a kind of biofeedback in the voice clinic.

Finally, the method can be expected to be rewarding also in future voice research, as the significance of vocal fold contact variations to phonation remains a widely open and challenging question.

Acknowledgments

The author gratefully acknowledges the contribution of valuable material to this chapter by a number of authors cited in the references and especially by Robert F Orlikoff. He also wants to thank Jan Olofsson and Johan Sundberg for their comments to earlier versions, and Anne Bindslev for reviewing the language.

References

1. Abberton E, Fourcin A. Electrolaryngography. In: Code C, Ball M, eds. *Experimental Clinical Phonetics*. London: Croom Helm, 1984: 62–78.
2. Anastaplo S, Karnell MP. Synchronized videostroboscopic and electroglottographic examination of glottal opening. *J Acoust Soc Am* 1988; **83:** 1883–90.
3. Aronson A, Heriksson I, Sandstedt E. *Jämförelse mellan elektroglottografisk analys av röstkvalitet och perceptuell röstbedömning före och efter röstterapi*. Thesis. Inst. För Logopedi och Foniatri, University of Göteborg, 1988.
4. Askenfelt A, Gauffin J, Sundberg J, Kitzing P. A comparison of contact microphone and electroglottograph for the measurement of vocal fundamental frequency. *J Speech Hear Res* 1980; **23:** 258–73.
5. Baer T, Löfqvist A, McGarr NS. Laryngeal vibrations: a comparison between high-speed filming and glottographic techniques. *J Acoust Soc Am* 1983; **73:** 1304–8.
6. Baken RJ. *Clinical Measurement of Speech and Voice*. London: Taylor & Francis Ltd, 1987.
7. Baken RJ. Electroglottography. *J Voice* 1992; **6:** 98–110.
8. Bartelt D. Das 'Laryngogramm des armen Mannes'. *Radiologe* 1991; **31:** 319–23.
9. Borden GJ, Baer T, Kay Kenney M. Onset of voicing in stuttered and fluent utterances. *J Speech Hear Res* 1985; **28:** 363–72.
10. Brasnu D, Strome M, Crevier Buchman L, *et al*. Voice evaluation of myomucosal shunt after total laryngectomy: comparison with esophageal speech. *Am J Otolaryngol* 1989; **10:** 267–72.
11. Carlson E. Accent method plus direct visual feedback of electroglottographic signals. In: Stemple JC, ed. *Voice Therapy: Clinical Studies*. St Louis: Mosby Year Book, 1993: 57–71.
12. Carlson E. Electrolaryngography in the assessment and treatment of incomplete mutation (puberphonia) in adults. *Eur J Disord Commun* 1995; **30:** 140–8.
13. Chevrie-Muller C, Arabia-Guidet C, Pfauwadel MC. Can one recover from spasmodic dysphonia? *Br J Disord Commun* 1987; **22:** 117–28.
14. Chevrie-Muller C, Dordain M, Decante P. Analyse automatisée des parametres acoustiques de la parole. In: *Union of the European Phoniatricians. IV Congress, Wroclaw*, 1975: 90–3.
15. Childers DG. Vocal quality factors: analysis, synthesis, and perception. *J Acoust Soc Am* 1991; **90:** 2394–410.
16. Childers DG, Krishnamurthy AK. A critical review of electroglottography. *Crit Rev Biomed Eng* 1985; **12:** 131–61.
17. Childers D, Larar JN. Electroglottography for laryngeal function assessment and speech analysis. *IEEE Trans Biomed Eng* 1984; **31:** 807–17.
18. Childers DG, Hicks DM, Moore GP, Eskenazi L, Lalwani AL. Electroglottography and vocal fold physiology. *J Speech Hear Res* 1990; **33:** 245–54.
19. Chouard CH, Meyer B, Chabolle F. The velo-impedancemetry. *Acta Otolaryngol (Stockh)* 1987; **103:** 537–45.
20. Colton RH, Conture EG. Problems and pitfalls of electroglottography. *J Voice* 1990; **4:** 10–24.
21. Comot C, Delaporte C. *Etude du fondamental laryngé dans la voix parlée chez l'adulte*. Thesis. Faculté Techniques de la Réadaptation, Lyon, 1987.
22. Conture EG, Rothenberg M, Molitor R. Electroglottographic observations of young stutterers' fluency. *J Speech Hear Res* 1986; **29:** 384–96.
23. Dejonckere PH. Control of fundamental frequency and glottal impedance with increasing sound pressure level in normal and pathological voices. *Voice* 1994; **3:** 10–16.
24. Dejonckere PH, Lebacq J. Electroglottography and vocal nodules – an attempt to quantify the shape of the signal. *Folia Phoniatr (Basel)* 1985; **37:** 195–200.
25. Dejonckere PH, Lebacq J. Differences in physiological mechanisms for producing vocal vibrato, trillo and tremolo. *Acta Phoniatr Latina* 1989; **11:** 43–53.
26. Dromey C, Stathopoulos ET, Sapienza CM. Glottal airflow and electroglottographic measures of vocal function at multiple intensities. *J Voice* 1992; **6:** 44–54.
27. Fabre P. Un procédé électrique percutané d'inscription de l'accolement glottique au cours de la phonation: glottographie de haute fréquence. Premiers résultats. *Bull Acad Nat Med* 1957; **141:** 66–9.
28. Fant G. Glottal source and excitation analysis. Speech transmission laboratory quarterly progress and status report. *R Inst Technol, Stockh* 1979; **4:** 1–13.
29. Fourcin AJ. Laryngographic assessment of phonatory function. In: Ludlow CL, Hart MO, O'Connell H, eds. *Proceedings of the Conference on the Assessment of Vocal Pathology. ASHA Reports* 1981; **11:** 116–27.
30. Fourcin AJ. Electrolaryngographic assessment of vocal fold function. *J Phonetics* 1986; **14:** 435–42.
31. Frøkjfr-Jensen B. Can glottography be used in the clinical practice? In: *Proceedings of the XIX Congress of the International Association of Logopedics and Phoniatrics, Edinburgh*. Perth, Scotland: College of Speech Therapists, 1983.
32. Gauffin J, Sundberg J. Data on the glottal voice source behaviour in vowel production. Speech transmission laboratory quarterly progress and status report. *R Inst Technol, Stockh* 1980; **2–3:** 61–70.
33. Gauffin J, Sundberg J. Spectral correlates of glottal voice source. *J Speech Hear Res* 1989; **32:** 556–65.
34. Gleeson MJ, Pearson RC, Armistead S, Yates AK. Voice changes following cricothyroidotomy. *J Laryngol Otol* 1984; **98:** 1015–19.
35. Guidet C, Chevrie-Muller C. Méthode de traitement du signal électroglottographique. Application au diagnostic automatisé des troubles de la phonation. *Innov Tech Biol Med* 1983; **4:** 617–35.
36. Hacki T. Klassifizierung von glottisdysfunktionen mit hilfe der elektroglottographie. *Folia Phoniatr (Basel)* 1989; **41:** 43–8.
37. Hacki T. Electroglottographic quasi-open quotient and amplitude in crescendo phonation. *J Voice* 1996; **10:** 342–7.
38. Hamlet SL. Ultrasound assessment of phonatory activity. In: Ludlow CL, Hart MO, eds. *Proceedings of the Conference on the Assessment of Vocal Pathology. ASHA Reports* 1981; **11:** 128–40.
39. Hanson DG, Gerratt BR, Wald PH. Glottographic

measurement of vocal dysfunction. A preliminary report. *Ann Otorhinolaryngol* 1983; **92:** 413–20.
40. Hanson DG, Gerratt BR, Karin RR, Berke GS. Glottographic measures of vocal fold vibration: an examination of laryngeal paralysis. *Laryngoscope* 1988; **98:** 541–9.
41. Hanson DG, Ward PH, Gerratt BR, Berci G, Berke GS. Diagnosis of neuromuscular voice disorders. In: Goldstein JC, Kashima HK, Koopman CF, eds. *Geriatric Otolaryngology*. Toronto: BC Decker BC, 1989: 71–9.
42. Hertegård S, Gauffin J. Glottal area and vibratory patterns studied with simultaneous stroboscopy, flow glottography, and electroglottography. *J Speech Hear Res* 1995; **38:** 85–100.
43. Hess W. *Pitch Determination of Speech Signals*. Berlin: Springer-Verlag, 1983.
44. Holmer N-G, Kitzing P, Lindström K. Echo glottography. *Acta Otolaryngol (Stockh)* 1973; **75:** 454–63.
45. Horiguchi S, Haiji T, Baer T, Gould WJ. Comparison of electroglottographic and acoustic waveform perturbation measures. In: Baer T, Sasaki C, Harris KS, eds. *Laryngeal Function in Respiration and Phonation*. San Diego: College-Hill Press, 1987: 509–18.
46. Karnell MP. Synchronized videostroboscopy and electroglottography. *J Voice* 1989; **3:** 68–75.
47. Kitzing P. *Glottografisk frekvensindikering*. Thesis, University of Lund, Malmö. [Condensed version in English: Glottal Frequency Analysis. Paper presented at The Society for Voice Research, Royal Society of Medicine, London, Sept. 1986.]
48. Kitzing P. Methode zur kombinierten photo- und elektroglottographischen registrierung von stimmlippenschwingungen. *Folia Phoniatr (Basel)* 1979; **29:** 249–60.
49. Kitzing P. Photo- and electroglottographical recording of the laryngeal vibratory pattern during different registers. *Folia Phoniatr (Basel)* 1982; **34:** 234–41.
50. Kitzing P. Simultaneous photo- and electroglottographical measurements of voice strain. In: Titze JR, Scherer RC, eds. *Vocal Fold Physiology*. Denver: The Denver Center for the Performing Arts, 1950: 221–9.
51. Kitzing P. Glottography the electrophysiological investigation of phonatory biomechanics. *Acta Otorhinolaryngol Belg* 1986; **40:** 863–78.
52. Kitzing P. Phoniatric aspects of microlaryngoscopy. *Acta Phoniatr Latina* 1987; **9:** 31–41.
53. Kitzing P. Clinical applications of electroglottography. *J Voice* 1990; **4:** 238-49.
54. Kitzing P, Löfqvist A. Clinical application of combined electro- and photoglottography. In: Buch NH, ed. *Proceedings of the 17th Congress of the International Association of Logopedics and Phoniatrics*. Part 1. Copenhagen: Special-paedagogisk forlag, 1977: 529–39.
55. Kitzing P, Sonesson B. A photoglottographical study of the female vocal folds during phonation. *Folia Phoniatr (Basel)* 1974; **26:** 138–49.
56. Krook MIP. Speaking fundamental frequency characteristics of normal swedish subjects obtained by glottal frequency analysis. *Folia Phoniatr (Basel)* 1988; **40:** 82–90.
57. Landman GHM. *Laryngography and Cinelaryngography*. Baltimore: Williams & Wilkins, 1970.
58. Lecluse FLE. *Elektroglottografie. An experimental study of the electrical impedance for the male human larynx*. Thesis, University of Rotterdam, Utrecht, 1977: 1–181.
59. Lesser THJ, William RG. Laryngographic investigation of postoperative hoarseness. *Clin Otolaryngol* 1988; **13:** 37–42.
60. Lesser THJ, Williams RG, Hoddinott C. Laryngographic changes following endotracheal intubation in adults. *Br J Disord Commun* 1986; **21:** 239–44.
61. Linders B, Massa GG, Boersma B, Dejoncker PH. Fundamental voice frequency and jitter in girls and boys measured with electroglottography: influence of age and height. *Int J Pediatr Otorhinolaryngol* 1995; **33:** 61–5.
62. Logeman JA. Non-imaging techniques for the study of swallowing. *Acta Otorhinolaryngol Belg* 1994; **48:** 139–42.
63. Mazzarella B, Macarone Palmieri A, Mastronardi P. Benzydamine for the prevention of pharyngo-laryngeal pathology following tracheal intubation. *Int J Tissue React* 1987; **9:** 121–9.
64. Motta G, Cesari U, Iengo M, Motta G Jr. Clinical application of electroglottography. *Folia Phoniatr (Basel)* 1990; **42:** 111–17.
65. Murty GE, Carding PN, Lancaster P. An outpatient clinic system for glottographic measurement of vocal fold vibration. *Br J Disord Commun* 1991; **26:** 115–23.
66. Neill WF, Wechsler E, Robinson JMP. Electrolaryngography in laryngeal disorders. *Clin Otolaryngol* 1997; **2:** 33–40.
67. Orlikoff RF. Assessment of the dynamics of vocal fold contact from the electroglottogram: data from normal male subjects. *J Speech Hear Res* 1991; **34:** 1066–72.
68. Orlikoff RF. Vocal stability and vocal tract configuration: an acoustic and electroglottographic investigation. *J Voice* 1995; **9:** 173–81.
69. Orlikoff RF. Scrambled EGG: the uses and abuses of electroglottography. *Phonoscope* 1998; **1:** 37–53.
70. Orlikoff RF, Kraus DH. Dysphonia following nonsurgical management of advanced laryngeal carcinoma. *Am Speech Lang Pathol* 1996; **5:** 47–52.
71. Painter C. Electroglottogram waveform types of untrained speakers. *Eur Arch Otorhinolaryngol* 1990; **247:** 168–73.
72. Pedersen MF, Kitzing P, Krabbe S, Heramb S. The change of the voice during puberty in 11–16 years old choir singers measured with electroglottographic fundamental frequency analysis and compared to other phenomena of puberty. *Acta Otolaryngol Suppl (Stockh)* 1982; **386:** 189–92.
73. Pedersen MF, Møller S, Krabbe S, Bennet P. Fundamental voice frequency measured by electroglottography during continuous speech. A new exact sex characteristic in boys in puberty. *Int J Pediatr Otorhinolaryngol* 1986; **11:** 21–7.
74. Rambaud-Pistone E. Place de l'étude instrumentale dans le bilan vocal. *Bull Audiophonol* 1984; **17:** 41–58.
75. Rothenberg M. Measurement of airflow in speech. *J Speech Hear Res* 1977; **20:** 155–76.
76. Rothenberg M. Some relations between glottal air flow and vocal fold contact area. *Proceedings of the Conference on the Assessment of Vocal Pathology, Bethesda*, 1979: 1–19.
77. Rothenberg M. A multichannel electroglottograph. *J Voice* 1992; **6:** 36–43.

78. Rothenberg M, Mahshie JJ. Monitoring vocal fold abduction through vocal fold contact area. *J Speech Hear Res* 1988; **31**: 338–51.
79. Roubeau B, Chevrie-Muller C, Arabia-Guidet C. Electroglottographic study of the changes of voice registers. *Folia Phoniatr (Basel)* 1987; **39**: 280–9.
80. Schoentgen J, de Guchteneere R. An algorithm for the measurement of jitter. *Speech Commun* 1991; **10**: 533–8.
81. Schultz JL, Perlman AL, van Daele DJ. Laryngeal movement, oropharyngeal pressure, and submental muscle contraction during swallowing. *Arch Phys Med Rehabil* 1994; **75**: 183–8.
82. Schutte HK, Seidner WW. Registerabhängige differenzierung on elektroglottogrammen. *Sprache-Stimme-Gehör* 1988; **12**: 59–62.
83. Sercarz JA, Berke GS, Gerratt BR, Kreiman J, Ming Y, Natividad M. Synchronizing videostroboscopic images of human laryngeal vibration with physiological signals. *Am J Otolaryngol* 1992; **13**: 40–4.
84. Sercarz JA, Berke GS, Ming Y, Gerratt BR, Natividad M. Videostroboscopy of human vocal fold paralysis. *Ann Otol Rhinol Laryngol* 1992; **101**: 567–77.
85. Slavit DH, Maragos NE, Lipton RJ. Physiologic Assessment of Isshiki type III thyroplasty. *Laryngoscope* 1990; **100**: 844–8.
86. Smith AM, Childers DG. Laryngeal evaluation using features from speech and the electroglottograph. *IEEE Trans Biomed Eng* 1983; **30**: 755–9.
87. Sonesson B. On the anatomy and vibratory pattern of the human vocal folds. *Acta Otolaryngol Suppl (Stockh)* 1960; **156**: 1–80.
88. Sopko J. *Die klinische Phoniatrie. Ergebnisse der vergleichenden Untersuchungen des gesunden und kranken Kehlkopfes beim Menschen mittels Photographie, Laryngostroboskopie und Elektroglottographie.* Habilitationsschrift (thesis), University of Basel, 1983; 1–126.
89. Sopko J. Zur Objektivierung der Stimmlippenschwingungen mittels synchroner elektroglottographischer und stroboskopischer Untersuchung. *Sprache-Stimme-Gehör* 1986; **10**: 83–7.
90. Sorin R, McClean MD, Ezerzer F, Meissner-Fischbein B. Electroglottographic evaluation of the swallow. *Arch Phys Med Rehabil* 1987; **68**: 232–5.
91. Sundberg J. Personal communication, 1997.
92. Theodoros DG, Murdoch BE. Laryngeal dysfunction in dysarthric speakers following severe closed-head injury. *Brain Inj* 1994; **8**: 667–84.
93. Vieira MN, McInnes FR, Jack MA. Analysis of the effects of electroglottographic baseline fluctuation on the F_0 estimation in pathological voices. *J Acoust Soc Am* 1996; **99**: 3171–6.
94. Vilkman E, Alku P, Laukkanen A-M. Vocal-fold collision mass as a differentiator between registers in the low-pitch range. *J Voice* 1995; **9**: 66–73.
95. Watson C. Quality analysis of laryngography in a busy hospital ENT voice clinic. *Eur J Disord Commun* 1995; **30**: 132–9.
96. Wechsler E. A laryngographic study of the voice disorders. *Br J Disord Commun* 1977; **12**: 9–22.
97. Zajac DJ. Voice perturbations of children with perceived nasality and hoarseness. *Cleft Palate J* 1989; **26**: 226–32.

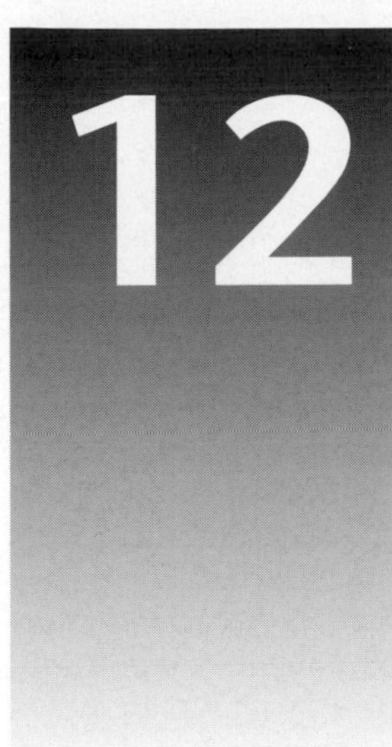

Spectrographic voice analysis

Satoshi Imaizumi

The sound spectrograph is a useful tool to visualize acoustic characteristics of voice signals.[3,7,13] Assessment of voice disorders and phonatory characteristics is best accomplished on the basis of the entire visual display rather than a single measure.[12] Potential clinical benefits are:

- to record vocal conditions which affect speech intelligibility and communication effectiveness;
- to gain insights into laryngeal health; and
- to test effectiveness of clinical treatment and vocal training.

Various forms of sound spectrograph can be easily generated using computerized voice analysis systems,[11] which are now available on a small personal computer or even on a laptop computer. Those software systems also supply automatically extracted parameters characterizing acoustic quality of pathological voice. For normal and subnormal voice samples which are nearly periodic, acoustic measures extracted by computer software systems are reliable and useful. For moderate to severe pathological cases, spectrographic qualitative observation is more suitable because computerized quantitative analyses may generate errors. For heavily damaged voices, such as aphonia, perceptual assessment may be useful.

Observable characteristics

The acoustic characteristics observable from sound spectrograms and relevant to the assessment of vocal function are:

- Fundamental frequency (F0) of vocal fold vibration: the average of a given phonation; the possible range of a given subject; regularity of a given phonation.
- Energy, intensity contour of the acoustic waveform: the average of a given phonation; the possible range of a given subject; regularity of a given phonation.
- Harmonic structure and noise (nonharmonic) components.
- Energy distribution within a frequency range: richness of harmonics.

Dynamic properties or stability of the above-listed measures are important for the assessment of voice disorders. Other characteristics relating to articulation and vocal tract configuration, such as formant frequencies, can also be visualized.

Voice samples

For the assessment of voice disorders, sustained vowel phonations are frequently used because such utterances are relatively easy to analyze. Sentences or paragraphs have also been used, particularly for the assessment of laryngeal adjustments in speech.

Recording should be carried out in a quiet room using a high quality tape recorder such as a digital audio recorder. Computerized spectrography installed on a multimedia personal computer provides a direct recording facility with a high precision. Sampling frequency (Fs, the number of data points recorded per second) should be higher than 10 kHz, which determines the upper limit of frequency information below the half of Fs. Volume has to be adjusted properly so that vocal amplitude is as largely recorded as possible within the maximum range.

Display formats and clinical significance

The sound spectrograph visualizes an input voice signal in a variety of display formats. Among those, the following formats are most fundamental and useful for the assessment of laryngeal function.

Sectioned display of power spectrum

Any voice signal can be separated into its partial tones or frequency components. The power of partials as a function of frequency is called a power spectrum, and is represented as a sectioned display in spectrography. As shown in Fig 12.1, a periodic voice signal, such as normal phonation of a vowel, consists of discrete components; a fundamental and its *n*th higher harmonics. The frequency of the fundamental corresponds to the number of vibrations of the vocal folds per second (the fundamental frequency denoted as F0), and that of the *n*th higher harmonic is $n \times$ F0. Female subjects have a higher F0 and fewer harmonics than do males. The height of harmonic peaks relative to the adjacent troughs correlates with nonharmonic components reflecting perturbation in vocal fold vibration and turbulence noise in glottal voice source. Therefore, the peak height in decibels is a good qualitative index of harmonic-to-noise ratio, which usually decreases for higher harmonics than for lower ones, even in normal phonation.

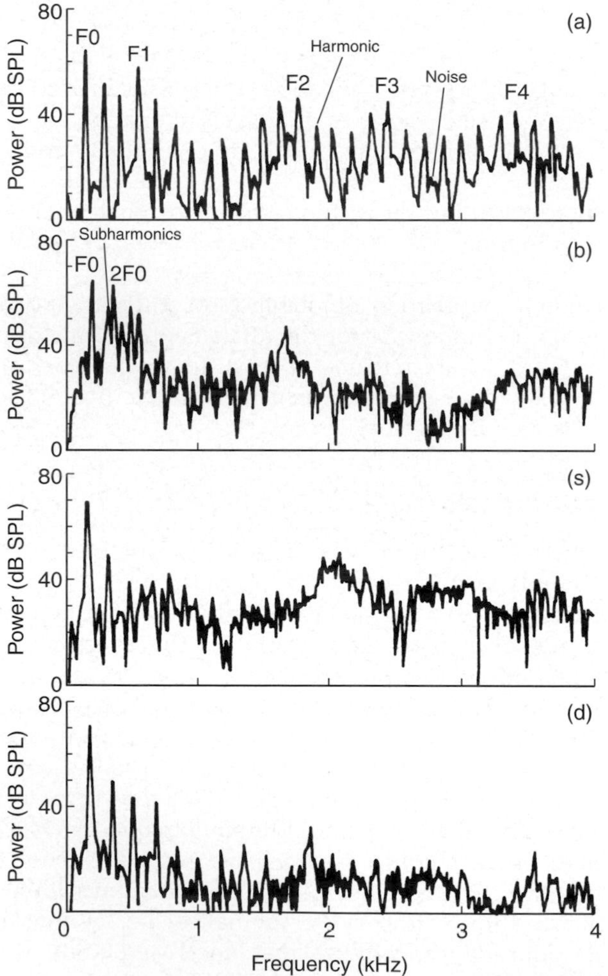

Figure 12.1 *The power spectrum of normal-sounding phonation of /e/ recorded from a healthy male (a), and a rough sample (b), a breathy sample (c) and an asthenic sample (d) recorded from patients with laryngeal disorders. A narrow-band analysis filter (24 Hz) with a long Hanning time window (102.4 ms) was used. F0, fundamental frequency; F1–F4, the first to fourth formant frequencies.*

Harmonics of pathologic voice samples tend to be unclear among noise components, particularly in the high-frequency range, due to several reasons. When vocal fold vibration fluctuates with modulation, in such a way that vibration varies, short-long-short-long in pitch or strong-weak-strong-weak in excitation, subharmonics appear between adjacent harmonics as shown in Fig 12.1b, and generate a 'rough' voice quality. Harmonics are replaced by nonharmonic noise components when turbulence noise in the glottal voice source increases, as shown in Fig 12.1c, whose resultant voice quality is noisy and breathy. Another possibility is a weak excitation of glottal voice source, which decreases significantly harmonic peaks in the high-frequency range, as shown in Fig 12.1d, with an asthenic or hypofunctional voice quality. Harmonic peaks which are significantly lower than the F0 peak, as shown in Figs 12.1c and d, reflect a breathy phonation with a weak excitation of glottal voice source.

Most modern spectrographic systems have several analysis parameters to generate a spectrograph suitable for the user's purposes. One of the most important parameters is 'the analysis filter', through which frequency components are extracted. The use of a narrower band analysis filter results in a higher frequency resolution with a lower temporal resolution. This parameter can be represented as an 'analysis time window', through which a temporal segment of voice signal is analyzed to calculate the power spectrum. The use of a longer analysis time window results in a lower temporal resolution with a higher frequency resolution. The shape of the time window is also important. For ordinal analyses, a rectangular time window should be avoided. Appropriate selection of these parameters is quite important for voice assessment.

The section displays the power spectrum at a particular time point of interest. Examples shown in Figs 12.1 and 12.2 are produced using a narrow-band analysis filter (24 Hz) with a long Hanning time window (102.4 ms), suitable to observe F0, harmonics and noise components. While section displays produced with a wide-band filter can be used to observe formant frequencies and overall spectral shapes, long-term average spectra (LTAS)[2] can be used for the quantitative assessment of overall spectral shapes for spontaneous speech as well for sentence or paragraph reading.

Narrow-band and wide-band spectrograms: three-dimensional display of power spectrum

Voice signals are dynamic; power and frequency of their partial tones vary with time, depending on various factors such as physiological properties of vocal folds, as well as respiratory, laryngeal and vocal tract adjustments. The dynamic properties of partial tones can be visualized by

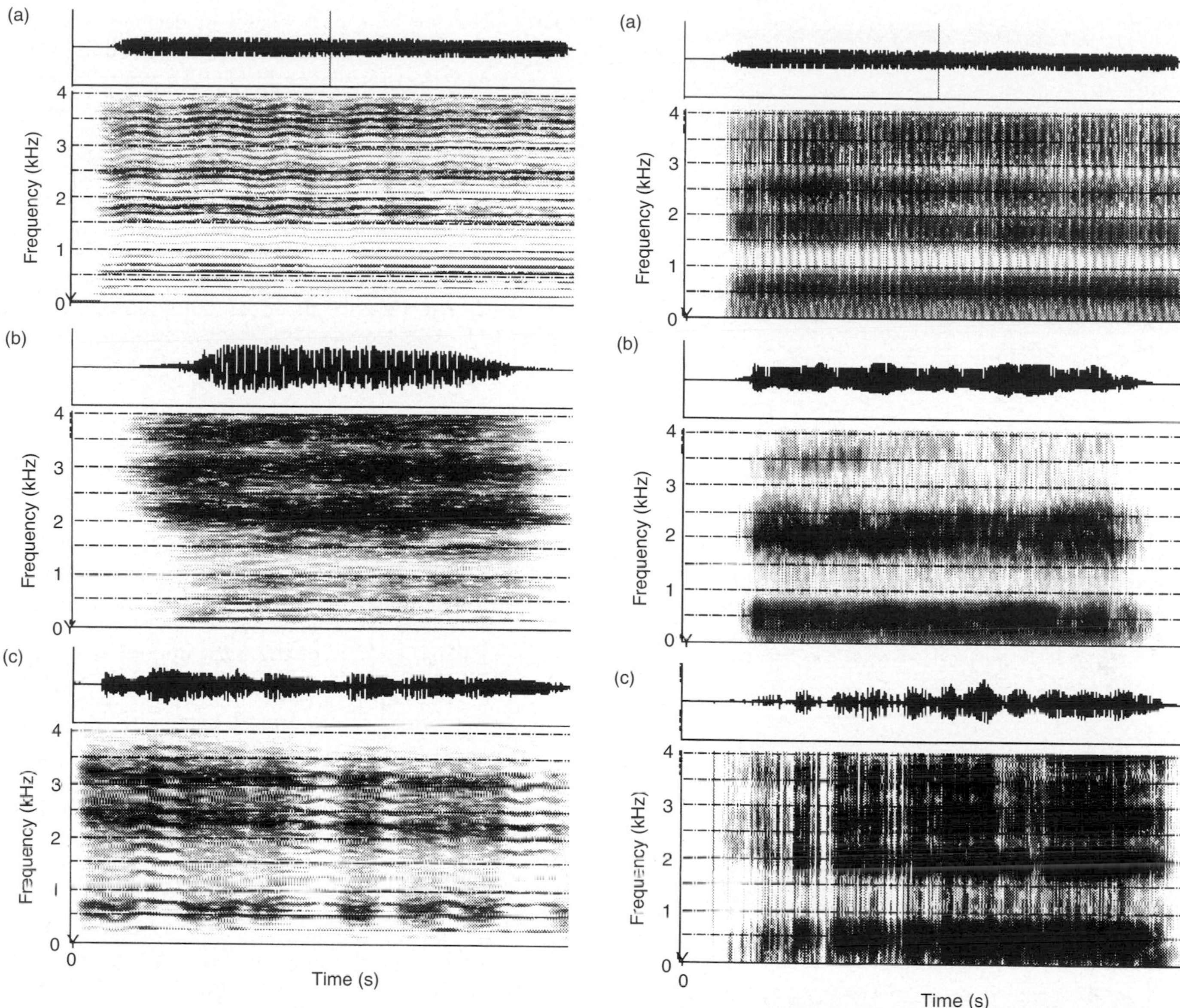

Figure 12.2 *Narrow-band spectrograms together with voice waveforms. (a) Normal phonation. (b) A pathologic case with significant noise above 0.5 kHz. (c) A pathologic case with repeated abrupt transitions to different phonatory regimens.*

Figure 12.3 *Wide-band spectrograms together with voice waveforms. (a) Normal phonation with regularly repeated glottal pulses. (b) A pathologic case with significant magnitude fluctuation in glottal pulses. (c) A pathologic case with repeated interruptions.*

three-dimensional spectrograms as shown in Fig 12.2. The power of partials is represented in darkness as a function of time (*x*-axis) versus frequency (*y*-axis). Darker is louder.

A narrow-band spectrogram, a pattern generated using a narrower filter (a longer time window), is suitable to visualize temporal variations in frequency components such as F0 contour, harmonic structure including noise and subharmonic components as well as abrupt transitions to different phonatory regimes.[12]

Three examples are shown in Fig 12.2 together with voice waveforms. Normal phonation (Fig 12.2a) consists of stable harmonics in all the frequency range displayed up to 4 kHz with least natural fluctuation. Very soft noise components can be observed mainly in high frequency range, although female voices tend to have louder noise components than male. While, pathological cases have different characteristics in several aspects. In the sample shown in Fig 12.2b, for instance, harmonics are not observable over the whole frequency range reflecting lack of periodic vibration of the vocal folds and significant turbulent noise. In Fig 12.2c, abrupt transitions to different phonatory regimens are observed reflecting spasmodic phonation. It shows unstable F0 fluctuation, which is more evident for higher harmonics, because the extent of fluctuation of the *n*th harmonic is *n* times larger than that of F0.

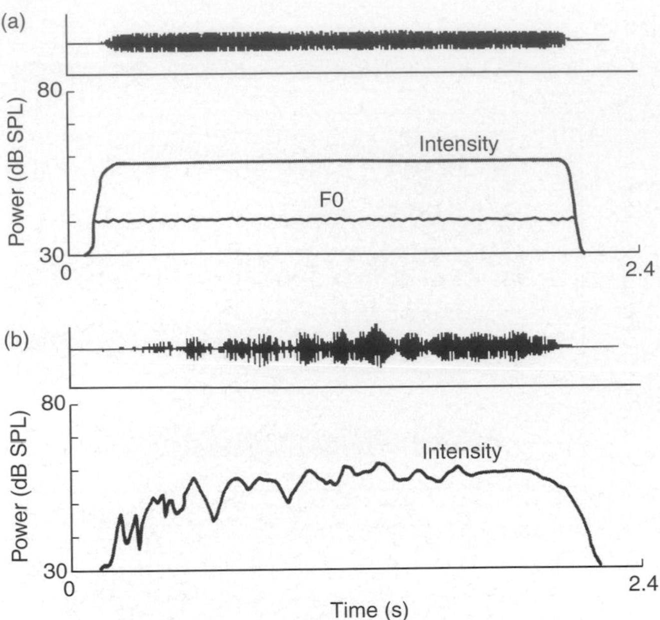

Figure 12.4 *Intensity contour display. (a) Normal phonation with natural and small fluctuation in intensity. F0 contour, which is stable, is also displayed. (b) A pathologic case with significant intensity fluctuation. F0 contour is not reliable in this case.*

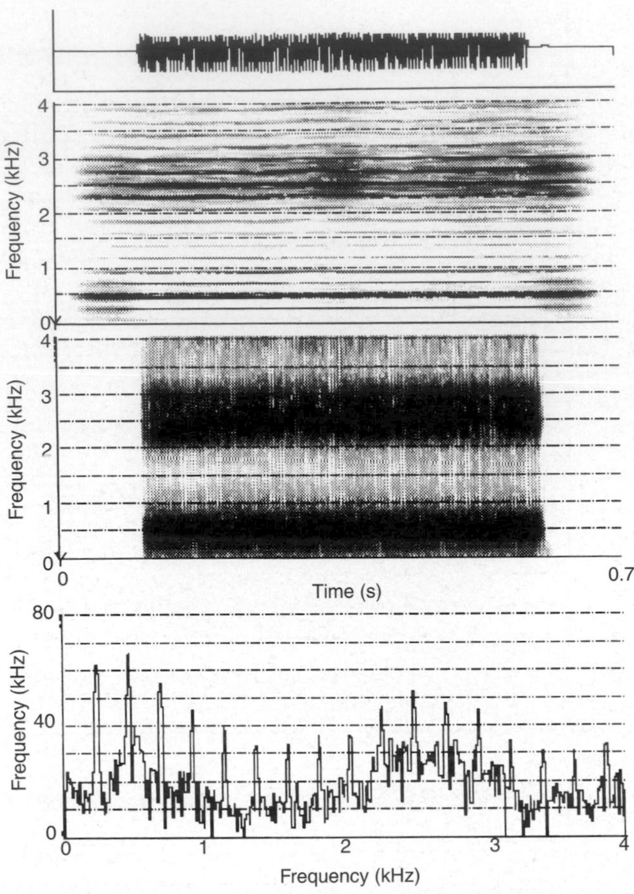

Figure 12.6 *Spectrographic characteristics of a voice sample recorded from a female subject with Reinke's edema after surgical treatment.*

A wide-band spectrogram, a pattern generated using a wide-band filter (a short time window), is best to visualize fast changes in frequency components, particularly articulation-related quantities, such as formant frequencies and their trajectories, frequency characteristics of consonants. This type of pattern is also useful for observing glottal pulses and their regularity. The glottal pulses observed in Fig 12.3a are regularly repeated, whilst those in Fig 12.3b show irregular glottal pulses and the case shown in Fig 12.3c had vocal interruptions or very low F0 particularly at the initial part of phonation.

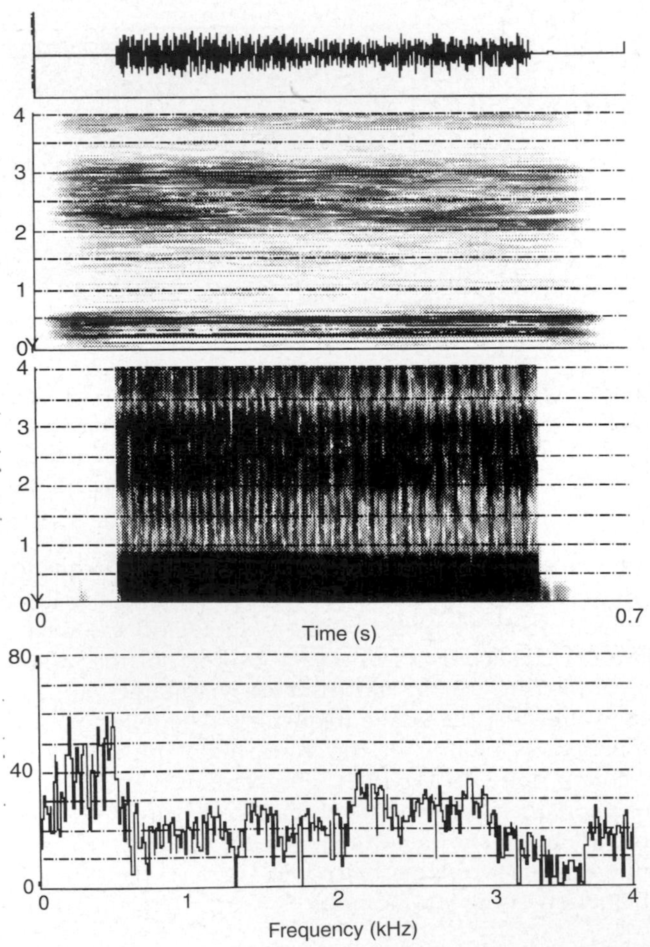

Figure 12.5 *Spectrographic characteristics of a voice sample recorded from a female subject with Reinke's edema before surgical treatment. Waveform, narrow-band spectrogram, wide-band spectrogram, and the power spectrum at the center of the voice sample. Only a central segment with a duration of 0.5 seconds was analyzed.*

Intensity contour display

Modern computerized spectrographic systems provide some other useful display formats, for instance the intensity contour and F0 contour. The intensity contour display produces a single trace representing temporal change of the total intensity (power). The intensity contour tends to fluctuate irregularly in pathologic voices, as shown in Fig 12.4b, reflecting unstable excitation of glottal voice source. The intensity contour display can be used to measure the possible intensity range of phonation and its approximate mean value.

Clinical application

As one possible clinical application, spectrographic voice analyses[7] supplemented by computerized analyses[6] are discussed in this section for patients with Reinke's edema[14] before and after surgical treatment.

The effects of surgical treatment on the voice characteristics were remarkable. One example of voice changes before and after the surgical treatment is shown in Figs 12.5 and 12.6 for a female subject. The harmonic peaks in the voice recorded after surgery are evident, even in the high-frequency range up to 4 kHz, reflecting remarkable reduction of F0 fluctuation and non-harmonic noise components compared to that recorded before surgery.

The average F0 can be a useful index to evaluate the effects of training and surgical treatment. For patients with Reinke's edema,[14] the surgical treatment significantly affected their average F0. As shown in Fig 12.7a, it increased particularly for female patients, although their average F0 remained lower than the normal controls even after the surgery.

The extent of F0 fluctuation is defined as the present score of the ratio of the peak-to-peak value of fluctuation to the mean fundamental frequency, which tends to be larger for pathologic voices, especially for ones perceived as rough, than for normal ones. Some perturbation measures such as jitter[4,12] and pitch perturbation quotient (PPQ)[9] are useful for quantitative assessment. For patients with Reinke's edema,[8] significant reduction in PPQ was found after surgery, particularly for female patients as shown in Fig 12.7b.

Noise level[5] was estimated on a section display as the difference between the value averaged over the peaks and that averaged over troughs within a certain frequency range. Pathologic voices, especially ones perceived as breathy, tend to contain a larger amount of noise. Noise level decreased drastically after surgery particularly for female subjects as shown in Fig 12.7c. Various sophisticated signal processing methods to estimate harmonics-to-noise ratio[1,8,10,15] have been proposed.

The spectrography is most appropriate for overall qualitative assessments of voice, which can be supplemented by quantitative analyses using computerized voice analysis systems.[11] It is important, however, to remember that many types of laryngeal pathologies yield similar resultant acoustic characteristics and the final judgments of vocal conditions should be an evaluation of all the parameters available to the clinician.

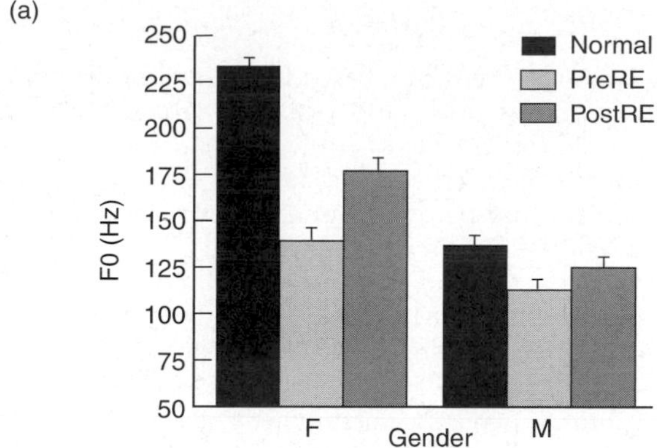

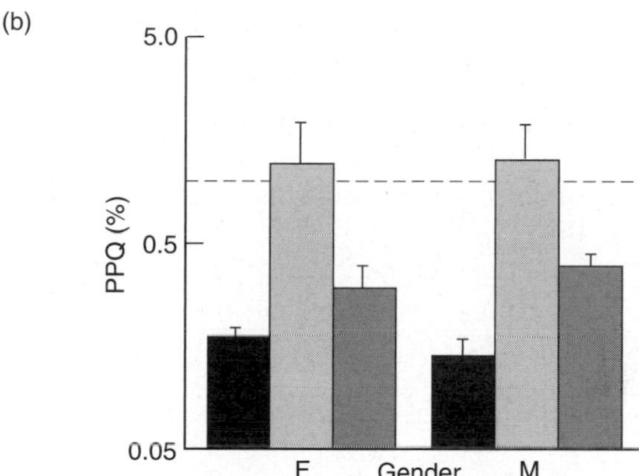

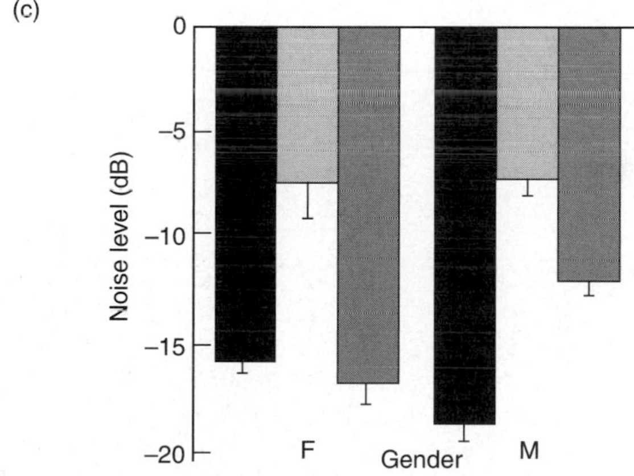

Figure 12.7 *Significant improvements in vocal characteristics of 72 patients with Reinke's edema compared with normal controls. (a) Average F0. (b) Pitch perturbation quotient (PPQ). (c) Noise level extracted by an adaptive comb filtering method. Normal, normal controls; PreRE, before surgery; PostRE, after surgery.*

References

1. de Krom G. A cepstrum-based technique for determining a harmonics-to-noise ratio in speech signals. *J Speech Hear Res* 1993; **36**: 254–66.
2. Hammarberg H, Fritzell B, Gauffin J, Sundberg J, Wedin L. Acoustic and perceptual analysis of vocal dysfunction. *J Phonetics* 1986; **14**: 533–47.
3. Hirano M. *Clinical Examination of Voice*. New York: Springer-Verlag, 1981.
4. Horii Y. Jitter and shimmer differences among sustained vowel phonation. *J Speech Hear Res* 1982; **25**: 12–14.
5. Imaizumi S. Acoustic measurement of pathological voice qualities for medical purposes. *Proc ICASSP* 1986; **1**: 677–80.
6. Imaizumi S, Hiki S, Hirano M, Matsushita H. Analysis of pathological voices with a sound spectrograph. *J Acoust Soc Jpn* 1980; **36**: 9–16.
7. Imaizumi S, Abdoerrachman H, Niimi S, Hirose H, Saida S, Shimura Y. Evaluation of vocal controllability by an object oriented acoustic analysis system. *J Acoust Soc Jpn* 1994; **15**: 113–16.
8. Kasuya H, Ogawa S, Mashima K, Ebihara S. Normalized noise energy as an acoustic measure to evaluate pathologic voice. *J Acoust Soc Am* 1986; **80**: 1329–34.
9. Koike Y. Application of some acoustic measures for the evaluation of laryngeal dysfunction. *Studia Phonetica* 1973; **7**: 17–23.
10. Qi Y, Hillman RE. Temporal and spectral estimations of harmonics-to-noise ratio in human voice signals. *J Acoust Soc Am* 1997; **102**: 537–43.
11. Read C, Buder EH, Kent RD. Speech analysis systems: an evaluation. *J Speech Hear Res* 1992; **35**: 314–32.
12. Titze IR. Summary statement. *Workshop on Acoustic Voice Analysis*. Iowa City: National Center for Voice and Speech, 1995: 26–30.
13. Yanagihara N. Significance of harmonic change and noise components in hoarseness. *J Speech Hear Res* 1967; **10**: 531–41.
14. Yonekawa H. A clinical study of Reinke's edema. *Auris Nasus Larynx* 1988; **15**: 57–78.
15. Yumoto E, Gould WJ. Harmonics-to-noise radio as an index of the degree of hoarseness. *J Acoust Soc Am* 1982; **71**: 1544–9.

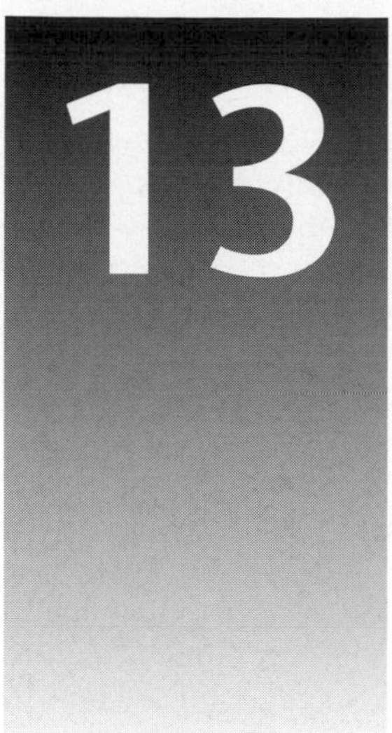

The phonetogram: measurement and interpretation

Harm K Schutte

In 1910, Gutzmann[11] wrote that there were actually three important aspects of the voice that needed to be investigated, as follows:

- the *fundamental frequency*, which as he wrote could easily be registered by just listening and comparing the pitch heard with a musical instrument;
- the *loudness* of the voice, which, in 1910, was very difficult to measure; and
- the *timbre* of the voice.

He evaluated the timbre by careful listening to the tone produced, and perceptually analyzing the different overtones. Of these three variables he also found pitch and timbre the easiest to measure, whereas he actually had no possibility of measuring the sound pressure level (SPL) or sound loudness. Since then, the approach to the investigation of vocal sound has changed drastically. Nowadays, nobody finds it difficult to measure the SPL; even the evaluation of timbre in its spectral components is an easy task with the proper, but mostly very expensive, instruments. Instrumental measurement of the pitch, or better – the fundamental frequency – appears to be more difficult. The composite vocal sound, as radiated from the mouth opening, is strongly influenced by the differentiating effect of the transition from mouth opening to the surroundings. This influences the strength of the upper partials, which then dominate in the sound being measured, giving rise to an incorrect data result for the fundamental frequency. The complexity of the instrumental determination of the fundamental frequency of vocal sound, as well as the costly instruments for spectral analysis, make it more difficult to use these kinds of instruments in most clinical settings.

Information about fundamental frequency and the SPL produced is of utmost importance for a proper evaluation of the voice of a patient. It was an idea of two Frenchmen, Calvet and Malhiac,[6] to use the combination of both variables to investigate the changes which go along with the changes of a boy's voice. They presented a diagram which was called 'courbe vocale'. A literature search revealed that even in one of the first issues of the *Journal of the Acoustical Society of America* such a diagram had been used to present data on the possibilities of the singing voice by Wolf *et al.* in 1935.[30]

After the first description of phonetogram-like profiles by Wolf *et al.*[30] and the early article by Calvet and Malhiac,[6] the method received sporadic attention in the literature.[7–9,13,18,29] In recent years, however, an increasing number of practical and theoretical articles on vocal function and voice use have dealt with phonetography. Recommendations were formulated to standardize procedures in the acquisition of phonetograms;[12,21] the potential of phonetography as a clinical tool was illustrated;[17,19,20] and the theoretical bases of voice range profiles were explored.[10,15,27,28]

The practical use of phonetography, as reflected in the literature, can be summarized as:

- assessing information about individual voice potentialities;
- investigating the influence of therapy or surgical intervention; and
- comparing phonetograms of selected groups.[1–3,7]

In 1968, Waar and Damsté[29] described tentatively the possibility of using phonetography in cases of voice patients. The method was further developed for routine clinical use by the present author. Since then the method has been used on a routine basis as an integral part of the work in the voice clinic in Groningen. Data of numerous cases were gathered and placed in relation to other data of voice patients. An extensive study on the characteristics of phonetograms in relation to voice training was done by Sulter *et al.*[25,26] The method was propagated in the DDR by Seidner and Schutte[23] and Seidner and Wendler.[24] For German-speaking countries they proposed the name 'Stimmfeld'. Nowadays, the term 'voice range profile' is more in use, after a decision of the Voice Committee of the International Association of Logopedics and Phoniatrics in 1992.[4]

Procedure of registering a phonetogram or voice range profile

A voice range profile can be defined as a graphical representation of the vocal potentialities, studying the attainable levels of sound pressure on different fundamental frequencies. To obtain a voice range profile, systematically the maximum and minimum SPLs are registered on several frequencies over the whole possible range of a voice.[18,21] To measure the SPL, a microphone is used at a constant mouth–microphone distance of 30 cm. Measurement of the pitch or fundamental frequency may be done by the easiest, and after our experience quite reliable, way by listening and comparing the tone sung with the known pitch of a musical instrument or custom-built pitch prompter. A certain procedure is followed in choosing the pitches after which the patient or test person has to sing. It appeared sensible to measure maximum and minimum SPL on about four pitches per octave, extending the number of prompted pitches at critical or interesting places over the frequency range. For instance, at the region of register change, it is worthwhile measuring at pitches closer together. Also at the very ends we use smaller steps. Since 1968, when we started, fundamental research has been done on the reliability of the voice range profile measurement, and a couple of investigators developed computer-assisted phonetographs, especially for solving the problem of the necessity of relying on the investigator's ear.

Therefore, a further contribution to the automatic registration of phonetograms has been the incorporation of a unit to determine fundamental frequency into the equipment.[5,14,16] The benefit of this unit is twofold: subjects or patients not able to sustain the given pitch can use an alternative (freely chosen) pitch. In addition, the occurrence of octave errors and other mistakes in determining the correct pitch, already small when the registration is performed by experienced investigators, will be minimal. The computer also makes it possible to create immediately processable phonetographic data files.

However, it is our considered opinion that in many pitch-measuring machines the probability of making errors is quite a possibility, although drastic measures have been undertaken to avoid these errors. In almost all cases this is noticeable in a registration of fewer potentialities of the voice investigated in the phonetogram. Also, much has already been said about the acoustic features of the room in which a voice range profile should be registered. For clinical purposes, however, the comparison of voice range profiles, intra-individual as well as inter-individual, is the most fundamental step.

Since a voice range profile reflects a person's voice capabilities, standardized measurement should provide a basis for a reliable comparison. It is therefore sufficient for clinical purposes to keep the registration conditions, also acoustical, the same between sessions. Aiming at a higher precision of the SPL measurement than 2–3 dB is not necessary, since a voice in a clinical situation shows that amount of variability. The same can be said about the frequency measurement, a precision of more than half a semitone, or even a semitone, is of no clinical significance. This practical approach often is neglected in exchange for a quasi-accuracy of the measurements, which is meaningless, but calls for a lot of effort. Involuntary changes of the same (2–3 dB) degree can be caused by the influence of microphone–mouth distance changes, acoustical influences of the room, and so on. Inaccuracies of this origin do not devale the clinical usefulness of a phonetogram registration. A mouth–microphone distance of 30 cm is usually practical. Small movements of the head or body, and therefore small changes in the distance, will have less influence on the SPL readings than with the microphone at a closer distance. A small head-mounted microphone will overcome the differences due to head movements to a certain extent, but the placement of the microphone near the mouth opening should be done very precisely, and therefore is more critical to small differences. A distance of 30 cm is, in a normal examination room, close enough to the microphone to be able to register the softest phonation of a voice, above the background noise in the room. Sometimes, background noise in the room from an air-conditioning machine or from adjacent rooms disturbs the reading of the softest phonations. These noises usually contain a considerable amount of low-frequency components. That explains why in such cases the use of a weighting filter might solve the problem in registering the soft SPL values of a voice.

Examples of voice range profiles

The following discussion presents some specific examples of normal and abnormal voice range profiles. To start with a normal healthy, but untrained voice, see Fig 13.1. Usually, the measured points of the softest and loudest phonation are connected by lines, which constitutes then the egg-like presentation. At a certain region, in males as well in females, there is a dip in the upper line of the phonetogram. This dip is closely related to the different registers of the voice.[22] In general terms, the part of lower frequencies is the region of the chest voice, whereas the high-frequency part is the region of the falsetto voice register. This dip in the line of the loudest phonation lies mostly around g^1, in American notation G4.

Figure 13.2 shows these two different areas corresponding with the two different registers indicated. To display

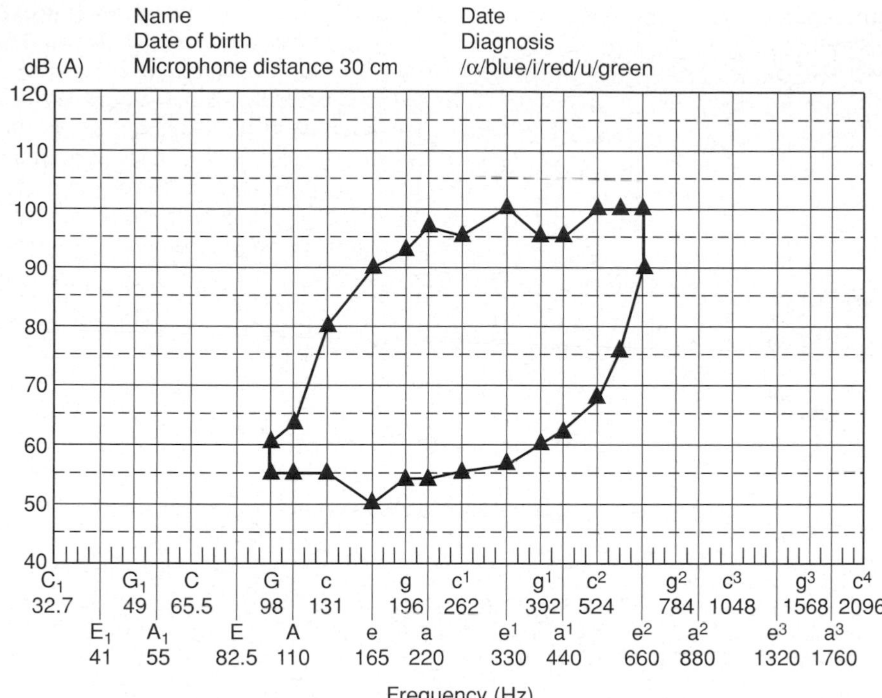

Figure 13.1 *Normal voice range profile of a not-exceptional, but healthy voice. Below, an indication of the musical note-names following the European (except France) standard.*

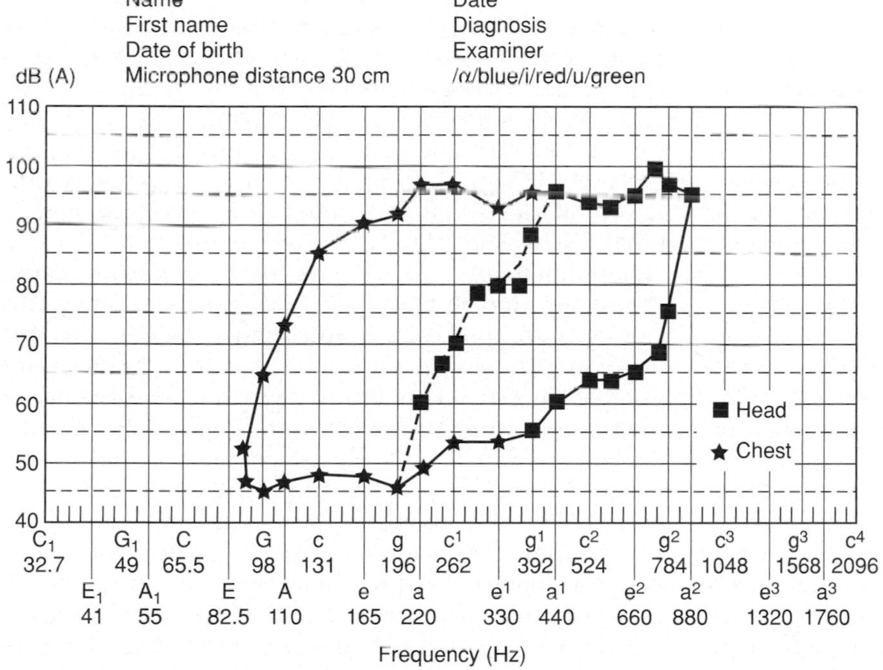

Figure 13.2 *Voice range profile of a singing voice (male) where the difference in quality between chest and head (falsetto) is indicated. The dotted line indicates the transition area, which was found by careful listening to the sound character change making a crescendo or decrescendo on the pitches between a (A3) and g^1 (G4).*

these register border lines in a voice range profile, the third voice characteristic, timbre, is included. This is done by listening to the quality of the vocal sound produced, also by extending the basic use of the phonetogram.

In most cases of voice patients it is not possible to make a clear, reliable distinction between registers. In patients' cases, in general, we may find one register, which may most appropriately be called 'the modal register'. More acoustical features measured by some instruments can be included in the voice range profile, like vocal jitter, vocal shimmer and spectral balance of the produced voice.[16] In this way the use of a voice range profile is extended, which makes sense for a deeper evaluation of the voice. For clinical use, the most basic form of a voice range profile with only the fundamental frequency versus the sound pressure level, can give essential information and

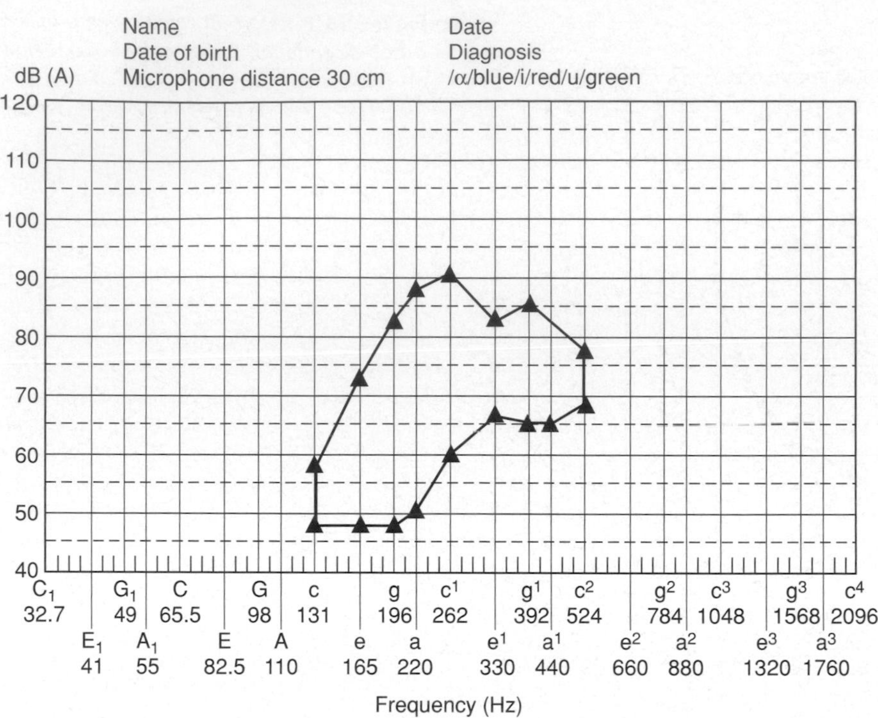

Figure 13.3 *A voice range profile from a female teacher with voice problems. The total possible sound pressure level – loudness capacity – is only 90 dB (A) on a too high pitch for ordinary use. In the speaking pitch level range only about 60–75 dB (A) can be obtained. This means in fact that the patient really will have problems in a noisy classroom.*

can make it easy to understand why a patient will have vocal complaints, especially in cases of vocally demanding professions. The next voice range profile (Fig 13.3) represents such a case.

This voice range profile shows the vocal potentialities of a female teacher. Even the loudest possible phonation, which is in fact screaming, just reaches 90 dB. A constant use of such a loud voice means vocal abuse and straining of the voice, and it may be assumed that this will rather soon lead to organic changes of the vocal folds. For a proper evaluation of the voice range profile we need to know the maximal capacities of the voice, to be able to compare this with the vocal demands. Therefore, and this must be stressed again, for clinical purposes, we can refrain from an evaluation of the voice quality during taking the voice range profile.

A normal voice range profile is characterized by a frequency range of at least 2 octaves and an intensity range of at least 30 dB at the mean speaking pitch level.

A voice range profile should be treated as a document of one specific patient and be evaluated in relation to other laryngeal evaluations. It is, in principle, an aid in comparing the vocal potentialities to the vocal demands, which makes sense especially in a voice-dependent profession. An evaluation of a voice range profile, and the interpretation of it, should be supported by a thorough visual examination of the larynx.

An acoustic-perceptual evaluation, sound recording and the registration of a voice range profile give, in general, sufficient information for daily clinical practice. The functional evaluation of vocal potentialities or capacities in relation to the vocal demands and the findings of the visual inspection give the medical doctor the basis for diagnosis and proper treatment. Although stroboscopy is most helpful for the evaluation of the larynx and studying the fast movements of the vocal folds, even without using the stroboscope, an incomplete dynamic glottis closure can easily be seen. This is an important aspect, because a larynx, showing an incomplete glottis closure, mostly at the dorsal part, means a larynx with limited possibilities. This fact is strongly corroborated by the establishment of a small voice range profile. It is our considered opinion that if one finds an incomplete glottis closure, and also a small voice range profile, this has important consequences for the prognosis of the voice disorder. In many, if not most cases, an improvement of the closure can hardly be expected, since it is an organic disturbance rather than a functional one.

The finding of low vocal potentialities can easily explain why the larynx also very often shows a slightly swollen aspect of the vocal folds, small epithelial changes, or vocal nodules. Even moderate vocal demands, put on a larynx with low capacity, lead to secondary organic changes of the vocal folds. A voice range profile helps us to understand the etiology of certain voice-use-related voice disturbances.

Voice range profiles may unravel more interesting aspects of the voice. For the interpretation of a voice range profile it is apparent from daily practice that implicit an evaluation is made of the total appearance of the profile. It is not only the frequency and dynamic range that are evaluated as such, but also the continuity, voice timbre equalization aspects, dips in the curves, which all constitute the shape, the curvature of the curve. All these aspects play an important role in the overall judgment.

References

1. Åkerlund L. Averages of sound pressure levels and mean fundamental frequencies of speech in relation to phonetograms: comparison of nonorganic dysphonia patients before and after therapy. *Acta Otolaryngol (Stockh)* 1993; **113:** 102–8.
2. Åkerlund L, Gramming P, Sundberg J. Phonetogram and averages of sound pressure levels and fundamental frequencies of speech: comparison between female singers and nonsingers. *J Voice* 1992; **6:** 55–63.
3. Awan SN. Phonetographic profiles and F0-SPL characteristics of untrained versus trained vocal groups. *J Voice* 1991; **5:** 41–50.
4. Bless DM, Baken RJ. International Association of Logopedics and Phoniatrics (IALP) Voice Committee Discussion of Assessment Topics. *J Voice* 1992; **6:** 194–210.
5. Bloothooft G. Nieuwe ontwikkelingen in de fonetografie. *Tijdschr Logoped Foniatr* 1982; **54:** 79–90.
6. Calvet PJ, Malhiac G. Courbes vocales et mue de la voix. *J Fr Otorhinolaryngol Chir Maxillofac* 1952; **1:** 115–24.
7. Coleman RF, Henn Mabis J, Kidd Hinson J. Fundamental frequency-sound pressure level profiles of adult male and female voices. *J Speech Hear Disord* 1977; **20:** 197–204.
8. Damsté PH. The phonetogram. *Pract Otorhinolaryngol* 1970; **32:** 185–7.
9. Dejonckere PH. Le phonetogramme, son interêt clinique. *ORL J Otorhinolaryngol Relat Spec* 1977; **12:** 865–72.
10. Gramming P. *The phonetogram: an experimental and clinical study*. Thesis, Lund University, Malmö, 1988.
11. Gutzmann H. Zur Messung der relativen Intensität der menschlichen Stimme. *Beitr Anat Physiol Pathol Ther Ohres Nase Halses* 1910, **3**: 233–60.
12. Hirano M. *Clinical Examination of Voice*. Berlin: Springer-Verlag, 1981.
13. Hollien H, Dew D, Philips P. Phonational frequency ranges of adults. *J Speech Hear Res* 1971; **14:** 755–60.
14. Jaroma M, Sonninen A, Hurme P, Toivonen R. Computer voice field observations of postmenopausal dysphonia. In: Frank F, ed. *Proceedings UEP Conference 1986, Vienna*. Vienna: Union of European Phoniatricians, 1986: 34–5.
15. Klingholz F, Martin F. Die quantitative Auswertung der Stimmfeldmessung. *Sprache-Stimme-Gehör* 1983; **7:** 106–10.
16. Pabon JPH, Plomp R. Automatic phonetogram recording supplemented with acoustical voice-quality parameters. *J Speech Hear Res* 1988; **31:** 710–22.
17. Schultz-Coulon H-J, Asche S. Das 'Normstimmfeld' – ein Vorschlag. *Sprache-Stimme-Gehör* 1988; **12:** 5–8.
18. Schutte HK. Over het fonetogram. *Tijdschr Logoped Foniatr* 1975; **47:** 82–92.
19. Schutte HK. *The Efficiency of Voice Production*. Thesis, University of Groningen. San Diego: Singular Publishing Group, 1980.
20. Schutte HK. Belastbaarheid van de stem en het fonetogram. *Ned Tijdschr Geneeskd* 1986; **130:** 2062.
21. Schutte HK, Seidner WW. Recommendation by the union of European phoniatricians (UEP): standardizing voice area measurement/phonetography. *Folia Phoniatr (Basel)* 1983; **35:** 286–8.
22. Schutte HK, van den Berg J. The efficiency of voice production. In: Urban BJ, ed. *Proceedings XVIIIth IALP*. Washington, DC: IALP Organizing Committee, 1980: 439–44.
23. Seidner WW, Schutte HK. Empfehlung der UEP: Standardisierung Stimmfeldmessung/Phonetographie. *HNO Praxis (Leipzig)* 1982; **7:** 305–7.
24. Seidner WW, Wendler J. Spektrales Stimmfeld. *HNO Praxis (Leipzig)* 1981; **6:** 187–91.
25. Sulter AM, Schutte HK, Miller DG. Differences in phonetogram features between male and female subjects with and without vocal training. *J Voice* 1995; **9:** 363–77.
26. Sulter AM, Wit HP, Schutte HK. Automatic evaluation of phonetograms. *Clin Otolaryngol* 1993; **18:** 86.
27. Titze IR. Acoustic interpretation of the voice range profile (phonetogram). *J Speech Hear Res* 1992; **35:** 21–34.
28. Vilkman EA, Sonninen A, Hurme P. Observations on voice production by means of computer voice fields. In: Kirikae I, ed. *Proceedings Logopedics and Phoniatrics: Issues for Future Research*. Tokyo: Organizing Committee of the XXth Congress IALP, 1986: 370–1.
29. Waar CH, Damsté PH. Het fonetogram. *Tijdschr Logoped Foniatr* 1968; **40:** 198–201.
30. Wolf SK, Stanley D, Sette WJ. Quantitative studies on the singing voice. *J Acoust Soc Am* 1935; **6:** 255–66.

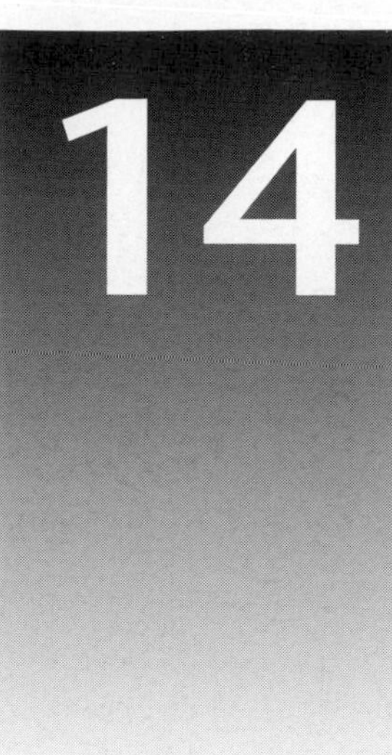

Diagnostic imaging of the larynx

Ian J Witterick, Arnold M Noyek and Edward E Kassel

Many benign laryngeal diseases have a typical clinical history and appearance and usually do not require any form of imaging. However, imaging is an important adjunct in the diagnosis and management of some laryngeal diseases, most importantly laryngeal neoplasms. The otolaryngologist evaluating a laryngeal mass can usually assess the surface limits by indirect and direct laryngoscopy.[91] Laryngeal imaging is most helpful in assessing the depth and extent of disease deep to the surface. This information is used in staging of disease and may help to guide surgeons or radiotherapists in their treatment plans. Imaging will rarely give a definitive diagnosis as this requires a biopsy. The information gained from both clinical surface evaluation and imaging will give the treating physician a better understanding of the extent of disease.

In the past, plain radiographs and complex motion tomography gave some useful information to clinicians but have been superseded by the technologic advances made by computed tomography (CT) and magnetic resonance imaging (MR). In a living, breathing and therefore moving person, the quality of laryngeal imaging has a major dependence on the speed of image acquisition. Patient movement (especially breathing and swallowing) during image acquisition will cause motion artifact which can make image interpretation difficult or impossible. However, with newer spiral CT scanners and fast MR techniques, this problem has been dramatically reduced, but not altogether eliminated.

Respiratory movements

In the past, diagnostic imagers asked patients to go through several respiratory maneuvers to highlight certain areas of the larynx and demonstrate vocal cord mobility. In the coronal plain with breath-holding and straining against a closed glottis (Valsalva maneuver), the cords are adducted and the subglottic arch squared off. In a modified Valsalva maneuver, the patient puffs his or her cheeks and allows air to escape slowly. This dilates the pyriform sinuses and the airway structures above the true vocal cord. Phonation (e.g. high-pitched ‘eeee’ sound) on expiration tenses the cords, leaving a narrow airway, whilst phonation on inspiration dilates it. Some maneuvers are expected to produce certain effects in the larynx but, in reality, the ‘effect’ may only show up with another maneuver. Therefore, most patients are put through all of the maneuvers.

These respiratory maneuvers were especially useful during contrast laryngography and multidirectional tomography. However, the maneuvers were difficult for patients to maintain during the acquisition times initially required for CT and MR and so were not useful and their popularity waned. With the advent of faster CT and MR imaging, these techniques may once again prove useful in highlighting some structure and movement of the larynx.

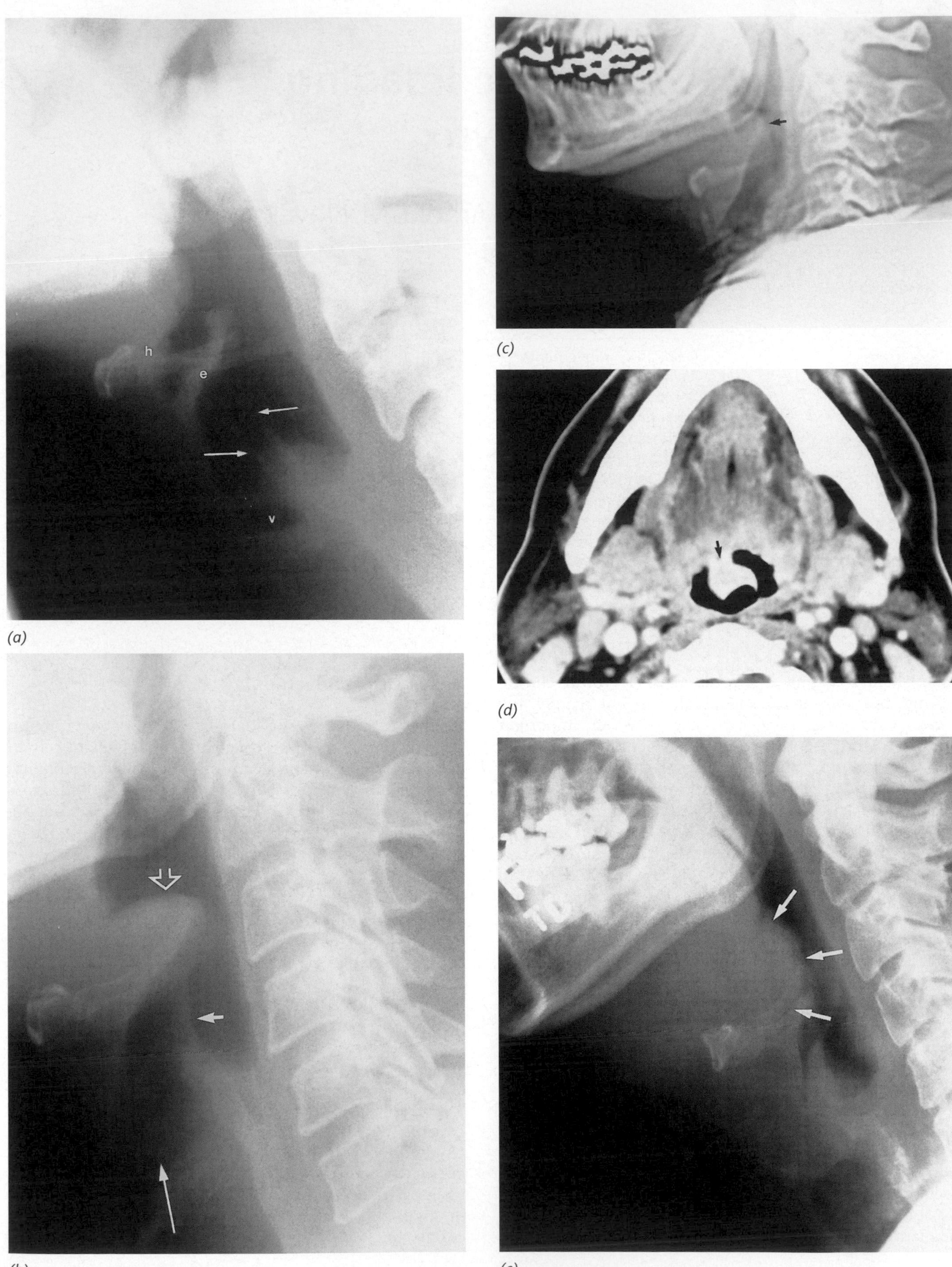

(a)

(b)

(c)

(d)

(e)

Figure 14.1 *Plain radiographs: upper airway, epiglottis, submandibular space, larynx. (a, b) Lateral plain film. (a) Normal anatomy. Epiglottis (e), aryepiglottic folds (horizontal arrows) and laryngeal ventricle (v) clearly defined; h, hyoid bone. (b) Acute epiglottitis. Note diffuse swelling of the epiglottis (open arrow). Aryepiglottic folds (short arrow) and ventricle (long arrow) also seen. (c, d) Same patient. (c) Lateral digital CT image shows enlarged epiglottis (arrow). Lateral image obtained for CT slice localization does not replace higher resolution characteristics of conventional or diagnostic computed/digital imaging. (d) Corresponding axial CT shows thickened epiglottis and glossoepiglottic fold (arrow). (e) Ludwig's angina. Lateral film shows prominence of soft tissues of submandibular space and base of tongue (solid arrows). Epiglottis and aryepiglottic folds have normal calibre.*

Plain radiographs

Plain radiographs give a crude appreciation of the larynx and pharynx using air as a differentiating contrast medium within soft tissues of the neck. Anteroposterior (AP) and lateral films are usually taken. AP views are limited in interpretive capabilities because the overlapping cervical spine obscures an adequate assessment in most instances. High-kilovolt filtered radiographs[45,46] and tomography to blur the image of the spine have been used to visualize the airway in the AP plain but are rarely necessary today with the advent of modern imaging techniques.

The lateral film gives the most useful information. Air in one or both ventricles marks the upper margin of the true cords and air extending below the larynx marks the tracheal air column. The epiglottis and aryepiglottic folds are usually visualized. The thickness of the retropharyngeal soft tissues can be a clue to inflammatory, infectious or post-traumatic events (Fig 14.1b–e).

An understanding of the normal variable ossification aging patterns of the laryngeal cartilages is important so a normally ossified laryngeal cartilage is not misdiagnosed as a foreign body. The superior margin of the cricoid lamina usually calcifies early, causing a linear radiopacity on plain films often mistaken for a foreign body by emergency room personnel. The signet portion of the cricoid then ossifies and may be asymmetric, giving the false impression of a foreign body. Calcification in arytenoid cartilage, thyroid cartilage and the tretaceous cartilage in the posterior thyrohyoid ligament may also masquerade as a foreign body.

The radiographic imaging should not alter the decision for surgical intervention since not all foreign bodies are radiopaque. In one study by Silva *et al.* of 93 patients with an airway foreign body, the sensitivity and specificity of conventional radiography in identifying the presence of a foreign body was 73% and 45%, respectively.[75]

Xeroradiography

Xeroradiography enhances the soft tissue edges to help define the anatomy of the larynx and trachea, including soft tissues, fat planes and cartilage.[16] It was a good technique to evaluate the subglottis, trachea and to search for foreign bodies. It is rarely available today due to the three to five times higher exposure to radiation compared with conventional plain films and the availability of superior imaging modalities, namely CT and MR.

Tomography

Conventional linear and multidirectional tomography (Fig 14.2) help view the anatomy of the larynx by blurring out the adjacent cervical spine. The technique involves moving the x-ray tube in a specific motion over the desired target (the patient on a table) and moving the film in the opposite direction. The exposures can be done over several seconds which is long enough for most patients to perform the respiratory maneuvers discussed above to help delineate certain areas of the larynx, especially in the coronal plain. However, the radiation exposure can be very high since multiple slices are taken, often with and without respiratory maneuvers.

Tomography of the larynx is most helpful in the frontal projection because it blurs out the superimposed cervical spine seen on plain AP images. Tomography in the lateral plain adds little additional information to standard lateral plain film radiographs.

Tomography visualizes the surface topography of laryngeal deformities well but does not show the deeper extension or invasive nature of a lesion. Deeper extent/invasion can be estimated by looking at distortion of the soft tissues but for this reason, tomography has been replaced by CT and MR imaging.

Fluoroscopy

Fluoroscopy is seldom required today with the advent of fiberoptic telescopes to visualize the larynx. However, in the past it was used in a select group of patients to assess vocal cord mobility. If the otolaryngologist was unable to assess vocal cord mobility due to a strong gag reflex or obstructing tumor and the patient was thought to be unfit or it was deemed unsafe to perform direct clinical examination of the larynx without general anaesthesia, then this technique had an application. It has also been used for research purposes to measure the movements of the epiglottis during respiration in humans.[1] It requires the patient to be able to lie still on an examination table with the fluoroscopy machine over their neck and to be able to follow verbal commands. The resulting images are viewed in real time and can be recorded for more detailed assessment or discussion at a later date.

Contrast laryngography

Contrast laryngography is a technique of coating the larynx with a non-toxic contrast material, e.g. oil-based propyliodone (Dionosil). The oral cavity, pharynx and larynx are first anesthetized topically and the contrast

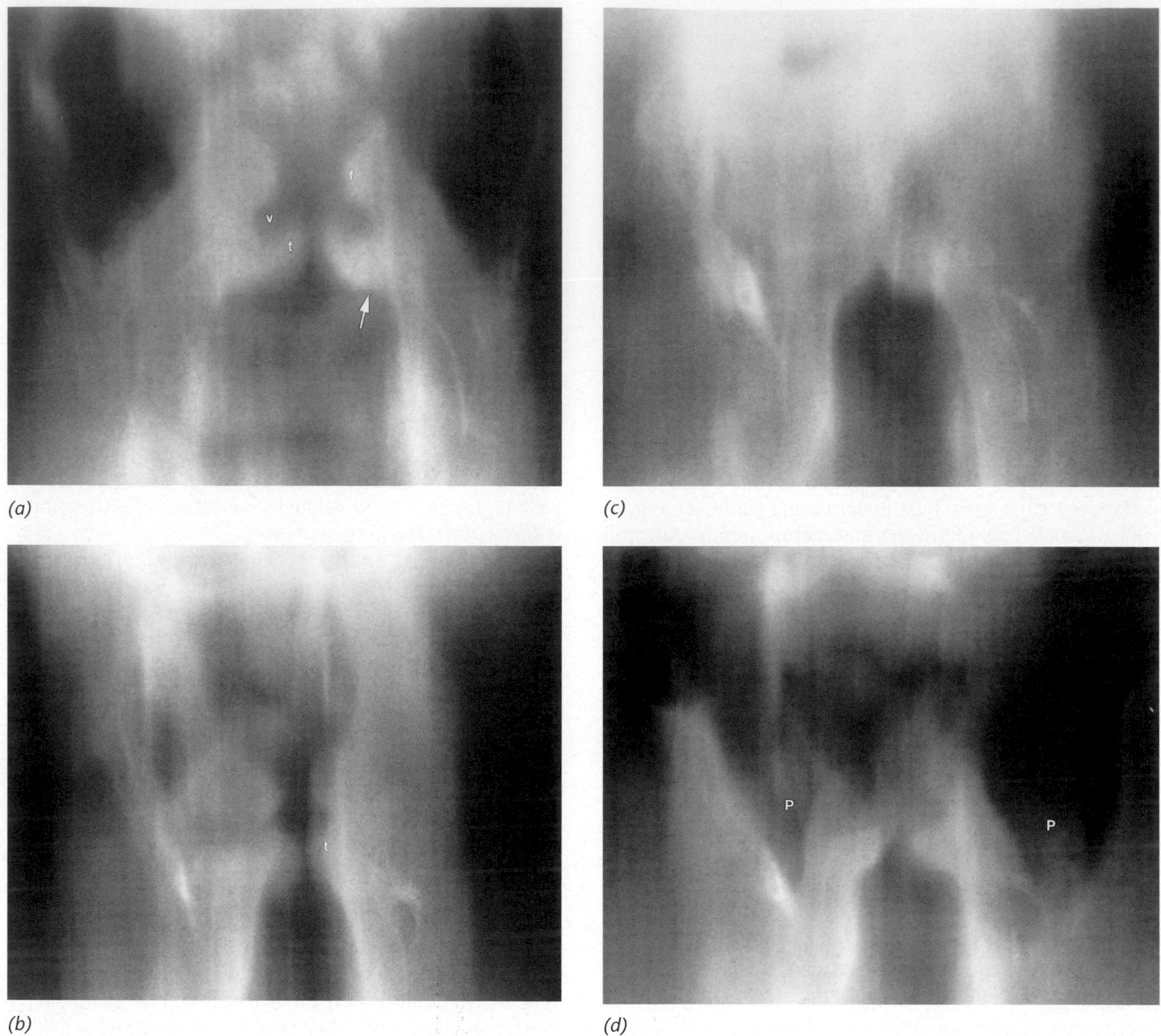

(a) (c) (b) (d)

Figure 14.2 *Conventional tomography of the larynx. (a) Coronal tomogram during phonation ('eeee' maneuver) demonstrates the true cord (t), false cord (f) and laryngeal ventricle (v) very well. The vocal cords tense and approach the midline with a narrow airway at the level of the true cords. The flat upper surface and downward sloping lower surface (subglottic arch) of the vocal cords (arrow) are best seen on phonation. (b–d) Different patient. Alteration and configuration of larynx noted with various respiratory maneuvers during imaging. (b) Quiet breathing. The vocal cords (t) are abducted from the midline and less sharply contoured than noted in phonation. With slow inspiration, the true and false cords would abduct further. (c) Valsalva maneuver. The cords have moved to the midline (adducted) and no airway is seen at the level of the true cords. The false cords may also approximate in the midline. The subglottic arch is squared off. (d) Modified valsalva (puffed cheeks). This maneuver dilates the pyriform sinuses (P) and all structures above the level of the true cords. Since any specific maneuver may not offer the desired result, the tomographic study typically includes the full set of maneuvers. No information is offered regarding the depth of tissue involvement, a significant limitation of this modality.*

material is dripped in by a laryngeal cannula or nasal tube. The patient coughs gently to distribute the contrast and the effect can be monitored by fluoroscopy. After there is sufficient coating of the laryngeal structures, various projections of the larynx (frontal, lateral, oblique) are taken with or without respiratory maneuver.

In the past, the contrast laryngogram was considered useful to visualize the ventricle and anterior commissure regions, especially if obscured by a neoplasm. If the lateral view shows the thin line of contrast in the ventricle and if the line reaches the anterior commissure, then this is evidence that the region is free of tumor. The anterior projection is checked to ensure that both ventricles fill as they could be superimposed on the lateral projection. The pyriform sinuses and postcricoid areas can also be defined with contrast but are more easily visualized with barium swallow.

Contrast laryngography helps to define surface mucosal irregularities but not deeper submucosal pathology.[53,59,63] Unfortunately, the patients in whom it could be most helpful are also the ones on whom it would be the most dangerous to perform the procedure. These patients have large laryngeal neoplasms in which the extent of disease is difficult to define. The anesthesia and contrast material may precipitate upper airway obstruction and even with topical anesthesia, atropine to dry secretions and codeine or other cough suppressant, the procedure is poorly tolerated by many patients. For these reasons as well as the advent of better endoscopic instruments to visualize surface pathology and CT/MR to evaluate submucosal pathology, contrast laryngography is seldom used or required today.

Ultrasound

Ultrasound has limited applications for imaging the larynx due to the cartilaginous framework which reflects most of the sound before it reaches the interior of the larynx. Nonetheless, it is possible to image the larynx using high resolution and high-frequency probes.[64,87] The mobility of vocal cords can be assessed but are usually amenable to examination clinically.[64] The cystic nature of a mass adjacent to the larynx can be confirmed by ultrasound suggesting a laryngocele. It is also possible to assess the external surface of the thyroid and cricoid cartilages with ultrasound to look for extension of malignant disease through cartilage or perichondritis.[68] However, CT and MR are superior at defining these areas.

Arens *et al.* used high-frequency ultrasound for diagnosing diseases of the endolarynx using small, high-resolution, real-time ultrasound transducers (10 and 20 MHz) placed on the tip of endoluminal catheters in 20 autopsied larynges and five laryngectomy specimens.[2] Depending on the frequency used, the endolaryngeal anatomy was visualized well up to a depth of 2 cm. In the five laryngectomy specimens, the cancer's depth and its relationship to the surrounding laryngeal framework were clearly seen. It may be possible to apply this technology in the assessment of living patients.

The greatest usefulness of ultrasound may lie in prenatal and pediatric assessment. The laryngeal cartilages in these age groups are not ossified and permit assessment of the anterior portions of the larynx. It is difficult to see the posterior portions of the larynx including the subglottis through the acoustic signal of the airway, limiting ultrasound's usefulness for glottic and subglottic pathology. Ultrasound can be used to assess mobility of the vocal cords and invasion of lesions such as lymphangiomas and hemangiomas.[23,24,86]

In the prenatal period, the airway is full of fluid, allowing better through transmission of the ultrasound signal. This has been used in the prenatal period to predict laryngeal and tracheal problems prior to delivery.[36] Criteria for diagnosis of a laryngotracheoesophageal cleft during prenatal ultrasound scans include:

- polyhydramnios;
- absent stomach; and
- presence of a lung cyst.[70]

These findings should alert clinicians to the problem and institute appropriate counselling and management.

Nuclear medicine imaging

There are very limited and selected indications for nuclear medicine imaging of the larynx. Red blood cell tagged scans have been used to accurately identify the vascular nature of laryngeal hemangiomas.[21] Noyek *et al.* have also described the usefulness of nuclear medicine imaging in diagnosing inflammatory arthropathies and relapsing chondritis of the larynx.[58,59]

Positron emission tomography

Positron emission tomography (PET) scanning is a relatively new radiologic imaging technique based on the difference in uptake and metabolism of substances such as glucose between normal and abnormal tissues. Its use is limited by the relatively few centers that have this technology and the intense demand for study time in facilities that do have one. It has not been used extensively to evaluate laryngeal pathology. Kostakoglu *et al.* studied the physiologic uptake of [^{18}F]fluoro-2-deoxyglucose (FDG) by the laryngeal muscles during speech in 24 patients randomized into a talking group and a no talking group.[41] FDG uptake in the laryngeal muscles correlated with speech and increased with increasing levels of speech during the uptake period. Subjects who remained silent had no detectable increase in uptake in the region of the larynx. This may provide a basis to allow differentiation of physiological from pathological uptake in the neck.

Greven *et al.* found PET with labeled FDG to be useful in distinguishing benign from malignant changes in the larynx after radiation therapy.[28] A follow-up study by McGuirt *et al.* evaluated 38 patients with laryngeal cancer; 25 prior to treatment and 13 patients who were previously radiated with curative intent but presented with edema and a diagnostic dilemma between the effects of radiation or cancer recurrence.[50] The PET scans using a glucose analog were compared with clinical examination, CT and MR. The PET scans were as accurate as the other methods of evaluation in identifying primary tumors (88% correct) and metastatic lesions (82% correct). However, the PET scans were most helpful in differentiating recurrent tumor from postirradiation tissue sequelae. PET scans were found to lack anatomic detail compared with CT and MR as to the extent of disease for staging and therapeutic planning. More studies evaluating the utility of PET in laryngeal neoplasia are required to corroborate these findings.

Angiography

Angiographic evaluation of the larynx has very limited application and is seldom performed unless the vascular nature of a mass needs to be confirmed. Another indication for angiography includes embolization of a vascular mass (e.g. hemangioma, paraganglioma) either preoperatively or as an attempt to 'stabilize' it.[40]

Barium swallow

Barium is a contrast agent, swallowed by the patient, and followed by fluoroscopy into the pharynx, esophagus and stomach. The motility, pliability and mucosal surfaces of these areas are assessed and recorded. A swallowing study uses a similar but more complex procedure where patients swallow contrast-coated liquids and solids of various consistencies with or without specific maneuvers to identify and make recommendations regarding an individual's ability to swallow safely and effectively. If aspiration is a possibility, barium is a better contrast medium since water-soluble agents cause a chemical pneumonitis. On the other hand, if a perforation of the pharynx or esophagus is suspected, a water-soluble contrast agent is preferable as it is less toxic to the mediastinal structures compared with barium.

When the patient swallows the barium, it is normally deflected around both sides of the vallecula into both pyriform sinuses and then joins again in the postcricoid region to enter the esophagus. The larynx normally acts as a filling defect but if there is asymmetry to the columns of barium as they flow around the larynx, then a mass is suspected. After coating the mucosal surfaces with contrast and using some of the respiratory maneuvers discussed above, surface irregularities can be defined. The postcricoid region is evaluated on lateral films but can be difficult to interpret due to the small irregularities frequently seen in normal patients from mucosal redundancy and a venous plexus. In these cases it may be difficult to distinguish an early carcinoma from a normal mucosal variation on barium swallow.

In the hypopharynx, the barium swallow can be used to assess for mucosal irregularities or lack of normal pliability/distensibility suggestive of a neoplastic process. If a foreign body is suspected in the hypopharynx or esophagus, the barium swallow may help to define its presence and location. The cricopharyngeus muscle is assessed for abnormal relaxation or contraction. Esophageal diverticula and spontaneous gastroesophageal reflux are looked for. The patient can also be placed in the Trendelenburg position with abdominal pressure over the stomach to look for gastroesophageal reflux.

Computed tomography scanning

In the past, the abbreviation 'CAT' scan, standing for computer-assisted or computerized axial tomography, was used. With the advent of modern computerized tomographic imaging, other plains can be imaged directly or indirectly via computerized reformations/reconstructions. Hence the 'A' has been dropped from 'CAT' scan and the modality is simply referred to as CT by most diagnostic imagers. However, the axial plain is still the most frequently used CT imaging plain, including laryngeal imaging. Although the axial plain gives very useful information, the coronal plain seems ideal for understanding the depth and extent of many laryngeal tumors. Unfortunately, coronal images usually need to be reconstructed after the fact from images taken in the axial plain and rarely give the same high-quality sharp images seen with axial imaging. The major advantage of CT imaging is in the evaluation of structures deep to the mucosa.[44,47,59,81]

Technique

The patient is placed supine with the head stabilized on a sliding table top which moves into the large central aperture of a circular 'donut' (gantry) housing the x-ray source and detectors. The patient is positioned to orientate the slices through the larynx parallel to the laryngeal ventricle. The imaging sequence starts at the epiglottis or hyoid bone and proceeds inferiorly to below the level of the cricoid cartilage (i.e. to include the subglottis and upper trachea). If a laryngeal malignancy is known or suspected, then the neck is imaged at the same time to look for metastatic nodal disease.

There are several choices for slice thickness. Generally thinner slices closer together will give the most detail but add increased imaging time and resources. Many institutions set up their own policies to try to maximize diagnostic information and patient 'throughput'. Some imagers take 1 mm slices every 3 mm whereas others use 3 mm slices every 3–5 mm. Thin 1 mm slices every 1 mm through an area of interest can be taken if deemed to be necessary or helpful. The patient moves the desired distance through the gantry for each slice. The scan can be done with the patient breath-holding for each slice or breathing quietly throughout the scan. This type of conventional CT scan can usually be completed in 10–20 minutes.

Spiral CT scanners acquire images much faster than conventional CT scanners with as little as 10–20 seconds required for laryngeal imaging. Instead of moving the patient repeatedly for incremental images at each desired slice distance, the spiral CT scanner moves the patient continuously through the x-ray apparatus, which continuously circles the patient and acquires the volume

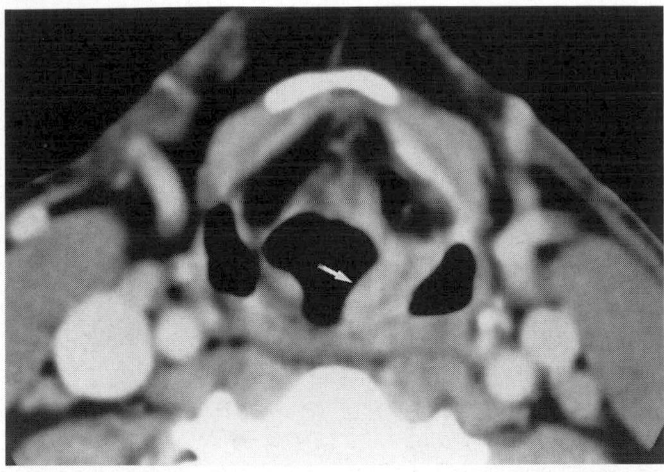

(a)

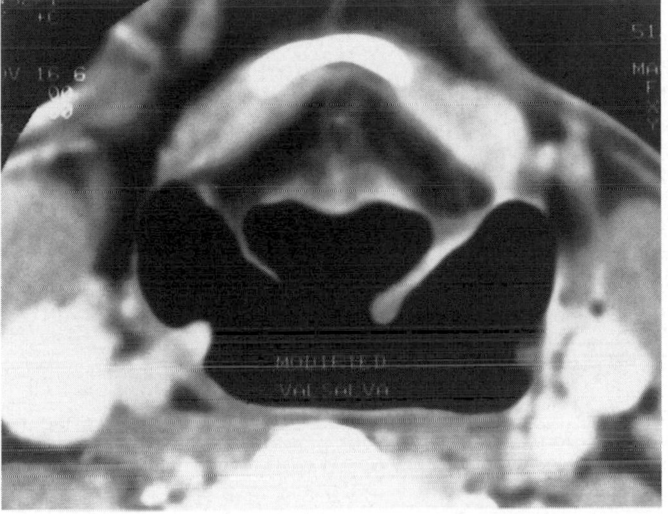

(b)

(c)

Figure 14.3 *Imaging techniques: airway distensibility/tissue measurements. (a, b) Same patient, CT at same level at rest and during modified Valsalva. (a) At rest. Left aryepiglottic fold prominent (arrow). (b) Slice level repeated with modified Valsalva to better visualize pyriform sinus and aryepiglottic fold. Although high-resolution CT usually demonstrates tissues well at rest, imaging with the airway distended may help assess or rule out mass lesions. (c) Use of wide windows and Hounsfield tissue measurement (square box) allows low density lipoma (minus 70 HU) to be more easily distinguished from air. Density reading is specific for adipose tissue. Patient presented with stridor.*

acquisition imaging data. Figuratively speaking, the acquired data set looks like a spiral or like the peel of an apple on stretch. The same data can be used to generate coronal, sagittal and three-dimensional images.

The image quality of spiral CT scanners is comparable to conventional CT scanners. The obvious advantage of spiral CT scanners is the rapid acquisition time which minimizes motion artifact.[65,76,81] Theoretically, spiral CT scanners could allow the reintroduction of respiratory maneuver to delineate some areas of the larynx, although to our knowledge this has not been extensively investigated (Fig 14.3).

Using helical CT scanners, a three-dimensional (3D) virtual endoscopy of the larynx and trachea can be performed.[67,76] Sakakura *et al.* used reconstructed 3D images in one dissected human larynx and 10 patients with laryngeal cancer.[69] The larynges were scanned in 1–2 mm slices and reconstructed using a slice thickness of 0.5–1.0 mm. The macroscopic or endoscopic findings were compared with the 3D CT images. The 3D images were very helpful in understanding laryngeal anatomy, especially in the subglottic area. Yumoto *et al.* found, in the patients with laryngeal cancer, axial images which showed that the extent of tumor gave more information than 3D endoscopic images.[94] However, in patients with recurrent laryngeal nerve paralysis, the combination of 3D endoscopic and cross-sectional images offered more diagnostic information than axial images alone.

The volume of various structures and tumors can be measured using spiral CT. The normal volume estimation of the pre-epiglottic and paraglottic spaces is highly variable and must be taken into context with the body area and more importantly the gender of the patient. In a study by Hermans *et al.*, the mean estimated volume of the pre-epiglottic and paraglottic space was 2.8 ml (standard deviation 1.7 ml, range 0.7–5.9 ml).[31] Volume estimation has been found to be helpful in predicting local control for T3 glottic cancers[61] but not T2 glottic cancers.[54]

Intravenous (IV) contrast is not usually required for imaging of the larynx itself but is beneficial to better delineate a neoplasm or to differentiate lymph nodes from blood vessels.

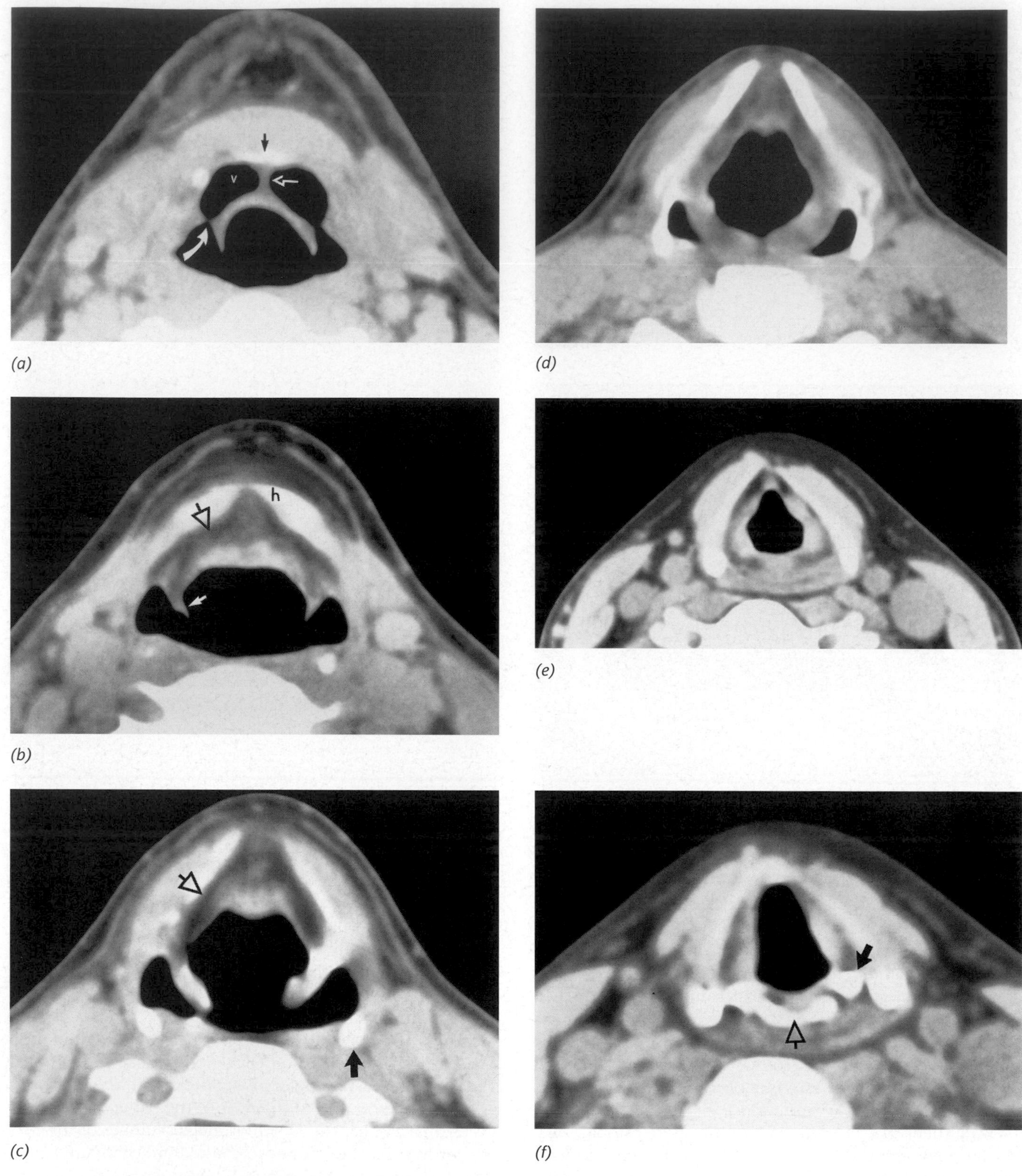

Correct timing of the IV bolus of contrast in relation to image acquisition is essential. If the contrast is given too early or too late, there will not be a high enough concentration in the blood vessels to adequately delineate the vessels from lymph nodes. If a vascular neoplasm of the larynx is suspected, contrast may be helpful to corroborate this.[40]

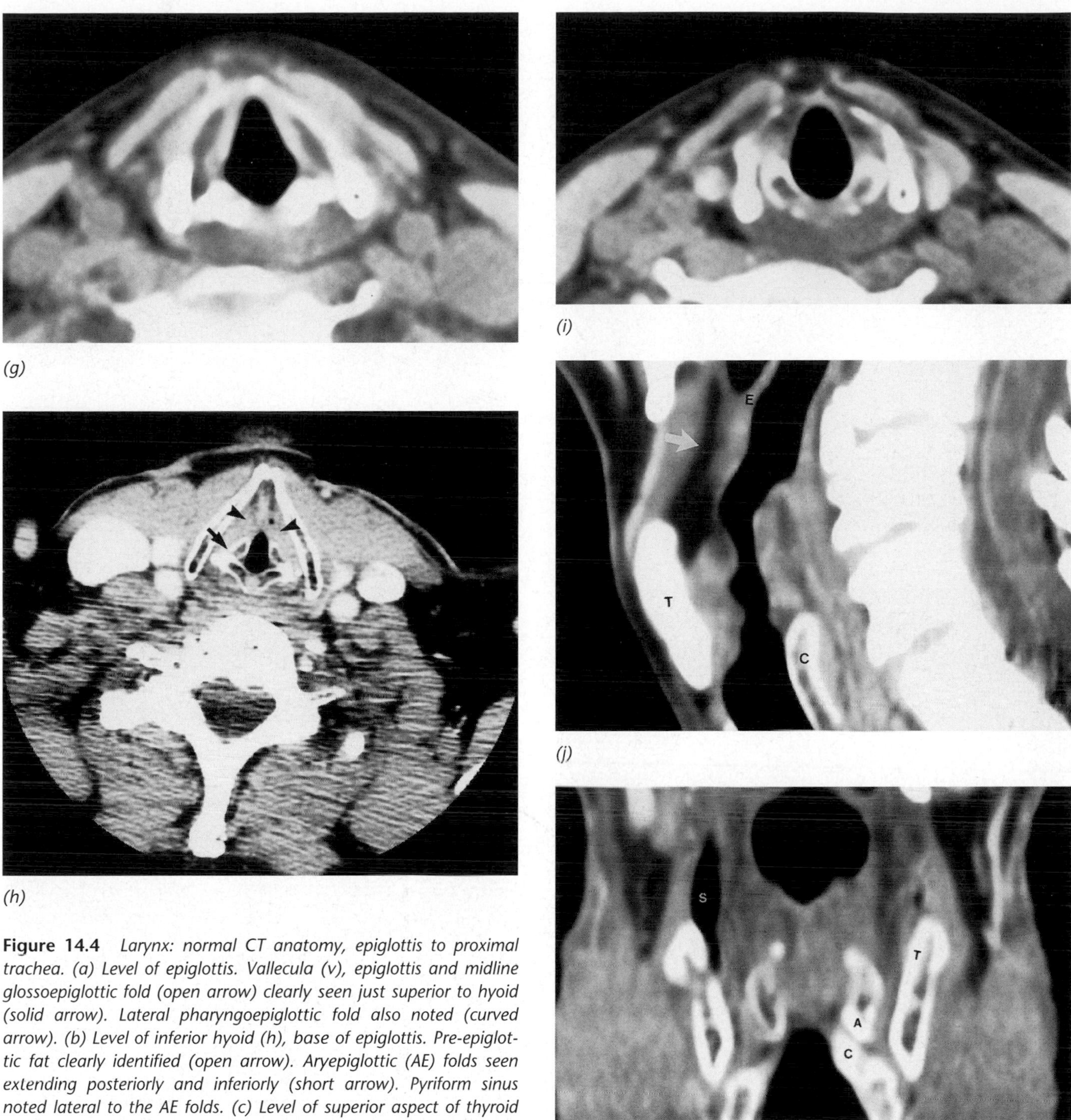

(g)

(h)

(i)

(j)

(k)

Figure 14.4 *Larynx: normal CT anatomy, epiglottis to proximal trachea. (a) Level of epiglottis. Vallecula (v), epiglottis and midline glossoepiglottic fold (open arrow) clearly seen just superior to hyoid (solid arrow). Lateral pharyngoepiglottic fold also noted (curved arrow). (b) Level of inferior hyoid (h), base of epiglottis. Pre-epiglottic fat clearly identified (open arrow). Aryepiglottic (AE) folds seen extending posteriorly and inferiorly (short arrow). Pyriform sinus noted lateral to the AE folds. (c) Level of superior aspect of thyroid cartilage. AE folds more prominent, separating the pyriform sinus from larynx. Paraglottic fat tissue plane (open arrow) noted anterolateral to AE fold. Superior thyroid cornu noted posterior to pyriform sinus (solid arrow). (d) AE folds approach each other posteriorly. Normal paralaryngeal fat tissue plane seen bilaterally. Note normal prevertebral and retropharyngeal tissue thickness at posterior hypopharyngeal wall. (e) Supraglottic larynx just above level of false cord. Paraglottic fat still present. (f) Level of upper true cord. Normal relationship of arytenoid (solid arrow) and cricoid (open arrow) cartilages seen. Paraglottic fat plane becomes effaced by prominence of thyroarytenoid muscle. (g) Level of true cord one slice inferior to (f) shows normal configuration of anterior commissure, cricoarytenoid joints. (h) Thinner slice (1 mm), detail algorithm better displays muscle density attenuation of thyroarytenoid muscles bilaterally (arrowheads) with absence of paraglottic fat. Cricoarytenoid joints better displayed (arrow). (i) Level of subglottic larynx shows normal minimal thickness of subglottic mucosa/submucosa. (j) Sagittal reformation just off midline clearly demonstrates pre-epiglottic fat tissue space (white arrow). Epiglottis (E), thyroid cartilage (T) and cricoid cartilage (C) also seen. (k) Posterior coronal reformat shows arytenoid (A), thyroid (T) and cricoid (C) cartilages, as well as posterior aspect of right pyriform sinus (S).*

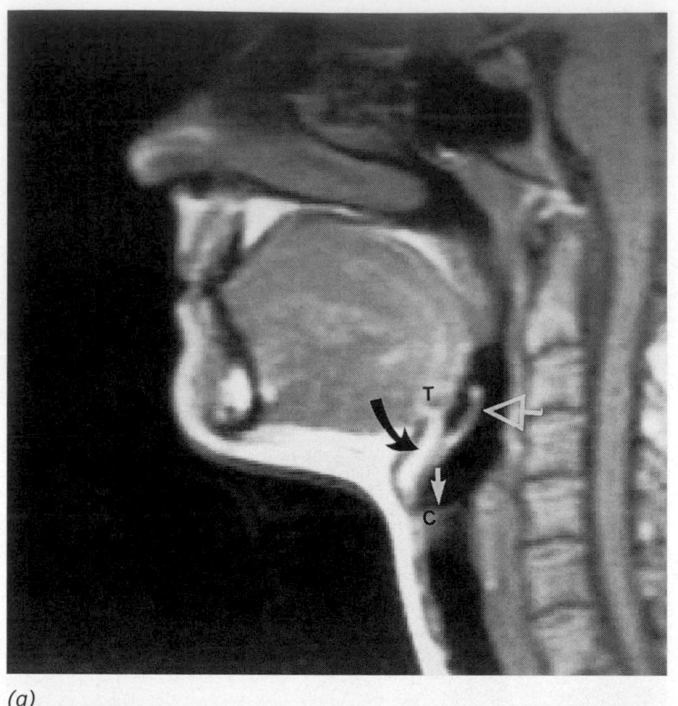

(a)

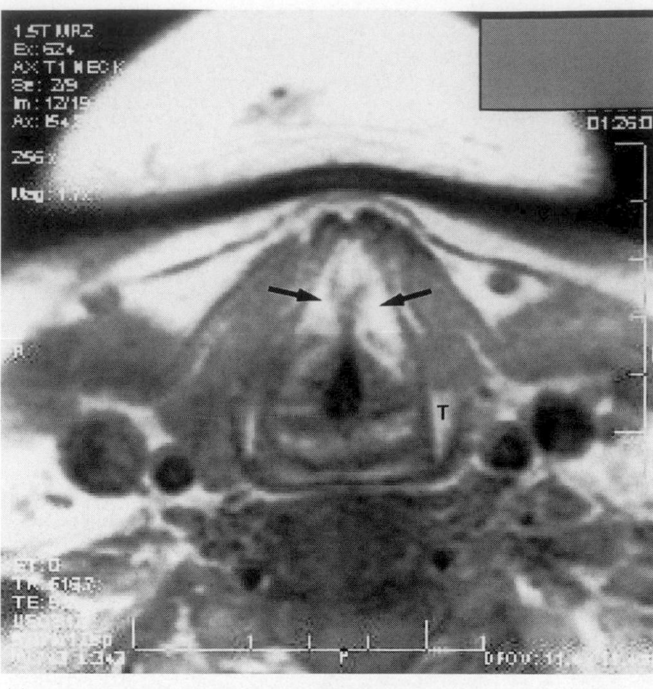

(c)

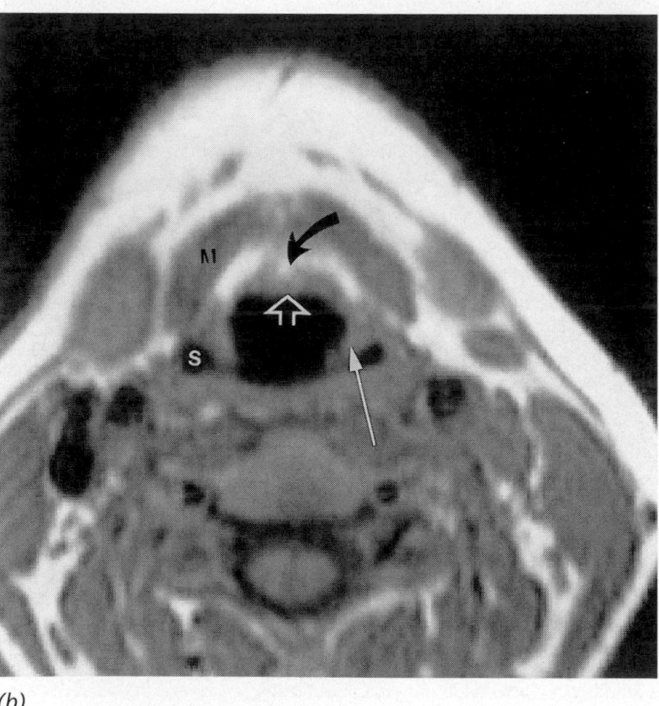

(b)

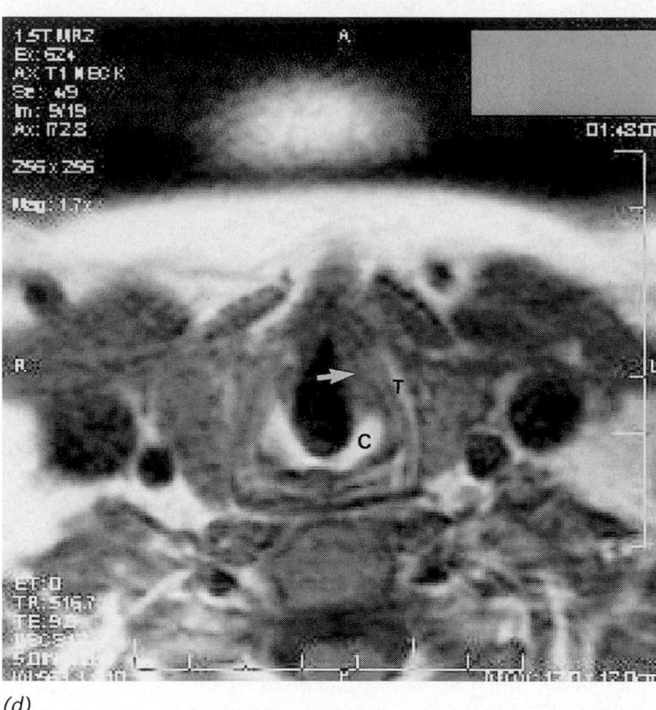

(d)

CT: normal anatomy (Fig 14.4)

The upper axial slices show the vallecula, epiglottis and connecting ligaments. Proceeding inferiorly, the lateral margins of the epiglottis merge with the aryepiglottic folds. The shape of the black air column progressively narrows to a slit at the level of the true vocal cords but then widens again in the subglottis. The pharyngeal constrictors have an elongated flattened appearance due to their attachments laterally to the thyroid and cricoid cartilages. The transition from the hypopharynx to the esophagus is at the level where the muscle takes on a more rounded appearance, denoting the level of the cricopharyngeus muscle.

The pre-epiglottic space bounded by the hyoepiglottic ligament superiorly, the thyrohyoid ligament anteriorly and the anterior surface of the epiglottic cartilage posteriorly appears as a low attenuation space as the principal

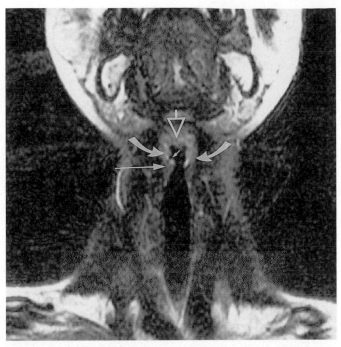

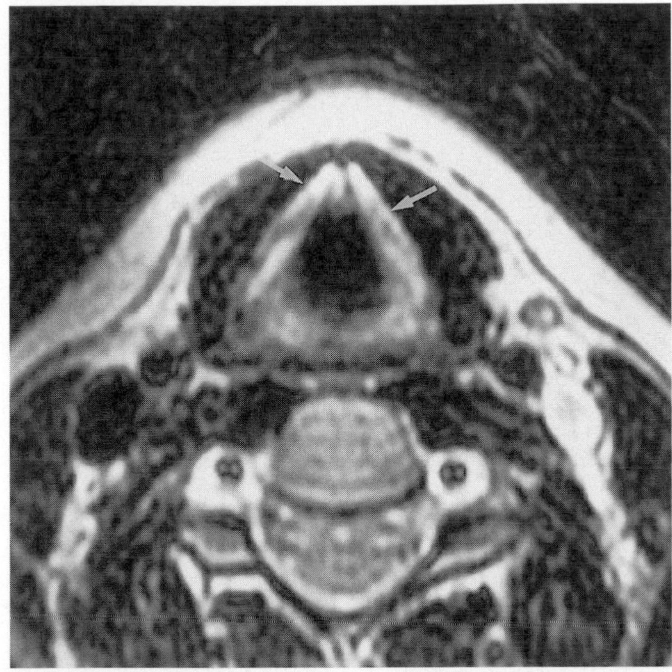

(e)

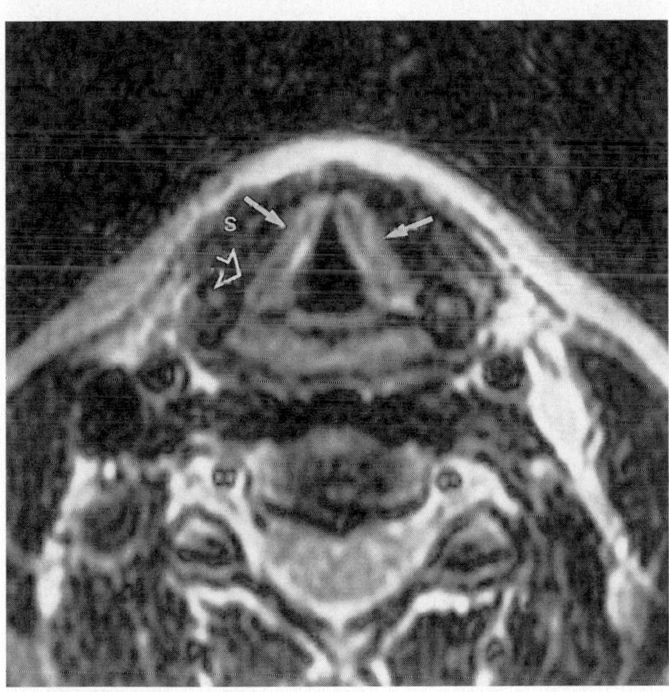

(f)

(g)

Figure 14.5 *Normal MR anatomy. (a) Sagittal T1 image. Sagittal images are excellent for displaying relationship of epiglottis (open arrow), pre-epiglottic fat (curved arrow), tongue base (T). Ventricle faintly seen (short arrow) just above true cord (C). (b) Axial T1 image level of epiglottis (open arrow). Pre-epiglottic fat (curved arrow), aryepiglottic fold (thin arrow), pyriform sinus (S) and strap muscles (M) clearly identified. (c) Axial T1 image at level of false cords shows fat in paraglottic space (arrows). T, thyroid lamina. (d) Axial T1 image at level of true cords. Note absence of paraglottic fat. Thyroarytenoid muscle (arrow), thyroid lamina (T), cricoid (C). (e, f) Fast spin-echo (FSE) T2 images at level of false cord (e) and true cords (f) show the increased paraglottic fat content (arrows, e) compared to the lower intensity signal at the level of the true cords (solid arrows, f). Note decreased signal of thyroid ala (open arrow, f), difficult to distinguish from overlying strap muscles (S). (g) T1 coronal image shows increased signal of pre-epiglottic fat (open arrow) and paraglottic space fat extending to the false cords (curved arrows). Signal intensity of thyroarytenoid muscle (horizontal thin arrow) noted at level of true cords. Anterior aspect of ventricle noted (oblique thin arrow).*

content is fat. The pre-epiglottic space opens laterally to be continuous with the paraglottic spaces. The paraglottic space on each side also contains predominantly fat and is of low attenuation lateral to the airway which appears black. Breath-holding during each slice will usually make the true cords come together and can improve visualization of the paraglottic fat. When the axial slices pass through the ventricle, the paraglottic space changes to muscle density (thyroarytenoid muscle). More inferiorly, the paraglottic space ends at the upper margin of the cricoid cartilage as it is limited by the conus elasticus. Therefore, there should be no soft tissue thickening within the ring of the cricoid cartilage.

The laryngeal cartilages have considerable variation in their appearance. Women in general have a wider angle between the two thyroid alae and men have a more prominent thyroid notch or 'Adam's apple'. Normally, in children and younger individuals there is not much 'calcification'

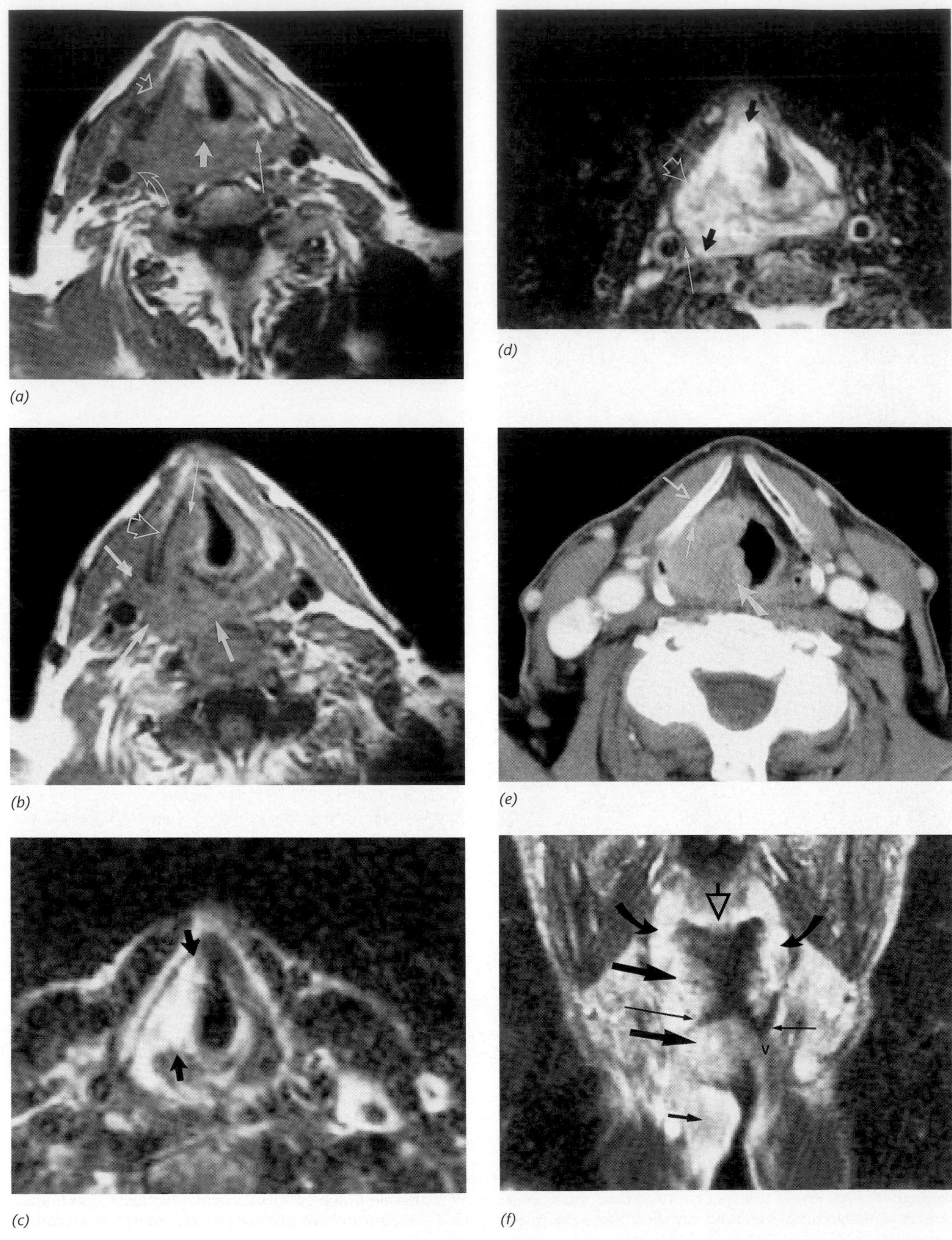
(a)
(b)
(c)
(d)
(e)
(f)
V

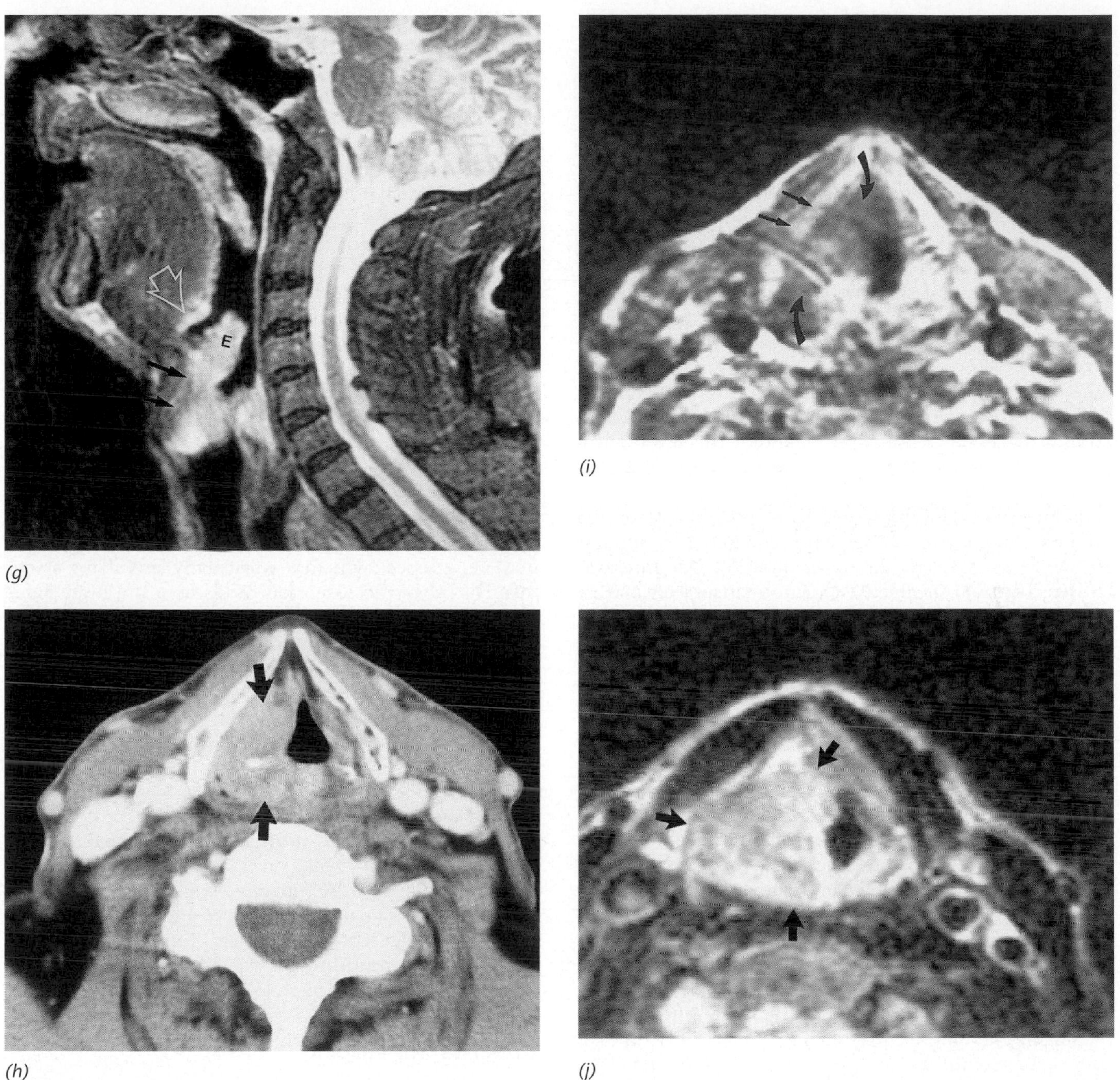

Figure 14.6 *MR of laryngeal carcinomas. (a–d) Same patient. Right supraglottic carcinoma. (a) Axial T1 image shows large mass as intermediate signal intensity extending to the retrolaryngeal tissues and abutting the right carotid artery (curved open arrow), loss of signal in the right thyroid ala (short open arrow) posteriorly, as well as destruction of right arytenoid (short solid arrow). Left arytenoid present (thin arrow). (b) Adjacent T1 axial image shows continued loss in normal thyroid lamina signal (open arrow) as well as extralaryngeal (including retrolaryngeal) extension (solid arrows). Right glottic neoplasm (thin arrow). (c, d) Axial T2 images show the altered increased signal due to increased water content within the right supraglottic neoplasm (solid arrows, c, d) and extent of spread (d). Note tissue plane between mass and carotid artery (thin arrow) and loss of signal posterior right thyroid ala (open arrow). (e–g) Same patient. Right supraglottic mass. (e) Axial CT shows involvement of paralaryngeal tissue plane (thin arrow) and sclerosis of right thyroid lamina (open arrow); mass (solid arrow). (f) Fast spin-echo (FSE) coronal T2 image shows extensive right supraglottic–glottic carcinoma (large straight arrows) with extension to subglottic tissues (small arrow). Increased signal of pre-epiglottic fat (open arrow) and paraglottic fat (curved arrows) extending to false cords noted. Ventricles (thin arrows) seen bilaterally. Tumor has extended around ventricle to reach glottis and subglottis. V, true cord. (g) Sagittal T2 image shows extension to involve epiglottis (E) and loss of normal pre-epiglottic fat tissue plane (solid arrows). Tongue base involvement (open arrow) better seen on adjacent sagittal images. (h–j) Same patient. Right supraglottic carcinoma (arrows) with subtle sclerosis right thyroid ala (h). Despite motion artifact, axial T1 image (i) shows mass (curved arrows) and altered signal of right thyroid ala (straight arrows). Axial T2 image (j) shows tumor extent (arrows) more clearly.*

(really ossification) but there is tremendous variability. As the cartilages progressively ossify, they become more radiopaque. Interpreting invasion of the laryngeal cartilage is difficult due to differential ossification and so an area that is not ossified may mimic invasion when in fact there is no invasion. In addition, the ossified areas may contain fatty low-attenuation marrow spaces, which may also mimic invasion and further complicate the differentiation of normal cartilage from tumor invasion.

The thyroid and cricoid cartilages are identified easily but identification of the arytenoid cartilages is critical to the relationships of the true and false vocal cords. The first superior slices identifying the triangular-shaped arytenoid cartilages are usually at the level of the false vocal cords. Proceeding inferiorly, the arytenoid cartilages take on a more pointed anterior projection representing the vocal process identifying the level of the true vocal cords. The cricoarytenoid joint is also at this level. There is no definite cartilaginous landmark identifying the laryngeal ventricle.

Kallmes and Phillips found the mean width of the anterior commissure to be approximately 1.0 mm as measured by CT.[38] If an upper limit of 1.6 mm was chosen, it would include 92% of normal subjects and an upper limit of 2.1 mm would have included the mean plus two standard deviations. Normally the anterior commissure should have air density (i.e. black) closely approximating the thyroid cartilage. If this appearance is seen, there is little chance of any significant disease at the anterior commissure. If it is not black, the anterior commissure could be involved by tumor or alternatively there could be cord edema or the cords may have been adducted because of the phase of respiration during acquisition of the particular slice. Hence the normal air density close to the cartilage is more helpful to exclude disease at the anterior commissure than obliteration is to prove disease.

Magnetic resonance imaging

MR imaging (Figs 14.5, 14.6) has the capability of multiplanar high-resolution imaging and can provide superior soft tissue definition compared with CT.[10–12,29,42,43,47,49,79] However, due to the relatively long image acquisition times, laryngeal imaging with MR can be difficult due to motion artifact from patients breathing and swallowing. The pulsatile flow from the carotid arteries can also present imaging artifacts. Patients are asked to breathe quietly without moving and to swallow as infrequently as possible, which may be difficult for many patients in the claustrophobic and noisy confines of most MR machines. Motion artifact can also be reduced by using fast spin-echo (FSE) techniques, which acquire images much faster than conventional spin-echo images and still provide valuable T2-weighted (T2W) information.

Patients are placed supine on the MR table with the airway parallel to the tabletop. Different imaging protocols are used by different institutions and diagnostic imagers. A sagittal T1-weighted (T1W) series from one sternocleidomastoid muscle to the opposite side is commonly performed as an initial localization sequence followed by thin section (3–5 mm) axial (parallel to the vocal cords) and coronal (perpendicular to the vocal cords) T1W images. Axial T2W sequences also include primary node-bearing areas. Fat-suppression techniques lower the signal from fat and allow better definition of high signal intensity coming from abnormal soft tissues from that of adjacent fat. Contrast imaging with gadolinium is controversial. It may improve the differentiation of a neoplasm from the surrounding normal soft tissues but FSE T2W images frequently offer comparable information without requiring gadolinium.

Sagittal views show the epiglottis, valleculae, base of tongue and pre-epiglottic space well. The epiglottis can be followed down to the anterior commissure and the arytenoids can be visualized superior to the cricoid cartilage.

Coronal views are ideal for assessing the superior to inferior extent of neoplasms. In particular, the mucosal and submucosal extent of disease not apparent clinically may be assessed, which is particularly useful for assessment of subglottic extension of disease. The high signal of the fatty tissue in the normal paraglottic space offers an excellent anatomic landmark on coronal (or axial) T1W sequences. If the ventricle is not seen well, the false cord can be differentiated from the true cord on T1W images by the fatty signal of the false cord versus the intermediate density thyroarytenoid muscle signal of the true cord.

Axial views are best for evaluating cartilage invasion but the appearance is quite variable depending on the degree of ossification. Ossified cartilage which has medullary fat will have a bright signal on T1W images and a lower (darker) signal on T2W images. Non-ossified cartilage is usually of low signal on both T1W and T2W sequences. Ossified cartilage cortex looks black on both sequences. The cervical lymph nodes can be assessed on either sequence.

CT versus MR imaging

The advantages of CT include wider availability, lower cost, faster image acquisition (and therefore less motion artifact), and better ability to demonstrate calcifications and cortical bone detail.[90] Disadvantages include the use of ionizing radiation, poorer soft tissue resolution compared with MR, streak artifacts from metallic objects, and more difficult multiplanar imaging. CT usually requires the use of iodinated contrast for laryngeal imaging which some patients may be allergic to.

The advantages of MR include no ionizing radiation, superb soft tissue contrast, multiplanar views without the need for repositioning, and information about vascularity and blood vessels without necessarily needing contrast (gadolinium).[90] MR disadvantages include increased expense, and in many areas less accessibility than CT, and longer examination time. Five to ten percent of patients are claustrophobic such that they cannot complete the study. MR is more sensitive to patient motion and less sensitive to cortical bone erosion and calcifications than CT. Absolute contraindications to MR include ferromagnetic cerebral aneurysm clips, orbital metallic foreign bodies, cardiac pacemakers, and cochlear implants.

Laryngeal imaging should help to define the extent of disease and concentrate on features that could influence therapy. Some centres prefer to use MR as the imaging modality of choice in patients with laryngeal carcinoma.[9,26,62] The choice between CT and MR imaging is determined largely by the availability of the two modalities and the experience of the radiologist and treating physician with these two modalities. We agree with Williams[90] in preferring CT as the initial examination of laryngeal carcinoma because it usually provides the necessary information about tumor size, extent and nodal status such that treatment decisions can be made. MR is used more selectively to determine cartilage invasion in some cases, to further identify extent of disease when disease approximates structures important in surgical decision-making (e.g. laryngeal ventricle in supraglottic carcinoma) and for most nonepithelial neoplasms. MR also plays an important role in evaluating the tongue base in large supraglottic carcinomas because of its sagittal imaging capabilities.

Pathologic conditions

Laryngologists usually have some idea of the disease process affecting patients prior to requesting laryngeal imaging. Frequently a diagnosis is known or suspected and laryngeal imaging is requested to assess the extent of a disease process. Good communication between the laryngologist and diagnostic imager is essential to gather the most information from the imaging consultation. This communication can be through a detailed written requisition, phone call or copy of a consultation letter. If the imager is given few details of a particular patient problem or specific questions that need to be addressed, then the quality of the images and report will reflect this. If specific questions are asked, specific imaging protocols and detailed examination of certain targeted areas can be performed to try to answer the clinical questions. The categories of conditions that may need diagnostic imaging include congenital lesions, infection and inflammation, trauma, vocal cord paralysis, and neoplasms. These problems will be covered in the subsequent sections of this chapter.

Congenital lesions

Diagnostic imaging can be useful in the evaluation of some congenital lesions. However, many are diagnosed on the basis of clinical signs and symptoms.[85] Plain x-rays or tomography can assess the size of the airway or the length of a stenosis. However, CT in the axial plain gives the best cross-sectional view. Volume acquisition CT scanners allow reformations to better characterize abnormalities in different plains.

The collapse of the supraglottic airway in laryngomalacia can be demonstrated but it is difficult to demonstrate subglottic stenosis because the cricoid has not calcified in infants.[34] Likewise, due to the small size of the airway, webs, clefts and atresias are difficult to visualize well with diagnostic imaging techniques and are therefore not very useful for this purpose.[25,89]

Cysts and laryngoceles

Mucosal cysts can occur anywhere in the larynx where submucosal glands are located[30,45] but are most common in the supraglottic region. These cysts are usually superficial and may protrude into the airway. Vallecular cysts are seen anterior to the epiglottis.

The saccule of the ventricle is a tubular structure that normally extends superiorly into the paraglottic region and the false cord. If the saccule enlarges with air it is called a laryngocele and if it fills with secretions it is called a saccular cyst.[27,33] A normal air-filled ventricular appendix can often be seen on CT or MR axial images and should not be called a laryngocele/saccular cyst unless there is deformity of the ipsilateral supraglottic larynx.

A laryngocele can be diagnosed on plain films, CT or MRI (Figs 14.7, 14.8). A supraglottic air- or fluid-filled mass is identified and followed inferiorly through the paraglottic space to the level of the ventricle. The internal consistency of fluid-filled cysts varies on CT and MR depending on their protein content. A laryngocele may be associated with a malignancy in the region of the ventricle which may be suggested on CT or MR.

Thyroglossal duct remnants occur adjacent to the larynx. At the level of the larynx, thyroglossal duct cysts usually occur on either side of midline between the thyroid ala and strap muscles. They are distinguishable from laryngoceles because of their more anterior location outside of the larynx and lack of intralaryngeal component. Long-standing thyroglossal duct cysts have been rarely reported to cause deossification of the thyroid cartilage and push into the larynx itself (Fig 14.9).

Infection and inflammation

Imaging is not commonly required in infectious or inflammatory conditions of the larynx but may be required to evaluate the extent of disease or rule out other diagnostic possibilities.

Croup is usually diagnosed clinically but plain films may be used to confirm the diagnosis or exclude a foreign body. There is inflammation of the mucosa of the subglottic larynx, resulting in the characteristic 'steeple-shaped' airway seen on plain AP films.

Epiglottitis, or supraglottitis, show characteristic swelling of the epiglottis and loss of the vallecula on plain lateral films. However, if epiglottitis is suspected, the risk

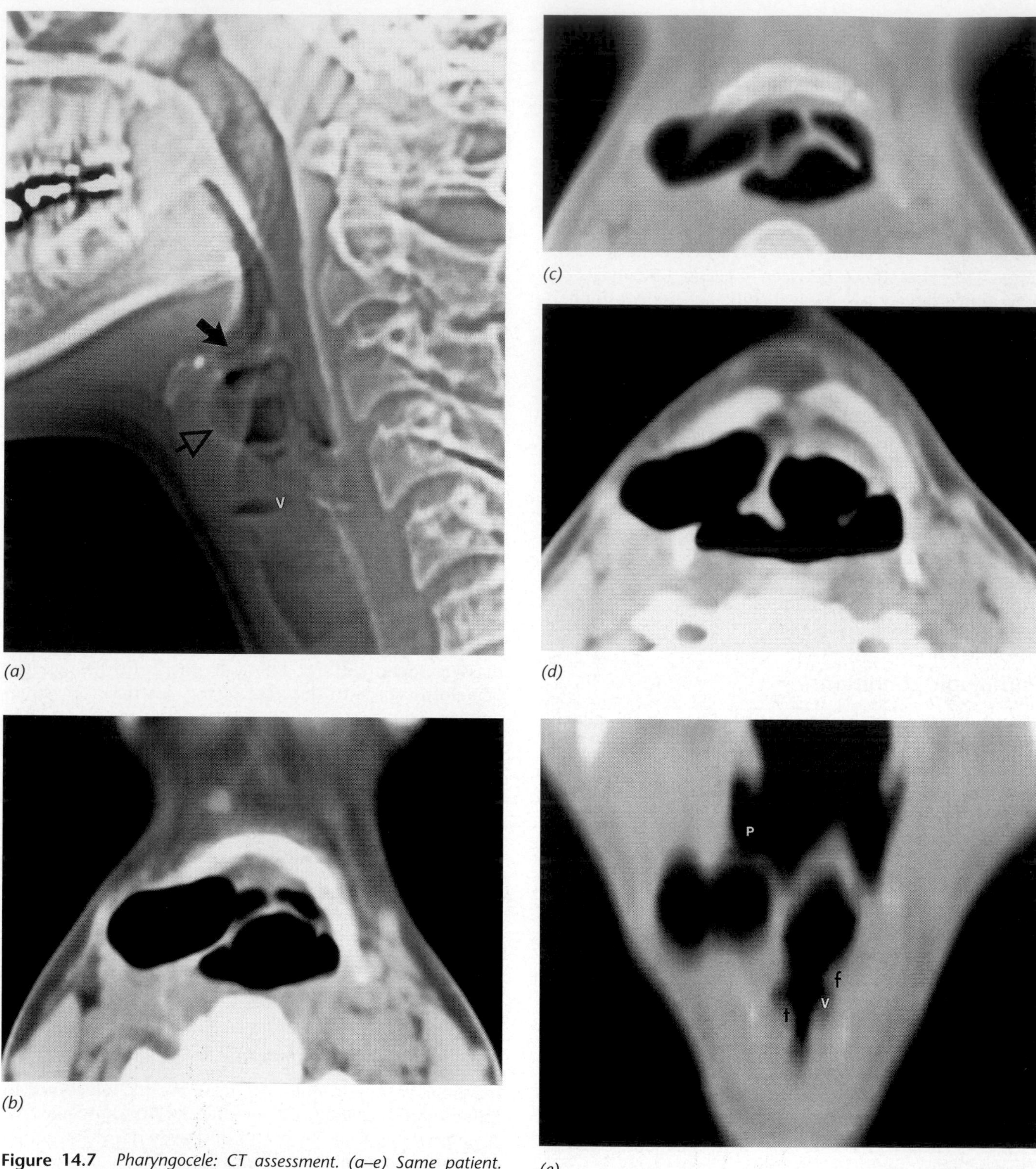

Figure 14.7 *Pharyngocele: CT assessment. (a–e) Same patient. (a) Lateral digital image shows prominent collection of air (open arrow), just inferior to the hyoid and vallecula (solid arrow). Ventricle (v). (b) Axial CT shows large air collection lateral to right vallecula at level of base of epiglottis. (c) Thin membrane between vallecula and pharyngocele better seen with wider window setting. (d) More inferior image shows relationship of pharyngocele to pyriform sinus. (e) Coronal reformation shows relationship of pharyngocele to laryngeal airway. Pyriform sinus (P), false cord (f), ventricle (v), true cord (t) all seen.*

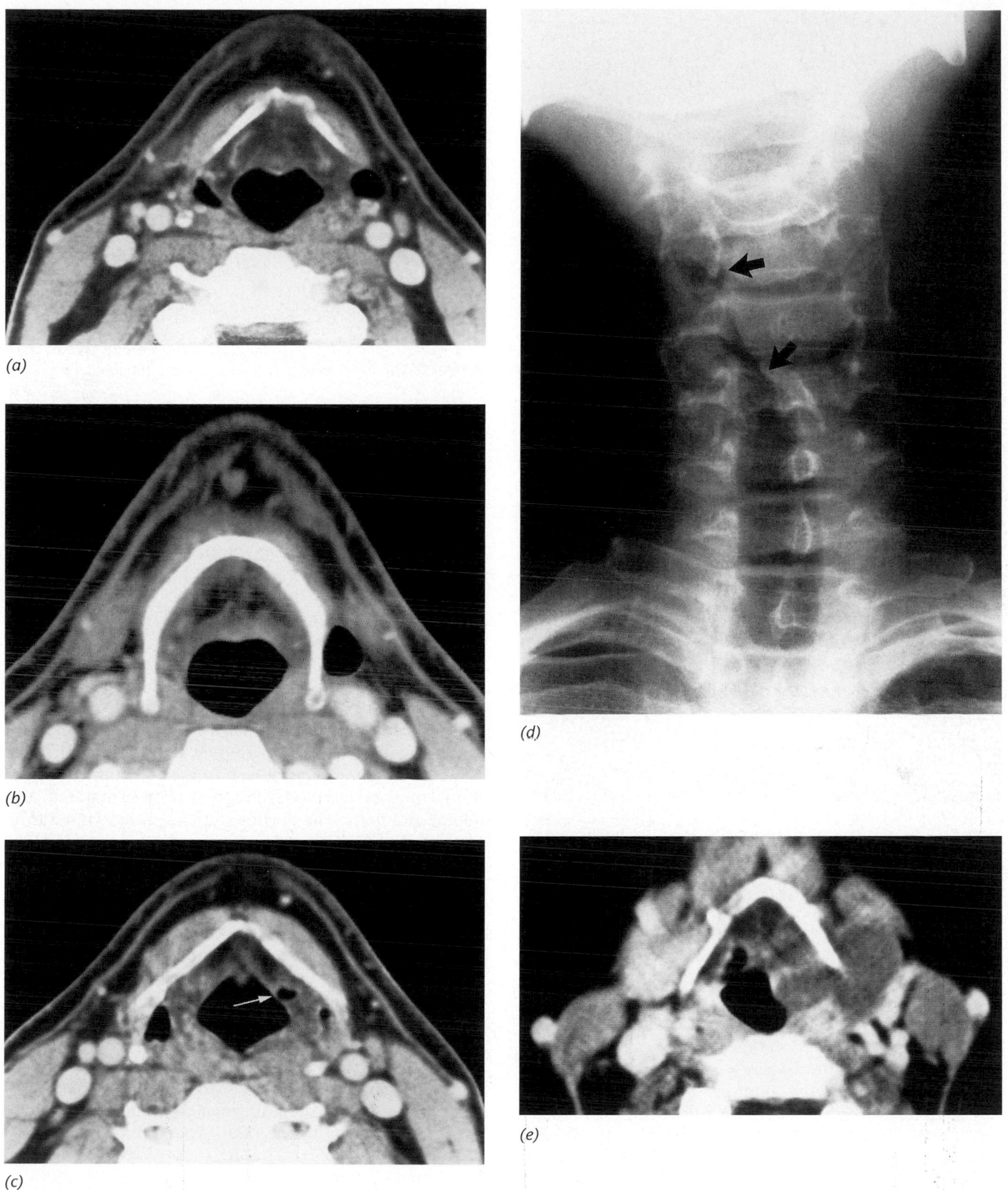

(a)

(b)

(c)

(d)

(e)

Figure 14.8 *Laryngocele: CT definition. (a–c) Same patient. (a) Air lateral to most superior aspect of left thyroid ala is more laterally located than pyriform sinus seen on right. (b) Collection of air is seen lateral to hyoid bone traversing thyrohyoid membrane. (c) More inferiorly, just superior to laryngeal ventricle, air is noted in soft tissues (arrow) medial to thyroid lamina. (d–g) Same patient (different from patient a–c). (d) Frontal projection film shows laryngeal airway displaced to right (arrows) by large mass.* continued

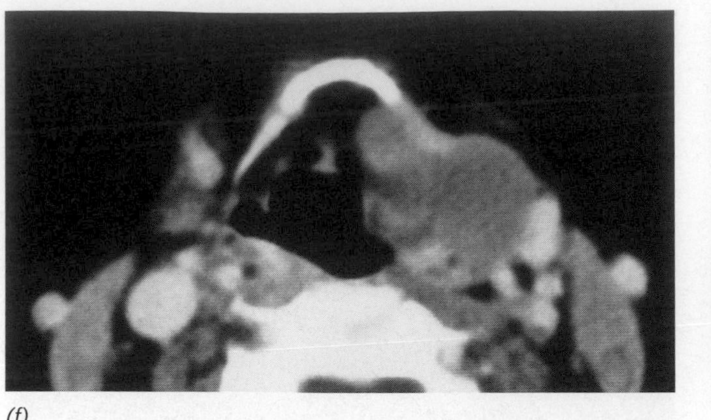

(f)

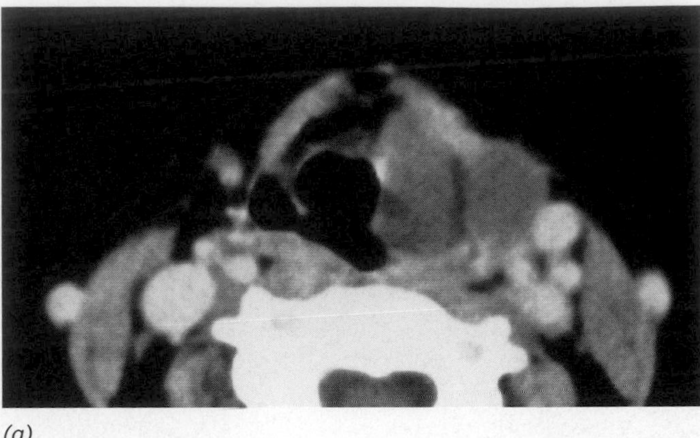

(g)

Figure 14.8 *(e–g) Axial CT images (e, f, g) show lobulated mass with both intrinsic and extrinsic components hypodense relative to cervical musculature, suggesting cystic content. Note motion artifact on (e). Intrinsic component largest and least defined superiorly (e).*

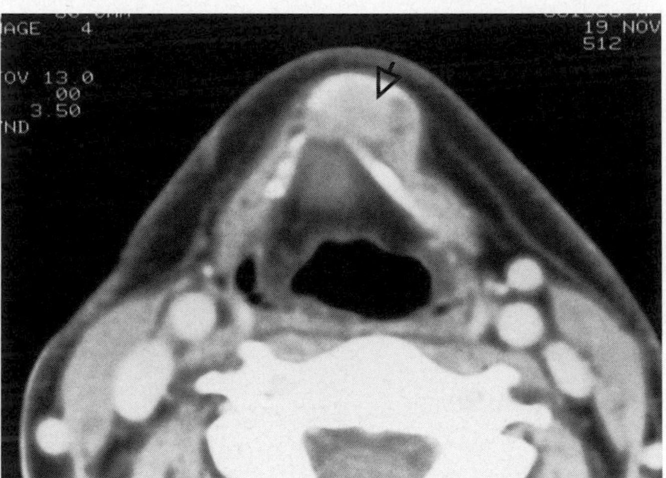

Figure 14.9 *CT: thyroglossal duct cyst. Mass lesion (open arrow) intimately associated with and deep to strap muscles just to left of midline.*

of transportation of the patient, especially a child, to the radiology department may not be warranted due to the possibility of rapid deterioration from airway obstruction.

Granulomatous diseases rarely affect the larynx. There are no specific imaging findings but most can cause nodular lesions, diffuse laryngeal thickening or localized infiltrative lesions. Characteristic findings of laryngeal tuberculosis on CT include bilateral involvement, thickening of the free margin of the epiglottis, and preservation of the pre-epiglottic and paralaryngeal fat spaces even in the presence of extensive mucosal involvement.[39] With carcinoma, there is usually invasion of the fat spaces and/or cartilage with comparable degrees of mucosal disease as seen with tuberculosis.

Trauma

Motor vehicle and recreational vehicle accidents account for the majority of injuries to the larynx (Fig 14.10). The most common mechanism of trauma occurs when the laryngeal cartilages are compressed against the cervical spine.[92] In children the larynx is relatively protected by its higher position in the neck relative to the mandible.

CT gives the best delineation of the laryngeal framework (thyroid and cricoid cartilages) following trauma, particularly when the cartilages are calcified.[6,72,73] Axial scans with fine 1–1.5 mm cuts are analyzed for evidence of breaks in the cartilaginous framework, particularly if impinging into the airway. There is usually associated soft tissue swelling. Air may be seen in the adjacent soft tissues if the mucosa has been breached or a hematoma may appear as a mass. The epiglottis may appear avulsed from the petiole or torn[17] and the hyoid bone may also be fractured.

Vertical fractures occur when the larynx is splayed against the spine and are usually easily detected on CT. Horizontal fractures may be more difficult to detect if fine CT cuts with multiplanar reformations are not used. Cricoid fractures may cause collapse of the normal cricoid ring. The normal subglottic airway appears slightly oval but after fracture it may appear more rounded with increased soft tissue swelling. Patients with previous trauma to their larynx may show inward bowing of the thyroid cartilage on axial CT scans.[7]

If patients with laryngotracheal separation make it to the imaging department, the separation may not be obvious due to the associated soft tissue edema and hematoma. When the arytenoid cartilage is dislocated relative to the cricoid cartilage, this fact can usually be detected on CT scan but may be subtle. Rodenwaldt *et al.* recommend a collimation of 1 mm with a pitch of 2 to improve the quality of CT imaging of the arytenoid cartilages since the quality of images depends greatly on the

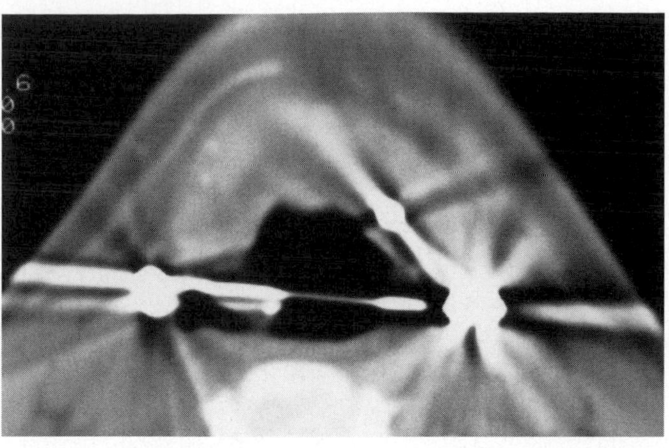
(a)

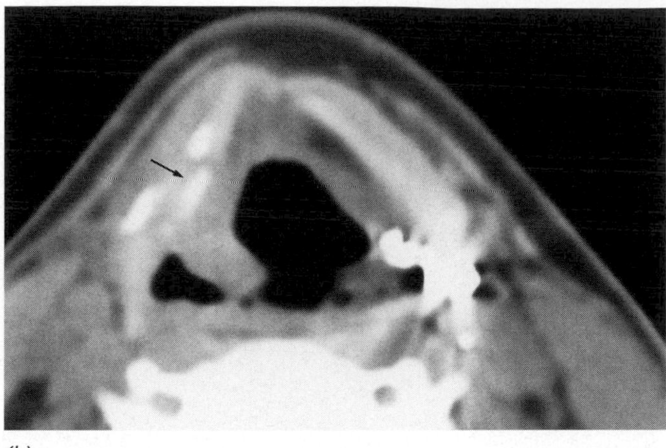
(b)

Figure 14.10 *CT laryngeal trauma: gunshot wound. (a, b) Same patient with multiple 'pellets' in region of left pyriform sinus. Artifact from metallic foreign body obscures image information (a). Note associated fracture of right thyroid ala with medial displacement of fragment (arrow) and loss of right paraglottic tissue plane (b).*

scanning parameters, compliance of the patient and mineralization of the arytenoid cartilages.[66] If the cricothyroid joint is dislocated, the thyroid cartilage usually appears rotated to one side relative to the cricoid cartilage.[71]

Vocal cord paralysis (Fig 14.11)

Enhanced CT scans of the neck and mediastinum are often performed to look for the cause of unexplained vocal cord paralysis. The course of the vagus nerve from the brainstem as it exits the skull base in the jugular foramen, to the posterior carotid sheath must be followed through the neck into the mediastinum. On the left side the scans are continued down inferior to the aortic arch and on the right inferior to the level of the subclavian artery as these are the structures that the respective recurrent laryngeal nerves curve around. The course of the recurrent laryngeal nerves are then followed back along the tracheoesophageal grooves into the larynx.

The superior laryngeal nerves supply the cricothyroid muscles and the recurrent laryngeal nerves supply the rest of the laryngeal musculature. If one superior laryngeal nerve is not functioning, the normal contracting cricothyroid muscle rotates the posterior cricoid to the contralateral side. However, this is very difficult to appreciate by imaging and usually the appearance of the larynx is normal unless there is a neoplasm along the course of the nerve.

Recurrent laryngeal nerve paralysis may be identified on plain films, tomography and CT.[18] The major finding with time is atrophy of the thyroarytenoid muscle. Associated findings related to this atrophy include flattening of the normal subglottic arch and relative enlargement of the ipsilateral ventricle and pyriform sinus.

In the treatment of vocal cord paralysis, Teflon or other foreign materials (e.g. collagen, Gelfoam) may be injected into the paralyzed cord. Teflon is radiopaque and its position can usually be easily seen on CT. Most other materials are not radiopaque and cannot be assessed well by imaging. Type I thyroplasty is more commonly performed for this problem now with plastic/silastic prostheses placed beside the paralyzed vocal cord through a window cut in the adjacent thyroid cartilage. It may be possible in some cases to visualize this prosthesis.

Neoplasms

Most laryngeal masses require biopsy and histopathologic examination for definitive diagnosis. If a neoplastic process is suspected from the history and physical examination and it is thought that laryngeal imaging will be required to help map out the extent of the neoplastic process, then it is useful to try to get the imaging done prior to the biopsy. The biopsy itself may cause edema and trauma, which may affect the ability of the diagnostic imager to discern the true extent of the disease. In addition, if other operations such as a tracheotomy are performed at the same sitting, there may be artifact created from the tube, neck edema and loss of tissue planes from the surgical procedure. In these circumstances, the quality of information may not be optimal and it can be difficult to discern what imaging findings are due to disease versus surgical trauma. The ability to get the appropriate imaging prior to biopsy will depend on the availability of equipment and scheduling issues but more importantly on the clinical circumstances, especially the ability of the patient to lie flat if the airway is compromised.

The majority of laryngeal masses or 'tumors' turn out to be neoplasms, usually malignant neoplasms. Patients with neoplastic disease affecting their larynx present with a variety of symptoms, most notably a change in the

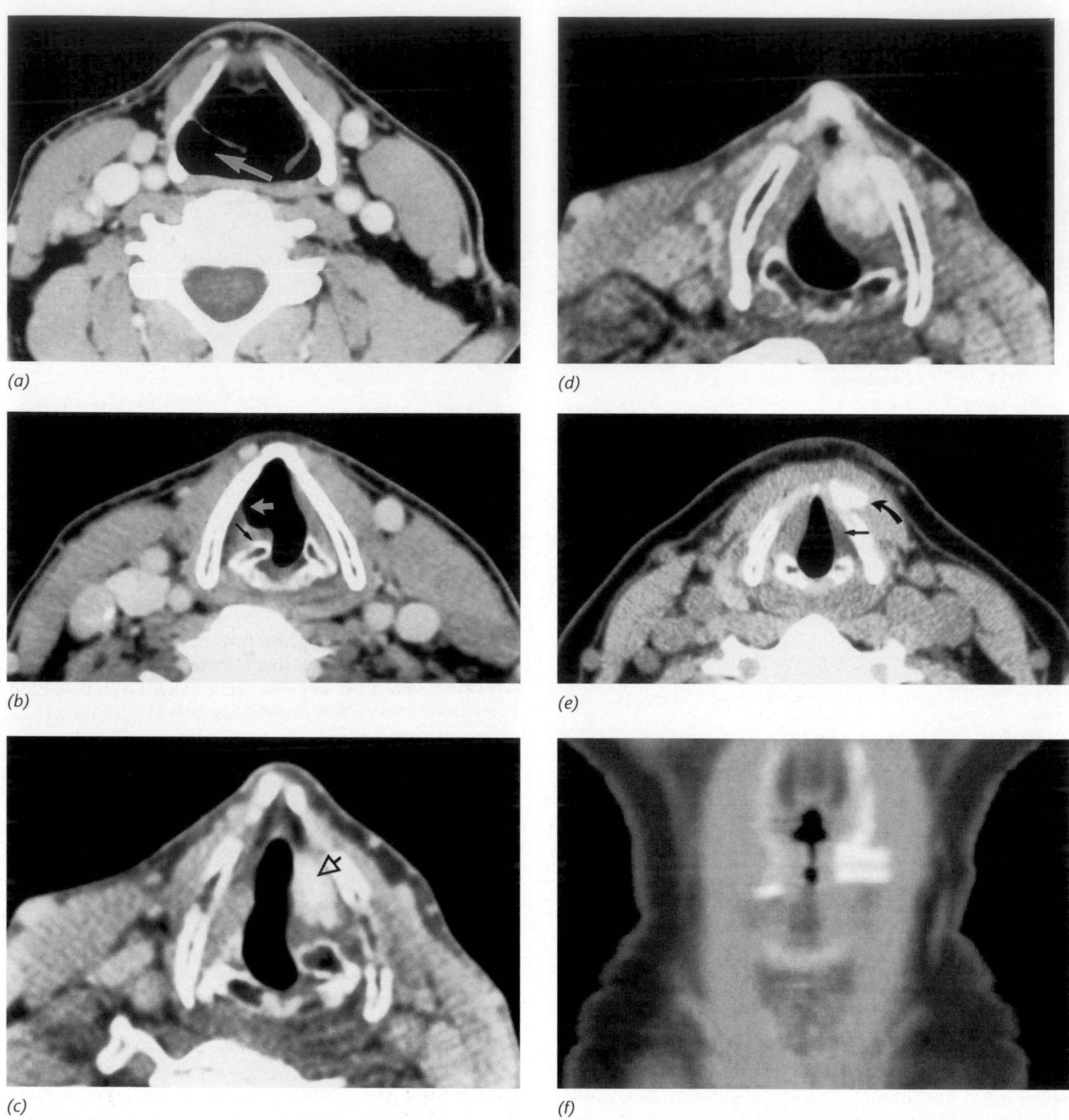

Figure 14.11 *Long-term vocal cord palsy. (a,b) Patient with long-term right vocal cord palsy. (a) Right pyriform sinus (arrow) larger than left. (b) More inferior scan shows the enlarged right ventricle (white arrow) and the arytenoid in a more anteromedial position (black arrow) than normal. (c, d) Same patient. Teflon injection left vocal cord. (c) Teflon (open arrow) positioned within left vocal cord, with adducted position of left vocal cord now present. (d) Teflon extending into left subglottic tissues with airway encroachment. (e, f) Same patient with thyroplasty for left vocal cord palsy. Axial CT (e) and coronal reformat (f) show extruded position of strut (curved arrow, e). Note fatty infiltration (thin arrow) of left thyroarytenoid muscle (e).*

quality of their voice, difficulty swallowing and sometimes shortness of breath, otalgia or hemoptysis. If there is a history of smoking and alcohol abuse, the laryngologist has a very high suspicion of finding a malignant neoplasm, usually squamous cell carcinoma.[3]

Squamous cell carcinoma

Most squamous cell carcinomas of the larynx present with a visible lesion in the larynx which can be mapped out by endoscopy. Small superficial carcinomas may be obvious clinically but missed on CT or MR. However, for larger lesions, imaging may pick up clinically unsuspected disease in the submucosa or deep extension into the paraglottic or pre-epiglottic spaces or disease extension into or through the laryngeal cartilages. This information could have important implications in the choice of therapy (e.g. partial laryngectomy versus total laryngectomy). Generally speaking, imaging may not be necessary for smaller T1 glottic carcinomas but in our opinion should be considered for most other carcinomas of the larynx. Diagnostic imagers must have an appreciation of what information physicians treating laryngeal cancer need in making their treatment decisions.

Cartilage involvement

Evaluation of the laryngeal cartilages, particularly the thyroid cartilage, is important because cartilage invasion has been thought of as portending a poorer prognosis.[8] However, in the TNM staging of laryngeal carcinoma, cartilage invasion is defined as full thickness invasion through the cartilage (making the cancer a T4). However, with CT and MR, more subtle cartilage involvement may be detected. In the past, laryngeal imaging may not have picked up on this cartilage involvement and currently the significance of this involvement is still open to debate, particularly with reference to the curability with radiation versus surgery.[22,51]

Carcinomas confined to the supraglottic larynx rarely invade cartilage but cartilage invasion is more common in glottic and subglottic carcinoma. The thyroid and cricoid cartilages are the important cartilages. Invasion of the epiglottis or minimal involvement of one arytenoid cartilage (e.g. vocal process) does not necessarily preclude partial laryngectomy.

The major problem with assessment of laryngeal cartilage is that the mineralization of the cartilage is inconsistent and frequently asymmetric. Cortical bone, marrow, and nonossified cartilage may all be present simultaneously. For example, islands of ossified and nonossified cartilage may be seen in the thyroid cartilage's alar surfaces. This normal phenomenon may look abnormal with CT and MR and must be interpreted with caution in relationship to a carcinoma. Knowledge of the usual ossification patterns is important in interpreting laryngeal images. The thyroid cartilages usually ossify from the inferior margin superiorly and from the posterior margin anteriorly. The cricoid cartilage usually ossifies first along the lamina and upper margin.

Sclerosis of cartilage adjacent to tumor does not necessarily mean invasion since there is frequently an inflammatory response at the outer edge of squamous cell carcinomas which can give a similar appearance.[57] Approximately 16% of patients (especially women) will have arytenoid sclerosis as a normal variant with no evidence of carcinoma.[74] In a study by Becker *et al.* evaluating several different CT criteria for cartilage invasion (extralaryngeal tumor, sclerosis, tumor adjacent to nonossified cartilage, serpiginous contour, erosion or lysis, obliteration of marrow space, cartilaginous blowout, and bowing), sclerosis was the most sensitive criteria in all cartilages but often corresponded to reactive inflammation in the thyroid cartilage.[5] Sclerosis of cartilages adjacent to tumor has been shown by Pameijer *et al.* to be a negative prognostic indicator in T3 glottic cancers.[61]

Using CT imaging, the only reliable sign of cartilage invasion is demonstration of tumor on the opposite side of the cartilage from the primary lesion. Nonossified cartilage and carcinoma usually have the same soft tissue attenuation so detecting minimal cartilage involvement is very difficult with CT.

MR may offer some advantage over CT because of the different pulse sequences that can be compared.[10–12] Nonmineralized cartilage is relatively dark on T1W and T2W images but not as black as cortical bone. The cortex of ossified cartilage appears black but fatty marrow, if present, will appear bright on T1W sequences and darkens on T2W sequences. Fast spin-echo with fat suppression allows highly detailed T2W images. Contrast enhancement with gadolinium generally increases the signal of carcinomas and by using T1W, fat-suppressed images, early cartilage invasion may be seen. However, high quality FSE T2W images may give the same information.

Squamous carcinoma is intermediate in intensity or relatively dark on T1W sequences and brightens on T2W sequences whereas nonmineralized cartilage does not.[10–12] Therefore, if the cartilage is relatively dark on T1W sequences and brightens on T2W sequences, cartilage invasion may be present. This finding has been questioned because the inflammatory component frequently seen adjacent to squamous cell carcinomas also gives a relatively high T2W signal. Furthermore, the T2W images of invaded and uninvolved cartilage may look similar if the uninvolved cartilage has a fatty medullary area. However, it is the change in appearance between T1W and T2W images that is important. Relative brightening between the T1W and T2W sequences suggests tumor invasion and little or no change in brightness suggests no cartilage involvement.

In summary, the most reliable sign of cartilage invasion with CT or MR is still the detection of tumor outside the laryngeal cartilages. If the cartilage has normal signal, it is likely not invaded. If the cartilage enhances on T2W sequences or with gadolinium on T1W fat-suppressed images, it is likely abnormal, especially if the tumor is adjacent to the enhancing area. Several authors believe that MR imaging is more sensitive than CT in detecting

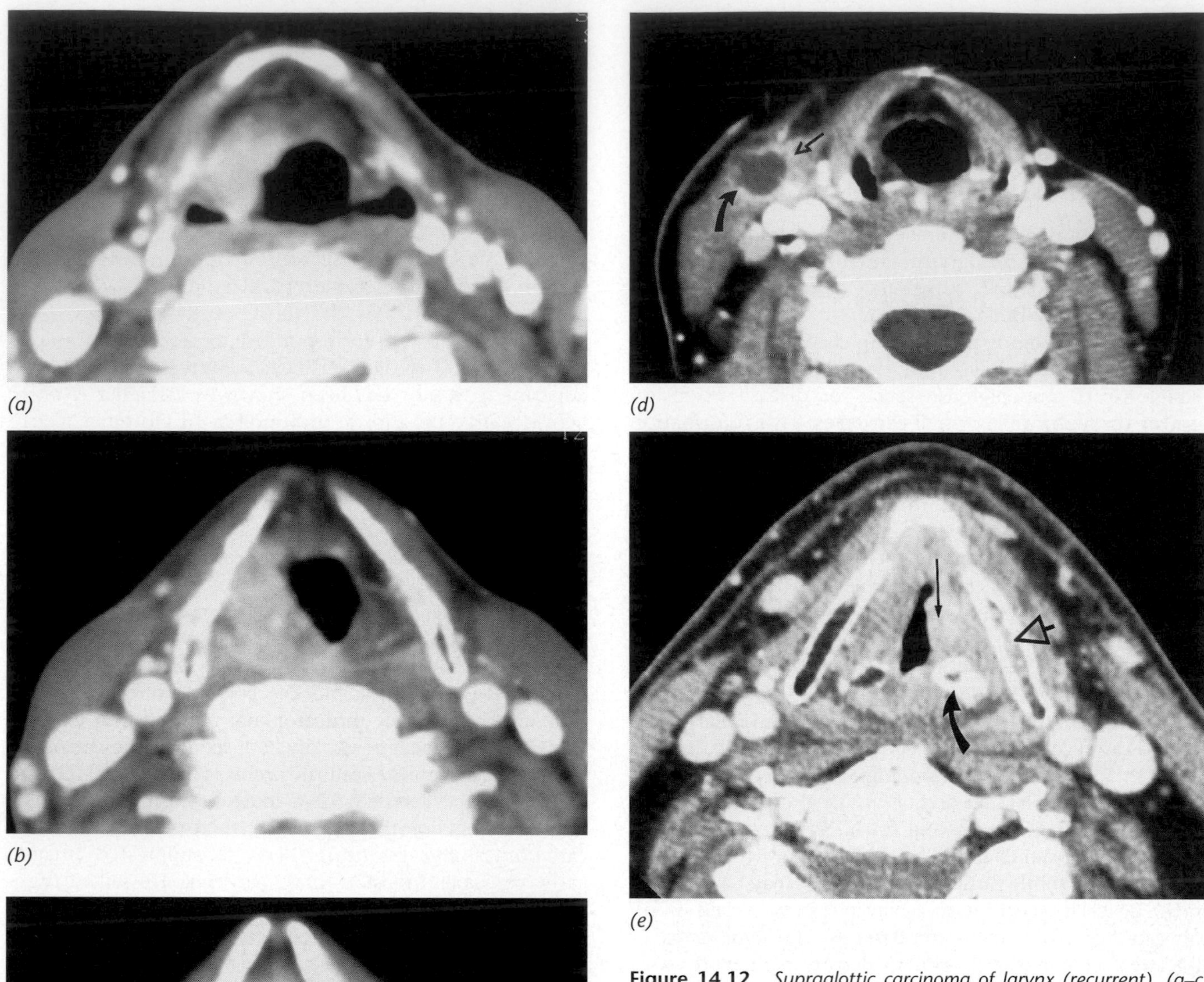

(a)

(b)

(c)

(d)

(e)

Figure 14.12 *Supraglottic carcinoma of larynx (recurrent). (a–c) Same patient. Recurrent supraglottic tumor 15 years postradiation treatment. (a) Soft tissue enhancing mass right aryepiglottic fold. (b) Enhancing soft tissue mass infiltrates right paralaryngeal supraglottic tissue. (c) Abnormal enhancement due to recurrent tumor in patient with long-term right vocal palsy (enlarged ventricle and paretic cord configuration). (d) Different patient with supraglottic carcinoma presented with necrotic lymph node (curved arrow) with extracapsular spread and infiltration of adjacent tissue plane (straight arrow). (e) Patient with left supraglottic mass (thin arrow) and sclerosis of left arytenoid cartilage (curved arrow). Note asymmetry of thyroid lamina, with sclerosis on the left (open arrow).*

pathologic involvement of the cartilages but there is also an overestimation of invasion because of the inability to differentiate between non-neoplastic inflammatory changes and carcinoma by MR.[4,9] CT is recommended in patients who have rapid breathing or coughing or in whom MR is contraindicated.[9]

Supraglottic larynx

Supraglottic carcinomas (Fig 14.12) may involve the suprahyoid region, the infrahyoid region or both. The true size of the lesion may be difficult to discern by endoscopy alone, especially in the region of the pre-epiglottic space, paraglottic spaces and base of tongue (Fig 14.13). Cancer

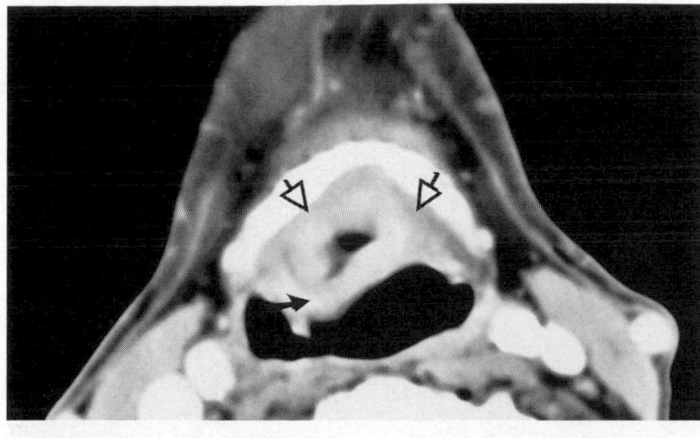

(a)

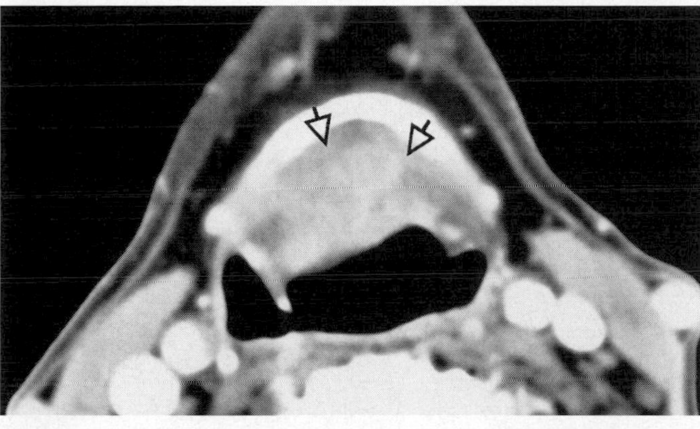

(b)

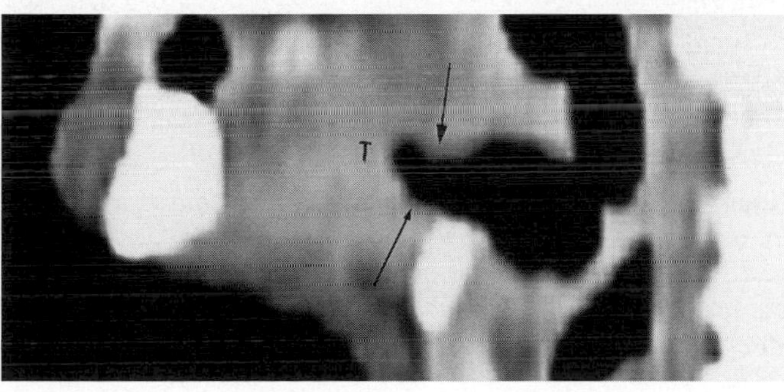

(c)

Figure 14.13 *Pre-epiglottic fat space: infiltration. (a–c) Same patient. (a) Axial CT shows loss of pre-epiglottic fat by carcinomatous infiltration (open arrows). Epiglottis diffusely involved (solid arrow). (b) Adjacent slice shows diffuse loss of fat attenuation in pre-epiglottic space (arrows). (c) Right parasagittal reformation shows deep sinus tract (arrows) into tongue base (T).*

extending anteriorly into the pre-epiglottic fat replaces the characteristic fat density seen on CT or the high signal intensity seen on T1W MR images. Tongue base extension is seen well on MR, especially with sagittal views.

Inferior extension of a supraglottic carcinoma in relationship to the anterior commissure, ventricle and arytenoids is important in determining the suitability for supraglottic laryngectomy if that is the preferred mode of therapy.[77,84] In trying to assess the inferior extent of a supraglottic carcinoma, the ventricle is the most important landmark. The ventricle is seen well on coronal MR sequences but on axial imaging with either CT or MR, the transition from the fat density of the false cord to the muscle density of the thyroarytenoid muscle is used to define the ventricle. On axial CT or MR images, there should be at least one and preferably more slices without cancer between the slice with the inferior border of the cancer and the slice with the superior surface of the true cord. If cancer is seen above and below the ventricle, a supraglottic laryngectomy is not feasible.

The difference between carcinoma and muscle signal/density is easier to define with MR than CT. Cancer frequently has the same density as muscle on CT and T1W MR images but on T2W images or fat-suppressed T1W images with gadolinium, the cancer has a relatively higher signal intensity than normal muscle. Inflammation around the cancer may also cause relative brightening of the T2W MR muscle signal; hence, muscle of normal signal is the most diagnostically useful information indicating the muscle is probably uninvolved by cancer.

The anterior commissure can be assessed by CT or MR axial imaging, but sagittal MR imaging is preferable. On sagittal imaging the presence of air against the lower epiglottis is a reliable indicator that tumor is not extending to the anterior commissure. If axial images are used to assess the anterior commissure, it is important to make sure the images are taken parallel to the ventricle to avoid any miscalculation about the relative positions of the true and false cords.

Glottic and subglottic larynx (Fig 14.14)

In glottic squamous cell carcinomas, imaging can provide useful information as to the degree of tumor extension, particularly as it relates to the anterior commissure, arytenoid, thyroid cartilage, and the paraglottic space at the level of the ventricle.

Tumor volume as measured by CT can be a significant predictor of local control. Pameijer *et al.* found in T3 glottic carcinomas with a volume of less than 3.5 cm^3 that the local control was 85% but with volumes greater than or equal to 3.5 cm^3 the local control was only 25%.[61] In a similar study of T2 glottic carcinomas from the same institution, they did not find a significant relationship between tumor volume and local control.[54] However, they did find that the pretreatment CT scan was helpful in detecting submucosal spread across the ventricle and subglottic extension in T2 glottic carcinomas which has implications for surgical treatment.

Laryngeal radiation

Laryngeal radiation (Figs 14.15, 14.16) causes mucosal changes which may confuse the post-treatment imaging assessment for persistent or recurrent disease.[55,56,83] Post-irradiation imaging needs to be closely correlated with clinical and endoscopic evaluations.[52] Even when there is

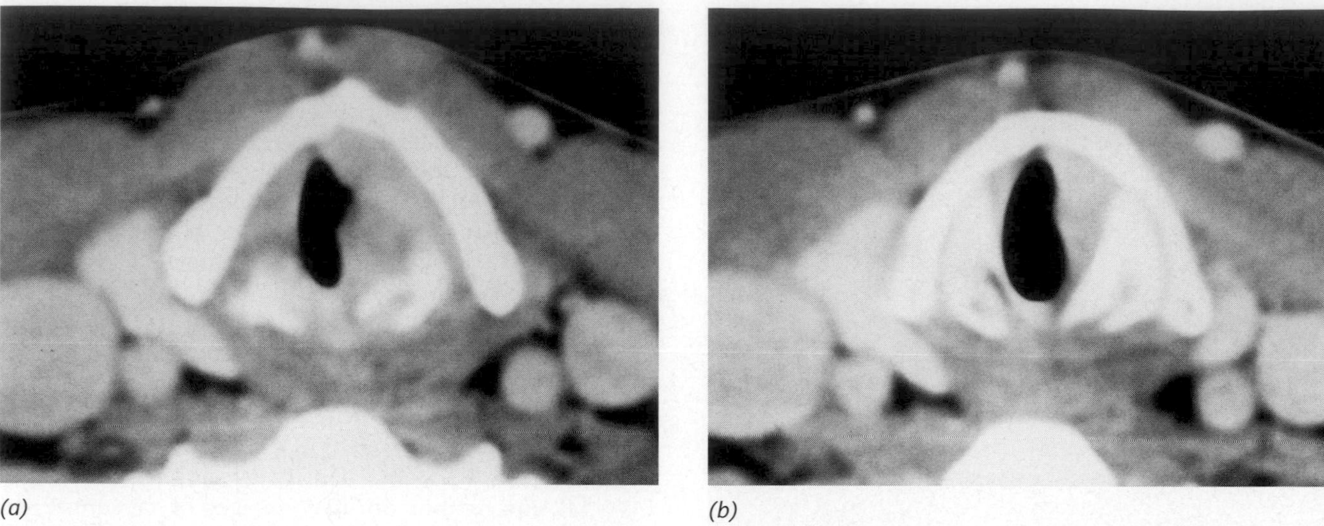

(a) (b)

Figure 14.14 *Laryngeal cancer: glottic–subglottic extension. (a, b) Same patient. Mass left vocal cord (a) encroaches on airway with left subglottic extension of neoplasm (b).*

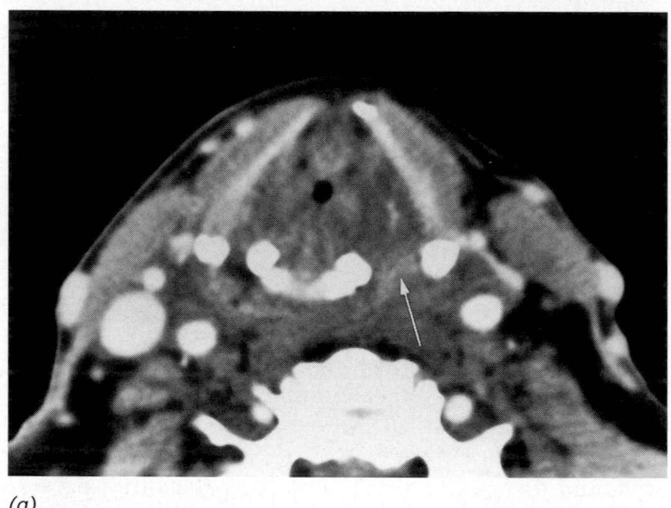

(a)

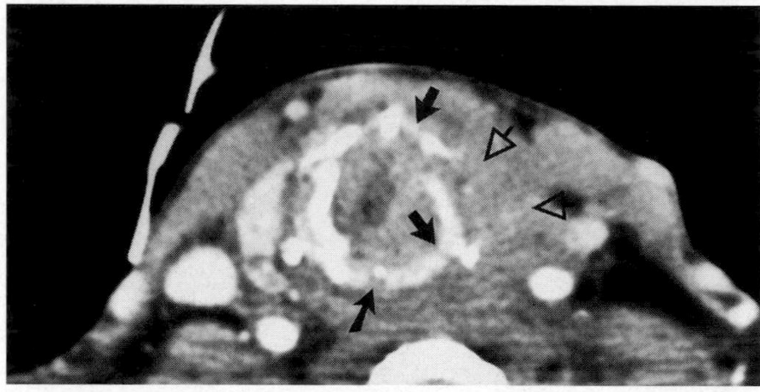

(b)

Figure 14.15 *Laryngeal cancer recurrence postradiation therapy. (a, b) Same patient. (a) Marked airway compromise. Diffuse laryngeal edema with soft tissue prominence causing left cricothyroid displacement (arrow). (b) Gross laryngeal cartilage destruction (solid arrows) with extralaryngeal soft tissue spread (open arrows).*

no carcinoma present, previous laryngeal radiation causes persistent symmetric thickening of the epiglottis, prominence of the aryepiglottic folds, false cords and arytenoids and streaky increased attenuation in the paraglottic and pre-epiglottic spaces.[55] The posterior pharyngeal wall is usually thickened and the mucosa enhanced. Glottic changes include thickening of the anterior and posterior commissures and in the subglottis, there is frequently thickening of the mucosa and submucosa. Soft tissue changes include thickening of the skin and platysma and increased attenuation of the subcutaneous fat.

O'Brien found that 50% of patients with severe edema or necrosis following radiotherapy for laryngeal carcinoma cancer had recurrent disease.[60] Mukherji *et al.* studied patients with serial CT scans every 4 months after completion of laryngeal radiation therapy and found that if the lesion was reduced in size by 50% or less there was a high likelihood of residual or recurrent carcinoma.[55] Ichimura *et al.* found 14 of 67 patients (20.9%) radiated for laryngeal carcinoma had moderate or severe laryngeal edema persisting or developing more than 3 months after completing radiotherapy.[35] Of the 14 patients, six (42.9%) had persistent or recurrent disease.

The CT findings of chondroradionecrosis of the larynx are non-specific. Hermans *et al.* found sloughing of the arytenoid cartilage, fragmentation and collapse of the thyroid cartilage, and/or gas bubbles around the cartilage to be highly suggestive of this diagnosis.[32]

Postsurgical imaging

CT and MR are both helpful in detecting local and/or regional disease recurrence after surgery, but neither one

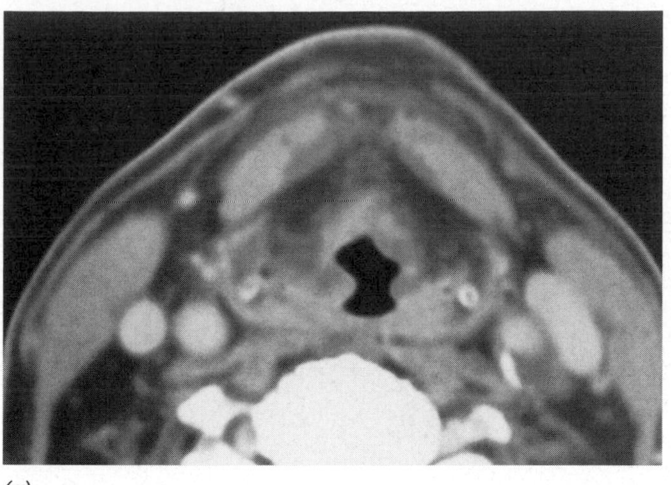

(a)

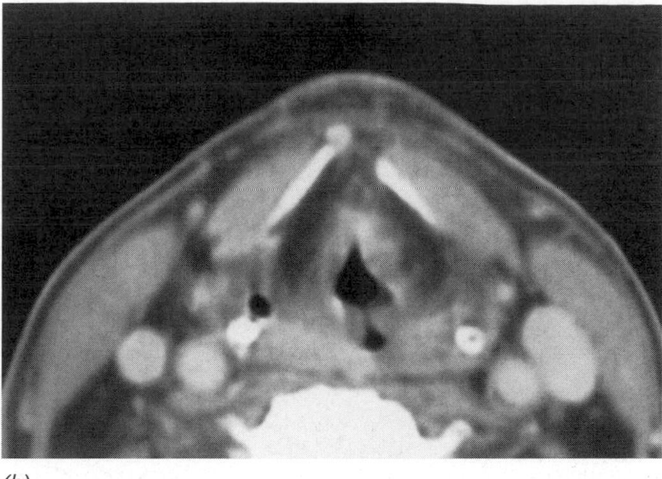

(b)

Figure 14.16 *Post-irradiation changes of the larynx: CT. (a, b) Same patient. Axial CT shows persistent diffuse soft tissue swelling of the supraglottic (a) larynx with laryngeal stenosis but no focal mass. Laryngeal stenosis more prominent posteriorly on more inferior image (b).*

is 100% accurate. Granulations, scar tissue and fibrosis can mimic recurrent tumor. Postsurgical changes depend on the type of surgery performed[14,15] and may be combined with postradiation changes if the patient received combined treatment. Furthermore, myocutaneous and free flaps may give an unusual CT or MR appearance and lead to confusion over tumor recurrence. A thorough knowledge of expected and unexpected postoperative findings is essential to proper interpretation of CT and MR images.

Maroldi *et al.* studied the postoperative CT appearance of 73 patients undergoing partial (52) and total (21) laryngectomies. Recognizable landmarks were changes in the laryngeal framework but the soft tissue resections often resulted in a more unpredictable appearance of the neolarynx.[48] There was significant thickening of the mucosa over the arytenoid cartilage(s) after horizontal supraglottic laryngectomy and supracricoid laryngectomies. A 'pseudocord' due to scar tissue was a consistent feature following vertical hemilaryngectomy and frequently after supracricoid laryngectomy. The most frequent findings and their respective percentages found in 28 recurrences were a mass larger than 10 mm spreading beyond the larynx (63.1%), thickening of the anterior commissure (57.9%), and erosion of residual cartilage (16.9%). CT detected one subclinical recurrence and in all the rest the recurrence was suspected clinically, calling into question the routine follow-up by CT scan of patients following partial or total laryngectomy. Others recommend routine follow-up imaging 6–8 weeks after surgery as a baseline for future studies. This time period is sufficient to allow the acute effects of surgery to resolve but is usually not enough time for significant regrowth of the cancer.

Nodal metastases

Bilateral metastatic spread to the upper cervical lymph nodes is common with supraglottic cancer, especially when the pre-epiglottic space, paraglottic spaces or base of tongue are involved. The upper cervical lymph nodes, as a minimum, should be imaged in supraglottic cancers, usually by axial scans. With MR imaging, coronal or sagittal images will also adequately show these nodal levels.

Glottic cancers confined to the true vocal cord rarely metastasize. If the cancer extends into the supraglottic or subglottic larynx, then there is a higher likelihood of cervical metastases. Subglottic cancers spread to the lymph nodes in the lower neck, paratracheal and pretracheal regions as well as to the mediastinum. Therefore the entire neck should be imaged in glottic cancers extending beyond the true vocal cords and in cases of supraglottic and subglottic cancers.

The value of imaging is in the detection of clinically occult metastatic disease. Size criteria to suggest a potentially malignant lymph node include diameters greater than 1 or 1.5 cm. In addition, central low attenuation within a lymph node of any size is usually a reliable sign of malignancy.[19,20] Many small positive lymph nodes go undetected by palpation and imaging and are found histologically (if surgery is performed on the neck lymph nodes). Ultrasound-guided fine-needle aspiration biopsy of small lymph nodes is another avenue which has shown good results in selected centres.[88] Extracapsular spread of nodal metastases is suggested by irregular margins or when there appears to be 'strandy' densities extending into the perinodal fat.[90]

Other malignant tumors

Squamous cell carcinoma is the most common malignant neoplasm of the larynx, accounting for approximately 90–95% of malignancies. Other malignancies include adenocarcinoma, verrucous carcinoma, anaplastic carcinoma, spindle cell carcinoma, sarcomas (Figs 14.17,

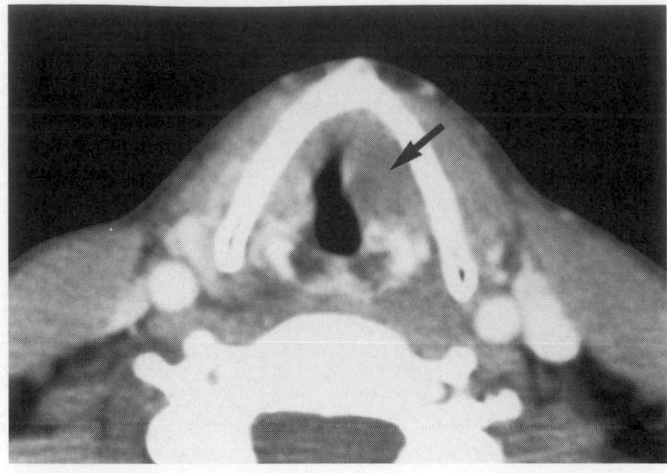
(a)

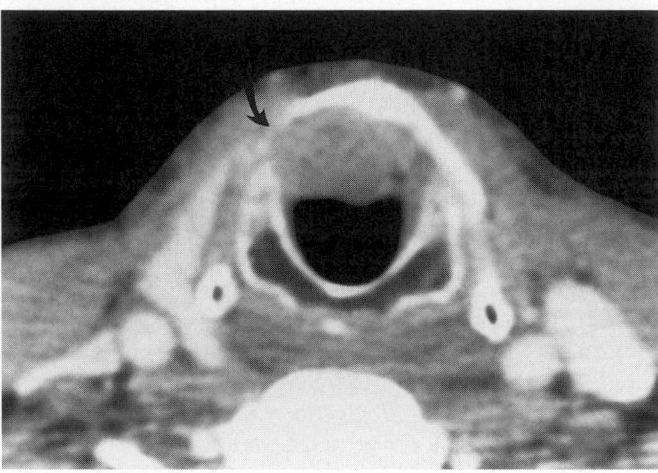
(b)

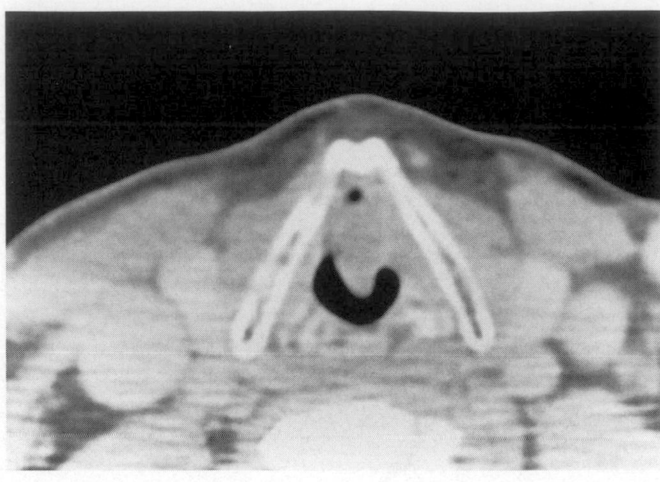
(c)

Figure 14.17 *Nonspecific tissue characterization of laryngeal masses. Malignant fibrous histiocytoma (MFH). (a, b) Same patient. (a) Mass lesion (arrow) left vocal cord, obscuring paralaryngeal tissue planes, encroaching on laryngeal airway and extending across anterior commissure. (b) Subglottic mass very extensive anteriorly with invasion of right thyroid lamina (curved arrow). (c) Different patient. Exophytic mass lesion (MFH) arising from left supraglottic laryngeal wall.*

14.18), melanomas, lymphoma, myeloma,[93] plasmacytoma and metastatic disease (Fig 14.19).

There are no particular imaging features which would lead one to suspect these diagnoses over squamous cell carcinoma in the majority of cases and biopsy is usually required for definitive diagnosis. When the lesion is completely submucosal, the radiologist may suggest to the clinician a diagnosis other than squamous cell carcinoma.

In general, the appearance of a laryngeal sarcoma is nonspecific but tends to be submucosal. Special mention is required of chondrosarcomas, which usually cause obvious defects in the cricoid and/or thyroid cartilages and have calcifications (often ring-like) more easily appreciated on CT than MR. The cartilage may be expanded rather than eroded, especially in low-grade lesions. It is usually impossible to distinguish benign from low-grade malignant chondroid lesions based on imaging characteristics unless there are aggressive features.

Benign tumors

Benign lesions of the larynx include vocal cord nodules, polyps, papillomatosis, and a variety of nonepithelial lesions. Imaging is hardly ever considered necessary for vocal cord nodules and polyps that are diagnosed clinically. However, they may be seen incidentally when imaging of the larynx is done for other reasons. The wart-like lesions of papillomatosis may give the appearance of nodules impinging on the airway on CT or MR.

Rare benign neoplasms of the larynx include hemangiomas, paragangliomas, neural tumors, lipomas, granular cell myoblastomas, leiomyomas, rhabdomyomas and chondromas. There are few imaging characteristics to distinguish between these tumors and other pathologies in the larynx. Exceptions include vascular tumors (hemangiomas and paragangliomas),[40] lipomas[78] and chondromas (see Fig 14.18d,e).

Hemangiomas enhance with contrast on CT and have intermediate signal intensity on T1-weighted MR images and high T2-weighted MR signal intensities. Occasionally, phleboliths are seen in older adults with large hemangiomas on CT or plain films. Hemangiomas in adults are usually localized and tend to be glottic or supraglottic. Pediatric hemangiomas occur most commonly in the subglottic

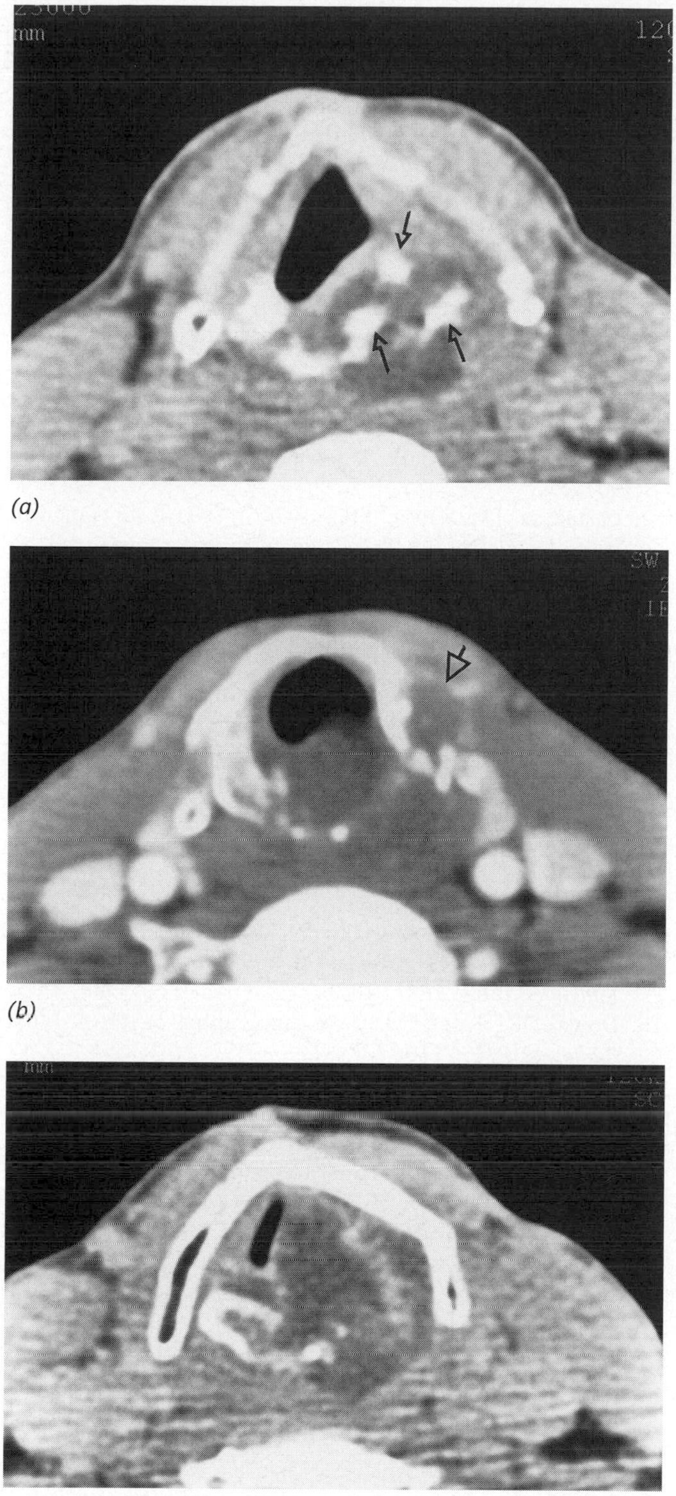

(a)

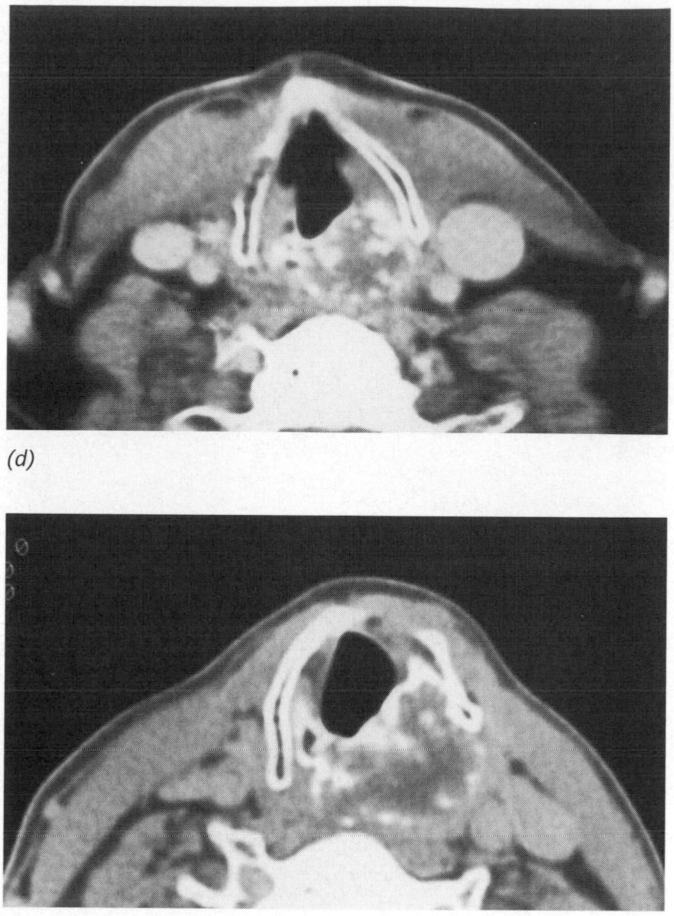

(d)

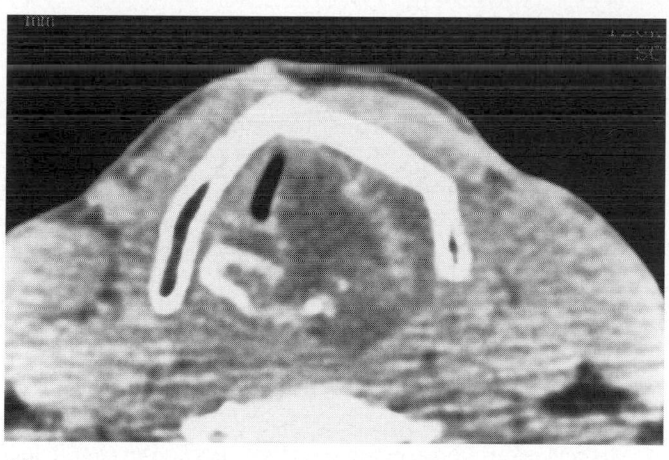

(b)

(e)

Figure 14.18 *Cartilaginous neoplasms of larynx. (a–c) Chondrosarcoma: same patient. (a) Axial CT. Soft tissue mass left posterior larynx with several punctate calcifications (open arrows) within mass. Note left thyroid lamina displaced laterally. (b) Soft tissue mass centered on left cricoid cartilage displacing airway anteriorly. Extralaryngeal involvement noted (open arrow). (c) Left cricoid destruction. Large heterogeneous left subglottic soft tissue mass. (d, e) Enchondroma: same patient. (d) Multiple punctate calcifications seen within mass at posterior left supraglottic larynx. (e) Heterogeneous soft tissue mass centered on left cricoid cartilage with multiple punctate calcifications. Appearance indistinguishable from chondrosarcoma.*

(c)

larynx. Subglottic hemangiomas typically display a localized protrusion or concentric narrowing adjacent to the cricoid cartilage inferior to the vocal cords. Paragangliomas occur rarely in the larynx, usually in a supraglottic location.[40] They have similar imaging characteristics as described for hemangiomas but do not show phleboliths.

Lipomas have a characteristic appearance on both CT and MR because of their high fat content (see Fig 14.3c).[37,78] Chondromas show a calcified matrix and relationship to one of the laryngeal cartilages. As mentioned earlier, it is almost impossible to distinguish a chondroma from a low-grade chondrosarcoma by imaging (see Fig 14.18).

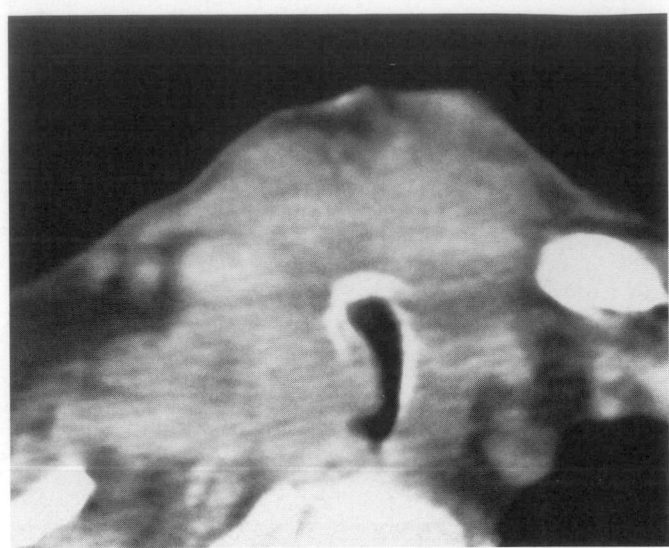

Figure 14.19 *Metastatic disease: airway encroachment. Extensive soft tissue mass in anterior neck compromising airway with invasion of tracheal cartilage and transverse collapse of trachea.*

Neurilemomas (schwannomas) rarely occur in the larynx as submucosal tumors. In patients with neurofibromatosis, isolated neurofibromas can occur in the larynx which have a nonspecific appearance on CT or MR. If the neurofibroma is of the plexiform variety, it may display a more infiltrative pattern suggesting malignancy.[80,82]

Although not strictly a neoplasm, osteophytes arising from the anterior cervical spine, if large, can cause significant mass effect on the posterior pharyngeal wall as well as anterior displacement of the larynx.[13]

Acknowledgment

This chapter was supported by the Saul A Silverman Family Foundation as a Canada International Scientific Exchange Program (CISEPO) project.

References

1. Amis TC, O'Neill N, Somma ED, Wheatley JR. Epiglottic movements during breathing in humans. *J Physiol (Lond)* 1998; **512:** 307–14.
2. Arens C, Eistert B, Glanz H, Waas W. Endolaryngeal high-frequency ultrasound. *Eur Arch Otorhinolaryngol* 1998; **255:** 250–5.
3. Barnes L, Gnepp DR. Diseases of the larynx, hypopharynx, and esophagus. In: Barnes L, ed. *Surgical Pathology of the Head and Neck.* New York: Marcel Dekker, 1985: 141–226.
4. Becker M, Zbären P, Laeng H, Stoupis C, Porcellini B, Vock P. Neoplastic invasion of the laryngeal cartilage: comparison of MR imaging and CT with histopathologic correlation. *Radiology* 1995; **194:** 661–9.
5. Becker M, Zbären P, Delavelle J *et al.* Neoplastic invasion of the laryngeal cartilage: reassessment of criteria for diagnosis at CT. *Radiology* 1997; **203:** 521–32.
6. Biller HF, Lawson W. Management of acute laryngeal trauma. In: Bailey BJ, Biller HF, eds. *Surgery of the Larynx.* Philadelphia: Saunders, 1985: 149–54.
7. Bouchayer M, Cornut G. Dysphonia in adults caused by unilateral pseudohypertrophy of the ventricular band with deformation of the thyroid cartilage. Apropos of three cases. *Ann Otolaryngol Chir Cervicofac* 1994; **111:** 343–6.
8. Castelijns JA, Becker M, Hermans R. Impact of cartilage invasion on treatment and prognosis of laryngeal cancer. *Eur Radiol* 1996; **6:** 156–69.
9. Castelijns JA, van den Brekel MW, Niekoop VA, Snow GB. Imaging of the larynx. *Neuroimag Clin North Am* 1996; **6:** 401–15.
10. Castelijns JA, Kaiser MC, Valk J, Gerritsen GJ, van Hattum AH, Snow GB. MR imaging of laryngeal cancer. *J Comput Assist Tomogr* 1987; **11:** 134–40.
11. Castelijns JA, Gerritsen GJ, Kaiser MC *et al.* MRI of normal or cancerous laryngeal cartilage: histopathologic correlation. *Laryngoscope* 1987; **97:** 1085–93.
12. Castelijns JA, Gerritsen GJ, Kaiser MC *et al.* Invasion of laryngeal cartilage by cancer: comparison of CT and MR imaging. *Radiology* 1988; **166:** 199–206.
13. Deutsch EC, Schild JA, Mafee MF. Dysphagia and Forrestier's disease. *Arch Otolaryngol* 1985; **111:** 400–3.
14. DiSantis DJ, Balfe DM, Hayden RE, Sessions D, Sagel SS. The neck after vertical hemilaryngectomy: computed tomographic study. *Radiology* 1984; **151:** 683–7.
15. DiSantis DJ, Balfe DM, Hayden RE, Sagel SS, Sessions D, Lee JK. The neck after total laryngectomy: CT study. *Radiology* 1984; **153:** 713–17.
16. Doust DB, Ting YM. Xeroradiography of the larynx. *Radiology* 1975; **110:** 727–31.
17. Duda JJ Jr, Lewin JS, Eliachar I. MR evaluation of epiglottic disruption. *AJNR Am J Neuroradiol* 1996; **17:** 563–6.
18. Farooq P. Recurrent laryngeal nerve paralysis: laryngographic and computed tomography study. *Radiology* 1983; **148:** 149–51.
19. Feinmesser R, Freeman JL, Noyek AM, Birt BD. Metastatic neck disease. A clinical/radiographic/pathologic correlative study. *Arch Otolaryngol Head Neck Surg* 1987; **113:** 1307–10.
20. Feinmesser R, Freeman JL, Noyek AM, Birt BD, Gullane P, Mullen JB. MRI and neck metastases: a clinical, radiological, pathological correlative study. *J Otolaryngol* 1990; **19:** 136–40.
21. Finkelstein DM, Noyek AM, Kirsh JC. Red blood cell scan in cavernous hemangiomas of the larynx. *Ann Otol Rhinol Laryngol* 1989; **98:** 707–12.
22. Freeman DE, Mancuso AA, Parsons JT, Mendenhall WM, Million RR. Irradiation alone for supraglottic larynx carcinoma: can CT findings predict treatment results? *Int J Radiat Oncol Biol Phys* 1990; **19:** 485–90.
23. Friedman EM. Role of ultrasound in the assessment of vocal cord function in infants and children. *Ann Otol Rhinol Laryngol* 1997; **106:** 199–209.
24. Garel C, Contencin P, Polonovski JM, Hassan M, Narcy P.

Laryngeal ultrasonography in infants and children: a new way of investigating. Normal and pathological findings. *Int J Pediatr Otorhinolaryngol* 1992; **23:** 107–15.

25. Garel C, Hassan M, Hertz Pannier L, François M, Contencin P, Narcy P. Contribution of MR in the diagnosis of 'occult' posterior laryngeal cleft. *Int J Pediatr Otorhinolaryngol* 1992; **24:** 177–81.
26. Giron J, Joffre P, Serres Cousine O, Senac JP. CT and MR evaluation of laryngeal carcinomas. *J Otolaryngol* 1993; **22:** 284–93.
27. Glazer HS, Mauro MA, Aronberg DJ, Lee JK, Johnston DE, Sagel SS. Computed tomography of laryngoceles. *AJR Am J Roentgenol* 1983; **140:** 549–52.
28. Greven KM, Williams DW III, Keyes JW Jr *et al.* Distinguishing tumor recurrence from irradiation sequelae with positron emission tomography in patients treated for larynx cancer. *Int J Radiat Oncol Biol Phys* 1994; **29:** 841–5.
29. Hanafee WN. Hypopharynx and larynx. In: Valvassori GE, Carter BL, Mafee MF, Buckingham RA, Hanafee WN, eds. *Head and Neck Imaging.* New York: Thieme Medical Publishers, 1988: 311–38.
30. Henderson LT, Denneny JC III, Teichgraeber J. Airway-obstructing epiglottic cyst. *Ann Otol Rhinol Laryngol* 1985; **94:** 473–6.
31. Hermans R, van der Goten A, Baert AL. Volume estimation of the preepiglottic and paraglottic space using spiral computed tomography. *Surg Radiol Anat* 1997; **19:** 185–8.
32. Hermans R, Pameijer FA, Mancuso AA, Parsons JT, Mendenhall WM. CT findings in chondroradionecrosis of the larynx. *AJNR Am J Neuroradiol* 1998; **19:** 711–18.
33. Hubbard C. Laryngocele: a study of five cases with reference to radiologic features. *Clin Radiol* 1987; **38:** 639–43.
34. Hudgins PA, Siegel J, Jacobs I, Abramowsky CR. The normal pediatric larynx on CT and MR. *AJNR Am J Neuroradiol* 1997; **18:** 239–45.
35. Ichimura K, Sugasawa M, Nibu K, Takasago E, Hasezawa K. The significance of arytenoid edema following radiotherapy of laryngeal carcinoma with respect to residual and recurrent tumour. *Auris Nasus Larynx* 1997; **24:** 391–7.
36. Isaacson G, Birnholz JC. Human fetal upper respiratory tract function as revealed by ultrasonography. *Ann Otol Rhinol Laryngol* 1991; **100:** 743–7.
37. Johnson J, Curtin HD. Deep neck lipoma. *Ann Otol Rhinol Laryngol* 1987; **96:** 472–3.
38. Kallmes DF, Phillips CD. The normal anterior commissure of the glottis. *AJR Am J Roentgenol* 1997; **168:** 1317–19.
39. Kim MD, Kim DI, Yune HY *et al.* CT findings of laryngeal tuberculosis: comparison to laryngeal carcinoma. *J Comput Assist Tomogr* 1997; **21:** 29–34.
40. Konowitz PM, Lawson W, Som PM, Urchen ML, Breakstone BA, Biller HF. Laryngeal paraganglioma: update on diagnosis and treatment. *Laryngoscope* 1988; **98:** 40–9.
41. Kostakoglu L, Wong JC, Barrington SF, Cronin BF, Dynes AM, Maisey MN. Speech-related visualization of laryngeal muscles with fluorine-18-FDG. *J Nucl Med* 1996; **37:** 1771–3.
42. Lufkin RB, Hanafee WN. Application of surface coil to MR anatomy of the larynx. *AJR Am J Roentgenol* 1985; **145:** 483–9.
43. Lufkin RB, Hanafee WN, Wortham D, Hoover L. Larynx and hypopharynx: MR imaging with surface coils. *Radiology* 1986; **158:** 747–54.
44. Mafee MF, Schild JA, Valvassori GE, Capek V. Computed tomography of the larynx: correlation with anatomic and pathologic studies in cases of laryngeal carcinoma. *Radiology* 1983; **147:** 123–8.
45. Maguire GH. The larynx: simplified radiological examination using heavy filtration and high voltage. *Radiology* 1966; **87:** 102–10.
46. Maguire GH, Beigue RA. Selective filtration: a practical approach to high kilovoltage radiography. *Radiology* 1965; **85:** 345–51.
47. Mancuso AA, Hanafee WN. *Computed Tomography and Magnetic Resonance of the Head and Neck*, 2nd edn. Baltimore: Williams & Wilkins, 1985: 241–357.
48. Maroldi R, Battaglia G, Nicolai P *et al.* CT appearance of the larynx after conservative and radical surgery for carcinomas. *Eur Radiol* 1997; **7:** 418–31.
49. McArdle CB, Bailey BJ, Amparo EG. Surface coil magnetic resonance imaging of the normal larynx. *Arch Otolaryngol Head Neck Surg* 1986; **112:** 616–22.
50. McGuirt WF, Greven KM, Keyes JW Jr *et al.* Positron emission tomography in the evaluation of laryngeal carcinoma. *Ann Otol Rhinol Laryngol* 1995; **104:** 274–8.
51. Million RR. The myth regarding bone or cartilage involvement by cancer and the likelihood of cure by radiotherapy. *Head Neck* 1989; **11:** 30–40.
52. Misiti A, Macori F, Caimi M *et al.* Computerized tomography in the evaluation of the larynx after surgical treatment and irradiation. *Radiol Med (Torino)* 1997; **94:** 600–6.
53. Momose KJ, MacMillan AS Jr. Roentgenologic investigation of the larynx and trachea. *Radiol Clin North Am* 1978; **16:** 321–41.
54. Mukherji SK, Mancuso AA, Mendenhall W, Kotzur JM, Kubilis P. Can pretreatment CT predict local control of T2 glottic carcinomas treated with radiation therapy alone? *AJNR Am J Neuroradiol* 1995; **16:** 655–62.
55. Mukherji SK, Mancuso AA, Kotzur IM *et al.* Radiologic appearance of the irradiated larynx. Part I. Expected changes. *Radiology* 1994; **193:** 141–8.
56. Mukherji SK, Mancuso AA, Kotzur IM *et al.* Radiologic appearance of the irradiated larynx. Part II. Primary site response. *Radiology* 1994; **193:** 149–54.
57. Muñoz A, Ramos A, Ferrando J *et al.* Laryngeal carcinoma: sclerotic appearance of the cricoid and arytenoid cartilage. CT–pathologic correlation. *Radiology* 1993; **189:** 433–7.
58. Noyek AM, Witterick IJ, Kirsh JC. Radionuclide imaging in otolaryngology – head and neck surgery. *Arch Otolaryngol Head Neck Surg* 1991; **117:** 372–8.
59. Noyek AM, Shulman HS, Steinhardt MI, Zizmor J, Som PM. The larynx. In: Bergeron RT, Osborne AG, Som PM, eds. *Head and Neck Imaging: Excluding the Brain.* St Louis: Mosby, 1983: 402–90.
60. O'Brien PC. Tumour recurrence or treatment sequelae

following radiotherapy for larynx. *J Surg Oncol* 1996; **63:** 130–5.

61. Pameijer FA, Mancuso AA, Mendenhall WM, Parson JT, Kubilis PS. Can pretreatment computed tomography predict local control in T3 squamous cell carcinoma of the glottic larynx treated with definitive radiotherapy? *Int J Radiat Oncol Biol Phys* 1997; **37:** 1011–21.
62. Phelps PD. Carcinoma of the larynx: the role of imaging in staging and pre-treatment assessments. *Clin Radiol* 1992; **46:** 77–83.
63. Powers WE, McGee HH, Seaman WB. The contrast examination of larynx and pharynx. *Radiology* 1957; **68:** 169–72.
64. Raghavendra BN, Horii SC, Reede DL, Rumancik WM, Persky M, Bergeron T. Sonographic anatomy of the larynx, with particular reference to the vocal cords. *J Ultrasound Med* 1987; **6:** 225–30.
65. Robert Y, Rocourt N, Chevalier D, Duhamel A, Carcasset S, Lemaitre L. Helical CT of the larynx: a comparative study with conventional CT scan. *Clin Radiol* 1996; **51:** 882–5.
66. Rodenwaldt J, Niehaus HH, Kopka L, Grabbe E. Spiral CT in arytenoid cartilage dislocation: the optimization of the study parameters with a cadaver phantom and its clinical evaluation. *Rofo Fortschr Geb Rontgenstr Neuen Bildgeb Verfahr* 1998; **168:** 180–4.
67. Rodenwaldt J, Kopka L, Roedel R, Margas A, Grabbe E. 3D virtual endoscopy of the upper airway: optimization of the scan parameters in a cadaver phantom and clinical assessment. *J Comput Assist Tomogr* 1997; **21:** 405–11.
68. Rothberg R, Noyek AM, Freeman JL, Steinhardt MI, Stoll S, Goldfinger M. Thyroid cartilage imaging with diagnostic ultrasound. Correlative studies. *Arch Otolaryngol Head Neck Surg* 1986; **112:** 503–15.
69. Sakakura A, Yamamoto Y, Uesugi Y, Nakay K, Takenaka H, Narabayashi I. Three-dimensional imaging of laryngeal cancers using high-speed helical CT scanning. *ORL J Otorhinolaryngol Relat Spec* 1998; **60:** 103–7.
70. Samuel M, Burge DM, Griffiths DM. Prenatal diagnosis of laryngotracheoesophageal clefts. *Fetal Diagn Ther* 1997; **12:** 260–5.
71. Sataloff RT, Rao VM, Hawkshaw M, Lyons K, Spiegel JR. Cricothyroid joint injury. *J Voice* 1998; **12:** 112–16.
72. Scaglione M, Romano L, Palumbo P, Giovine S, Rossi G, Muzj C. Blunt trauma of the larynx: comparative assessment of computerized tomography, conventional radiology, and laryngoscopy. *Radiol Med (Torino)* 1996; **92:** 575–80.
73. Schaefer SD. Use of CT scanning in the management of the acutely injured larynx. *Otolaryngol Clin North Am* 1991; **24:** 31–6.
74. Schmalfuss IM, Mancuso AA, Tart RP. Arytenoid cartilage sclerosis: normal variations and clinical significance. *AJNR Am J Neuroradiol* 1998; **19:** 719–22.
75. Silva AB, Muntz HR, Clary R. Utility of conventional radiography in the diagnosis and management of pediatric airway foreign bodies. *Ann Otol Rhinol Laryngol* 1998; **107:** 834–5.
76. Silverman PM, Zeiberg AS, Sessions RB, Troost TR, Davros WJ, Zeman RK. Helical CT of the upper airway: normal and abnormal findings on three-dimensional reconstructed images. *AJR Am J Roentgenol* 1995; **165:** 541–6.
77. Sinard RJ, Netterville JL, Garrett CG, Ossoff RH. Cancer of the larynx. In: Suen JY, Myers EN, eds. *Cancer of the Head and Neck*. Philadelphia: Saunders, 1996: 381–421.
78. Soliman AM, Matar SA. Imaging quiz case 3. Paraglottic laryngeal lipoma. *Arch Otolaryngol Head Neck Surg* 1997; **123:** 550, 552.
79. Stark DD, Moss AA, Gamsu G, Clark OH, Gooding GA, Webb WR. Magnetic resonance imaging of the neck. Part I. Normal anatomy. *Radiology* 1984; **150:** 447–54.
80. Stines J, Rodde A, Carolus JM, Perrin C, Becker S. CT findings of laryngeal involvement in von Recklinghausen disease. *J Comput Assist Tomogr* 1987; **11:** 141–3.
81. Suojanen JN, Mukherji SK, Wippold FJ. Spiral CT of the larynx. *AJNR Am J Neuroradiol* 1994; **15:** 1579–82.
82. Supance JS, Queneue DJ, Crissman J. Endolaryngeal neurofibroma. *Otolaryngol Head Neck Surg* 1980; **88:** 74–9.
83. Tartaglino LM, Rao VM, Markiewicz DA. Imaging of radiation changes in the head and neck. *Semin Roentgenol* 1994; **29:** 81–91.
84. Thawley SE, Sessions DG. Surgical therapy of supraglottic tumors. In: Thawley SE, Panje WR, eds. *Comprehensive Management of Head and Neck Tumors*. Philadelphia: Saunders, 1987: 959–90.
85. Tostevin PM, de Bruyn R, Hosni A, Evans JN. The value of radiological investigations in pre-endoscopic assessment of children with stridor. *J Laryngol Otol* 1995; **109:** 844–8.
86. Ueda D, Yano K, Okuno A. Ultrasonic imaging of the tongue, mouth, and vocal cords in normal children: establishment of basic scanning positions. *J Clin Ultrasound* 1993; **21:** 431–9.
87. Valente T, Farina R, Minelli S. The echographic anatomy of the larynx and the perilaryngeal structures. *Radiol Med (Torino)* 1996; **91:** 231–7.
88. van den Brekel MWM, Castelijns JA, Reitsma CRL, Leemans CR, van der Waal I, Snow GB. Outcome of observing the N0 neck using ultrasonographic-guided cytology for follow-up. *Arch Otolaryngol Head Neck Surg* 1999; **125:** 153–6.
89. Wilkinson AG, Mackenzie S, Hendry GM. Complete laryngotrachesophageal cleft: CT diagnosis and associated abnormalities. *Clin Radiol* 1990; **41:** 437–8.
90. Williams DW III. Imaging of laryngeal cancer. *Otolaryngol Clin North Am* 1997; **30:** 35–58.
91. Witterick IJ, Gullane PJ. Laryngoscopy. In: Pearson FG, Deslauriers J, Ginsberg RJ, Hiebert CA, McKneally MF, Urschel HC Jr, eds. *Thoracic Surgery*. New York: Churchill Livingstone, 1995: 183–90.
92. Witterick IJ, Gullane PJ, Irish JC. Trauma to the larynx. In: Pearson FG, Deslauriers J, Ginsberg RJ, Hiebert CA, McKneally MF, Urschel HC Jr, eds. *Thoracic Surgery*. New York: Churchill Livingstone, 1995: 1535–42.
93. Yoskovitch A, al-Abdulhadi K, Wright ED, Watters AK, Chagnon F. Multiple myeloma of the cricoid cartilage. *J Otolaryngol* 1998; **27:** 168–70.
94. Yumoto E, Sanuki T, Hyodo M, Yasuhara Y, Ochi T. Three-dimensional endoscopic mode for observation of laryngeal structures by helical computed tomography. *Laryngoscope* 1997; **107:** 1530–7.

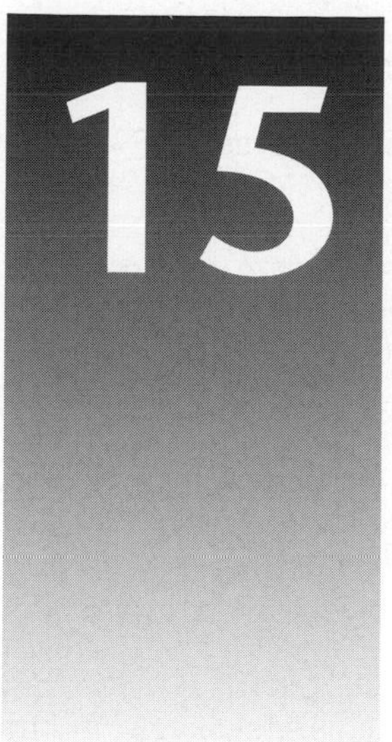

Anesthetic principles of airway management

Allan C D Brown

The larynx is a constrictor mechanism between the pharynx and the trachea. The framework of the organ is composed of hyaline cartilages suspended at the bottom of a midline 'funnel' of suspensory ligaments and muscles attached to the hyoid bone and ultimately to the mandible and skull base. The essence of laryngeal function is the plication of several folds of softer tissue lining, the funnel whose degree of folding or unfolding determines the function performed: a cavernous duct for ventilation, a vibratile slit for sound generation, an entrance barrier against potential contaminants and an exit plug for postural effort. Thus, the four prime functions of ventilation, phonation, protection and the glottal stop are all associated with different degrees of muscular folding.[7] Above all, the larynx is a powerful muscular organ.

The anesthesiologist has to overcome the powerful reflex closure of the glottis, whether it be to maintain a patent airway during mask general anesthesia or in order to pass an endotracheal tube in the awake or asleep patient. Simultaneously, the anesthesiologist must still provide effective protection against contamination of the airway. Endotracheal intubation is usually achieved in the awake patient with the use of topical anesthesia sometimes supplemented with conduction blockade of cranial nerves. In the anesthetized patient reliance is placed on deep surgical anesthesia or the use of muscle relaxant drugs in conjunction with lighter levels of general anesthesia. Continued protection for the airway while normal muscle activity is diminished or abolished is problematic, relying on a sequence of preventive measures, and cricoid pressure at induction of general anesthesia[23] in those patients considered to be at risk for aspiration.

When pathology or anatomic abnormality is located in the larynx itself, early resort may have to be made to a tracheotomy in order to control the airway and permit the intended operation. However, as a general principle, anesthesiologists attempt to control the airway from above the larynx rather than resorting to tracheotomy as patient morbidity with the former approach[12] tends to be of lesser frequency and severity than the complications associated with a tracheotomy.[4,24]

In order to achieve control of the larynx under general anesthesia, the supraglottic airway must permit one of three conditions:

- adequate spontaneous ventilation;
- artificial ventilation by mask;
- or effective anesthetic laryngoscopy and intubation.

The distinction between rigid laryngoscopy and anesthetic laryngoscopy is drawn here to denote the difference between rigid anesthetic laryngoscopes designed to facilitate the simultaneous manipulation of endotracheal tubes and those instruments used for other purposes. It is ideal that the glottis should be visible when using anesthetic laryngoscopy techniques. The ability to visualize the glottis directly with a standard rigid instrument is dependent on two prerequisites: the ability to gain access to the pharynx through the mouth and, having gained access, the ability to compress and deflect the tongue within the mandible. In some patients labeled as having difficult airways,[16] either or both of these two prerequisites may not be met.

Patients may have either congenital or acquired conditions that limit mouth opening or obstruct one or both nares. If access is available, in some patients displacement of the tongue and lifting the mandible with the usual laryngoscopic action may not bring the glottis into view. This appears to be a function of the relative volume of the base of tongue within the variable restriction of the arc of the mandible and the range of movement present in the cervical spine. The presence of friable or space-occupying lesions in the hypopharynx may make this problem of visualization worse. In some patients, access to and visualization of the anatomic area where the larynx is expected to be found does not pose a problem, but the glottis or 'target' for intubation may not be easily identified due to anatomic distortion from disease, scarring from previous surgery or the presence of pathologic lesions overhanging or occupying the glottis. Therefore, the requirements for anesthetic laryngoscopy and intubation are conveniently divided into access, visualization and target.[2] Absence or limitation in any one of these requirements may pose problems for controlling the airway and a combination of problems may make the safe conduct of anesthesia extremely difficult. Usually the problem highest in the airway dictates what may or may not be done. Thus access ranks before visualization and visualization ranks before target problems in planning anesthetic management.

The difficult airway

The truly difficult airway is rare[21] but since death or serious morbidity may result from mismanagement,[3] the anesthesiologist must master the techniques that are available to avert an hypoxic disaster. Anesthesiologists working in otorhinolaryngology gain considerable experience with difficult airways and have the advantage of working with surgeons who are skilled in tracheotomy when the need arises but, in spite of these advantages, patient safety is still dependent on well planned airway management.

It is useful to divide patients with airway problems into three distinct groups in order to discuss their management:

- *Patients in extremis* with severe airway obstruction and hypoxia will have accompanying hypercapnia, delirium, or unconsciousness. Cardiac arrest will occur if the airway is not cleared immediately.
- *Patients with respiratory distress* represent the largest group that present for anesthesia. They may exhibit stridor, tracheal tug, intercostal retraction, labored breathing and agitation. Although increasingly fatigued, they are able to compensate sufficiently to maintain adequate oxygenation and remain alert and cooperative.
- *Patients with occult impending obstruction* volunteer little information in their history to suggest airway difficulties and a cursory physical examination reveals little to warn of the management problems that are to follow the induction of anesthesia.

The management of the first group is clear-cut. Oxygenation must be reestablished immediately. If the patient is unconscious and relaxed, it is worth a few seconds to attempt mask ventilation and rapid laryngoscopy for intubation, but no time should be wasted. If intubation is obviously not going to be easy, the surgeon or anesthesiologist should perform an immediate cricothyrotomy to reestablish oxygenation before moving the patient to the operating room for formal tracheotomy. There is probably no longer any place for a so-called 'emergency' tracheotomy done under unfavorable conditions by an inexperienced surgeon in the hospital environment.

If the patient is still moving some air into his lungs, laryngoscopy should be omitted as this stimulus can lead to total obstruction. The patient should have his airway supported and be transferred to the operating room breathing 100% oxygen by mask and accompanied by the means of doing a cricothyrotomy and manual ventilation if his condition should deteriorate in transit.

The remaining two groups of patients permit the anesthesiologist and surgeon the opportunity to plan airway management in advance. In those patients with respiratory distress, it is the technical skill of the anesthesiologist that determines both the airway control plan and its success. In patients with occult impending obstruction, it is the anesthesiologist's diagnostic acumen in detecting that a problem is present in the first place which is paramount.

Most occult problems result from subtle congenital anatomic abnormalities for which the patient usually compensates with muscular effort. The only clue to the condition may be a history of obstructive sleep apnea. However, the patient may only admit to early waking under direct questioning and often the true sequence of events is obtained only from the patient's 'bedmate', who is awakened by heavy snoring and then hears the onset of obstruction or 'choking' followed by the patient's awakening. The normal anesthetic induction abolishes all muscle tone and promptly precipitates complete obstruction, which is frequently not amenable to the normal methods of reestablishing the airway due to the anatomic abnormalities involved. Premedication alone may be sufficient to precipitate this crisis. Besides congenital conditions, some carcinomas of the base of the tongue and

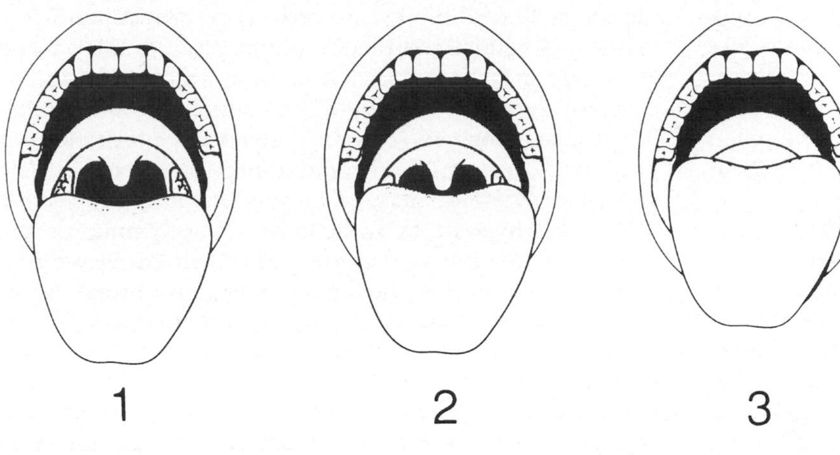

Figure 15.1 *Mallampati presentation.[18] This simple classification system gives an indication of tongue volume relative to the mandibular space available. The patient is examined sitting with the tongue protruding without phonation. Presentation 1 (Mallampati 1, etc.) is normal; the pillars of the fauces and uvula are clearly visible. Presentation 2 is less common; only part of the pillars, the uvula and soft palate are visible; difficulty with laryngoscopic visualization is sometimes encountered. Presentation 3 occurs in approximately 7% of adults; only a part or none of the soft palate is visible; approximately 30% of these patients are found to have a Grade IV laryngoscopy.*

supraglottic tumors behave in this manner, as may the patient with epiglottitis.

Evaluation of the airway

The problem with airway evaluation is deciding where to stop! It is unrealistic to expect a detailed evaluation in every patient for surgery when the vast majority will prove to be normal in all respects. However, unless every patient is screened for airway problems, those with difficulties will be missed. Therefore a quick clinical screening protocol is required and only those patients demonstrating abnormalities are selected for further detailed evaluation. Unfortunately, with the lack of sensitivity of our current methods of assessment, there is no general agreement on what such a protocol should include,[5] but some general guidelines can be suggested.

An airway screening protocol for all patients presenting for anesthesia

Patient's airway history

- Nasal patency?
- Voice changes: duration and progress?
- Dyspnea: effort or positional?
- Shortness of breath?
- Painful throat or difficulty swallowing?
- Masses noted in the neck or mouth?
- Any reflux complaints?
- Sleeping position and any history of sleep disturbance?
- Problems with previous anesthetics or intubations?
- Anesthetic problems in the family?
- Smoking history?
- Any extensive dental work?
- Anemia?
- Any musculoskeletal disease?
- Significant hypertensive or cardiac disease?
- Significant respiratory disease?
- Obesity: height and weight, any recent weight gain?
- Pregnancy?

Patient's external airway and functional anatomy examination

- Note the patient's posture: Is there obvious dyspnea or shortness of breath?
- Can the patient lie flat and adopt the anesthesia 'sniffing' position?
- What is the body habitus (obese, deformity, limited movement of head and neck)?
- External malformations suggesting possible branchial arch malformations?
- Do the nostrils each move air normally?

Full face view

- Are the larynx and trachea central and normally aligned?
- Do the larynx and trachea move normally on swallowing?
- Normal mouth opening (4 cm +)?
- Normal hard palate and dentition?
- Mallampati presentation (Fig. 15.1)?
- Visible masses and abnormalities in the mouth and oropharynx?
- Can the tongue be protruded?
- Does the width of mandible and maxilla appear normal?
- Short neck – tracheotomy external landmarks?

Lateral view

- Relative micrognathia or overbite?
- Vertical separation of thyroid cartilage from lower border of mandible (>3 cm)?
- Assessment of *effective* length of mandible (mentum to hyoid >6 cm)?

Although the list may seem long, the assessment only takes a few moments. A single minor abnormality does not usually indicate a difficult airway but as the number of abnormalities detected increases, the examiner's index of suspicion should rise until the point is reached when the examiner judges that a full airway evaluation is warranted.

Airway compromise is usually evident from the general history and examination. However, to detect occult impending airway compromise requires detailed examination of the airway. Congenital anomalies of the airway may involve any part of the respiratory tract, but the most commonly underestimated ones occur in structures arising from the first and second branchial arch structures. The classic syndromes such as Treacher Collins, Hallermann–Streif, etc., are obvious, but similar deformities of a lesser degree are not. These may occur in otherwise normal patients who compensate for their deformity with muscular effort. Premedication or induction of anesthesia modifies or abolishes this compensatory effort, leading to airway obstruction.

Full evaluation of the suspected difficult airway

The airway and all related factors should be assessed at a preoperative clinic visit when there is time for a thorough assessment of the problems involved. In particular, the patient's ability to deliver oxygen to the tissues should be evaluated in its broadest sense.

Airway and general anatomy require particularly careful assessment as these two factors are likely to impose limitations on surgical positioning, and the choice of technique for anesthetic induction and maintenance. An extremely obese patient may not only pose problems of access for the surgeon but also difficulty for the anesthetist in intubation and choice of technique to minimize well-recognized intraoperative problems and postoperative sequelae.[20]

Oxygen delivery to the tissues

The maintenance of oxygen delivery to the patient's tissues is one of the prime functions of the anesthesiologist. In the management of patients with difficult airways, both components of oxygen delivery – oxygen transport and oxygen reserve – must be considered. The patient's oxygen reserve is important because this is the major determinant of the time available for intubation maneuvers. The state of the patient's oxygen transport mechanisms is important because the response to even minor hypoxia may pose additional problems, particularly in those patients with significant cardiovascular disease.

The patient's oxygen reserve may be defined as the oxygen contained in the functional residual capacity (FRC) of the lungs and the oxygen contained in the patient's blood volume. Many conditions can diminish the available oxygen reserve by interfering with the normal state of these two oxygen stores. Anemia for any reason will reduce the blood volume store available. The FRC store may be reduced in a number of ways due to different respiratory diseases. The volume of the FRC may be reduced due to obesity, advanced pregnancy or prolonged bedrest with pulmonary atelectasis. The volume of the FRC may be increased, causing a relative 'dilutional' hypoxia as in advanced emphysema, or the delivery of oxygen to a normal FRC volume by spontaneous ventilation may be impaired by active bronchoconstriction or upper airway partial obstruction.

The patient's oxygen transport is a function of cardiac output, hemoglobin concentration and oxygen/hemoglobin combining power (usually a constant). In patients who smoke or who have hemoglobinopathies, the effective combining power is reduced. Similarly, anemia absolutely reduces transport ability. Such reductions are usually compensated for by a combination of increased oxygen extraction from oxyhemoglobin in the tissues and an increase in cardiac output achieved by a combination of increased heart rate and stroke volume. If a relative hypoxia is superimposed, these changes will be exaggerated. The stress of laryngoscopy and intubation will also contribute to these changes with hypertension and additional cardiac work. Under such circumstances the patients most at risk are those with ischemic heart disease. Unfortunately, many of the patients presenting with difficult airways fall into the age group where atherosclerotic heart disease is to be expected.

The evaluation of these risk factors is necessary to permit the optimization of the patient's condition and to determine the best approach to airway management. The patient's arterial oxygen saturation ($Sa\text{O}_2$) should be measured while breathing room air. Where any sort of impairment is suspected the arterial oxygen tension ($Pa\text{O}_2$) and blood gases should also be measured and improvement demonstrated with increases in the inspired oxygen concentration ($F\text{IO}_2$). Pulmonary function tests will be helpful in demonstrating any reversible bronchospasm and in some patients with airway obstruction improvement may be achieved with inspired oxygen/helium mixtures.

In the face of anemia little can be done to change the situation. The risks of blood transfusion are rarely justified unless there is a severe reduction in hemoglobin levels and patients with chronic anemias appear much more tolerant of insult than those with acute conditions. The hemoglobinopathies allow no more than the usual prospective precautions. Patients with ischemic heart disease and hypertension require careful evaluation, particularly where a history of effort angina or cardiac dysrhythmia is obtained, together with the optimization of any medications being taken.

External anatomy

Anatomic variations, scarring and tumor also contribute to technical difficulties with laryngoscopy and intubation.

Of particular interest in anticipating such problems is the presence of micrognathia, microstomia, macroglossia, or relative macroglossia, unusual angulation of the larynx, short thick neck or combinations thereof. In the clinical examination of the upper airway attention should be paid to the patency and size of the nasal passages for the potential use of nasal endotracheal tubes. The full face should be examined for symmetry and a full lateral view examined for the size and position of the mandible relative to the maxilla. The state and presentation of dentition should be noted, as should the presence of a narrow high-arched hard palate. A high-arched palate in association with closely spaced parallel upper alveolar ridges can make the simultaneous manipulation of laryngoscope and endotracheal tube impossible. The position of the larynx relative to the mandible should be identified. If the vertical distance between the prominence of the thyroid cartilage and the lower border of the mandible admits 1.5 finger-breadths (3 cm) or more, it is unlikely that a high larynx tucked under the base of the tongue will be encountered. The mobility of the larynx should be observed by asking the patient to swallow, and the presence of induration or scarring in the base of the tongue and hypopharynx should be sought by palpation of the soft tissues beneath the mandible. Palpation of the neck will confirm the midline position of the trachea and identify the possibility of an awkward laryngeal presentation due to edema or scarring, together with the presence of any tumors impinging upon the trachea, which might make the passage of an endotracheal tube difficult. Finally, the full and free movement of the cervical spine and the occipitoatlantal joints should be confirmed as well as the patient's ability to open the mouth without limitation. If the inability to intubate or ventilate the patient is encountered unexpectedly at anesthetic induction the presence of a short thick neck may make a safe rapid tracheotomy more difficult, thereby placing the patient's life in immediate jeopardy.

Radiologic evaluation

The use of radiologic studies to evaluate airway pathology is well established for diagnostic purposes. Plain films, tomography and the more recent and expensive coaxial scanning techniques all contribute useful information. However, there are two drawbacks to these techniques. All give a static view of the patient with no indication of the flexibility and mobility of the tissues visualized and they require the patient to visit the radiology department which is not the best place to handle airway emergencies. Some studies require the patient to lie flat, which is not always possible.

Recently the use of a C-arm image intensifier has proved more satisfactory for anesthetic airway evaluation.[17] The advantage of the technique is that a dynamic sequence of airway behavior may be viewed and captured on video tape in different postures to identify the most favorable presentation of the airway in each patient. Thus, easily

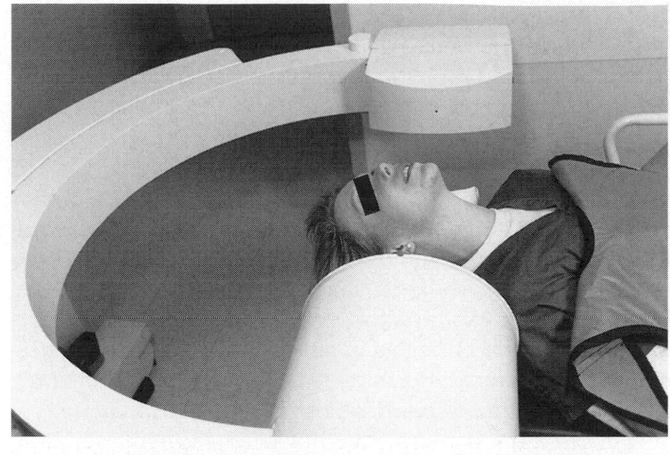

(a)

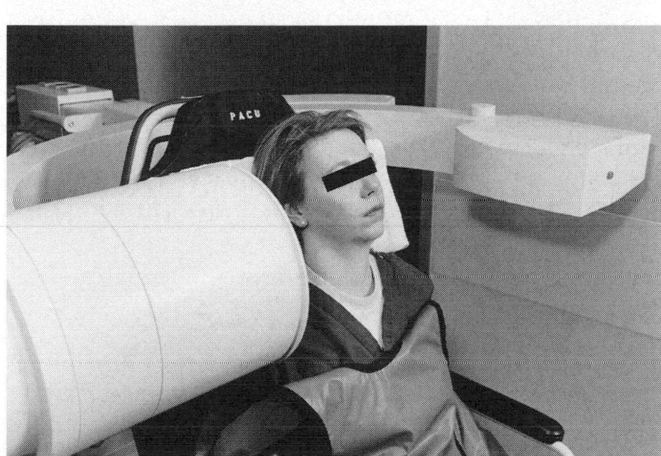

(b)

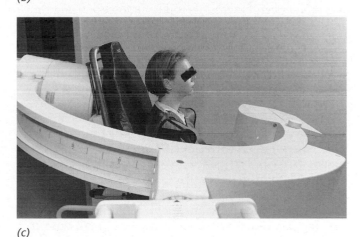

(c)

Figure 15.2 *Positions for C-arm examination of the extrathoracic airway. Illustration (a) demonstrates the lateral view of the supine anesthesia sniffing position. Only if significant abnormality is detected in this position does the examination progress to position (b), the lateral erect position, to see if airway diameters are improved by postural change. If a lateral erect view is required, position (c), an A-P erect view, is also obtained to visualize coronal plane diameters in the airway. All three views are recorded with a dynamic sequence including swallowing, tongue protrusion and phonation.*

demonstrating the full and free movement of the cervical spine, occipitoatlantal joints and temporomandibular joints (TMJ); variations in hypopharyngeal airway diameters with change of position from supine to erect; improvement of airway dimensions with tongue protrusion; and whether airway constrictions are fixed or variable with respiration. Of particular value is the ability to visualize the movements of coordinated swallowing and the mobility of the laryngotrachea, together with the movements of pathologic shadows associated with these structures. The examination may be done in the operating room for an emergency case or at the bedside in the preoperative preparation area within easy reach of effective intervention to control the airway if required.

The examination sequence has been refined over time to three basic views (Fig 15.2), the supine lateral anesthetic 'sniffing' position, the lateral erect position and the anterior–posterior erect position. Additional views to demonstrate abnormalities of TMJ movement and odontoid stability are sometimes useful in selected patients. Frequently, the information obtained in this noninvasive manner is sufficient to reassure the anesthesiologist and suggest the preferred management plan without proceeding further.

The awake look

Where significant distortion of normal airway anatomy is identified, there is usually no alternative to awake endoscopy in order to define the details of the problems to be overcome to achieve endotracheal intubation. This can be done effectively with indirect mirror laryngoscopy and more recently with fiberoptic endoscopy. One *caveat* must be emphasized; *satisfactory visualization of the glottis with an indirect or flexible instrument does not necessarily imply good visualization with a rigid laryngoscope.* The ability to compress and deflect the tongue base must be assessed by the palpation of tissues and the dynamic radiologic appearance of the structures.

With a cooperative and stoic patient, endoscopy may be achieved without local anesthesia but the majority of patients require effective topical anesthesia of the upper airway. If the airway is already compromised this should be done without sedation which can reduce muscle tone and make the situation worse. Most patients can be 'talked through' the examination with minimal discomfort, but for those with great anxiety, a small dose of a benzodiazepine followed by a small dose of ketamine gives adequate sedation and maintains blood pressure in the erect position. The patient sitting in an examination chair is ideal as this position usually produces the most widely patent airway for examination.

It is useful to regard the examination as a reconnaissance for the anesthesiologist and a learning experience for the patient. The anesthesiologist is exploring the patient's airway anatomy and identifying the problems to be overcome for intubation to be successful. The patient is becoming familiar with the experience and learning what to expect when the time for intubation arrives. These activities are best conducted in a quiet, private examination area with full resuscitation facilities if required for an emergency.

If the examination is for elective surgery the patient must be fully prepared. Topical anesthesia of the airway will impair normal protective reflexes; therefore it is advisable to starve the patient for the usual period (4–6 hours). Many laryngeal conditions are associated with the chronic reflux of stomach contents so the use of premedication to guard against this risk must be considered. H2-blockers, the dopamine antagonist metoclopramide and antacid preparations are all appropriate alone or in combination in the absence of specific contraindications. Topical anesthesia works best on dry mucous membranes; therefore one of the antisialagogue drugs is indicated in sufficient dose and time to ensure dry membranes, bearing in mind that the effective 'drying' dose of these drugs varies considerably from one patient to another.

Once prepared, several techniques are available to achieve adequate local anesthesia of the airway. The topical anesthetic of choice is lidocaine, although 4% cocaine solution is still popular for the topical preparation of the nasal passages. The use of benzocaine is diminishing due to increasing awareness of its propensity to induce significant methemoglobinemia. Three common techniques are as follows.

Local anesthesia techniques

Topical spray technique

Proprietary aerosol sprays of lidocaine (which can range up to a 10% concentration) and stock lidocaine (usually in the 2–4% range) applied with a reusable spray such as a DeVilbis varidirectional spray are both popular. Both have the disadvantage that most patients initially recoil from the idea of these devices being introduced far back into their airway. In addition, the proprietary sprays tend to foam on contact and taste unpleasant, diminishing the patient's confidence. Similar problems are encountered with ordinary lidocaine solutions in a standard spray. Although contact foaming is not a problem, the solution is cold and the patient is very aware of the spray. Both these drawbacks can be minimized by warming the solution to blood temperature and dissolving a small amount of artificial sweetener[1] in the solution.

Swish and swallow technique

This technique appears to be associated with a greater level of patient comfort and acceptance. After full preparation and drying the patient is given *10 ml of 4% warm aqueous* lidocaine solution with sweetener added and asked to swill it around his/her mouth and then gargle for 15 seconds with the residue before swallowing it. *After 10 minutes* the patient is given a second dose, this time, *10 ml of 2% warm viscous* lidocaine solution (without

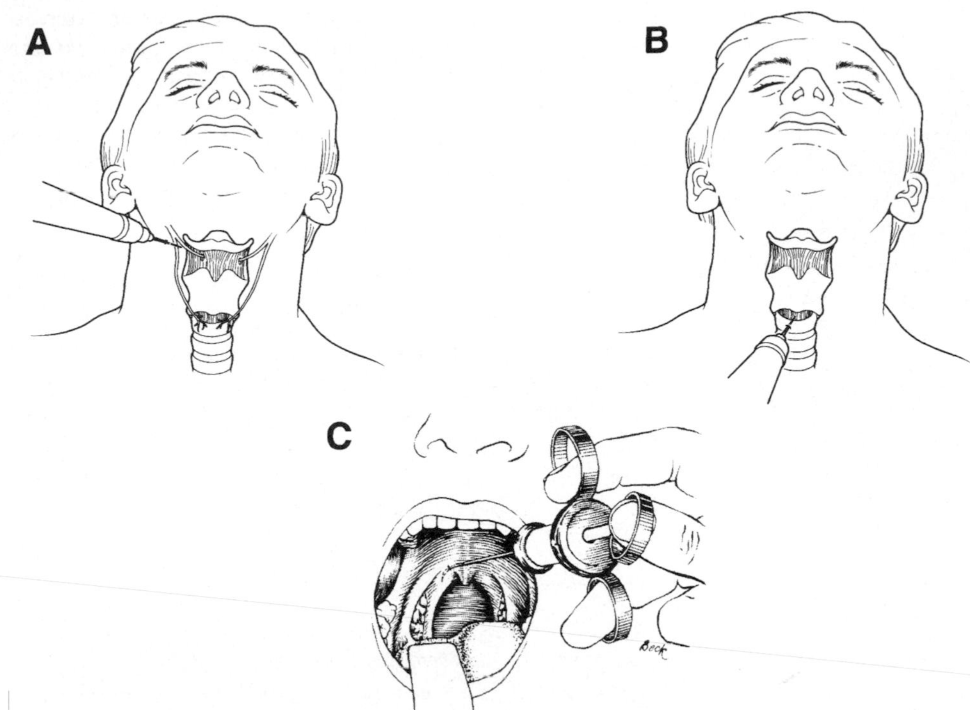

Figure 15.3 *Conduction blockade of the airway. The three illustrations in this figure show the common percutaneous/conduction blocks of the airway. (a) Shows the block of the superior laryngeal nerve where it divides into its internal and external branches adjacent to the posteroinferior aspect of the hyoid cornu major. This is to achieve anesthesia of the mucous membrane of the hypopharynx. (b) Shows the percutaneous instillation of local anesthetic through the cricothyroid membrane to achieve tracheal anesthesia and laryngeal intrinsic muscle relaxation. (c) Shows the use of a guarded needle and dental syringe to block the branch of the glossopharyngeal that enters the pillar of the fauces in order to anesthetize the base of the tongue and block the afferent arc of the gag reflex.*

sweetener) and asked to repeat the process. A further 5 minutes is allowed to pass before endoscopy is attempted. In patients who cannot swallow, the technique is still effective even if the residuum has to be spat out.

Conduction blockade

Excellent airway anesthesia can also be achieved with combined bilateral blocks of the superior laryngeal and glossopharyngeal nerves (Fig 15.3). The superior laryngeal nerve may be blocked percutaneously in the neck or its internal branch to the airway mucosa may be blocked topically by applying a pledget soaked in lidocaine solution with Krause (Jackson) forceps to the mucous membrane lining the pyriform fossae. The glossopharyngeal nerves may be blocked where they enter the pillars of the fauces by submucous injection using a guarded needle and a dental syringe. This latter block is also useful to supplement topical anesthesia in the occasional patient where a troublesome gag reflex persists after topical preparation.

Tracheal anesthesia

This is rarely required for airway evaluation unless the lesion is below the vocal folds. If the need arises and for intubation, three methods are available to achieve topical anesthesia of the trachea. Anesthetic solution (4 ml of 2% lidocaine is usually sufficient) may be introduced by percutaneous puncture and instillation through the cricothyroid membrane (Fig 15.3) or it may be instilled from above the larynx using indirect mirror laryngoscopy and a malleable cannula. An even more patient acceptable variation on the latter technique is to use an epidural catheter passed through the suction channel of the fiberoptic endoscope to instil the solution under direct vision (Fig 15.4). Again, warming the solution and gentle injection diminish patient irritability and the cough response.

The secret of consistent success with the topical preparation of the airway is the adequate drying of the mucous membranes and waiting sufficiently long for the topical drug to take full effect. Premature endoscopy is distressing to the patient and the loss of confidence and cooperation may make an adequate examination impossible.

If a nasal endotracheal tube is required for the proposed operation, both nasal passages must also be examined for adequate patency. They should be prepared at the same time as the oral airway. First, a proprietary vasoconstrictor nasal spray is applied, followed by the application of topical anesthetic by spray or on pledgets. It is unnecessary to execute a full surgical nasal block sequence with sphenopalatine ganglia injection, etc., as contact with both endoscope and endotracheal tube is limited to the area below the inferior turbinate.

The major risk of topical preparation of the airway is the toxic effects of drug overdose (see below). It is important to avoid overdose but also to be prepared to treat it should the need arise. The 'swish and swallow' technique described above apparently exceeds recommended doses for lidocaine but actually relies on 70% first-pass metabolism in the liver to avoid systemic toxicity (of importance in patients with liver function impairment).

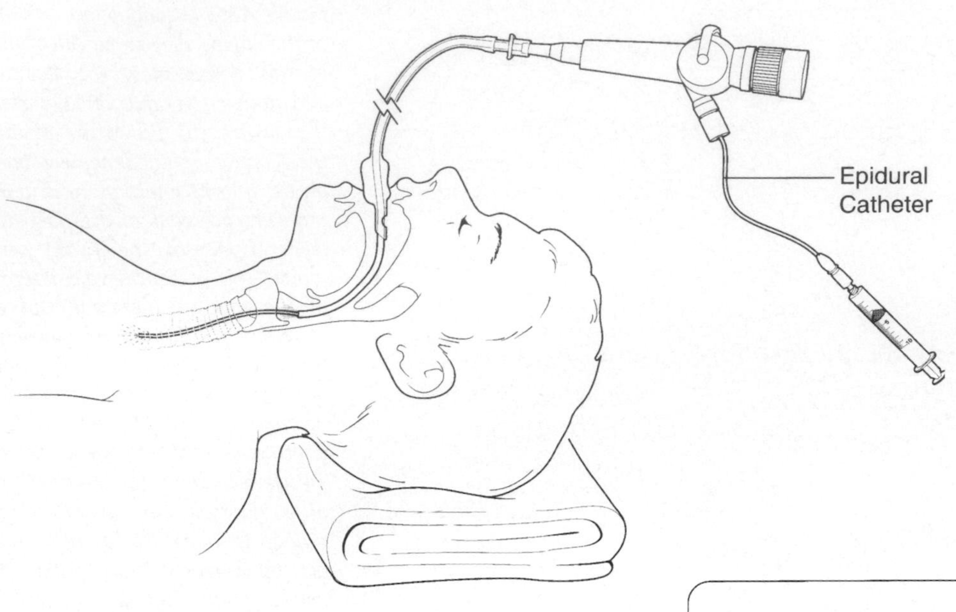

Figure 15.4 *Epidural catheter tracheal instillation. Most patients prefer an instillation technique, rather than a percutaneous block of tracheal sensation. This method, utilizing direct vision of the glottis through a fiberoptic endoscope to pass an epidural catheter from the suction channel into the trachea, has been found particularly useful, as careful positioning of the catheter causes little stimulation.*

Controlling the airway

The purpose of the detailed preoperative examination of the airway is to enable the formulation of an airway management plan with a good chance of success whilst limiting risk for the patient. The choices involved are threefold:

- How to make the intubation maneuvers tolerable for the patient by *choice of an anesthetic technique* which does not add to the patient's problems.
- Deciding on the *route of intubation*, bearing in mind the needs of the intended operation and the particular problems to be circumvented (Fig 15.5).
- Finally, deciding on the *technique of intubation* most likely to succeed under the circumstances.

Deciding on the choice of anesthetic

Given the choice, most patients would prefer to be asleep for endotracheal intubation. The normal sequence for inducing general anesthesia involves the use of an intravenous induction agent to block awareness and a muscle relaxant to facilitate laryngoscopy maneuvers and an atraumatic intubation. Both drugs once given intravenously cannot be retrieved and both usually abolish spontaneous respiration and the patient's ability to oxygenate. Therefore, the time available to secure the airway is limited by the patient's oxygen reserve. If there is any doubt at all concerning the ease of securing the airway, the dose of induction drugs should be reduced and succinylcholine should be used in preference to longer acting muscle relaxants in the hope that spontaneous respiration will return quickly in the event of failure to control the airway. To increase the time

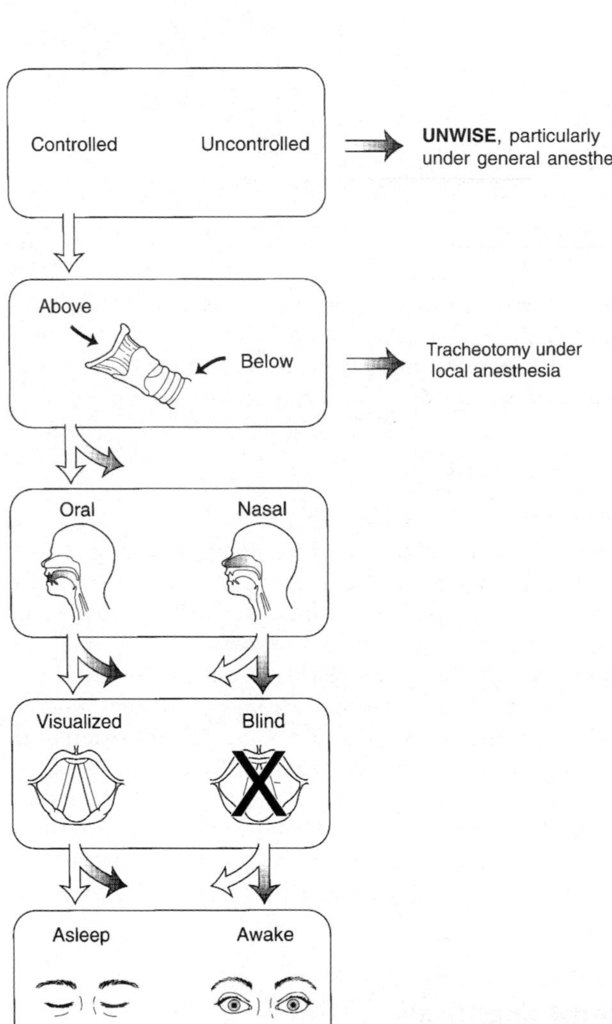

Figure 15.5 *Anesthetic intubation decision choices. This 'decision tree' summarizes the general approach to the choices available in terms of choice of anesthetic technique, intubation route and intubation problems to be anticipated. The more desirable choices are indicated by white arrows, the less desirable by dark arrows. The 'norm' is the sequence down the left margin.*

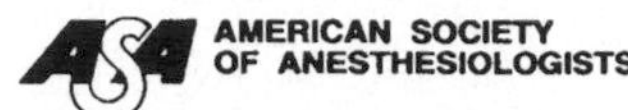

DIFFICULT AIRWAY ALGORITHM

1. Assess the likelihood and clinical impact of basic management problems:

A. Difficult Intubation

B. Difficult Ventilation

C. Difficulty with Patient Cooperation or Consent

2. Consider the relative merits and feasibility of basic management choices:

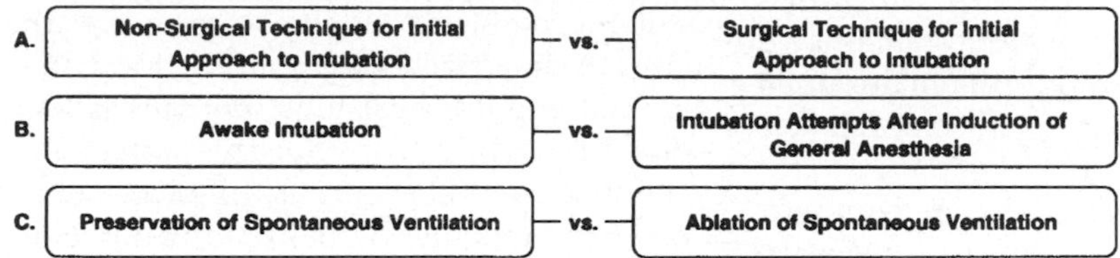

3. Develop primary and alternative strategies:

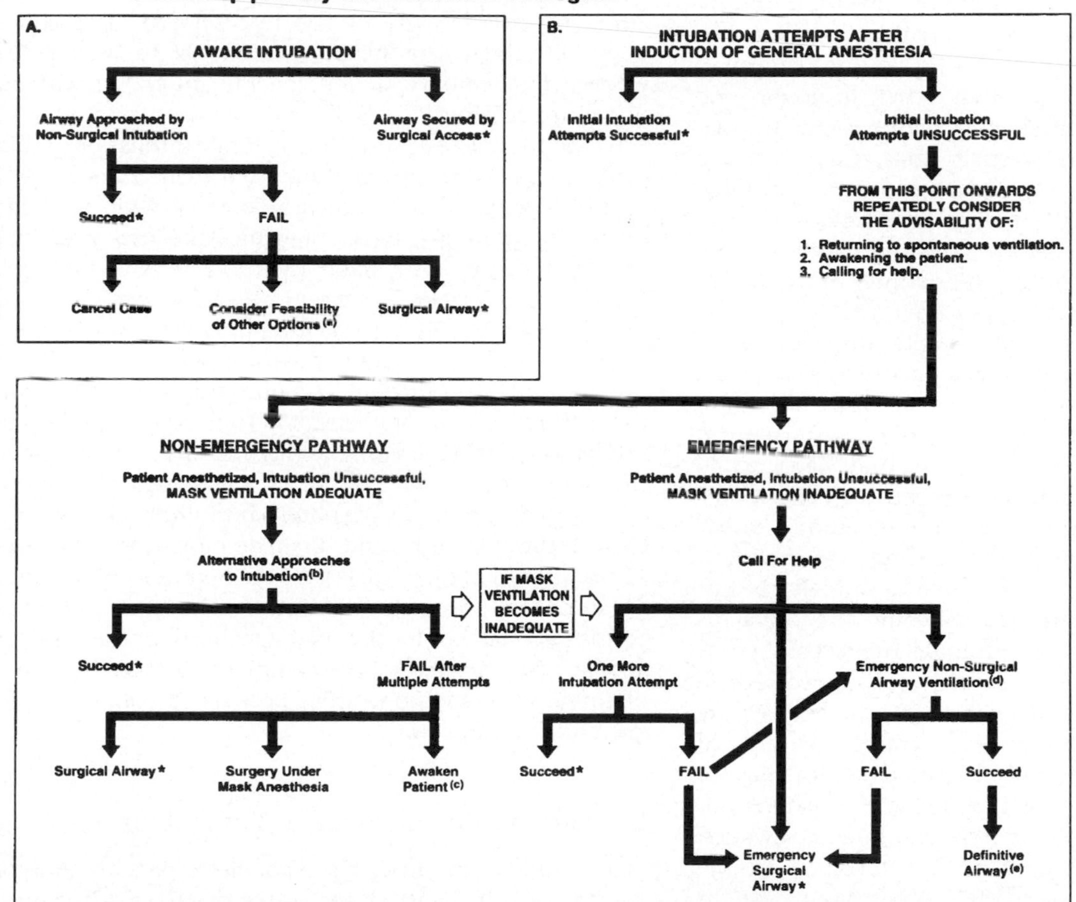

* CONFIRM INTUBATION WITH EXHALED CO_2

(a) Other options include (but are not limited to): surgery under mask anesthesia, surgery under local anesthesia infiltration or regional nerve blockade, or intubation attempts after induction of general anesthesia.

(b) Alternative approaches to difficult intubation include (but are not limited to): use of different laryngoscope blades, awake intubation, blind oral or nasal intubation, fiberoptic intubation, intubating stylet or tube changer, light wand, retrograde intubation, and surgical airway access.

(c) See awake intubation.

(d) Options for emergency non-surgical airway ventilation include (but are not limited to): transtracheal jet ventilation, laryngeal mask ventilation, or esophageal-tracheal combitube ventilation.

(e) Options for establishing a definitive airway include (but are not limited to): returning to awake state with spontaneous ventilation, tracheotomy, or endotracheal intubation.

Figure 15.6 *The ASA difficult airway algorithm. Is a useful consensus attempt to offer guidance to a rational sequence of management techniques for dealing with a difficult airway? It is NOT a protocol, but it does go some way to establishing a standard of care for anesthesiologists. (Reproduced from* Anesthesiology *1993;* ***78:*** *597–602, with the permission of Lippincott-Raven publishers)*

available, the patient's oxygen reserve should be maximized by breathing 100% oxygen for at least 3 minutes through a close-fitting mask before induction.

When significant airway problems are anticipated but a judgment has been made that the patient's airway may be safely maintained with a mask, it is prudent to avoid abolishing spontaneous ventilation. Induction of general anesthesia may be achieved with the patient breathing a standard anesthetic vapor. Once the third stage of anesthesia is achieved, laryngoscopy is feasible and intubation may be achieved with or without relaxants, depending upon an adequate view of the glottis. Should the problems involved be greater than anticipated, the option of awaking the patient remains as long as effective spontaneous ventilation is maintained to remove the anesthetic vapor excreted through the lungs.

If the airway problems faced are severe or complex, with serious coincident systemic disease, an awake intubation under topical anesthesia is indicated. This approach minimizes the possibility of apnea induced by anesthetic drugs at the expense of patient comfort, but does permit the erect position for intubation. However, there is a growing perception that, when in doubt, one is never wrong in attempting an awake fiberoptic intubation. This is not true. Drug toxicity may still precipitate an emergency as may laryngospasm in an irritable airway. There are still contraindications to the technique, such as severe active bleeding in the airway, and patients already on the borderline of profound hypoxia.

A failed intubation, in association with any of the three anesthetic techniques above, should be anticipated with a secondary plan to achieve intubation promptly (Fig 15.6). Should the secondary plan also fail, resort to a surgical airway must be made sooner rather than later while something is left in the patient's oxygen reserve.

In some clinical situations a formal tracheotomy under infiltration anesthesia may be the method of first choice, to ensure patient safety, if the anesthesiologist is not confident of his/her ability to overcome the problems posed with any intubation technique. However, there is one trap that should be carefully considered before attempting intubation, and that is the patient whose anatomy would make any form of emergency surgical airway time-consuming and technically difficult to achieve in the face of a failed intubation with developing hypoxia. Patients with severely deformed or swollen necks, or with severe fixed flexion deformities of the neck, together with those patients whose larynx lies in close proximity or behind the sternum, all fall into such a group; careful consideration of awake tracheotomy as the method of first choice for securing the airway is required.

As a general rule, all patients with identified airway problems should have their surgeon present and ready to secure a surgical airway in the face of a failed intubation before any type of anesthetic induction is begun.

Deciding on the route of intubation

Having assessed the patient, the route for achieving airway control must be considered. The purpose of the management plan is to achieve full control of the airway to guarantee oxygenation while sealing it against contamination. The ideal method is to achieve control from above the larynx by passing an oral endotracheal tube under direct vision in a relaxed anesthetized patient, with full aspiration precautions, if indicated.[25] This is assumed to cause the least trauma to both psyche and anatomy. When pathology intervenes, the patient's best interest may be served by deviations from the ideal.

If the problems involved are severe, the surgeon may elect to do a tracheotomy under local anesthesia without an oral endotracheal tube, but this is less desirable than doing a tracheotomy after the protection afforded by an endotracheal tube cuff is in place, even in an awake patient. Similarly, visualized manipulations are always preferable to blind approaches. The latter are associated with an increased risk of damage to the structures of either the nasal cavity or the hypopharynx and consequent bleeding. The height of folly is to attempt an elective tracheotomy under general anesthesia with an uncontrolled airway.

If the desirable condition is oral intubation under general anesthesia, alternatives have to be decided by a process of exclusion. Ludwig's angina, with its large, upwardly swelling tongue, precludes the use of an oral tube, but passage of a nasal tube awake, with fiberoptic visualization, may be feasible. However, a leukemic coagulopathy resulting in a large tongue would also render a nasal intubation attempt unwise. Similarly, although micrognathia may prevent visualization of the glottis and the passage of an oral endotracheal tube, blind nasal intubation might be easily achieved. Any friable hemorrhagic tumor above the glottis, or a large pointing abscess in the pharynx, is an absolute contraindication to any blind technique and could dissuade most from visualized techniques as well. This leaves tracheotomy under local anesthesia as the only alternative. The prerequisites of consistent success in the management of the difficult airway are thorough preoperative assessment, good planning and full cooperation between the anesthesiologist and the surgeon.

Deciding on the technique of intubation

Many different methods are available to pass an endotracheal tube in patients either awake or asleep. The choice of technique depends very much on the skill and experience of the anesthesiologist and the route of intubation required for the operation. However, some methods are more suited than others to overcome the problems associated with the particular problems of access, visualization or the target. Each anesthesiologist should master at least two alternative methods to address each of the three problems. This in turn implies that the methods chosen

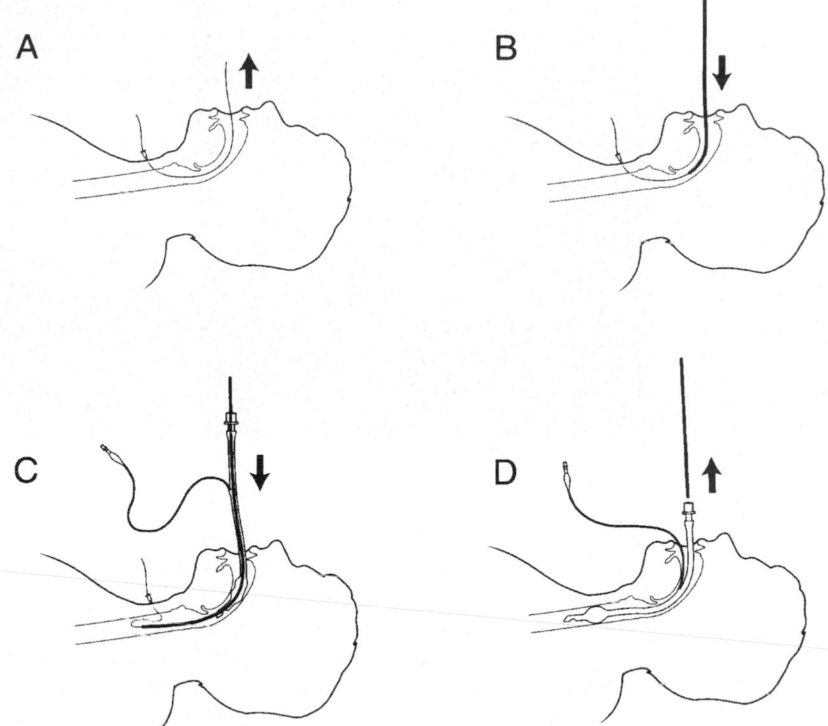

Figure 15.7 *Retrograde intubation. This illustration shows the principle of the technique using a proprietary retrograde intubation kit. (a) A soft wire is introduced via a cricothyroid needle puncture of the trachea, after instillation of local anesthetic, and passed gently cephalad until the end can be retrieved through the mouth. (b) A hollow tube guide is threaded over the wire which guides it into the trachea. (c) The guide is pushed below the point of insertion of the wire, and an endotracheal tube is 'railroaded' over the guide into the trachea. (d) The wire is then cut at the point of insertion, to prevent contamination of the airway, and the guide and the wire are withdrawn from the airway.*

should allow ethical practice on normal patients, so that facility is gained before they are needed in earnest.

The following is a list of selected techniques which are considered to meet these criteria; each may be used in some circumstances in both the asleep and the awake patient. The list is not exhaustive and the mention of these techniques does not imply their superiority over techniques that are not mentioned.

Problems of access

- Nasal access only available: *blind nasal or fiberoptic-guided nasal intubation.* Blind techniques require a stiff tube, which can be guided by manipulation from above. A guided technique requires a soft tube, which more easily follows the contour of the guide. The size of the tube is dictated by the size of the nasal passage, not the size of the glottis.
- No nasal access and limited oral access: *retrograde oral intubation over a cricothyrotomy guide* (Fig 15.7). Proprietary kits are available. This technique is particularly useful for reconstructive cases following burns or trauma to the face and neck where scarring with deformity is the problem rather than airway patency. This is the one technique that cannot be justified in normal patients for practice. On the other hand, problems of access should always be diagnosed preoperatively, allowing a controlled timely procedure rather than rapid execution.

Problems of visualization

- Grade III or IV laryngoscopy[6] or floppy epiglottis: *anesthetic straight-blade laryngoscope with tube guide.* A basic technique to overcome the shortcomings of a standard Macintosh laryngoscope. The tube guide is passed in the midline into the glottis, blindly if necessary. Usually the tracheal rings can be felt with the guide as it passes down the trachea. A tube is then 'railroaded' over the guide.
- Grade III or IV laryngoscopy with an incompressible tongue base: *light-wand intubation* (Fig 15.8). A simple technique that requires practice but is easily mastered. It is not only of value for difficult airways, but is also useful for routine intubations where the state of the patient's dentition is poor, or where extensive (and expensive) dental restoration work is present. The largest instrument to pass between the teeth with this technique is the tube, and that is soft!

Problems with the target

- The obscured glottis: *standard laryngoscope of choice with a tube guide used as a probe* (Fig 15.9). This is the situation where the rough position of the glottis is known but the entrance can only be found by gentle probing. Once found, a tube can be 'railroaded' over the probe.
- The deformed or constricted larynx: *rigid pediatric ventilating bronchoscope.* This is for the situation where some

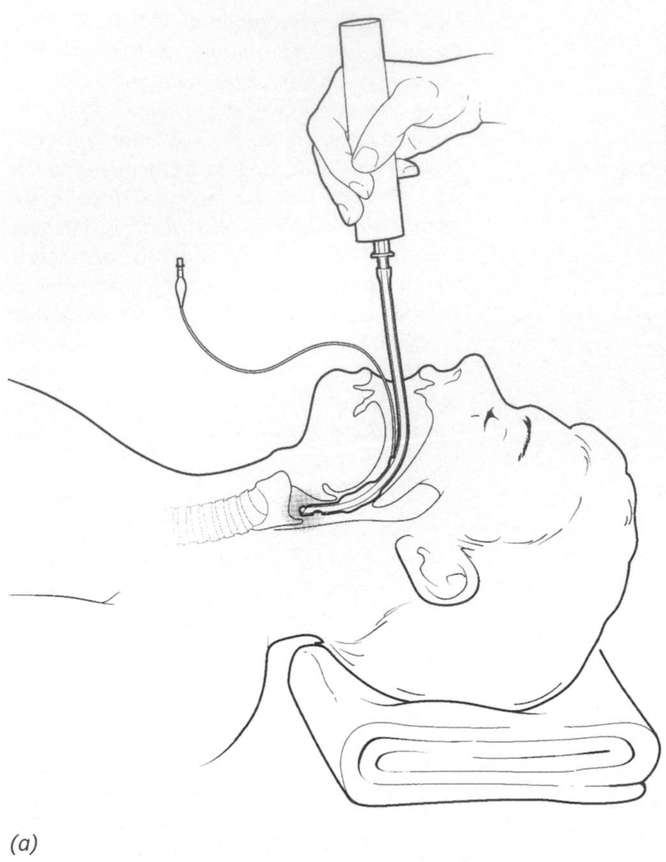

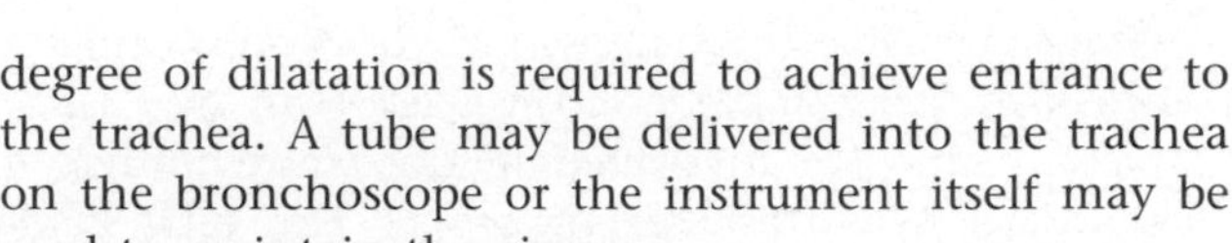

(a)

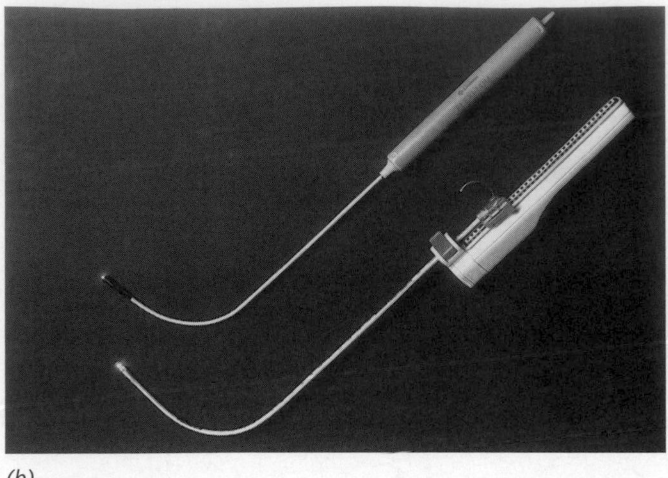

(b)

Figure 15.8 *Light-wand intubation. Illustration (a) shows the light wand in use. The tube is placed over the wand, which is then introduced to the midline hypopharynx with the patient in the standard 'sniffing position'. The wand is then manipulated until a 'flare' of light down the trachea is seen transilluminating the neck. The tube is then slid off the wand into the trachea. Illustration (b) shows two examples of proprietary light wands. The upper wand (Flexilum™) is cheap and robust but its use requires the tube to be cut to length, so is better suited to planned use with standard tubes. The lower wand (Trachlight™) is more expensive but it permits the rapid use of uncut or preformed tubes by virtue of its adjustable wand section.*

degree of dilatation is required to achieve entrance to the trachea. A tube may be delivered into the trachea on the bronchoscope or the instrument itself may be used to maintain the airway.

Fiberoptic intubation

Nasal or oral fiberoptic technique is a viable alternative for managing all three types of problems in most patients. However, it does not perform well in the presence of a significant amount of secretions, blood or pus in the airway as the view is quickly obscured. When fiberoptic intubation technique is being considered, it should be used first rather than as a secondary technique, since some degree of bleeding is not uncommon after failed attempts at intubation with other techniques.

Intermediate devices

The laryngeal mask

The laryngeal mask (Fig 15.10) is a device used in routine anesthesia when endotracheal intubation is not indicated. It has proved life saving as a temporizing measure for oxygenation while a surgical airway is secured. A variation will be available shortly that is designed to permit intubation through the mask after placement.[13]

The Combitube™

The Combitube™ (Fig 15.11) is a double-cuffed, double-lumen tube designed to isolate the esophagus from the trachea, providing a sealed airway for ventilation and a preferential channel for any regurgitated material. It is a development from the old esophageal obturator devices originally introduced for the use of paramedics in the field. It is a useful temporizing measure and is easier to place in edematous airways than the laryngeal mask.

Anesthetic techniques available for laryngeal operations

There are four main groups of anesthetic techniques, all of which may be suitable for operations on the larynx in different situations.

Topical anesthesia

Topical anesthesia is used mainly for endotracheal intubation and diagnostic or therapeutic endoscopy, particularly where patient cooperation is required as with Teflon injection of the vocal cords. Attention to total drug dosage is important, as is the careful selection of patients who will tolerate the experience. The secret of consistent success is to take sufficient time at each step to allow full analgesia

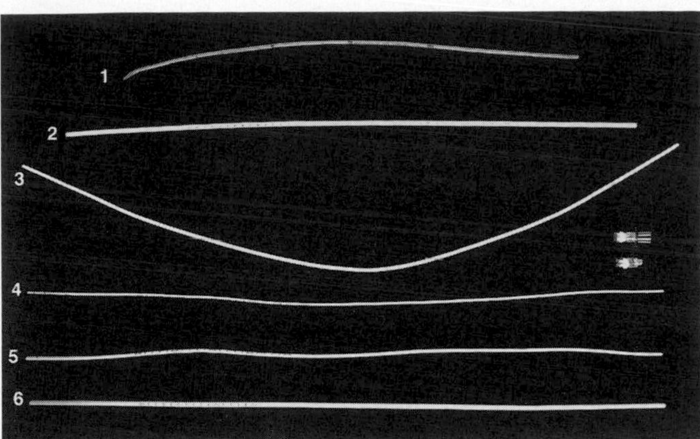

Figure 15.9 *Examples of tube guides. 1, The gum-elastic bougie with its 'ski-tip' to the left is a long-established aid to intubation. 2, The original hollow 'Tube-changer™', first introduced for managing tube changes in the ICU environment. 3, A home-made device comprising a solid Teflon rod in different diameters developed for use with double-lumen tubes and laser tubes. 4,5,6, Examples of the different diameters of 'Cook airway exchange catheters™' that are now available for use even in pediatric situations. The catheters are hollow and, by use of the attachments illustrated on the right of the picture, may be used for both low-pressure gas insufflation and jet ventilation in situations other than just tube changes.*

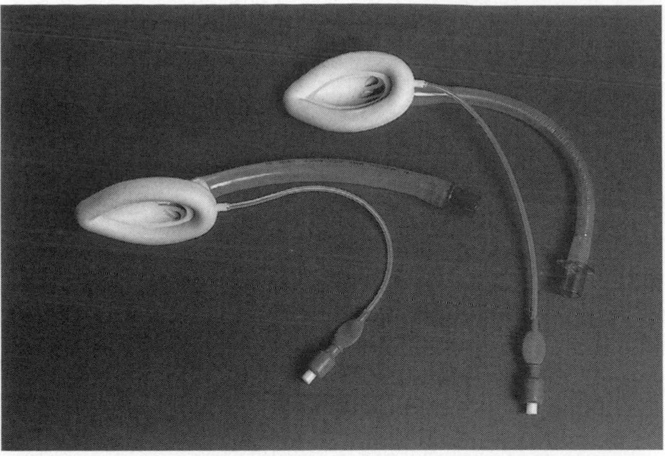

Figure 15.10 *Laryngeal masks. Two examples illustrating the design of the laryngeal mask. The cuff is inflated in the hypopharynx so the lumen is held over the laryngeal inlet. The mask below is the original design for routine use when intubation is not indicated, but has proved life saving with failed intubations. The upper mask is a more recent refinement, with a flexible armored tube extension more suited to head and neck surgery.*

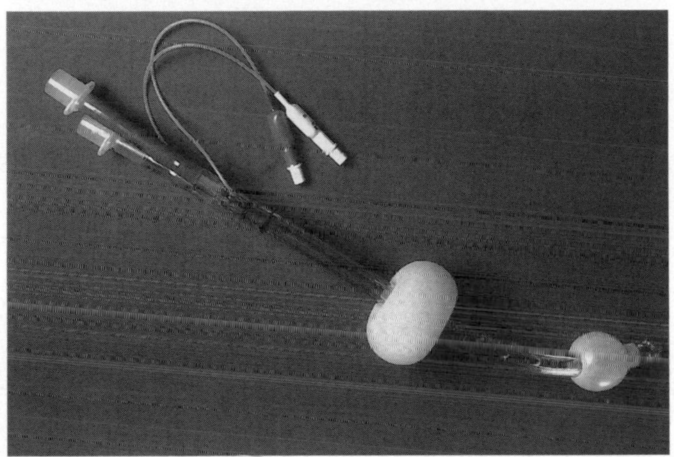

Figure 15.11 *The Combitube™. This device is a double-lumen tube with two cuffs. It is placed with its tip in the esophagus and the lower small cuff is inflated. The upper larger cuff is then inflated behind the base of the tongue. One tube lumen passes through the lower cuff and provides a route for regurgitation; the other lumen ends blindly above the lower cuff but has side holes between the two cuffs that permit ventilation through the second lumen by virtue of the cuff seals above and below the hypopharynx.*

to develop. An important contribution to success is a dry airway mucosal lining, to permit optimum contact with the local anesthetic drug. This is best achieved with an individually titrated dose of an antisialagogue to the point where the patient is actually dry, rather than stopping at an arbitrary dosage which is not fully effective. This may require a dose of atropine, for example, in excess of 2 mg in some adults. If tachycardia is of concern in a 'cardiac' patient, scopolamine may prove a more appropriate choice. The details of the technique were described earlier in relation to examination of the difficult airway. However, in patients with a normal airway the whole process will be more comfortable with sedative premedication.

Cocaine, an alkaloid of *Erythroxylon coca*, is still a popular agent for topical anesthesia, particularly for the topical preparation of the nose, as it is the only local anesthetic with vasoconstrictor properties. Its analgesia precedes the vasoconstrictor effects by approximately 5 minutes and may last as long as 90 minutes without reapplication. It is absorbed from mucosal surfaces and, if applied to the pyriform fossae, blood levels equivalent to an intravenous injection are quickly achieved. Peak levels are usually reached within the first hour and first-order kinetics are followed with a serum half-life of 60–80 minutes. Most of the absorbed drug is metabolized by hydrolysis by plasma pseudocholinesterase. Cocaine inhibits the reuptake of endogenous norepinephrine, and blocks the uptake of exogenous epinephrine, suggesting the reason for cocaine's ability to sensitize various end organs to catecholamine effects. It is recommended that no greater than a 4% solution be used with the maximum safe dose in an adult being 3 mg/kg. Although severe toxic reactions have been reported with a total dose as low as 20 mg in adults, the usual fatal dose is approximately 1 g cocaine.[9] Cocaine toxicity is manifest by a diphasic reaction in the central nervous system: first excitement, then depression with convulsions and unconsciousness. Respiratory and cardiovascular signs will be evident and death can occur rapidly without treatment. The best protection is to avoid toxic doses but if treatment is required, intravenous injections of thiobarbiturates or benzodiazepines, together with labetalol to block both α- and β-adrenergic responses, are usually rapidly effective.

Infiltration anesthesia

Infiltration anesthesia, with or without *monitored anesthesia care* for sedation and/or resuscitation by the anesthesiologist, is most commonly used in our context for tracheotomy or for operations on the body of the larynx itself, such as thyroplasty. The surgeon is solely responsible for the use and dosage of whatever local anesthetic agent is selected and should ensure that the safe total dose, with or without epinephrine, is not exceeded.[22] However, the anesthesiologist should nevertheless keep a running check on the cumulative doses that have been given. Care should be exercised in selecting patients to ensure that the procedure as planned can be completed in the time made available by the technique and the patient can tolerate the experience. The safety of the technique depends on not exceeding safe drug dosages and frequent aspiration during injection with a constantly moving needle to minimize the risk of inadvertent intravenous injection. This is not a second-best technique to get away with surgery on inadequately prepared patients already rejected for general anesthesia. Therefore, the anesthesiologist should be fully aware of what is to be attempted.

Conduction anesthesia

Conduction anesthesia is the technique whereby a local anesthetic agent is introduced via a needle to the immediate proximity of a specific nerve, series of nerves, or a nerve trunk in order to produce analgesia over the sensory distribution. The technique is used infrequently and, in the context of the larynx, is used primarily for supplementing topical anesthesia, or in its own right to achieve anesthesia of the larynx before endoscopy. The commonly used blocks have been described earlier. There are two fundamental disadvantages to conduction blockade. The duration of surgical analgesia depends upon the accuracy of the initial injection, the properties of the drug and the concentration injected. Therefore, if the surgical procedure takes longer than anticipated and the block wears off, general anesthesia with its concomitant risks usually has to be superimposed. The other major drawback is the time required for the block to be executed and for analgesia to develop. It is because of the relative inflexibility of the 'one-shot' technique that these blocks are not used more frequently.

General anesthesia

In spite of the availability of a rapidly increasing variety and number of anesthetic drugs, general anesthetic techniques can still be divided into two basic categories: single-agent techniques and balanced techniques. The fundamental difference between the two categories lies in the use of muscle relaxants to diminish or abolish muscle tone in balanced anesthesia.

A single agent may be an inhaled agent or a drug given by injection, depending on circumstances. The use of a single agent without muscle relaxants does not preclude the full control of ventilation if required. A single agent can achieve all three properties of the general anesthetic triad: narcosis, relaxation, and reflex suppression. However, profound degrees of muscle relaxation are achieved only by relative overdose of the drug compared with that required for adequate narcosis or reflex suppression. This means that the maintenance of the circulation becomes more difficult with greater degrees of muscle relaxation. The problem is overcome with muscle relaxant drugs. However, these drugs mandate full control of the patient's ventilation, converting the normal negative intrathoracic pressure to positive, with the associated implication for venous pressure and surgical field blood

Table 15.1 Comparison of the two basic techniques of general anesthesia

Single-agent technique	*Balanced technique*
Simple: reduces number of potential adverse reactions to drugs	Complex: more drugs, more potential adverse reactions
Control of circulation more difficult: patient usually requires fluid loading	Can be tailored to maintain the circulation more easily
Cardiac dysrhythmia with exogenous catecholamines more common	Can be tailored to minimize catecholamine dysrhythmias
Nerve stimulator use unaffected	Response to nerve stimulator abolished or diminished
Suited to initial management of some difficult airways	Contraindicated for the initial management of most difficult airways
Awareness during anesthesia extremely rare	Awareness may occur
Muscle relaxant reversal not required	Muscle relaxant reversal required; may be incomplete and 'recurarization' can occur postoperatively
Involves use of halogenated hydrocarbon agents	Volatile agents can be excluded with hepatitis or hyperthermia risk
Anesthetic effects completely reversible as long as patient is breathing with a clear airway	Clearance of intravenous drugs depends primarily on liver and renal excretion, which may be impaired

oozing. With single-agent anesthesia, spontaneous breathing through a mask or tracheal tube can be maintained, albeit with some intermittent support of ventilation during the longer surgical procedures to minimize peripheral lung atelectasis. However, even with spontaneous breathing, the problem with oozing in the surgical field is not completely overcome, as the anesthetized respiratory center requires a higher driving tension of carbon dioxide than normal (5.9–7.2 kPa versus 5.0–5.5 kPa), and hypercapnia leads to increased oozing in its own right. Since many of the operations on the larynx require a secure airway, an endotracheal tube is indicated for most procedures no matter which type of technique is to be used, so the choice of preferred technique, in the absence of specific patient medical problems, is reduced to the consideration of a few general advantages and disadvantages in different surgical situations. The list in Table 15.1 is not exhaustive as a specific medical condition may favor the choice of a technique different from that which might have been chosen for a generally healthy patient undergoing the same surgical procedure. The use of muscle relaxants is further governed by the possible need for nerve stimulator use or sensory evoked potentials during the operation. If a nerve stimulator is to be used, then muscle relaxants are contraindicated, but if evoked potentials are desired, muscle relaxants may be required in order to block background muscle noise from interfering with the measurements.

One of the problems faced by the anesthesiologist is the use of vasoconstrictors by the surgeon when the patient is anesthetized with a volatile anesthetic. It has long been recognized that the halogenated volatile anesthetics 'sensitize' the myocardium to catecholamine-induced cardiac dysrhythmias with the possible risk of ventricular fibrillation and circulatory arrest. Sensitization of the myocardium is defined as a state in which the dose of epinephrine required to produce an arrhythmia is less than the dose in the awake state when the myocardium is free of drug effects.[8] Halothane has a far greater sensitizing effect than the other commonly used agents. Johnston and colleagues measured the dose of epinephrine that produces ventricular arrhythmia in 50% of patients (ED50) at 1.25 MAC with a $Paco_2$ controlled at 3.9–5.3 kPa. They found the arrhythmogenic ED50 for halothane at 2.1 mg/kg, the ED50 for isoflurane at 6.7 mg/kg and the ED50 for enflurane at 10.9 mg/kg.[11] Children, however, seem to be much less susceptible to sensitization for reasons that are still unclear.[14] The clinical implications of this work are not as obvious as they might seem because many factors can modify the degree of sensitization observed. Joas and Stevens demonstrated that deepening anesthesia in dogs raises the arrhythmogenic threshold as did the use of lidocaine/epinephrine mixtures.[10] The role of $Paco_2$ is not clear. Joas and Stevens[10] observed an increased threshold with hypocapnia whereas Katz and Katz describe the opposite.[15] However, the latter authors have made three suggestions for clinical precautions that have stood the test of time:

- Only solutions of epinephrine of 1 in 100 000 to 1 in 200 000 should be used, as greater concentrations offer little additional vasoconstriction.[22]
- The dose in adults should not exceed 10 ml of 1 in 100 000 epinephrine in any 10 minute period.
- The dose in adults should not exceed 30 ml of 1 in 100 000 epinephrine in any given 60 minute period.

Microsurgery of the larynx

When a laryngologist has declined to operate on a conscious patient, several methods are available for the management of general anesthesia. The major problem is the difficulty of securing the airway and guarding against contamination because of the close proximity of surgical activity. If a small standard cuffed endotracheal tube is used, normal inhalation techniques are feasible. However, the surgeon's access to the structures of the larynx is restricted, which may be unacceptable if work is to be done on or near the posterior commissure, where the tube comes to lie naturally. If laryngeal polyps or papillomata are the reason for surgery, difficulty in working around the tube may be insurmountable, and some consider the risk of passing a standard tube through such a glottis in the first place to be unacceptable.

An alternative is the use of Venturi jet ventilation as part of a balanced technique. Jet ventilation may be achieved by using a rigid injector (Fig 15.12) above or protruding below the glottis attached to the laryngoscope or by using the cuffed Carden tube (Fig 15.13) placed below the larynx independent of the laryngoscope. Each is attached to a high-pressure gas source, either oxygen or a nitrous oxide/oxygen mixture from a high-pressure blender, and intermittent pulses of gas are used to inflate the patient's lungs by means of a manual or automatic pneumatic switch (Fig 15.14) under full muscle relaxation. The high-pressure gas stream in theory entrains room air from the pharynx. In practice, entrainment is slight if the injector orifice is below the cords, and when a nitrous oxide/oxygen mixture is used, anesthetic tensions can be achieved. The patient must be fully paralyzed to facilitate ventilation, and the surgeon must ensure a clear expiratory pathway at all times to prevent pressure injury to the lungs. Intravenous adjuvants are used to ensure an adequate depth of anesthesia as standard vaporizers cannot be used in high-pressure systems.

The rigid injector used in modifications of the Toronto ventilating laryngoscope improves access in comparison with a standard endotracheal tube, but is still inflexible. The advantage of the Carden tube is that only the small cuff inflation tube and the jet tube protrude above the larynx (Fig 15.15), and since both are made of soft flexible material, the surgeon can lift them out of the way if necessary. With Venturi jet techniques, when the injector orifice is above the cords, the surgeon must remember the risks of blowing blood and particulate matter into the unprotected tracheobronchial tree.

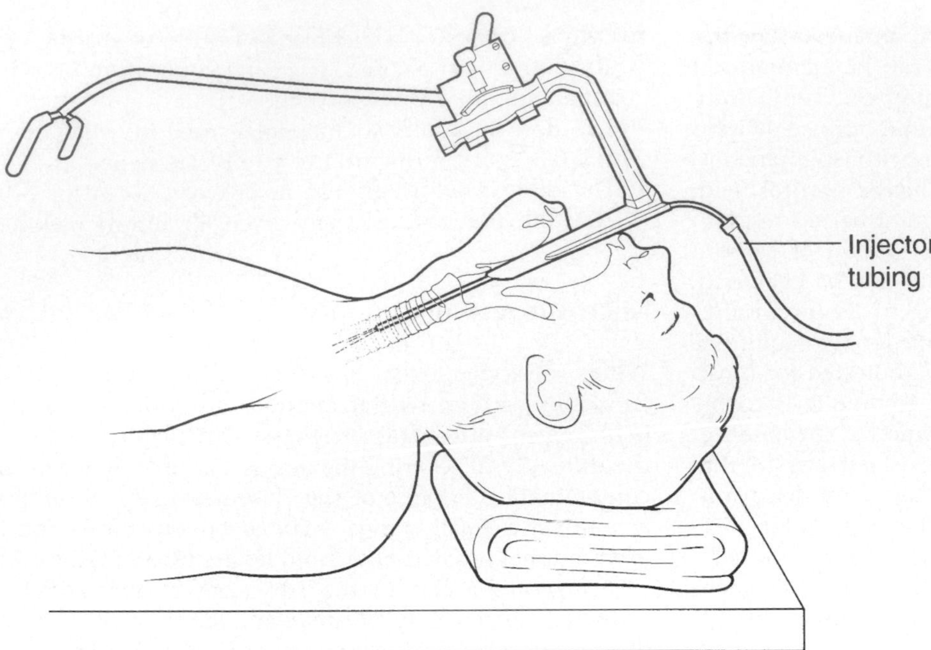

Figure 15.12 *Jet ventilation with rigid injector. The use of a rigid metal injector with a suspension laryngoscope for Venturi jet ventilation is illustrated. The surgeon places the injector below the cords and aligns it with the axis of the trachea. The suspension arm should NOT be placed on the patient's chest, as this will interfere seriously with ventilation. The same principles apply if the surgeon's preference is to use a shoulder role for positioning.*

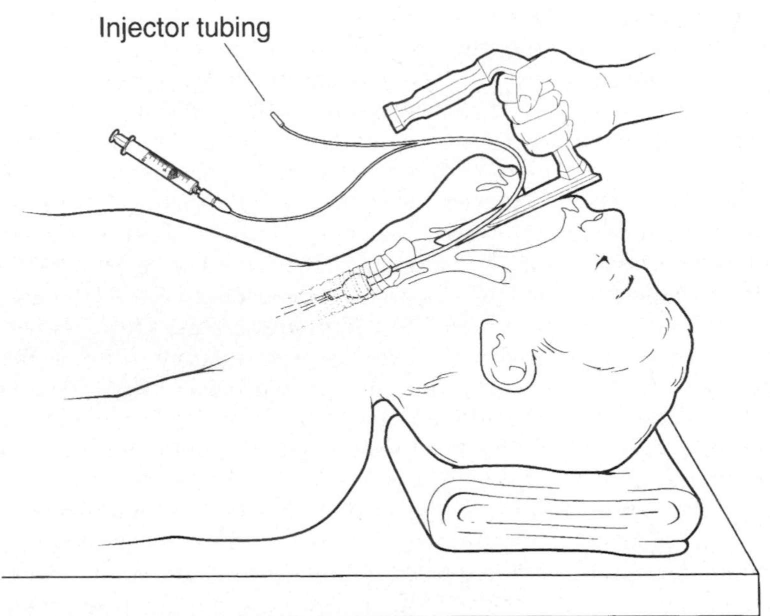

Figure 15.13 *Jet ventilation with the Carden tube. The Carden tube's cuffed section is placed below the vocal folds (medium biopsy forceps work well) and the cuff is inflated to hold it in position. Its use permits the surgeon better access to the posterior third of the cords and the posterior commissure. It also allows some flexibility to move the laryngoscope, but a view of the glottis must be maintained at all times while jet ventilation is in progress to ensure an expiratory pathway.*

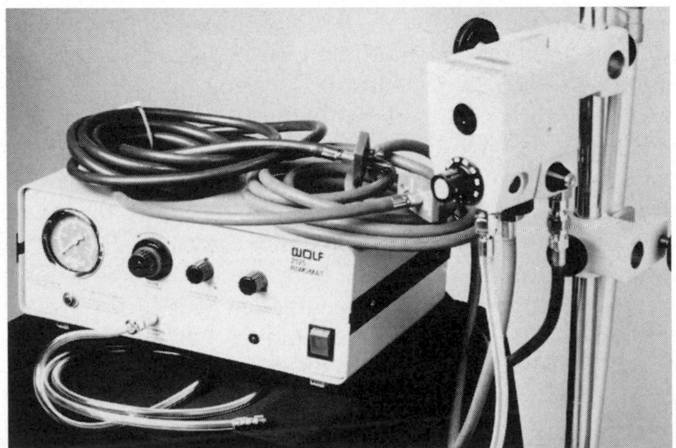

Figure 15.14 *Jet ventilation equipment. The illustration shows equipment setup for automatic jet ventilation. To the right is a Bird high-pressure nitrous oxide/oxygen blender feeding a Wolf Injectomat™ on the left. The Injectomat is connected to the patient injector, via the tube on the front panel, and permits the setting of inflation pressure, frequency and the inspiration/expiration time ratio required for automatic ventilation.*

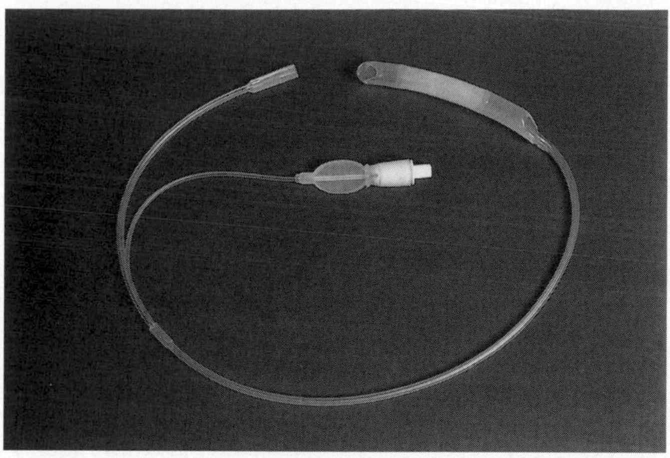

Figure 15.15 *The Carden tube. The Carden tube is a jet-ventilation device in a range of sizes made of a soft flexible material. The cuffed section, which is placed completely below the vocal folds, is seen to the upper right of the picture. The cuff inflation tube with its white valve and pilot balloon is seen towards the center of the picture. The injector tube is seen on the left. Only the two small flexible tubes come to lie between the vocal folds, and they are easily moved out of the way by the surgeon.*

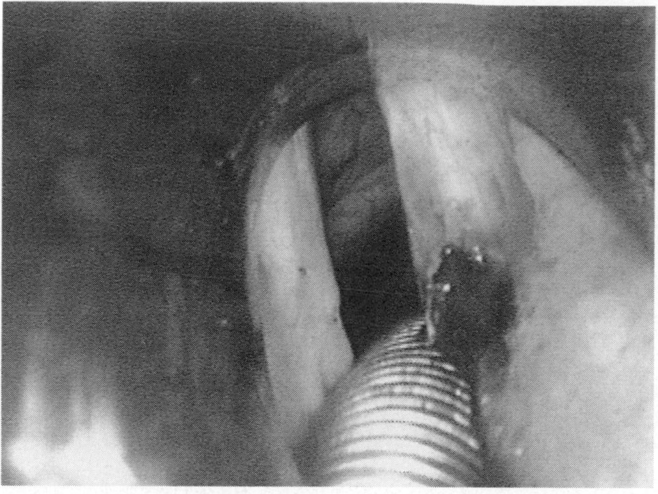

Figure 15.16 *Surgical access with a laser tube. The cuffed laser tube comes to lie naturally in the posterior commissure, obstructing access to the posterior third of the glottis. This picture illustrates the tube position clearly, following the removal of a tumor on the middle third of the right vocal fold.*

Laser surgery

The laser (the word is an acronym for *light amplification by stimulated emission of radiation*) is finding an increasing number of applications as a tool for surgery. The laser of particular interest in laryngeal surgery is the carbon dioxide laser. The requirements for anesthetic management may be summarized:

- complete patient immobility to ensure that normal tissue is not hit accidentally;
- unencumbered surgical access to and visualization of the target area;
- protection of the patient from stray laser radiation or reflection;
- protection of the airway against blood and the products of vaporization;
- removal of smoke and debris; and
- prevention of airway fires.

Applications in the airway have already established the laser as an important treatment modality. The need for absolute immobility demands the use of muscle relaxants and hence general anesthesia. The choice of methods for ventilation and maintaining the airway depend on the site of the target lesion. The carbon dioxide laser is used with an operating microscope for susceptible lesions in the larynx and access for the surgeon is difficult. Two methods of ventilation are available: use of a small cuffed endotracheal *laser tube* or, if that restricts access to the lesion (Fig 15.16), Venturi ventilation with the orifice of a *metal injector* sited below the glottis and attached to the laryngoscope (Fig 15.12). The positioning of the injector below the target minimizes the risk of blowing blood into the lungs, and the expired gases are very effective in removing smoke. However, the relaxed vocal cords 'balloon' with ventilation, necessitating synchronization of any surgical activity on the cords with the ventilatory cycle so as not to have to hit a moving target.

The use of an endotracheal tube introduces the risk of intratracheal fires. Early efforts to minimize this risk involved wrapping standard tubes with dampened muslin or metallic tape to disperse or reflect the aberrant laser strike. This approach was not particularly successful because tubes still ignited. Energy would be transferred from the laser beam to the tube in the form of heat, and once the flashpoint for the material constituting the tube was reached, ignition occurred. The subsequent fire was fed by the anesthetic carrier gases, creating a reasonable facsimile of a blowtorch within the trachea. Different tube materials and coatings have been tried to minimize this risk, but it now seems clear that the silicone-coated metal tube (Fig 15.17) is the instrument of choice for ventilation. The risk of cuff ignition is minimized by inflation with 1% aqueous lidocaine rather than air, so that if the cuff ignites and ruptures, the escaping liquid will tend to quench the fire and minimize any local tissue burn reaction. The metal spiral is designed to distribute heat away from the laser impact point. Unlike earlier all-metal tubes,[19] the silicone-coated metal tubes are gas tight but have a very small lumen relative to external diameter which can lead to ventilation pressure problems as well as limiting the choice of method for placement with a difficult airway.

For palliative procedures to relieve neoplastic obstruction of the trachea and larynx, when getting below the laser target is not possible, Venturi ventilation with a

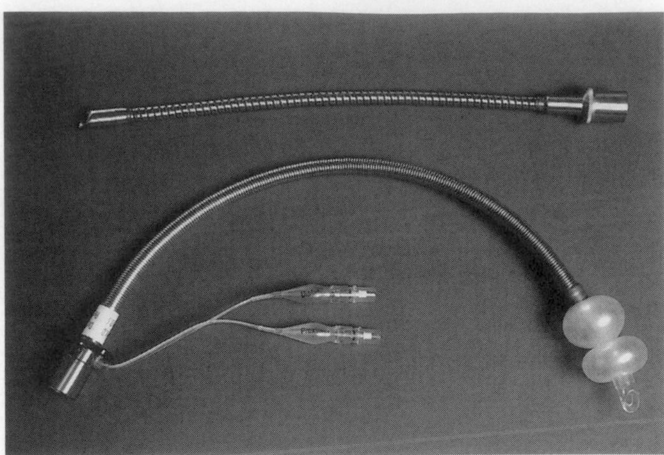

Figure 15.17 *Examples of laser tubes. The picture shows above, one of the original metal spiral uncuffed laser tubes, and below, a Laserflex™ metal spiral reinforced, double-cuffed, silicon laser tube, which has overcome many of the drawbacks of the former. The proximal cuff is inflated with saline or lidocaine solution, rather than air, while the distal cuff is kept in reserve to deal with a laser strike on the proximal cuff.*

Sanders Venturi ventilation attachment secured to a laryngoscope or a rigid bronchoscope is an alternative approach. If the patient already has a tracheostomy, the tube should be exchanged for a laser tube or a *metal tracheostomy tube* that is suitably protected.

Additional general precautions are required for the conduct of laser surgery. Care should be exercised to ensure that the patient is electrically grounded. The patient's eyes should be protected with wet eye patches secured with canvas tape (plastic tapes should be avoided as they can melt into the skin!). The immediate area surrounding the operative site should be draped with wet linen towels. Instrumentation should have stippled surfaces to minimize the risk of coherent beam reflection. All personnel in the operating room should wear protective eyeglasses with side guards appropriate to the laser.

If in spite of precautions taken, a laser fire still occurs, all personnel should be informed immediately and the following actions taken:

- the flow of anesthetic gases should be cut off;
- the endotracheal tube should be removed; and
- the laser discontinued.

The fire should be quenched with water held in readiness on the instrument table for such an eventuality. The patient should be reintubated immediately and then standard therapeutic and respiratory support measures for severe airway burns should be instituted.

General endoscopy

The topical techniques discussed earlier for intubating the larynx in the awake patient are equally suited to laryngoscopy and bronchoscopy although less so for esophagoscopy, because of patient discomfort. Therefore it only remains to add here a few points that can facilitate the technique. When the procedure is to be undertaken electively, starving the patient is a wise precaution because his or her protective airway reflexes will be obtunded. Light premedication with a benzodiazepine or barbiturate will facilitate the procedure if not contraindicated by an airway already compromised by disease. When the surgeon's practice requires large planned endoscopy clinics, the services of an anesthesiologist in preparing the second and subsequent patients, while the surgeon is working, speeds matters considerably.

When the use of a topical technique is inappropriate, the following methods for management under general anesthesia are available.

Laryngoscopy

As far as the anesthesiologist is concerned, laryngoscopy involves two types of surgical technique, suspension and manual. When the laryngoscope is suspended and manipulation kept to a minimum, Venturi ventilation with or without a Carden tube may be used, since it gives the surgeon the best possible access. The patient must be fully paralyzed, and maximum driving pressures must be monitored with care. The surgeon should place the axis of the injector parallel to the axis of the trachea to avoid a pneumatic cut in the mucosa and must ensure a clear expiratory pathway at all times to avoid barotrauma to the lungs. Anesthesia may be induced intravenously in the usual way, but anesthesia and relaxation are maintained with intravenous agents, since standard vaporizers cannot be used in high-pressure systems.

Should a manual laryngoscopic technique be used for diagnostic work, particularly when the surgeon is exploring the hypopharyngeal area, Venturi ventilation should not be used, because intermittent interruption of the expiratory pathway occurs too frequently. If biopsies are being taken when the larynx is not in view continuously, the additional risk of blood contaminating the tracheobronchial tree has to be recognized. In this situation, a small cuffed endotracheal tube is a better choice for securing the airway, with anesthesia being maintained by means of inhaled vapors or a balanced technique.

Bronchoscopy

Bronchoscopy allows four main variations in technique:

- The rigid ventilating bronchoscope allows maintenance of anesthesia with an anesthetic vapor through a side arm with a 15 mm connector, which permits attachment to and ventilation with standard anesthetic circuits. Surgeons derive some protection from anesthetic gases by using a glass eyepiece, but it must be firmly attached during positive-pressure ventilation, otherwise it can blow off into the surgeon's face! An

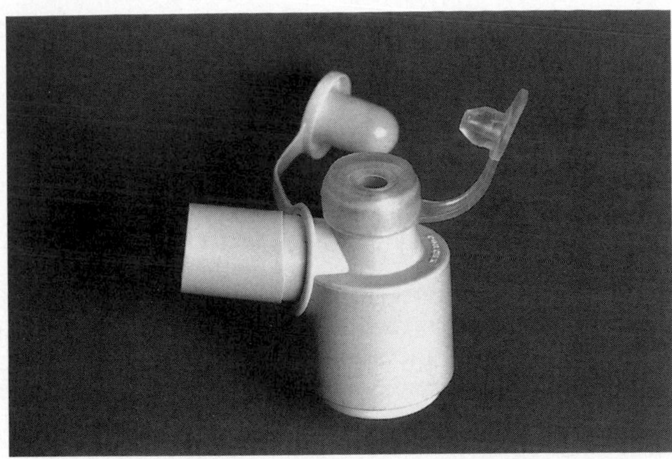

Figure 15.18 *Swiveltrach™ connector. The connector, of the type illustrated, connected to an endotracheal tube, permits uninterrupted ventilation with standard equipment attached to the side arm on the left during fiberoptic endoscopy through the tube. The fiberoptic bundle is passed through the perforated diaphragm, visible on top, which gives a sufficient gas seal. However, resistance to ventilation may be increased significantly.*

alternative is to use a Sanders Venturi attachment and proceed with a balanced intravenous technique and jet ventilation.

- Fiberoptic bronchoscopy permits the passage of the instrument through the lumen of a standard endotracheal tube. This allows the airway to be secured against aspiration at all times while permitting standard anesthetic maintenance techniques. The connection between the circuit and tube is made with a right-angled swivel connector with a perforated rubber diaphragm that permits access for the bundle while maintaining a gas-tight seal (Fig 15.18).
- The limitation of the approach is the resistance to expiration, which is determined by the cross-sectional area of the instrument relative to the area of the lumen of the tube. Anatomy dictates the size of the tube lumen, but the size of the bundle is a matter of technology. The ability to manufacture ever-smaller fiberoptic bundles with satisfactory optical properties is improving rapidly, and now the technique may be considered even in small children.
- Apneic oxygenation uses the principle of oxygenation by diffusion in a fully paralyzed patient. Intravenous drugs are used to maintain anesthesia. Once anesthesia is induced, profound hypocapnia is achieved with hyperventilation by mask. A small-gauge catheter is passed through the larynx to the carina under direct vision. A 1–3 l/min flow of oxygen is attached to the catheter, and the patient is presented to the surgeon. The duration of uninterrupted access is limited only by the rate of rise of endogenous carbon dioxide to significant levels, as long as the patient remains fully paralyzed. The technique works well in patients without significant pulmonary disease, but the surgeon must be sparing and careful in the use of suction through the bronchoscope.
- Deep inhalation anesthesia is another established technique; it is particularly helpful in small children. Anesthesia is induced, and the patient is allowed to breathe an anesthetic vapor in oxygen spontaneously. Any of the standard agents is suitable, but the most prolonged uninterrupted access to the airway is achieved with the highly blood-soluble, potent analgesic vapor of methoxyflurane. Anesthesia is taken to the deepest safe level. When the mask is removed, the surgeon applies topical lidocaine to the larynx and trachea and then proceeds with bronchoscopy while the patient lightens slowly, still breathing spontaneously. This technique is equally suited to rigid or flexible bronchoscopy provided an oral airway is used with the flexible instrument.

Esophagoscopy

This procedure requires the full control of the airway when performed under general anesthesia. With a large rigid esophagoscope, some difficulty may be experienced in passing the instrument past the posterior tracheal bulge of the tube cuff. Therefore the anesthesiologist should be ready to deflate the cuff transiently to assist the surgeon. As the instrument passes the arch of the aorta, an occasional patient will develop profound reflex bradycardia requiring intervention. The major risk is perforation of the esophagus, so the patient must remain immobile (deep anesthesia) with muscle relaxants if necessary. Some surgeons maintain that if the patient is breathing spontaneously, the residual muscle tone, particularly in the inferior pharyngeal constrictor, permits them to judge more accurately the amount of force that they are using to pass the instrument.

Management for supraglottic lesions

The major anesthetic considerations related to supraglottic lesions concern their bulk and friability. If the lesion is large, it may obstruct the patient's breathing and make intubation difficult. If it is friable, intubation maneuvers may result in profuse hemorrhage into the airway. The risk of bleeding increases if the lesion involves the tongue base and the vallecula. Control of the airway may require anything from standard laryngoscopy and intubation under general anesthesia, to elective tracheotomy under local infiltration anesthesia, depending on the findings at the preoperative airway evaluation. A potential trap for the unwary is the patient who has already undergone surgery and/or radiation therapy who now presents for a recurrence. With the scarring and anatomic distortion that usually follows the previous therapy, there is no assurance that the management plan that worked well for the first operation will work at all for the second! The method of maintaining anesthesia usually poses no particular problems, once intubation is achieved, and the usual choices are available, governed by the patient's general medical condition.

Management for glottic lesions

The management of glottic lesions depends primarily on the nature of the lesion and the operation that is planned. The anesthesiologist and the surgeon are competing directly for a very small space in the airway, so full cooperation is the prime requirement. Frequently the use of even a small standard endotracheal tube will block the surgeon's access to the lesion, and access requirements can also change during the course of the operation. This requires flexibility and preparation on the part of the anesthesiologist in order to facilitate the surgeon's activities. It is important that the management of such patients be discussed in detail before the operation begins, and any limitations posed by the patient's medical condition understood.

Tumor invading the glottis may render any attempt to pass an endotracheal tube dangerous due to the risk of avulsion of tissue with bleeding that is then carried down the tracheobronchial tree with the further risk of peripheral obstruction or obstruction of the lumen of the tube itself. Such a situation may require the application of low-pressure jet ventilation or deep general anesthesia with spontaneous ventilation without a tube until part of the lesion has been excised, after which a small cuffed tube may be passed to protect against bleeding during definitive resection. In severe cases an elective tracheotomy under a local anesthetic may be the safest course.

A profuse crop of papillomata can pose similar problems and in addition disguise the location of the glottis itself. This is a classic difficult airway target problem, but having successfully probed for the tracheal entrance, many consider the passage of a tube to be contraindicated by the risk of seeding papillomata further down the airway. To avoid this, a subglottic jet injector may be used as the initial probe. It is introduced gently into the trachea and ventilation is maintained initially with low-pressure jet ventilation under balanced anesthesia. As resistance to expiration is increased by the crop of papillomata, a careful watch is kept to ensure that sufficient gas is escaping from the lungs to avoid barotrauma and inflation settings are adjusted accordingly. However, as the surgeon starts to excise papillomata, this resistance progressively decreases, requiring continual adjustment of pressure settings upward, to maintain adequate ventilation.

The advent of the thyroplasty operation poses a number of interesting problems for the anesthesiologist. The operation requires a patient who is conscious and cooperative at different points during the procedure, in order to test the varying quality of the voice with fine adjustments to the implant. Since the operation is quite extensive, infiltration anesthesia of the neck alone is rarely sufficient, requiring the addition of quickly reversible sedation or general anesthesia. The presence of a cuffed endotracheal tube would negate the whole purpose of the operation, posing a dilemma for the anesthesiologist who now has an obtunded patient with an uncontrolled airway, where the damage to the patient's larynx, necessitating the operation, is frequently related to chronic gastric reflux! Anesthesiologists have spent most of their training learning how to avoid getting into just this situation!

The answer to the dilemma is not yet clear. In the author's institution several techniques have been tried to satisfy surgical requirements while minimizing the very real anesthetic risks. The need for a quickly reversible sedation or general anesthesia has been well satisfied by a single-agent intravenous technique utilizing a continuous infusion of propofol. The absence of a controlled airway has been addressed with the usual precautions of preoperative starvation and premedication with an H2-blocker which diminishes acid production, metoclopramide which stimulates gastric motility and emptying, and an antacid preparation to raise intragastric pH. We have gone one step further in that with the known risk of reflux, it seemed important to know if and when reflux actually occurred intraoperatively. The patient is prepared with an antisialagogue and a 'swish and swallow' topical technique and a fiberoptic nasopharyngoscope is then placed via the nose to maintain continuous surveillance of the larynx throughout the procedure on a video screen. If reflux occurs in spite of these precautions and the patient's slight reverse Trendelenburg position on the table, the anesthesiologist can then intervene to suction the pharynx. Previously, we passed the nasopharyngoscope through a laryngeal mask, which worked well. However, during some of the operations, an apparently progressive glottic edema was noted to develop, which was attributed to the increased inspiratory resistance caused by the fiberoptic bundle inside the laryngeal mask, so the laryngeal mask was abandoned. Since then, without any airway device in place, several patients have also developed a similar, visible but less severe, progressive glottic edema, which suggests that the cause may also be related to surgical manipulation and interference with venous or lymphatic drainage from the area.

Management for tracheotomy

Tracheotomy has many indications whether it be part of a major operation such as laryngectomy or in isolation for prolonged endotracheal intubation. Tracheotomy done for any reason is usually best managed with a cuffed endotracheal tube already in place to control and protect the airway irrespective of whether the patient is awake or asleep. The anesthetic problems with the procedure usually occur at the point of incising the trachea. The cuff of the endotracheal tube frequently lies below the point of incision and is vulnerable to incision with the wall of the trachea. If the cuff is damaged, controlled ventilation becomes difficult and it can no longer afford any protection to the patient in the event of technical difficulties and bleeding into the airway during the remainder of the procedure. The tube itself is flammable and carries an oxygen-containing atmosphere, usually enriched, so is therefore at risk for ignition by diathermy. This risk is sometimes forgotten and fires have resulted, but the problem is easily avoided by achieving hemostasis before the wall of the trachea is incised with a knife. To protect the tube cuff for later use, a series of tube position changes is recommended as illustrated in (Fig 15.19).

Management for subglottic lesions

Deciding the management for subglottic lesions is heavily dependent on preoperative examination and radiologic studies. If the patient can breathe adequately when awake, it is likely that control of the airway under anesthesia will produce adequate ventilation as well. If the patient already has severe dyspnea, there is no guarantee that an artificial airway of sufficient size to improve the situation can be created quickly from above the larynx. In the latter situation an elective tracheotomy under a local anesthetic is indicated.

Separating these two groups of patients is an uncertain business heavily dependent on clinical judgment. The basis of the problem is airway narrowing due either to external compression or intrinsic stenosis in the subglottic area or further down the trachea. Narrowing may take the form of an orifice or a segment. First, the precise position and extent of narrowing must be determined. Next, the nature of the narrowing must be defined, whether it is fixed or varies with respiration. Finally, the maximum diameter of the lumen in the narrowed area *and whether it is straight or tortuous* must be estimated as this defines the limit of what may be passed through it.

If the patient is severely dyspneic with a small fixed orifice (<4 mm) or has a narrowed segment with a small tortuous lumen, an elective awake tracheotomy is a wise precaution. In patients with a less severe condition, a number of methods can be used to maintain oxygenation after induction of anesthesia. The method chosen may be only temporarily effective provided the surgeon is sure that he can immediately improve gas dynamics with his intervention. Patients with severe dyspnea are usually badly fatigued by the time they arrive for operation and the inhalation induction of anesthesia will abolish spontaneous respiration before an adequate depth of anesthesia is achieved. Those patients without severe dyspnea usually tolerate an inhalation induction well and in fact their condition may be considerably improved when the respiratory efforts engendered by anxiety are suppressed by anesthesia. The gentle manual support of ventilation will also help in overcoming the resistance to inspiration.

Once anesthetized, oxygenation and anesthesia have to be maintained, preferably with spontaneous respiration, until a satisfactory airway has been created. If the lumen diameter is fixed, this can be achieved for varying lengths of time simply by insufflating a mixture of anesthetic

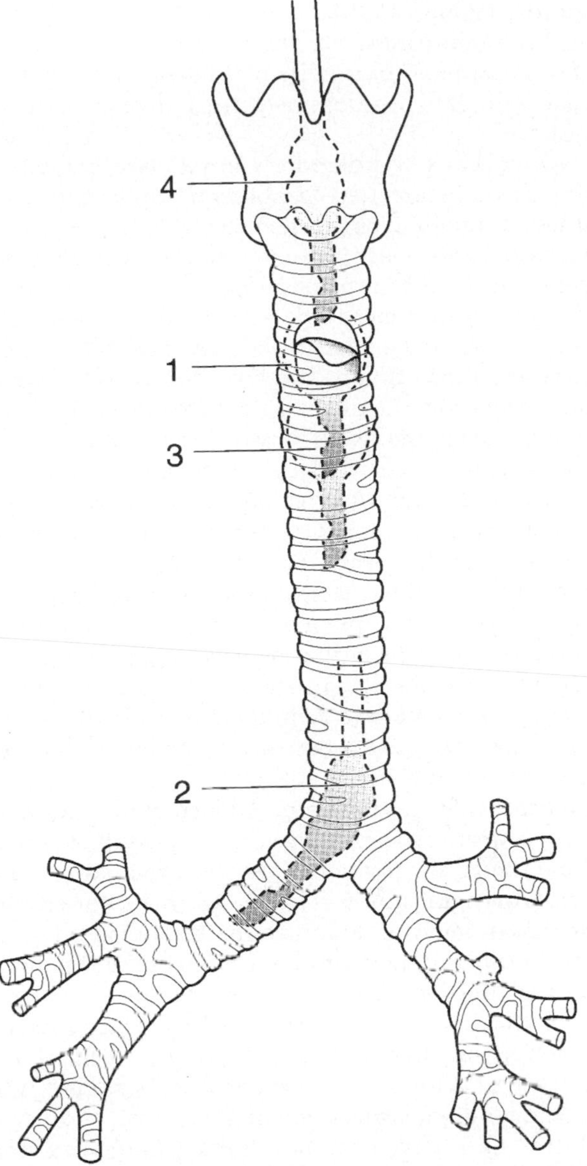

Figure 15.19 *Airway control technique for tracheotomy. An endotracheal tube tends to lie with its cuff below the point of tracheal incision for tracheotomy (position 1). To avoid losing the cuff early in the operation, when the surgeon is ready to incise the trachea, the cuff is deflated and the tube is advanced as far down the trachea as possible (position 2). After the window is created, the tube is drawn back up the trachea and the cuff reinflated at the lower border of the window (position 3), sealing the airway against contamination, permitting normal ventilation and preventing blood spraying from the window. Once the window is fully fashioned and the surgeon is ready to place the tracheostomy tube, the cuff is deflated and the endotracheal tube is withdrawn slowly, under the direction of the surgeon, until the tip is level with the upper border of the window (position 4). The tracheostomy tube is then placed and tested, but the endotracheal tube is not removed from position 4 until after undraping the patient and the final tying of the tracheostomy tube tapes, so that the endotracheal tube is still available if an accident befalls the tracheostomy tube.*

vapor in oxygen through a long catheter with its tip near the carina, taking care that intrathoracic pressure is not allowed to rise progressively due to inadequate gas escape around the catheter in the narrowed area. The technique is made smoother if lidocaine is first instilled into the trachea.

If spontaneous ventilation cannot be maintained, careful low-pressure jet ventilation under balanced anesthesia through a long, fine injector with its tip below the narrowed area is an alternative, albeit a dangerous one as there is high risk for barotrauma.

If the lumen diameter is variable, there is a reasonable chance that it may be dilated either by passage of a small standard endotracheal tube (try both cuffed and uncuffed for each size) or by the use of a rigid ventilating bronchoscope. This technique is also usually successful in those rare cases of true tracheomalacia. Sometimes an unusually long tube is required in order to get below the area of narrowing. Although standard tubes may not have the length, a nasal RAE tube passed through the mouth usually suffices. If the area of narrowing is well down the trachea, and as long as there is 4–5 cm available between the vocal folds and the beginning of the narrowing, a tube may be passed with enough room to inflate the cuff to maintain positive pressure ventilation, without the lumen of the tube becoming obstructed by the abnormal anatomy.

The insufflation technique mentioned above, although very old, is worth remembering as it has proved life saving in some unusual situations. As an example, in two patients a laryngeal stint was lost down the trachea during the process of removal. Both became firmly lodged at the carina, obstructing the right main bronchus and partially obstructing the left after an initial attempt at retrieval failed. A small suction catheter was then passed rapidly into the left main bronchus through the tracheostomy and oxygen at 2 l/min was insufflated. This bought sufficient time for different instruments to be made ready and the stint to be retrieved without the $Sa\text{O}_2$ in either patient falling below 90%. Both patients recovered without incident.

A final variation on this theme, which goes contrary to what has been recommended so far, is the management of those unfortunate patients with abnormal storage diseases such as mucopolysaccharidosis and amyloidosis. If deposition occurs in the trachea, the narrowed segment may involve the whole length of the trachea with a narrow tortuous lumen throughout. In such patients even awake tracheotomy may not be viable, as the lumen in the trachea is not easy to identify. If such a patient presents as an emergency, the best course is to pass a rigid ventilating bronchoscope under general anesthesia down to the carina or where normal rings can be identified and use this as a marker for effecting a rapid surgical airway while ventilation is maintained. In an elective situation one should remember the alternative of veno–veno bypass oxygenation, which is rarely available in time for an airway emergency.

Management for trauma to the larynx

Trauma to the larynx may be thermal, chemical or physical. All three sources are usually associated with airway edema and respiratory embarrassment. When first seen, if dyspnea is not evident but significant trauma is suspected, the patient should be intubated anyway, in anticipation of later deterioration when intubation may be more difficult. The one exception to this is where laryngeal fractures are suspected in association with physical trauma. In these patients there may also exist a disruption of the continuity of the larynx with the trachea. Here standard laryngoscopy and intubation may result in ventilating the tissues of the neck and mediastinum, resulting in severe subcutaneous emphysema and a technically impossible tracheotomy. These patients are best managed with an awake tracheotomy in the first instance, but if severe hypoxia requires immediate action, it is better to establish an airway from above the larynx with a rigid ventilating bronchoscope and avoid any attempt at ventilation until after the rings of the trachea have been identified with certainty. The airway may then be controlled with the bronchoscope while a tracheotomy is completed in a less hurried fashion.

Management of the postoperative airway

Patients recovering from general anesthesia traverse the stages of anesthesia in reverse and must be watched closely throughout the process. If the patient is still in the third stage, without an endotracheal tube, laryngeal mask or tracheostomy, continued airway support is needed. As the second stage is traversed, muscle tone progressively returns and the patient becomes irritable and salivates, which can lead to coughing and swallowing. External stimulation should be kept to a minimum to avoid the risk of laryngospasm or vomiting (which are not mutually exclusive). The effects of the continued accumulation of secretions, blood or pus in the airway may be minimized by facilitating drainage from the pharynx by placing the patient in the 'tonsil position' for recovery (Fig 15.20). In the first stage the patient is able to be roused but in a state of analgesia. However, some time may elapse before normal mental faculties and spatial and temporal orientation are regained. It is during this period that the perception of postoperative pain first intrudes.

All forms of anesthesia potentially reduce cardiac output and peripheral vascular resistance. This leads to increased ventilation/perfusion mismatch in the lungs and a reduced $Pa\text{O}_2$. Therefore, all postoperative patients must have their $Sa\text{O}_2$ monitored and be supported with supplemental oxygen administered by mask (nasal prongs are not reliable without $Pa\text{O}_2$ determination), giving an inspired oxygen concentration of at least 30–35% until consciousness returns. This is equally true for patients who are still intubated and being ventilated. All patients benefit from humidification of the inspired gas, particularly those with an irritable airway. Patients who have had

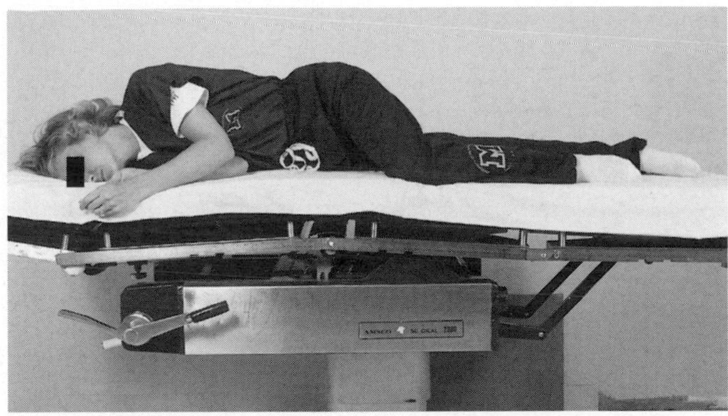

Figure 15.20 *Right tonsil position. It should be noted that there is no support under the head, thereby inclining the neck downwards. This position facilitates the drainage of pharyngeal contents away from the larynx and out of the dependent mouth. The position is maintained by flexing the upper hip and knee and both arms. The right tonsil position is illustrated, as this can facilitate emergency laryngoscopy, for those who hold the instrument in their left hand.*

operations on the larynx and associated structures may be assumed to have an irritable airway.

Postoperative supraglottic edema

Extensive instrumentation of the airway by either the surgeon or the anesthesiologist will frequently lead to supraglottic edema postoperatively. Surgical interference with the normal lymphatic drainage of the upper airway can also contribute to this condition, as will large volumes of intravenous crystalloid given by the anesthesiologist during the course of the procedure. The condition is usually manifest by the onset of dyspnea and signs of obstruction in the postanesthesia recovery unit. If the patient has not fully recovered from general anesthesia, the first signs of trouble may be the appearance of patient irritability and restlessness. It is best to reintubate the patient as soon as the condition is suspected, as the passage of time will make intubation more and more difficult. The diagnosis, once suspected, may be confirmed by rapid fiberoptic endoscopy of the hypopharynx, which can usually be achieved without a full topical anesthesia preparation. Once the diagnosis has been confirmed, if the degree of edema is not so advanced as to obscure laryngeal landmarks, intubation should be undertaken using standard anesthetic laryngoscopy following preoxygenation and a general anesthetic intravenous induction. However, if the degree of edema is already severe, laryngoscopy with an anesthetic laryngoscope is usually unsuccessful, as the edematous tissue tends to flow in over the flange of the laryngoscope, preventing visualization of the glottis. As such a situation constitutes an emergency, immediate preparation should be made to establish a surgical airway below the larynx. However, if the patient shows no sign of desaturation, the use of an anterior commissure laryngoscope may enable intubation from above. In this situation, the laryngoscope is placed with reference to the externally palpated position of the larynx and once the glottis is visualized down the axis of the cylinder of the instrument, a tube guide may be passed into the trachea. The instrument is then withdrawn over the tube guide and an endotracheal tube, usually one full size smaller than that originally used for the operation, is then railroaded over the tube guide into the trachea and the airway is secured. Obviously, in the presence of this degree of supraglottic edema with obstruction, the ability to implement this technique depends on the immediate availability of the instrumentation required.

Extubation protocol for the difficult airway

If a difficult intubation has been encountered at induction of anesthesia, it is usual to transfer the patient from the operating room with the endotracheal tube in place if a tracheotomy is not already present. The patient is allowed to awaken fully before any consideration is given to removing the tube. If the patient fights the tube during second-stage emergence, it must not be removed but rather the patient sedated and his vital signs controlled as appropriate. Once the patient is fully conscious and oriented, and the anesthesiologist is satisfied with the adequacy of the patient's spontaneous ventilation, a standard protocol for extubation should be followed.

If reintubation is required and fails, what is the emergency management plan?

- Prepare equipment for reintubation, including an endotracheal tube one full size smaller.
- Suction tracheal and pharyngeal secretions if necessary and preoxygenate the patient.
- Instil 4 ml of 2% lidocaine down the endotracheal tube into the patient's trachea.
- Deflate the tube cuff and 'stop' the tube (obstruct the lumen with thumb) to see if the patient can breathe around the tube.

If the patient can breathe around the tube:

- Pass a tube guide (e.g. Teflon guide, Cook catheter or gum elastic bougie) through the tube into the trachea (Fig 15.21).
- Withdraw the tube over the guide leaving the guide in place.
- Secure the guide through an oxygen mask and observe the patient for developing obstruction.

Patients will tolerate the presence of a guide for extended periods and can talk around it (Fig 15.22). If there is no evidence of developing obstruction it is usually safe to remove the guide after 30 minutes. However, if there is any suggestion of deterioration in the function of the patient's airway, the guide is used to immediately 'railroad' a new tube of similar size or smaller back into the trachea. *If the patient cannot breathe around the original tube when 'stopped', airway obstruction after extubation is more likely so the patient's surgeon should be consulted before*

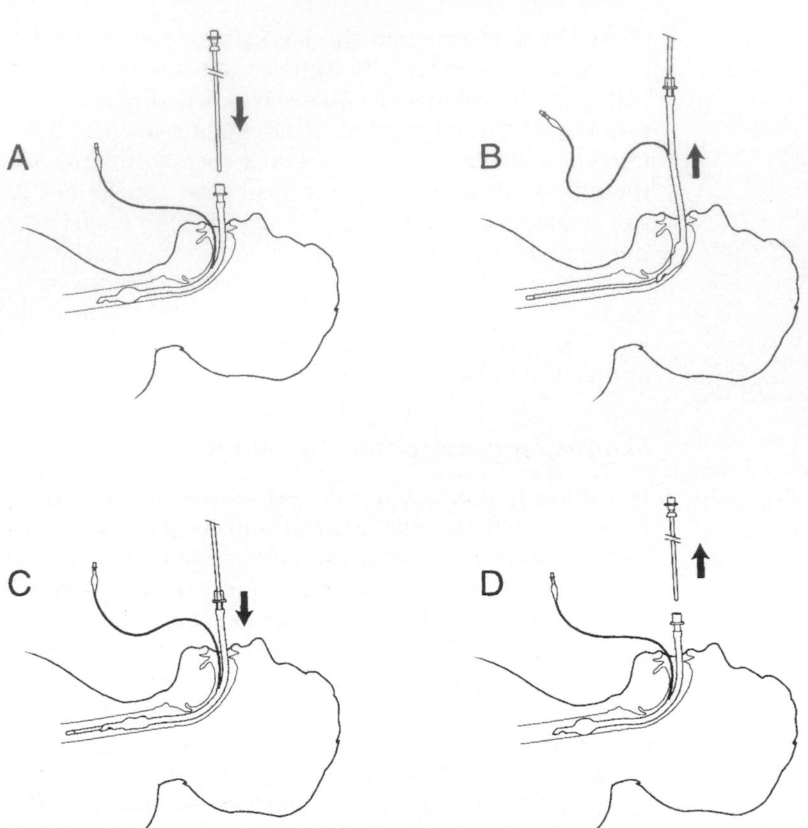

Figure 15.21 *Technique for tube guide use in extubation protocol. The choice of a hollow tube guide permits the insufflation of oxygen during the following maneuvers. (a) After preparation of the patient, the tube guide is inserted into the original endotracheal tube, so that its tip protrudes a centimeter beyond its bevel in the trachea. (b) The tube is then withdrawn over the guide, leaving the guide in place, ensuring that the guide's extent of insertion relative to the teeth is not changed. The patient is then observed for a period with the guide taped in place. (c) If spontaneous ventilation deteriorates and reintubation is necessary, a new tube is 'railroaded' over the guide into the trachea. If the new tube will not pass the larynx, the guide permits the continuation of oxygenation by insufflation until a smaller tube can be placed. (d) Once the patient is safely reintubated the guide is removed and the tube secured.*

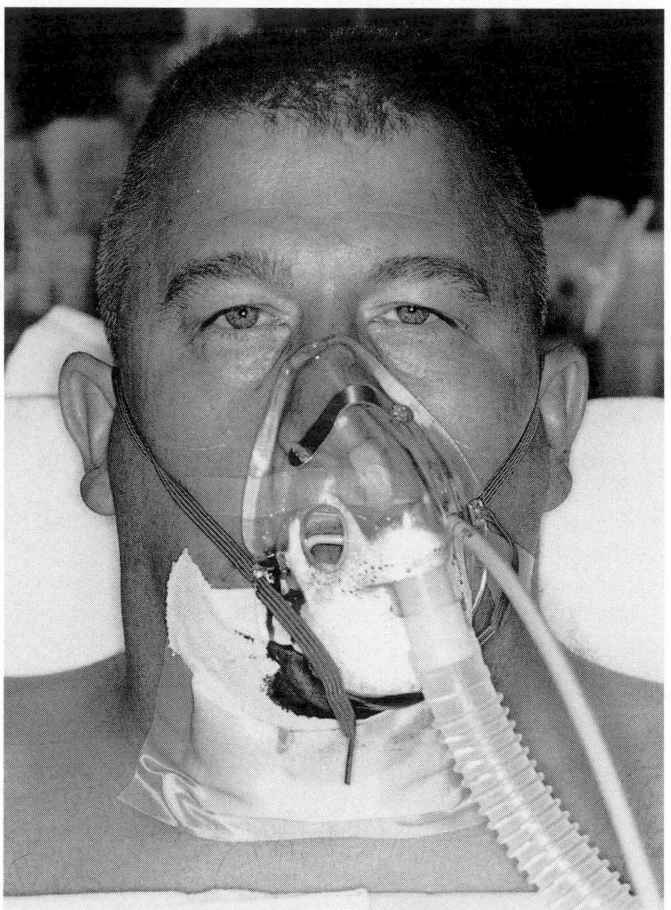

Figure 15.22 *Well tolerated by the patient! A patient, with severe airway edema associated with extensive cellulitis of the anterior neck and floor of mouth, undergoing trial of extubation per protocol. The patient is awake, comfortable and talking with tube guide in place. Supplementary humidified oxygen is being delivered via mask rather than the guide (Cook airway exchange catheter in this case).*

proceeding further. The surgeon may wish to be present during extubation attempts or may decide to return the patient to the operating room for an elective tracheotomy with the existing endotracheal tube in place.

These precautions are no protection against the occasional late airway obstruction that does occur. If the patient has been a difficult intubation, this fact should always be communicated to the postoperative ward medical and nursing staff and clearly noted on the patient's chart, whether the patient is transferred intubated or extubated. It is hoped that this knowledge will prevent any ill-considered inappropriate intervention in the event of an airway emergency on the ward!

References

1. Benumof JL. Lidocaine to topically anesthetize the mucosal lining of the airway. *Anesthesiology* 1997; **87:** 1598–9.

2. Brown ACD. Anesthetic management. In: Norton ML, Brown ACD, eds. *Atlas of the Difficult Airway.* St Louis: Mosby Year Book, 1991: 169–98.
3. Caplan RA, Posner KL, Cheney FW. Adverse respiratory events in anesthesia: a closed claims analysis. *Anesthesiology* 1990; **72:** 828–33.
4. Chew JY, Cantrell RW. Tracheostomy complications and their management. *Arch Otolaryngol* 1972; **95:** 538–45.
5. Cobley M, Vaughan RS. Recognition and management of difficult airway problems. *Br J Anaesth* 1992; **68:** 90–7.
6. Cormack RS, Lehane J. Difficult tracheal intubation in obstetrics. *Anaesthesia* 1984; **39:** 1105–11.
7. Fink BR, Demarest RJ. *Laryngeal Biomechanics.* Cambridge: Harvard University Press, 1978: 1–13.
8. Gallo JA. Catecholamine anesthetic interaction in ENT surgery. In: Brown BR, ed. *Anesthesia and ENT Surgery.* Philadelphia: FA Davis Company, 1987: 7–30.
9. Gay GR, Inaba DS, Rappolt RT Sr, Gushue GF Jr, Perkner JJ. 'An' ho, ho, baby, take a whiff on me.' La dama blanca cocaine in current perspective. *Anesth Analg* 1976; **55:** 582–7.
10. Joas TA, Stevens WC. Comparison of arrhythmic doses of epinephrine during Forane, halothane and fluroxene anesthesia in dogs. *Anesthesiology* 1971; **35:** 48–53.
11. Johnston RR, Eger EI II, Wilson C. A comparative interaction of epinephrine with enflurane, isoflurane and halothane in man. *Anesth Analg* 1976; **55:** 709–12.
12. Kambic V, Radsel Z. Intubation lesions of the larynx. *Br J Anaesth* 1978; **50:** 587–90.
13. Kapila A, Addy EV, Verghese C, Brain AI. The intubating laryngeal mask airway: an initial assessment of performance. *Br J Anaesth* 1997; **79:** 710–13.
14. Karl HW, Swedlow DB, Lee KW, Downes JJ. Epinephrine–halothane interactions in children. *Anesthesiology* 1983; **58:** 142–5.
15. Katz RL, Katz GJ. Surgical infiltration of pressor drugs and their interaction with volatile anaesthetics. *Br J Anaesth* 1966; **38:** 712–18.
16. Latto IP. Management of difficult intubation. In: Latto IP, Rosen M, eds. *Difficulties in Tracheal Intubation.* Eastbourne: Baillière Tindall, 1985: 99–141.
17. Londy F, Norton ML. Radiologic techniques for evaluation and management of the difficult airway. In: Norton ML, Brown ACD, eds. *Atlas of the Difficult Airway.* St Louis: Mosby Year Book, 1991: 55–66.
18. Mallampati SR, Gatt SP, Gugino LD *et al.* A clinical sign to predict difficult tracheal intubation: a prospective study. *Can Anaesth Soc J* 1985; **32:** 429–34.
19. Norton ML, de Vos P. A new endotracheal tube for laser surgery of the larynx. *Ann Otol* 1978; **87:** 554–7.
20. Putnam L, Jenicek JA, Allen CR, Wilson RD. Anesthesia in the morbidly obese patient. *South Med J* 1974; **67:** 1411–17.
21. Samsoon GLT, Young JRB. Difficult tracheal intubation: a retrospective study. *Anaesthesia* 1987; **42:** 487–90.
22. Scott DB, Jebson PJ, Ortengren B, Frisch P. Factors affecting plasma levels of lignocaine and prilocaine. *Br J Anaesth* 1972; **44:** 1040–9.
23. Sellick BA. Cricoid pressure to prevent regurgitation of gastric contents during induction of anaesthesia. *Lancet* 1961; **2:** 404–5.
24. Stauffer JL, Olson DE, Petty TL. Complications and consequences of endotracheal intubation and tracheostomy. A prospective study of 150 critically ill adult patients. *Am J Med* 1981; **70:** 65–76.
25. Wraight WA, Chamney AR, Howells TH. The determination of an effective cricoid pressure. *Anaesthesia* 1983; **38:** 461–6.

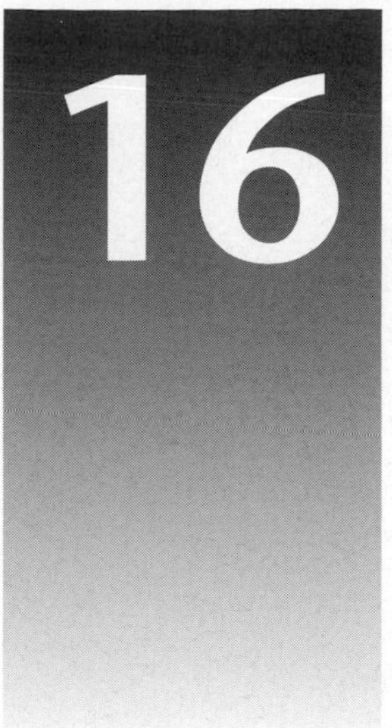

16 Congenital anomalies of the larynx

Trevor J McGill

Congenital laryngeal anomalies are important causes of respiratory distress in the neonate or infant. Clinicians managing these patients should have an organized approach to diagnosis and management. The diagnostic approach should focus on the distinction between the self-limited lesions and conditions that are life threatening.

Comparison of the infant and adult larynx

Several factors distinguish the infant larynx from the adult larynx and may contribute to diagnostic difficulties. The infant larynx lies higher in the neck just under the posterior one third of the tongue, and the inferior aspect of the cricoid lamina descends during childhood from the level of C-4 to the level of C-6. The infant epiglottis projects into the oropharynx, and its shape may vary considerably (Fig 16.1). The infantile epiglottis is longer and narrower and more tubular. This omega-shaped epiglottis is seen often in laryngomalacia but is not a pathognomonic feature. The thyroid cartilage overrides the cricoid such that the cricothyroid membrane is thus only a slit. The operation of cricothyrotomy is not feasible in the infant.

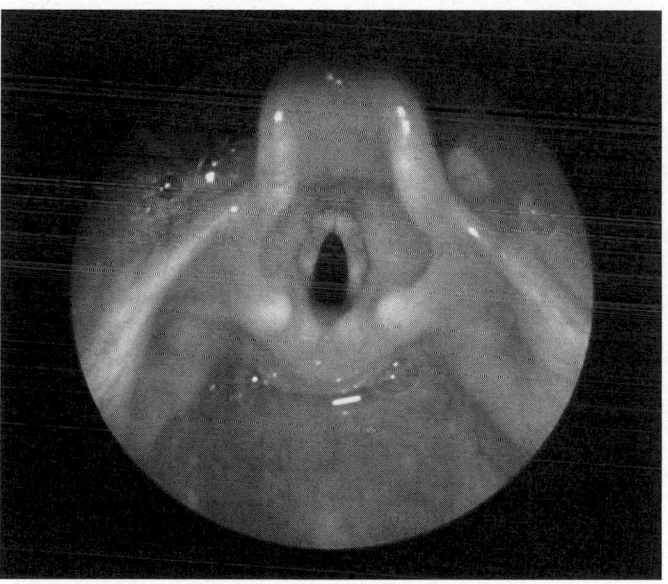

Figure 16.1 *The normal infant larynx.*

Stridor

The cardinal sign of laryngeal obstruction is stridor. Most laryngeal lesions present with some form of stridor, defined as noisy breathing produced by turbulent airflow through an obstructed airway. Most laryngeal lesions cause inspiratory obstruction due to the negative pressure produced by the turbulent airflow and its effect on the soft tissues of the larynx. Intrathoracic lesions cause obstruction that is worse in the expiratory phase and improved during inspiration because inspiration causes a widening of the airway due to the effects of thoracic excursion. These factors allow the site of obstruction to be localized according to the pattern of the presenting stridor. Inspiratory stridor usually indicates supraglottic obstruction, biphasic stridor suggests obstruction at the level of the vocal cords or subglottis, and expiratory stridor suggests a tracheal or pulmonary lesion. Other associated signs and symptoms include hoarseness (glottic web, vocal cord paralysis), feeding difficulties (laryngomalacia, vocal cord paralysis, and laryngeal cleft), cough, apnea and other signs of respiratory compromise including cyanosis, nasal flaring, and chest retractions.

The evaluation of any child with a suspected congenital laryngeal lesion depends on a thorough analysis of the nature of the stridor, including its quality and timing, positional change, and association with feeding or crying. Additionally, one must be aware of the multiplicity of lesions that may cause airway obstruction in children in order to expedite a rapid yet thorough evaluation of the child with upper airway obstruction.

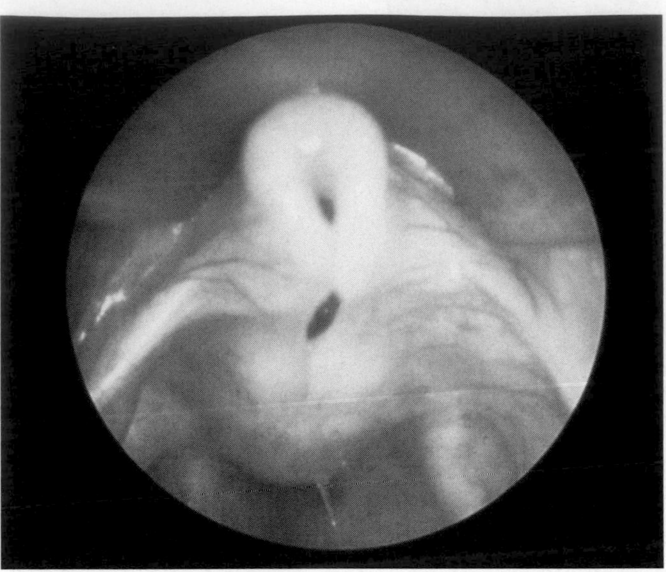

Figure 16.2 *Laryngomalacia: on inspiration the hypermobile arytenoids and the aryepiglottic folds are sucked into the supraglottic area. The posterior edges of the epiglottis coming together are contributing to inspiratory obstruction and stridor.*

Laryngomalacia

The characteristic feature of laryngomalacia is the intermittent low-pitched crowing inspiratory stridor which is due to abnormal flaccidity and collapse of the supraglottic structures caused by the inspiratory tide of air. The inspiratory stridor is not present at birth but usually presents within the first 4 weeks of life. This crowing inspiratory stridor may change with positioning, being worse while supine and relief while prone. The stridor is worse when the infant is excited or feeding.

The cause of laryngomalacia is not known, although most theories suggest either an intrinsic abnormality in the supraglottic larynx or hypotonicity of the airway. Three abnormalities in the supraglottis have been described in laryngomalacia:

- an omega-shaped epiglottis;
- short aryepiglottic folds; and
- redundant bulky arytenoids.

Because these findings can be seen in normal neonates, a cause and effect relationship has not been well established. Similarly, intrinsic weakness of the cartilages has been described in laryngomalacia; however, comparative studies have shown no histologic difference between the cartilages of children with laryngomalacia and normal children.

Other studies have shown a relationship between laryngomalacia and neurologic disease, suggesting that laryngomalacia may be part of a generalized hypotonicity that manifests with inspiratory collapse due to weakness of the muscular support of the laryngeal cartilages. In a review of laryngomalacia, Grundfast found that children with laryngomalacia had associated neurologic findings, including gastroesophageal reflux, hypothermia, obstructive and central apnea and failure to thrive.[20] Most likely, laryngomalacia is due to both localized cartilaginous weakness and hypotonicity. Gastroesophageal reflux has been implicated in the pathophysiology of laryngomalacia; however, it is unclear whether they are merely associated findings as part of a generalized dysfunction or whether reflux itself worsens the obstruction seen in laryngomalacia.

The diagnosis of laryngomalacia must be made only by direct endoscopic examination of the dynamic movements of the larynx. If the stridor is purely inspiratory and not severe, a flexible fiberoptic examination of the supraglottic larynx may be sufficient to confirm the diagnosis. Radiographic studies of the lower airway and esophagus should also be performed to avoid missing a coexistent lesion. Children with more severe stridor or with the suggestion of a coexistent lesion on radiographic studies should undergo microlaryngoscopy and rigid bronchoscopy under general anesthesia. Whether direct laryngoscopy or flexible laryngoscopy is performed, the typical finding is that of collapse of the supraglottic structures on inspiration (Figs 16.2, 16.3). The epiglottis may be tubular or omega-shaped, but these findings alone do not confirm the diagnosis and may indeed be seen in neonates without stridor.

The majority of children with laryngomalacia improve by 12–18 months; thus watchful waiting is the treatment of choice. Holinger, in a review of 650 patients with laryngomalacia, found that only two required surgical intervention because of significant respiratory distress during feeding and the need for hospitalization.[28] Other studies have shown the incidence of severe laryngomalacia to be 5–22%.[15,17,31] These children have associated feeding diffi-

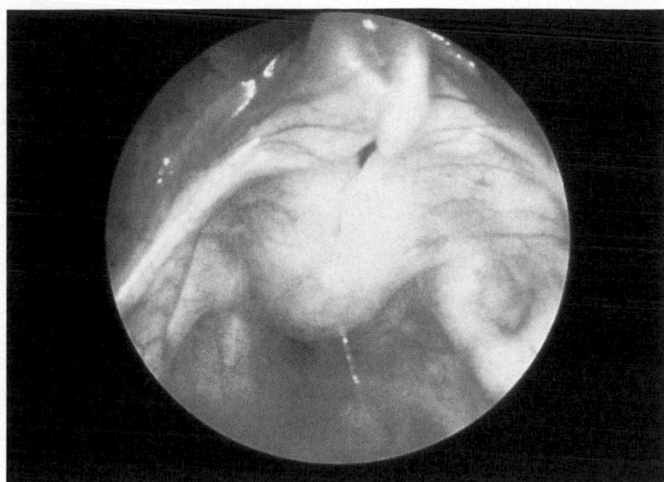

Figure 16.3 *Laryngomalacia: almost complete laryngeal obstruction caused by collapse of the supraglottic structures at the end of inspiration.*

culties, respiratory compromise, apnea, or cor pulmonale and are candidates for surgical intervention.

Most cases of laryngomalacia can be managed with simple observation and reassurance. If the infant shows progressive stridor associated with minimal feeding difficulties, home monitoring may be helpful to reassure the parents. When there are cases where laryngomalacia is associated with progressive respiratory distress, cyanosis and failure to thrive, surgical intervention may be necessary. The operation of choice is a surgical division of the taut aryepiglottic folds preferably with a carbon dioxide laser.[29,30,34,38] This procedure must be carefully indicated since the majority of children with laryngomalacia will have spontaneous resolution of their airway compromise.

Vocal cord paralysis

Vocal cord paralysis (VCP) is the second most common congenital anomaly of the infant larynx and may be unilateral or bilateral.

Vocal cord paralysis can result from a lesion anywhere along the vagus nerve, from nucleus ambiguous to the neuromuscular junction of the larynx.

Causes include central nervous system lesions, birth trauma, surgery, idiopathic paralysis and other less common conditions. Neoplasm is a rare cause of VCP in newborns.

Cohen *et al.*[8] reviewed 100 cases of children with VCP and found that the vast majority presented within 4 weeks of birth. Birth trauma and Arnold–Chiari malformation were the most common causes; however, 36% of cases were thought to be idiopathic. Children with extensive CNS disease, such as cerebral dysgenesis, and those with birth trauma presented within the first week of life. Those with meningomyelocele and Arnold–Chiari presented later at a mean of 47 days.

Arnold–Chiari malformation is the most common cause of bilateral VCP in newborns. The precise cause of VCP in Arnold–Chiari malformation is unknown. The Arnold–Chiari malformation is seen in 90% of children with meningomyelocele and is characterized by caudal displacement of the cerebellum or brainstem into the foramen magnum.[3] This displacement is due to either a primary brain dysfunction or intrauterine hydrocephalus and results in hydrocephalus due to brainstem compression at the fourth ventricle with resultant collection of cerebrospinal fluid.[33] VCP in children with Arnold–Chiari malformation may be due to stretching of vagal nerve rootlets, altered vascular supply to the brainstem, dysplastic changes in the vagal nuclei, or a lack of afferent input from carotid bodies.[20] Once the diagnosis of Arnold–Chiari malformation is made, prompt neurosurgical correction of the elevated intracranial pressure usually results in improvement of the VCP. The return of stridor in a patient with a VP shunt is often an indication of shunt malfunction and the need for revision. Arnold–Chiari syndrome may be associated with other respiratory complications, including abnormal ventilatory drive, apnea and swallowing difficulties, all of which may contribute to aspiration and the necessity for airway control. In addition to Arnold–Chiari syndrome, any neurologic disorder with associated hydrocephalus may be associated with VCP, and thus VCP must be considered in any child with a known neurologic disorder who develops stridor.[4]

Birth trauma has been cited as a cause in approximately 20% of cases of congenital VCP and is most likely due to traction of the recurrent laryngeal nerves during vaginal delivery or cesarean section, although it is most common following complicated deliveries.[8,18] These patients are symptomatic soon after birth, and the paralysis may be unilateral or bilateral. The prognosis of laryngeal paralysis associated with birth trauma is excellent, with most recovering within the first year of life.

Regardless of cause, children with bilateral VCP typically present with stridor and respiratory compromise due to the paramedian location of the vocal cords. The stridor may be biphasic or inspiratory alone and the voice is usually normal. The respiratory distress may become more obvious with increasing age due to the increased oxygen requirement seen with elevated activity levels. Unilateral VCP typically presents with a weak breathy voice and signs of aspiration, such as coughing, feeding difficulties, and aspiration pneumonia. Usually there is no respiratory compromise, leading to a possible delay in diagnosis.

Once suspected, the diagnosis of VCP requires endoscopic visualization of the larynx. The endoscopist must be careful not to immobilize the larynx by placing the laryngoscope on the glottic fold or the false cord. The laryngoscope is inserted into the vallecula, thus exposing the larynx and permitting observation of the dynamic movement of the vocal cords. Flexible fiberoptic laryngoscopy may also give excellent visualization of the vocal cords without the need for general anesthesia. It also allows for an undistorted view of the larynx, without any vector of force exerted on the larynx or its associated structures. Under these circumstances, however, the endoscopist is not able to palpate the arytenoids to rule out fixation of the cricoarytenoid joint and is not able to assess the remainder of the upper respiratory tract.

Ultrasound evaluation of the larynx has been found to be an accurate, reproducible method for the evaluation of VCP in children. Although not intended to replace direct visualization of the larynx, it may be useful in the ongoing evaluation of the child with known VCP and in the diagnosis of the very sick child who may be unstable for endoscopic evaluation.

Because of the association of VCP with CNS lesions such as the Arnold–Chiari malformations, radiographic evaluation of the CNS with either computed tomography and magnetic resonance imaging is imperative. Another useful radiographic technique is barium swallow, which can help for further evaluation of the aerodigestive tract.

Many children with bilateral VCP require a tracheotomy, whereas few or none with unilateral VCP require one.[18,36] In patients with bilateral VCP due to Arnold–Chiari malformation, tracheostomy should be delayed until a shunt procedure is performed. Nasotracheal intubation may be temporarily used following shunt placement, and only those children who do not demonstrate return of vocal cord function after several weeks should be considered for tracheotomy.

Although many patients with VCP have return of function within the first few years of life, those who demonstrate permanent paralysis may require further therapy. The goals of surgical correction of bilateral VCP are establishing an adequate airway, while preserving an acceptable voice and preventing aspiration. The treatment of unilateral VCP involves improving glottic closure and thus improving both voice and airway protection. Although work has been done on the surgical correction of VCP in adults, the treatment of this entity in children is more controversial regarding the timing for intervention and the nature of the surgical repair.

Because many children with VCP recover, and because this recovery may take up to several years, many authors recommend a conservative approach with maintenance of the tracheotomy and observation.[8] Procedures for bilateral VCP include endoscopic or open arytenoidectomy, open arytenoidopexy and transverse cordotomy. All procedures should be delayed until the child is 4–5 years of age.

Congenital subglottic stenosis

Subglottic stenosis is the third most common congenital anomaly of the larynx and the most common resulting in a tracheotomy in children under 1 year of age. Subglottic stenosis is present when the diameter of the subglottic space is less than 4 mm or when it does not admit a 3.0 mm bronchoscope (Fig 16.4). Congenital subglottic stenosis is due to a defect in the development of the cricoid cartilage or the conus elasticus.[25] This may result in a cartilaginous deformity, such as a small or elliptical-shaped cricoid, or in a soft tissue abnormality with excessive submucosal fibrosis.[24] Although severe subglottic stenosis presents soon after birth with biphasic stridor and respiratory compromise, milder cases may not present until later with recurrent episodes of croup.[21] These episodes are more protracted than typical croup and do not respond to standard medical therapy.[10,14,16] Severe cases with airway compromise may require airway intervention in the form of endotracheal intubation, which may cause further edema of the subglottic space, possibly necessitating a tracheotomy after failed extubation.

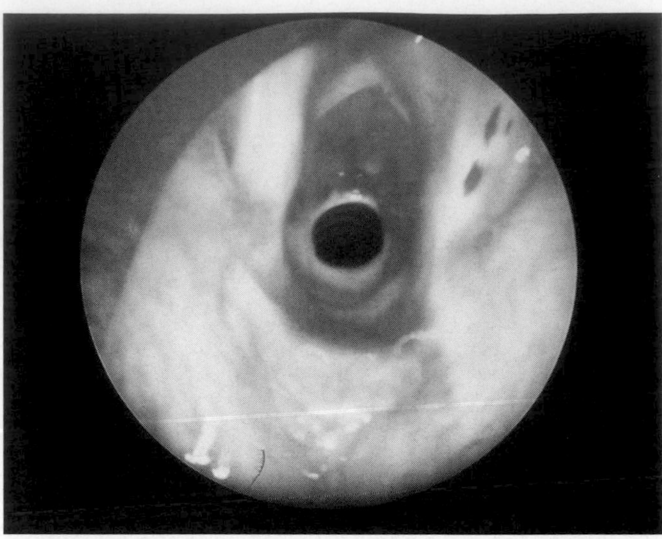

Figure 16.4 *Congenital subglottic stenosis.*

The diagnosis of congenital subglottic stenosis is strongly suggested by the clinical presentation, although lateral and anteroposterior soft tissue radiographs of the neck may be helpful in establishing the diagnosis, and airway fluoroscopy with barium swallow evaluates for other coexistent lesions, such as vascular compression. Endoscopy under general anesthesia is necessary to confirm the diagnosis, plan further therapy, and evaluate for other coexistent lesions. Studies show that children with one lesion of the airway have a second lesion in 18.8–58% of cases, emphasizing the need for careful evaluation of the entire upper aerodigestive tract.[10] Airway endoscopy includes flexible laryngoscopy while awake, direct microlaryngoscopy with a telescope, and rigid bronchoscopy using either a telescope or a ventilating bronchoscope. This evaluation is best performed using deep inhalational anesthesia. The subglottic area should be visualized, and further instrumentation should be avoided.

The management of congenital subglottic stenosis in patients who require intubation and fail subsequent extubation involves either a tracheotomy or a cricoid

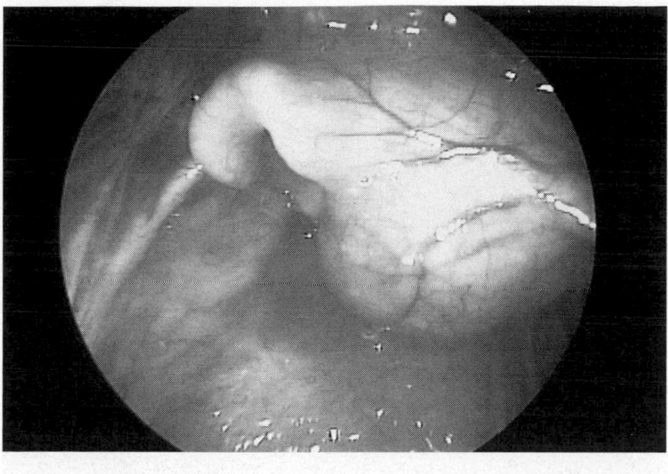

(a)

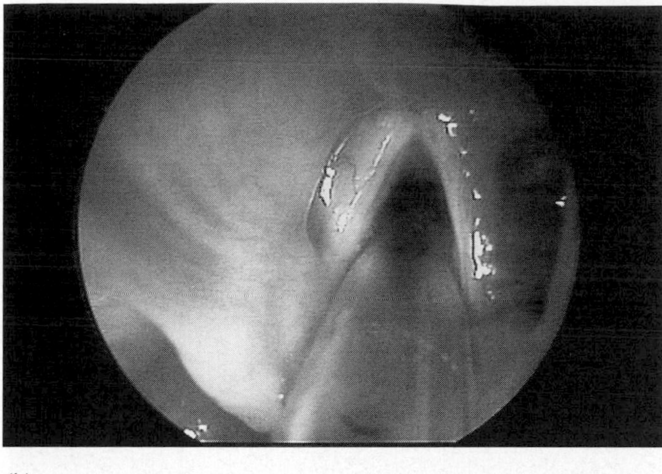

(b)

Figure 16.5 *(a) A large lateral saccular cyst in the right hemilarynx of a newborn causing inspiratory stridor and severe respiratory distress. (b) Larynx following aspiration and surgical excision of saccular cyst.*

split.[9,26,35] The anterior cricoid split has been used over the last decade in those neonates with stenosis who fail attempted extubation. This procedure can be effectively performed in neonates weighing over 1500 g, in those with only subglottic pathology, and in those with no contraindication to steroid usage. Additionally, vocal cord mobility must be assessed before attempted cricoid split, and gastroesophageal reflux should be evaluated and properly treated.[19] The cricoid split should be performed using an open procedure, making a vertical incision through the lower thyroid cartilage, cricoid cartilage, and first two tracheal rings. The patient is intubated nasally for approximately 5 days before a trial of extubation is considered. Steroids should only be used before extubation, and antibiotics should be continued for several days after extubation. A statistical survival analysis of children with congenital subglottic stenosis concluded that the anterior cricoid split is associated with less hospitalization, less morbidity, and possibly less mortality than long-term tracheotomy.[35]

Cotton[9] has proposed a staging system for subglottic stenosis:

- grade 1, 0–50% obstruction;
- grade 2, 50–70% obstruction;
- grade 3, 71–99% obstruction; and
- grade 4, 100% obstruction.

Patients with grades 2 and 3 may be candidates for single-stage laryngotracheal reconstruction (LTR). The airway is maintained through a small nasotracheal tube. The tracheotomy stoma is excised and a cartilage graft is harvested from the rib. An anterior midline incision is made through the cricoid up to the tracheal rings and the lower one-third of the cricoid cartilages. In some cases the posterior lamina of the cricoid is also divided. The graft is sutured to the divided anterior ends of the cricoid cartilage. The patient remains intubated and sedated in the ICU for at least 7–10 days until a leak occurs around the endotracheal tube. Steroids are administered prior to extubation. The timing of extubation is based on the clinical assessment at the primary surgery and presence of a leak. In carefully selected patients, more than 90% of these patients have been successfully extubated.

Laryngeal cysts and laryngoceles

Laryngeal saccular cysts arise from the mucous glands of the saccular appendage, an area that begins at the anterior ventricle and courses posteriorly deep to the false cords.[12] Its orifice empties into the ventricle, and it is involved in lubrication of the vocal cords. Lateral cysts are located in the aryepiglottic fold, epiglottis, or lateral larynx, whereas anterior cysts extend directly into the laryngeal inlet (Fig 16.5a).[27] These children typically present with stridor that begins soon after birth, and 20% require emergent airway intervention. Whilst these cysts may be treated using endoscopic aspiration (Fig 16.5b), incision and drainage, or unroofing, one study found that early excision via an open laryngofissure may be associated with a better outcome.

Laryngoceles are distinguished from saccular cysts in that they are dilatations of the saccule that contain air and communicate with the laryngeal lumen. Laryngoceles are also different from saccular cysts in that they typically cause intermittent symptoms only during acute inflammation or infection.[5] They most likely are due to a congenital weakness that is exacerbated by excessive intralaryngeal pressure and are most commonly of the mixed type, both involving the laryngeal lumen and extending into the neck through the thyrohyoid membrane. The recommended treatment for internal

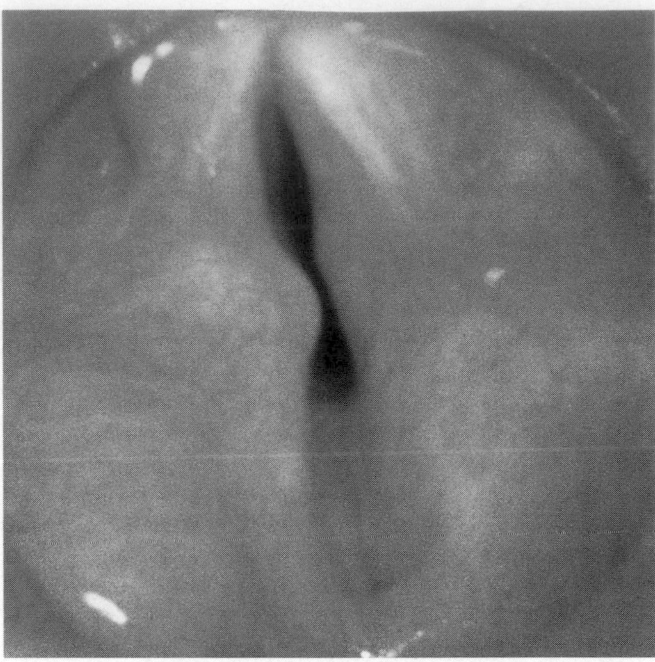

Figure 16.6 *Type 1 supraglottic interarytenoid cleft above the vocal cords. This patient did not aspirate.*

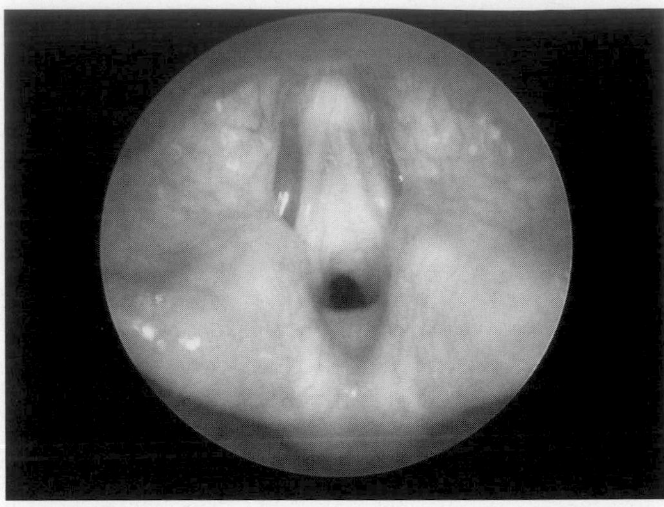

Figure 16.7 *Thick glottic web with subglottic stenosis.*

laryngoceles in children is that of endoscopic deroofing only if symptomatic, although surgical treatment is usually not required. External and mixed laryngoceles require open excision.

Laryngeal clefts

Posterior laryngeal clefts are an extremely rare cause of neonatal feeding difficulty and respiratory obstruction. They can involve the entire tracheoesophageal septum or be isolated to the posterior larynx (Fig 16.6).

Laryngeal clefts are part of the spectrum of arrested medial fusion of the lateral aspects of the laryngotracheal groove, and the stage of development determines the extent of cleft formation. Benjamin and Inglis more recently classified type I as a supraglottic interarytenoid cleft above the vocal cords, type II as a partial cricoid cleft, and type III completely involving the cricoid.[2]

Infants with laryngeal clefts present with feeding difficulties and aspiration or with signs of airway obstruction due to inspiratory collapse of redundant arytenoid.[13] The diagnosis may be missed if the stridor is attributed to laryngomalacia alone. Barium swallow strongly suggests the diagnosis in extensive clefts where contrast material enters the trachea and esophagus simultaneously. However, a small type I cleft confined to the larynx may be very difficult to diagnose on barium swallow. A rare type of cleft involving the anterior larynx has been described, and these children demonstrate aphonia or other voice changes.

A suspected laryngeal cleft requires direct microlaryngoscopy and esophagoscopy for definitive diagnosis. The edges of the laryngeal cleft can be sucked in; thus the diagnosis can be easily missed on laryngoscopy. A laryngeal probe should be used to separate the redundant mucosa between the arytenoids, palpating for a possible cricoid defect. An operating microscope or laryngeal telescope is helpful for this evaluation.

Cohen, in 1975, presented a series of laryngeal clefts and suggested that minor clefts did not require surgical repairs.[6] Clefts are approached through an anterior laryngofissure, though recent work has been done using endoscopic repair with endoscopic suture techniques. More extensive clefts may require a lateral cervical approach and thoracotomy. A tracheotomy should be avoided to prevent the possibility of erosion of the party wall suture line, and intubation should be used instead.

Laryngeal webs and atresia

These lesions result from varying degrees of incomplete recanalization of the primitive larynx during the tenth week of embryogenesis. The most common web is at the level of the glottis and extends across the anterior one-third of both vocal cords (Fig 16.7). This type of web presents with a weak, hoarse voice and varying degrees of respiratory distress, depending on the area of involvement. Rare supraglottic webs may cause feeding difficulties or respiratory compromise, posterior intra- arytenoid webs present with respiratory compromise, and posterior interarytenoid webs present with respiratory obstruction without alteration in voice or cry. Complete atresia of the laryngeal inlet is the rarest of these lesions and causes immediate respiratory obstruction at birth unless there is a concomitant tracheoesophageal fistula or if the obstruction is relieved by tracheotomy. A laryngeal cleft may be the presenting feature of velocardiofacial syndrome.

The diagnosis of laryngeal webs or atresia is made by direct laryngoscopy under general anesthesia. Proper evaluation includes an evaluation of the thickness of the web and the presence of other lesions, such as subglottic stenosis. Only 60% of children with webs require surgical intervention, and the treatment depends on the thickness of the web. A thin anterior web is amenable to endoscopic treatment with either the CO_2 laser or a cold knife.[31] These excisions must be staged in order to prevent the formation of opposing raw areas with resultant stenosis of the anterior commissure. A thick anterior laryngeal web or one extending into the subglottic space requires a tracheotomy, followed by a laryngofissure and insertion of a keel at the anterior commissure. Posterior interarytenoid webs are much more difficult to treat, and there is presently no accepted method of treatment. Similarly, supraglottic webs are difficult to treat, leaving tracheotomy as the safest option. Laryngeal atresia requires an emergent tracheotomy at birth, unless the child can be ventilated via a concomitant tracheoesophageal fistula until a definitive airway can be established.

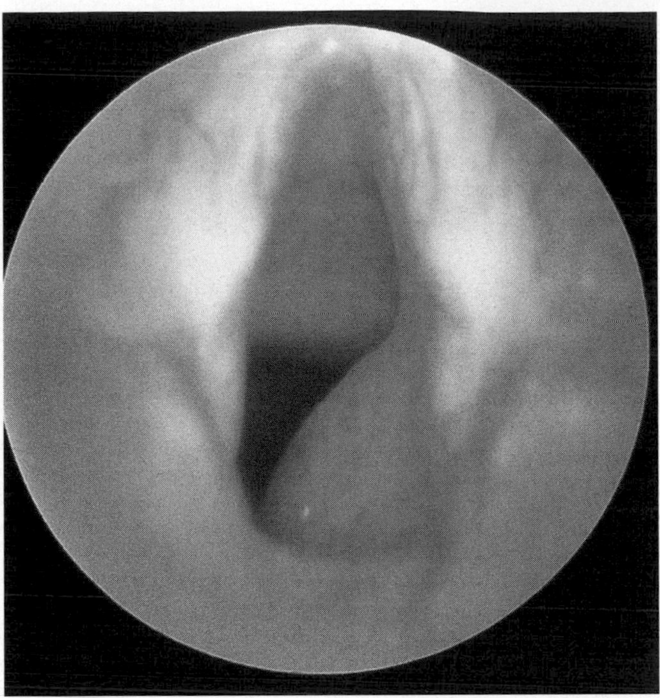

Figure 16.8 *Subglottic hemangioma. A pink mass covered by mucosa seen in the posterolateral wall of the subglottic space.*

Congenital subglottic hemangioma

Subglottic hemangioma appears as a smooth, compressible mass immediately below the posterior commissure with possible extension along the lateral wall of the subglottic space (Fig 16.8).[1] Overlying mucosa and submucosa may cause a pink or even white color, and the typical appearance usually precludes biopsy, which may be dangerous in an already obstructed airway. Subglottic hemangiomas are rare but are important because of their ability to severely compromise the pediatric airway. Characteristically, they are asymptomatic at birth; however, at about 6 weeks of age the child will develop a biphasic stridor associated with varying degrees of respiratory distress.[22] Commonly the clinical presentation is that of a protracted episode of croup. Subglottic hemangiomas proliferate rapidly for 12 months and then slowly involute over 3 years. Approximately 50% of patients with subglottic hemangiomas have cutaneous lesions.

Many treatment options have been described for the management of subglottic hemangiomas. Although subglottic hemangioma typically involutes spontaneously, expectant management is associated with an unacceptable mortality rate and is not recommended. Tracheotomy is a safe method of ensuring a stable airway, but it may have to remain in place for 3–4 years and has the associated morbidity. Radiation therapy and radioactive gold implantation have been used in the past, but the risk of secondary malignancies and other more acceptable alternatives now preclude their general use. External surgical approaches have been used with success but run the risk of causing subglottic stenosis. Systemic steroid therapy was introduced by Cohen and Wang in 1972 as a possible medical therapeutic approach to subglottic hemangioma.[7] Whilst steroid therapy can reduce the size of subglottic hemangioma and may hasten their involution, steroid use has been associated with retardation of growth and susceptibility to infection. Additionally, steroids alone rarely are effective in causing sufficient involution of the large, obstructing hemangioma. Direct intralesional steroid injection has also been suggested, although further experience is needed before it can be recommended. Embolization has been used in a case of extensive hemangioma of the larynx and trachea, although it is recommended only for those lesions refractory to conventional therapy. Interferon-a2A has been used with success in 15 patients with life-threatening airway hemangiomas, but is recommended at present only for those that are unresponsive to conventional treatment.[32]

The unique advantages of the CO_2 laser in the pediatric airway make it ideal for use in managing the obstructing subglottic hemangioma.[22,23] The CO_2 laser has been used in the treatment of 31 patients with subglottic hemangiomas with an overall success rate of 94%.[37] General anesthesia is maintained via jet ventilation with a Venturi apparatus, and laser surgery is performed in the intermittent mode with low-power settings. This technique should be performed only in conjunction with anesthesiologists who are comfortable with jet ventilation in the young child. Laryngeal stenosis has been reported in three patients with subglottic hemangiomas who underwent CO_2 laser therapy, emphasizing the need for careful patient selection, the avoidance of circumferential laser surgery, and the staged treatment of the rare concentric hemangioma.[11]

Miscellaneous abnormalities

Bifid epiglottis is a rare laryngeal anomaly often associated with other laryngeal abnormalities. The presenting symptoms are usually feeding difficulties due to aspiration and respiratory compromise due to enfolding of the two epiglottic halves. Diagnosis is confirmed by endoscopy, and described treatment options include tracheotomy and amputation of the epiglottis.

Cri du chat syndrome is due to partial deletion of the short arm of chromosome 5. The newborn infant has a cry similar to that of a cat's mew. On phonation, the posterior larynx remains open, possibly due to paresis of the interarytenoid muscles, giving a diamond-shaped appearance to the larynx. Other associated anomalies include hypertelorism, mental retardation, hypotonia, and low-set ears.

Cystic hygromas or lymphatic malformations may occur in the supraglottic larynx and histologically consist of malformed dilated lymph vessels. Lymphatic malformations of the supraglottic larynx are typically extensions of the adjacent neck lesion, although they may rarely be located primarily in the larynx. Endoscopic measures to remove cystic hygromas of the larynx are often unsuccessful, and external surgical excision of the neck lesion is usually required.

Conclusions

The diagnosis and management of the newborn or young child with a congenital malformation of the larynx requires knowledge of the embryology and anatomy of the pediatric airway, in addition to an understanding of the normal physiology and pathophysiology of the obstructed airway. The evaluation of these lesions should be performed only by one who is comfortable with pediatric endoscopy and in a center where appropriate support is available.

References

1. Benjamin B, Carter P. Congenital laryngeal hemangioma. *Ann Otol Rhinol Laryngol* 1983; **92:** 448–55.
2. Benjamin B, Inglis A. Minor congenital laryngeal clefts: diagnosis and classification. *Ann Otol Rhinol Laryngol* 1989; **98:** 417–20.
3. Charney EB, Rorke LB, Sutton LN, Schut L. Management of Chiari II complications in infants with myelomeningocele. *J Pediatr* 1987; **111:** 364–71.
4. Chaten FC, Lucking SE, Young ES, Mickell JJ. Stridor: intracranial pathology causing postextubation vocal cord paralysis. *Pediatrics* 1991; **87:** 39–43.
5. Civantos FJ, Holinger LD. Laryngocele and saccular cysts in infants and children. *Arch Otolaryngol Head Neck Surg* 1992; **118:** 296–300.
6. Cohen SR. Cleft larynx. A report of seven cases. *Ann Otol* 1975; **84:** 747–56.
7. Cohen SR, Wang CI. Steroid treatment of hemangioma of the head and neck in children. *Ann Otol* 1972; **81:** 584–90.
8. Cohen SR, Geller KA, Birns JW, Thompson JW. Laryngeal paralysis in children: long-term retrospective study. *Ann Otol* 1982; **9:** 417–24.
9. Cotton RT, Richardson MA. Congenital laryngeal anomalies. *Otolaryngol Clin North Am* 1981; **14:** 203–18.
10. Cotton RT, Tewfik TL. Laryngeal stenosis following carbon dioxide laser in subglottic hemangioma. Report of three cases. *Ann Otol Rhinol Laryngol* 1985; **94:** 494–7.
11. Davidoff AM, Filston HC. Treatment of infantile subglottic hemangioma with electrocautery. *J Pediatr Surg* 1992; **27:** 436–9.
12. Donegan JO, Strife JL, Seid AB, Cotton RT, Dunbar JS. Internal laryngocele and saccular cysts in children. *Ann Otol* 1980; **89:** 409–13.
13. Evans JNG. Management of the cleft larynx and tracheoesophageal clefts. *Ann Otol Rhinol Laryngol* 1985; **94:** 627–30.
14. Fearon B, Cotton RT. Subglottic stenosis in infants and children: the clinical problem and experimental correction. *Can J Otolaryngol* 1972; **1:** 281–9.
15. Fearon B, Ellis D. The management of long term airway problems in infants and children. *Ann Otol* 1971; **80:** 669–77.
16. Fearon B, Crysdale WS, Bird R. Subglottic stenosis in the infant and child. Methods of management. *Ann Otol* 1978; **87:** 645–8.
17. Friedman EM, Vastola AP, McGill T, Healy GB. Chronic pediatric stridor: etiology and outcome. *Laryngoscope* 1990; **100:** 277–80.
18. Gentile RD, Miller RH, Woodson GE. Vocal cord paralysis in children 1 year of age and younger. *Ann Otol Rhinol Laryngol* 1986; **95:** 622–5.
19. Gray S, Miller R, Myer CM III, Cotton RT. Adjunctive measures for successful laryngotracheal reconstruction. *Ann Otol Rhinol Laryngol* 1987; **96:** 509–13.
20. Grundfast KM, Harley E. Vocal cord paralysis. *Otolaryngol Clin North Am* 1989; **22:** 569–97.
21. Healy GB. Subglottic stenosis. *Otolaryngol Clin North Am* 1989; **22:** 599–606.
22. Healy GB, McGill T, Friedman EM. Carbon dioxide laser in subglottic hemangioma. An update. *Ann Otol Rhinol Laryngol* 1984; **93:** 370–3.
23. Healy GB, Fearon B, French R, McGill T. Treatment of subglottic hemangioma with the carbon dioxide laser. *Laryngoscope* 1980; **90:** 809–13.
24. Holinger LD. Histopathology of congenital subglottic stenosis. *Ann Otol Rhinol Laryngol* 1999; **108:** 101–11.
25. Holinger LD, Oppenheimer RW. Congenital subglottic stenosis: the elliptical cricoid cartilage. *Ann Otol Rhinol Laryngol* 1989; **98:** 702–6.
26. Holinger LD, Stankiewicz JA, Livingston GL. Anterior cricoid split: the Chicago experience with an alternative to tracheotomy. *Laryngoscope* 1987; **97:** 19–24.
27. Holinger LD, Barnes DR, Smid LJ, Holinger PH. Laryngocele and saccular cysts. *Ann Otol* 1978; **87:** 675–85.
28. Holinger PH. Clinical aspects of congenital anomalies of the larynx, trachea, bronchi and esophagus. *J Laryngol Otol* 1961; **75:** 1–44.
29. Katin LI, Tucker JA. Laser supraarytenoidectomy for

laryngomalacia with apnea. *Trans Pa Acad Ophthalmol Otolaryngol* 1990; **42:** 985–8.

30. McClurg FLD, Evans DA. Laser laryngoplasty for laryngomalacia. *Laryngoscope* 1994; **104:** 247–52.
31. McGill T. Congenital diseases of the larynx. *Otolaryngol Clin North Am* 1984; **17:** 57–62.
32. Ohlms LA, Jones DT, McGill T, Healy GB. Interferon alfa-2a therapy for airway hemangiomas. *Ann Otol Rhinol Laryngol* 1994; **103:** 1–8.
33. Oren J, Kelly DH, Todres JD, Shannon DC. Respiratory complications in patients with myelodysplasia and Arnold–Chiari malformation. *Am J Dis Child* 1986; **140:** 221–4.
34. Polonovski JM, Contencin P, Francois M, Viala P, Narcy P. Aryepiglottic fold excision for the treatment of severe laryngomalacia. *Ann Otol Rhinol Laryngol* 1990; **99:** 625–7.
35. Rosenfeld RM, Bluestone CD. Does early expansion surgery have a role in the management of congenital subglottic stenosis? *Laryngoscope* 1993; **103:** 286–90.
36. Rosin D, Handler SD, Potsic WP, Wetmore RF, Tom LW. Vocal cord paralysis in children. *Laryngoscope* 1990; **100:** 1174–9.
37. Sie KC, McGill T, Healy GB. Subglottic hemangioma: ten years experience with the carbon dioxide laser. *Ann Otol Rhinol Laryngol* 1994; **103:** 167–72.
38. Zalzal GH, Anon JB, Cotton RT. Epiglottoplasty for the treatment of laryngomalacia. *Ann Otol Rhinol Laryngol* 1987; **96:** 72–6.

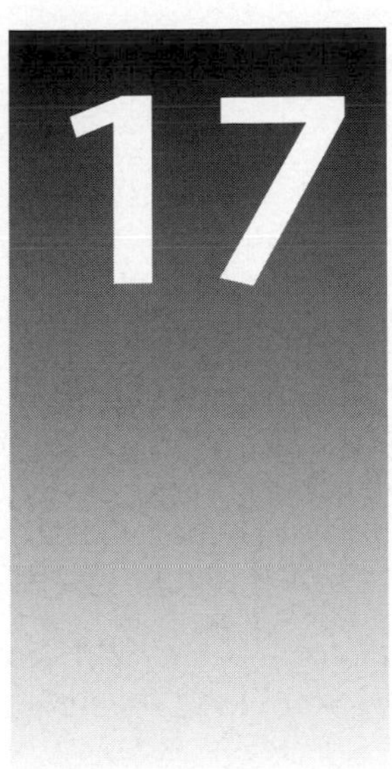

Acquired diseases of the pediatric larynx

Frank L Rimell

Before one begins to study disease processes that affect the pediatric larynx, it is important to understand anatomic characteristics which distinguish the pediatric larynx from the adult. Size is the most important factor with the normal term newborn subglottic circumference of 5.7 mm. Because of this relatively small size, there is little room for accommodation secondary to injury, or surgical repair in early childhood. A second difference is the lack of calcification and soft pliable cartilage which forms the pediatric laryngotracheal complex. Although this factor allows for accommodation of an intrinsic abnormality, it is less resilient to extrinsic compression and makes the pediatric larynx more vulnerable during blunt force trauma. A third important factor is positioning of the laryngotracheal complex at the level of the second cervical spine with its descent to a more inferior position throughout early childhood. The tip of the epiglottis is at the level of the nasopharynx at birth and this position protects an infant from aspiration while drinking in the recumbent position. This position also requires the child to have a patent nose and nasopharynx for airflow to occur behind the soft palate and epiglottis.

Viral infections of the pediatric larynx

Recurrent respiratory papillomatosis (RRP)

This is the most common tumor of the pediatric airway and shows extreme variation in clinical course. The human papilloma virus (HPV) is the cause of this lesion and the virus will only live in squamous epithelium. The initial infection begins on the true vocal cords or where there has been squamous metaplasia. The cause is almost always HPV type 6 or HPV type 11. We have now found one case of HPV 16 that later degenerated to squamous cell carcinoma.[54,58] Infecting HPV type may be of importance because those children who are infected by HPV 11 are statistically more likely to suffer from an airway obstructive course and more likely to require a tracheotomy than those infected by HPV 6 (Fig 17.1).[45,60] Typing is most effective and accurate if done by the polymerase chain reaction technique. The fact that HPV 11 is associated with a more virulent clinical course initially has no bearing on eventual clinical outcome. In

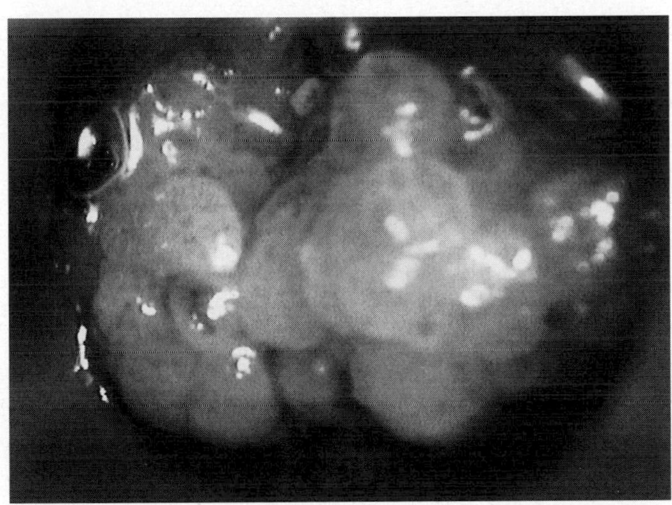

Figure 17.1 *Supraglottic larynx of a 10-month-old child infected by HPV type 11. There is complete obstruction of the airway with all aspects of the larynx involved.*

fact, those children infected by HPV 11 were just as likely to go into clinical remission as those infected by HPV 6.[60]

It is our approach to classify children infected by HPV into a benign or aggressive clinical course. Those with an aggressive disease course have disease persistence past puberty or spread of disease to the carina or beyond. Obviously those with an aggressive clinical course are far more likely to succumb to disease than reach a point of remission, whereas those with a benign course should eventually achieve remission. It should also be noted that those children who eventually achieve remission may present in adulthood with recurrent disease.[20]

Viral transmission

It has been theorized that childhood disease is acquired through the birth canal from the mother. This theory, however, has not been scientifically substantiated. The disease tends to affect first-born children from young mothers (teenagers or early 20s) and subsequent children from the same mother seem not to be affected. It has also been reported from the database maintained by the Recurrent Respiratory Papilloma Foundation that 13 of 220 cases of laryngeal papillomas occurred in children delivered by cesarean. Therefore a cesarean birth is not recommended unless there are gross cervical lesions that cannot be removed prior to delivery.

Surgical management

Anesthetic management is far more difficult in a child than in an adult, because of the size of the airway and the fact that a child is more likely to present with airway obstruction. Choices of anesthesia include endotracheal intubation, Venturi, jet and apnea. We make a distinction between Venturi ventilation, which places a needle above the vocal cords and entrains room air plus oxygen into the airway, from that of jet ventilation, which places a needle below the vocal cords into the trachea. It has been our preference to use Venturi ventilation to manage these patients. Arguments against Venturi ventilation are that it may insufflate HPV distally into the trachea. Knowing that HPV needs squamous mucosa to implant and grow, we are more concerned about the use of the apneic technique with multiple intubations as this can cause squamous metaplasia distal to the vocal cords and implant HPV. Venturi ventilation has been used in over 80 patients with HPV in our experience with no higher rate of distal spread than one would normally expect. Obviously a laser protected endotracheal tube is another option but in the small pediatric larynx our preference is not to have a tube in the way of our surgical field. When a child presents in extremis with airway obstruction, our current technique utilizes an inhalational anesthetic for induction, followed by propofol given intravenously and topical lidocaine to the laryngeal area allowing for spontaneous respiration. Gross disease is quickly debulked with the child spontaneously breathing and the patient is ventilated once an airway is visible. This is the same anesthetic technique we use for removal of a laryngeal foreign body. Hemostasis is obtained with topical oxymetazoline hydrochloride applied by cotton pledget.

The main technique used for debulking is with carbon dioxide vaporization or manual removal of gross disease. It is important to remember that debulking is not a cure, so do no harm. The virus, once present in the larynx, is there for the life of the patient whether it is producing active lesions or in remission. Overzealous removal results in significant damage to the larynx which is also lifelong once the patient achieves disease remission.[51,61]

When distal spread beyond the larynx in a child occurs, our preference is to use a laser delivered by a fiberoptic source such as potassium titanyl phosphate (KTP). The disadvantage of carbon dioxide is that it has to be coupled to a bronchoscope so visualization is from the top of the bronchoscope and not at the tip as occurs when a laser fiber is coupled with the Hopkins rod telescope. We typically use the standard pediatric bronchoscope and place a 400 nm or 600 nm fiber through the suction port alongside the Hopkins rod telescope for superior visualization and airway control during vaporization of distal papilloma lesions.[59]

Tracheotomy

The use of a tracheotomy to control the airway in children with obstructive papillomas has been condemned because it is thought to promote distal tracheal spread. Our experience shows that those children who required a tracheotomy have a more aggressive disease process with an earlier age of presentation (21 months versus 52 months) and required more surgery prior to tracheotomy (0.95 procedures per month versus 0.62) than those children who did not require a tracheotomy.[63] Thus the problem may not be the tracheotomy but the variability of the disease course. Two of 22 children in the nontracheotomy group developed distal tracheal disease whilst one of 13 in the tracheotomy group developed distal tracheal disease. Although, papillomas will grow around the tracheotomy site, they will disappear as the disease goes into remission. Ten of 13 children with tracheotomies were decannulated at an average age of 6 years. Our current recommendation is to consider a tracheotomy if a child is presenting with laryngeal obstruction every 6 weeks or less.

Medical management

The only drug that has been adequately studied for the treatment of juvenile RRP is interferon-α. Interferons are polypeptides produced by white cells in response to various protein stimuli, particularly viral particles. The best known studies of interferon treatment in RRP are by Leventhal, Healy and colleagues.[28,33,36] Leventhal, Kashima and colleagues[36] clearly showed a benefit of using interferon-α-n1 (Wellferon) with a significant decrease in laryngeal disease. Healy showed no benefit from human leukocyte interferon. The Healy study[28] is criticized because of its lower dosing and its use of interferon from the New York Blood Bank as opposed to the recombinant form. An important aspect of the Healy paper, however, is that it was the only study to have a distinct control group that never received medical therapy. This control group improved over time negating any positive effect by interferon. This is typical for RRP where the amount of physical lesions can vary over time and the natural history of the disease is eventual remission in most cases. One needs to keep this fact in mind when judging articles on a few patients given a new drug to treat RRP without a control group. We will consider the use of interferon in certain cases as a means to avoid a tracheotomy or as a trial when disease has spread to the carina or beyond. Although we currently use interferon-α-2β on an experimental basis, the current standard is α-n1 at a dose of 2 million units per square meter per day or 4 million units per square meter per every other day for 6 months.

Other medications that have been described as adjuvant therapy for RRP include acyclovir, indol-3-carbinol, isotretinoin, ribavirin and methotrexate.[1,39,40,42] All of the reports on the use of these agents in the treatment of RRP have been preliminary and uncontrolled. It has been our policy not to use these agents unless the patient is formally enrolled in a study as there is currently no known benefit to any of these agents.

Croup

Croup or laryngotracheobronchitis is one of the more common conditions affecting the larynx of a child. Croup is characterized by edema and vascular engorgement of the immediate subglottic region, giving it a deep red color. This process can also affect the true and false vocal cords. The classic presentation is that of a brassy cough which sounds much like the bark of a dog. The child will typically have a low-grade fever, respiratory infectious symptoms such as rhinorrhea but a normal white blood cell count. The child presenting to the emergency room usually has inspiratory stridor with or without expiratory rhonchi. It is helpful to classify these children and document their severity with the use of a croup score (Table 17.1). Children with scores that are stable and equal to or under 3 are likely to do well at home. Those that remain above 3 should probably be admitted for observation and those with scores above 8 are likely to be intubated. It is the inspiratory stridor with retractions that signals significant subglottic edema in the patient and a life-threatening event. The subglottic edema is acute and soft and therefore dilatable with passage of an endotracheal tube if necessary. Management of these children is with short-term endotracheal intubation as opposed to tracheotomy.

The use of cool mist air in mild cases (scores under 3) comes from the observation that the symptoms of many children improved or disappeared as they were heading to the hospital in the cool night air. There is a lack of scientific evidence to support that cool mist air is of any benefit and that 'croup tents', although still occasionally used, are of questionable benefit and may be more dangerous than helpful. Cool mist is still used in emergency rooms as first-line therapy in the treatment of croup.

Table 17.1 Modified Westley Croup Score[14,22]

Inspiratory stridor	
None	0
At rest, with stethoscope	1
At rest, without stethoscope	2
Retractions	
None	0
Mild	1
Moderate	2
Severe	3
Air entry	
Normal	0
Decreased	1
Severely decreased	2
Cyanosis	
None	0
With agitation	4
At rest	5
Level of consciousness	
Normal	0
Altered mental status	5

Most children who present to the emergency room with scores above 3 can be managed with racemic epinephrine (Vaponefrin) and systemic steroids.[74] The dose of racemic epinephrine given by nebulization is 0.05 ml/kg of a 2.25% solution to a maximum of 1.5 ml (usual dose is 0.5 ml). The dose of dexamethasone is 0.6 mg/kg (maximum 15 mg) by mouth, intramuscularly or intravenously, although lower dosages to 0.15 mg/kg have been found to be equally effective.[23] The use of these agents has been shown in clinical trials to be effective in the treatment of croup.[54,66,68,69] Currently debate exists about the safe use of these agents on an outpatient basis and the role of a rebound effect. Currently, children receiving only one to two treatments of racemic epinephrine and a single dose of dexamethasone and who maintain a croup score under 3 for a period of 2–4 hours following treatment can be discharged home provided there is a reliable caregiver.[35] Need for repeated treatment and rapid rebound indicates significant obstruction by edema and probably the need for admission and/or intubation. Steroids can take several hours before they are effective and there can also be a rebound effect 24–36 hours later. In addition to systemic steroids, the use of inhaled steroids has gained in popularity. Commonly 2 mg of budesonide is given by inhalation and has been found to be as effective as systemic steroids and possibly as effective as racemic epinephrine.[22] Although often not discussed in the literature, Heliox can be used to ease the work of breathing until systemic steroids become effective and help avoid intubation in severe cases.

The causative organisms of croup are influenza A and B and parainfluenza 1 and 3 as well as respiratory syncytial virus, which accounts for the majority of cases particularly in the winter. There have also been sporadic cases of croup caused by herpes simplex types 1 and 2.[41] It was felt these cases occurred in children on steroids or who had herpetic oral stomatitis. Children under the age of 3 years are typically affected with an estimated incidence of 60 cases per 1000 child-years in those aged between 1 and 2 years.[14,16] Croup occurs in clustered outbreaks that typically occur in fall or spring with a reported hospitalization rate from 1 to 15% and with 1–5% of hospitalized children requiring intubation.[3,17,71] However, we have seen croup outbreaks in the middle of summer and therefore one must never assume a diagnosis based on the season. It is important to elicit a full history to rule out underlying subglottic stenosis, foreign body or other anatomic obstructive problems such as subglottic hemangioma or glottic webs. A child who repeatedly presents with croup or does not respond to conventional treatment should be suspected of having one of these other conditions and strong consideration given to diagnostic endoscopy.

Spasmodic croup and croup in the older child

There are those children with croup episodes unrelated to an antecedent fever or signs of upper respiratory infection. They tend to occur at night and because of the recurrent nature it is called 'spasmodic croup'. It is thought to result from spasms of the larynx in a child older than 2 years of age. When a child is labeled with the diagnosis of spasmodic croup, it implies that there are no anatomic lesions narrowing the airway. It has been our approach to perform a full workup before the diagnosis of spasmodic or recurrent croup is made. We have found on occasion various anatomic lesions that were surgically correctable. In the case where there are no anatomic abnormalities, one should rule out whether a problem with irritation of the airway by gastroesophageal reflux, allergens or idiopathic reactions, such as a C1 esterase inhibitor deficiency, exists. Gastroesophageal reflux has been associated with recurrent episodes of croup in infants as well as in older children.[72] It has been our experience that one can often find the answer to the cause of spasmodic croup. A workup may include endoscopy and if so our opinion is that an esophagoscopy with biopsy be performed at the time of airway endoscopy to rule out the possibility of associated gastroesophageal reflux.[65]

Herpes

Herpetic infections of the larynx will typically occur in the 1–5 years age group and more than likely are encountered in those who are immunosuppressed or have a chronic disease. In the majority of cases they are an extension of oral pharyngeal lesions.[62,77] Because of the mucositis and edema associated with a herpetic infection, these children may require intubation to bypass laryngeal edema and obstruction. It is important to biopsy and culture these lesions to make sure they are not aciclovir resistant (Fig 17.2).

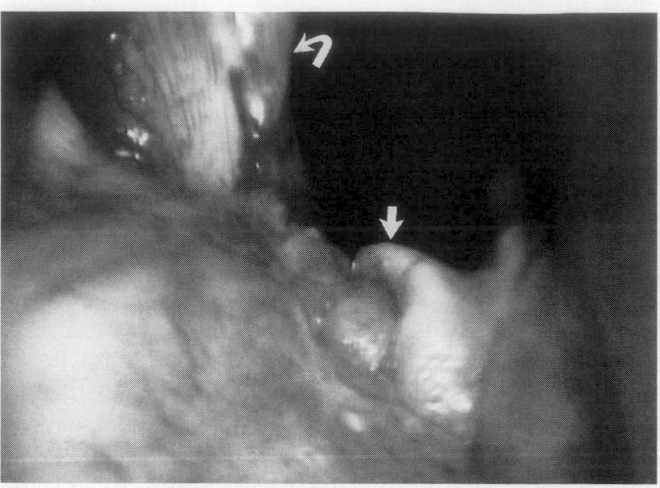

Figure 17.2 *This adolescent female with cystic fibrosis presented with hemoptysis. On laryngoscopy, a lesion was noted in the posterior glottic region that later proved to be herpetic and acyclovir resistant. Straight arrow denotes herpetic lesion; curved arrow denotes left true cord.*

Bacterial infections of the pediatric larynx

There is somewhat of a debate as to the usefulness of laryngeal and tracheal cultures in children for diagnostic purposes. Pathogenic bacteria such as *Haemophilus influenzae* and *Streptococcus pneumoniae* are found routinely on culture in the normal pediatric larynx.[30]

Epiglottitis

No disease is probably more feared by the on-call otolaryngologist than a child with suspected epiglottitis. Fortunately, the number of children affected by this life-threatening infection has declined significantly. Traditionally the most common cause was *Haemophilus influenzae* type B (HIB), although there are multiple infectious causes for epiglottitis. The rate of epiglottitis has dropped 80–90% with the development of conjugated vaccines.[25] In Quebec, Canada, routine vaccinations of HIB began in 1988, with the older PRP-D vaccine. In 1992, the more effective conjugates (PRP-T, HbOC, PRP-OMPC) were introduced and since this introduction 15 children in Quebec suffered acute epiglottitis in 1993 as opposed to 97 cases per year between 1984 and 1987.[76]

The majority of cases seen today are vaccine failures but one needs to be suspicious for other infecting organisms, including group A b-hemolytic streptococcus, group B streptococcus, candida, and epiglottitis as an initial presentation of AIDS.[4,78]

The diagnosis and management of epiglottitis has also changed over the past 30 years from primary management by tracheotomy to intubation and management by a pediatric intensivist without the need for otolaryngologic consultation. The child who presents with epiglottitis usually has inspiratory stridor of acute onset, retractions and drooling. The child will lean forward to allow the red and swollen epiglottis to pull away from the laryngeal inlet and thereby reduce airway obstruction. However, there is great variation in clinical presentation and the variation is directly related to cause as well as to the degree and location of epiglottic edema.

The child typically will present to the emergency room and upon receiving a consultation, the managing otolaryngologist will need to immediately assess airway stability. A child in extremis needs an immediate laryngoscopy in a controlled setting so that a diagnosis is made and the airway controlled. The child who is stable and swallowing secretions can undergo high kilovoltage lateral neck films prior to physical examination if the diagnosis is in doubt. Flexible nasopharyngoscopy can also be performed and is our preference. In the past such manipulations were condemned but in the proper setting of today's modern pediatric emergency center such an examination for the evaluation of epiglottitis in the stable child has become more routine.[13] If edema is mild to moderate and if one is practicing in a tertiary pediatric center with a skilled in-house intensivist, these children can be observed and treated with intravenous antibiotics with or without steroids. Heliox may be used to decrease the work of breathing and allow for the time needed for antibiotics and steroids to decrease the supraglottic edema. A differential diagnosis includes retropharyngeal abscess, bacterial tracheitis and foreign body. In a retropharyngeal abscess there is drooling but usually there is no stridor or retractions. Bacterial tracheitis is similar for high fevers and airway distress but is without drooling or dysphagia typical of supraglottic pathologies, whilst laryngeal foreign bodies typically present with stridor but without fevers or drooling.

In the case of extremis, the child is best handled in an operating room setting. The child should be allowed to sit up and breathe oxygen mixed with an inhalational anesthetic. Once the child has passed the excitement phase, an IV can be placed and the child should be able to be intubated. Supraglottic edema can be handled easily with a jaw thrust and positive-pressure mask ventilation. The child can undergo diagnostic laryngoscopy and intubation, preferably by a nasotracheal approach. Once the airway is controlled, biopsies for culture can be taken from the epiglottis as well as blood cultures.

Postoperative management is again influenced by the comfort level of the pediatric intensive care unit. At our institution we would keep the patient sedated and comfortable but not necessarily paralyzed. Usually 3–4 days is enough for the edema to resolve and the patient extubated at bedside following a laryngoscopy.

Tracheitis

Bacterial tracheitis, also known as membranous or pseudomembranous croup, is so name because of the membrane seen on endoscopy from sloughed tracheal epithelium. Diagnosis is more difficult to make and the differential diagnosis includes epiglottitis, croup and foreign body. One should be suspicious of bacterial tracheitis in a previously healthy child with fever, elevated white count, a brassy cough and retractions, although not all of these signs may be present. Classically one will see an outline of the pseudomembrane on chest radiograph or fluoroscopy. The best way to make the diagnosis is by endoscopy and any child with retractions and fever who is in danger of needing endotracheal intubation should undergo endoscopy and culture. The most common infecting organisms include *Staphylococcus aureus*, *Streptococcus pneumoniae* and *Moraxella catarrhalis*. These children can be managed by endoscopy only in less severe cases or endotracheal intubation with daily rigid or flexible bedside bronchoscopy. The need for tracheotomy is rare and it is imperative that a culture is taken for culture and sensitivities as well as fungal and viral organisms.

Tuberculosis

Laryngeal tuberculosis is exceedingly rare in children with only a handful of cases reported in the world literature. It is thought that, unlike the adult form in which laryngeal involvement is usually secondary to a pulmonary infection, pediatric laryngeal tuberculosis tends to be a primary infection.[55] Reported cases show that the same anatomic areas affecting adults are involved in children, i.e. the posterior glottis or the superior portion of the laryngeal surface of the epiglottis. Treatment is the same and consists of control of the airway with tracheotomy, if needed, for airway obstruction as well as endoscopy with biopsy for culture and sensitivities. The patient is empirically begun on triple or quadruple antibiotic therapy based on the acid-fast bacterial stain. The final treatment regimen will depend on mycobacterial sensitivities.

Diphtheria

This is a condition, because of vaccination, that is rare to see in developed countries; however, resurgence is being seen in Eastern Europe.[53] The disease process is caused by the release of bacterial exotoxins from *Corynebacterium diphtheriae*. These exotoxins result in epithelial degeneration and a pseudomembrane that can affect any portion of the upper or lower airway and in particular the larynx, resulting in significant airway obstruction. In fact, the word 'croup' was originally associated with the white membrane over the larynx associated with diphtherial infection. Diagnosis is made by cultures of the membranous debris on Loffler or tellurite media. Treatment consists of airway control by endotracheal intubation or tracheotomy followed by penicillin or erythromycin and 20 000–60 000 units of diphtheria antitoxin intravenously. Recently, it has been suggested that the use of systemic dexamethasone may help to avoid tracheotomy or intubation in some cases of diphtherial croup.[26]

Fungal infections

Coccidiomycosis

Coccidiomycosis is a soil organism that primarily results in a pulmonary fungal infection seen in the south-western United States and northern Mexico. In the majority of cases it is isolated to the lungs and asymptotic. In less than 1% of cases there is life-threatening dissemination. Spread to the larynx is rare but there have been a handful of pediatric cases reported in endemic areas. Appearance is that of granulomas reported in various laryngeal sites including the subglottis. There does not have to be pulmonary involvement and the diagnosis is made on histology by the identification of spherules with or without endospores.[7] Confirmation is seen with a positive skin test and IgM- and IgG-specific antibodies provided the patient is immunocompetent. Treatment consists of supportive airway care including tracheotomy and amphotericin.

Aspergillosis

Aspergillosis of the laryngotracheal complex is fortunately rare and similar to that of the sinuses in that two forms may be seen: invasive and noninvasive. Although, presently all reported cases have been in adults, we have treated a 13-year-old with an invasive infection acquired during chemotherapy for acute lymphocytic leukemia. Endoscopically the appearance is that of an invasive squamous cell carcinoma when the disease is in the invasive form. The diagnosis is confirmed on histology and culture where the classic finding of hyphae with right-angle branches are seen on sliver stains. Treatment for invasive aspergillosis has consisted of laryngectomy.[56] In our patient we were able to debride the necrotic areas, treat with systemic amphotericin and reconstruct the larynx in order to avoid laryngectomy for invasive disease.

Candidiasis

Candidiasis is probably the most common of all fungal infections to involve the larynx and is seen in those children who are immunocompromised. Unlike the adult form, young children with a significant infection can present with airway obstruction due to the small size of the larynx and edema that occurs secondary to the infection.[21] These children are begun on systemic agents effective against *Candida* and the airway controlled by intubation if needed.

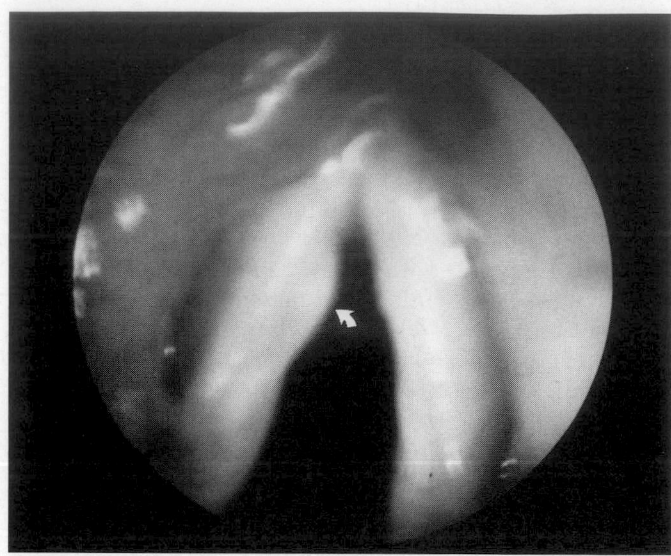

Figure 17.3 *Five-year-old male child evaluated for hoarseness with a classic finding of vocal cord nodules. Arrow denotes right true vocal cord nodule.*

Acquired inflammatory lesions

Vocal cord nodules

The most common cause of hoarseness in a child are vocal cord nodules which are typically seen in the male child (Fig 17.3). These always occur at the junction of the anterior and middle third of the vocal folds. This is because the maximal point of trauma occurs in this area as the vocal folds collide during forceful phonation. The swelling on the vocal cords is secondary to stress and results in vascular congestion and edema that later becomes fibrotic, similar to a callous.[2]

Diagnosis is made easily in the clinic with fiberoptic or indirect laryngoscopy. It is important that any child with hoarseness for greater than 2 weeks receives a laryngoscopic examination, which can be done in the office. The nodules can easily be seen on examination and other more potentially life-threatening conditions such as respiratory papillomatosis ruled out. It has been our experience that almost any child or infant can tolerate a flexible fiberoptic examination in the office and we routinely perform this in any age infant or child without difficulty. Newer fiberoptic scopes have an outer diameter as small as 1.8 mm, although we prefer the resolution of the 2.2 mm scope. Many older children (5 years of age or older) will tolerate the use of the rigid endoscope with a full stroboscopy if performed with patience and careful explanation.

The cause of vocal nodules is typically forceful voice projection by the child and the treatment is conservative therapy. One should obtain a full history to make sure that certain medications such as decongestants that can result in drying of the laryngeal mucosa are not exacerbating the condition. Treatment consists of voice therapy where the voice therapist works with both parent and child to try and discourage poor vocal habits such as yelling and habitual throat clearing as well as to encourage the use of good vocal technique.

Failure to modify this behavior can result in progression of the nodules to the point where they impair vocal cord function and result in severe hoarseness or near aphonia and therefore need to be treated surgically. This is seen rarely but often occurs when there is persistence of this process into adolescence. Surgical removal is done with the aid of a microscope and strict adherence to the principles of a microsurgical dissection as outlined in previous chapters. It is important when considering a surgical procedure to correct nodules, that the child and parents both understand preoperatively the importance of voice therapy postoperatively.[64]

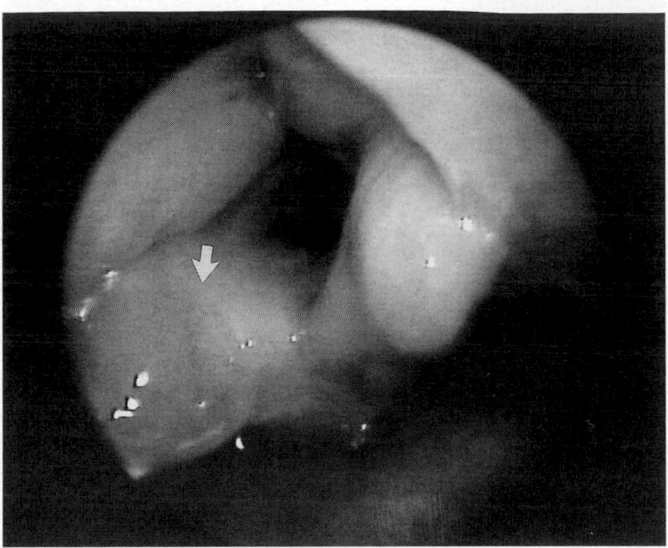

Figure 17.4 *Caustic ingestion with severe laryngeal edema. This child required prolonged intubation but a tracheotomy was avoided. Arrow denotes posterior glottic edema.*

Thermal and caustic injury

Children account for a significant number of patients admitted to burn units in the USA and roughly 20% of these children have suffered some type of inhalational injury.[29] The vast majority of children who suffer significant airway injury are those involved in close space trauma and there is little correlation to orofacial burns and airway injury.[32] Although there may be little evidence of airway edema on initial evaluation, this will change 12–24 hours later with intravenous rehydration. The vast majority of these children are best managed by endotracheal intubation. However, a small number may require tracheotomy because of difficult intubation or multiple failed attempts at extubation.[8]

Lye and other corrosive chemicals ingested either accidentally or as a suicide attempt can result in significant laryngeal and subglottic damage (Fig 17.4). There is little information published on the management of this problem. An initial dilemma that confronts the surgeon is prolonged intubation with the endotracheal tube acting as a stent versus the use of a tracheotomy early to avoid pressure and additional inflammation to the larynx. Our approach is to make an assessment after 2–3 weeks of intubation. Depending on the clinical state and whether, on endoscopy, there appears to be consistent edema and/or stricture, a tracheotomy is performed. The patient is followed clinically for the resolution of inflammation and the maturation of scar prior to laryngotracheoplasty. In rare instances the supraglottis and/or glottis is so severely injured that reconstruction is impossible and one must consider a laryngectomy or separation secondary to a nonfunctional larynx that is allowing chronic aspiration.[43]

Mucositis

Severe oral and laryngeal mucositis is often encountered in children undergoing chemotherapy for malignancy or bone marrow transplantation. Most of the time it is self-limited and resolves. Occasionally a child has a severe mucosal response resulting in marked edema and oral or pharyngeal bleeding. These children often require intubation to control the airway. Laryngoscopy performed often reveals severe supraglottic edema and blood clots, resulting in airway obstruction. These intubations are quite challenging and it is best to be prepared with other alternatives to achieve airway control, including a tracheotomy. Once intubated, bleeding will often continue until the marrow is able to produce white blood cells. To control bleeding in these children, we have tried carbon dioxide laser coagulation of the oral pharynx and packing of the oral pharynx once the child is intubated with gauze soaked in 0.25% phenylephrine. These measures, if successful, are at best temporary until the patient is able to produce an adequate number of white blood cells (> 500). Tracheotomy has been performed in these patients but the bleeding from the oral and hypopharynx will continue. It has been our experience that tracheotomy offers little help in these patients and that those who go on to require a tracheotomy because of the length of intubation often do not survive.

Acquired neurologic injury of the pediatric larynx

Vocal cord paralysis

Vocal cord paralysis in the newborn is not uncommon and noted by Holinger *et al.* to be the second most

Table 17.2 Differential diagnosis for an infant presenting with vocal cord paralysis

Congenital
CNS
Arnold–Chiari malformation
Hydrocephalus
Encephalocele
Meningomyelocele
Meningocele
Congenital absence nucleus ambiguus
Cardiovascular
Tetralogy of Fallot
Vascular ring
Dilated aorta (Ortner's)
Aortic arch anomalies (double arch, right arch with aberrant subclavian)
Transposition
Acquired
Non-infectious
Cardiothoracic procedure
Birth injury
Kernicterus
Infectious
Diphtheria
Polio
Rabies
Syphilis
Tuberculosis
Tetanus
Whooping cough

common pediatric laryngeal lesion following laryngomalacia.[31] One may suspect a unilateral lesion with a 'breathy' or 'soft cry' and a bilateral lesion with substernal and costal retractions as well as stridor. This will, however, vary by site as well as causation as not all unilateral lesions are an adductor paralysis and not all bilateral lesions result in an abductor paralysis. Acquired lesions in the pediatric age group are primarily unilateral, left-sided and result from cardiac surgery such as a patent ductus arteriosus ligation.[37] Other common acquired causes include birth trauma and central neurologic injury.

Diagnosis

The true clinical dilemma one encounters is sorting out a congenital lesion from an acquired one. It is important to elucidate the etiology as it often impacts on treatment.[9,15] The differential diagnosis for an infant presenting with vocal cord paralysis is large and presented in Table 17.2. One should initially begin with the history, including the child's delivery, to assess for associated birth trauma as well as a review of systems. Physical examination includes a bedside flexible laryngoscopy, which, in our experience, is quite easy to do even with a newborn. It may be of benefit to video record the flexible examination for frame-by-frame analysis as the infant examination is often hampered by rapid laryngeal motion.[73] It has been our experience that occasionally a stroboscopy through the flexible nasopharyngoscope in the infant or young child may be of benefit in helping to determine pathology. In the older child (5 years of age or older) it is possible to perform a stroboscopy using the standard size adult rigid laryngeal telescope.

Technique for direct laryngoscopy in the infant or child

If the cause of a weak cry or stridor in the newborn is unclear by bedside flexible endoscopy, then there should be a low threshold to follow through with a direct examination in the operating room. Anesthetic technique for rigid or flexible endoscopy in the infant or small child is difficult and best performed by experienced personnel. It is important that there be spontaneous ventilation and vocal cord movement and at the same time laryngospasm avoided or handled so as not to endanger the child. Our preference currently is to mask ventilate the child into a light plane of anesthesia with sevoflurane followed by an intravenous catheter placement. The inhalational agent is then turned off or reduced and propofol is titrated intravenously to the child's need so that he/she is spontaneously breathing but not responsive to painful stimuli. The usual starting dose begins at 200 μg/kg delivered with an infusion pump. The vocal cords are sprayed with 1% lidocaine without epinephrine prior to manipulation to help prevent laryngospasm. A rigid laryngoscope is inserted and oxygen or oxygen and an inhalational agent are insufflated through the laryngoscope or via a nasopharyngeal tube. The laryngoscope can be suspended and a rigid telescope passed to examine the subglottis and trachea. Additionally, a microscope can be used to examine and manipulate the glottis under finer detail. Vocal cord motion is noted and the arytenoid joint palpated. It is not uncommon in our experience for posterior glottic stenosis to be misdiagnosed as unilateral or bilateral vocal cord paralysis.[10,57] If it is unclear an electromyography (EMG) can be performed in any age child. Small hook electrodes are placed under direct visualization into the vocalis muscle. Electrical silence within the first 2 weeks of birth would indicate congenital absence of innervation. A normal EMG may indicate posterior glottic stenosis as opposed to neurologic injury.

Additional workup

In addition to a thorough history and physical examination, an important question remains as to causation in order to make the diagnosis. If a child has had a thoracic procedure, the cause is obvious. In the infant and small child where the cause is not so obvious, central pathology should be carefully ruled out and magnetic resonance imaging of the head considered, particularly in the child with bilateral vocal cord paralysis.[5]

Management

The management of acquired unilateral or bilateral vocal cord paralysis in the infant or child is difficult due to the limited size of the airway as well as neurologic immaturity. All initial approaches should be conservative as over 70% of these cases will spontaneously resolve within the first 6 months of injury but possibly even years later.[67,70,73] Unilateral adductor paralysis is often asymptotic but can result in problematic aspiration, particularly when other cranial nerve palsies are involved. In cases of aspiration, it may be beneficial to perform an initial Gelfoam injection. This can be followed up with a more permanent substance in the future.[31] If the vocal cord is permanently damaged then in our opinion this substance should be fat in children. Gelfoam injection in the infant has not been discussed in the literature but is performed by the author in order to avoid a tracheotomy in an aspirating child. It is technically more challenging with an increased risk for airway obstruction. An open approach thyroplasty with implant placement has not been discussed in children and is not used by this author. Although technically easy to do, one should worry about unfavorable migration of the implant in the growing laryngotracheal complex over the long term.[44] There is also the issue of accurate implant placement because the procedure would be done under general anesthesia in this age group.

In the case of acquired bilateral vocal cord paralysis with marked airway obstruction the standard of care today is still a tracheotomy.[49] If the child is clinically doing well, despite a reduced glottic airway and follow-up is good, then it is reasonable to do nothing but follow the patient.[46] If one is unsure whether the injury is temporary or permanent then one should wait 2 years before undertaking corrective surgical intervention or performing serial laryngeal EMG to document total deinnervation. In the case of a permanent injury in a child with significant airway obstruction and tracheotomy dependence, three main surgical options exist for the child:

- arytenoidectomy and/or cordectomy;
- vocal cord lateralization; and
- laryngeal reinnervation.

Laryngeal reinnervation by both the nerve muscle pedicle technique or by an ansa cervicalis to recurrent nerve anastomosis has been described in young children with varying degrees of success.[11,50] Arytenoidopexy through a lateral external approach has also been reported in children, also with varying degrees of success.[48] Arytenoidectomy, with or without posterior cordotomy, has also been reported in young children.[6,10] There is no single best way to manage this problem in children. Our current preference in a tracheotomy-dependent child is to be convinced that the lesion is permanent. For us this is a minimum of 2 years followed by EMG documentation of denervation. In consultation with the parents, our current preference is an ansa cervicalis nerve to recurrent laryngeal nerve anastomosis as described by Crumley.[11] If this fails, we would follow with a destructive technique such as an arytenoidectomy with posterior cordotomy as described by Ossoff *et al.*[52]

Chronic aspiration in the pediatric patient

One of the more challenging problems encountered in pediatric otolaryngology is the management of a child with chronic aspiration. Acquired forms are usually the result of trauma and central neurologic injury with multiple cranial nerve palsies. It is important in these children to understand the neuropathology as well as the social situation and parental desires so that one can have an adequate treatment plan.

In the case of severe aspirations, secondary to multiple cranial neuropathies, placement of a tracheotomy tube for deep suctioning has been the traditional approach. Often one will place a cuffed tube in the child in the hope of trapping secretions above the cuff. Often there is soiling around the rim of the cuff with continued aspiration. In addition, there is damage over time to the tracheal walls, which become softer and more pliable secondary to cuff pressure. These children often need aggressive pulmonary toilet which is labor intensive and therefore less than an ideal method of management.

Other options include a tracheal diversion, tracheal separation or salivary reduction surgery. The first two options are the procedures of choice if the child is unable to communicate verbally. Although a narrow field laryngectomy is an additional option, we do not use it because of the rare chance of recovery in even the most severely injured child. The procedures proposed by Lindeman and colleagues are the most widely used and our preference is a modification of the type II.[19] Essentially, our approach is to separate the trachea between the third and fourth tracheal rings, removing the third ring but saving the perichondrium as the first layer of closure for the proximal pouch. The second tracheal ring is then closed over this perichondrial pouch and the proximal laryngotracheal complex is left as a blind stump in the neck while the distal tracheal end is brought out as a stoma. In all cases done to date there has been a total relief of aspiration and improvement in pulmonary function. The procedure is reversible by an end-to-end tracheal anastomosis, which we have performed in a few cases.

In cases where the child is verbally communicating and laryngotracheal separation is less desirable, salivary reduction may be of great benefit in either preventing the need for a tracheotomy or in reducing tracheal soiling. Pharmacologic salivary reduction by scopolamine or glycopyrrolate is usually of temporary benefit. Bilateral tympanic neurectomy is an additional option but also usually of temporary benefit as, over time, salivary production returns. Bilateral submandibular gland excision with bilateral parotid duct ligation will usually reduce salivary production enough to avoid the need for a tracheotomy or allow the use of a cuffless tube in cases where a cuffed tube was used previously.[24]

Pediatric tracheotomy

Many of the laryngeal disorders discussed above require placement of a tracheotomy tube at some point. The performance and care of a tracheotomy in the infant and small child is different from that in the adult and because of the increased risk of mortality following a tracheotomy in children it is important to understand these differences.

Technique

The preferred technique is described by Myers *et al.*[47] Although, it is ideal to have the child intubated, it is not always possible and therefore performance over a masked airway or laryngeal masked airway may be required. It is optimal for the child to be in a position where the neck is extended if possible. This is accomplished by the placement of a shoulder roll and by the anesthesiologist holding two fingers under the chin or by using tape to pull the chin up. The pediatric larynx is softer and covered by fat and therefore the identification of landmarks can be difficult. The suprasternal notch is a reliable landmark and the incision whether horizontal or vertical should be one finger breadth above the sternal notch or higher. Because of the higher incidence in small children of innominate arteries that run above the manubrium it is safer in our opinion to stay high with the dissection. The distal tracheal rings can easily be pulled upward into the neck of a small child if needed.

After the initial skin incision, the next step is to remove fat. Unlike the normal adult neck, the infant neck has a lot of subcutaneous fat and removal is best accomplished with a pick-up and needle tip electrocautery. Fat is removed until strap muscles are encountered. Blunt or electrocautery dissection is then continued in the midline as in a standard adult tracheotomy until the tracheal rings are encountered. The thyroid gland can also be approached similarly to an adult by retraction or ligation of the thyroid isthmus. The tracheal rings in a small child are very soft and can be mistaken for the esophagus or carotid artery. In fact an esophagus with a feeding tube can feel similar to an infant trachea. It is important that the surgeon recognizes tracheal cartilage prior to any incision.

Once the trachea is encountered, it is important that stay sutures be placed lateral to the proposed vertical tracheal wall incision. Using 3-0 or 4-0 permanent sutures and a small curved needle, sutures are placed around two tracheal rings in a vertical direction. Once these are placed, they are used as traction for the tracheal wall incision. This is an important maneuver as it is easy to cut through the posterior membranous wall of an infant trachea. The stay sutures pull the anterior wall away and provide countertraction. The stay sutures are brought out and taped to the anterior chest wall and removed one week later following the first tracheotomy tube change.

Table 17.3 ISO sizes for neonatal and pediatric tracheotomy tubes

Internal diameter (mm)	*Length (mm)*
Neonatal tracheotomy tube	
3.0	30
3.5	32
4.0	34
4.5	36
Pediatric tracheotomy tube	
3.0	39
3.5	40
4.0	41
4.5	42
5.0	44
5.5	46

The system for choosing a pediatric tracheal tube size has often led to confusion. Recently there has been agreement by most manufacturers to use the ISO designation of internal diameter for labeling pediatric tracheal tubes (Table 17.3). Also available in the smaller internal diameters are neonatal tubes that are a few millimeters shorter than their pediatric counterpart. It is important in a small child that either an endoscopic or radiographic assessment be made at the time of the tracheotomy tube placement to determine that it is the proper distance from the carina. In all cases a postoperative chest radiograph should be taken to rule out a pneumothorax.

Postoperative care varies from the adult in that there is no inner cannula and therefore the tube must be changed at certain intervals. The exact timing of changes vary by institution. We recommend changes every 2 weeks depending on the needs and past history of the child. Institutional recommendations can vary from a nightly change to every 4 weeks. It is imperative that multiple caregivers be trained in pediatric tracheotomy care and that the child never be left in the care of someone who is unable to change a tracheotomy tube. Overall mortality rates of children with a pediatric tracheotomy tube vary from 11% to 40%. The mortality rate directly related to the tracheotomy tube is reported at 0–3.4%.[18,27,75] Those children who are at high risk of mortality with a tracheotomy tube are mechanically ventilated, have pulmonary disease, usually under 1 year of age and tend to be preterm.[12,34,38]

References

1. Avidano MA, Singleton GT. Adjuvant drug strategies in the treatment of recurrent respiratory papillomatosis. *Otolaryngol Head Neck Surg* 1995; **112:** 197–202.
2. Bastian RW. Benign mucosal disorders, saccular disorders, and neoplasms. In: Cummings CW, ed. *Otolaryngology Head and Neck Surgery*, 1st edn. St Louis: Mosby, 1986: 1965–86.

3. Baugh R, Gilmore BB. Infectious croup: a critical review. *Otolaryngol Head Neck Surg* 1986; **95**: 40–6.
4. Berg S, Trollfors B, Nylen O, Hugosson S, Prellner K, Carenfelt C. Incidence, aetiology, and prognosis of acute epiglottitis in children and adults in Sweden. *Scand J Infect Dis* 1996; **28**: 261–4.
5. Boey HP, Cunningham MJ, Weber AL. Central nervous system imaging in the evaluation of children with true vocal cord paralysis. *Ann Otol Rhinol Layrngol* 1995; **104**: 76–7.
6. Bower CM, Choi SS, Cotton RT. Arytenoidectomy in children. *Ann Otol Rhinol Laryngol* 1994; **103**: 271–8.
7. Boyle JO, Coulthard SW, Mandel RM. Laryngeal involvement in disseminated coccidiomycoses. *Arch Otolaryngol Head Neck Surg* 1991; **117**: 433–8.
8. Calhoun K, Deskin R, Garza C *et al.* Long term airway sequelae in a pediatric burn population. *Laryngoscope* 1988; **98**: 721–5.
9. Cavanaugh F. Vocal palsies in children. *J Laryngol Otol* 1955; **69**: 399–402.
10. Cohen SR, Geller KA, Birns JW, Thompson JW. Laryngeal paralysis in children. *Ann Otol Rhinol Laryngol* 1982; **91**: 417–24.
11. Crumley RL. Update: ansa cervicalis to recurrent laryngeal nerve anastomosis for unilateral laryngeal paralysis. *Laryngoscope* 1991; **101**: 384–7.
12. Crysdale WS, Feldman RI, Naito K. Tracheotomies: a 10 year experience in 319 children. *Ann Otol Rhinol Laryngol* 1988; **97**: 439–43.
13. Damm M, Eckel HE, Jungehulsing M, Roth B. Airway endoscopy in the interdisciplinary management of acute epiglottitis. *Int J Pediatr Otorhinolaryngol* 1996; **38**: 41–51.
14. DeBoeck K. Croup: a review. *Eur J Pediatr* 1995; **154**: 432–6.
15. Dedo DD, Dedo HH. Neurogenic diseases of the larynx. In: Bluestone CB, Stool SE, eds. *Pediatric Otolaryngology*, 2nd edn. Philadelphia: Saunders, 1990: 1172–7.
16. Denny FW, Clyde FW, Clyde WA Jr. Acute lower respiratory tract infections in nonhospitalized children. *J Pediatr* 1986; **108**: 635–45.
17. Denny FW, Murphy TF, Clyde WA, Collier AM, Henderson FW. Croup: an 11-year study in a pediatric practice. *Pediatrics* 1983; **71**: 871–6.
18. Dutton JM, Palmer PM, McCulloch TM, Smith RJH. Mortality in the pediatric patient with tracheotomy. *Head Neck* 1995; **17**: 403–8.
19. Eisele DW, Yarington CT Jr, Lindeman RC, Larrabee WF Jr. The tracheoesophageal diversion and laryngotracheal separation procedures for treatment of intractable aspiration. *Am J Surg* 1989; **157**: 230–6.
20. Erisen L, Fagan JJ, Myers EN. Late recurrences of laryngeal papillomatosis. *Arch Otolaryngol Head Neck Surg* 1996; **122**: 942–4.
21. Fisher EW, Richards A, Anderson G, Albert DM. Laryngeal candidiasis: a cause of airway obstruction in the immunocompromised child. *J Laryngol Otol* 1992; **106**: 168–70.
22. Geelhoed GC, MacDonald WBG. Oral and inhaled steroids in croup. *Pediatr Pulmonol* 1995; **20**: 355–61.
23. Geelhoed GC, MacDonald WBG. Oral dexamethasone in the treatment of croup. *Pediatr Pulmonol* 1995; **20**: 362–8.
24. Gerber ME, Gaugler MD, Myer CM III, Cotton RT. Chronic aspiration in children. When are bilateral submandibular gland excision and parotid duct ligation indicated? *Arch Otolaryngol Head Neck Surg* 1996; **122**: 1368–71.
25. Gonzalez Valdepena H, Wald ER, Rose E, Ungkanont K, Casselbrant ML. Epiglottitis and *Haemophilus influenzae* immunization: The Pittsburgh experience – a five year review. *Pediatrics* 1995; **96**: 424–7.
26. Havaldar PV. Dexamethasone in laryngeal diphtheritic croup. *Ann Trop Paediatr* 1997; **17**: 21–3.
27. Hawkins DB, Williams EH. Tracheostomy in infants and young children. *Laryngoscope* 1976; **86**: 331–40.
28. Healy GB, Gelber RD, Trowbridge AL. Treatment of recurrent respiratory papillomatosis with human leukocyte interferon. *N Engl J Med* 1988; **319**: 401–6.
29. Herndon D, Thompson P, Linares H, Niehaus G. Postgraduate course: respiratory injury. Part I: Incidence, mortality, pathogenesis and treatment of pulmonary injuries. *J Burn Care Rehabil* 1986; **7**: 184–91.
30. Hjuler IM, Hansen MB, Olsen B, Renneberg J. Bacterial colonization of the larynx and trachea in healthy children. *Acta Paediatr* 1995; **84**: 566–8.
31. Holinger LD, Holinger PC, Holinger PH. Etiology of bilateral abductor vocal cord paralysis: a review of 389 cases. *Ann Otol* 1976; **85**: 428–31.
32. Jones J, Rosenberg D. Management of laryngotracheal thermal trauma in children. *Laryngoscope* 1995; **105**: 540–2.
33. Kashima H, Leventhal B, Clark K *et al.* Interferon alfa-N1 (Wellferon) in juvenile onset recurrent respiratory papillomatosis: results of a randomized study in twelve collaborative institutions. *Laryngoscope* 1988; **98**: 334–40.
34. Kenna MA, Reilly JS, Stool SE. Tracheotomy in the preterm infant. *Ann Otol Rhinol Laryngol* 1987; **96**: 68–71.
35. Kunkel NC, Baker D. Use of racemic epinephrine, dexamethasone, and mist in the outpatient management of croup. *Pediatr Emerg Care* 1996; **12**: 156–9.
36. Leventhal BG, Kashima HK, Weck PW *et al.* Randomized surgical adjuvant trial of Alfa-n1 in recurrent papillomatosis. *Arch Otolaryngol Head Neck Surg* 1988; **114**: 1163–9.
37. Levine BA, Jacobs IN, Wetmore RF, Handler SD. Vocal cord injection in children with unilateral vocal cord paralysis. *Arch Otolaryngol Head Neck Surg* 1995; **121**: 116–19.
38. Line WS Jr, Hawkins DB, MacLaughlin EF, Kahlstrom EJ, Ensley JL. Tracheotomy in infants and young children: the changing perspective 1970–1985. *Laryngoscope* 1986; **96**: 510–15.
39. Lippman SM, Donovan DT, Frankenthaler RA *et al.* 13-cis-retinoic acid plus interferon alpha-2a in recurrent respiratory papillomatosis. *J Natl Cancer Inst* 1994; **86**: 859–61.
40. Lopez Aguado D, Perez Pinero B, Betancor L, Mendez A, Campos Banales E. Acyclovir in the treatment of laryngeal papillomatosis. *Int J Pediatr Otolaryngol* 1991; **21**: 269–74.
41. Mancao MY, Sindel LJ, Richardson PH, Silver FM. Herpetic croup: two case reports and a review of the literature. *Acta Paediatr* 1996; **85**: 118–20.

42. McGlennen RC, Adams GL, Lewis CM, Faras AJ, Ostrow RS. Pilot trial of ribavirin for the treatment of laryngeal papillomatosis. *Head Neck* 1993; **15**: 504–13.
43. Miller R, Gray S, Cotton R, Myer CM III. Airway reconstruction following laryngotracheal thermal trauma. *Laryngoscope* 1988; **98**: 826–9.
44. Mitskavich MT, Rimell FL, Shapiro AM, Post CJ, Kapadia SB. Laryngotracheal reconstruction using microplates in a porcine model with subglottic stenosis. *Laryngoscope* 1996; **106**: 301–5.
45. Mounts P, Kashima H. Association of human papillomavirus subtype and clinical course in respiratory papillomatosis. *Laryngoscope* 1984; **94**: 28–33.
46. Murty GE, Shinkwin C, Gibbin KP. Bilateral vocal fold paralysis in infants: tracheostomy or not? *J Laryngol Otol* 1994; **108**: 329–31.
47. Myers EN, Stool SE, Johnson JT. Technique of tracheotomy. In: Myers E, Stool S, Johnson J, eds. *Tracheotomy*. New York: Churchill Livingstone, 1985: 113–24.
48. Narcy P. Arytenoidopexy for laryngeal paralysis in children. *Int J Pediatric Otorhinolaryngol* 1995; **32(Suppl)**: S101–2.
49. Narcy P, Contencin P, Viala P. Surgical treatment for laryngeal paralysis in infants and children. *Ann Otol Rhinol Laryngol* 1990; **99**: 124–8.
50. Nunez DA, Hanson DR. Laryngeal reinnervation in children: the Leeds experience. *Ear Nose Throat J* 1993; **72**: 542–3.
51. Ossoff RH, Werkhaven JA, Dere H. Soft tissue complications of laser surgery for recurrent respiratory papillomatosis. *Laryngoscope* 1991; **101**: 1162–6.
52. Ossoff RH, Duncavage JA, Shapshay SM, Krespi YP, Sisson GA Sr. Endoscopic laser arytenoidectomy revisited. *Ann Otol Rhinol Laryngol* 1990; **99**: 764–71.
53. Popovic T, Wharton M, Wenger ID, McIntyre I, Wachsmuth IK. Are we ready for diphtheria? A report from the Diphtheria Diagnostic Workshop. *J Infect Dis* 1995; **171**: 765–7.
54. Pou AM, Rimell FL, Jordan JA *et al.* Adult respiratory papillomatosis: human papillomavirus type and viral coinfections as predictors of prognosis. *Ann Otol Rhinol Laryngol* 1995; **104**: 758–62.
55. Ramadan HH, Wax MK. Laryngeal tuberculosis. *Arch Otolaryngol Head Neck Surg* 1995; **121**: 109–12.
56. Richardson BE, Morrison VA, Gapany M. Invasive aspergillosis of the larynx: case report and review of the literature. *Otolaryngol Head Neck Surg* 1996; **114**: 471–3.
57. Rimell FL, Dohar JE. Endoscopic management of pediatric posterior glottic stenosis. *Ann Otol Laryngol Rhinol* 1998; **107**: 285–90.
58. Rimell FL, Maisel R, Dayton V. In situ hybridization and laryngeal papillomas. *Ann Otol Rhinol Laryngol* 1992; **101**: 119–26.
59. Rimell FL, Shapiro AM, Mitskavich MT, Modreck P, Post JC, Maisel RH. Pediatric fiberoptic laser rigid bronchoscopy. *Otolaryngol Head Neck Surg* 1996; **114**: 413–17.
60. Rimell FL, Shoemaker DL, Pou AM, Jordan JA, Post JC, Ehrlich GD. Analysis of pediatric respiratory papillomatosis: prognostic role of viral typing and cofactors. *Laryngoscope* 1997; **107**: 915–18.
61. Saleh EM. Complications of treatment of recurrent laryngeal papillomatosis with the carbon dioxide laser in children. *J Laryngol Otol* 1992; **106**: 715–18.
62. Schwenzfeier CW, Fechner RE. Herpes simplex of the epiglottis. *Arch Otolaryngol* 1976; **102**: 374–6.
63. Shapiro AM, Rimell FL, Shoemaker D, Pou A, Stool SE. Tracheotomy in children with juvenile-onset recurrent respiratory papillomatosis: the Children's Hospital of Pittsburgh experience. *Ann Otol Rhinol Laryngol* 1996; **105**: 1–5.
64. Shapshay SM, Rebeiz EE, Bohigian RK, Hybles RL. Benign lesions of the larynx: should the laser be used? *Laryngoscope* 1990; **100**: 953–7.
65. Stroh BC, Faust RA, Rimell FL. Results of esophageal biopsies performed during triple endoscopy in the pediatric patient. *Arch Otolaryngol Head Neck Surg* 1998; **124**: 545–9.
66. Super DM, Cartelli NA, Brooks LJ, Lembo RM, Kumar ML. A prospective randomized double-blind study to evaluate the effect of dexamethasone in acute laryngotracheitis. *J Pediatr* 1989; **115**: 323–9.
67. Swift AC, Rogers J. Vocal cord paralysis in children. *J Laryngol Otol* 1987; **101**: 169–71.
68. Taussig LM, Castro O, Beaudry PH. Treatment of laryngotracheitis (croup). *Am J Dis Child* 1975; **129**: 790–3.
69. Tibbals J, Shann FA, Landau LI. Placebo-controlled trial of prednisolone in children intubated for croup. *Lancet* 1992; **340**: 745–8.
70. Tucker HM. Vocal cord paralysis in children, principles in management. *Ann Otol Rhinol Layrngol* 1986; **95**: 618–21.
71. Wagener JS, Landay LI, Olinsky A, Phelan PD. Management of children hospitalized for laryngotracheobronchitis. *Pediatr Pulmonol* 1986; **2**: 159–62.
72. Waki EY, Madgy DN, Belenky WM, Gower VC. The incidence of gastroesophageal reflux in recurrent croup. *Int J Pediatr Otorhinolaryngol* 1995; **32**: 223–32.
73. Waters KA, Woo P, Mortelliti AJ, Colton R. Assessment of the infant airway with videorecorded flexible laryngoscopy and the objective analysis of vocal fold abduction. *Otolaryngol Head Neck Surg* 1996; **114**: 554–61.
74. Westley CR, Cotton EK, Brooks JG. Nebulized racemic epinephrine by IPPB for the treatment of croup. *Am J Dis Child* 1978; **132**: 484–7.
75. Wetmore RF, Handler SD, Potsic WP. Pediatric tracheostomy: experience during the past decade. *Ann Otol Rhinol Laryngol* 1982; **91**: 628–32.
76. Wurtele P. Acute epiglottitis in children: results of a large-scale anti-*Haemophilus* type B immunization program. *J Otolaryngol* 1995; **24**: 92–7.
77. Yeh V, Hopp ML, Goldstein NS, Meyer RD. Herpes simplex chronic laryngitis and vocal cord lesions in a patient with acquired immunodeficiency syndrome. *Ann Otol Rhinol Laryngol* 1994; **103**: 726–31.
78. Young N, Finn A, Powell C. Group B streptococcal epiglottitis. *Pediatr Infect Dis J* 1996; **15**: 95–6.

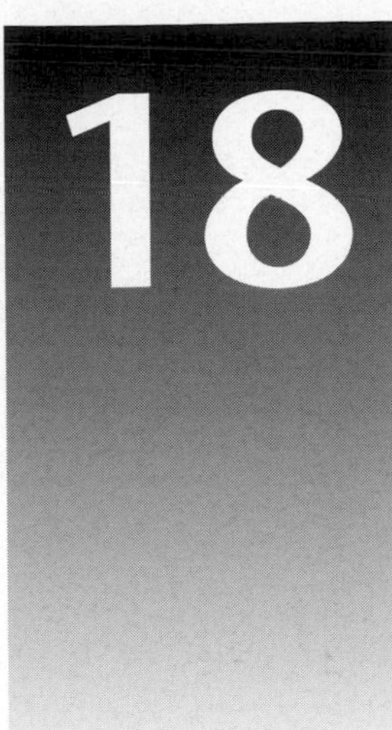

Childhood inhalation of laryngotracheal foreign bodies

David Albert

Modern society is less likely to accept any adverse incident as a true accident or 'act of God' but is fond of finding and apportioning blame. The circumstances that lead up to a child inhaling something are multiple and only some are under our control. Careful study of the epidemiology of choking and inhalation does, however, offer some hope that modification of our environment and behavior can reduce the incidence of choking deaths and nonfatal choking incidents. Choking is usually due to food blocking the larynx and is sometimes fatal. Almost anything of an appropriate size can be inhaled into the tracheobronchial tree but this is usually nonfatal. The three main groups of inhaled objects in children are toy parts, food and everyday objects such as coins. Parental awareness via education needs to go hand in hand with regulation for toys and foodstuffs.

The education of parents and child carers in the first aid management of a choking incident is at present sporadic. A more coordinated education policy could save a few lives per year. There also needs to be heightened awareness amongst medical personnel of the veiled nature of many of the signs and symptoms of inhaled foreign bodies and the complexities and challenges of bronchoscopic removal. Good history-taking and targeted examination as well as radiology and bronchoscopy are all clinical skills needed in the management of foreign body inhalation.

This chapter discusses the epidemiology and avoidance of foreign body inhalation and choking in children before focusing on the medical presentation, assessment and management of the child.

Incidence

In 1995 the UK Department of Trade and Industry commissioned a report on Choking Hazards for Children in the European Community (EC), which reported 400 deaths from choking each year in the EC.[19] There were also 50 000 nonfatal choking accidents per year, with higher accident rates in the south (see Table 18.1).

In the EC, the death rate from inhalation in children has fallen from 18 per million children to 9 per million between 1982 and 1993, mostly due to a reduction in nonfood-related inhalation, presumably as a result of toy regulation and heightened awareness. Food accounts for 84% of choking deaths and 46% of nonfatal choking incidents.

The very young child is particularly at risk with 73% of food deaths occurring in the first year of life and 90% in the first 3 years. Nonfatal inhalations are more evenly spread throughout the first 10 years with a smaller peak aged 2 years.

Geographic incidence

The same report[19] demonstrated that the death rate showed an increase from the north to the south areas within the EC with lowest rates in Sweden and highest in Greece. However, the report also stressed that the quality of data varied between different countries so that interpretation required care. Differing diets, toys or parental supervision could explain geographic differences.

Table 18.1 Choking deaths and accidents involving children under 10 in the European Community

	Deaths		*Accidents*	
	Rate (no. per year per million)	*Number per year*	*Rate (no. per year per million)*	*Number per year*
Austria	12	11	1020	969
Belgium	11	13	1640	1990
Denmark	6	4	1480	907
Finland	5	3	1190	713
France	5	41	*1230**	9244
Germany	12	94	*1230**	9995
Greece	34	36	*1230**	1294
Ireland	10	5	1250	610
Italy	10	55	*1230**	7123
Netherlands	5	11	850	1672
Portugal	24	28	3590	4221
Spain	21	81	1230	4819
Sweden	4	4	1230	1287
UK	5	34	880	6140
Average	**10**	**418**	**630**	**50 984**

*Approximate figures

Types of foreign body

Foods

Whether a food will lodge in the larynx, causing spasm and asphyxia, or pass through the cords into the tracheobronchial tree depends largely on the size of item (Fig 18.1a,b). Sweets, and pieces of hotdog or other meat are particularly likely to lodge in the larynx, whilst peanuts and seeds tend to cause nonfatal inhalation into the tracheobronchial tree. Hotdog inhalation as a fatal choking episode is a particular problem in the USA because of the vast numbers eaten, often when moving about, thus increasing the chance of accidental inhalation. Peanuts are commonly inhaled[13] and are very irritant to the tracheobronchial mucosa but do not in general cause fatal choking.

Toys and toy parts

A lot of effort has been spent in regulating the construction of toys so that they do not contain small parts that can be inhaled (Fig 18.2a,b). Nonetheless, there are numerous toys, such as construction kits, which rely on small parts for their very complexity and challenge. These are sold as not suitable for children below a certain age.

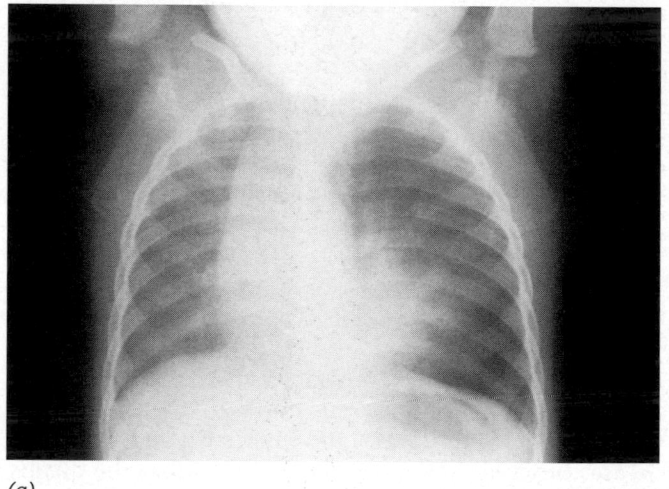
(a)

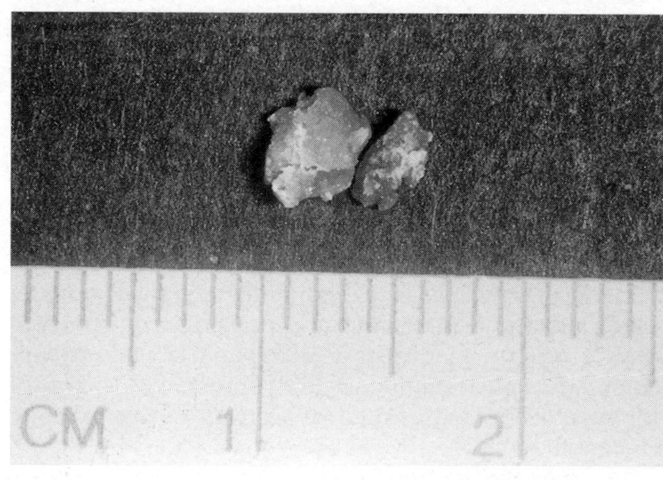

(b)

Figure 18.1 *Organic foreign body – peanut inhalation. (a) Radiograph, obstructive emphysema. (b) Peanut removed in two pieces.*

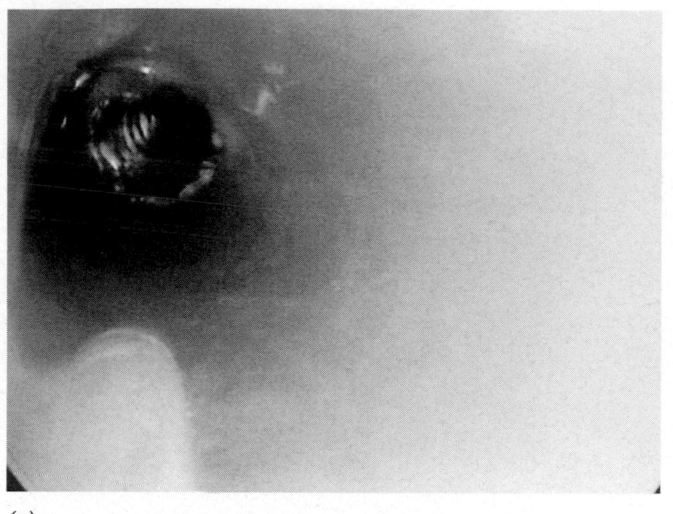

(a)

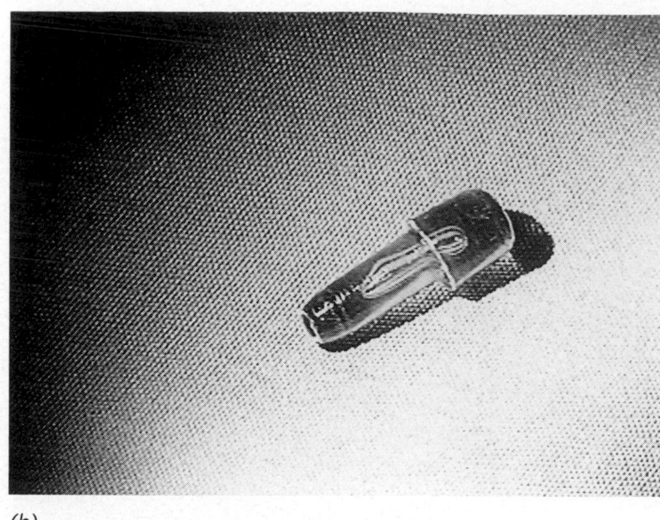

(b)

Figure 18.2 *Plastic foreign body inhalation: (a) bronchoscopic view; (b) peg from child's board game.*

However, in a family with children of multiple age groups it requires great vigilance from parents to ensure that each child is playing with age-appropriate toys.

Everyday objects

There are numerous papers describing bizarre and unusual inhaled foreign bodies (Fig 18.3a,b,c). For an object to feature highly in the list of commonly inhaled foreign bodies, it must be itself common, it must again be of the right size and finally, it is usually one that is often placed in the mouth for 'safe keeping'. Examples would include sewing pins, turban pins,[28] headscarf pins in the Middle East,[26] jewelry, pens, ring pulls, drawing pins, nails, screws, buttons and hair clips.[19] Plastic pen tops were a problem but simply making a hole or airway through the pen tops has been effective in reducing deaths. Insect inhalation must rank highly as a true accident or 'act of God'; certainly it would be difficult to know whom else to blame unless the insect is perceived as the guilty party.

Anatomic considerations

At 1 year of age the trachea has a diameter of 7 mm and the cricoid about 6 mm, by 4 years the trachea is 9 mm and the cricoid 10 mm and by 9 years the airway has grown a further 1–2 mm. A 3–4-year-old open mouth can just accept objects of 25 mm. For children below this age the critical size range for laryngeal obstruction as opposed to tracheobronchial inhalation is 5–25 mm. In simple terms, any foreign body within the range 5–25 mm presents a risk of laryngeal obstruction and death with items smaller than 5 mm presenting a risk of inhalation.

Legal issues

As stated earlier, 84% of EC choking deaths are due to aspirated food such as nuts, sweets and meat. The remaining nonfood deaths are due to a wide variety of objects such as coins, conkers and stones, as well as toys such as marbles, plastic balls and toy figures. Legislation and regulation aimed at making toys safer will hopefully reduce the number of nonfatal choking accidents but may have little impact on deaths.

At present the European Directive on the Safety of Toys (88/378/EEC) defines the size of toys, their components and any parts of them which can be detached with a specified force. Toys that do not pass these tests must be labeled as unsuitable for children less than 36 months old.

The test designed to assess whether detachable components of a toy or the toys themselves are small enough to present a hazard for children under 36 months is the truncated cylinder test. The cylinder has an internal diameter of 31.7 mm (larger than the 25 mm opening of a 3-year-old's mouth). The cylinder is 57.1 mm long and is truncated obliquely in its lower half (Fig. 18.4). No toy (or removable, liberated component, or fragment of toy) should be small enough to fit entirely within the cylinder without being compressed.

A historical perspective – changes in bronchoscopic practice over the last 40 years

Paul Holinger *et al.*,[12] writing in the *Illinois Medical Journal* in 1948, analyzed 1026 patient records following foreign body removal from the tracheobronchial tree and esophagus. He described the complications of pneumothorax,

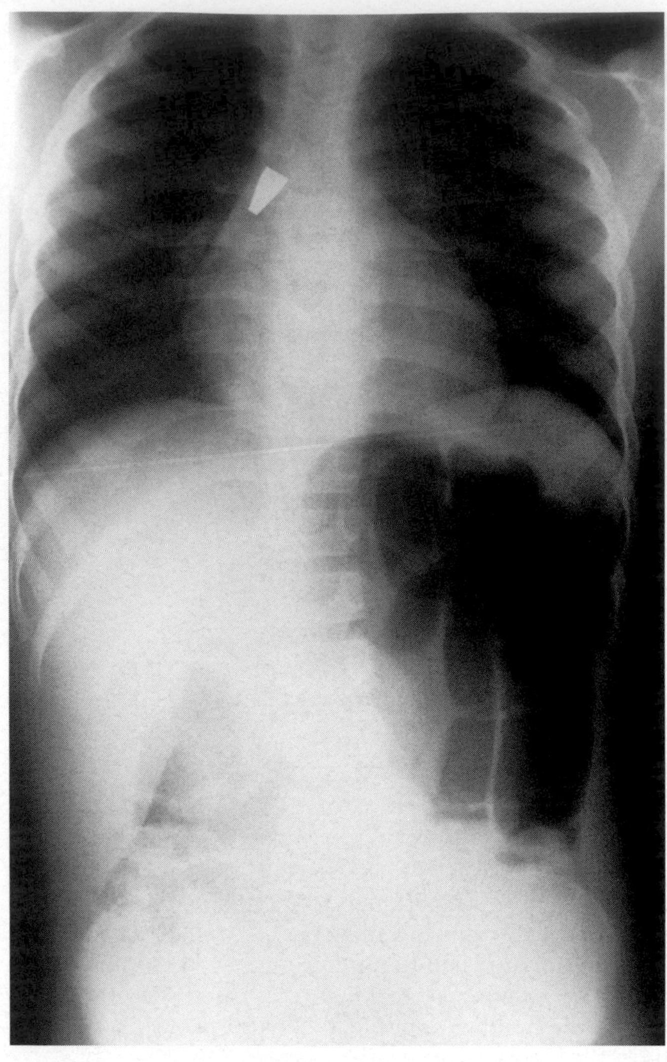

(a)

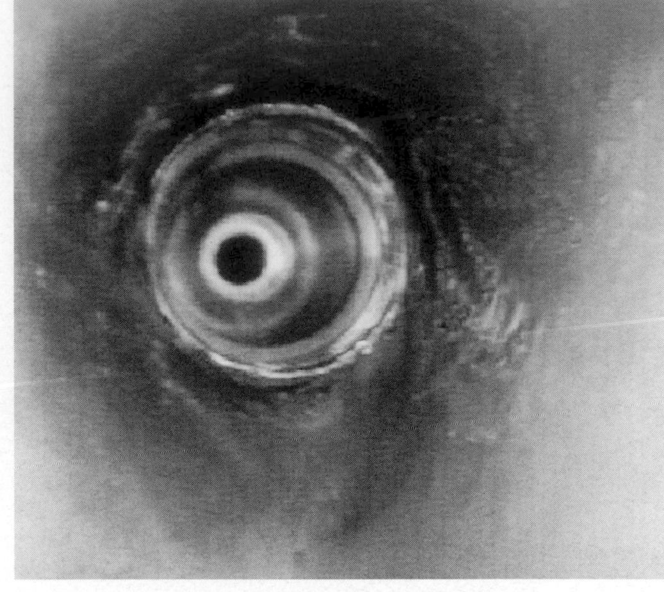

(b)

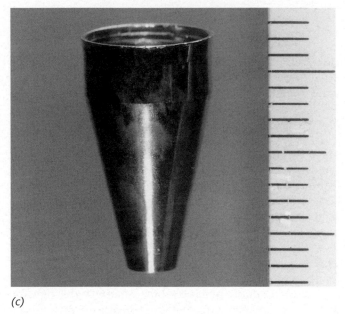

(c)

Figure 18.3 *Metal foreign body inhalation. (a) Radiograph, radiopaque foreign body. (b) Bronchoscopic view, metal end of ball point pen. (c) Foreign body removed.*

obstructive emphysema, atelectasis and lung abscess. Laryngeal edema was a feared complication of bronchoscopic removal so, following Jackson's dictum, the duration of each bronchoscopy was limited. He comments (with masked gratification) that in his series tracheotomy was not required because of laryngeal edema. However, four patients had required tracheotomies at other institutions.

Inglis and Wagner[14] reported a reduction in the complication rate over a 20-year period associated with bronchial foreign bodies at the Children's Hospital, Seattle due to improved anesthesia and endoscopic equipment.

Some authors[21–23] who currently have a major interest in paediatric foreign body inhalation, stress the need for medical familiarity with the condition and for parental education to help with prevention.

Assessment of the child with a suspected foreign body (Table 18.2)

History

Awareness is the key to prompt diagnosis, both in near-death choking episodes with a foreign body in the larynx and in nonfatal inhalation with a foreign body in the tracheobronchial tree. In either case the parent should be closely questioned for a history of possible foreign body inhalation. This can range from a well-remembered

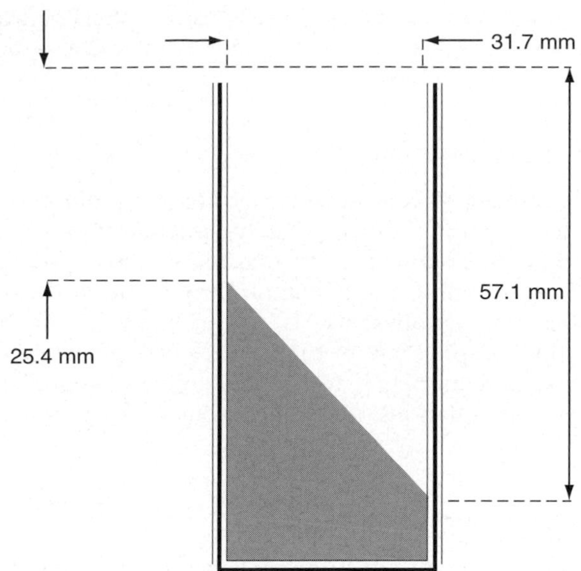

Figure 18.4 *Truncated cylinder to test size of toys: 'small parts cylinder'.*

observed choking episode, to a missing toy or a recollection of the child playing with something in his mouth. This information is often not volunteered.

With a foreign body impacted in the larynx, the airway will be obstructed to a variable degree from the foreign body itself and from secondary laryngospasm. Inspiratory *stridor* will be present so long as there is sufficient airflow to be turbulent to generate the noise. Parents may notice transient stridor that improves. This is not necessarily a good sign as the foreign body may have moved distally or the airway become so minimal that the noise is inaudible. With an obstructed airway, the child will initially be making *violent inspiratory efforts* with recession, though once the child loses consciousness the movements will cease and irreversible brain damage occurs soon after. If, however, the laryngeal foreign body allows a reasonable airway around it, a *cough* or *change in voice* may be the only symptoms.

With an inhaled foreign body in the tracheobronchial tree there is often a short-lived spell of coughing, choking, gagging or wheezing. Short-lived cyanosis can occur immediately after aspiration and was found in nearly 30% in one series.[16] This often settles, as the airway becomes relatively tolerant of even organic foreign bodies. There may be tachypnea, temperature and malaise, indicating pneumonia, but the key to the diagnosis is that the *pneumonia* is *resistant* to treatment or *recurs* after treatment. Tracheal foreign bodies can cause audible stridor, usually expiratory or biphasic. The symptoms, however, are often very slight or even absent, raising few suspicions in the minds of parents and doctors alike. Many cases are mistakenly treated as asthma, as both conditions occur in the same age group.[5,10]

Examination (Table 18.3)

In an emergency situation, the larynx needs to be cleared prior to any history or examination. However, in the non-acute situation, *observing* the child at rest provides not only an initial assessment of the degree of respiratory distress and the characteristics of any stridor but also gives time to gain the child's confidence prior to any further examination.

Typically, inspiratory *stridor* is due to an extrathoracic obstruction such as larynx or high trachea with bronchial obstruction producing an expiratory stridor. Biphasic stridor can occur with obstruction anywhere in the tracheobronchial tree. Expiratory stridor may be absent but a prolonged expiratory phase may be present, indicating an intrathoracic obstruction. The site of the abnormal vibration can rarely be tracked down with the aid of a stethoscope, because of the variable transmission of sound through the thorax.

Subcostal, intercostal and suprasternal *recession* may occur separately or together and also be associated with

Table 18.2 Presenting symptoms

Immediate and transient symptoms
Coughing attack
Dyspnea
Vomiting
Cyanosis
Stridor
Hoarseness
Delayed and persistent symptoms
Dyspnea
Cough
Stridor/Wheeze
Hoarseness
Asymptomatic (30%)

Table 18.3 Differential diagnosis

Acute presentation
Asthma
Angioedema
Pneumothorax
Persistent or recurrent pneumonia
Bronchial mass or compression
Cystic fibrosis
Immotile cilia
Immunological deficiency
Stridor
Any cause of upper airway obstruction

Table 18.4 Radiological abnormalities

Radio-opaque foreign body
Pneumonia
Atelectasis/diffuse
Recurrent/resistant
Obstructive emphysema
Shifted mediastinum
Reduced diaphragmatic movement
Pneumothorax
Pneumomediastinum

seesaw respiration. The severity of recession is a better indicator of the severity of airway compromise than the degree of stridor, which can paradoxically become less obvious as obstruction worsens due to the diminishing airflow. *Pyrexia* is more likely if the presentation is delayed. *Cyanosis* is usually a late event and no comfort should be taken from the fact that a child still looks pink!

The ears, nose and throat should be examined last, with the usual caution not to examine the throat of child in whom epiglottitis is suspected. The ears and nose may harbor other foreign bodies, whilst in the throat there may be scratches, suggesting abortive parental attempts to remove a foreign body.

Finally it must be remembered that up to 30% may be asymptomatic.[16]

Special investigations (Table 18.4)

A *plain chest radiograph* may show air-trapping with obstructive emphysema (see Fig 18.1a) and mediastinal shift but will rarely demonstrate the foreign body (see Fig 18.1b) as most are radiolucent. Air trapping is due to a ball-valve effect in which air bypasses the foreign body on inspiration but is trapped distally as the airway collapses and is compressed on expiration by the increased intrathoracic pressure. With complete obstruction the air distal to the obstruction is absorbed and the lung collapses (atelectasis). Healy[10] describes decubitus views of the chest with the 'downside' of the chest not emptying on expiration if it is the affected side. Older children will cooperate with *inspiratory and expiratory views*[7] on a plain radiograph, which may show reduced diaphragmatic movement. In younger children, diaphragmatic screening with *videofluoroscopy* is indicated. If the foreign body is radiolucent and there is no significant obstruction to the airway, it is easy for diagnosis to be delayed. The radiograph may be normal in up to 30%[16] even with fluoroscopy.[27]

In *acute* airway obstruction, *O_2 saturation monitoring* is extremely helpful as it is noninvasive (unlike arterial blood gases) and yet much more sensitive than clinical estimation, as cyanosis is a very late event as described above.

Unusual presentations

Inhaled foreign bodies can be responsible for a number of pulmonary complications.[12] Rarely, pneumothorax can occur prior to endoscopy,[4,25,31] due to increased pressure or a collapsed lung, the pneumothorax *ex vacuo* theory. Subcutaneous emphysema is occasionally a result. Mediastinal emphysema in the absence of a pneumothorax suggests a bronchial tear.[3,24] Hemoptysis[6] represents infection, granulations or trauma from a sharp foreign body.

Summary of assessment

Awareness, a detailed history and examination and the help of an experienced radiologist should protect most children from an incorrect or delayed diagnosis of foreign body aspiration. If doubt exists after assessment, bronchoscopy should be performed. Indeed, some would argue that a proportion of endoscopies should be negative![17]

Management of the child with an inhaled foreign body

Emergency measures

Acute management at home

If a child is found unconscious, it is imperative to think of the possibility of a foreign body and clear the *A*irway before progressing to the *B*reathing and *C*irculation (the *ABC* of first aid).

The *Heimlich maneuver* (an abdominal squeeze to force the diaphragm up) has become established as the best technique for expelling an impacted laryngeal or subglottic foreign body[11] in adults and is now taught as part of a number of first aid resuscitative programs. Obviously care needs to be taken in smaller children to prevent abdominal damage so back slaps or chest thrusts with the child lying down along one's arm are preferable. Smaller children can be inverted so that gravity will assist the back slaps.

A *finger sweep* in the pharynx used to be taught as part of resuscitation, but can cause laryngospasm and pharyngeal tears.[15] A physician caught in that nightmare situation of a choking child and no laryngoscope could try to improvise with a flashlight (torch) and a spoon in an attempt to visualize the larynx.

Emergency cricothyrotomy is a straightforward surgical procedure but for the inexperienced physician or layman without the benefit of anesthesia, good light or proper equipment is hazardous. It may, however, be the only option if all else has failed.

Acute management in hospital

In the acute situation assessment, history-taking and active resuscitation will often proceed in parallel to stabilize the airway as expeditiously as possible. In the example of a child arriving in the emergency room with airway obstruction, the physician will be assessing the child for the degree of airway obstruction, at the same time as asking the mother for the length of history and whether there is any possibility of foreign body inhalation. The nurse will be checking the oxygen saturation and setting up humidified oxygen. Another member of the team may have to call and alert the operating room that the child may need intubation as well as calling the anesthesiologist and otolaryngologist. This situation clearly benefits from careful planning with most units having a protocol for how to deal with the stridulous airway-compromised child. The protocols vary considerably, some units insisting on the presence of an otolaryngologist at intubation in case a tracheotomy is needed whilst others have managed for many years without.

If a foreign body is suspected from the history and the child is desaturating significantly, the larynx will need to be examined urgently to exclude or remove a foreign body by whoever is available in the emergency room. If possible, however, it is better to wait for an experienced pediatric anesthetist to take the child to the operating room. This more controlled environment allows a careful examination and intubation (e.g. for epiglottitis) if required. The Heimlich maneuver, cricothyroidotomy and tracheotomy are alternatives that should be considered.

Medical and supportive therapy

In long-standing foreign bodies presenting with pneumonia, 24 hours of intensive antibiotics may be helpful in stabilizing the child prior to surgery and perhaps improving the surgical field. Physiotherapy should be avoided as the foreign body may be dislodged. This is a particular danger if the child has very poor respiratory function in the affected lung due to pneumonia or obstructive emphysema, and is therefore managing on virtually one lung alone. Rapid deterioration will occur if the foreign body is dislodged into the unaffected lung.

Endoscopy

Intubation and anesthesia[29]

Pediatric airway anesthesia for the extraction of foreign bodies is particularly challenging, especially if the foreign body has been present for some time with poor respiratory function in the affected lung. Any intubation has to be conducted with great care not to dislodge the foreign body further into the bronchus or into the unaffected lung. This can occur with high-pressure hand ventilation by mask, or during intubation, the tube itself can dislodge a tracheal foreign body. Jet ventilation should not be used for obvious reasons.

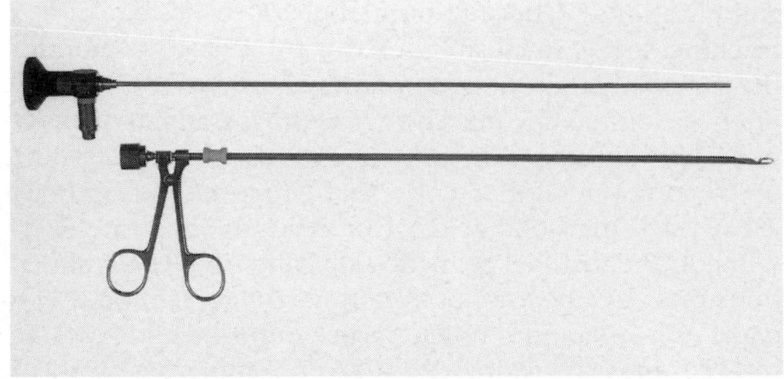

Figure 18.5 *Operating equipment: Storz peanut extraction forceps.*

The presence, in a small child, of a ventilating bronchoscope with the lumen partially occluded by the bronchoscopic forceps raises the airways resistance significantly and makes desaturation a hazard. This risk is heightened by the potential for shunting of poorly oxygenated blood from the affected lung.

Fiberoptic endoscopy

Flexible endoscopy[20] under sedation in an endoscopy suite is widely practiced by pediatricians and pulmonologists and is becoming more popular with otolaryngologists as an adjunct to rigid endoscopy. Grasping forceps and wire baskets[18] are used for foreign body extraction. The gold standard for foreign body extraction is, however, rigid endoscopy because it allows greater control. Despite this, a fiberscope also needs to be available in the operating room even if rigid endoscopy is planned, in case the rigid 'scope cannot reach. This can happen if there is distal tracheal stenosis, a small distal foreign body, or if the child is very small.

Rigid endoscopy[30]

A full range of bronchoscopic equipment is required with differing lengths and diameters of bronchoscope to suit the individual child. The 3.5 mm bronchoscope will only just accept the usual size of spaghetti sucker so, if possible, a 4 mm bronchoscope should be used (Storz have recently produced ultra-slim foreign body grasping forceps that will fit down a 2.5 mm bronchoscope). Several patterns of bronchoscopic grasping forceps may be required. The flexible side-arm forceps can be used if there is a distal foreign body or the child is very small. Whichever technique is employed, a high level of experience of normal pediatric endoscopy is required in the endoscopist, anesthesiologist and nursing staff.[2] If in doubt, it is better to refer to a center with sufficient experience as bronchoscopic removal is seldom an emergency. The equipment is all-important as the latest Hopkins rod telescopes passed through grasping forceps (Fig 18.5) give a superb view and are associated with fewer complications.[8] The addition of a video system allows teaching and is invaluable for the anesthetist to monitor the surgical progress. Long-standing foreign bodies[1] are often surrounded by pus and act as plugs trapping copious pus behind them. There is a real danger of bleeding obstructing the view and also that when the foreign body is extracted the flood of pus can affect the opposite lung. Epinephrine instilled bronchoscopically onto the granulations prior to any attempt to remove the foreign body can make the operation much more controlled.[9] Lidocaine sprayed onto the carina can make coughing less likely.

Tracheotomy

This is rarely needed now for foreign body extraction unless there is some reason why a normal bronchoscope cannot be passed through the larynx, such as stenosis or mandibular hypoplasia. Otherwise any foreign body that passed through the laryngeal inlet should be removable via the same route so long as it is extractable from the bronchus. Historically, tracheotomy was required not to remove the foreign body but to cope with the laryngeal edema that followed.

Open surgical procedures

Thoracotomy is rarely needed nowadays. Occasionally a long-standing foreign body is so embedded in granulations that bronchoscopic removal is not possible. Lobectomy may be required because of damage to the lung from chronic infection and collapse.

Postoperative medical treatment

Systemic steroids can be used to reduce laryngeal and tracheobronchial edema but may reduce the body's ability to fight infection. Unless the foreign body is clean and inorganic and has been present for less than 24 hours, prophylactic antibiotics should be used. Without this there is a high incidence of postoperative pyrexia due to pneumonia. Postoperative physiotherapy is advisable.

Complications after removal

Pneumothorax and pneumomediastinum

Pneumothorax occurs due to high pressure ventilation during the procedure or a cough against a resistance such as a bronchoscope. Sharp foreign bodies can disrupt the integrity of the tracheal or bronchial wall, leading to pneumomediastinum, emphysema and pneumothorax. Minor changes in respiratory function are demonstrable for some time after removal, presumably due to bronchiectasis.

Conclusions

Death from choking (usually laryngeal obstruction) is most often due to food and is common under 3 years of age. It seems to be reducing, presumably related to increased awareness and toy regulation. Parent education about the risks of food inhalation and greater control of the use of toys designed for older children by siblings may offer the best route to a further reduction in deaths. 'Sit down and don't rush your food' may sound like rules from a Victorian era but could save lives. Greater education in, and awareness of, the Heimlich maneuver are needed.

Foreign body aspiration (into the tracheobronchial tree), which is seldom fatal, is due to food and toys equally. Here legislation and parental awareness may reduce the incidence.

Medical awareness is also important, to avoid missing the diagnosis of inhaled foreign body due to the relatively silent presentation that occurs particularly with nonorganic foreign bodies.

Improved endoscopic instruments with Hopkins rod telescopes attached to a video camera have greatly simplified removal of most foreign bodies by skilled endoscopists. Long-standing organic foreign bodies with profuse granulations still, however, provide a surgical and anesthetic challenge.

Complications can occur prior to endoscopy but should occur rarely as a result of endoscopy, which is a significant change from the situation only some 50 years ago.

References

1. Barbato A, Novello A Jr, Tormena F, Corner P. Problems with the retrieval of long-standing inhaled foreign bodies in children. *Monaldi Arch Chest Dis* 1996; **51**: 419–20.
2. Black RE, Johnson DG, Matlak ME. Bronchoscopic removal of aspirated foreign bodies in children. *J Pediatr Surg* 1994; **29**: 682–4.
3. Blazer S, Naveh Y, Friedman A. Foreign body in the airway. *Am J Dis Child* 1980; **134**: 68–71.
4. Burton EM, Riggs W Jr, Kaufman RA, Houston CS. Pneumomediastinum caused by foreign body aspiration in children. *Pediatr Radiol* 1989; **20**: 45–7.
5. Caglayan S, Erkin S, Coteli I, Oniz H. Bronchial foreign body vs asthma. *Chest* 1989; **96**: 509–11.
6. Fabian MC, Smitheringale A. Hemoptysis in children: the hospital for sick children experience. *J Otolaryngol* 1996; **25**: 44–5.
7. Griffiths DM, Freeman NV. Expiratory chest x-ray examination in the diagnosis of inhaled foreign bodies. *Br Med J* 1984; **288**: 1074–5.
8. Hamilton AH, Carswell F, Wisheart JD. The Bristol Children's Hospital experience of tracheobronchial foreign bodies 1977–87. *Bristol Med Chir J* 1989; **104**: 72–4.
9. Harries ML, Albert DM. Bronchoscopic foreign bodies: overcoming granulation tissue. *J Otolaryngol* 1993; **22**: 134.
10. Healy GB. Management of tracheobronchial foreign bodies in children: an update. *Ann Otol Rhinol Laryngol* 1990; **99**: 889–91.
11. Heimlich HJ, Patrick EA. The Heimlich maneuver. Best

technique for saving any choking victim's life [see comments]. *Postgrad Med* 1990; **87:** 38–48, 53.

12. Holinger PH, Andrews AH, Anison GC. Pulmonary complications due to endobronchial foreign bodies. *Illinois Med J* 1948: 19–24.
13. Hughes CA, Baroody FM, Marsh BR. Pediatric tracheobronchial foreign bodies: historical review from the Johns Hopkins Hospital. *Ann Otol Rhinol Laryngol* 1996; **105:** 555–61.
14. Inglis AFJ, Wagner DV. Lower complication rates associated with bronchial foreign bodies over the last 20 years. *Ann Otol Rhinol Laryngol* 1992; **101:** 61–6.
15. Kabbani M, Goodwin SR. Traumatic epiglottis following blind finger sweep to remove a pharyngeal foreign body. *Clin Pediatr (Phila)* 1995; **34:** 495–7.
16. Laks Y, Barzilay Z. Foreign body aspiration in childhood. *Pediatr Emerg Care* 1988; **4:** 102–6.
17. Mantor PC, Tuggle DW, Tunell WP. An appropriate negative bronchoscopy rate in suspected foreign body aspiration. *Am J Surg* 1989; **158:** 622–4.
18. McCullough P. Wire basket removal of a large endobronchial foreign body [letter]. *Chest* 1985; **87:** 270–1.
19. Metra Martech. Anonymous. *Consumer Safety Research: Choking Hazards for Children in the European Community.* 1996; 6722/1800/96: 1 p.
20. Monden Y, Morimoto T, Taniki T, Uyama T, Kimura S. Flexible bronchoscopy for foreign body in airway. *Tokushima J Exp Med* 1989; **36:** 35–9.
21. Reilly JS. Prevention of aspiration in infants and young children: federal regulations. *Ann Otol Rhinol Laryngol* 1990; **99:** 273–6.
22. Reilly JS, Cook SP, Stool D, Rider G. Prevention and management of aerodigestive foreign body injuries in childhood. *Pediatr Clin North Am* 1996; **43:** 1403–11.
23. Rimell FL, Thome A Jr, Stool S *et al.* Characteristics of objects that cause choking in children [see comments]. *JAMA* 1995; **274:** 1763–6.
24. Rothman BF, Boeckman CR. Foreign bodies in the larynx and tracheobronchial tree in children. *Ann Otol* 1980; **89:** 434–6.
25. Saoji R, Ramchandra C, D'Cruz AJ. Subcutaneous emphysema: an unusual presentation of foreign body in the airway. *J Pediatr Surg* 1995; **30:** 860–2.
26. Shabb B, Taha AM, Hamada F, Kanj N. Straight pin aspiration in young women. *J Trauma* 1996; **40:** 827–8.
27. Svensson G. Foreign bodies in the tracheobronchial tree. Special references to experience in 97 children. *Int J Pediatr Otorhinolaryngol* 1985; **8:** 243–51.
28. Ucan ES, Tahaoglu K, Mogolkoc N *et al.* Turban pin aspiration syndrome: a new form of foreign body aspiration. *Respir Med* 1996; **90:** 427–8.
29. Versichelen L, Herregods L, Donadoni R, Vermeersch H. Anesthesia for foreign bodies in the tracheo-bronchial tree in children. *Acta Anaesthesiol Belg* 1985; **36:** 222–9.
30. Witt WJ. The role of rigid endoscopy in foreign body management. *Ear Nose Throat J* 1985; **64:** 70–4.
31. Woodring JH, Baker MD, Stark P. Pneumothorax ex vacuo. *Chest* 1996; **110:** 1102–5.

Traumatic disorders of the pediatric larynx and subglottis

Robert F Yellon

Significant external trauma to the laryngotracheal complex in the pediatric population can be life-threatening. The treating physician must give consideration to maintenance of the airway, stability of the cervical spine, possible major hemorrhage, as well as other associated traumatic injuries. The small caliber of the pediatric airway makes any narrowing significant in terms of airway obstruction, whether the narrowing results from edema or structural injury. Although the relatively superior location of the larynx and cricoid in the neck of a small child often allows it to be protected by the mandible from direct trauma, these injuries still occur when trauma is severe or when the neck is extended. The flexibility of the cartilage in children decreases the incidence of traumatic fractures, whilst the immature connective tissue membranes increase the incidence of traumatic separations and tears. Expertise in the diagnosis and treatment of significant laryngotracheal injuries in children is critical to correctly manage life-threatening injuries as well as those that can later lead to cicatricial stenosis to prevent the need for major reconstructive surgery.

Incidence and mechanisms of injuries

Significant laryngotracheal injuries in children less than 2 years of age are usually the result of internal trauma from endotracheal intubation, foreign bodies, caustic ingestion or iatrogenic causes, and the management of these injuries is discussed elsewhere.[12] External trauma to the laryngotracheal complex usually occurs in older children, and may be divided into blunt and penetrating varieties. Blunt trauma to the laryngotracheal complex usually results from motor vehicle accidents. Minibike, snowmobile or bicycle accidents commonly involve neck contact with a clothesline or tree branch. Contact with the object compresses the laryngotracheal complex against the vertebral column, usually resulting in separation of the soft tissues from the cartilage, which often results in intralaryngeal hematoma. Laryngotracheal separation may also occur more commonly than fractures of the cartilaginous structures. Traumatic tracheoesophageal fistulas may occur as well as injury to the recurrent laryngeal nerves.[1] Arytenoid cartilage dislocation may occur. Penetrating injuries may result from assaults, falls on sharp objects or iatrogenic causes such as tracheotomy.[7,12] Air dissection may lead to pneumothorax or pneumomediastinum. Associated cervical spine or vascular injuries may occur, and must be treated concomitantly.

Diagnosis

The diagnosis of traumatic airway injury in children may be easily overlooked because of the presence of concomitant severe injuries and the unfamiliarity of pediatricians with this type of injury.[16] A thorough history should be taken from the patient and any possible witnesses, noting in particular the exact mechanism of injury. A history of hoarseness, stridor, apnea, hemoptysis, odynophagia and dysphagia should be sought. On physical examination, progression of stridor or respiratory distress may indicate impending complete airway obstruction and stabilization of the airway must be a priority. Lacerations and contusions on the anterior neck should be noted as well as loss of the prominence of the laryngeal and cricoid cartilages. Crepitus indicates air dissection into the soft tissues. A neurologic examination and cervical spine clearance is mandatory, and if the status of the cervical spine is uncertain, the patient should be managed as if a fracture is present. Flexible laryngoscopy is useful to assess the status of the supraglottis, vocal cords and laryngeal airway.

Radiographic tests

If significant injuries are suspected, chest radiographs and cervical spine films are indicated. Pharyngeal or esophageal tears and foreign bodies may be identified by a non-barium esophagram. Lateral neck soft tissue radiographs or anteroposterior high-kilovolt xeroradiographs may help delineate the injured airway. Computed tomography[20] or magnetic resonance imaging are the best imaging modalities to assess for cartilaginous fractures, stenoses, hematomas and edema. In the presence of massive airway edema or massive hematoma found at endoscopy, the use of the CT scan to show intact cartilaginous structures may obviate the need for open neck exploration.[21] Schaefer and Brown[20] suggest use of the CT scan selectively for patients in whom the findings would influence outcome. Scanning would not be necessary for patients with normal flexible laryngoscopies and head and neck examinations, nor for those with massive injuries obviously requiring open repair. The use of contrast with these imaging modalities helps to delineate significant vascular injuries, but formal angiography may be required.

Classification of extent of injury

Schaefer and Close[21] devised a four-level severity grouping in order to classify external laryngotracheal injuries. This initial classification has been modified by Fuhrman *et al.*[9] to include the fifth group and is shown in Table 19.1.

Group 1 injuries are usually managed with conservative and medical management. *Group 2* injuries are managed with direct laryngoscopy, rigid bronchoscopy and conservative management. *Group 3* patients are managed with rigid endoscopy and open surgical repair. Finally, *groups 4 and 5* patients are managed with rigid endoscopy and open surgical repair with intraluminal airway stenting to prevent uncontrolled wound healing and stenosis that may occur with massive injuries or loss of cartilaginous support.[3]

Conservative and medical management

For children with a stable airway and milder injuries, once the diagnostic testing has been completed, these children may be managed conservatively. Humidified air and close monitoring should be provided in a setting in which the airway can be controlled if it deteriorates, such as an intensive care unit. The head of the bed should be elevated to enhance lymphatic drainage and decrease edema.

The factors that are known to contribute to airway granulation tissue and stenosis are trauma, infection and gastroesophageal reflux. Therefore antimicrobial agents are administered to treat or prevent infection when mucosal disruption has occurred.[13,18,22,25] Treatment or prevention of possible gastroesophageal reflux is also believed to minimize reflux-induced injury to traumatized airway mucosa.[14,25,26] Additionally, corticosteroids are useful to decrease edema and limit the inflammatory and cicatricial response in the airway mucosa. Prospective, controlled studies are lacking in this area.

Table 19.1 Classification of extent of injury by groups

Group	*Extent of injury*
Group 1	Minor endolaryngeal hematoma or laceration without detectable fracture
Group 2	Edema, hematoma, minor mucosal disruption without exposed cartilage, nondisplaced fractures noted on CT scan
Group 3	Massive edema, mucosal tears, exposed cartilage, cord immobility, displaced fractures
Group 4	Same as group 3 with more than two fracture lines or massive trauma to laryngeal mucosa
Group 5	Complete laryngotracheal separation

Endoscopic evaluation and treatment

If the history and physical examination indicate a significant upper aerodigestive tract injury, the direct laryngoscopy, rigid bronchoscopy and esophagoscopy should be performed prior to the administration of barium, which may make visualization of the airway more difficult. If there is severe airway obstruction, establishment of the airway by rigid bronchoscopy or tracheostomy is safer than endotracheal intubation because the airway can be visualized. Although Gussack and Jurkovich[10] recommend careful endotracheal intubation, Schaefer[19] and Fuhrman *et al.*[9] advocate tracheostomy because if laryngotracheal separation is present there may be a false passage of the endotracheal tube and small airway mucosal lacerations may be enlarged by passage of the endotracheal tube. Rigid endoscopy also allows full characterization of airway caliber, hematomas, edema, lacerations, granulation tissue, stenoses, disruptions, arytenoid dislocation and the need for tracheostomy. In adults with laryngeal trauma, tracheotomy under local anesthesia has been recommended, but for children it is recommended that the airway be established prior to tracheotomy, using a rigid bronchoscope, because children are less cooperative than adults, more susceptible to laryngospasm and tolerate airway narrowing poorly as the pediatric airway is already narrow.

In general, surgical therapy, whether it be performed by endoscopic or open methods, is required when it is felt that the injuries are unlikely to resolve spontaneously. The goal of surgery is to restore a normal airway, voice and protection from aspiration. Suspension microlaryngoscopy will provide the best visualization for repair of laryngeal lacerations and for repositioning of a dislocated arytenoid cartilage. The CO_2 or KTP lasers may be used via suspension microlaryngoscopy or rigid bronchoscopy to excise limited scars or granulation tissue.[5,6] Rigid esophagoscopy may show esophageal perforation or tracheoesophageal fistulae.

The maximal cicatricial narrowing of airway mucosa usually occurs approximately 6 weeks after the injury and therefore the child must be observed closely during this period. If a significant injury occurs and a tracheostomy is performed, the follow-up endoscopy should be performed at least 6 weeks following the injury and any surgical repair, to see if decannulation is then possible.

Open surgical therapy

Significant laryngeal, cricoid and tracheal fractures and separations should be repaired via an open approach through the tracheotomy incision when possible. Open surgical repairs should be done as soon as possible after the injury, and preferably within 1 week.[1,15,17] Significant laryngeal injuries may be approached via midline thyrotomy or explored via paramedian fracture lines. Fractures should be stabilized with nonabsorbable suture material. Since some fractures of the larynx will flatten even with suturing, some authors have advocated more stable fixation alternatives. Austin *et al.*[2] have advocated the use of a wire-tube fixation technique and Woo[24] has advocated the use of mini-plates. Mucosal lacerations should be repaired with absorbable sutures. Suturing the mucosa of the anterior vocal cord to the external perichondrium of the thyroid cartilage will help to avoid blunting at the anterior commissure.[21] If the caliber of the airway lumen has been compromised or if loss of cartilaginous support of the airway has occurred, stenting of the lumen is required until healing has occurred. Costal cartilage or hyoid bone may be used to augment the caliber of the airway and provide rigid support. Severe crush injuries of the trachea or complete stenoses may be managed by end-to-end anastomosis with laryngeal mobilization with infrahyoid release to achieve a tension-free closure.[1,4,15,17] Historically, nondisplaced fractures have been managed conservatively; however, it is possible that subtle voice changes do occur when nondisplaced fractures are not repaired.[11] Austin *et al.*[2] reported a series of moderately displaced or angulated laryngeal fractures without airway compromise, and suggested that open reduction and internal fixation was superior to observation of such fractures based on outcomes of phonatory testing. Vocal cord mobility should be assessed and documented prior to open repairs.

For penetrating injuries to the neck, stable patients with zone I or III injuries should undergo angiography. For penetrating zone II injuries to the neck that are associated with a foreign body, a pulsatile or expanding hematoma or significant bleeding, the neck should be explored.[8]

Cricoarytenoid joint displacement

The cricoarytenoid joint may be displaced by blunt or penetrating trauma to the neck, although it usually occurs as a result of endotracheal intubation. This diarthrodial joint may be totally dislocated or only subluxed, which implies partial separation. The clinical signs and symptoms include a change in voice, odynophagia and possible difficulty breathing if the displaced arytenoid prolapses into the airway. A subluxed joint may reposition spontaneously, whilst a dislocated joint will not. An attempt at endoscopic or open repositioning should be undertaken as soon after the injury as possible to try to minimize the adverse long-term effects of joint ankylosis on voice. Mucosal lacerations should be carefully closed. Open therapeutic modalities include vocal fold medialization, arthrodesis, or pin fixation.[23]

Complications

Complications include airway obstruction, hoarseness or aphonia, laryngotracheal stenosis, tracheoesophageal fistula and aspiration. Vocal cord paralysis with poor voice or aspiration should not be definitively treated for 1 year, pending the spontaneous return of function, although Gelfoam injection may be useful as a temporizing measure to improve voice or decrease aspiration. Tracheoesophageal fistulae may require open repair with flap interposition. Posterior glottic and subglottic stenosis may require laryngotracheal reconstruction with costal cartilage grafting and stenting for severe lesions, although laser therapy may be useful for smaller lesions. At least 6–8 weeks should be allowed until the injured airway is reassessed for the need for reconstruction to allow the lesion to mature fully.

Outcomes

In an adult series, Schaefer and Close[21] reported no difference in outcomes related to blunt versus penetrating trauma, with outcomes in both groups being related to severity of injury. This is in contrast to the pediatric series reported by Ford *et al.*[8] who reported more severe injuries and poorer outcomes in children with blunt rather than penetrating injuries. In their series, children with blunt trauma required rigid endoscopy and open neck exploration more often than did those with penetrating injuries.

References

1. Alonso WA, Pratt LL, Zollinger WK, Ogura JH. Complications of laryngotracheal disruption. *Laryngoscope* 1974; **84:** 1276–90.
2. Austin JR, Stanley RB, Cooper DS. Stable internal fixation of fractures of the partially mineralized thyroid cartilage. *Ann Otol Rhinol Laryngol* 1992; **101:** 76–80.
3. Bent JP III, Silver JR, Porubsky ES. Acute laryngeal trauma: a review of 77 patients. *Otolaryngol Head Neck Surg* 1993; **109:** 441–9.
4. Dedo HH, Fishman NH. Laryngeal release and sleeve resection for tracheal stenosis. *Ann Otol* 1969; **78:** 285–96.

5. Duncavage JA, Ossoff RH, Toohill RJ. Carbon dioxide laser management of laryngeal stenosis. *Ann Otol Rhinol Laryngol* 1985; **94**: 565–9.
6. Duncavage JA, Piazza LS, Ossoff RH, Toohill RJ. The microtrapdoor technique for the management of laryngeal stenosis. *Laryngoscope* 1987; **97**: 825–8.
7. Fitz Hugh GAS, Powell JB II. Acute traumatic injuries of the oropharynx, laryngopharynx, and cervical trachea in children. *Otolaryngol Clin North Am* 1970; **3**: 375–93.
8. Ford HR, Gardner MJ, Lynch JM. Laryngotracheal disruption from blunt pediatric neck injuries: impact of early recognition and intervention on outcome. *J Pediatr Surg* 1995; **30**: 331–5.
9. Fuhrman GM, Stieg FH III, Buerk CA. Blunt laryngeal trauma: classification and management protocol. *J Trauma* 1990; **30**: 87–92.
10. Gussack GS, Jurkovich GJ. Treatment dilemmas in laryngotracheal trauma. *J Trauma* 1988; **28**: 1439–44.
11. Hirano M, Kurita S, Terasawa R. Difficulty in high-pitched phonation by laryngeal trauma. *Arch Otolaryngol* 1985; **111**: 59–61.
12. Holinger PH, Schild JA. Pharyngeal, laryngeal and tracheal injuries in the pediatric age group. *Ann Otol* 1972; **81**: 538–45.
13. Johnson JT, Myers EN, Thearle PB, Sigler BA, Schramm VL Jr. Antimicrobial prophylaxis for contaminated head and neck surgery. *Laryngoscope* 1984; **94**: 46–51.
14. Little FB, Koufman JA, Kohut RI, Marshall RB. Effect of gastric acid on the pathogenesis of subglottic stenosis. *Ann Otol Rhinol Laryngol* 1985; **94**: 516–19.
15. Montgomery WW. *Surgery of the Upper Respiratory System*, Vol. 2. Philadelphia: Lea and Febiger, 1973: 373–435, 543–95.
16. Myer CM III, Orobello P, Cotton RT, Bratcher GO. Blunt laryngeal trauma in children. *Laryngoscope* 1987; **97**: 1043–8.
17. Ogura JH, Biller HF. Reconstruction of the larynx following blunt trauma. *Ann Otol* 1971; **80**: 492–506.
18. Sasaki CT, Horiuchi M, Koss N. Tracheostomy-related subglottic stenosis: bacteriologic pathogenesis. *Laryngoscope* 1979; **89**: 857–65.
19. Schaefer SD. The acute management of external laryngeal trauma. A 27-year experience. *Arch Otolaryngol Head Neck Surg* 1992; **118**: 598–604.
20. Schaefer SD, Brown OE. Selective application of CT in the management of laryngeal trauma. *Laryngoscope* 1983; **93**: 1473–5.
21. Schaefer SD, Close LG. Acute management of laryngeal trauma. Update. *Ann Otol Rhinol Laryngol* 1989; **98**: 98–104.
22. Squire R, Brodsky L, Rossman J. The role of infection in the pathogenesis of acquired tracheal stenosis. *Laryngoscope* 1990; **100**: 765–70.
23. Stack BC Jr, Ridley MB. Arytenoid subluxation from blunt laryngeal trauma. *Am J Otolaryngol* 1994; **15**: 68–73.
24. Woo P. Laryngeal framework reconstruction with miniplates. *Ann Otol Rhinol Laryngol* 1990; **99**: 772–7.
25. Yellon RF, Parameswaran M, Brandom BW. Decreasing morbidity following laryngotracheal reconstruction in children. *Int J Pediatr Otorhinolaryngol* 1997; **41**: 145–54.
26. Yellon RF, Szeremeta W, Grandis JR, Diguisseppe P, Dickman PS. Subglottic injury, gastric juice, corticosteroids, and peptide growth factors in a porcine model. *Laryngoscope* 1998; **108**: 854–62.

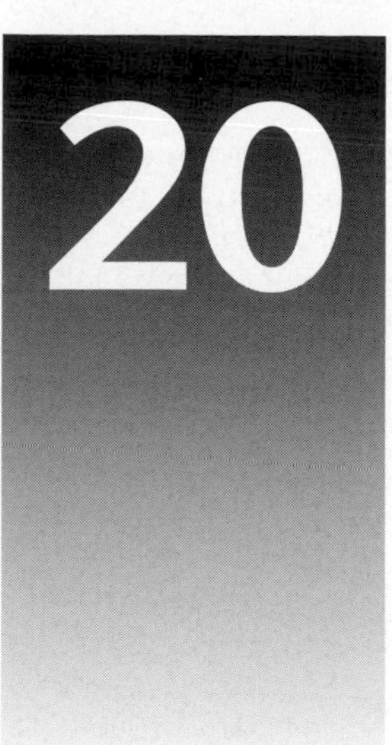

20 The evaluation and management of laryngotracheal trauma

James C Alex, John K Joe and Clarence T Sasaki

Injury to the laryngotracheal complex can result from either external or internal trauma, or both. The primary mechanisms of external trauma are blunt and penetrating, while intubation accounts for the majority of internal trauma. However, regardless of the mechanism, the goals of laryngotracheal trauma management are always the same: preservation of an effective airway and normal vocal function. In order to achieve these goals, early accurate diagnosis of laryngeal injuries and proper initial management are imperative. Proper evaluation and management of laryngotracheal trauma begins with an understanding of the larynx's complex anatomy and physiology together with the different physical mechanisms of injury.

External laryngeal injuries

Blunt trauma

External laryngeal trauma is a relatively rare occurrence with only 1 in 30 000 patients presenting to the emergency room with this injury.[26,55] The most common causes of blunt laryngeal trauma include motor vehicle accidents, personal assaults, sporting injuries, and strangulation injuries.

Anterior blunt injuries are most commonly the result of motor vehicle accidents.[44,47] However, with the introduction of lap and shoulder seat belt laws, lower speed limits, child seat restraints and air bags, the incidence of this type of injury is declining.

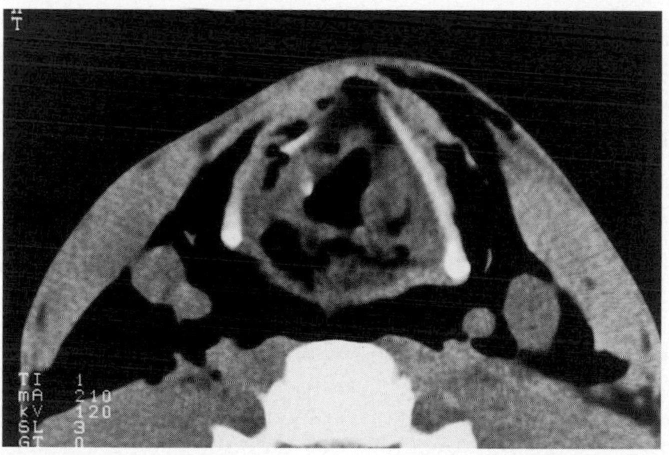

(a)

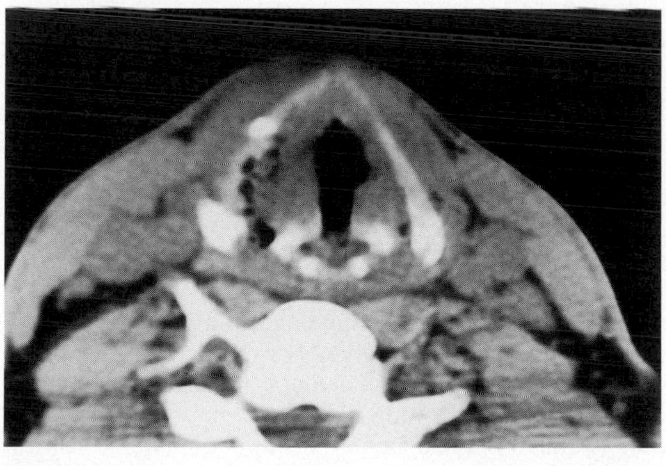

(b)

Figure 20.1 *(a) Thyroid cartilage fracture. In this computer tomographic image of a left paramedian thyroid cartilage fracture, there is effacement of the left piriform sinus by air pockets trapped in this region. The region of the false cords is noticeably swollen, producing asymmetry of the airway. (b)Thyroid cartilage fracture. In the same patient, the arytenoid and cricoid cartilages appear normal. There is the suggestion of swelling in the true cord region bilaterally. Multiple small gas pockets are also apparent on the fracture side of the piriform sinus.*

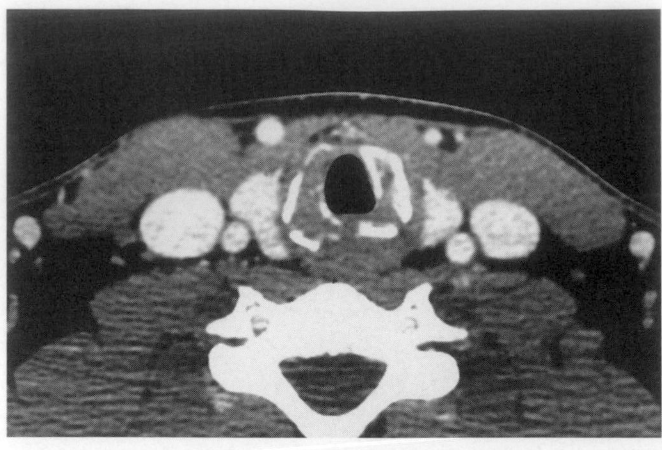
(a)

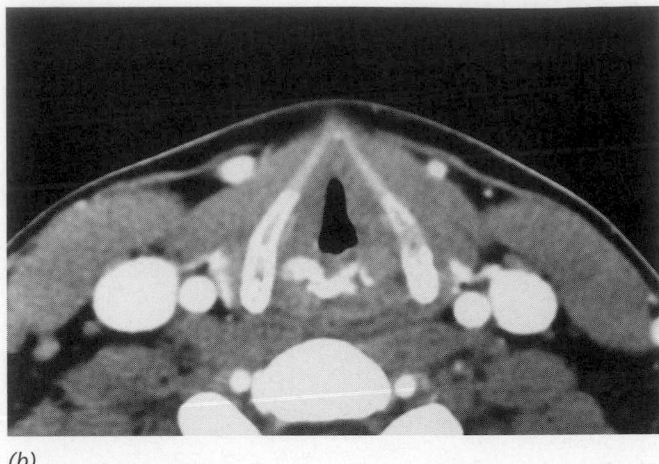
(b)

Figure 20.2 *(a) Cricoid cartilage fracture. A computer tomographic scan of a comminuted fracture of the cricoid cartilage with fractures anteriorly and posteriorly. On the left, the cricoid is displaced posterolaterally. Small gas pockets are noted anteriorly. (b) Cricoid cartilage fracture. In the same patient, the thyroid cartilage and laryngeal soft tissues are symmetric and normal in appearance. There is, however, the suggestion of a posteromedial displacement of the right arytenoid.*

A classic vehicular-induced laryngeal injury involves an unrestrained occupant who hyperextends his neck after contact with the windshield and strikes the anterior laryngotracheal complex against the dashboard or steering wheel.[44,59] As the exposed larynx is compressed against the cervical spine it fractures. The extent of injury depends on the size, type and vector force of the impacting object. Usually the thyroid cartilage is fractured in the paramedian/parasymphyseal area as the thyroid alae are spread laterally by the spine (Figs 20.1a,b).[40,45] The cricoid cartilage, in addition to fracturing anteriorly (paramedian/parasymphyseal), also fractures posteriorly and splits open (Figs 20.2a,b).[36,40]

With a glottic and supraglottic impact, the thyroepiglottic ligament can also rupture, dislocating the epiglottis posteriorly.[47] Sharp blows to the anterior neck from sporting injuries or personal assault produce similar injuries.

The so-called, 'clothesline injury' is seen when the rider of a recreational vehicle, such as a motorcycle, snowmobile, or minibike, strikes a stationary object such as a rope, chain, or wire fence with neck extended. This type of mechanism frequently results not only in laryngeal fracture but also in laryngotracheal separation due to the shearing force tearing the cricoid and thyroid cartilages off the trachea. Although asphyxiation often occurs at the scene of such accidents, patients can present several hours after injury to the emergency room.[10] A helpful radiographic finding indicative of laryngotracheal separation is that of hyoid bone elevation on lateral cervical spine x-ray.[50] Emergency tracheotomy should be considered when this finding is present.

Strangulation injuries are produced by a relatively static and low-velocity injuring force. As a result, multiple cartilage fractures may occur without obvious mucosal laceration, fracture displacement, or submucosal hematoma. A patient with this mechanism of injury should be observed closely because airway compromise may be delayed in onset.[48]

Laryngotracheal trauma in children is rare. The reasons for this are several.[24,43] Mandatory child car seat laws have reduced pediatric motor vehicle trauma. Children are less likely to be involved in high-impact injury or assault. Physically the immature larynx is located higher in the neck relative to the adult and thus is more protected by the mandibular arch. The cartilage of the pediatric larynx also has greater pliability, reducing the incidence of fracture and severe injury.[41,43] However, this same increased cartilaginous pliability of the larynx combined with the relative looseness of overlying mucous membrane leads to increased soft tissue damage. As a result, the pediatric patient can have significant endolaryngeal swelling with minimal external manifestation of injury. Accurate evaluation of traumatic injury in the relatively small pediatric larynx is critical in order to avoid loss of airway control.

Penetrating trauma

Unlike blunt trauma, which is on the decline due to improved motor vehicle safety, the incidence of penetrating head and neck trauma is increasing with the rise in personal assaults. The most common presenting forms of penetrating trauma are knife and gunshot wounds. Injuries commonly involve blood vessels, nerves, cartilage, esophagus, hypopharynx and the laryngotracheal complex.

The most critical factor determining the degree of injury from a gunshot is the velocity of the projectile shot from the firearm. The equation $KE = mv^2$ determines the kinetic energy of any mass moving at a particular velocity. As the equation demonstrates, the kinetic energy of a given projectile is proportional to the size of its mass but exponential to its velocity. Thus, a 0.22 caliber pistol which has a muzzle velocity of 300 ft/s (approx. 90 m/s) causes less tissue destruction than a 0.270 caliber hunting rifle which has a muzzle velocity of 2200 ft/s (approx. 660 m/s).

In addition to producing less tissue damage, the pathway of slow-velocity projectiles is much more erratic as it tends to be deflected by structures such as vessels, nerves and fascial planes. High-velocity projectiles typically make a straight pathway through bone and tissue and produce a zone of tissue damage extending beyond the area of obvious necrotic tissue. Other ballistic factors that influence the degree of injury are the flight stability of the projectile, the angle of projectile impact, and the design of the bullet.[65]

Knife wounds have comparatively negligible kinetic energy and cause less adjacent soft tissue damage and tissue necrosis. The challenge in evaluating these injuries is that the depth of penetration is unclear and injury to deepest structures can occur a distance from the site of the entrance wound.

Diagnostic assessment

Primary survey

The initial part of the patient evaluation is the patient history. Facts should be sought from the patient and/or the family members, witnesses, or rescue personnel who have knowledge of the circumstances surrounding the patient's injury. Clearly, the extent of the history will be largely determined by the patient's neurologic, respiratory and hemodynamic stability but should minimally include mechanism of injury, time of injury, and duration of symptoms. In the absence of impending airway or hemodynamic compromise, the presence of the signs and symptoms presented in Table 20.1 should be thoroughly evaluated. If the patient is unstable, the physician should follow the advanced trauma life support protocol as outlined by the Committee on Trauma of the American College of Surgeons.[66]

The foremost initial management concern is airway stabilization and airway management. Patients who present to the ER with evidence of laryngeal trauma and impending airway compromise receive a controlled emergent tracheotomy under local anesthesia at our institution. Orotracheal intubation and cricothyroidotomy both have a strong potential for exacerbating laryngeal injuries. Intubation may even result in the total loss of a compromised airway.[26,57] In addition, tracheotomy allows the neck to be completely immobilized in the neutral position until an occult cervical spine fracture can be ruled out.

Some physicians believe that experienced personnel can perform intubation with a small endotracheal tube under direct vision without adverse sequelae.[26] This is one of the several controversies that are explored further in the discussion section. Once the airway is established, breathing must be evaluated and evidence of hypoventilation (usually secondary to pneumothorax) must be recognized and treated rapidly. Finally, the patient's hemodynamic function is evaluated. If the patient presents clinically with shock, a review of the signs and symptoms will help determine whether it is hypovolemic, neurogenic, or cardiogenic in nature. Hypovolemia is the most common cause of shock following trauma and hemorrhage should be the assumed etiology until proven otherwise. Fluid resuscitation through two large peripheral bore IVs is initiated and excess bleeding can often be controlled with manual pressure and compressive packing.

Secondary survey

Once the patient is stable, the secondary survey, consisting of a detailed examination with the patient fully exposed, is performed. The extent of this examination is determined by the degree of the patient's injuries and the need for surgical intervention. The patient's history is expanded and should include preexisting medical conditions, previous surgeries, medications, known allergies, history of substance abuse and the time the patient last ate. Blood count, C-spine film, chest radiograph and urinalysis are obtained as well as toxicology studies, blood typing and cross-matching as deemed appropriate. A comprehensive physical examination should include evaluation of neurologic deficits and injuries to the head and neck region, thorax, abdomen and extremities. The otolaryngologist is responsible for a focused and detailed evaluation of the head and neck region during the secondary survey. Typically the examination includes endoscopic evaluation of the larynx, hypopharynx, piriform sinus, vallecula and tongue base region.

Management

After identifying and endoscopically evaluating the relevant signs and symptoms noted in Table 20.1, patients can be grouped (Table 20.2) according to the severity of their laryngotracheal injuries.[5,23,57,70]

Based on this laryngotracheal trauma grouping, the most appropriate management protocol is then initiated (Fig 20.3).

Discussion

There are three goals of management: acute airway control and restoration of long-term airway and vocal function. Although these goals are universally accepted, there is still controversy as to the best method to achieve them. The first area of management controversy concerns the method of providing an adequate airway. Lambert and McMurry[35] and Gussack *et al.*[26] believe that, if performed under direct visualization by experienced personnel with a small endotracheal tube, elective intubation can be performed on patients with severe laryngeal tracheal injuries without adverse sequelae. Fuhrman *et al.*,[23] Snow[60]

Table 20.1 Signs and symptoms of blunt and penetrating neck trauma

Airway	**Nervous system**
Respiratory distress	Hemiplegia
Stridor	Quadriplegia
Cyanosis	Coma
Hemoptysis	Cranial nerve deficit
Hoarseness	Change of sensorium
Tracheal deviation	Hoarseness
Subcutaneous emphysema	Thrill
Sucking wound	
Vascular system	**Esophagus/Hypopharynx**
Hematoma	Subcutaneous emphysema
Persistent bleeding	Dysphagia
Neurological deficit	Odynophagia
Absent pulse	Hematemesis
Hypovolemic shock	Hemoptysis
Bruit	Tachycardia
Thrill	Fever
Change of sensorium	

Table 20.2 Laryngotracheal injury classifications

Group I	Minor endolaryngeal hematoma without detectable fracture
Group II	Edema, hematoma, minor mucosal, disruption without exposed cartilage, nondisplaced fractures noted on CT scan
Group III	Massive edema, mucosal tears, exposed cartilage and cord immobility
Group IV	As with group III, with more than two fracture lines or massive trauma to laryngeal mucosa
Group V	Complete laryngotracheal separation

and Schaefer and Close[57] disagree, preferring tracheotomy instead. Exacerbation of tracheal injuries and airway compromise is the primary reasons for this preference.

With the introduction of flexible fiberoptic laryngoscopy and computed tomographic (CT) scanning, the care of patients with laryngotracheal trauma has improved significantly. Flexible fiberoptic endoscopy allows for minimally invasive and accurate assessment of endolaryngeal injury. Its main application has been in the examination of those patients with a stable airway. The information from this examination allows the patient to be successfully triaged to observation, CT evaluation, or surgery.

Computed tomography has also further refined the ability to identify which patients can be treated conservatively versus those requiring surgical intervention and repair. Bent *et al.*[5] advocate the use of CT scans not only to rule out occult injuries to the larynx but also as a means of operative planning in cases with severe trauma. Other investigators feel that CT scans should be used selectively when the CT results will alter specific management plans. Accordingly, they suggest that only patients classified as group 2 should receive CT scans.[54,56]

The decision to operate should be based on the likelihood that spontaneous resolution of a laryngeal injury will occur. Injury groups 1 and 2 (laryngeal edema, hematoma without mucosal interruption, small lacerations of the endolarynx not involving the anterior commissure or vocal cord free margin, nondisplaced laryngeal fractures and small lacerations of supraglottic larynx) typically have full recovery without operative intervention.[14]

However, certain nondisplaced fractures may be an exception to medical management alone. Although single nondisplaced thyroid fractures are typically managed conservatively, work by Stanley *et al.*[63] suggests that nondisplaced fractures that change thyroid cartilage angulation produce measurable alterations in vocal quality. As such, several authors have advocated open reduction in internal fixation without open thyroidotomy in these cases.[4,55] Further objective study with such fractures will determine the true efficacy of such a management approach.

Groups 3 and 4 (massive laryngeal edema, mucosal tears, exposed cartilage, cord immobility, displaced fractures, and more than two fracture lines in the laryngeal cartilage) are typically managed with tracheotomy, endoscopy and laryngeal exploration through a midline thyroidotomy or through a laryngofissure at the site of the paramedian fracture. Mucosal injuries are carefully sutured with 5-0 or 6-0 sutures with the knots placed outside the endolarynx. The normal anatomic configuration of the vocal fold, the anterior commissure and laryngeal cartilage must be reconstituted. Although suture or wire can be used to immobilize the fractures, Woo[74] points out that such fixation restricts movement in only two planes. He advocates the use of mini-plates to restrict cartilage movement in all three planes, thereby maintaining proper laryngeal angulation and relationships throughout the wound healing process.

Group 4 patients tend to have more severe injuries to the anterior larynx with an increased risk of endolaryngeal adhesions and overriding or collapse of cartilage fragments. For such cases, an endolaryngeal splint is advocated. In addition to supporting the fracture fixation, laryngeal stents maintain the lumen of the larynx, prevent the formation of adhesions and maintain the scaphoid shape of the anterior commissure needed for normal vocalization. However, although all investigators acknowledge the importance of stenting for such severe cases,[70] stenting can lead to increased incidence of infection and granulation.[69] The optimal time for stent removal, which would minimize inflammatory responses while maximizing the structural supportive functions of

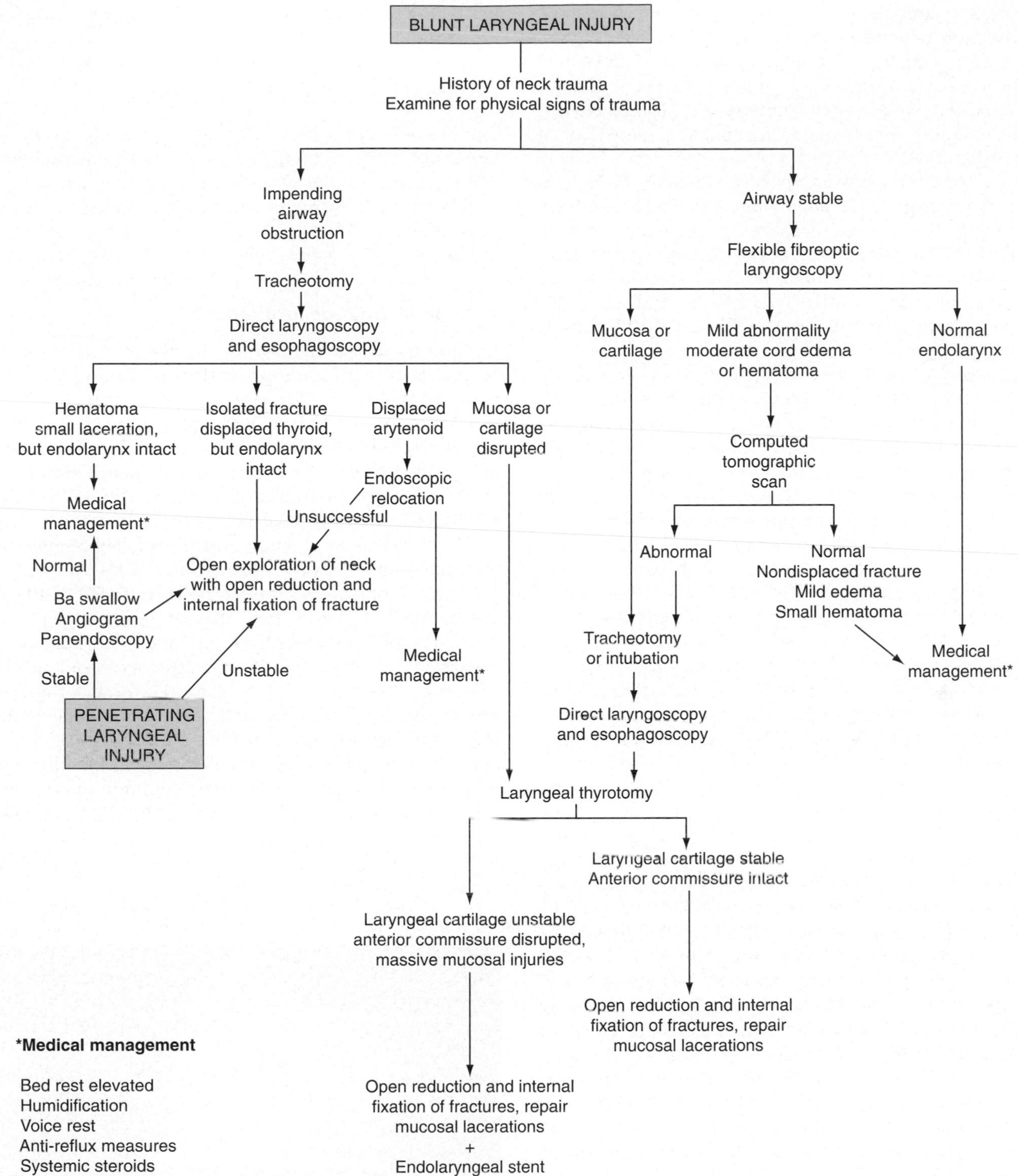

Figure 20.3 *Diagnostic protocol for the treatment of blunt laryngeal injury (adapted from Schaefer[55] and Gussack* et al.*[26]).*

stenting noted above, has been debated over the years.[28,37,46,57,69,70] Current recommendations from several authors indicate that adequate structural healing occurs in 2–3 weeks and removal of the stent at that time will minimize inflammatory complications.[37,47]

The patient with penetrating trauma has two other major concerns in addition to those mentioned above: vascular injury and esophageal perforation. Esophageal perforation must be recognized early in order to avoid neck abscess or mediastinitis. Signs include tachycardia, fever, or radiographic evidence of an enlarged mediastinum or retropharyngeal space. Esophagoscopy is the most widely advocated diagnostic procedure. However, because a wide range of false-negative rates have been reported, we prefer to combine esophagoscopy with barium swallow which has a documented sensitivity of greater than 90%.

The second concern is that of vascular injury. In penetrating trauma, an angiogram should be routinely obtained if the patient is stable. If hemodynamically unstable, the patient should proceed to open exploration and repair. In blunt trauma, formation of a massive hematoma in stable patients is also an indication for angiogram. Unstable patients should proceed directly to the operating room for surgery.

The timing of operative intervention has only recently reached some consensus. Currently most authors urge early surgery because it allows primary closure of mucosal lacerations, early reduction of cartilage fractures and reduces the incidence of inflammatory complications. Recently, several authors reported improved long-term functional results with early intervention.[23,25,37,57]

Traditionally, investigators proposed that diagnosis and repair may be easier after waiting 3 or 4 days for laryngeal swelling to subside.[44,46] However, even Olsen recognized the need for healing by primary intention:

> *We are searching here for a technique that will give us the equivalent of a 'fine scar' which is the ultimate goal of cosmetic surgeons. The fine scar has great functional importance and if ever the surgeon needed it, this is the place.*[46]

Further down in his article Olsen mentions healing by secondary intention only to be condemned. Harris and Tobin[28] and Leopold[37] support this principle of basic wound healing. In Leopold's review of 200 cases, early intervention and primary closure had a substantial effect on airway and voice results. When treated within 24 hours, 87% of patients achieved good airway stabilization and 84% achieved excellent (58%) or fair (26%) voice. This compares to 69% of patients achieving a good airway after 24 hours and 69% of patients achieving excellent (50%) or fair (19%) vocal function. Schaefer and Close's[57] study of 123 patients over a 20-year period also confirmed that immediate operative treatment within 24 hours facilitated primary closure of the injured larynx and resulted in overall good return of voice and airway function in their patients.

Conclusion

Management of acute blunt and penetrating laryngeal trauma mandates that the physician performs a comprehensive and accurate early diagnosis. In the short term this guarantees proper airway stabilization and avoidance of airway catastrophe and provides the patient with the best long-term chance of normal airway and vocal function.

Laryngeal trauma from intubation

The use of endotracheal intubation for mechanical ventilation has led to an increased awareness of potential iatrogenic trauma to the larynx. Such endolaryngeal injury may occur at the time of intubation, or may result from early or late changes in the larynx as a reaction to the indwelling endotracheal tube.

Trauma at time of intubation

Complications associated with the act of intubation may be associated with improper patient positioning, aberrant patient anatomy, inexperience with the intubation technique, or emergency blind intubation. Such complications include pharyngeal laceration, laryngeal abrasion and resultant vocal cord hematoma,[49] perforation of the airway with potential deep space neck abscess, paresis of the lingual or hypoglossal nerves from excessive pressure on the tongue,[34] or disruption of the cricoarytenoid joint.

Cricoarytenoid joint disruption may present as arytenoid subluxation, in which the arytenoid cartilage is abnormally displaced but still in contact with the cricoarytenoid joint space, or as arytenoid dislocation, involving complete separation of the arytenoid cartilage from the cricoarytenoid joint space (Fig 20.4).[32] Arytenoid dislocation may be associated with submucosal hemorrhage with subsequent scarring and vocal fold stiffness, and patients may complain of hoarseness, breathy voice, dysphagia, or dyspnea.[53] The most common and diagnostic symptom is odynophagia. Joint injury may be evalu-

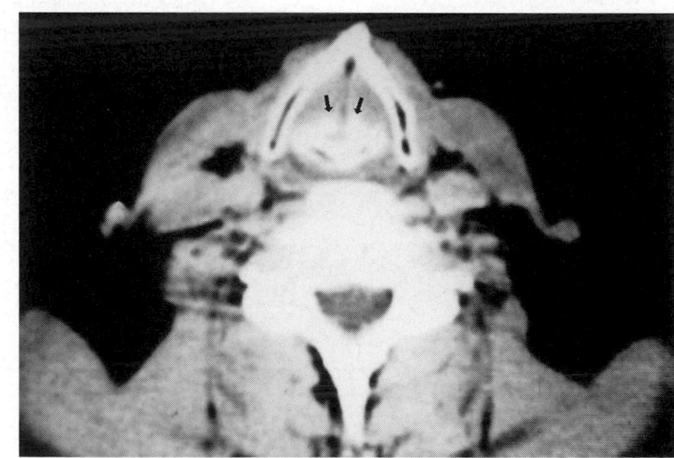

Figure 20.4 *Cricoarytenoid dislocation. This computed tomography scan demonstrates anteromedial displacement of both cricoarytenoid joints at the posterior larynx. Both true vocal folds are fixed in a paramedian position.*

ated by computed tomography (CT), but in pediatric patients insufficient cricoarytenoid mineralization may result in a non-diagnostic study. In order to differentiate vocal fold immobility secondary to cricoarytenoid joint injury versus laryngeal nerve injury, laryngeal electromyography (EMG) in association with laryngoscopy may provide information regarding function and symmetry.[75] During laryngoscopic examination, it may be difficult to ascertain direction of arytenoid displacement because the arytenoid may be dislocated in any direction.[53] Early diagnosis of joint disruption is important, in that arytenoid cartilage fixation may occur as early as 24–48 hours following injury. Treatment involves reduction of the dislocated joint, followed by vocal fold medialization if reduction fails to restore adequate laryngeal function.[32]

Trauma from prolonged intubation

Complications of prolonged intubation may arise from changes in the larynx secondary to pressure from the indwelling endotracheal tube. The acute and chronic changes observed in the larynx following extubation represent a spectrum of healing patterns in response to ischemic injury caused by pressure from the endotracheal tube.

One of the early changes observed in the larynx following extubation includes erythema of the true vocal folds which usually resolves spontaneously.[51]

Vocal fold irritation may progress to mucosal edema after periods of intubation longer than 48 hours.[11] Symptoms of glottic edema include hoarseness, dysphagia, cough and dyspnea, and these complaints often resolve within 72 hours after extubation.[34]

Pressure from an indwelling endotracheal tube may result in areas of ulceration, particularly at the posterior larynx and subglottis.[8] The curvature of the endotracheal tube results in ischemic pressure injury at the posteromedial aspect of the arytenoids and posterolateral cricoid cartilage.[31] Microscopic examination of these cartilaginous structures demonstrates complete or focal loss of epithelium with episodes of intubation as brief as 3 hours.[18] The depth of ulceration increases with longer periods of intubation,[73] with deeper mucosal ulceration demonstrating microscopically more pronounced inflammation.[38]

Depth of mucosal injury is critical, for deep ulceration and perichondrial inflammation may result in cartilaginous exposure with chronic changes as healing occurs. Perichondritis of the vocal processes of the arytenoids may be severe following periods of intubation longer than 96 hours.[18] Granulation tissue may form as acute inflammation resolves, and laryngeal surfaces at particular risk include the posterior commissure, the medial surface of the arytenoid vocal processes, the inner, posterolateral cricoid, and subglottic region in contact with the endotracheal tube cuff.[9] Granulation tissue at these sites may lead to scar tissue formation and potential stenosis of the airway.

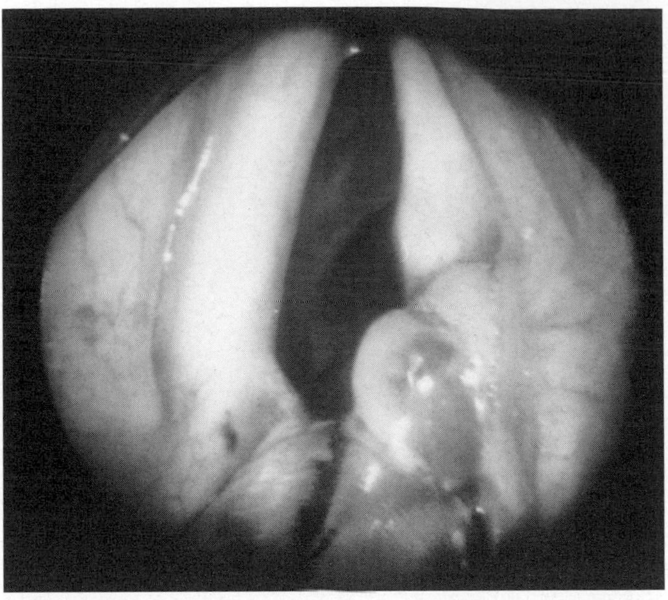

Figure 20.5 *Intubation granuloma. Note the fleshy, pedunculated mass may be seen at the posterior vocal process of the right arytenoid cartilage.*

Intubation granuloma

Localized maturation of granulation tissue may give rise to a pedunculated mass usually situated at the vocal process of the arytenoid cartilage (Fig 20.5).[38] Often unilateral, intubation granulomas may result in hoarseness, sore throat, globus sensation, stridor, or dyspnea, especially if large in size.[1] These masses are usually treated by surgical removal with a laser or microlaryngeal scissors. In a further attempt to minimize injury and contamination, we institute strict anti-reflux measures and long-term antibiotics to suppress quantitative bacteriology.

Interarytenoid adhesion

Interarytenoid adhesion may occur if opposing ulcerated surfaces of the arytenoid vocal processes heal to one another, resulting in a transverse fibrous band (Fig 20.6).[29] Often mistaken for bilateral vocal cord paralysis because of limited abduction of the tethered vocal cords, interarytenoid adhesions may be divided with a laser or microlaryngeal scissors.[3]

Posterior glottic stenosis

The mucosa covering the arytenoid cartilages and interarytenoid region overlies thin mucoperichondrium with very little submucosa, and so ischemic necrosis secondary to pressure from an indwelling endotracheal tube may result in granulation tissue maturing into a thick, contracted scar filling the posterior larynx (Fig 20.7).[13] The sites involved with scar tissue include the posterior one-third of the true vocal folds, the posterior commissure,

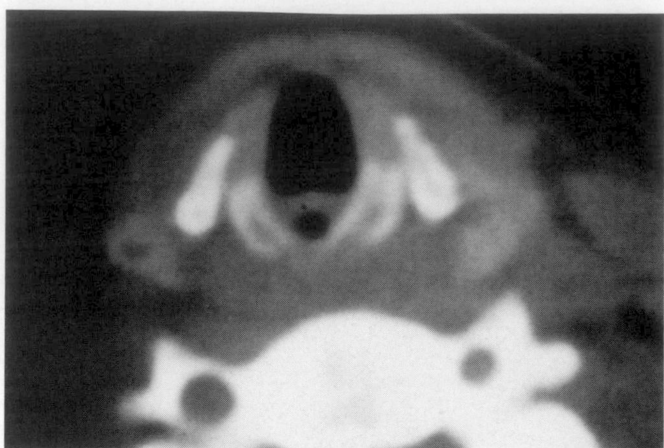

Figure 20.6 *Interarytenoid adhesion. A transverse band is illustrated on this computed tomography scan extending across the arytenoid cartilages.*

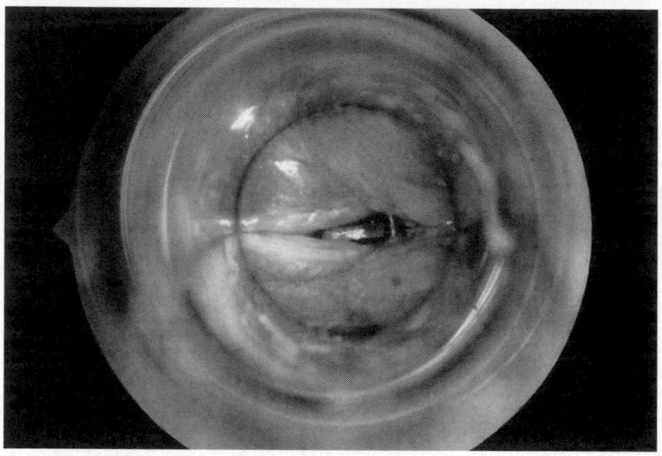

Figure 20.7 *Posterior glottic stenosis. In addition to a thin interarytenoid adhesion, a thick fibrotic scar is present at the posterior larynx.*

and the interarytenoid region, with more extensive scarring resulting in ankylosis of the cricoarytenoid joints.[6] Posterior glottic stenosis may be associated with fixation of the true vocal folds in adduction with inability to abduct.[42,72] Because of the adducted position of the true vocal folds, the patient's voice quality is often normal.[6] The diagnosis of posterior glottic stenosis may be confirmed with direct laryngoscopy, and mobility of the cricoarytenoid joints should be assessed by palpating the arytenoids.

Posterior glottic stenosis may be treated with laryngofissure, incorporating scar excision and mucosal grafting, combined with arytenoidectomy if both cricoarytenoid joints are fixed.[6] Posterior glottic stenosis with less extensive scarring and without cricoarytenoid joint fixation may be endoscopically incised with a laser or microlaryngeal instruments.

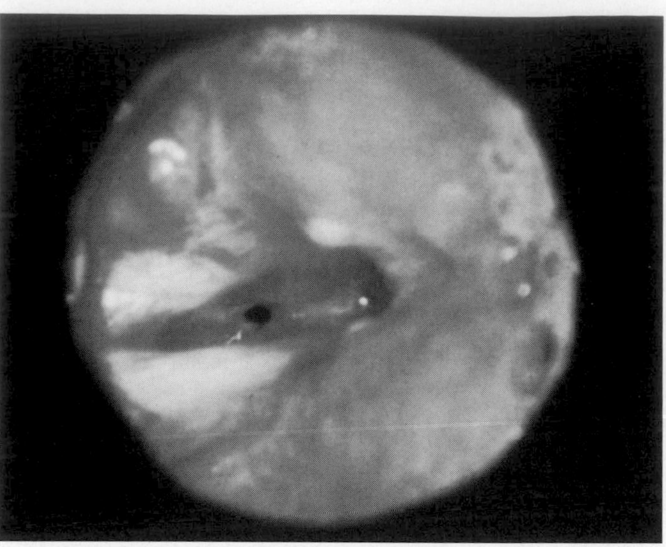

Figure 20.8 *Subglottic stenosis. Extensive subglottic scarring nearly obliterates the airway lumen.*

Subglottic stenosis

Ulceration in the subglottis may lead to granulation tissue and subsequent fibrous thickening, resulting in narrowing of the subglottic airway following extubation (Fig 20.8).[30] Subglottic ulceration may become secondarily infected from mucociliary stasis,[52] and severe cicatricial injury has been observed following 14–21 days of intubation.[67]

Acquired subglottic stenosis following prolonged intubation often results in loss of cartilaginous support and a greater degree of airway obstruction than does congenital subglottic stenosis.[15] Furthermore, acquired subglottic stenosis from prolonged intubation is less likely to be outgrown in children than is congenital subglottic stenosis.[16]

The goals of treatment for subglottic stenosis include maintaining airway patency, glottic competence and voice quality. Unfortunately, no treatment option has been completely satisfactory.[27] Permanent tracheotomy bypasses airway stenosis, but requires stomal occlusion to phonate and limits participation in water sports. Endoscopic dilatation is less successful with advanced scar formation.[15] Open surgical techniques for severe stenoses are more invasive and include epiglottic flap reconstruction,[61] autogenous grafts with cartilage,[15] myoperiosteal flaps,[21] and myo-osseous flaps.[68] The success of such procedures may be limited, as a result of difficulty in reestablishing the structural integrity and mucosal lining of the airway. During healing, reepithelialization must continually compete with scar formation.[17] The complex nature of multistaged traditional approaches to laryngotracheal repair have led to single-stage reconstructive procedures with cartilage grafting[39,58] or with primary anastomosis[64] for selected patients. Endoscopic placement of expandable mesh stents for subglottic stenosis has demonstrated favorable results with initial canine trials.[27]

Complete stenosis

Complete stenosis from extensive fibrosis and scarring at the glottis and subglottis may result in near-total or total obliteration of the airway lumen. Such stenoses are difficult to manage, since iatrogenic trauma from surgical dilatation or excessive laser excision may inadvertently result in further damage.[3]

Subglottic ductal retention cysts

Arising from obstruction of subepithelial mucinous gland ducts, subglottic ductal retention cysts may occur in infants following prolonged intubation. These cysts may require no treatment if small, for they may resolve spontaneously. Larger cysts may be removed by laser excision or microlaryngeal forceps.[2]

Vocal cord paralysis

Vocal cord immobility may result from cricoarytenoid joint ankylosis, as described earlier in this chapter. Vocal cord paralysis may also result from neurogenic injury following intubation. Compression injury of the anterior ramus of the recurrent laryngeal nerve may occur between the endotracheal tube and laryngeal cartilages.[7,12,20] Spontaneous recovery can be expected within 4 months.[71]

Risk factors for intubation trauma

Intubation technique

Proper positioning of the patient with intubation performed by personnel experienced in its technique is optimal. Flexible fiberoptic endoscopic guidance may be useful when a difficult intubation is anticipated.[19] Repeated intubation attempts should be avoided.

Endotracheal tube characteristics

The pathogenesis for injury from prolonged intubation described earlier in the chapter involves mucosal ischemia induced by pressure exerted by the endotracheal tube. Ideally, the endotracheal tube utilized should be nonirritating, of appropriate size and conform easily to the natural curvature of the cervical airway, with a low-pressure, high-volume cuff.

Constitutional health of patient

Patients in poor medical condition may be at particular risk for mucosal changes from prolonged intubation, including patients with multiorgan failure, hypoxemia, perfusion deficits, or head injury.

The risk of intubation trauma is increased in cases of preexisting laryngeal disease, including laryngeal trauma or inflammation secondary to infection or gastroesophageal reflux.

The presence of nasopharyngeal instrumentation such as feeding tubes may predispose to injury by inducing arytenoid edema, possible cricoid perichondritis and even postcricoid abscess.[22,33,62]

Movement of endotracheal tube

Pressure on the larynx by the endotracheal tube is constant and exacerbated by laryngeal movement during coughing, swallowing, or straining.[1,71] Adequate sedation of intubated patients is necessary to minimize movement against the endotracheal tube.

Length of intubation period

It has been suggested that endoscopic laryngeal examination should be considered for adults after 5–7 days of intubation, for children after 1–2 weeks of intubation, and for infants only when attempted extubation has been unsuccessful.[3] Tracheotomy may then be considered if deep ulceration or perichondritis of the laryngeal structures is present. Although the risk of injury may be significant when intubation time is longer than 10 days,[73] neonates may be able to sustain longer periods of intubation due to the resilience of the laryngeal cartilages at this young age.[30] Absolute time limits for periods of intubation, however, are difficult to establish. The evaluation and assessment for tracheotomy should be made on an individual basis, with consideration for predicted length of intubation, patient's medical condition and associated laryngeal injury.

Conclusions

Laryngeal trauma sustained during the act of intubation or resulting from prolonged intubation has been well documented. Risk factors that predispose individuals to such trauma should be considered, to prevent such injury from occurring. Prevention is, in fact, the most important determinant of patient outcome. When assessing the need for tracheotomy secondary to prolonged intubation, each patient's case should be evaluated individually and independently. Successful surgical management must also control for occult gastroesophageal reflux injury and bacterial contamination.

References

1. Balestrieri F, Watson CB. Intubation granuloma. *Otolaryngol Clin North Am* 1982; **15:** 567–79.
2. Bauman NM, Benjamin B. Subglottic ductal cysts in the preterm infant: association with laryngeal intubation trauma. *Ann Otol Rhinol Laryngol* 1995; **104:** 963–8.
3. Benjamin B. Prolonged intubation injuries of the larynx: endoscopic diagnosis, classification and treatment. *Ann Otol Rhinol Laryngol Suppl* 1993; **102:** 1–15.
4. Bent JP III, Porubsky ES. The management of blunt fractures of the thyroid cartilage. *Otolaryngol Head Neck Surg* 1994; **110:** 195–202.

5. Bent JP III, Silver JR, Porubsky ES. Acute laryngeal trauma: a review of 77 patients. *Otolaryngol Head Neck Surg* 1993; **109:** 441–9.
6. Bogdasarian R, Olson NR. Posterior glottic laryngeal stenosis. *Otolaryngol Head Neck Surg* 1990; **88:** 765–72.
7. Brandwein M, Abramson AL, Shikowitz MJ. Bilateral vocal cord paralysis following endotracheal intubation. *Arch Otolaryngol Head Neck Surg* 1986; **112:** 877–82.
8. Bryce DP, Briant TD, Pearson FG. Laryngeal and tracheal complications of intubation. *Ann Otol* 1968; **77:** 442–61.
9. Burns HP, Dayal VS, Scott A, van Nostrand AW, Bryce DP. Laryngotracheal trauma: observations on its pathogenesis and its prevention following prolonged orotracheal intubation in the adult. *Laryngoscope* 1979; **89:** 1316–25.
10. Camnitz PS, Shepherd SM, Henderson RA. Acute blunt laryngeal and tracheal trauma. *Am J Emerg Med* 1987; **5:** 158–62.
11. Campbell D. Trauma to larynx and trachea following intubation and tracheotomy. *J Laryngol Otol* 1968; **82:** 981–6.
12. Cavo JW. True vocal cord paralysis following intubation. *Laryngoscope* 1985; **95:** 1352–9.
13. Cohen SR. Pseudolaryngeal paralysis: a postintubation complication. *Ann Otol* 1981; **90:** 483–8.
14. Cohn AM, Larson DL. Laryngeal injury: a critical review. *Arch Otolaryngol* 1976; **102:** 166–70.
15. Cotton RT. Pediatric laryngotracheal stenosis. *J Pediatr Surg* 1984; **19:** 699–704.
16. Cotton RT, Evans JN. Laryngotracheal reconstruction in children: five-year follow-up. *Ann Otol* 1981; **90:** 516–20.
17. Delaere PR, Liu Z, Hermans R. Laryngotracheal reconstruction with tracheal patch allografts. *Laryngoscope* 1998; **108:** 273–9.
18. Donnelly WH. Histopathology of endotracheal intubation. An autopsy study of 99 cases. *Arch Pathol* 1969; **88:** 511–20.
19. Edens ET, Sia RL. Flexible fiberoptic endoscopy in difficult intubations. *Ann Otol* 1981; **90:** 307–9.
20. Ellis PD, Pallister WK. Recurrent laryngeal nerve palsy and endotracheal intubation. *J Laryngol Otol* 1975; **89:** 823–6.
21. Friedman M, Grybauskas V, Toriumi DM, Skolnik E, Chilis T. Sternomastoid myoperiosteal flap for reconstruction of the subglottic larynx. *Ann Otol Rhinol Laryngol* 1987; **96:** 163–9.
22. Friedman M, Baim H, Shelton V *et al.* Laryngeal injuries secondary to nasogastric tubes. *Ann Otol* 1981; **90:** 469–74.
23. Fuhrman GM, Stieg FH III, Buerk CA. Blunt laryngeal trauma: classification and management protocol. *J Trauma* 1990; **30:** 87–92.
24. Gold SM, Gurber ME, Shott SR, Myer CM III. Blunt laryngotracheal trauma in children. *Arch Otolaryngol Head Neck Surg* 1997; **123:** 83–7.
25. Gussack GS, Jurkovich GJ. Treatment dilemmas in laryngotracheal trauma. *J Trauma* 1988; **28:** 1439–44.
26. Gussack GS, Jurkovich GJ, Luterman A. Laryngotracheal trauma: a protocol approach to a rare injury. *Laryngoscope* 1986; **96:** 660–5.
27. Hanna E, Eliachar I. Endoscopically introduced expandable stents in laryngotracheal stenosis: the jury is still out. *Otolaryngol Head Neck Surg* 1997; **116:** 97–103.
28. Harris HH, Tobin HA. Acute injuries of the larynx and trachea in 49 patients. Observations over a 15-year period. *Laryngoscope* 1970; **80:** 1376–84.
29. Hawkins DB. Glottic and subglottic stenosis from endotracheal intubation. *Laryngoscope* 1977; **87:** 339–46.
30. Hawkins DB. Hyaline membrane disease of the neonate: prolonged intubation in management: effects on the larynx. *Laryngoscope* 1978; **88:** 201–24.
31. Hilding AC. Laryngotracheal damage during intratracheal anesthesia. *Ann Otol* 1971; **80:** 565–84.
32. Hoffman FT, Brunberg JA, Winter P, Sullivan MJ, Kileny PR. Arytenoid subluxation: diagnosis and treatment. *Ann Otol Rhinol Laryngol* 1991; **100:** 1–9.
33. Holinger PH, Schild JA, Maurizi DG. Internal and external trauma to the larynx. *Laryngoscope* 1968; **78:** 944–54.
34. Keane WM, Denneny JC, Rowe LD, Atkins JP. Complications of intubation. *Ann Otol Rhinol Laryngol* 1982; **91:** 584–7.
35. Lambert GE Jr, McMurry GT. Laryngotracheal trauma: recognition and management. *JACEP* 1976; **5:** 883–7.
36. Lee SY. Experimental blunt injury to the larynx. *Ann Otol Rhinol Laryngol* 1992; **101:** 270–4.
37. Leopold DA. Laryngeal trauma. A historical comparison of treatment methods. *Arch Otolaryngol* 1983; **109:** 106–11.
38. Lindholm CE. Prolonged endotracheal intubation: a clinical investigation with special reference to its consequences for the larynx and trachea and to its place as an alternative to intubation through a tracheostomy. *Acta Anaesthesiol Scand Suppl* 1969; **33:** 1–131.
39. Lusk RP, Gray S, Muntz HR. Single-stage laryngotracheal reconstruction. *Arch Otolaryngol Head Neck Surg* 1991; **117:** 171–3.
40. Mancuso AA, Hanafee WN. Computed tomography of the injured larynx. *Radiology* 1979; **133:** 139–44.
41. Merritt RM, Bent JP III, Porubsky ES. Acute laryngeal trauma in the pediatric patient. *Ann Otol Rhinol Laryngol* 1998; **107:** 104–6.
42. Montgomery WW. Posterior and complete laryngeal (glottic) stenosis. *Arch Otolaryngol* 1973; **98:** 170–5.
43. Myer CM III, Orobello P, Cotton RT, Bratcher GO. Blunt laryngeal trauma in children. *Laryngoscope* 1987; **97:** 1043–7.
44. Nahum AM. Immediate care of acute blunt laryngeal trauma. *J Trauma* 1969; **9:** 112–25.
45. Ogura JH, Heeneman H, Spector GJ. Laryngo-tracheal trauma diagnosis and treatment. *Can J Otolaryngol* 1973; **2:** 112–18.
46. Olson NR. Surgical treatment of acute blunt laryngeal injuries. *Ann Otol* 1978; **87:** 716–21.
47. Pennington CL. External trauma of the larynx and trachea: immediate treatment and management. *Ann Otol* 1972; **81:** 546–54.
48. Peppard SB. Transient local paralysis following strangulation injury. *Laryngoscope* 1982; **92:** 31–4.
49. Peppard SB, Dickens JH. Laryngeal injury following shortterm intubation. *Ann Otol Rhinol Laryngol* 1983; **92:** 327–30.

50. Polansky A, Resnick D, Sofferman RA, Davidson TM. Hyoid bone elevation: a sign of tracheal transection. *Radiology* 1984; **150:** 117–20.
51. Santos PM, Afrassiabi A, Weymuller EA. Risk factors associated with prolonged intubation and laryngeal injury. *Otolaryngol Head Neck Surg* 1994; **111:** 453–9.
52. Sasaki CT, Horiuchi M, Koss N. Tracheostomy-related subglottic stenosis: bacteriologic pathogenesis. *Laryngoscope* 1979; **89:** 857–65.
53. Sataloff RT, Bough ID, Spiegel JR. Arytenoid dislocation: diagnosis and treatment. *Laryngoscope* 1994; **104:** 1353–61.
54. Schaefer SD. The treatment of acute external laryngeal injuries. *Arch Otolaryngol Head Neck Surg* 1991; **117:** 35–9.
55. Schaefer SD. The acute management of external laryngeal trauma: a twenty-seven year experience. *Arch Otolaryngol Head Neck Surg* 1992; **118:** 598–604.
56. Schaefer SD, Brown OE. Selective application of CT in the management of laryngeal trauma. *Laryngoscope* 1983; **93:** 1473–5.
57. Schaefer SD, Close LG. Acute management of laryngeal trauma: update. *Ann Otol Rhinol Laryngol* 1989; **98:** 98–104.
58. Seid AB, Pransky SM, Kearns DB. One-stage laryngotracheoplasty. *Arch Otolaryngol Head Neck Surg* 1991; **117:** 408–10.
59. Shumrick DA. Trauma of the larynx. *Arch Otolaryngol* 1967; **86:** 691–6.
60. Snow JB Jr. Diagnosis and therapy for acute laryngeal and tracheal trauma. *Otolaryngol Clin North Am* 1984; **17:** 101–6.
61. Sobol SM, Levine H, Wood B, Tucker HM. Epiglottic laryngoplasty for complicated laryngeal stenosis. *Ann Otol* 1981; **90:** 409–11.
62. Sofferman RA, Hubbell RN. Laryngeal complications of nasogastric tubes. *Ann Otol* 1981; **90:** 465–8.
63. Stanley RB Jr, Cooper DS, Florman SH. Phonatory effects of thyroid cartilage fractures. *Ann Otol Rhinol Laryngol* 1987; **96:** 493–6.
64. Stern Y, Gerber ME, Walner DL, Cotton RT. Partial cricotracheal resection with primary anastomosis in the pediatric age group. *Ann Otol Rhinol Laryngol* 1997; **106:** 891–6.
65. Stiernberg CH, Jahrsdoerfer RA, Gillenwater A, Joe SA, Alcalen SV. Gunshot wounds to the head and neck. *Arch Otolaryngol Head Neck Surg* 1992; **118:** 592–7.
66. Subcommittee on Advanced Trauma Life Support of the American College of Surgeons Committee on Trauma 1993–1997 and American College of Surgeons Committee on Trauma. *Advanced Trauma Life Support Student Manual*, 6th edn. Chicago, IL: American College of Surgeons.
67. Supance JS, Reilly JS, Doyle WJ, Bluestone CD, Hubbard J. Acquired subglottic stenosis following prolonged endotracheal intubation: a canine model. *Arch Otolaryngol* 1982; **108:** 727–31.
68. Thawley SE, Ogura JH. Use of the hyoid graft for treatment of laryngotracheal stenosis. *Laryngoscope* 1981; **91:** 226–32.
69. Thomas GK, Stevens MH. Stunting in experimental laryngeal injuries. *Arch Otolaryngol* 1975; **101:** 217–21.
70. Trone TH, Schaefer SD, Carder HM. Blunt and penetrating laryngeal trauma: a thirteen-year review. *Otolaryngol Head Neck Surg* 1980; **88:** 257–61.
71. Whited RE. Laryngeal dysfunction following prolonged intubation. *Ann Otol* 1979; **88:** 474–8.
72. Whited RE. Posterior commissure stenosis post long-term intubation. *Laryngoscope* 1983; **93:** 1314–18.
73. Whited RE. A prospective study of laryngotracheal sequelae in long-term intubation. *Laryngoscope* 1984; **94:** 367–77.
74. Woo P. Laryngeal framework reconstruction with miniplates. *Ann Otol Rhinol Laryngol* 1990; **99:** 772–7.
75. Yin SS, Qiu WW, Stucker FJ. Value of electromyography in differential diagnosis of laryngeal joint injuries after intubation. *Ann Otol Rhinol Laryngol* 1996; **105:** 446–51.

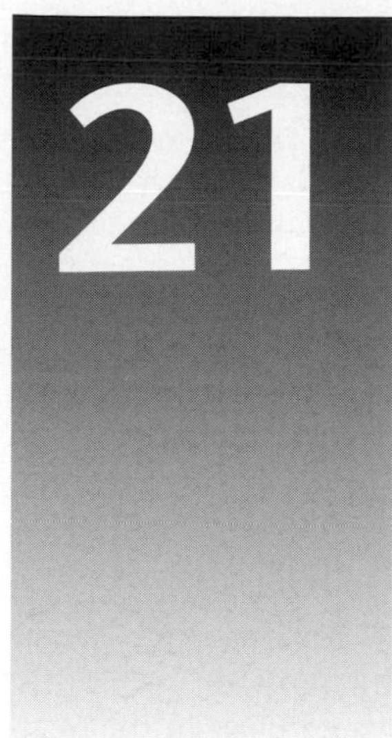

Infectious and inflammatory disorders of the larynx

Mark C Witte and H Bryan Neel III

This chapter was formulated as a working text to aid the laryngologist in the evaluation primarily of chronic infectious and inflammatory lesions of the larynx. Therefore, an attempt has been made to review all known infectious and inflammatory laryngeal diseases (with the exception of rheumatoid arthritis and associated diseases) that have been published in the English literature. It is hoped that the contents of this chapter will help the clinician to narrow the diagnostic search when faced with a chronic laryngeal lesion that defies diagnosis or is unexpectedly resistant to treatment.

Considerable effort has been exercised in an attempt to be both complete and concise in this chapter's contents. Therefore, emphasis has been placed on categorizing and detailing the diverse clinical manifestations and heterogeneous physical appearances of various laryngeal diseases. The coverage of other head and neck manifestations is somewhat narrower in scope, with descriptions of prominent, disease-characteristic head and neck signs and symptoms to aid in refining the differential diagnosis of a given disease presentation. Manifestations outside of the head and neck will be touched upon only insofar as they tend to aid in the diagnosis of the laryngeal process. The primary focus of this chapter is on disease entities that are most likely to be referred for subspecialist evaluation; accordingly, the reviews of laryngotracheobronchitis and epiglottitis are relatively less detailed than other sections as they are most often seen and initially treated by the primary caregiver. Within these two sections, emphasis will focus on details of urgent diagnostic or treatment considerations and unusual or recurrent manifestations, situations in which the laryngologist is likely to be consulted.

Due to the often diverse, gross manifestations of many disorders affecting the larynx, histologic identification of organisms or characteristic pathologic features is a cornerstone of diagnosis of these illnesses. Accordingly, efforts have been made to concisely categorize the histologic features of the disease entities and to emphasize those features that are characteristic or pathognomonic of the disease.

The chapter is organized into two broad categories: infectious diseases, and inflammatory disorders that have not been conclusively linked to a pathogenic organism. Within the category of infectious diseases, sections have been ordered from lower to higher phylogenetic levels; within these taxonomic categories, attempts have been made to order the sections from acute to chronic, from more to less common disease entities and, when appropriate, from broader to narrower host range. Within the category of noninfectious disorders, the diseases are ordered generally from more common to less common disease entities, although this is from the perspective of a 'first-world' observer.

Although many of the diseases are uncommon or rare, knowledge of these entities will become increasingly important in the future. It is anticipated that granulomatous infectious diseases, in particular, will be seen with increasing frequency due to improved support of susceptible patients (including a growing population with immunologic disease or on immunosuppressive therapy), increasing numbers of patients at the extremes of age, and increasing global travel.[28]

Laryngotracheobronchitis (croup)

Acute laryngotracheobronchitis (LTB) or croup is an upper airway infection of viral etiology. Seventy-five percent of all laryngotracheobronchitis cases are due to parainfluenza types I, II and III,[53] with disease due to parainfluenza type I the most common.[102] Other etiologic viral agents include influenza types A and B, which usually cause more severe disease,[53] as well as respiratory syncytial virus, rhinovirus and others.[8,102] The overall peak incidence of LTB is in autumn and spring, whilst that caused by the influenza viruses tends to peak in the winter months.[53] The upper respiratory symptoms of the typical viral prodrome predominate during the 2–6-day incubation period preceding the onset of laryngotracheal symptoms. The disease is spread by direct contact and infected individuals are capable of shedding infectious virus for 2 weeks.

LTB typically affects children between the ages of 6 months and 3 years; the peak incidence is at 2 years[102] within an age range from infancy to 10 years old.[8] There is a slight male-to-female predominance ratio of 1.5:1. LTB is one of the more common pediatric inpatient illnesses, affecting 1.5% of all children less than 6 years old,[102] and in 1979, 20 000 hospitalizations in the USA occurred due to LTB.[8]

The frequent history of antecedent rhinitis-type symptoms has been taken as evidence that the nasopharynx is the initial site for viral infection. With extension to the subglottis, the patient develops the typical signs and symptoms of LTB.[8] The pediatric airway is narrowest at the subglottis where the tissues are held rigidly within the cricoid ring;[102] even mild edema in this region can significantly reduce the nominal subglottic cross-sectional area. Also, the subglottic mucosa is relatively loosely adherent to underlying structures and readily allows the development of significant edema.

The typical patient with LTB presents with hoarseness, a 'barky' or 'seal-like' cough and biphasic stridor which may be accompanied by systemic signs and symptoms such as a moderate fever (more than 100°F) or leukocytosis to 15 000/mm^3.[8,25,102] In marked contrast to epiglottitis, drooling and marked odynophagia are characteristically absent and the patient does not assume the classic 'tripod' sitting position of epiglottitis.[102] Fifteen percent of all cases of 'LTB' are subcategorized as 'spasmodic croup' which is differentiated from traditional LTB by decreased severity, tendency to lack a viral prodrome, and sudden nocturnal onset.[8,102] The patient with spasmodic croup also tends to be afebrile and generally has a mild disease course and rapid resolution. Nevertheless, the need for airway support occasionally arises even in spasmodic croup.[8] It has been suggested that allergy can be a factor in the development of spasmodic croup.[102]

Because laryngeal examination is difficult in very young patients, the mainstay of diagnosis of LTB is the clinical assessment.[8] The classic radiographic characteristic in croup is symmetrical subglottic narrowing which is worse on expiration, the so-called 'steeple sign'. Hypopharyngeal distension and irregular thickening of the true vocal folds in the presence of a normal supraglottis are also suggestive features in neck films. Because the 'steeple sign' occurs in up to 30% of patients with epiglottitis, neck radiographic studies may 'have no place in the treatment of uncomplicated LTB'.[8]

The differential diagnosis of LTB includes spasmodic croup, epiglottitis, foreign body aspiration, congenital subglottic stenosis, laryngomalacia, and bacterial tracheitis.[8] In bacterial tracheitis, the subglottic appearance is similar to LTB but there are purulent subglottic secretions, pseudomembranes made up of necrotic debris, fibrin and sloughing epithelium, and submucosal congestion.[8] Patients with bacterial tracheitis tend as well to have a higher fever, a more toxic appearance, and a higher elevation of their white blood count.[8] Finally, patients with bacterial tracheitis do not respond to conventional treatment for LTB.

The characteristic appearance of LTB on endoscopic examination is remarkable for velvety, reddened subglottic tissues, a deep reddening of the laryngeal mucosa and rounded and intensely red semi-elliptical folds of edematous tissue below each true vocal fold; secretions are not prominent in LTB and the mucosa is not as friable as it is in bacterial infections.[8] In contrast to LTB, spasmodic croup is characterized by pale-appearing mucosa.

Much of the therapy for LTB is based on empirical treatment measures. Humidified air, for example, is nearly universally advocated yet has only anecdotal support. Presumably by moistening the larynx and subglottis, the inflamed mucosa is soothed and secretion clearance is improved.[102] Studies in kittens demonstrate that nebulized saline or water causes slowing of respiration and improved airflow.[25] Although small studies have shown no improvement in outcome over placebo,[102] it is still recommended that greater than 50% humidity be maintained in the patient's room. In contrast to humidified air, there is strong evidence that inhaled epinephrine is beneficial in temporarily reducing tracheal airway resistance. Although the 'racemic' form is commonly advocated, regular epinephrine at a strength of 1/1000 may be used with equal efficacy. The inhaled epinephrine is believed to exert a direct local action on the laryngeal and tracheal mucosa; studies have indicated that there is no substantial effect on airway dynamics by giving epinephrine subcutaneously.[8] Epinephrine's effects appear to be mediated through α-adrenergic stimulation of vasoconstriction within the edematous subglottic mucosa and possibly to β-adrenergic stimulation of bronchodilatation.[8] Epinephrine works rapidly after inhalation with a typical onset of activity within 10 minutes of treatment. Its effects last approximately 2 hours and rebound is possible thereafter; therefore, its use is not recommended unless the patient is going to be admitted for observation.[8,25] Despite the short-term positive effects, epinephrine has not resulted in any significant reduction in the length of hospitalization, the need for airway support, or any change in the natural history of the LTB disease process.[8]

The use of steroids in LTB is controversial. Of 14 studies that have been published, one-half demonstrated the benefits from steroid use whilst the other half did not. It has been more recently suggested by advocates of steroid use that these latter studies failed to use sufficient quantities of glucocorticoids to induce a measurable beneficial effect.[102] In order to investigate this question, a meta-analysis of nine carefully designed trials was instituted. This meta-analysis concluded that the use of high dose steroid (at least one dose of 125 mg of cortisone-equivalent) resulted in significantly increased clinical improvement at 12 and 24 hours and could markedly decrease the risk of endotracheal intubation.[53] It has been noted anecdotally that steroid use seems to decrease symptom severity and the need for epinephrine treatments.[25] A consensus seems to be emerging that, at least in severely affected children, a single dose of steroids at a dose of 0.6–1.5 mg/kg dexamethasone-equivalent is beneficial.[8,102]

Airway support is needed in less than 6% of patients with LTB. Nasotracheal intubation or tracheotomy may become necessary until the patient's airway stabilizes. Patients less than 1 year old are at particularly high risk of developing post-traumatic subglottic stenosis and an endotracheal tube at least two sizes smaller than normal is recommended.[8,25]

The guiding principle is the establishment of an adequate but not maximal airway.[102] Criteria for extubation include defervescence, decreased secretions and development of a large air leak around the tube as evidenced by the development of a cough, vocalization, or gurgling of secretions.[102] A tracheotomy should be considered when the functioning nasotracheal tube fails to relieve the signs of airway distress, if the nursing staff is inadequate to properly maintain a pediatric nasotracheal tube, if no one skilled in intubation will be available should the patient self-extubate, and if there is an absence of an air leak once the endotracheal tube is in place.[8] Endoscopic examination of the pediatric laryngeal airway should be considered in recurrent LTB in a patient less than 1 year old, or atypical, severe, or recurrent LTB,[8,102] or if the patient responds poorly to conventional therapy, or if there is a suspicion of foreign body aspiration.[8] When possible, it is recommended that endoscopy be delayed for 3–4 weeks following the acute illness until the reversible laryngeal changes subside; in such circumstances, open tube endoscopy under anesthesia is likely to yield the most valuable information.[102]

The prognosis for the vast majority of cases with LTB is quite good. Obstructive symptoms typically resolve after an average of 4 days.[53] There is a 15% complication rate consisting primarily of pneumonia and development of laryngeal obstruction.[53] It has been suggested that a vaccination program against parainfluenza types I, II and III would be valuable as it could reduce the disease incidence by at least 50%.[8]

Epiglottitis

Epiglottitis or 'supraglottitis' is a disease characterized by supraglottic or epiglottic edema secondary to bacterial infection. A significant proportion of the numerous cases of culture-negative epiglottitis may be of viral origin. In the context of the relatively subjective nature of the diagnosis of epiglottitis, which rests primarily on the appearance of the epiglottis, this seems a not unreasonable supposition. Early investigators felt that epiglottitis was most typically a sequel to infection of Waldeyer's ring or to a traumatic event. Anecdotal evidence for this theory is provided by case reports that describe pharyngitis or upper respiratory symptoms preceding the onset of airway compromise and epiglottitis by up to 3 weeks.[118] The organism most commonly associated with epiglottitis is *Haemophilus influenzae* type B (HIB), a Gram-negative coccobacillus. Prior to the institution of effective vaccination regimens, this organism was believed to be the 'sole agent' of epiglottitis in children;[76] indeed, in studies of populations prior to the initiation of widespread vaccination, positive blood cultures in pediatric patients identified HIB in 80–97% of cases.[13,25] Even today, in adults HIB still appears to be the most common pathogenic agent in epiglottitis.[37] Other pathogens that are commonly implicated in adult epiglottitis include *Streptococcus pyogenes* (group A β-hemolytic streptococcus), and viridans streptococci.[22,37] In the immunocompromised host, typically a patient with AIDS or a hematogenous malignancy, the clinician is cautioned to be more circumspect about unusual organisms such as *Aspergillus*, *Candida*, *Klebsiella* and even cytomegalovirus and herpes simplex virus as possible etiologic agents.[22] It has been speculated that the decreasing reservoir of HIB in children following widespread vaccine use will ultimately lead to a decrease in the rate of adult HIB epiglottitis.[37]

Epiglottitis classically affects children between 2 and 6 years of age. This is a considerably older age range than is characteristic of laryngotracheobronchitis (croup), the chief entity from which epiglottitis must be distinguished. Other factors that are more specific for epiglottitis include typical lack of a viral prodrome, prominent dyspnea and odynophagia, a 'toxic' appearance, and the tendency of the patient to assume a 'tripod' sitting position to facilitate air exchange. The incidence of epiglottitis in children has fallen from 11–14 per 100 000,[46,75] to an incidence of about 0.6–1.4 per 100 000 following the effective introduction of HIB vaccine.[25,37] By contrast, the incidence of adult epiglottitis has remained stable at 1.8–2.3 per 100 000.[22,46] This has resulted in a shift in the clinical spectrum in that epiglottitis is now more prevalent in adults than in children. A male predominance of about 2–3:1 is commonly noted in literature reviews.[37,54] The typical age of onset in adults is approximately 40 years. Prior to the widespread knowledge of epiglottitis as an entity affecting adults, the adult mortality rate was 30%.[41] Current adult mortality rates are 6–7% whereas the pediatric mortality rate is about 1%. A frequently cited factor contributing to mortality is lack of early clinical suspicion of epiglottitis in patients presenting with pharyngeal symptoms.[25] A seasonal variation has been documented, with relatively increased rates in the summer and winter.[37] Predisposing factors for epiglottitis include immunodeficiencies including neutropenia, acquired immunodeficiency, multiple myeloma, and HIV infection, diabetes mellitus, alcoholism and asthma.[37]

The pediatric presentation of epiglottitis is characterized by fever, irritability, lethargy and sore throat which may rapidly progress to dysphagia, drooling and respiratory distress.[75] The child develops inspiratory stridor which paradoxically decreases with disease progression, as increasing obstruction and fatigue combine to reduce airflow. The use of suprasternal and intercostal accessory muscles is also a classic sign in children.[75] Airway obstruction can progress unpredictably and often suddenly in pediatric patients.[13] In adults the presenting picture is somewhat more heterogeneous, typically with a slower onset of progressive disease;[46,76] in about half of patients more than 24 hours pass between the first symptoms and presentation.[54,76] Symptoms include a gradually progressive, severe sore throat, dysphagia, odynophagia, fever and, finally, dyspnea and shortness of breath with or without tachycardia.[22,25] The 'most constant and important' finding is that of increasing painful dysphagia over the course of several days.[118] Anterior cervical tenderness with or without lymphadenopathy and a stiff neck are also fairly frequent findings.[22,37,75] More worrisome symptoms include drooling, a muffled voice, stridor, and the assumption of an erect sitting posture.[37,54] The latter two signs have been associated with a five- to sixfold increased likelihood of requiring subsequent aggressive airway management, i.e. intubation or tracheotomy.[37] It has been suggested that one's clinical suspicion should be increased in adults who complain of a severe sore throat yet have a normal oropharyngeal examination.[37] Occasionally a macular rash over the face and arms has been described in association with epiglottitis.[54] Not surprisingly, disease progression in the AIDS patient is generally more aggressive.[22]

The diagnosis of epiglottitis in the pediatric patient is made based on direct supraglottic inspection in a setting in which the clinician is prepared for immediate intubation. The operating suite is typically considered the optimal location for this examination. One protocol that is recommended entails the use of mask-induction anesthetic with the patient breathing spontaneously followed by airway inspection and intubation as necessary.[75] Because of impaired gas exchange due to obstruction, induction time may be prolonged to as long as 30 minutes.[75] The characteristic finding on examination is 'cherry red' erythema and edema of the epiglottis with or without spread to the aryepiglottic folds and arytenoid mucosa.[54,75] During examination and subsequent intubation, the location of the laryngeal introitus is sometimes facilitated by gentle pressure on the chest while examining the pharynx for the expulsion of an air bubble from the larynx.[75] If intubation is deemed necessary, the nasotracheal route is preferred in pediatric patients as it may allow the patient to remain awake and spontaneously breathing while in place over the next several days; in such a patient the airway must be carefully secured and arm splints should be applied to minimize the opportunity for self-extubation.[75] Intubation is preferred over tracheotomy in children in that typically a relatively short period of intubation will be necessary, the complications of tracheotomy can be avoided, and the hospital stay can be shortened.[13] It is recommended that a tube one size smaller than would normally be used be selected, and that an appropriate size tube will be characterized by a definite air leak at a pressure of 20–25 cmH_2O.[13,75]

In adults, presumably due to higher airway reserve as a result of a much larger tracheal cross-sectional area, a less aggressive approach is considered appropriate. Numerous authors maintain that it is safe to inspect the larynx of an adult with suspected epiglottitis in the office setting; flexible fiberoptic endoscopy affords the best possible examination whilst minimizing the risk of provoking laryngospasm.[22,75,76] Needless to say, such examination should be performed expeditiously. The appearance of the supraglottic larynx in the adult with epiglottitis is similar to that of the pediatric patient. In the adult patient with no signs of respiratory distress and a respiratory rate of less than 20/min, observation in an intensive care setting is considered an appropriate measure. The need for an intensive setting is based on the case reports of rapid airway obstruction in adults requiring emergency intubation. If the patient has a respiratory rate of greater than 30/min, is cyanotic, retaining CO_2 or otherwise appears in extremis, it is considered appropriate that the patient be intubated in the operating room or at the bedside.[22] Overall, about 15% of adults with epiglottitis will ultimately require endotracheal intubation or tracheotomy.[37]

Other clinical data that may be obtained to help establish a diagnosis of epiglottitis include a white blood cell count of greater than or equal to 15 000/mm^3.[75] Lateral airway radiography may also be useful in young children with minimal airway symptoms in whom the diagnosis is in doubt or in older children or adults in whom observation is the planned first treatment.[75] The radiogram should be performed with the patient in an upright posture to facilitate air exchange.[75] Neither blood work nor radiological studies is considered appropriate if the index of suspicion for epiglottitis is high; this is particularly relevant in young children in whom aggressive handling may precipitate laryngospasm.[25] Characteristic radiographic findings include a thickened or 'thumb-shaped' epiglottis with obliteration of the valleculae and pyriforms, hypopharyngeal ballooning, tracheal narrowing and prevertebral soft tissue swelling.[75]

Once the airway is secured, blood culture should be obtained to aid in the diagnosis and to tailor antibiotic treatment. Of note, in children, only about 50% and in adults only 15–30% of blood cultures are positive. As previously stated, HIB is the usual pathogen in children's blood cultures; in adults pneumococcus, *Haemophilus parainfluenzae* and *Streptococcus pyogenes* have also been isolated.[54]

The differential diagnosis of epiglottitis includes laryngitis, croup and diphtheria. In children, croup usually affects an earlier age group of 6 months to 3 years old, and is not typically associated with throat pain or drooling. Diphtheria is characterized by severe dysphagia or hoarseness with the formation of a gray pharyngeal pseudomembrane and polyneuritis.[75] Other possible etiologies for airway obstruction in the pediatric patient include laryngomalacia, burns, or foreign body aspiration.

The critical component in treatment of epiglottitis is securing the airway. While settling on a course of action, it is recommended that all patients be started on 100% humidified oxygen.[75] Once the airway has been addressed and appropriate laboratory studies have been obtained, antibiotic therapy is instituted. Cefuroxime is considered the current drug of choice for pediatric epiglottitis.[76] In adults, a second- or third-generation cephalosporin with activity against β-lactamase-producing HIB is the drug of choice.[22] Further recommendations for treatment of adult epiglottitis include assurance of adequate coverage against HIB, *Staphylococcus aureus*, group A β-hemolytic streptococcus, and pneumococcus.[17] The classic treatment for epiglottitis is ampicillin and chloramphenicol and this is still considered a useful drug combination. In the pediatric patient in whom *Haemophilus* is found to be chloramphenicol-resistant, gentamicin or trimethoprim–sulfamethoxazole (TMP-SMX) therapy is an option.[75] Intramuscular epinephrine may have some role as a temporizing agent in adults with suspected epiglottitis.[22] Although glucocorticoids have often been used, there is currently no conclusive evidence that they have any substantial benefit in the treatment of epiglottitis.[37] In cases of recurrent epiglottitis a further workup to rule out collagen vascular diseases, sarcoid and occult carcinoma has been advocated.[22] In patients in whom *Haemophilus influenzae* type B is identified as the causative organism, rifampicin prophylaxis has been advocated for all close contacts. This should be administered at 20 mg/kg/day to a maximum dose of 600 mg/day for a total of 4 days.[22,118] Overall, the prognosis for epiglottitis is good if the airway is successfully secured. Typically, intubation is only required for 36–48 hours;[5] one large study reported an average 42 hour intubation span.[13] Daily direct supraglottic inspection in intubated adults is recommended; with a decrease in edema, erythema and reestablishment of the normal supraglottic landmarks, it is appropriate to attempt extubation.[13] Signs that the pediatric patient may be ready for extubation include cessation of fever, improved overall appearance, and the ability of the patient to swallow secretions.[75]

One insidious prognostic finding is the development of an epiglottic abscess. Such a condition is quite rare, nearly always occurs as a result of epiglottitis, and nearly always occurs in adults.[41] Epiglottic abscess occurs in about 15% in series of adults with epiglottitis.[54] The predilection for its occurrence in adults may reside in its overall rarity secondary to HIB infection; the most common pathogen found in epiglottic abscesses is streptococcus.[41] A typical presentation is in a patient receiving antibiotic treatment for epiglottitis who, after 10–72 hours of improvement, begins to complain of increased dysphagia and develops increased vocal muffling and inspiratory stridor. Although in the past many abscesses have been drained under local anesthetic, it is considered most prudent to attempt to secure the airway in the operating room prior to direct laryngoscopic inspection. Most commonly the abscess involves the lingual surface of the epiglottis; this is believed to be a more susceptible area due to the relative laxity of the submucosal connective tissue compared with that of the laryngeal epiglottic surface. If possible, attempts should be made to endotracheally intubate the patient prior to drainage to avoid the possibility of aspiration of purulent abscess material; if intubation is not possible, a tracheotomy should be strongly considered to secure the airway prior to drainage. One case presentation reports that, following drainage of an epiglottic abscess, subsequent epiglottic collapse necessitated urgent tracheotomy.[41] Once the airway is secured, incision and drainage is performed, and the patient is closely observed while intravenous antibiotic therapy is continued. The overall mortality rate from epiglottic abscesses is 30%.[11]

On a historical note, it has been plausibly asserted that George Washington, the first president of the USA, succumbed to epiglottitis rather than pneumonia.[22]

Scleroma

Scleroma, or rhinoscleroma, occurs after infection with *Klebsiella rhinoscleromatis*, an immotile Gram-negative diplobacillus.[107] This organism has a worldwide distribution, with primary foci of infections occurring in Eastern, Central and Southern Europe, North Africa, India, Indonesia and central South America.[20] Infection with the organism is facilitated by poor hygiene and low socio-economic conditions, and clinical infection probably requires periods of prolonged contact with infectious airborne secretions.[107] The typical patient is 20–40 years old.

There is a predilection for primary infection to occur at mucocutaneous boundaries. By far the most common site of primary infection is the nasal vestibule; the resultant nasal infection is the origin of the more common designation 'rhinoscleroma'; however, in reference to nonnasal disease, 'scleroma' is perhaps more appropriate. From the nose the disease frequently spreads to the nasopharynx and finally to the subglottis at the junction of the true vocal fold epithelium and the subglottic mucosa.[106] It has been postulated that three distinct phases of disease development exist in scleroma. The first is described as a catarrhal or exudative stage characterized by purulent rhinorrhea or foul-smelling green crusts.[3,51,100] After weeks or months the nasal mucosal lining may become atrophic and undergo squamous metaplasia.[87] This frequently coincides with the second or granulomatous stage of disease. In this stage, small, soft, granulomatous nodules may be seen studding the nasal turbinates and septum and other areas of involvement. Eventually these nodules coalesce into large friable nodules and in the larynx these may present as symmetrical nodular subepithelial infiltrates.[51] Following years of infection, the cicatricial or sclerotic stage of the disease ensues. This is characterized by fibrosis with collagen deposition, histiocytic and plasmacytic aggregates and airway narrowing.[51,87]

The patient with scleroma most commonly presents with complaints of nasal obstruction, epistaxis and nasal deformity. A classic presentation may commence with persistent large volume rhinorrhea (catarrh) followed by the gradual onset of nasal obstruction with crusting and scarring.[20] Oropharyngeal, tracheal and bronchial involvement have been reported, as well as lacrimal gland and orbital lesions.[51] With laryngeal involvement, hoarseness, biphasic stridor, and ultimately airway obstruction ensue.[51,106] The patient may complain of hoarseness that gradually leads to aphonia;[19] later dyspnea, chronic cough and expectoration of crusts may occur.[106]

The patient presenting with laryngeal scleroma nearly always displays evidence of concomitant nasal involvement,[51] typified by scarred nasal vestibules and marked crusting.[107] The disease is often of insidious onset and may take 3 or more years to progress to laryngeal infection.[100] Physical examination of the larynx may reveal large granulomatous masses, subglottic nodules, diffuse infiltrating lesions, and areas of ulceration and crusting with purulent exudate.[20,106] The most typical area of subglottic involvement is at the glottic–subglottic interface.[1] Also described are pale lesions with 'diffuse nodular thickening'[1] and circumferential subglottic stenoses with marked epithelial hypertrophy similar in appearance to verrucous carcinoma.[20,51,107] Finally, edematous granular subglottic masses[87] and granulomas at the glottic level[1] have been described. Although supraglottic lesions are uncommon, one patient was found to have epiglottic edema and a broad-based exophytic granulomatous mass arising from the laryngeal epiglottic surface with uninvolved vocal folds.[1] In epiglottic manifestations, involvement of the laryngeal surface is 'characteristic'.[51] Serial examinations suggest that progression of laryngeal disease begins with superior spread of an initial subglottic lesion. Untreated subglottic lesions may spread superiorly with subsequent glottic webbing, progressing to concentric stenosis.[3] In conjunction with laryngeal disease, bilateral shotty anterior cervical lymphadenopathy has been noted.[51]

As *K. rhinoscleromatis* is always a pathogen, its identification in diseased tissue warrants the diagnosis of scleroma. This organism must, however, be distinguished from *Klebsiella ozaenae*, which may exist in nasal biopsy specimens. Immunostaining using specific antibodies to the 'O' or smooth somatic antigen, and 'K' or capsular antigen, allow this distinction to be made; although not widely available, the O2 K3 antibody stain is the 'most specific' for *K. rhinoscleromatis*.[1,100] It has been suggested that *K. rhinoscleromatis* may be found in tissue both early in the disease and during the granulomatous stage of disease.[20,51] Culture of biopsy specimens is also a useful adjunct for diagnosis, although only 60% of these will typically prove positive.[20]

Histologic examination of typical biopsy specimens demonstrates 'bloated plasmacytes' or 'Russell bodies,' large homogenous eosinophilic bodies which are felt to represent degenerating plasmacytes.[20,107] Although characteristic, these are not pathognomonic of scleroma unless filled with Gram-negative diplobacilli.[87] Also, Mikulicz cells, foamy vacuolated histiocytes with centrally placed nuclei, may be seen. The *Klebsiella* located within the vacuoles do not stain, giving them their characteristic 'foamy appearance'[1,20] Finally, lymphocytes and plasmacytes may be found among the infiltrates. Examination of more advanced lesions often reveals irregular connective tissue bands and collagen aggregates in the submucosa which generally fail to resolve following successful eradication of the disease organisms; this is the origin of the extensive scarring that is often found after severe scleroma infection.[1]

The mainstay of treatment for early scleroma has traditionally been 2 g/day of tetracycline for at least 2 months;[20,100] this regimen results in a 60–70% cure rate.[87] Others have recommended that treatment be carried out for 6 months to 2 years or until nasal mucosal biopsies are negative for *K. rhinoscleromatis*.[1] Other antibiotics that may be useful include the fluoroquinolones,[87] clofazimine, streptomycin and aminoglycosides, such as gentamicin or amikacin combined with an antimetabolite such as TMP-SMX.[3,51] In pregnant women, first-generation cephalosporins may prove useful although they are not as effective as the first-line agents. Long-term follow-up is considered requisite to effective treatment as the disease may persist for decades with long periods of remission.

Several particulars of the organism contribute to the difficulty in trying to eradicate the disease. First, *K. rhinoscleromatis* is spore-forming under anaerobic conditions, and such spores may remain dormant for months to years prior to subsequent reactivation.[1] Even while dormant, the spores release small amounts of exotoxin which potentiate the inflammatory response even in the absence of propagating bacteria. Further, the propagating bacterium's mucopolysaccharide slime coat may cause osmotic rupture of phagocytizing histiocytes with premature release of viable bacteria.[51] Surgical treatments that have been advocated for laryngeal scleroma include dilatation of subglottic stenosis although this is of limited success, laser excision of discrete subglottic lesions, and tracheal resection and reanastomosis.[1]

As may be inferred from the above factors, the prognosis of laryngeal scleroma depends upon early recognition of the disease and judicious long-term use of appropriate antibiotics. The severe scarring which typically results from protracted disease may require extensive surgical treatment in attempts to improve airway and vocal function; the prognosis in such patients is guarded.

Syphilis

Syphilis is a disease of considerable notoriety, and was first described in the sixteenth century in the shepherd for whom the disease is named. Although still a matter of some dispute, many historians believe the German Emperor Frederick III was a victim of laryngeal syphilis.[72] Syphilis, caused by the spirochete *Treponema pallidum*, is surprisingly not highly contagious; there is only a 10% chance of being infected through sexual contact with an infected partner.[70] Worldwide, there are certain endemic forms of syphilis such as bejel. This is endemic among the Bedouin Arabs in whom over one-quarter are infected by disease; bejel is also endemic in some portions of sub-Saharan Africa and the Pacific Islands. Infection with such forms of syphilis is often clinically occult, as the patient typically does not develop a primary lesion and spread is by sharing of drinking vessels with household contacts in the highly infectious mucous patch stage of disease.[70]

There are four stages of syphilitic disease. Primary syphilis is characterized by a painless chancre with rolled borders that occur at the site of penetration of the organism following an incubation period of 10 90 days. After a variable quiescent period, the lesions of secondary syphilis may become evident in the head and neck as highly infectious, macerated, eroded mucous patches or grayish-white papules on the lips, tongue, and buccopharyngeal mucosa in a patient whose symptoms may range from none to severe pharyngitis.[20,64] Secondary nasal syphilis may present with acute rhinitis with a scant mucopurulent discharge.[70] There is a predilection for treponemal infection of the membranous bone of the maxilla which may result in the formation of bony sequestra in the lateral nasal wall with associated foul-smelling nasal discharge and hard and soft palate perforations.[64] Following primary infection, one-third of patients affected by syphilis will spontaneously cure themselves, one-third will go into a life-long latent period following secondary syphilis, and one-third will go on to develop the cardiac, neurologic and osteocutaneous sequelae of late syphilis.[70]

Laryngeal involvement with primary syphilis is considered doubtful or rare. One case report describes a grayish depressed zone with surrounding induration which healed spontaneously within 3–6 weeks.[64] Laryngeal lesions of secondary syphilis are commonly characterized by diffuse mucosal hyperemia, particularly over the epiglottis, sometimes accompanied by a maculopapular rash coalescing into mucous patches. Progression of the disease may lead to development of marked epithelial hypertrophy or hyperplasia and formation of condyloma lata.[70] Laryngeal lesions of tertiary syphilis include diffuse nodular infiltrates representing multiple small gummata which may coalesce and ulcerate, leaving deep necrotic ulcers and exposing underlying cartilage. This allows perichondritis and chondritis to develop; subsequent healing leads to late fibrosis, vocal fold adhesions, arytenoid fixation and cicatricial subglottic stenosis.[20] It is possible, however, that vocal fold paralysis may occur subsequent to tertiary neurosyphilis rather than by direct gummatous invasion or fibrosis; such a presentation is typically accompanied by other lower cranial nerve deficits.[70]

Many tests have been developed to aid in the diagnosis of syphilis. Darkfield examination may be performed on scrapings from lesions of primary and secondary syphilis; however, the standard darkfield test is not recommended for examination of oropharyngeal lesions as there is cross-reactivity with commensal treponemes which are often normal oral flora. The fluorescent antibody darkfield test labels the treponemes with fluorescent-tagged antibodies specific against *Treponema pallidum* and is therefore a much more useful test.[64] Standard serologic tests include the VDRL (venereal disease research laboratory) test, which detects a cardiolipin-cholesterol-lecithin antibody and, whilst inexpensive, is somewhat nonspecific. The TPHA (treponemal hemagglutination assay) and an FTA-ABS (fluorescent treponemal antibody absorption) are very specific for antibodies against treponemes but cannot distinguish between various species.[77]

The histology of secondary syphilitic lesions of the larynx is characterized by a patchy, dense perivascular aggregation of plasmacytes and lymphocytes and varying degrees of vasculitis.[20] The vasculitic processes trigger endothelial proliferation and obstruction of submucosal small vessels.[20] With the onset of secondary bacterial infection, perichondritis, ulceration and cartilage necrosis may be present. In some lesions the development of pseudoepitheliomatous hyperplasia can lead to confusion of the lesion with carcinoma. The gummatous lesions of tertiary syphilis are characterized by nodules and plasmacytes, lymphocytes, epithelioid cells and fibroblasts interspersed with variable numbers of giant cells.[64,70] A core of coagulated necrotic material is nearly always found at the center of larger gummatous nodules.[70] The vasculitis of tertiary syphilis is characterized by an obliterative endarteritis involving all three vessel layers. Other tertiary lesions have been described as demonstrating diffuse tissue infiltrates of plasmacytes and fibroblasts.[70]

In patients who have not been previously treated, high-dose penicillin therapy is recommended which should lead to the timely resolution of epithelial hyperplasia.[20] A typical dose is 2.4 million units of benzathine penicillin G given in two doses 1 week apart.[70,94] Slower microbe replication characteristic of latent disease necessitates more protracted treatment schedules using higher antibiotic dosages.[77] Higher doses are also recommended in central nervous system (CNS) disease. If the patient is allergic to penicillin, doxycycline 100 mg twice a day for 14 days or erythromycin 500 mg three to four times a day for 14 days is recommended.[77,94] There is also evidence that ceftriaxone may have utility in the treatment of syphilis.[94] During the initiation of antibiotic therapy, the clinician must watch carefully for the development of a Jarisch–Herxheimer reaction which typically occurs within 12 hours of the first antibiotic dose. This reaction, which is believed to be due to an increased local inflammatory reaction to the products of spirochete lysis, can lead to marked local erythema, edema, pain and possible airway compromise. Other characteristic symptoms include the onset of fever, chills, headache and malaise. In such an event, high-dose glucocorticoid therapy is recommended to control the inflammatory process.[70] As in many of the chronic infectious diseases of the larynx, surgical treatment is only instituted in an attempt to improve voice or airway in the case of late-stage fibrotic sequelae of the inflammatory process.

Tuberculosis

Historically, laryngeal tuberculosis or phthisis (Gk – 'wasting'),[18] was a common malady of the larynx. Prior to the advent of specific antibiotic therapy, laryngeal infection with tuberculosis was a fairly typical terminal, or near terminal, event in a course of pulmonary tuberculosis. Physicians at the turn of the century noted that few, if any, patients with laryngeal tuberculosis ever recovered, and one retrospective review indicates the mortality associated with laryngeal tuberculosis was about 70%.[89]

Since the advent of isoniazid and other antituberculous therapies, the incidence of laryngeal tuberculosis has fallen to much lower levels than in previous centuries; nevertheless, it is still considered by some the most common granulomatous disease of the larynx.[20] During the past decade, the incidence of laryngeal tuberculosis has risen, largely due to a growing number of immunocompromised individuals (typically HIV-infected) and the advent of multidrug-resistant organisms. The World Health Organization declared tuberculosis a global emergency in 1993,[121] whilst in the USA between the years 1986 and 1991 a 12% increase was seen in the number of reported cases.[121] Following the advent of effective tuberculosis chemotherapy, the mean age of presentation tended to rise initially. In the pre-antibiotic era patients more typically presented in the 20–39 years age range,[4,112] whereas following the introduction of isoniazid the average patient age increased to 45–60 years old.[4,59] With the advent of HIV and its tendency to affect a younger age group, this trend toward increasing patient age has begun to reverse; in a 1992 review the mean age of patients presenting with laryngeal tuberculosis was 38.7 years.[89]

The great majority of cases of laryngeal tuberculosis appear to occur as a result of seeding of the larynx following a primary pulmonary infection. Coughing episodes propel mycobacteria from cavitary lesions where they reside in large numbers, showering organisms upon the supraglottic laryngeal mucosa. Autopsy studies suggest that most of these lesions that subsequently form occur as mycobacteria pass through the intact epithelium via the ducts of mucous glands.[4] In the pre-antibiotic era this bronchogenic spread of tuberculous organisms represented a preterminal event because caseating laryngeal lesions which quickly developed would allow seeding of the opposite lung and rapid dissemination of the organism.[18] In a study initiated prior to the antibiotic era, over 99% of autopsy specimens had patterns of infection consistent with direct seeding of the larynx from a primary pulmonary focus.[4] In a more recent study, 80% of the patients with laryngeal tuberculous lesions were found to have concomitant pulmonary tuberculosis.[89] It is believed that laryngeal tuberculosis may rarely occur from hematogenous or lymphatogenous spread.[23,47,89] The evidence for such theories includes small but significant numbers of patients without concomitant active pulmonary tuberculosis and the demonstration of positive early morning urine cultures in up to one-third of patients tested (prima facie evidence of hematogenous spread).[47,121]

Most series note an increased incidence of laryngeal tuberculosis in males in about a 2:1 ratio.[4,89] The typical patient is in the 40–45 years age range, and heavy tobacco abuse is so common that some have suggested this may be a predisposing factor.[89] Hoarseness is universal among patients presenting with laryngeal tuberculosis; typically, the onset is insidious, and the patient is aware of progressive symptoms for several months prior to presentation. Other frequent symptoms that are seen are productive or nonproductive cough and odynophagia. This 'painful dysphagia' is a characteristic feature of laryngeal tuberculosis with discomfort out of proportion to the laryngeal findings.[47,59,121] Small numbers of patients also present with hemoptysis or stridor, and one-third of patients present with systemic symptoms including weight loss, fatigue, fever and night sweats. Careful questioning may elicit a history of previous (often under-treated) pulmonary tuberculosis.[89]

The appearance of the tuberculous larynx varies markedly depending upon the disease stage encountered. This may range from simple mucosal edema and hyperemia to painful local ulcerations. It has been suggested that areas of tightly adherent mucosa are more subject to ulceration than those in which there is more submucosal elasticity.[112] The stages of clinically visible lesions may at first be only marked by hyperemia, edema and erythema. As the mucosa breaks down, the clinician may note one or several 1–5 mm diameter, shallow, irregular ulcers. As the tuberculous ulcer cavity deepens, cartilage may be left exposed. Over time the ulcers may become confluent with local extension to adjacent structures including the base of tongue and trachea, leaving large patches of denuded cartilage. Before merging, the thickened borders of adjacent ulcers may give the larynx a characteristic 'geographic appearance'.[4] In a pre-chemotherapy autopsy series, 15% of specimens with laryngeal tuberculosis demonstrated ulceration of nearly the entire laryngeal surface with extensive destruction of the true vocal folds. Progression of tuberculous lesions may also lead to the formation of exophytic fungating masses which, depending on location, may cause airway obstructive symptoms and occasionally cord fixation due to bulk. Such lesions are especially subject to being misdiagnosed as carcinoma,[5] a situation made more difficult by case reports of concomitant laryngeal tuberculous and squamous cell carcinoma.[59] The 'lupus' form of the disease is characterized by edematous-appearing but palpably firm pale, fleshy swellings scattered throughout the supraglottic larynx.

Laryngeal tuberculous lesions in the pre-antibiotic era tended to concentrate around the posterior larynx;[5] however, this predilection for posterior lesions has not been borne out in more recent years. Studies of modern tuberculosis indicate that the most commonly affected locations include scattered areas of the supraglottis and the true vocal folds (40–70%) with an even distribution between the anterior and posterior glottis. The epiglottis is typically involved in 20–30% of cases, although in some series this may occur in as many as 75% of patients.[89,104,112] Finally, the false vocal folds, ventricles and mucosa overlying the arytenoids are involved in 30–50% of cases of laryngeal tuberculosis.

Cervical lymphadenopathy is a presenting feature in approximately 5% of all patients with tuberculosis and is bilateral in up to one-third.[121] Most commonly this presents as a matted mass of nodes in the posterior triangle of the neck which may be clinically indistinguishable from lymphoma. One study describes a matted, mobile, non-tender, firm, 3 by 6 cm right middle deep cervical lymph node infected with tuberculosis. In a small percentage of patients with long-standing lymphadenopathy, an abscess may develop in the affected node with development of a discharging sinus through the skin.

Tuberculosis may present in other head and neck sites, including the palate, tongue, gums and floor of the mouth; the lesions are often clinically indistinguishable from squamous cell carcinoma. Nasopharyngeal, oropharyngeal and hypopharyngeal tuberculous nodules appear as pink nodules with 'apple jelly' centers. Similar nodules may be seen on the nasal septal mucosa, and with progression may lead to perforation of the cartilaginous septum. In contradistinction to syphilis, nasal tuberculosis purportedly never perforates the bony septum. Lesions of the parotid and submandibular gland and Pott's cervical spinous abscess are other manifestations.[121]

Several routine laboratory examinations may be obtained to facilitate the diagnosis of tuberculosis. In 80–90% of patients with laryngeal tuberculosis, chest radiograms are abnormal.[5,47,59,89,112] Typical findings include apical infiltrates and fibrosis frequently with cavitation and a tendency towards symmetrical bilaterality.[47] A miliary or micronodular pattern may also be present.[104] The tuberculin skin test (purified protein derivative, PPD) is a highly specific diagnostic tool in the non-immunocompromised.[121] However, in some series a positive PPD has been found in only about 50% of patients.[89]

More direct methods for diagnosing tuberculous laryngitis include sputum and urine culture samples in the appropriate context and histologic examination and culture of laryngeal biopsies. Sputum cultures have a high diagnostic yield in patients with a productive cough, whilst early morning urine cultures are positive in up to a third of patients presenting with tuberculosis. The newer microbiological assays allow rapid identification of *Mycobacterium* organisms; in particular the Bactec 460, which utilizes radiolabeled probes to identify small amounts of mycobacterial DNA, is capable of producing definitive results within 3–7 days of sample collection. Other new highly sensitive procedures utilize PCR to amplify and detect conserved segments of mycobacterial DNA. One caveat of this identification procedure is that it cannot differentiate between live and dead mycobacteria and therefore it has no utility in monitoring drug efficacy.[121] In patients with cervical lymphadenopathy, fine needle aspiration is a useful modality. Studies indicate that fine needle aspiration of cervical nodes in tuberculosis is over 75% positive and over 90% specific; this procedure also has obvious utility in distinguishing laryngeal tuberculosis from a laryngeal malignancy.[121]

Finally, the most direct method of diagnosis of laryngeal tuberculosis is biopsy of the laryngeal lesion itself. However, in patients who have suggestive chest radiograms and positive PPD and sputum cultures, some authors advocate presumptively initiating appropriate antibiotic therapy for 3–4 weeks before considering direct laryngoscopy and biopsy. The rationale behind this more conservative approach is to reduce exposure risk to operating room personnel.

The histology of the classic tuberculous lesion is characterized by granulomas with caseating necrotic centers and prominent Langhans-type giant cells. In optimal specimens, demonstration of mycobacteria may also be possible, although the numbers are often too scanty for microscopic identification. An autopsy study of more than 300 patients attempted to define various histologic stages of tuberculosis infection. The earliest lesions of laryngeal tuberculosis are tuberculous foci that are seeded submucosally at varying depths. These foci are characterized by large numbers of epithelioid macrophages and giant cells with variable degrees of fibroblastic and lymphocytic infiltration. These cells tend to be concentrically arranged around a central focus, which becomes caseated as the granuloma enlarges. Typically, ulceration occurs when the expanding granuloma contacts the mucous membrane either via direct enlargement of the lesion with caseous envelopment of the mucosa or by pressure atrophy on the overlying mucosa. In the former state, liquefaction necrosis at the caseating center triggered by the release of proteolytic neutrophilic enzymes causes destruction of the adjacent mucosa. In the 'pressure atrophy' scenario, the expansion of the submucosal lesion leads to a progressive thinning of the mucosa and eventual ischemia and breakdown of the mucosa. After an ulcer is formed, fibrin and neutrophils are exuded onto the ulcerated area to form a 'pyogenic membrane'. Finally, the laryngeal cartilage is destroyed by either direct liquefaction necrosis or when ulceration results in exposure of underlying cartilage with perichondrial breakdown and granulation tissue formation.[4]

Mucosal ulcers may heal at any stage regardless of treatment, and the clinician may be witness to progression of lesions in some areas while others appear to be receding. Healing of the defect commences with the formation of granulation tissue covering. Over time, hyalinized connective tissue replaces the granulation tissue and remucosalization by hyperplastic squamous-type epithelium occurs. This type of epithelium tends to persist even in areas that nominally are covered with ciliated respiratory epithelium. Extensive lesions may heal with significant degrees of scarring, thickening of the laryngeal lumen and clinically significant airway narrowing.

Treatment of laryngeal tuberculosis, as in all obstructive laryngeal lesions, begins with securing the airway. Occasionally a patient may need a tracheotomy prior to initiating antibiotic therapy. The standard chemotherapeutic regimen includes isoniazid, rifampicin and ethambutol. Multidrug therapy is mandated by the increasing numbers of isoniazid- and rifampicin-resistant organisms which currently affect 9% of all patients with pulmonary tuberculosis.[121] Some authors have advocated the acute use of steroids for relief of dysphagia and in an attempt to decrease subsequent fibrosis of the larynx.[104] In the appropriately treated patient, one may be confident of improvement in appearance and symptoms within several weeks. Typically, dysphagia is relieved within 3–7 days of treatment onset and most laryngeal lesions can be expected to resolve within 2 months of initiation of therapy.[5,112] Biopsy of persistent laryngeal lesions is mandated in order to rule out concomitant laryngeal carcinoma.[59] Surgical treatment of tuberculosis is limited to treatment of residual fibrotic lesions to improve airway or laryngeal function.

Leprosy (Hansen's disease)

Leprosy is a disease caused by infection with *Mycobacterium leprae*. Skin testing in endemic areas suggests that leprosy is in fact highly contagious, as seroconversion is common.[20] Aerosolized droplets from infected nasal secretions are rich in bacteria and constitute one of the primary sources of human-to-human transmission.[123] Skin infection is believed to be transmitted through breaks in the epidermis.[95] Despite widespread exposure in endemic areas, the relative infrequency of clinical leprosy has led to the widely accepted doctrine that prolonged contact with infected individuals is necessary to contract the disease. More recently, it has been speculated that clinical leprosy may represent reactivation of latent disease following an immune perturbation in a previously exposed individual.[119] It is similarly believed that host factors such as genetic susceptibility, immunologic status and nutrition may in part determine susceptibility to infection. It is believed that up to 75% of patients who are exposed to *M. leprae* will clear the disease spontaneously without ever developing clinical signs or symptoms.[95] It is widely accepted that the host immunologic status has a decisive role in the presentation of clinical leprosy; this factor will be discussed in the disease presentation section below.

It is estimated that 12–15 million cases of leprosy exist worldwide; approximately one-third of these cases are in India.[105] Approximately 3000 cases have been registered in the USA, the majority resulting from exposure outside the country.

Lepromatous infection has a predilection for skin, peripheral nerves and the mucosa of the upper respiratory tract.[95] A patient presenting with laryngeal leprosy typically has suffered from clinically apparent cutaneous leprosy for many years. In one study the duration of symptoms was up to 20 years in those patients presenting with otolaryngological manifestations of leprosy.[40] More than 90% of these will present with advanced nasal disease.[105,123] Despite clinically evident disease elsewhere, a delay in the diagnosis of laryngeal leprosy of 6–12 months is typical in patients presenting in the USA; presumably this is due to the infrequency of the disease presentation.[119] Cervical adenopathy is a frequent finding in leprosy; in one study, 85% of autopsy cases of lepromatous leprosy demonstrated pathologically involved cervical lymph nodes.[61] The cutaneous presentations of leprosy are dependent on the host immune status and include lepromatous, tuberculoid and an intermediate or dimorphic form. The patient with tuberculoid lesions has a positive lepromin reaction (an intradermal inoculum of a homogenate of leprous tissue); this paucibacillary form affects only the peripheral nerves and skin and is characterized by small numbers of macular lesions. The lepromatous patient, however, does not respond to intradermal lepromin, and this relative immune impairment allows the mycobacteria to invade other tissues. In these patients the bacilli are numerous and highly infectious.[95]

Virtually all individuals who develop laryngeal leprosy are afflicted with lepromatous cutaneous disease;[40,123] in some studies 30–55% of all patients with lepromatous leprosy will develop concomitant laryngeal involvement.[61,105] In concordance with *M. leprae*'s predilection for cooler body areas, the epiglottic tip is the area of the larynx most frequently involved with leprosy, where the projection of the epiglottis into the inspired airstream causes air temperature to be approximately 2°C cooler than other areas of the larynx.[105] Although some authors believe that true vocal fold nodules of leprosy are rare, other studies have cited the true cords as the second most frequent location for leprous laryngeal disease; the aryepiglottic fold is less frequently involved. No involvement of the false vocal folds, pyriform apertures or vallecula have been reported.[40,105] The location of the disease determines the presenting symptoms. Specifically, large lesions of the supraglottis may lead to voice muffling or a 'leprous huskiness,' a peculiar vocal quality characteristic of laryngeal leprosy.[105] A patient with vocal fold involvement most frequently presents with hoarseness followed by dyspnea and/or dry cough; the patient may also complain occasionally of a foreign body sensation, throat pain, or hemoptysis.[20,105] In contradistinction to laryngeal tuberculosis, odynophagia and odynophonia are typically absent.[20]

The appearance of laryngeal leprosy varies considerably. This may consist of simple edema or 'congestion', diffuse thickening, subtle discrete pale yellow to pink nodules, or 'punched-out' ulcers surrounded by inflammation. Severe fibrosis following a prolonged inflammatory response may lead to a slowly progressive decrease in vocal fold mobility.[40,95,105] The classic pattern of laryngeal disease begins first with the appearance at the epiglottic dip of discrete nodules, which, as they continue to develop, enlarge and coalesce into a diffuse, irregular thickening, giving the epiglottis a 'mulberry appearance'.[40,95,105] In later stages the disease may spread to involve the 'entire larynx';[40,105] this may account for the common presentation of laryngeal lesions as 'diffuse swelling or thickening'.[40] Other less common presentations include punched-out ulcers over the arytenoid cartilages and unilateral or bilateral vocal fold thickening with decreased mobility.[40,105]

Other areas of the head and neck affected by lepromatous leprosy include the nose, oral cavity, oropharynx, skin and peripheral nerves. Nasal lesions that have been described range from 4 to 6 mm yellow-gray nodules on the nasal alae and turbinates to septal and turbinate ulceration and crusting with a yellowish, blood-tinged discharge, to complete nasal septal destruction and dorsal collapse.[95,123] Nodular lesions over the soft palate and tonsillar pillars and maculopapular rashes involving the tonsil, palate and facial skin have been reported.[119,123] The skin may be involved with hyperpigmented papular lesions, whilst diffuse infiltration of the facial skin may lead to thickening and a coarsened appearance known as 'leonine facies'.[119] Finally, lepromatous invasion of peripheral nerves, particularly the great auricular, often leaves them palpably stringy and knotted.[123]

The diagnosis of laryngeal leprosy is secured by the identification of the organism in tissue biopsies. The histology of active lepromatous lesions is characterized by marked edema and infiltration by large numbers of epithelioid cells, lymphocytes and nests of 'foamy' histiocytes containing the non-staining lepra bacilli. Compact, globular masses of free bacilli may also be found scattered throughout the infected tissue. Atrophic stratified squamous epithelium typically overlies the affected areas,[20] and inspection of small nerve bundles and blood vessels and the vocal musculature may reveal bacillus invasion.[61] In unchecked disease, fibrosis with nerve destruction develops, whilst the overlying epithelium may become hypertrophied and dysplastic. In a large autopsy series of patients with leprosy, 9% were found with cervical vagal nerve involvement; this suggests a possible neuropathic rather than direct infiltrative route of vocal fold paralysis.[61] Following the initiation of treatment, affected tissue is characterized by dense infiltrates of chronic inflammatory cells (largely mononuclear cells and plasmacytes) and occasional fibroblastic infiltrates in the absence of granuloma formation.[40]

The treatment of leprosy as outlined in 1982 by the World Health Organization stratifies patients according to type of presentation. Specifically, for paucibacillary or tuberculoid forms, treatment consists of dapsone 100 mg by mouth every day for 6 months and rifampicin 600 mg by mouth once per month for 6 months. In a patient with multibacillary or lepromatous leprosy, the suggested treatment consists of 2 weeks of dapsone 100 mg/day, rifampicin 600 mg/day and clofazimine 100 mg/day. Following this 2 week course, the patient is maintained on a regimen of dapsone 100 mg/day, clofazimine 50 mg/day and rifampicin 600 mg once per month for a minimum of 2 years.[105] Other authors have recommended that chemotherapy continue until all disease has ceased for at least 3 years or at least 2 years for tuberculoid and 5 years for lepromatous forms of leprosy.[95] During the commencement of chemotherapy, the clinician must be vigilant for the onset of erythema nodosum leprosum, an antigen–antibody mediated reaction which can trigger rapid generalized airway edema. It is speculated that this reaction occurs secondary to immune complex deposition in affected areas and often presents with disseminated painful nodular subcutaneous lesions. Treatment consists of glucocorticoids, thalidomide, clofazimine and occasionally tracheotomy for erythema nodosum leprosum.[95,119] Relapses are common, particularly in patients with lepromatous forms of leprosy, and the patient may require lifelong antibiotic therapy.[95] Typically, early lesions will respond to treatment within a few weeks.[95] Healing occurs with variable amounts of fibrosis and subsequent airway impairment may require a tracheotomy.[95] Unless there is significant scarring, surgical intervention is usually not necessary in the treatment of laryngeal leprosy.

Actinomycosis

Actinomycosis of the head and neck is the result of infection by *Actinomyces israelii*, a commensal saprophyte of the normal oral flora.[45] This organism is taxonomically classified with *Nocardia* in a niche that places it intermediately between the true fungi and the true bacteria.[31] It is an anaerobic or microaerophilic Gram-positive organism that grows and reproduces by forming an elongate monocellular mycelium. The delicate 0.5–1 μm hyphae that form these mycelia frequently fragment into bacillary and coccoid forms that often resemble diphtheroids.[31,115]

A. israelii is indigenous to the human oral cavity and has been found in the crypts of up to 15% of all excised tonsils.[115] The initial step in the pathogenesis of actinomycosis is believed to be penetration of the organism through mucosal barriers damaged by oral trauma; dental surgery is classically cited as an inciting cause. The penetration of the mucous membrane allows the organism access to a microaerophilic environment which is essential to its proliferation.[31] On occasion, paralaryngeal and parapharyngeal spread has been theorized to occur from a tonsillar crypt focus with extension in the lateral pharyngeal wall along the inferior constrictor.[99]

Multiple patient factors may increase the likelihood of actinomycotic infection. These were felt to include diabetes mellitus, systemic malignancy and generalized debility.[45] Presumably, tissues with impaired immune surveillance such as those that have been irradiated are also at increased risk; three of eight reported cases of laryngeal actinomycosis occurred in previously irradiated larynges often many weeks following the completion of radiation therapy. As only one case has been reported,[45] it is unclear whether heavy tobacco smoking or alcohol intake represent risk factors for actinomycotic infection; presumably any increased risk depends on weakened mucosal barrier function as a result of damage from exposure to these agents.

Actinomycosis of the head and neck may present acutely as an abscess with pain, fever, or leukocytosis and airway obstructive symptoms or it may progress in a more indolent fashion associated with chronic disease and the appearance of a slowly enlarging, painful, neck mass that is characterized by woody induration and a red-blue or violet discoloration of the overlying skin.[45] Accordingly, among the many initial manifestations are cervical facial pain, edema, erythema, a jaw mass, or with laryngeal involvement, a month-long history of dyspnea, hoarseness, or nocturnal stridor.[16] It is peculiar to actinomycosis that it tends to spread without regard to fascial planes, anatomic barriers or the lymphatics;[16,31] thus there often is a characteristic absence of lymphadenopathy in the presence of an indurated lesion. The typical mass of actinomycoses presents in proximity to the mandible, which may then become an abscess. Spontaneous rupture of the abscess or surgical drainage may lead to the formation of a sinus tract into the neck skin – a frequent occurrence in actinomycotic infection.[31,81,115]

Actinomyces infection is relatively frequent in the head and neck, particularly in relation to the mandible, but is quite rare in the endolarynx.[16] Manifestations include an abscess located external to the larynx and within the true vocal fold.[99] Less commonly, actinomycosis perichondritis has been described, and one case describes a polypoid subglottic mass 1.5 by 1.5 cm in size due to actinomycosis infection.[16,45]

Few cases of laryngeal actinomycosis have been reported in the literature.[45,81] The various appearances of these lesions include yellowish, exophytic, ulcerative lesions of the epiglottis, true cords, ventricles, aryepiglottic folds and pyriform sinuses, with occasional development of sinus tracts into the neck, and multiple small pharyngeal, arytenoid or vocal cord lesions.[45,81] One 'thickened' true vocal fold lesion was incised and drained of 10 ml of pus, revealing an abscess cavity lined with a thick rind of granulation tissue.[16] Another laryngeal lesion appeared as a gray, ulcerative, exophytic mass filling the pyriform with extension to the lateral hypopharynx and a fistulous tract extending into the anterior neck. This presentation was accompanied by marked epiglottic and ipsilateral false vocal fold edema and severe narrowing of the glottic airway.[45]

Histologic examination of infected tissues classically yields 1–2 mm diameter, yellow, friable masses[31] known as 'sulfur granules' which are aggregates of *Actinomyces*. Grossly it is often difficult to differentiate sulfur granules from necrotic debris in an abscess cavity.[31] Staining of such structures may reveal lobulated, basophilic masses of slender, beaded, branching organisms radiating from a central focus with club-like eosinophilic extensions.[31,81,99,115] The inflammatory infiltrate surrounding the granules is comprised chiefly of neutrophils, plasmacytes, epithelioid macrophages and occasionally giant cells.[31]

Histologically these granules are Gram-positive and also positive to Grocott's methenamine silver stain. Intense neutrophilic infiltrates may be intermixed with the granule in a zone of granulation tissue and may be seen to surround pockets of purulence. Frequently other bacteria may superinfect *Actinomyces* abscesses.[31] In a subacute or chronic infection, caseating granulomas may form.[16,31]

Several features of actinomycosis make its diagnosis as a pathogen difficult. Because it exists as a commensal in the oral cavity, biopsy and culture specimens must be interpreted with caution;[81] it has been suggested that it is helpful if one can identify a cuff of inflammatory cells surrounding the clumps of actinomyces as these are more suggestive of an invasive infectious process.[45] Additionally, actinomyces is an anaerobe that needs 2–4 weeks to grow on specialized media. Typically, only free pus and not tissue samples or sulfur granules will produce positive cultures.[99] Nevertheless, it is recommended that biopsies of abscess walls be performed to histologically identify the organism.[99] Serologic or fluorescent antibody techniques may also be helpful in the diagnosis of actinomycosis.[31]

Treatment of actinomycosis consists of surgical incision and drainage of abscesses, debridement of necrotic tissues, excision of sinus tracts, and appropriate antibiotic therapy.[16,45] If only soft tissue infection has occurred without an abscess or sinus tract, antibiotic therapy alone is usually effective.[45] In general, actinomyces are susceptible to any antibiotic with significant activity against Gram-positive bacteria.[31] Classic treatment has included intravenous penicillin 2–20 million units for 2–6 weeks followed by oral penicillin for 3–6 months.[16,45,99] Other antibiotics that have successfully been used include intravenous clindamycin 600 mg three times a day for 2 weeks followed by oral therapy for 4 weeks,[81] intravenous cefazolin for 5 days followed by 4 months of oral cephalexin[45] and tetracycline.[99] Disease-free follow-ups in patients treated with these alternate regimens range from 6 months to 2.5 years.[45,81]

The prognosis for actinomycosis infection depends largely on the institution of adequate therapy early in the course of disease. Typically, actinomycosis infection is a subacute granulomatous disease characterized by late abscess development with spontaneous drainage via sinus tracts and subsequent dense fibrous scarring.[31] In the larynx this may lead to permanent airway or phonatory compromise.

Nocardiosis

Nocardia asteroides is an aerobic higher bacterium which propagates in soil, its natural habitat, in a filamentous pattern with true branching growth. Fragmentation of these fragile branches produces the bacillary and coccoid forms often seen in infected tissues. Of the human pathogens it is most closely related to *Actinomyces*.[115]

As common to many pathogens in this chapter, the primary route of infection with *Nocardia* is via the respiratory tract,[19,115] although a dental source of infection has, rarely, been reported.[115] No known human-to-human or animal-to-human transmission has been described.[19] The symptoms of pulmonary *Nocardia* infection include a dry cough, dyspnea, anorexia, weight loss, pleuritic chest pain and occasionally hemoptysis. Progression of pulmonary disease may result in the development of lung abscess or empyema.[115] It has been suggested that a carrier state for *Nocardia* exists, as patients have been identified with positive sputum culture but with no clinical evidence of disease. It is theorized that dissemination may occur following deterioration of the immune status of the subject.[19] In the immunocompromised host, the incubation period has been estimated at 16–24 days.[24]

Dissemination of pulmonary nocardiosis is believed to occur primarily through the hematogenous route. Nocardial abscesses are generally poorly walled off, a feature which facilitates the spread of disease.[115] The expanding infection culminates in erosion of adjacent blood vessels and subsequent bacteremia.[19] The most common sites of hematogenous dissemination are CNS structures including the brain, spinal cord and meninges.[19] Other frequent sites of involvement include the gastrointestinal and upper and lower respiratory tracts.[115] The immunocompromised host is believed to be particularly sensitive to acute dissemination.[19,115] The most common immunocompromising factor is the presence of a hematogenous malignancy: in nearly all reported pediatric cases, patients suffered from underlying acute lymphocytic leukemia or Hodgkin's lymphoma and all developed disseminated nocardial laryngeal infection following 16–100 months of chemotherapy.[24] Other factors of immunocompromise that have been reported include chronic granulomatous disease, hypogammaglobulinemia, systemic lupus erythematosus (SLE), malnutrition and immunosuppression following renal transplant.[24,84] Despite such data, up to 50% of reported patients with disseminated nocardiosis were without known immunocompromise or predisposing factors.[19] Disseminated disease may vary from a mildly symptomatic localized infection to a fulminant fatal process.[19]

Laryngeal lesions of nocardiosis are exceedingly rare, and only a handful of cases have been reported.[24] Symptoms that have been described include hemoptysis, dysphagia and a sensation of a lump in the throat.[24,84] Lesions which have been described include an asymptomatic 3 by 3 cm nocardial vallecular cyst,[19] a granulomatous true vocal fold lesion[24] and extreme edema of the pyriform sinus, false vocal fold and ipsilateral epiglottis in the presence of freely mobile vocal folds.[84] Tracheitis, bronchitis and bronchopleural fistulae have also been described.[115]

Little has been written about the histological appearance of nocardial abscesses of the larynx. Descriptions detail the presence of microabscesses, intense inflammatory infiltrates, and scattered giant cells. In the case of the vallecular cyst, incision and drainage revealed thick, purulent material that was heavily infiltrated with *Nocardia*.[19] Diagnosis of nocardial lesions may be obtained through Gram stain or culture of purulent exudates.[84] Other stains are helpful in the diagnosis of this unusual organism as it is both weakly acid fast and Fite-stain positive.[19]

Various chemotherapeutic agents have been employed against nocardial infections with good success. *N. asteroides* is highly sensitive to TMP-SMX or sulfonamide alone. A 6 week course of TMP-SMX or a 2–12 month course of sulfonamide has been advocated.[19,115] One case reports the use of minocycline daily maintenance and that the patient was symptom free 8 months after commencement of treatment.[84] The aforementioned vallecular lesion was treated with incision and drainage and marsupialization and only 1 week of an oral cephalosporin; at 1-year follow-up examination the patient was free of recurrent disease.[19] Other surgical interventions that have been deemed necessary in the treatment of laryngeal nocardiosis include surgical debulking of necrotic tissue[19] and placement of a tracheotomy in a patient whose larynx became severely edematous following nocardial infection.[84]

The prognosis of disseminated nocardiosis varies widely as the disease may present with manifestations ranging from a mildly symptomatic, localized infection to widely disseminated fulminant disease.[19] It is possible for disseminated nocardial disease to involve every organ system in the body.[19] Patients with localized extrapulmonary *Nocardia* infection are said to have an 'excellent' prognosis.[19] A 15–20% mortality rate has been cited as typical in patients not receiving steroids or antineoplastic agents,[115] whereas the prognosis for immunocompromised hosts is considerably worse.[19] Patients who manifest dissemination to multiple sites, present with a rapidly advancing course of disease (less than 3 weeks), and patients on steroids have an 80% or greater mortality from disseminated nocardial infection.[19]

Histoplasmosis

Histoplasmosis is a disease caused by the dimorphic fungus, *Histoplasma capsulatum*, which grows in its natural soil environment in a branched hyphal form. These hyphae develop spores known as tuberculate conidia that after inhalation begin propagation in budding yeast form in the pulmonary bed.[35] *H. capsulatum* is a widespread organism that is endemic to the Ohio and Mississippi River valleys. Birds and bats have been identified as vectors of histoplasmosis; the high nitrogen content of bat and bird droppings appears to stimulate the growth of *H. capsulatum* and elevated risks of clinical infection have been identified in cave explorers, chicken farmers and pigeon breeders. In endemic regions, the rate of seropositivity to histoplasmosis is 80–90%.[28]

A patient presenting with clinically evident histoplasmosis is typically over 40 years old, although many cases in the literature describe patients in their 20s and 30s.[38,55] The clinical presentation of a primary histoplasmosis infection depends on the size of the inoculum and the host's immunity. A normal host with mild exposure to histoplasmosis may be completely asymptomatic.[115] It is estimated that 95% of all patients affected with histoplasmosis undergo some degree of clinical infection.[10] A normal host exposed to a heavy inoculum of the microbe typically develops flu-like symptoms from which he will spontaneously recover. The weakened or immunocompromised host, who is unable to eradicate the primary infection, may develop chronic pulmonary histoplasmosis which clinically resembles pulmonary tuberculosis,[10] and which may subsequently evolve into chronic progressive disseminated histoplasmosis. In this state, the patient's pulmonary focus of infection may undergo spontaneous flares and remissions even without treatment, but eventually dissemination is believed to occur.[10] Host immune responsiveness may be a key factor in dissemination, as 50% of patients who develop dissemination are anergic to histoplasmin compared to only 20% anergy in those with localized pulmonary lesions. These data suggest that a breakdown of cellular immunity may be a critical precipitating factor in the dissemination of disease.[10] Although histoplasmosis has a predilection for affecting organs of the reticuloendothelial system, it may affect nearly all of the body tissues in disseminated disease.[55] Depending on the organs of involvement, the symptoms of histoplasmosis may be as varied as fever, weight loss, rhinitis, pharyngitis, cough, dyspnea, anorexia, nausea, vomiting, diarrhea, hepatomegaly, or splenomegaly.[55] Eventually, adrenal glandular involvement and extensive tissue destruction lead to the development of an Addisonian crisis; this was the typical mode of death in histoplasmosis prior to the development of effective chemotherapy.

Mucosal involvement in head and neck lesions of histoplasmosis is common.[10] Oral cavity and oropharyngeal lesions may present as shallow ulcers on the palate or uvula that may resemble aphthous ulcers which are common in pediatric presentations.[97] These may evolve into deeply indurated lesions, firm, painful ulcers with a predilection for the palate or maxillary gingival mucosa. Erosion of the bone underlying such ulcers may lead to an initial presentation as an oral antral fistula. Multiple lesions have been described on the tongue including indurated tender nodules, indurated ulcers, and large firm sessile masses. Buccal mucosa and lip involvement has also been reported. Uncommonly, oral cavity lesions may appear as verrucous or granular masses suggestive of carcinoma.[10,38]

Laryngeal symptoms of histoplasmosis may develop for weeks or months prior to presentation. These consist of hoarseness and variable amounts of dysphagia, odynophagia, dyspnea, and cough productive of scanty blood-tinged sputum. The patient may also present in florid airway compromise due to massive laryngeal lesions.[28,38,85] Early laryngeal lesions of histoplasmosis most typically affect the true vocal folds and epiglottis.[10] The true cords may be erythematous and thickened with perforations of the false cords and a moth-eaten epiglottis with thickened irregular mucosa.[10,55] As in the oral cavity, with progression, such lesions may ulcerate and fibrose, leading to vocal fold fixation.[10,35,38] Other lesions that have been described include polypoid true vocal fold and extensive ulcerations covering the vocal folds, arytenoids and pyriforms. Bilateral true and false cord fixation have been described.[10,55]

In the pre-antifungal era, one case report documented the slow progression of the disease which was characterized by steadily enlarging ulcerative lesions that eventually destroyed the entire epiglottis.[38]

Laryngeal histoplasmosis occurs only in the setting of disseminated disease.[10,115] The spread of histoplasmosis to the larynx probably does not occur via direct implantation (from showering of infectious sputum); this theory is based upon the observation that 50% of patients with laryngeal histoplasmosis have no evidence of active pulmonary disease. It is suggested, therefore, that hematogenous spread from a pulmonary focus leads to laryngeal seeding.[10] Eventually two-thirds of patients with chronic disseminated histoplasmosis and one-third with subacute histoplasmosis progress to develop laryngeal lesions.[115]

The diagnosis of histoplasmosis relies primarily upon identification of the organism in biopsy specimens and culture results, although serological examinations are sometimes helpful. Characteristic biopsy specimens show noncaseating granulomata with occasional Langhans giant cells. Grocott silver stains may demonstrate single scattered or short chains of rounded yeast organisms; occasionally, one may be identified in the process of producing a characteristically narrow-based daughter cell by budding.[10,35,88] Culture swabs taken from the center of an ulcerative lesion may demonstrate growth of *Histoplasma* after appropriate incubation on Sabouraud's agar.[55] The complement fixation test is the most valuable serologic tool for the diagnosis of histoplasmosis, with the understanding that only patients with ≥1–16 titers are considered true positives.[28] Typically titers become detectable 1 month following initial exposure to the organism and tend to follow the disease course; therefore, they are useful in tracking therapeutic response. Although this test is helpful, the complement fixation test is not specific in that a negative test does not mean that a patient does not have an active histoplasmosis infection. Also, false-positive results in patients infected with blastomycosis, coccidioidomycosis and cryptococcus have been reported.[28] Immunodiffusion assays which detect the M and H antibodies to histoplasmosis are useful in detecting ongoing active disease. These first become detectable 3–4 weeks after initial infection. The histoplasmin skin test is not very useful, as it has little utility in the diagnosis of patients in endemic areas, whilst patients with disseminated histoplasmosis frequently have negative histoplasmin skin tests.

Histologic examination of the lesions may demonstrate hyperkeratotic thickened epithelium and extensive surrounding ulceration. The ulcer may penetrate into the underlying skeletal muscle, and the tissue is infused with a pleomorphic, chronic inflammatory infiltrate. In some cases, abundant histiocytes containing large numbers of histoplasma organisms may be identified. The lesions may exhibit a highly variable microscopic appearance with the degree of granulomatous response related to the host defenses. In the 'histiocytic' response, often seen in acute disseminated disease, lesions frequently contain no tubercles or true granulomas. Overall, tissue inflammatory reaction appears slight and the number of organisms numerous. In such a context, a fulminant disease course is quite probable. In patients with a less impaired immune response, such as in chronic slowly progressive histoplasmosis, a diffuse pleomorphic cellular infiltrate containing variable amounts of well defined noncaseating nodular granulomas is apparent. Uncommonly these granulomas may enlarge and develop necrotic centers.[55] The more granulomatous the reaction the more difficult it is for the pathologist to locate microbes within the specimen; those that are located are typically found within histiocytes or Langhans giant cells or free-floating in the tissue specimen.

The differential diagnosis of histoplasmosis includes tuberculosis, blastomycosis, syphilis and leishmaniasis.[38] Like blastomycosis, laryngeal lesions can also be easily confused with carcinoma. The patient presentation and chest radiograph findings are frequently indistinguishable from those of tuberculosis.[88] One distinguishing factor is that histoplasmosis frequently affects the oral cavity whereas tuberculosis does not.[10] In addition, biopsies of tuberculous lesions typically show caseating granulomas, whereas histoplasmosis typically does not. The clinical appearance of blastomycotic lesions is marked by pronounced pseudoepitheliomatous hyperplasia, which is infrequent in histoplasmosis. In addition, blastomycosis more typically presents with concurrent cutaneous lesions.[53]

The mainstay of treatment of histoplasmosis is intravenous amphotericin B to a total dose of 35 mg/kg or 2–4 g total.[28,115] A single case report has demonstrated regression of disease without recurrence using 400 mg/day of ketoconazole for 6 months.[35]

The prognosis for laryngeal histoplasmosis varies depending upon stage of disease and host immune factors. Cutaneous anergy tends to be a very poor prognostic factor.

Coccidioidomycosis

Coccidioidomycosis occurs following infection with *Coccidioides immitis*, a fungal pathogen that prefers environments with long hot summers, short winters and little rainfall. This preference is reflective of the fungus' tolerance of pH, temperature and salinity extremes and its inclination to grow in soils with little competition from other soil fungi or bacteria.[92] In soil, the vegetative phase of *Coccidioides* produces pathogenic chlamydospores and arthrospores. Once exposed to the elevated temperatures of pulmonary tissue, the inhaled spores convert to the spherules commonly identified in clinical disease.

Coccidioidomycosis is widespread throughout the New World in climates favoring the above growth criteria. Highly endemic areas include the San Joaquin Valley, the south-western USA and the adjacent portion of north-west Mexico, Argentina and Paraguay.[92,115] Previous large studies have suggested that the disease effects darker-skinned races more commonly than lighter-skinned; specifically, Filipinos are more commonly affected than blacks who are more commonly affected than Mexicans, whilst Caucasians are least affected.[115] The disease has a tendency to peak in summer and autumn, drier months which are conducive to the development of dust aerosols that can be inhaled.[117] Not only natural winds, but also human means of soil disruption can increase exposure to the organism; identified high-risk groups include construction workers and archeology students.[92]

Coccidioides is a highly infectious organism and a 50–70% seropositive rate is typical of endemic areas.[92] Of those exposed, two-thirds will never become symptomatic from their infection.[14,117] Following an incubation period of 8–30 days, the one-third that do become symptomatic may present with malaise, fever, pharyngitis, cough uncommonly associated with hemoptysis, chest pain, night sweats, or erythema nodosum.[117] Of those infected, 5% will progress to the development of pulmonary residua including cavitary lesions, lung nodules, or coccidioidomas.[86,115] Of all individuals exposed to coccidioidomycosis, 0.5–1% will ultimately develop disseminated extrapulmonary granulomatous disease.[14,92,115] Extrapulmonary coccidioidomycosis may manifest as single or multiple lesions involving the upper aerodigestive tract, skin, organs of the reticuloendothelial system (including bone marrow), endocrine glands and eye.[117] Of those who developed disseminated disease, 7% will exhibit head and neck manifestations.[14]

Clinical coccidioidomycosis is more frequent in males, probably resulting from increased exposure related to occupational status.[117] Clinical and disseminated disease are also more common in the darker complexioned races;[92,117] it is estimated that blacks and Filipinos have a tenfold higher rate of dissemination compared to whites.[92] Patients with type B blood and HLA haplotype A9 are at increased risk for dissemination of disease; both genetic types are more common in blacks and Filipinos.[92] Immunodeficient hosts are susceptible to reactivation of their disease years after initial exposure;[117] dissemination has also been reported up to 1 year after exposure in a non-immunocompromised host.[14]

Laryngeal involvement with coccidioidomycosis nearly always occurs by dissemination of concomitant pulmonary disease.[117] Lesions have been described on all parts of the larynx.[115] Patients may complain of weeks of hoarseness, odynophagia, pain, stridor, or the appearance of cervical lymphadenopathy.[14,115]

The appearance of laryngeal coccidioidomycosis varies considerably. Lesions described include markedly erythematous subglottic mucosa,[14] finely granular subglottic and supraglottic masses and granular irregular patches over the aryepiglottic and true vocal folds with impaired vocal cord motion.[63] Granulomatous lesions of the false vocal fold, arytenoid and aryepiglottic fold mucosa and extensive fungating endolaryngeal granulomas with epiglottic thickening have also been reported.[117] Granular subglottic and anterior commissure lesions and obstructive tracheal granulomas have been described in infants with laryngeal disease.[117]

The diagnosis of coccidioidomycosis is confirmed by the identification of thick-walled non-budding spherules containing multiple endospores.[115,117] Characteristic tissue reactions to invasion by *Coccidioides* include focal 'dyskeratosis' or pseudoepitheliomatous hyperplasia with an intense inflammatory infiltrate consisting largely of mononuclear cells and giant cells in a fibrous stroma. Spherules of *Coccidioides* may be found within these giant cells and scattered throughout the surrounding tissue.[86,92,117] A 10% KOH preparation of biopsy tissue, pus, sputum, or joint fluid may also demonstrate the characteristic spherules. Finally, serological tests including the coccidioidin skin test may be useful in identifying coccidioidomycosis. Initially the coccidioidin reaction may be positive but frequently becomes negative with the onset of disease dissemination;[14,117] this event may be a marker of failing cell-mediated immunity that enables the dissemination of disease.[14] Titers of complement-fixing antibody become measurable 1–3 weeks following exposure and are useful in following the disease course and treatment responsiveness.[14,117] The spherulin antigen test is less useful because of a high false-positive rate.[92]

Treatment of coccidioidomycosis has traditionally been amphotericin B at 1–1.5 mg/kg/day to a total dose of 0.5–2.5 g.[14,115] The wide variation in recommended total dosage reflects the use of other clinical criteria for concluding amphotericin therapy, including normalization of the erythrocyte sedimentation rate, and a decrease of the complement fixation titer to ≤1:32.[117] In cases of meningitis, intrathecal amphotericin B is indicated.[14] Fluconazole and itraconazole show promise as candidates for treatment of coccidioidomycosis but as yet no large studies have been performed.[115]

Paracoccidioidomycosis

Paracoccidioidomycosis, formerly known as South American blastomycosis, results from infection by the dimorphic fungus *Paracoccidioides brasiliensis*, which exists in nature in a filamentous form but propagates as a budding yeast in its pathogenic state at body temperature. Its natural habitat is believed to be the soil, from which it has rarely been isolated; however, its ecological niche has not been clearly defined. Endemic areas include those with humid, subtropical climates, particularly in regions with rivers banked by woods.[80] It has not been observed in semi-arid regions above 2000 ft (615 m). The epidemiologic center of disease is Brazil[115] with its northernmost distribution in Mexico stretching south to Argentina and Uruguay.[80,115] Infrequent cases have been identified in the Caribbean.[80] The disease tends to affect middle-aged male agricultural workers, particularly those who work on coffee plantations. Although serologic studies indicate that exposure occurs early (10–20 years), clinical disease is rare in children. The great preponderance of clinical disease in males (15:1) despite lack of intersex differences in exposure may be in part explained by the finding that 17β-estradiol inhibits the conversion of the filamentous form to the more pathogenic yeast phase.[80] There have been no known epidemics of paracoccidioidomycosis, nor has any human-to-human transmission ever been documented.[80] Some 250 or more new cases of clinically manifest paracoccidioidomycosis occur per year.

The pathophysiological presentation of disease depends on a number of factors including host immune capabilities, the virulence of the strain of *Paracoccidioides* and the inoculum. The lungs are the primary portal of entry of disease and lymphatic or hematogenous dissemination to organs of the reticuloendothelial system occurs in susceptible patients.[80] The typical exposure in a patient with normal immunity results in subclinical disease. Very uncommonly, a patient may develop a mild respiratory syndrome. This primary infection may result in the formation of a pulmonary lymph node complex, which may heal with calcification or become dormant spontaneously. After a latent period of perhaps years, development of impaired host immunity may allow reactivation of disease.[80,115]

Laryngeal manifestations of paracoccidioidomycosis only occur in the context of progressive disease; up to 70% of all patients with progressive disease will develop oropharyngeal and/or laryngeal ulcerations.[97] Oropharyngeal manifestations may vary from simple stomatitis to extensive indurated ulcerations involving the oral cavity and nose. Oral cavity ulcers are shallow with a granulomatous base and occur in conjunction with punctate hemorrhages and microabscesses. Untreated chronic lesions have a propensity to spread, forming extensive ulcers with 'vegetating' bases.[80] Extensive soft tissue destruction of the soft palate and uvula may occur, and ulcerative gingivitis may lead to tooth loss. Laryngeal lesions of paracoccidioidomycosis are characterized by dysphonia, dysphagia and severe dyspnea; up to 70% of patients will present with anterior cervical adenopathy. Hemoptysis, chest pain and draining sinus tracts from chronic lesions of the upper aerodigestive tract may also be seen. Laryngeal examination may reveal ulcerated or crusted, granulomatous lesions often located in the 'upper part' of the larynx.[80,115] The laryngeal mucosal disease may vary from diffuse infiltrates to granulomas which may subsequently ulcerate. Other targets of disseminated disease include the skin, gastrointestinal tract (manifesting with diarrhea, abdominal pain and weight loss), the adrenal glands (in 40% of patients with disseminated disease) and the CNS.[80]

Diagnosis may be approached via several different methods. In 80% of cases, a sputum smear, bronchial washings, exudates, or pus reveal typical yeast forms of paracoccidioidomycosis.[80,115] These are 5–25 μm diameter multinucleated spherical cells with thick, doubly refractile cell walls. Paracoccidioidomycosis reproduces by throwing off multiple narrow-based buds, giving the organism a characteristic 'pilot-wheel' appearance. Biopsy samples of suspect lesions may be examined by Gomori methenamine silver stain or direct immunofluorescence using specific antibodies to paracoccidioidomycosis.[80,97] Sputum and biopsy samples may be grown on Sabouraud medium containing chloramphenicol over 3–4 weeks. Typical colonies are whitish and cotton-like,[80] and microscopic examination reveals branched, septate, 2–3 μm hyphae with spherical intercalated and terminal chlamydoconidiae. In relatively nutrient-depleted media, the organisms will sporulate to form the infectious aleuroconidiae and arthroconidiae.[80] Serological studies may also be helpful in making the diagnosis of paracoccidioidomycosis.[97] Over 90% of patients with disseminated disease will develop detectable specific antibodies to the organism.[80] Complement fixation and immunodiffusion tests to paracoccidioidin antigens frequently become positive several weeks following exposure to disease, with titers tending to parallel disease activity.[80] In 50% of patients with advanced disease, the paracoccidioidin skin test is negative. This relative host anergy may be a significant prognostic factor,[80,97] and it is noteworthy that the paracoccidioidin skin test tends to become positive when the disease is adequately treated, suggesting an active immunosuppressive mechanism associated with the organism or its antigens.[80] It has been found that cell wall polysaccharides of some strains of paracoccidioidomycosis activate CD8-positive T-suppressor lymphocytes which can presumably down-regulate the immune response.

Histologic examination of biopsy specimens may also reveal pseudoepitheliomatous hyperplasia, epithelioid and granulomatous changes and epithelial abscesses. The typical granulomas of *Paracoccidioides* are characterized by central aggregates and macrophages surrounded by a thick cuff of numerous T-cells. In severe disease, suppuration and necrosis may appear at the center of the granulomas, and many fungi may be seen on tissue staining. Progressive disease may also result in cryptosporulation, which is characterized by the formation of blastoconidiae surrounding the mother cells.[80] Less virulent disease states may be characterized histologically by the presence of 'compact' granulomas.[80]

Treatment of paracoccidioidomycosis traditionally relies on the use of sulfa drugs. Sulfadiazine at a dose of 4–6 g/day for up to 3–5 years may be required, although once a clinical response has been documented, this dose may be decreased to a maintenance of 2–3 g/day.[97,115] More slowly eliminated sulfa drugs such as sulfamethoxypyridazine may be administered at a dose of 1 g/day for at least 3 years.[80] Finally, in patients with organisms that show resistance to sulfa drugs, TMP-SMX may have some use; the recommended dose is one double-strength tablet twice a day for 12 months.[80] In patients who present with severe disease, amphotericin B may be added to the sulfa agent of choice; however, amphotericin B alone is inadequate against paracoccidioidomycosis. The recommended dosage is 0.8 mg/kg/day to a total dose of 1.5 g or until clinical remission is achieved; thereafter, maintenance of the sulfa agent must be continued for 3 or more years.[80] Ketoconazole and itraconazole may become the first-line agents in the treatment of paracoccidioidomycosis. *P. brasiliensis* is extremely sensitive *in vitro* to ketoconazole and 200–400 mg daily doses for 1 year have been shown to achieve a 90% clinical cure rate. Therapy may be held once the paracoccidioidin skin test becomes positive, in the face of a complete clinical response, and with the development of low titers of specific antibody. In the event of a relapse, resumption of ketoconazole therapy is usually effective in halting the disease.[80] When available, itraconazole at 100 mg/day for 4–12 months may be the agent of choice. A study using daily itraconazole for 6 months and treating relapses for an additional 12 months resulted in an overall 95% cure.[80]

The prognosis in patients who develop disseminated paracoccidioidomycosis is guarded. Such cases are almost always fatal without antimicrobial therapy, and even in adequately treated patients a 20% relapse rate is typical.[80] Even in patients in whom treatment is appropriately instituted, healing of the involved mucosal lesions often results in intense fibrotic scarring which may lead to tracheal or laryngeal stenosis. Healing of extensive pulmonary lesions may culminate in severe interstitial fibrosis with subsequent cardiorespiratory failure. Adverse prognostic factors in addition to cutaneous anergy to paracoccidioidin include the acute onset of disseminated disease in young patients and the development of CNS or adrenal lesions.

Blastomycosis

Blastomycosis is a disease process caused by the fungus *Blastomyces dermatitidis*, a thermal dimorphic fungus, which, in common with all pathogenic fungi, exists in a mycelial form in nature and as a yeast at human body temperature. It is nominally a soil saprophyte and prefers soils of high organic content and low pH and is found in highest concentrations in geographic proximity to bodies of water.[15,92,115] Under natural conditions the mycelia produce dumbbell-shaped infectious spores.[115]

Despite its widespread geographic distribution throughout the USA, far fewer individuals will present with clinical evidence of blastomycosis as they will with the similarly widespread histoplasmosis.[108] The geographic distribution of blastomycosis includes south-eastern and south-central USA, particularly along the Mississippi River valley and along the Great Lakes and St Lawrence Seaway. Epidemics of blastomycosis have been reported in northern Wisconsin and Minnesota, the greater Chicago area, and North Carolina.[15,83] Interests and occupations which place individuals at particular risk are those that bring them into prolonged contact in wooded areas, particularly in the autumn months.[29] Such individuals include forest workers and avid hunters[15] and bird hunters in particular;[83,108] chicken farming may also confer increased exposure risk.[83] As one of the true pathogenic fungi, blastomycosis has the capacity to infect non-immunocompromised hosts; due to their comparatively large numbers the immunocompetent are the most frequent victims of the organism.[15] Curiously, the immune status of infected individuals does not seem to markedly alter the presentation of disease.[115]

As with most other pathogenic fungi, the primary portal of infection is following the inhalation of spores. With exposure to the increased body temperature, the spores begin reproducing as budding yeasts.[29] After an incubation period of 4–6 weeks, the symptomatic individual may present with alveolar, miliary, or nodular infiltrates on chest radiograph, with or without cavitation,[15,115] that tend to be apically located.[15] The patient may present with a picture of an acute or pneumonic process with fever, chills, productive cough, night sweats and chest pain with or without hemoptysis.[15] In approximately 5% of all patients with clinical blastomycosis, the larynx will be infected by hematogenous spread.[15,29] Despite the frequent concurrence of pulmonary and laryngeal blastomycosis, the chest radiograph appears negative in half of patients with laryngeal lesions.[15,29] Although isolated laryngeal, tongue, gingival and hard palate involvement has been reported, it is the rule rather than the exception that most patients with laryngeal blastomycosis will present with concurrent pulmonary infection.[97]

The most common sites of involvement in blastomycosis are, in decreasing order of incidence; lung, skin, bone (particularly long bones) and genitourinary tract.[15] Therefore, frequent concomitant skin lesions are often present in patients with laryngeal lesions. These may be verrucous plaques with raised, sharp, irregular borders, nodular pustules, or exudative ulcerating lesions with heaped up edges.[15,29] The most common head and neck sites of blastomycotic involvement are the larynx, the oral cavity and the nasal cavity.[71]

The presentation of laryngeal blastomycosis is marked by persistent hoarseness of duration 2 months to 8 years,[29,115] which may progress to aphonia.[11] Cough, indicative of concurrent pulmonary involvement, is common and may be dry or productive of clear or occasionally blood-streaked sputum.[11,83] Dysphagia, dyspnea, shortness of breath, and dull pharyngeal and laryngeal pain with foreign body sensation have also been reported.[11,115] A survey of the literature suggests that the true vocal folds are the most common areas of the larynx to be infected by focal blastomycotic lesions followed by the supraglottis; in one study, 100% of the patients with laryngeal blastomycosis demonstrated true vocal fold lesions; 50% showed ventricular fold or other supraglottic areas of involvement, and only about 15% showed subglottic involvement.[29]

The appearance of laryngeal blastomycosis varies depending upon the stage of disease. It often mimics other more common diseases, particularly laryngeal squamous cell carcinoma.[71,83] Appearances range from erythematous, granulomatous, irregularly bordered lesions to exophytic, verrucous-appearing lesions to bulky, irregular lesions of the true vocal folds. As lesions advance, the verrucous growth may become extensive and subsequent fibrosis can lead to vocal fold fixation.[97,115] Less commonly, laryngeal blastomycosis may present with cervical lymphadenopathy.[108] Abscessing nodes may lead to the formation of laryngocutaneous fistulae.[115]

The approach to diagnosing laryngeal blastomycosis depends in part upon the clinical picture. If the patient is producing sputum, a KOH wet preparation will frequently demonstrate the characteristic yeast forms of blastomycosis. Scrapings or exudate from skin or mucous membrane lesions may also demonstrate the yeasts.[15,97] Culture of sputum for 3–4 weeks on Sabouraud's agar at 25°C is often positive because of the high frequency of concurrent pulmonary disease in laryngeal blastomycosis. Complement fixation, immunodiffusion and blastomycin skin tests are considered of insufficient sensitivity and specificity to be of diagnostic utility.[15]

The characteristic histologic feature of blastomycosis is the presence of doubly refractile broad-based budding yeast forms contained either within Langhans giant cells or scattered throughout the affected tissue. Periodic acid–Schiff (PAS) or Gomori methenamine silver are taken up by the yeast cell wall and may facilitate identification of fungal elements in tissue.[115] In addition to the typical 10–15 μm, thick-walled *Blastomyces* yeast forms, 2–3 μm yeast forms resembling histoplasmosis have been described in tissue specimens of blastomycotic infection.[108] Depending upon the severity and chronicity of the disease process, tissue specimens may demonstrate neutrophils in microabscesses, infiltrates of chronic inflammatory cells, or noncaseating granulomas.[29,71,115] Common histologic findings in blastomycosis include the presence of pseudoepitheliomatous hyperplasia and acanthosis, chronic inflammatory changes, and the presence of giant cells and microabscesses.[83] Pseudoepitheliomatous hyperplasia is a typical finding in those lesions that resemble squamous cell carcinoma.[29] The differential diagnosis of laryngeal blastomycosis includes histoplasmosis and squamous cell carcinoma.[97] Histoplasmosis much more commonly affects the oropharynx than does blastomycosis, and its lesions are more frequently ulcerative.

The treatment strategy for blastomycosis has changed in recent years following advances in antifungal therapy. The drug of choice for invasive blastomycosis is itraconazole 400 mg/day for 6 months[96] and should result in improvement of laryngeal symptoms within 1–4 weeks.[11] Ketoconazole at doses of 400–800 mg/day for the same duration is also typically effective. If, however, the patient suffers from life-threatening or CNS (meningeal) infection, intravenous amphotericin B is recommended to a total dose of 500–1000 mg, followed by a 6 month course of itraconazole or ketoconazole.[96] If the patient can not tolerate ketoconazole or itraconazole, amphotericin B monotherapy can be employed at a dose of 0.8 mg/kg three to four times a week to a total dosage of 2000 mg.[97] Surgical treatment for blastomycosis, if indicated, requires incision and drainage or debridement of large blastomycotic abscesses.[15]

Candidiasis

In contradistinction to the pathogenic fungi, *Candida albicans* is a saprophytic fungus, the natural environment of which is the mucosal surfaces of the human body, and it is common to the alimentary tract of almost all mammals and birds.[92] *Candida* exists as a yeast form in its commensal state and as a branching hyphal form in its pathogenic state. Its blastospore or yeast form is able to adhere to the mucosal surfaces of the acrodigestive tract and vagina.[92] The yeast stage of the fungus is considered necessary for initiation of a candidal lesion and is in itself an invasive organism; the formation of mycelia occurs when host environmental factors combine to cause inhibition of cell division without halting progression of growth. This results in elongate hyphae without budding.[92]

Certain host factors facilitate the development of candidiasis. These include extreme youth, prolonged administration of antibiotics, general debility and impaired host cell-mediated immunity.[92,115] Specific host factors which are associated with immunocompromised and pathogenic overgrowth of *Candida* include AIDS, diabetes mellitus, post-organ transplantation, hematogenous malignancy (in particular acute myelogenous leukemia), systemic lupus erythematosus and severe burns.[115] Radiation therapy-exposed tissues are susceptible to invasive *Candida* infection; the impaired blood flow which occurs as a late effect of radiation therapy presumably results in weakened local host immunity and increased susceptibility of such tissues to invasive disease.[44] In addition, local factors such as preexisting cartilage damage from tumor invasion, infection, or trauma or mucosal damage from continued smoking may allow such tissues to be more easily infiltrated with *Candida*.[44] Despite the key role that immunocompromise plays in the pathogenesis of candidiasis, case reports exist of patients with 'no significant underlying predisposing conditions'.[43]

In the pre-AIDS era, the typical patient presenting with laryngeal candidiasis was most commonly afflicted whilst on antibacterial medications,[111] although chemotherapy, diabetes, extensive burns and preceding endotracheal intubation with presumed mucosal damage have been reported as predisposing factors.[122] Since the advent of widespread HIV infection, the most common presentation is in the context of depressed cell-mediated immunity as a result of the AIDS virus.[49]

The typical appearance of laryngeal candidiasis is one of white painful patches over an erythematous friable surface; this patient will usually also be suffering from obvious oropharyngeal disease. In addition to severe pharyngeal pain which may progress to dysphagia and drooling,[98,115,122] hoarseness is a prominent feature and may be the first symptom in adults with laryngeal candidiasis.[111] In infants presenting with laryngeal candidiasis, the thick exudative patches often contribute to an initial presentation with upper airway obstruction.[50,111,115] The white to grayish-green or yellowish adherent exudate may be so extensive as to form a pseudomembrane covering the entire supraglottis with spread to both false cords or pyriforms.[98,122] Scraping of the pseudomembrane reveals a rugose, brightly erythematous mucosal base.[122] This bright erythema is indicative of mucosal invasion.[122] A variable amount of submucosal edema may give the underlying tissue an irregular appearance.[122] The most typical location of laryngeal candidiasis is in the supraglottic larynx where it may infrequently form large ulcerations,[111,115] although such lesions can be limited to the true vocal folds.[116] Finally, the exophytic or thickened whitish lesions may be suggestive of a glottic carcinoma.[43] Epiglottitis secondary to *Candida* invasion is more slowly developing and less virulent than bacterial epiglottitis.[49] Finally, some papillomatous lesions which were found histologically to contain *Candida* have been described in infants.[50]

The diagnosis of laryngeal candidiasis is secured by biopsy specimens obtained by direct laryngoscopy. The histology of a typical candidal laryngeal infection commonly demonstrates a reactive epithelial hyperplasia, superficial ulceration, and a variable inflammatory reaction that may be extremely intense.[115,122] Inflammatory exudates may consist largely of neutrophils or may demonstrate lymphocyte-predominate mixtures.[111,122] Infected tissues demonstrate the typical Gram-positive oval budding cells 5–7 μm in diameter with tubular hyphae.[115] Invasive candidal disease is most reliably indicated by the precedence of mycelia and pseudomycelia penetrating the underlying tissue.[115] Finally, the demonstration of pseudocarcinomatous hyperplasia has been reported.[43]

The treatment of simple mucosal candidiasis consists of either nystatin gargle (800 000 units) three to four times a day for 7–10 days or clotrimazole troches five times a day for 7–10 days. It has been noted that daily gentian violet application to laryngeal lesions can lead to the resolution of laryngeal candidiasis in absence of other antifungal therapy.[43] When systemic infection is suspected, ketoconazole 400 mg/day for 3 days followed by 200 mg/day for 10 days is frequently effective and should result in the complete resolution of signs and symptoms of laryngeal candidiasis. Recurrent disease is amenable to short-course retreatment with ketoconazole; this is reportedly always effective.[98] In patients with invasive disease, fluconazole or amphotericin B is recommended; these two drugs are felt to be equally efficacious in the presence of candidemia.[49] Compared to other fungal infections, doses of amphotericin B that are required are relatively low.[115] Finally, oral amphotericin B rinses or aerosolized amphotericin B has been used as effective treatment;[111] miconazole has also been advocated as a newer treatment with fewer side effects.[98]

Although uncommonly fatal,[111] chronic untreated candidiasis can lead to laryngeal scarring, necessitating subsequent surgical attempts to improve voice or airway.[111,115]

Cryptococcosis

Cryptococcosis is caused by infection with *Cryptococcus neoformans*, a fungus which maintains a worldwide distribution. *Cryptococcus* is found in great quantities in pigeon excreta[48,115] and one case of laryngeal cryptococcosis has been linked to exposure to chicken manure.[91]

Infection with cryptococcosis occurs via inhalation of the unencapsulated airborne yeast buds which are 2–7 μm in diameter.[48] Of all infections, 25–40% are said to occur in non-immunocompromised patients and relative degrees of immunocompromise such as heavy oral steroid use or the abnormal pulmonary anatomy of the chronic obstructive pulmonary disease (COPD) patient may predispose to infection.[48] Immunocompromised hosts, and particularly those with AIDS, are particularly susceptible to extrapulmonary spread of cryptococcosis. The organism is strongly neurotropic which accounts for its propensity for CNS spread; this may be due to a lack of protective factors which are found in blood serum but not in cerebrospinal fluid (CSF).[48,115]

Laryngeal cryptococcosis is extremely rare; only five cases have been reported in the literature, and only two of these have been in immunocompetent hosts.[48,115] The presentation of laryngeal cryptococcosis includes a dry cough and hoarseness that progresses over months and is refractory to standard antibiotic therapy.[103] One case reports the gradual onset of progressive hoarseness and dyspnea over 2 years in a patient presenting with acute upper airway obstruction.[91] Laryngeal cryptococcosis is most commonly presented in association with AIDS and this disease manifestation should therefore prompt appropriate serologic testing.[115] It is notable that dissemination of cryptococcosis may occur in the presence of a subclinical or already healed pulmonary infection.[91] Spread to the CNS is associated with irritability, headache, and memory and personality changes.[115]

The physical appearance of laryngeal cryptococcosis is quite varied. Cases described include that of an 'exudative lesion' on the anterior true vocal folds with edema and erythema of the surrounding vocal folds bilaterally, multiple raised exudative lesions 'circumferentially' around the larynx, and punctate tracheal ulcers with exudate.[91] A less distinctive lesion has been described as simple erythema and edema of the true vocal cords.[17] Finally a 'warty' 5 by 5 mm subglottic lesion of cryptococcosis has been described.[103]

The histologic appearance of a cryptococcal laryngeal lesion is characterized by pseudoepitheliomatous hyperplasia with associated submucosal inflammation and edema and infiltration by eosinophils, neutrophils and giant cells containing 4–15 μm diameter ovoid fungal bodies.[48,91,103,115] Close inspection may reveal yeast cells forming narrow-based 'teardrop' buds. There is a tendency for the organisms to aggregate into small submucosal collections.[48,115] Identification of *Cryptococcus* may be aided by the use of mucicarmine dyes which stain the thick polysaccharide capsule.[115]

The diagnosis of laryngeal cryptococcosis is secured by demonstration of the organisms on biopsy samples. However, there are multiple other findings that are suggestive of cryptococcal dissemination. Sputum cultures may be positive for *Cryptococcus* even without organ involvement.[115] The rapid capsular antigen agglutination test is also helpful in narrowing the differential diagnosis. It has been noted that chest radiograms are frequently negative even in the presence of florid tracheobronchial cryptococcal disease;[91] however, positive biopsy specimens have been obtained from cavitary pulmonary lesions.[17] Dissemination to the CNS is best demonstrated by examination of the CSF; typical findings are increased opening pressure on lumbar puncture, and elevated white count (largely lymphocytes), elevated protein and decreased glucose levels. Urine cultures may also be positive in disseminated cryptococcal disease.

Treatment of cryptococcal disease is evolving with the continued emergence of new antifungal agents. One suggested regimen is fluconazole 400 mg/day for 2 months; this drug is a particularly appropriate agent against *Cryptococcus* because it demonstrates excellent CNS penetration.[48,115] In the face of aggressive disease or in a severely immunocompromised host, amphotericin B with or without flucytosine is an appropriate regimen. An earlier study recommends treating to a total dose of 2 g,[91] whilst later studies recommend instituting amphotericin B at 0.3 mg/kg/day plus flucytosine at 37.5 mg/kg/day for 6 weeks.

The prognosis for disseminated cryptococcosis, the presumptive diagnosis in laryngeal cryptococcosis, depends largely on whether or not the CNS becomes affected. One successfully treated laryngeal lesion was described as demonstrating complete resolution of the pseudo-epithelial hyperplasia, with only mild residual edema of the false cords.[91] Yet in the face of CNS infection, a 30% mortality is expected and a 20–25% relapse rate is typical. Patients who have AIDS are rarely, if ever, cured of cryptococcosis. In those patients with CNS involvement, 40% will, even if cured, be left with significant residual neurologic sequelae.[115]

Leishmaniasis

Leishmaniasis is a disease with worldwide distribution caused by a number of protozoal parasites of the genus *Leishmania*. These parasites have been broken down into four main groups:

- *Leishmania donovani* complex, an Old World variety, which causes visceral leishmaniasis (kala-azar);
- *Leishmania mexicana* and *Leishmania brasiliensis*, the primary pathogens in New World cutaneous and mucocutaneous leishmaniasis; and
- the *Leishmania tropica major* and *minor* Old World varieties of cutaneous leishmaniasis.[124]

The most frequent manifestations of leishmaniasis are cutaneous whereas leishmaniasis of the larynx is extremely rare and occurs only in the context of mucocutaneous disease.[78,97] Laryngeal leishmaniasis is by far most common amongst the parasites of the *L. brasiliensis* group, whereas the few Old World cases of laryngeal leishmaniasis are typically of the *L. donovani infantum* type, and the *L. tropica* subtypes only very rarely cause mucous membrane infection.[62,97,124]

The leishmaniasis parasites are transmitted by vectors of the sandfly (*Phlebotomus*) species. These parasites exist as promastigotes in the digestive tract of the sandfly and are transmitted by its bite. In humans or other susceptible mammals, the parasite converts to an amastigote form which multiples by binary fission.[21] Uncommon vectors include human-to-human modes of transmission such as blood transfusion, sexual contact, or transplacental passage of the organism.[78] Patients at increased risk for development of disease include those with relative or absolute degrees of immune impairment; predisposing factors include chronic ethanol abuse, severe malnutrition, chronic steroid use, old age, diabetes mellitus, tuberculosis and HIV infection.[62,116]

Laryngeal leishmaniasis represents an uncommon subtype of mucocutaneous leishmaniasis or espundia.[62] The disease develops by hematogenous spread from a long-standing cutaneous ulcer[62,97] and only rarely represents a primary mucosal infection.[63] The location and duration of cutaneous lesions are felt to influence the risk of mucosal spread. Of patients who develop mucosal disease, 50% will do so within 2 years of primary cutaneous infection; also, there appears to be an increased likelihood of mucosal disease in patients with multiple or long-standing lesions above the waistline.[62] Mucosal involvement may ensue months to years after primary cutaneous inoculation with half the patients developing mucosal spread within 2 years of their primary skin infection;[62] however, mucosal dissemination has been reported as late as 24 years following primary cutaneous exposure.[78,116] Most typically, however, in patients in whom an extensive period of latency exists, it has been speculated that the mucosal disease represents activation of a dormant infection triggered by a subsequent mucosal trauma or systemic illness.[62] In those with mucosal involvement, one-third will be affected in multiple mucosal sites and of these, 40% will have laryngeal involvement. In a series of 189 patients, only 1.6% were found to have isolated laryngeal lesions, and these were all secondary to *L. brasiliensis* infection.[62]

The patient with laryngeal leishmaniasis presents with progressive hoarseness, dysphagia, and odynophagia which may be accompanied by a brassy cough.[21,78] The lesions of laryngeal leishmaniasis tend to localize in the supraglottis or glottis.[78] Many physical appearances have been described depending in part upon the state of development of the lesion. These include generalized edema involving the pharynx, epiglottis and pyriforms, granular, friable epiglottic and hypopharyngeal erythema, widespread transglottic granulations and leukoplakia of the true vocal fold.[124] Also described are extensive ulcerations covered with a gray, fibrinous exudate involving the epiglottis, hypopharynx, pharynx and true vocal folds,[21] glottic and epiglottic granulomas leading to subsequent fibrosis, and a solitary broad-based polypoid lesion covering the majority of one true vocal fold with normal mobility.[21,32,39,78,116,124]

Other sites of upper airway mucosa are more commonly involved with leishmaniasis than is the larynx. The nasal septal mucosa in particular is the most common site of mucous spread of cutaneous leishmaniasis. It is felt that the specialized venules of the septal blood supply may trap or act as a reservoir for the blood-borne parasite.[62] In addition, it has been postulated that *Leishmania* prefer a low temperature such as afforded by the exposure of the anterior septum to the nasal airstream, for their growth.[62] The patient with nasal leishmaniasis frequently complains of obstruction, epistaxis, excessive amounts of nasal secretions, and occasionally passage of pieces of granulomatous tissue from the nose. In a study of 47 patients with nasal leishmaniasis, 70% were found to have active, friable granuloma, 40% had septal perforation, 10% presented with polypoid nasal mucosal changes and vestibular collapse. Inferior turbinate lesions are said to be infrequent.[62] Infectious spread to the lateral cartilages and inferior turbinates can lead to subsequent collapse of the nasal tip with the development of a 'tapir nose'.[62] The next most common sites of involvement are the pharynx and palate followed by the larynx and lips. Notably, the tongue is usually spared in mucosal leishmaniasis.

On close examination, 85–90% of patients presenting with mucosal leishmaniasis will be found to have an old scar of a primary cutaneous infection. Such lesions may appear as slightly depressed, hypopigmented, 'puckered' scars, macules, plaques, papules, or nodules.[62,78] It has also been described as similar in appearance to a large burn scar. The patient typically relates a history of a chronic skin ulcer which took several months to heal; the most common location for cutaneous New World leishmaniasis is on the lower anterior tibia.[62]

The definitive diagnosis of leishmaniasis is by biopsy and identification of the amastigotes. These are frequently found within macrophages on hematoxylin and eosin or Giemsa stains; 40% or more of appropriate biopsy specimens will demonstrate identifiable parasites.[62,97] Nasal mucosal scrapings of clinically affected areas are often adequate for diagnosis. In addition, bone marrow biopsy has been advocated as the 'safest diagnostic procedure' and reportedly yields a 55–85% positive rate on smears.[21] The leishmanin skin reaction (Montenegro skin test), which utilizes an intradermal extract of killed promastigotes, is typically positive in mucosal disease.[62,97] Patients with leishmaniasis that fail to react with at least 5 mm of induration within 48 hours are considered to be anergic. Other serologic tests that have been developed include an immunofluorescence and ELISA assays.[62] Attempts to culture *Leishmania* are only successful 45% of the time because of the difficulty in isolating and maintaining the organisms.

Histologic examination of biopsy specimens is dominated by an exudative cellular reaction. Typically the overlying epithelium demonstrates squamous change with pseudoepitheliomatous hyperplasia and moderate dysplasia.[21,32] Ulceration with necrosis or progression to granulomatous tubercle formation may occur.[62,124] A diffuse inflammatory infiltrate consisting largely of lymphocytes, plasmacytes and histiocytes is present surrounding the lesions. Staining with Giemsa may reveal 'Leishman–Donovan bodies', red-staining 2–4 μm granules that represent the amastigote kinetoplast.[62,78,124] Of note, these bodies are PAS-negative, helping to distinguish leishmaniasis from fungal infections.

The differential diagnosis for mucocutaneous leishmaniasis includes paracoccidioidomycosis, which shares the similar New World distribution, histoplasmosis (both of which stain PAS-positive), and laryngeal carcinoma.[62]

The pentavalent antimonials constitute the primary treatment for leishmaniasis. These are believed to impair oxidative phosphorylation or the citric acid cycle or glycolysis in the parasites, with subsequent inhibition of ATP/GTP synthesis.[12] The two pentavalent antimonials currently available are sodium stibogluconate (Pentostam) and meglumine antimonate (Glucantime). The dose should be adjusted to 20 mg/kg of pentavalent antimony intravenously once a day for 30 days or for at least 1 week following the cessation of all disease activity.[62] The most notable side effects of antimonial therapy are ECG abnormalities; although typically minor, occasional life-threatening arrhythmias have been reported.[62] On this regimen, drug resistance is typically 10%, although this increases to 15% in HIV-positive patients;[78] this latter group may require long-term, low-dose prophylaxis.[21] Should the patients fail antimonial therapy, amphotericin B is an appropriate second-line agent. This is typically highly effective, although a total dose of 2.5 g is recommended (one patient was cured with only a 1.5 g total dose).[62] Another study reported a cure using 3 mg/kg/day of amphotericin B for 32 days.[39] Liposomal amphotericin B, although expensive, is better tolerated by patients and may be considered when available. Pentamidine has also been studied in the use of leishmaniasis, although its efficacy remains to be determined. Experimental vaccination programs against leishmaniasis are currently being developed.[62]

The course of mucosal leishmaniasis is unpredictable. Mucosal lesions are more resistant forms of infection than simple cutaneous lesions. However, even in the absence of antibiotic therapy, the infection may smolder for years, being held in check by the host immune system, and the patient may present with only small septal granuloma. In other patients, however, the disease may rapidly spread, causing extensive necrosis and tissue loss within weeks. Typically, such aggressive disease is heralded by marked edema and erythema over the sites of subsequent necrosis. Cutaneous anergy to histoplasmin is considered a poor prognostic factor, and such patients have a high relapse rate regardless of therapy.[62,97] Because even healed lesions of laryngeal leishmaniasis tend to be characterized by scarring, it is rare for the voice to return to normal even following successful treatment of the disease. Even in cases where the larynx appears normal on examination, dysphonia is often noted.[39,62]

Wegener's granulomatosis

Wegener's granulomatosis (WG) is a syndrome of unknown etiology characterized by necrotizing vasculitis affecting diffuse areas of the respiratory tract, kidneys, skin, eyes and joints.[120] It has been postulated that a transiently present infectious agent may act as a trigger for onset of disease. Others have speculated that the c-ANCA antibody itself is a critical factor in the pathogenesis of disease.[52] The specific antigen for the c-ANCA antibody is a 29 kDa serine proteinase, proteinase III (Pr-III) located within neutrophil azurophilic granules.[30] It has been determined that neutrophil and monocyte activation leads to translocation of Pr-III from its normal location in the intracytoplasmic department to the cell surface where it is exposed to the c-ANCA antibody. It has also been demonstrated that tumor necrosis factor alpha (TNF-α) can lead to translocation of Pr-III to the cell surface. c-ANCA antibodies enhance neutrophil activation, degranulation, respiratory burst and adherence.[30] The predilection of WG lesions to involve the respiratory tract has led to speculation that the inflammatory process has an affinity for ciliated respiratory epithelium.[58]

The prevalence of WG is estimated at 3 per 100 000 population. The mean age of patients presenting with WG is about 40 years, range 9–78 years. Although WG is believed to affect both sexes equally,[30] several studies of laryngeal WG lesions suggest that there is a strong female predominance for this disease appearance. In one citation, 12 of 13 patients with subglottic lesions were women,[68] whilst in another study 10 of 10 patients presented were female.[2]

Seventy-five percent of presentations in Wegener's granulomatosis will include head and neck manifestations.[58] These may include nasal obstruction, crusting and epistaxis, infrequent sore throat and, with laryngeal lesions, stridor, shortness of breath, and less frequently hoarseness or hemoptysis.[69,120] The percentage of patients with WG who will have concurrent laryngeal involvement has ranged between 8 and 48% in series. In adult populations, this typically ranges between 8 and 25%.[30,58,113,120] However, nearly half of pediatric and adolescent patients who present with WG will be affected with laryngeal disease.[30,58] Due to a propensity for subglottic involvement, the stridor associated with laryngeal Wegener's is typically biphasic, and flow–volume analysis will indicate a fixed extrathoracic lesion.[120] In three-quarters of patients with laryngeal Wegener's, the onset of laryngeal lesions follows other manifestations of disease.[58] It may take from several months to 10 years for laryngeal lesions to develop after the initial symptoms of WG.[68,69,120]

The characteristic lesion of Wegener's granulomatosis is a subglottic mass or eccentric, circumferential stenotic segment 2–4 cm in length.[57,69] Hoarseness ensues when the stenotic segment extends superiorly to involve the undersurface of one or both vocal folds. The lesions of laryngeal Wegener's have been variously described as reddish friable masses, polypoid lesions, ulcerative lesions which are occasionally quite extensive, weblike lesions, and healed areas of scarring.[30,110,113] The infrequent destructive epiglottic lesion has been described as well, although the vast majority of lesions are subglottic.[113]

The diagnosis of Wegener's granulomatosis relies on demonstration of characteristic pathologic features in the absence of an underlying infectious etiology. The histologic features of WG lesions are variable. A classic description is that of necrotizing and non-necrotizing granulomata in the context of a vasculitis involving small arteries and veins. Those granulomata that undergo degeneration demonstrate fibrinoid central necrosis with microabscess formation.[68] Others have described necrotizing inflammatory foci and necrotic vessels surrounded by foreign body and Langhans-type giant cells.[110] Other patterns include polypoid masses of granulomatous tissue with a core of fibroblasts, lymphocytes, neutrophils and occasional giant cells and eosinophils or granulation tissue with significant fibrotic scarring and abundant eosinophilia.[68,110] Biopsies obtained during treatment demonstrate healing vasculitis with intramural fibrosis,[68] or granulation tissue with marked fibrosis and small amounts of obliterative endarteritis.[110]

The most diagnostic serologic test for Wegener's granulomatosis is the c-ANCA or cytoplasmic pattern antinuclear cytoplasmic antibody which is 90–97% specific in the appropriate context.[30] c-ANCA is positive in 90% of patients with active WG and in 40% of those in remission.[30] In patients with WG, the rheumatoid factor is usually positive and the sedimentation rate is sometimes markedly elevated.[69,120] A complete workup of a patient for WG should include a chest radiogram, serum creatinine and urinalysis to screen for occult fulminant glomerulonephritis.[30]

Glucocorticoids are the mainstay of treatment for Wegener's granulomatosis. These act through inhibition of inflammatory mediators and adhesion, activation, and proliferation of various types of leukocytes. They are typically started at a dose of at least 1 mg/kg/day; if the patient faces life-threatening complications, several days of massive dose pulse steroids (1000 mg of methylprednisolone) may be indicated.[30] Steroids are generally insufficient to halt disease progression in generalized Wegener's granulomatosis.[30] In these patients, cyclophosphamide, which induces B- and T-cell lymphopenia and decreases immunoglobulin production, is started at an initial dose of 2 mg/kg/day and may be increased to 3–5 mg/kg/day in life-threatening disease. The dose is tapered to maintain the patient's white blood cell count above $3500/mm^3$. In patients requiring multimodality therapy, it is deemed appropriate to attempt to wean the patient off the steroid prior to discontinuing the cyclophosphamide. The cyclophosphamide is continued for at least 1 year after remission has been achieved, and is tapered at 25 mg/day increments every 2–3 months as tolerated. More recently, methotrexate has been advocated as substitute for cyclophosphamide as it has less inherent oncogenicity.[30] A dose of 0.15–0.30 mg/kg/week with concomitant glucocorticoids results in clinical improvement in about 80% of patients.[30] Finally, trimethoprim–sulfamethoxazole and cyclosporin A are still considered controversial as monotherapy for WG.[30]

Surgical treatment for Wegener's granulomatosis is indicated in cases of airway compromise. A tracheotomy may need to be performed at the initiation of chemotherapy, and residual stenotic narrowing and fibrosis post-treatment may require surgical intervention. Treatments that have been employed range from simple dilatation with steroid injections to laser resection or laryngotracheoplasty.[58] Some authors advocate no surgical intervention at all in a stable airway that is at least 6–7 mm in diameter. With progressive disease, it is deemed appropriate to attempt to dilate non-inflamed lesions with biopsy of any visible granulations prior to the definitive procedure to assess disease activity. Typically, steroids may be injected in any friable or polypoid subglottic tissues that are evident. CO_2 laser treatment has been tried in eight patients in one series with 'uniformly poor results', leading to increased postoperative scarring; all of these patients required other procedures to improve and stabilize their airways.[58] Tracheal reconstructions including end-to-end anastomoses and laryngotracheoplasty enjoy a high degree of success in patients with subglottic WG.[58,69]

[illegible]ler lesions may be subject to end-to-end reanasto[illegible]otic procedures whilst larger lesions may require anterior and posterior cricoid split laryngotracheoplasty with cartilage-graft insertion. In such cases, a Montgomery T-tube stent is placed for 3–6 months to allow the airway to stabilize. This technique was successful in three of five patients in one series.[58] One of those who failed standard laryngotracheoplasty required a subsequent laryngotracheoplasty with a microvascular repair (an intercostal vessel-based rib-free flap); this patient healed well.[58]

The prognosis for Wegener's granulomatosis is variable and difficult to predict from patient to patient. In some patients, even while receiving nominally adequate drug treatment, some lesions rapidly regress whilst other areas continue to progress relentlessly.[120] The larynx in particular is one area that is frequently resistant to treatment.[120] A correlation has been suggested between the time of presentation of laryngeal disease and the prognosis for voice and airway. It has been noted that late-developing laryngeal lesions are less responsive to treatment, and up to 50% of patients will experience disease progression despite cyclophosphamide and steroid therapy.[120] Overall, cicatricial subglottic healing is common and a significant number of patients will require long-term tracheotomy despite aggressive therapy. Finally, the disease course of WG follows waxing and waning pattern, with reactivation seen up to 2 years following initial disease control.[69] The leading causes of death in WG are renal failure and infection (sepsis).[68]

Sarcoidosis

Sarcoidosis is a chronic inflammatory condition of unknown etiology. It has been postulated that sarcoidosis may represent a primary autoimmune disease or a host response to an as yet unidentified infectious agent or inhaled chemicals. Exposure to inhaled metals such as zirconium and beryllium has been noted to cause a pulmonary sarcoidosis-like syndrome.[79,82] Community outbreaks of sarcoid-like pulmonary lesions have been reported, suggesting a mode of person-to-person spread or the shared environmental exposure as important etiologic factors. It has also been noted that sarcoidosis has been transmitted via bone marrow in cardiac transplants. There is a significant genetic association with HLA class I groups A1 and B8 as well as those of HLA class II DR3; these HLA classes parallel those in other autoimmune disorders such as SLE and rheumatoid arthritis. A genetic predisposition to sarcoidosis is suggested by familial clustering with a 19% incidence in black families and a 5% incidence in white.[82]

The proposed pathogenetic mechanism of disease has been divided into three events; an antigen exposure, followed by a specific cell-mediated immune response, which then becomes broadened pathologically into a nonspecific and self-perpetuating inflammatory response.[82] Sarcoidosis tends to present in the winter and spring.[82] Sarcoidosis is a multiorgan system disease and 9% of patients with sarcoidosis will develop head and neck manifestations. In the head and neck region the eyes and the lacrimal glands are the most frequently affected areas followed by cutaneous manifestations such as erythema nodosum, nasal and laryngeal lesions. All patients who suffer from sarcoidosis demonstrate impairment of cell-mediated and elevation of hormonally mediated immune function. The evidence for this resides in the observation that many patients with sarcoidosis mount a delayed-type hypersensitivity reaction to certain antigens, and that elevated levels of circulating immune complexes are found in their blood.[82] African and Hispanic patients have a higher incidence of sarcoidosis estimated at 35 per 100 000 whilst in the Caucasian population it is about 10 per 100 000.[82] The typical patient is female and 20–40 years old on presentation.[56,79] Although pediatric patients in the 12–20 years age range have been described with sarcoidosis, overall the disease is much less common in the pediatric population and is very rare under age 12.[74,93]

The patient presenting with sarcoidosis typically complains of dysphagia, dyspnea and, less commonly, sore throat and hoarseness. It has been proposed that voice problems are uncommon in sarcoidosis because the true vocal folds are infrequently involved with disease due to their lack of intrinsic lymphoid tissue.[56] Constitutional symptoms such as fatigue, cough, fever, weight loss, migratory polyarthralgia, lymphadenopathy and splenomegaly are common. The typical disease course is waxing and waning, slowly progressive, with a tendency to 'burn out' over many years.[79] Other head and neck manifestations include the presence of erythema nodosum over the nose and cheeks[56,82] or lupus pernio, a skin lesion characterized by disfiguring violaceous plaques and nodules that tend to affect cooler skin areas.[42,82] Finally, isolated cases of bilateral cervical adenopathy in association with sarcoidosis have been reported.[9]

The larynx is involved in 1–5% of patients with sarcoidosis.[56] The supraglottic larynx tends to be affected more often than the subglottis with conspicuous skipping of the glottis and a lack of transglottic lesions. The vocal cords are normally mobile.[79] The typical laryngeal lesion of sarcoidosis is a pale pink, edematous fullness that diffusely involves the supraglottic laryngeal structures. In general the mucosa is completely intact, and ulceration is quite uncommon.[79] The mass effect associated with the smooth swelling of the epiglottis and aryepiglottic folds results in a downward and backward pull on the epiglottis, giving the appearance of a widened vallecula.[56] Pediatric lesions have been described with a similar 'glassy edema and pallor' of the epiglottis.[93] Less commonly the lesions of sarcoidosis appear as inflamed nodular laryngeal mucosal distortions,[9] or as large supraglottic granulomas or edema associated with yellowish supraglottic ulcerations.[56] Occasionally vocal fold paralysis may occur secondary to neuropathic involvement of the recurrent laryngeal nerve.[56]

The diagnosis of sarcoidosis is one of exclusion, although several features help to narrow the diagnostic possibilities. The radiographic finding of bilateral hilar adenopathy and mild symptoms disproportionate to the clinical findings are quite suggestive of sarcoidosis. Multiple laboratory values are also suggestive but nonspecific for the diagnosis. These include the serum angiotensin converting enzyme, levels of which tend to parallel the clinical course, immunoglobulin levels, C-reactive protein levels, sedimentation rate, serum and urine calcium, and alkaline phosphatase.[56,74,93] Cutaneous anergy is also frequently associated with sarcoidosis.[93] Finally, biopsy of the involved tissue is helpful in the diagnosis. Noncaseating granulomas are necessary but not sufficient to diagnose sarcoidosis. Lymphoma, cartilaginous tumors and other granulomatous diseases must be ruled out.

Characteristics of the noncaseating granulomas of sarcoidosis are 'abundant' numbers of CD4-positive oligoclonal T-cells. As a result of this T-cell stimulation, fibroblasts and mast cells are drawn into the region of the granuloma and due to their fibrotic response cause collagen fiber encasement of the granuloma and surrounding tissue damage.[82] Histologic examination of sarcoid granulomatous lesions demonstrates clumps of epithelioid cells and occasional Langhans-type giant cells with a conspicuous absence of necrosis. In later stages, affected areas may be replaced with large amounts of hyalinization and fibrosis.

The primary treatment for sarcoidosis is glucocorticoid therapy. Typically oral steroids are initiated at a dose of 30–40 mg/day,[82] and reversal and resolution of disease manifestations may take several months.[56,74] In the event that oral steroids fail to halt the disease progression, intralesional steroid injection has been advocated. Triamcinolone at a dose of 80–160 mg has been injected in supraglottic sarcoid lesions with marked improvement in patient symptomatology within 2–7 days of injection; occasionally repeat injections are required to reverse the disease course. These patients are reportedly free of airway symptoms 1–4.5 years following treatment.[56] In patients unresponsive to or intolerant of steroids, methotrexate may be initiated; a dose of 10 mg/week has been found effective in clearing cutaneous and laryngeal lesions.[42] An early article described treatment of a subglottic lesion using surgical excision and split-thickness skin graft placement with good long-term results.[27]

Relapsing polychondritis

Relapsing polychondritis is an episodic inflammation of the cartilaginous structures of the body, resulting in their progressive destruction and subsequent replacement with fibrotic scar. Recurrent inflammation of various special sense organs is also characteristic of some presentations of relapsing polychondritis. Necessary and sufficient diagnostic criteria include characteristic histologic changes as well as three or more of the following manifestations:

- recurrent bilateral auricular chondritis;
- nasal chondritis;
- respiratory tract chondritis;
- audiovestibular symptoms (sensorineural);
- ocular inflammation;
- non-erosive inflammatory polyarthritis.[66]

Some authors have suggested liberalizing these criteria to not include histologic confirmation,[26] although the diagnosis can be made with considerably more confidence if a tissue biopsy is available that demonstrates focal inflammatory destruction of cartilage.[7]

The etiology of relapsing polychondritis remains unknown. It has been postulated that cell-mediated immune mechanisms are pivotal in the pathogenesis of this disease, and *in vitro* assays have demonstrated T-lymphocyte proliferation following exposure to cartilage preparations. Although originally this disease was felt to be characterized by a 'paucity of humoral immune aberrations' and infrequent anti-cartilage antibodies,[66] some more recent studies have suggested that humoral mechanisms may play a significant role in the pathogenesis of this disease. One study of serum from patients with relapsing polychondritis demonstrated antibodies to type II collagen in 5 of 15 patients with active disease.[36] There is also evidence that immune complexes may have a role in the pathogenesis of relapsing polychondritis. Specifically, granular deposits of IgG, IgA and IgM and complement component C3 have been demonstrated at the fibrochondral junctions of lesions of relapsing polychondritis.[36,66] Despite such suggestive findings, none of the above studies has been able to determine if antibodies to collagen represent active components of the disease process or simply epiphenomena of primary cartilage destruction with antigen release.

The average age of onset of disease is 40–45 years; there appears to be no gender, racial, or familial predilection.[7,66,67] However, in one study of 10 patients, a 4:1 female-to-male ratio was noted.[26]

Laryngeal involvement in relapsing polychondritis occurs in 40–55% of patients[26,66] and is a serious manifestation of this disease. This patient typically presents with a cough rarely productive of blood-tinged sputum and hoarseness, which may progress to aphonia, dyspnea, or inspiratory stridor. Patients usually present with airway compromise in the active, inflammatory stages of the disease with such compromise secondary to intense inflammatory edema of the glottis and subglottis rather than the tracheomalacia of long-standing inactive disease.[66] Such a patient may present with tenderness over the thyroid cartilage and trachea or absent thyroid cartilage bulge. Laryngeal examination may reveal firm, swollen false vocal folds and a diffuse inflammatory process. Subglottic inflammation is more likely to result in airway symptoms. Over time, dissolution of any or all of the laryngeal and bronchial cartilages may occur. This may result in the disruption of normal cricoid and tracheal cartilage architecture[26] and tracheobronchial ndromalacia with inspiratory collapse. Tracheal volvement is characterized by diffuse circumferential involvement of the cartilages of the central airway (i.e. trachea and mainstem bronchi) with sparing of the small airways;[65] diffuse bronchial cartilage involvement may result in chronic obstructive pulmonary disease.[66]

The ear cartilages are the most frequently involved site in relapsing polychondritis, occurring in about 90% of cases. Auricular inflammation is characterized by the sudden onset of episodes of erythema, edema and extreme tenderness over the cartilaginous pinna. These attacks, which are frequently bilateral, tend to resolve spontaneously within 5–10 days. Succeeding attacks tend to be less severe as the cartilage undergoes progressive lysis and replacement.[66] The joints of the extremities and central thoracic joints are the next most commonly involved areas in relapsing polychondritis, with manifestations in approximately 80% of patients. This is characterized as an inflammatory oligo- or polyarthritis that is seronegative, nonerosive, non-nodular, and often asymmetrical. It often initially presents with migratory joint pains accompanied by effusions, closely mimicking early rheumatoid arthritis. Nasal chondritis, which occurs in 70% of patients with relapsing polychondritis, is characterized by extreme dorsal tenderness, fullness, and erythema of sudden onset, and spontaneously resolves within several days. Other serious but less frequent symptoms include audio-vestibular complaints (sensorineural hearing loss, vertigo), cardiovascular manifestations (aortitis, valvular damage, myocardial infarction, vasculitis), CNS dysfunction (facial nerve paralysis), erythema nodosum-like cutaneous lesions, and ocular manifestations (iritis, episcleritis).[26,66] Autoimmune diseases, particularly rheumatoid arthritis, may be seen in up to 30% of patients with relapsing polychondritis. Case reports of patients with concurrent relapsing polychondritis and Crohn's disease have also been reported.[66,114]

The characteristic histologic features of an early lesion of relapsing polychondritis consist of a loss of basophilic staining of the cartilage matrix corresponding to the loss of the matrix acid mucopolysaccharides and perivascular cellular infiltrates consisting primarily of lymphocytes and plasmacytes. All forms of cartilage including hyaline cartilage, fibrocartilage and elastic cartilage may be involved; this feature distinguishes relapsing polychondritis from rheumatoid arthritis.[7] Progression of the lesions is marked by fibroblastic and capillary endothelial proliferation. The cartilage destruction is marked by the death of chondrocytes with vacuolation and pyknosis of the nuclei, followed by disruption of lacunae and cellular outlines. Finally, the dead chondrocytes are phagocytized by macrophages and replaced with fibrous tissue.[7]

The diagnosis of relapsing polychondritis relies on a significant confluence of characteristic symptoms as indicated by the first paragraph of this section. In addition to those features mentioned, some hematologic and serologic indicators of disease include an elevated sedimentation rate in the range of 50–100, which typically occurs during acute manifestations of the disease, a mild to moderate elevation of the leukocyte count, and mild anemia.[26,66]

Prolonged corticosteroid therapy remains the cornerstone of treatment in relapsing polychondritis. A typical maintenance dose consists of 20–25 mg/day of prednisone,[26,66] with a boost to 1 mg/kg or more during flares (80–100 mg/day of prednisone is typical). One-third of McAdam's series were able to reduce their maintenance steroid dose to less than or equal to 15 mg every other day and 25% of his patients were able to be maintained only on nonsteroidal anti-inflammatory drugs.[66] If disease flares cannot be controlled with high-dose corticosteroid, more intensive therapy using cyclophosphamide or azathioprine may be indicated, although in some series this has only been shown to be of 'moderate value'.[26,66] Seven of seven patients treated with dapsone demonstrated clinical improvement in one series.[26] This drug may act through inhibition of the lysosomal enzyme release or interference with the myeloperoxidase-halide mechanism of neutrophil cytoxicity. Patients whose involvement causes severe tracheomalacia may require a permanent tracheotomy.

The prognosis for relapsing polychondritis is somewhat variable. Respiratory tract involvement appears to be the best predictor of serious morbidity from relapsing polychondritis, and the time of onset of respiratory tract involvement has prognostic significance. A literature review indicated that of those who demonstrated early respiratory tract symptoms, 75 ultimately required permanent tracheotomy, and 30% ultimately died of respiratory complications. Of those who had later onset involvement, 25% ultimately required tracheotomy, and none succumbed to the disease. When followed up for several years, 20–30% of patients with relapsing polychondritis die of disease.[66] The cited causes of death are, in order of frequency, airway collapse or obstruction, pneumonia and ruptured arterial aneurysm. Of note, most of these studies are of older patient groups and newer immunosuppressive therapies may have a favorable impact on prognosis.

Amyloidosis

Amyloidosis is a group of disorders characterized by deposition of acellular proteinaceous material in tissues.[90] Amyloid aggregates are composed of homogenous subunits of different proteins which share several common features: all demonstrate a similar tertiary protein structure, the twisted β-pleated sheet; all amyloid deposits contain amyloid P protein which is identical to serum amyloid P; and all of the primary protein structures are rich in aspartic acid and glutamic acid residues. The resulting structure has a highly polyanionic surface which may predispose the formation of a β-pleated structure and presumably contributes to the great stability of the protein aggregates. This characteristic, in turn, allows amyloid to accumulate as a nonreactive proteinaceous deposit that causes structural damage simply by pressure effects on adjacent tissues.[34]

Several subtypes of amyloidosis have been defined based on the protein makeup of the amyloid deposits and the clinical characteristics of the patient. AL or primary amyloid is a product of an immunocyte (plasmacyte) dyscrasia. The proteins in AL amyloid are derived exclusively from immunoglobulin λ and κ chains. This type of amyloidosis occurs in patients with primary systemic amyloidosis, myeloma-associated amyloid, and in most cases of localized amyloidosis such as those involving the larynx.[60,90] There is significant evidence that suggests that the λ chains in AL amyloid are more amylogenic then the κ chains.[33] Whereas primary amyloidosis is characterized by the deposition of amyloid in mesenchymal tissues such as the tongue, heart and gastrointestinal tract, secondary or AA amyloidosis is associated with deposits mainly in reticuloendothelial organs such as the liver and spleen.[33] AA amyloidosis is associated with chronic destructive inflammatory and infectious diseases such as long-standing tuberculosis and rheumatoid arthritis and inherited disorders such as familial Mediterranean fever. A third type of amyloid, AF, is a familial variant in which the amyloid subunits are derived from a genetic variant of prealbumin.[101] The protein deposits in AS, 'senile', or age-related amyloidosis are derived from the plasma protein transthyretin. Finally, other variants of amyloidosis include one associated with chronic dialysis in which β2-microglobulin is the protein which forms the protein aggregates.[60]

Laryngeal involvement in amyloidosis is rare, accounting for <1% of all benign laryngeal tumors.[33] Only about 200 cases have been reported in the literature. Those laryngeal lesions that are reported typically are of primary amyloidosis although a few cases exist of laryngeal involvement as a result of generalized secondary amyloidosis.[33] Prognostic significance has been attached to the appearance of laryngeal amyloidosis as a presenting symptom versus its appearance later in the course of systemic amyloidosis.

The typical patient who presents with laryngeal amyloidosis is in the 40–60 year age range and there is a male-to-female predominance of approximately 2:1.[27,33] Amyloidosis is a chronic, slowly progressive disease of insidious onset characterized by hoarseness, dyspnea, cough, stridor or odynophagia[101]and, rarely, hemoptysis.[34] The typical lesion of laryngeal amyloidosis is a firm, nonulcerated, orange-yellow to gray submucosal nodule. Less commonly it may present as one or multiple discrete pedunculated polypoid lesions which may involve any part of the larynx. Several series have noted that the location of amyloid deposits tends to be highest on the ventricles and false cords, somewhat less common in the subglottis and on the aryepiglottic folds, and least common on the true vocal cords.[27,60] The most common clinical presentation is, however, for multiple sites of the larynx to be involved.[60] It is extremely rare for vocal fold fixation or cicatricial stenosis to occur in the context of laryngeal amyloidosis unless other predisposing factors are also present.[20] Various clinical descriptions of amyloidosis include that of a cystic lesion on the true vocal fold,[109] an infiltrating tumor of the true vocal folds and subglottis,[101] multinodular deposits in the subglottis, trachea and mainstem bronchus,[101] a diffuse infiltrative subglottic narrowing,[33] and an ulcerative process of the anterior commissure with submucosal posterior commissure fullness extending into the subglottis.[33]

The diagnosis of amyloidosis is based on biopsy specimens that characteristically demonstrate amorphous sheets or globules of homogenous eosinophilic (hyaline) material that forms the matrix of the protein fibril deposits. x-Ray diffraction studies and electron microscopy have demonstrated the repetitive fibrillar pattern of the amyloid ultrastructure.[20] Inspection of the Congo Red-stained deposits under polarized light demonstrates the characteristic 'apple green' birefringence,[33,60] and as well allows the pathologist to distinguish between laryngeal amyloidosis and the grossly similar hyalinized laryngeal polyp, which does not stain with Congo Red.[34] Plasmacytes tend to aggregate around the periphery of amyloid deposits; immunohistochemical staining demonstrates their polyclonal origin.[60] Four histologic patterns of amyloidosis have been described. These include amorphous random masses, deposits around blood vessel walls, deposits in continuity with the basement membrane of seromucinous glands, and deposits within adipose tissue.[6,33] Finally, in one series where the laryngeal deposits were carefully subtyped, the amyloidosis was found to be exclusively of the AL type with more than 60% of the laryngeal deposits displaying a λ light chain staining pattern and 25% with a κ pattern.[60]

In the rare instances of laryngeal amyloidosis secondary to a chronic disease, management focuses upon control of the primary disease. In the much more common isolated laryngeal amyloidosis, the primary treatment is endoscopic surgical removal of nodules that interfere with laryngeal or airway function. In many series it has been demonstrated that if the lesion can be completely excised, there is little or no tendency for recurrence. Because the likelihood of recurrent or residual disease is significant, special care must be taken to avoid traumatization of adjacent normal laryngeal tissues.[109] Removal of amyloid lesions may be complicated by bleeding because of the propensity of amyloid to infiltrate blood vessels. Advocates of CO_2 laser excision cite improved control of blood flow as one advantage of the laser. However, it is cautioned that laser use should be avoided in more extensive lesions because of the significant likelihood of extensive scarring postoperatively.[101,109] In large lesions it often becomes necessary to use external approaches. Although an early study indicated that 'coring out' a subglottic lesion was a lasting and effective treatment,[27] more recent series employ laryngofissure for treatment of diffuse subglottic and tracheal amyloidosis. In such studies, excision and curettage of gross lesions has been used, and some have found that repeated curettage as necessary

…nately allows stabilization of the lesions and subse-…ent decannulation of tracheotomy-dependent patients.[33] Local or systemic steroids are ineffective in controlling or reversing the lesions of amyloidosis.[33,34,73]

In patients with significant subglottic amyloid deposits, bronchoscopy may be merited to determine the extent of the lesions. In addition, pulmonary function tests including flow–volume loops provide a helpful baseline of the patient's airway obstruction as well as differentiating between upper and lower airway obstruction.[34]

Overall, the prognosis for laryngeal amyloidosis is quite good. The need for a tracheotomy is rare,[20] although extensive subglottic lesions may require such measures until they can be controlled or resected.[33] Rarely, death has been reported secondary to amyloidosis; this typically occurs from diffuse tracheobronchial disease and pulmonary failure.[60]

Conclusions

The majority of these disease entities share many common pathologic and pathophysiologic features which allow some useful generalizations to be made. Several features of disease presentation are common to the majority of chronic infectious and inflammatory laryngeal disorders. For example, because of the particulate, aerosolizable nature of most microbes, the most common portal of entry in infectious diseases is the lungs. Other frequently involved areas of the head and neck include the nasal cavity and skin. Microbes preferring cooler mucosal sites typically spread from the nose to the epiglottic tip and then to the free edges of the true vocal folds, structures which are more subject to cooling by respiratory air currents.

The appearances associated with the majority of the chronic infectious and inflammatory disorders of the larynx are diverse. In advanced granulomatous or ulcerative laryngeal lesions, lack of lymphadenopathy is conspicuous and helpful in differentiating from laryngeal squamous cell carcinoma.

The appearance of lesions on histologic examination frequently bears prognostic significance. In general, granuloma formation is suggestive of a more indolent, slowly progressive disease process whereas lack of granulomatous response is more often associated with fulminant disease dissemination, often implicitly in the context of impaired cell-mediated immunity. Indeed, for several infectious disorders, the development of cutaneous anergy parallels the dissemination of the disease process. Conversely, the presence of the laryngeal lesion itself is a frequent indicator of widespread disease dissemination. In addition, most chronic inflammatory disorders of the larynx are by nature systemic and the degree of involvement of extralaryngeal sites often reflects poorly on prognosis. Accordingly, a thorough, careful evaluation of a patient with a chronic laryngeal lesion should include a number of laboratory investigations to assess the degree of systemic involvement by the disease.

For many of these disorders, the indications for surgery are infrequent and typically focus on attempts to palliate the fibrosis of long-standing destructive laryngeal disease in an attempt to improve voice or airway. Common to all presentations is the need for early diagnosis and treatment, not only to avoid the obvious complications of airway compromise, but also to minimize the permanent laryngeal damage from chronic inflammation, ulceration, perichondritis, ankylosis and fibrosis.

References

1. Amoils CP, Shindo ML. Laryngotracheal manifestations of rhinoscleroma. *Ann Otol Rhinol Laryngol* 1996; **105:** 336–40.
2. Arauz JC, Fonseca R. Wegener's granulomatosis appearing initially in the trachea. *Ann Otol Rhinol Laryngol* 1982; **91:** 593–4.
3. Armstrong WB, Peskind SP, Bressler KL, Crokett DM. Airway obstruction secondary to rhinoscleroma during pregnancy. *Ear Nose Throat J* 1995; **74:** 768–73.
4. Auerbach O. Laryngeal tuberculosis. *Arch Otolaryngol* 1946; **44:** 191–201.
5. Bailey CM, Windle Taylor PC. Tuberculous laryngitis: a series of 37 patients. *Laryngoscope* 1981; **91:** 93–100.
6. Barnes EL, Zofar T. Laryngeal amyloidosis: clinicopathological study of seven cases. *Ann Otol* 1977; **86:** 856–62.
7. Batsakis JG, Manning JT. Relapsing polychondritis. *Ann Otol Rhinol Laryngol* 1989; **98:** 83–4.
8. Baugh R, Gilmore BB. Infectious croup: a critical review. *Otolaryngol Head Neck Surg* 1986; **95:** 40–6.
9. Becker GL, Tenholder MF, Hunt KK. Obligate mouth breathing during exercise: nasal and laryngeal sarcoidosis. *Chest* 1990; **98:** 756–7.
10. Bennett DE. Histoplasmosis of the oral cavity and larynx: a clinicopathological study. *Arch Intern Med* 1967; **120:** 417–27.
11. Bennett M. Laryngeal blastomycosis. *Laryngoscope* 1964; **74:** 498–512.
12. Berman JD, Waddell D, Hanson BD. Biochemical mechanisms of the antileishmanial activity of sodium stibogluconate. *Antimicrob Agents Chemother* 1985; **27:** 916–20.
13. Bottenfield GW, Arcinue EL, Sarnaik A, Jewell MR. Diagnosis and management of acute epiglottitis. Report of 90 consecutive cases. *Laryngoscope* 1980; **90:** 822–5.
14. Boyle JO, Coulthard SW, Mandel RM. Laryngeal involvement in disseminated coccidioidomycosis. *Arch Otolaryngol Head Neck Surg* 1991; **117:** 433–8.
15. Bradsher RW. Blastomycosis. *Clin Infect Dis* 1992; **14:** S82–90.
16. Brandenburg JH, Finch WW, Kirkham WR. Actinomycosis of the larynx and pharynx. *Otolaryngol Head Neck Surg* 1978; **86:** 739–42.
17. Browning DG, Schwartz DA, Jurado RL. Cryptococcosis of the larynx in a patient with aids. *South Med J* 1992; **85:** 762–4.
18. Burns JL. Laryngeal tuberculosis. *J Otolaryngol* 1993; **22:** 398.
19. Burton DM, Burgess LPA. Nocardiosis of the upper aerodigestive tract. *Ear Nose Throat J* 1990; **69:** 350–3.

20. Caldarelli DD, Freidberg SA, Harris AA. Medical and surgical aspects of the granulomatous diseases of the larynx. *Otolaryngol Clin North Am* 1979; **12:** 767–81.
21. Cánovas DL, Carbonell J, Torres J, Altés J, Buades J. Laryngeal leishmaniasis as initial opportunistic disease in HIV infection. *J Laryngol Otol* 1994; **108:** 1089–92.
22. Carey MJ. Epiglottitis in adults. *Am J Emerg Med* 1996; **14:** 421–4.
23. Cleary KR, Batsakis JG. Mycobacterial disease of the head and neck: current perspective. *Ann Otol Rhinol Laryngol* 1995; **104:** 830–3.
24. Cox F, Hughes WT. Contagious and other aspects of nocardiosis in the compromised host. *Pediatrics* 1975; **55:** 135–8.
25. Cressman WR, Myer CM. Diagnosis and management of croup and epiglottitis. *Pediatr Clin North Am* 1994; **41:** 265–76.
26. Damiani JM, Levine HL. Relapsing polychondritis: report of ten cases. *Laryngoscope* 1979; **89:** 929–46.
27. Djalilian M, McDonald TJ, Devine KD, Weiland LH. Nontraumatic, nonneoplastic subglottic stenosis. *Ann Otol* 1975; **84:** 757–63.
28. Donegan JO, Wood MD. Histoplasmosis of the larynx. *Laryngoscope* 1984; **94:** 206–9.
29. Dumich PS, Neel HB. Blastomycosis of the larynx. *Laryngoscope* 1983; **93:** 1266–70.
30. Duna GF, Galperin C, Hoffman GS. Wegener's granulomatosis. *Rheum Dis Clin North Am* 1995; **21:** 949–86.
31. Everts EC. Cervicofacial actinomycosis. *Arch Otolaryngol* 1970; **92:** 468–74.
32. Ferlito A, Pesavento G, Visonà A, Recher G, Meli S, Bevilacqua P. Leishmaniasis donovani presenting as an isolated lesion in the larynx. *ORL J Otorhinolaryngol Relat Spec* 1986; **48:** 243–8.
33. Fernandes CMC, Pirie D, Pudifin DJ. Laryngeal amyloidosis. *J Laryngol Otol* 1982; **96:** 1165–75.
34. Finn DG, Farmer JC. Management of amyloidosis of the larynx and trachea. *Arch Otolaryngol* 1982; **108:** 54–6.
35. Fletcher SM, Prussin AJ. Histoplasmosis of the larynx treated with ketoconazole: a case report. *Otolaryngol Head Neck Surg* 1990; **103:** 813–16.
36. Foidart JM, Abe S, Martin GR *et al.* Antibodies to type II collagen in relapsing polychondritis. *N Engl J Med* 1978; **299:** 1203–7.
37. Frantz TD, Rasgon BM, Quesenberry CP. Acute epiglottitis in adults: analysis of 129 cases. *JAMA* 1994; **272:** 1358–60.
38. Gammell EB, Breckenridge RL. Histoplasmosis of the larynx. *Ann Otol* 1949; **58:** 249–59.
39. Grant A, Spraggs PD, Grant HR, Bryceson AD. Laryngeal leishmaniasis. *J Laryngol Otol* 1994; **108:** 1086–8.
40. Gupta OP, Jain RK, Tripathi PP, Gupta S. Leprosy of the larynx: a clinicopathological study. *Int J Lepr Other Mycobact Dis* 1984; **52:** 171–5.
41. Heeneman H, Ward KM. Epiglottic abscess: its occurrence and management. *J Otolaryngol* 1977; **6:** 31–6.
42. Henderson CA, Ilchyshyn A, Curry AR. Laryngeal and cutaneous sarcoidosis treated with methotrexate. *J R Soc Med* 1994; **87:** 632–3.
43. Hicks JN, Peters GE. Pseudocarcinomatous hyperplasia of the larynx due to *Candida albicans*. *Laryngoscope* 1982; **92:** 644–7.
44. Hollis LJ, Montgomery PQ, Hern JD, Mahada U, Tolley NS. Invasive candidiasis of a late presentation laryngeal chondroradionecrosis. *J Laryngol Otol* 1996; **110:** 789–92.
45. Hughes RA, Paonessa DF, Conway WF. Actinomycosis of the larynx. *Ann Otol* 1984; **93:** 520–4.
46. Hugosson S, Olcén P, Ekedahl C. Acute epiglottitis: aetiology, epidemiology and outcome in a population before large-scale *Haemophilus influenzae* type B vaccination. *Clin Otolaryngol* 1994; **19:** 441–5.
47. Hunter AM, Millar JW, Wightman AJA, Horne NW. The changing pattern of laryngeal tuberculosis. *J Laryngol Otol* 1991; **95:** 393–8.
48. Isaacson JE, Frable MAS. Cryptococcosis of the larynx. *Otolaryngol Head Neck Surg* 1996; **114:** 106–9.
49. Israel L. *Candida* epiglottitis in an adult with acquired immunodeficiency syndrome treated with oral fluconazole. *J Laryngol Otol* 1995; **109:** 337–9.
50. Jacobs RF, Yasuda K, Smith AL, Benjamin DR. Laryngeal candidiasis presenting as inspiratory stridor. *Pediatrics* 1982; **69:** 234–6.
51. Jay J, Green RP, Lucente FE. Isolated laryngeal rhinoscleroma. *Otolaryngol Head Neck Surg* 1985; **93:** 669–74.
52. Jennette JC, Ewert BH, Falk RJ. Do antineutrophil cytoplasmic antibodies cause Wegener's granulomatosis and other forms of necrotizing vasculitis? *Rheum Dis Clin North Am* 1993; **19:** 1–14.
53. Kairys SW, Olmstead EM, O'Connor G. Steroid treatment of laryngotracheitis: a meta-analysis of the evidence from randomized trials. *Pediatrics* 1989; **83:** 683–93.
54. Khilanani U, Khatib R. Acute epiglottitis in adults. *Am J Med Sci* 1984; **287:** 65–70.
55. King HC, Cline JFX. Histoplasmosis involving the larynx. *Arch Otolaryngol* 1958; **67:** 649–54.
56. Krespi YP, Mitrani M, Husain S, Meltzer CJ. Treatment of laryngeal sarcoidosis with intralesional steroid injection. *Ann Otol Rhinol Laryngol* 1987; **96:** 713–15.
57. Lampman JH, Querubin R, Kondapalli P. Subglottic stenosis in Wegener's granulomatosis. *Chest* 1981; **79:** 230–2.
58. Lebovics RS, Hoffman GS, Leavitt RY. The management of subglottic stenosis in patients with Wegener's granulomatosis. *Laryngoscope* 1992; **102:** 1341–5.
59. Levenson MJ, Ingerman M, Grimes C, Robbett WF. Laryngeal tuberculosis: review of twenty cases. *Laryngoscope* 1984; **94:** 1094–7.
60. Lewis JE, Olsen KD, Kurtin PJ, Kyle RA. Laryngeal amyloidosis: a clinicopathologic and immunohistochemical review. *Otolaryngol Head Neck Surg* 1992; **106:** 372–7.
61. Liu TC, Qiu JS. Pathological findings on peripheral nerves, lymph nodes, and visceral organs of leprosy. *Int J Lepr Other Mycobact Dis* 1984; **52:** 377–83.
62. Marsden PD. Mucosal leishmaniasis. *Trans R Soc Trop Med Hyg* 1986; **80:** 859–76.
63. Marsden PD, Sampaio RN, Gomes LF *et al.* Lone laryngeal leishmaniasis. *Trans R Soc Trop Med Hyg* 1985; **79:** 424–5.
64. Martinez SA. Treponemal infections of the head and neck. *Otolaryngol Clin North Am* 1982; **15:** 613–20.

asaoka A, Yamakawa Y, Niwa H *et al*. Pediatric and adult tracheobronchomalacia. *Eur J Cardiothorac Surg* 1996; **10:** 87–92.

66. McAdam LP, O'Hanlan MA, Bluestone R, Pearson CM. Relapsing polychondritis: prospective study of 23 patients and a review of the literature. *Medicine (Baltimore)* 1976; **55:** 193–215.
67. McCaffrey TV, McDonald TJ, McCaffrey LA. Head and neck manifestations of relapsing polychondritis: review of 29 cases. *Otolaryngol Head Neck Surg* 1978; **86:** 473–8.
68. McDonald TJ, DeRemee RA. Wegener's granulomatosis. *Laryngoscope* 1983; **93:** 220–31.
69. McDonald TJ, Neel HB, DeRemee RA. Wegener's granulomatosis of the subglottis and the upper portion of the trachea. *Ann Otol Rhinol Laryngol* 1982; **91:** 588–92.
70. McNulty JS, Fassett RL. Syphilis: an otolaryngologic perspective. *Laryngoscope* 1981; **91:** 889–905.
71. Mikaelian AJ, Varkey B, Grossman TW, Blatnik DS. Blastomycosis of the head and neck. *Otolaryngol Head Neck Surg* 1989; **101:** 489–95.
72. Minnegerode B. The disease of emperor Frederick III. *Laryngoscope* 1986; **96:** 200–3.
73. Mittrani M, Biller HF. Laryngeal amyloidosis. *Laryngoscope* 1985; **95:** 1346–7.
74. Mochizuki H, Morikawa A, Tokuyama K, Tajima K, Kuroume T, Imamura J. Laryngeal sarcoidosis in a young child. *Clin Pediatr (Phila)* 1987; **26:** 486–8.
75. Munro HM, Castilla L, Taylor BL, Smith GB. Epiglottitis: a disease of all ages. *Br J Hosp Med* 1994; **52:** 443–9.
76. Murrage KJ, Janzen VD, Ruby RR. Epiglottitis: adult and pediatric comparisons. *J Otolaryngol* 1988; **17:** 194–8.
77. Nandwani R. Modern diagnosis and management of acquired syphilis. *Br J Hosp Med* 1996; **55:** 399–403.
78. Navarro Cunchillos M, Villanueva Marcos JL, Torre Cisneros J, Ostos Aumente P, López Rubio F, López Villarejo P. Isolated laryngeal leishmaniasis in an immunocompetent patient: successful treatment with surgery. *J Laryngol Otol* 1994; **108:** 249–51.
79. Neel HB, McDonald TJ. Laryngeal sarcoidosis: report of 13 patients. *Ann Otol Rhinol Laryngol* 1982; **91:** 359–62.
80. Negroni R. Paracoccidioidomycosis. *Int J Dermatol* 1993; **32:** 847–59.
81. Nelson EG, Tybor AG. Actinomycosis of the larynx. *Ear Nose Throat J* 1992; **71:** 356–8.
82. Newman LS, Rose CS, Maier LA. Sarcoidosis. *N Engl J Med* 1997; **336:** 1224–34.
83. Payne J, Koopman CF Jr. Laryngeal carcinoma – or is it laryngeal blastomycosis? *Laryngoscope* 1984; **94:** 608–11.
84. Petri M, Katzenstein P, Hellman D. Laryngeal infection in lupus: report of nocardiosis and review of laryngeal involvement in lupus. *J Rheumatol* 1988; **15:** 1014–15.
85. Pickard RE, Kotzen S. Histoplasmosis of the larynx. *South Med J* 1973; **66:** 1311–13.
86. Platt MA. Laryngeal coccidioidomycosis. *JAMA* 1977; **237:** 1234–5.
87. Postma GN, Wawrose S, Tami TA. Isolated subglottic scleroma. *Ear Nose Throat J* 1996; **75:** 306–8.
88. Rajah V, Essa A, Path FF. Histoplasmosis of the oral cavity, oropharynx, and larynx. *J Laryngol Otol* 1993; **107:** 58–61.
89. Ramadan HH, Tarazi AE, Baroudy FM. Laryngeal tuberculosis: presentation of 16 cases and review of the literature. *J Otolaryngol* 1993; **22:** 39–41.
90. Raymond AK, Sneige N, Batsakis JG. Amyloidosis in the upper aerodigestive tracts. *Ann Otol Rhinol Laryngol* 1992; **101:** 794–6.
91. Reese MC, Colclasure JB. Cryptococcosis of the larynx. *Arch Otolaryngol* 1975; **101:** 698–701.
92. Rippon JW. *Medical Mycology: the Pathogenic Fungi and the Pathogenic Actinomycetes*, 3rd edn. Philadelphia: Saunders, 1988.
93. Rybak LP, Falconer R. Pediatric laryngeal sarcoidosis. *Ann Otol Rhinol Laryngol* 1987; **96:** 670–3.
94. Sanchez MR. Infectious syphilis. *Semin Dermatol* 1994; **13:** 234–42.
95. Sandberg P, Shum TK. Lepromatous leprosy of the larynx. *Otolaryngol Head Neck Surg* 1983; **91:** 216–20.
96. Sarosi GA, Davies SF. Therapy for fungal infections. *Mayo Clin Proc* 1994; **69:** 1111–17.
97. Schlech WF, Carden GA. Fungal and parasitic granulomas of the head and neck. *Otolaryngol Clin North Am* 1982; **15:** 493–513.
98. Selkin SG. Laryngeal candidiasis and ketoconazole. *Otolaryngol Head Neck Surg* 1985; **93:** 661–3.
99. Shaheen SO, Ellis FG. Actinomycosis of the larynx. *J R Soc Med* 1983; **76:** 226–8.
100. Shum TK, Crockett DM, Hawkins DB. An unusual case of laryngeal scleroma. *Otolaryngol Head Neck Surg* 1985; **93:** 663–5.
101. Simpson GT II, Strong MS, Skinner M, Cohen AS. Localized amyloidosis of the head and neck and upper aerodigestive and lower respiratory tracts. *Ann Otol Rhinol Laryngol* 1984; **93:** 374–9.
102. Skolnik N. Croup. *J Fam Pract* 1993; **37:** 165–70.
103. Smallman LA, Stores OPR, Watson MG, Proops DW. Cryptococcosis of the larynx. *J Laryngol Otol* 1989; **103:** 214–15.
104. Soda A, Rubio H, Salazar M, Ganem J, Berlanga D, Sanchez A. Tuberculosis of the larynx: clinical aspects in 19 patients. *Laryngoscope* 1989; **99:** 1147–50.
105. Soni NK. Leprosy of the larynx. *J Laryngol Otol* 1992; **106:** 518–20.
106. Soni NK. Scleroma of the larynx. *J Laryngol Otol* 1997; **111:** 438–40.
107. Stiernberg CM, Clark WD. Rhinoscleroma: a diagnostic challenge. *Laryngoscope* 1983; **93:** 866–70.
108. Suen JY, Wetmore SJ, Wetzel WJ, Craig RD. Blastomycosis of the larynx. *Ann Otol* 1980; **89:** 563–6.
109. Talbot AR. Laryngeal amyloidosis. *J Laryngol Otol* 1990; **104:** 147–9.
110. Talerman A, Wright D. Laryngeal obstruction due to Wegener's granulomatosis. *Arch Otolaryngol* 1972; **96:** 376–9.
111. Tashjian LS, Peacock JE. Laryngeal candidiasis: report of seven cases and review of the literature. *Arch Otolaryngol* 1984; **110:** 806–9.
112. Thaller SR, Gross JR, Pilch BZ, Goodman ML. Laryngeal tuberculosis as manifested in the decades 1963–1983. *Laryngoscope* 1987; **97:** 848–50.
113. Thomas K. Laryngeal manifestations of Wegener's granuloma. *J Laryngol Otol* 1970; **84:** 101–6.

114. Touma DJ, Gross EJ, Karmody CS, Fawaz KA. Relapsing polychondritis in association with Crohn's disease. *Am J Otolaryngol* 1996; **17:** 424–6.
115. Vrabec DP. Fungal infections of the larynx. *Otolaryngol Clin North Am* 1993; **26:** 1091–114.
116. Walton BC, Chinel LV, Eguia O. Onset of espundia after many years of occult infection with *Leishmania braziliensis*. *Am J Trop Med Hyg* 1993; **22:** 696–8.
117. Ward PH, Berci G, Morledge D, Schwartz H. Coccidioidomycosis of the larynx in infants and adults. *Ann Otol* 1977; **86:** 655–660.
118. Warshawski J, Havas TE, McShane DP, Gullane PJ. Adult epiglottitis. *J Otolaryngol* 1986; **15:** 362–5.
119. Wathen PI. Hansen's disease. *South Med J* 1996; **89:** 647–52.
120. Waxman J, Bose WJ. Laryngeal manifestations of Wegener's granulomatosis: case reports and review of the literature. *J Rheumatol* 1986; **13:** 408–11.
121. Williams RG, Douglas-Jones T. Mycobacterium marches back. *J Laryngol Otol* 1995; **109:** 5–13.
122. Yonkers AJ. Candidiasis of the larynx. *Ann Otol* 1973; **82:** 812–15.
123. Younus M. Leprosy in ENT. *J Laryngol Otol* 1986; **100:** 1437–42.
124. Zaitoun AM, Mady SM. Leishmaniasis of the larynx. *Histopathology* 1995; **26:** 79–81.

Nodules, polyps, Reinke edema, metabolic deposits and foreign body granulomas

Frederik G Dikkers

Primary disorders of the vocal folds can be either true neoplasms (malignant or benign) or pseudotumors. True benign tumors of the vocal folds are encountered infrequently.[54]

Many of the more common benign conditions involving the vocal folds, including vocal cord nodules, polyps, cysts and hyperplastic changes,[35] are pseudotumors. Metabolic deposits and foreign body reactions in the larynx can also lead to distension of the vocal folds.

The most frequently diagnosed benign lesions of the vocal folds are polyps, Reinke edema and vocal fold nodules.[54] Their clinical appearances do partly overlap, which leads to small inter- and intraobserver agreement in diagnosis.[16,19]

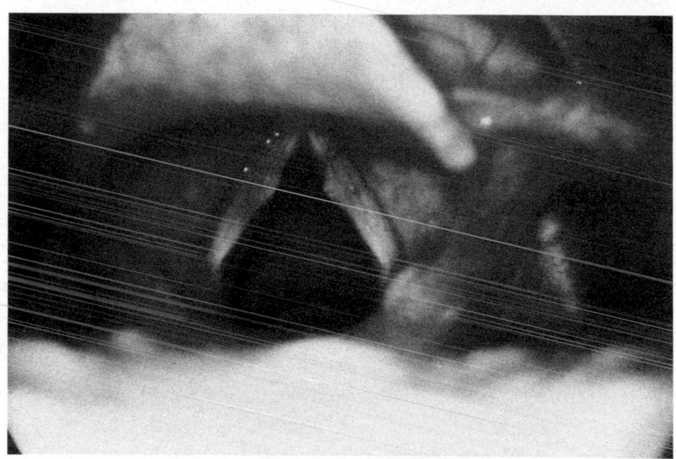

Figure 22.1 *Vocal fold nodules.*

Nodules

Vocal fold nodules (Fig 22.1) have been described in a considerable variety of ways, concerning size, composition, location on the vocal fold, and their effect on vibratory pattern and the resulting vocal quality. Grossly, two main groups of observers can be distinguished. The first main group favors the concept that vocal fold nodules are round neoplasms, 1–2 mm in diameter, located bilateral symmetrically on the free edge of the true vocal fold, on the junction of the anterior and middle third of the fold, i.e. halfway from the membranous portion of the fold. The second main group states that the nodules may be either unilateral or bilateral. In our view, nodules should be defined as small lesions occurring on both sides of the larynx, strictly symmetric on the border of the anterior and middle third of the vocal folds, macroscopically immobile during phonation.[18]

The nodules may be either whitish or grayish white, like the adjacent squamous mucosa, or slightly pink, except in the case of 'acute' (inflamed) nodules. Especially among singers, nodules take on an almost pointed appearance and are very white and small.[6] The surface is smooth. The size varies from one to several millimetres in diameter. Microwebs in the anterior commissure ('micropalmures') are present in 10–23% of the cases.[6,12,24]

In vocal fold nodules, the voice is frequently hoarse, breathy (with a waste of air) and easily fatigued. The size of the nodule does not necessarily bear direct relationship to the extent of vocal disability: sometimes, small nodules disproportionately impair the voice.

Adult women suffering from vocal fold nodules usually show hoarseness for more than half a year.[38] The nodules are smaller in singers than in non-singers, probably because a change in maximum vocal performance is a reason for singers to note problems at an earlier stage than non-singers.[56]

An open posterior chink is present in 95% of the patients.[50,51] This chink is thought to have a causative relation with the lesion.[18]

The consistency of the nodules can be observed laryngostroboscopically. Amplitudes and mucosal wave pattern are small, but symmetric and regular.[32]

Nodules are very common benign lesions of the vocal folds, occurring in 17–24% of the cases in very large series.[12,33] In singers the lesion is even more common, occurring in 28% of 101 professional singers.[13] However, these data provide insufficient evidence for defining these lesions as singer's nodules.

Nodules are frequently seen in (predominantly male) children.[3,14,44,50,51,59,72] The incidence in children varies from 1 to 23% of all children, with peaks between 5 and 10 years;[68] in another group the peak age is slightly higher.[3] The incidence among children with voice problems varies from 16 to 95%.[68] The onset of symptoms is gradual in 95% of the children.[68]

In adults, the condition is seen more frequently or exclusively in women.[11–13,33,38,44,50,51,73,75] When appearing in women, their age is predominantly the early 20s[50] or up to 10 years older.[12,73] Psychological or psychosomatic facets of etiology have been said to be of paramount importance, when these facets lead to excessive voice use or misuse.[13]

Epithelial changes in the epithelium of vocal fold nodules are nonspecific.[9,21,58] However, the subepithelial combination of epithelial basement-membrane thickening, absence of hemorrhage and absence of edematous lakes histologically confirms the clinical diagnosis of vocal fold nodules.[18]

Therapy consists primarily of speech therapy. In refractive disease, suspension microlaryngoscopic surgery under general anesthesia, or indirect microlaryngostroboscopic surgery under local anesthesia, both followed by 2 days of voice rest, provides good results.[20]

Polyps

Polyps (Fig 22.2) are small pedunculated or sessile lesions on the anterior third of the free edge (or phonating edge) of the true vocal fold.[28,36,44] They are mobile during phonation when pedunculated.[18,36]

Polyps occur mostly singularly and unilaterally,[44,63] but bilateral cases have also been reported.[18,28,33,39,40] In the majority of the cases, stroboscopic vibratory movements are asymmetrical, glottic closure is incomplete, and the amplitude and mucosal wave are decreased to varying degrees.[32]

Polyps differ in size from only a few millimetres in diameter to nearly occluding the glottis. The macroscopic aspect of polyps can vary. There is no correlation between the macroscopic aspect and histopathologic findings of polyps.[18]

In 82% of the cases, persistent hoarseness (existing for a few weeks) is the presenting symptom.[75] The hoarseness can occur intermittently. In case of extreme growth, vocal fold polyps sometimes lead to dyspnea, stridor and even choking spells[28,65] or intubation difficulties.[41]

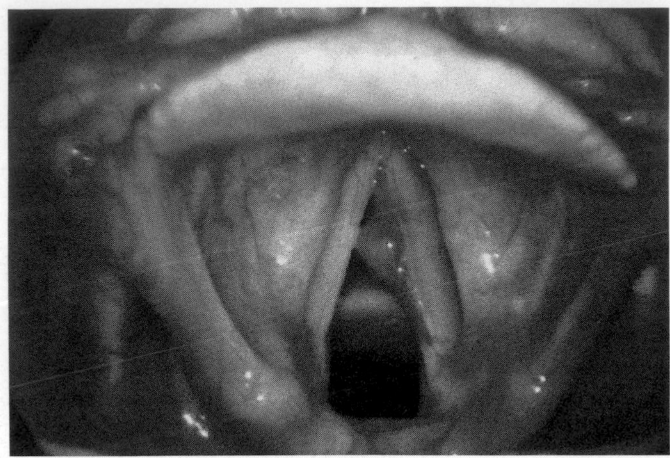

Figure 22.2 *Polyp of the right vocal fold.*

Polyps are very common benign non-neoplastic tumors of the vocal folds, occurring in 11–51% of reported cases of benign lesions of the vocal folds.[12,18,33,54] There is a significant male preponderance in polyps.[6,38,40,44,75] Most patients are smokers, many use their voice professionally.[39,59] The age peak is between 30 and 50 years.

The stratified squamous epithelium that covers the polyps can vary considerably. Atrophic, acanthotic, normal, hyperplastic and keratinized epithelium have been described.[25,36,45] This implicates that epithelial changes are aspecific.[9,18,58] Subepithelially, the combination of signs of recent bleeding, depositions of iron and fibrin, and thrombosis confirms the clinical diagnosis vocal fold polyp.[18]

Therapy consists of suspension microlaryngoscopic surgery under general anesthesia, or indirect microlaryngostroboscopic surgery under local anesthesia, both followed by 2 days of complete voice rest. Results of either surgical modality are good.[20]

Reinke edema

Reinke edema (Fig 22.3) is a unilateral or bilateral bleach-white swelling of the vocal fold, filled with fluid, sessile and in advanced stages very mobile during phonation. The lesion is bilateral in 62–85% of the cases.[27,33,48] The classic form, with 'diffuse spindle-shaped edema of both vocal folds along their entire length and with unchanged epithelium with fluid shining through',[43] is seen in 25%.

Many synonyms exist for Reinke edema. In English literature the lesion is also known as polypoid chorditis, polypoid degeneration, cordal polyposis, polypoid hypertrophy and polypoid vocal cord. In French literature the lesion is described as chronic edema of the vocal folds, pseudomyxoma or pseudomyxomatous laryngitis. The first time the lesion was described in American literature, it was called smoker's larynx,[53] suggesting a correlation with tobacco consumption.

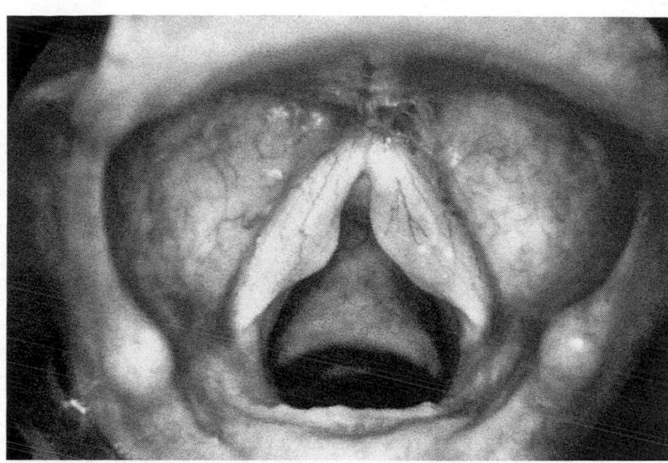

Figure 22.3 *Reinke edema of the vocal folds. Right vocal fold grade III, left vocal fold grade II.*

Table 22.1 Reinke edema grading and corresponding laryngostroboscopic findings

Grade	*Macroscopy*	*Laryngostroboscopy*
Grade I	Lesion almost undetectable; marginal edema	Blunt mucosal wave, large amplitudes
Grade II	Obvious swelling, sessile, thrown over vocalis muscle during phonation	Irregular blunt mucosal waves, decreased at lesion
Grade III	Large swelling, filled with fluid, 'plastic bag'. Sometimes dyspnea during exercise	Mucosal wave not recognizable, irregular amplitudes
Grade IV	Hyperemic cavity, filled with fluid. Often dyspnea during exercise	Same as grade III

Savic has proposed staging the lesion in four consecutive grades.[62] Table 22.1 shows these grades, including laryngostroboscopic findings.[32] Tillmann and Rudert describe a progression in size during the course of months to years,[67] corresponding to Savic's observation.

In 97% of the cases, persistent hoarseness is the initial symptom. It generally lasts one year or longer before the patient is referred to the laryngologist.[48] The voice pitch is low: 80 Hz and lower for men and an average of 108 Hz for women.[2,4,49] The pitch drops due to the increasing weight of the vibrating part of the vocal fold when edema develops.[26,64] Pain is a very unusual symptom. In extreme cases dyspnea and even stridor can occur,[27,67] for which at least one patient was reported to require a tracheotomy.[53]

Reinke edema appears only in heavy smokers.[4,46] The relationship between smoking and Reinke edema is suggested by many authors.[26,44,48,49,61] Chronic voice strain has also been reported as the cause of Reinke edema,[38,61] or as an important cofactor.[27] However, others stated the contrary.[48]

The predilection age of Reinke edema is 40–60 years, with a range of 14–78 years. The reported distribution over sexes shows wide variation. A meta-analysis of 1538 cases provided 49% male and 51% female patients.[17]

As in other benign lesions of the vocal folds, epithelial changes are nonspecific.[9,18,21,58] Subepithelially, the combination of epithelial basement-membrane thickening, edematous lakes, extravascular erythrocytes and increased thickness of subepithelial vessel walls confirms the clinical diagnosis of Reinke edema. In 50% of the cases inflammation is present.[18]

Therapy consists of surgical intervention after cessation of smoking. During suspension microlaryngoscopy under general anesthesia, a chordotomy is performed in the most affected vocal fold. A caudally based epithelial flap is prepared, the edematous contents excised and the flap is folded back. The size of the epithelial redundancy, which should be reduced, can thus be estimated. The flap is glued to the vocal ligament using fibrin glue. If the anterior commissure is left unaffected, the second vocal fold can be treated in the same intervention. A postoperative voice rest of at least 5 days in indicated after chordotomy.[7] Indirect microlaryngostroboscopic surgery and stripping of the vocal fold are contraindicated.[20,47]

Metabolic deposits

The larynx can be the target organ for several metabolic diseases. A wide variety of metabolic products are – sometimes preferentially – deposited in the larynx. This leads to either compromised airway, or voice complaints, or both.

Amyloidosis

Laryngeal amyloidosis may be either localized or systemic disease. However, in most instances amyloidosis of the larynx is localized and is not associated with or followed by systemic disease. Laryngeal amyloidosis appears as a diffuse gray-to-yellow mass. It may affect any part of the glottis, supraglottis, or subglottis.[66] In most cases, hoarseness is the predominant symptom. In glottic localization, the voice is strained, and laryngostroboscopy reveals a very small mucosal wave with almost absent amplitudes.

Laryngeal amyloidosis is a rare condition. It accounts for approximately 1% of all benign laryngeal lesions. Men and women are equally affected. Primary localized and primary disseminated laryngeal amyloidosis in a family have been described.[31,52]

The classification of amyloidosis is dependent on the biochemical nature of its protein deposits.[42] Biopsy specimens show amorphous material consistent with amyloid deposits with a plasmacytic infiltrate. Both plasma cells and amyloid deposits stain positively by immunohistochemistry for κ light chains.[5]

Laryngeal amyloidosis is treated, when indicated, by local surgical excision, often repeatedly because of persistence or multifocal deposits. Left unaffected, the amyloid tumors show a slowly progressive growth pattern.

Gout

Gout is a disorder of purine metabolism characterized by hyperuricemia with rare involvement of the head and neck. Macroscopy resembles a lesion suspicious for carcinoma of the larynx in the older age groups. The presenting symptom is hoarseness. Histology shows characteristic birefringent crystalline deposits and giant cell granuloma.[30]

There have been limited reports of gouty involvement of the larynx, more commonly involving cricoarytenoid arthritis. Tophi of the laryngeal soft tissues are exceedingly rare. Therapy consists of local excision, and treatment of the underlying cause.

Tracheobronchopathia osteochondroplastica

Tracheobronchopathia osteochondroplastica is a rare disease characterized by osseocartilaginous subepithelial nodules projecting into the lumen of the larynx, trachea and bronchi. Its etiology is unknown. Most cases are asymptomatic and frequently diagnosed incidentally during intubation or endoscopy. The diagnosis is made on the basis of endoscopy, CT scan and histopathology.

In the mucosa, fragments of adipose tissue, deposits of calcification and ossification often with foci of bone marrow and active hemopoiesis are present. Surgical treatment is indicated for airway obstruction and recurrent infections.[1]

Hereditary diseases

Urbach–Wiethe syndrome (hyalinosis cutis et mucosae) is a rare, probably autosomal recessively inherited disease. A characteristic symptom, already present in the first weeks of life, might be hoarseness. Later on, manifestations with hyalin deposits in the larynx, oral cavity and oropharynx might occur as well as yellowish-white papular deposits in the skin.

The most significant histopathologic alterations are lesions of the vessel walls.[37] The overall prognosis of this disease is good. Therapeutic intervention is symptomatic for functional purposes (narrowing of the laryngeal lumen).[29]

Foreign body granulomas and distensions

Numerous substances have been used to medialize a vocal fold on the side of vocal fold immobility in case of neurogenic lesions of the larynx. The most generally used materials that are applied endoscopically are Teflon, collagen, fat and room temperature vulcanizing silicone. Among others, silicone and hydroxyapatite implants are used in external medialization techniques. In due course these foreign bodies can induce reactions in laryngeal tissue.

Another foreign body responsible for diseases of the larynx is chronic exposure to asbestos.

Teflon

Endolaryngeal injection of Teflon paste has been used for decades to augment and medialize the paralyzed hemilarynx to improve dysphonia and relieve aspiration. After an initial short-lived inflammatory reaction in the laryngeal tissues, a classic foreign body granuloma forms around the Teflon.[23]

In most cases the voice results are good, but it may occasionally be necessary to consider removal of the granuloma if over-injection took place, if it is inappropriately placed, or if the paralyzed hemilarynx subsequently recovers. Surgical removal is difficult and the results are unpredictable. Laser chordotomy followed by vaporization and preservation of a margin of mucosa of the cord medially has led to subsequent improvement of voice.[71]

Local and regional migration of Teflon has been demonstrated.[22,23] Occasionally, a 'teflonoma' develops. Surgical removal of the mass alleviated all symptoms.[74]

Collagen

Unilateral hemilarynx immobility treated by glutaraldehyde-cross-linked (GAX) collagen showed no long-term local or systemic reaction to the collagen. Collagen, unlike Teflon, does not cause an inflammatory reaction. The partial maintenance of the improvement achieved, which is to be compared with the instability of the effects produced by resorbable substances, is said to make it the 'least objectionable' injectable for the treatment of unilateral hemilarynx immobility. One must overcompensate 20–30%, given the results of the long-term stability studies.[57]

Fat

Autogenous fat, harvested by suction from the abdominal wall, has been described as an alternative to alloplastic substances for vocal cord augmentation and medialization. It can be applied under local anesthesia under guidance of laryngostroboscopy.[10]

Autogenous fat, which has not been damaged during harvesting or microinjection, can survive transplantation into the vocal cord.[8] The bulk of the vocal cord is maintained by microlipocytes and fibrous connective tissue, both of which partly replace the damaged fat cells that are gradually being reabsorbed.

Silicone

Silicone has been used in the USA since the 1960s in a variety of forms as a replacement for soft tissue. Contrary to what was once thought, silicone is not biologically inert. In due course particles of silicone encapsulated by thin fibrous tissue develop, with few multinucleated giant cells and little cell infiltration.[70] With respect to soft tissue response, silicone is less reactive than Teflon.[23]

Silicone elastomer used in the larynx has not been implicated in the development of systemic immune disease or carcinogenesis. The evidence to date supports the continued use of silicone elastomer implants in the larynx.[60] It is clear, however, that continued investigation into the basic biologic properties and mechanisms of the host–silicone implant interaction is warranted.

Hydroxyapatite

Preliminary data evaluating the use of preformed hydroxyapatite laryngeal implants have been published.[15] In animals implanted with hydroxyapatite, histologic findings include limited acute inflammatory response, thin fibrous encapsulation, and osteogenesis in the region of the fenestra, with lamellar bone bridging the space between the implant and thyroid lamina.[23]

Advantages include a readily available implant selection, rapid determination of correct size and position, and improved implant stabilization with a hydroxyapatite shim due to osteogenesis. Conversely, the presence of bone growth may limit the reversibility of medialization procedures performed with hydroxyapatite.

Asbestos

Asbestos exposure may act as an irritant, and induce laryngitis.[55] In a group consisting of employees who had a minimum of 1 year of employment in jobs with potential exposure to asbestos at a refinery and petrochemical plant, the observed number of deaths for cancer of the larynx was virtually the same as expected.[69] The association between laryngeal cancer and asbestos exposure showed a tendency towards a nonsignificant increase in odds ratios in the highest cumulative exposure categories in a large French study; this tendency disappeared when adjusting for occupational confounders.[34]

References

1. Akyol MU, Martin AA, Dhurandhar N, Miller RH. Tracheobronchopathia osteochondroplastica: a case report and a review of the literature. *Ear Nose Throat J* 1993; **72:** 347–50.
2. Baarsma EA. Reinke's oedeem. *Logoped Foniatr* 1977; **49:** 2–9.
3. Benjamin B, Croxson G. Vocal nodules in children. *Trans Am Laryngol Assoc* 1987; **108:** 80–4.
4. Bennett S, Bishop S, Lumpkin SMM. Phonatory characteristics associated with bilateral diffuse polypoid degeneration. *Laryngoscope* 1987; **97:** 446–50.
5. Berg AM, Troxler RF, Grillone G *et al.* Localized amyloidosis of the larynx: evidence for light chain composition. *Ann Otol Rhinol Laryngol* 1993; **102:** 884–9.
6. Bouchayer M, Cornut G. Microsurgery for benign lesions of the vocal folds. *Ear Nose Throat J* 1988; **67:** 446–66.
7. Bouchayer M, Cornut G. Instrumental microscopy of benign lesions of the vocal folds. In: Ford CN, Bless DM, eds. *Phonosurgery: Assessment and Surgical Management of Voice Disorders.* New York: Raven Press, 1991: 143–65.
8. Brandenburg JH, Unger JM, Koschkee D. Vocal cord injection with autogenous fat: a long-term magnetic resonance imaging evaluation. *Laryngoscope* 1996; **106:** 174–80.
9. Cervera-Paz FJ, Dikkers FG. Ultraestructura y patogenia de las lesiones fonatorias de las cuerdas vocales. *Acta Otorrinolaringol Esp* 1994; **45:** 261–5.
10. Chang HP, Chang SY. Autogenous fat intracordal injection as treatment for unilateral vocal palsy. *Chung Hua I Hsueh Tsa Chih Taipei* 1996; **58:** 114–20.
11. Cornut G, Bouchayer M. Apport de la microchirurgie laryngée dans le traitement du nodule de la corde vocale. *Folia Phoniatr (Basel)* 1973; **24:** 431–7.
12. Cornut G, Bouchayer M. Bilan de quinze années de collaboration entre phoniatre et phonochirurgien. *Bull Audiophonol Ann Sc Univ Franche-Comté* 1988; **4:** 7–50.
13. Cornut G, Bouchayer M. Phonosurgery for singers. *J Voice* 1989; **3:** 269–76.
14. Cornut G, Bouchayer M, Witzig É. Indications phoniatriques et résultats fonctionnels de la microchirurgie endo-laryngée chez l'enfant et l'adolescent. *Bull Audiophonol* 1984; **17:** 473–95.
15. Cummings CW, Purcell LL, Flint PW. Hydroxylapatite laryngeal implants for medialization. Preliminary report. *Ann Otol Rhinol Laryngol* 1993; **102:** 843–51.
16. Dikkers FG. Intraobserver variation in diagnosis of benign non-neoplastic lesions of vocal folds. *Lancet* 1991; **337:** 866.
17. Dikkers FG. The pathological larynx: a review. In: *Benign Lesions of the Vocal Folds – Clinical and Histopathological Aspects.* Groningen: Thesis, 1994: 17–37.
18. Dikkers FG, Nikkels PGJ. Benign lesions of the vocal folds: histopathology and phonotrauma. *Ann Otol Rhinol Laryngol* 1995; **104:** 698–703.
19. Dikkers FG, Schutte HK. Benign lesions of the vocal folds: uniformity in assessment of clinical diagnosis. *Clin Otolaryngol* 1991; **16:** 8–11.
20. Dikkers FG, Sulter AM. Suspension microlaryngoscopic surgery and indirect microlaryngostroboscopic surgery for benign lesions of the vocal folds. *J Laryngol Otol* 1994; **108:** 1063–7.
21. Dikkers FG, Hulstaert CE, Oosterbaan JA, Cervera-Paz FJ. Ultrastructural changes of the basement membrane zone in benign lesions of the vocal folds. *Acta Otolaryngol (Stockh)* 1993; **113:** 98–101.
22. Ellis JC, McCaffrey TV, DeSanto LW, Reiman HV. Migration of Teflon after vocal cord injection. *Otolaryngol Head Neck Surg* 1987; **96:** 63–6.
23. Flint PW, Corio RL, Cummings CW. Comparison of soft tissue response in rabbits following laryngeal implantation with hydroxylapatite, silicone rubber, and Teflon. *Ann Otol Rhinol Laryngol* 1997; **106:** 399–407.
24. Ford CN, Bless DM, Campos G, Leddy M. Anterior commissure webs associated with vocal fold nodules: detection, prevalence, and significance. *Laryngoscope* 1994; **104:** 1369–75.

25. Frenzel H, Kleinsasser O, Hort W. Licht- und elektronenmikroskopische Untersuchungen an Stimmlippenpolypen des Menschen. *Virchows Arch A Pathol Anat Histol* 1980; **389:** 189–204.
26. Fritzell B, Hertegård S. A retrospective study of treatment for vocal fold edema: a preliminary report. In: Kirchner JA, ed. *Vocal Fold Histopathology, a Symposium.* San Diego: College-Hill Press, 1986: 57–64.
27. Fuchs B. Zur Pathogenese und Klinik des Reinke-Ödems: Langzeitstudien. *HNO* 1989; **37:** 490–5.
28. Gilman RH, Karmody CS, Fried MP, Speth R. Gigantic obstructing laryngeal polypi. *J Laryngol Otol* 1982; **96:** 167–72.
29. Grevers G. Zur Manifestation des Urbach-Wiethe Syndroms im HNO-Bereich. *Laryngorhinootologie* 1994; **73:** 543–4.
30. Guttenplan MD, Hendrix RA, Townsend MJ, Balsara G. Laryngeal manifestations of gout. *Ann Otol Rhinol Laryngol* 1991; **100:** 899–902.
31. Hashimoto H, Itami S, Kurata S, Takayasu S, Yokota T. Primary localized amyloidosis in one family. *Int J Dermatol* 1991; **30:** 632–4.
32. Hirano M. Objective evaluation of the human voice: clinical aspects. *Folia Phoniatr (Basel)* 1989; **41:** 89–144.
33. Holinger PH, Johnston KC. Benign tumors of the larynx. *Ann Otol Rhinol Laryngol* 1951; **60:** 496–509.
34. Imbernon E, Goldberg M, Bonenfant S *et al.* Occupational respiratory cancer and exposure to asbestos: a case-control study in a cohort of workers in the electricity and gas industry. *Am J Ind Med* 1995; **28:** 339–52.
35. Jones SR, Myers NM, Barnes L. Benign neoplasms of the larynx. *Otolaryngol Clin North Am* 1984; **17:** 151–78.
36. Kambic V, Radsel Z, Zargi M, Acko M. Vocal cord polyps: incidence, histology and pathogenesis. *J Laryngol Otol* 1981; **95:** 609–18.
37. Kautzky M, Schenk P, Bigenzahn W, Rappersberger K, Konrad K. Hyalinosis cutis et mucosae im Hals-Nasen-Ohren-Bereich. *Laryngorhinootologie* 1989; **68:** 602–6.
38. Kitzing P. Phoniatric aspects of microlaryngoscopy. *Acta Phoniatr Lat* 1987; **9:** 31–41.
39. Kleinsasser O. Pathogenesis of vocal cord polyps. *Ann Otol Rhinol Laryngol* 1982; **91:** 378–81.
40. Kleinsasser O. Microlaryngoscopic and histologic appearances of polyps, nodules, cysts, Reinke's edema, and granulomas of the vocal cords. In: Kirchner JA, ed. *Vocal Fold Histopathology, a Symposium.* San Diego: College-Hill Press, 1986: 51–5.
41. Kloss J, Petty C. Obstruction of endotracheal intubation by a mobile pedunculated polyp. *Anesthesiology* 1975; **43:** 380.
42. Knobber D, Niehaus H, Jautzke G. Die lokalisierte Amyloidose im HNO-Bereich. *HNO* 1994; **42:** 750–3.
43. Kosokovic F, Cepelja J, Vecerina S, Krajina Z. Experience with Reinke's edema. *Acta Otolaryngol (Stockh)* 1974; **78:** 150–4.
44. Kotby MN, Ghaly AF, Barakah MA, Abu El-Ezz AE, Bassiony SS. Pathology of voice. In: Singh W, ed. *Proceedings of International Voice Symposium.* Edinburgh: Miniprint, 1989: 5–8.
45. Loire R, Bouchayer M, Cornut G, Bastian RW. Pathology of benign vocal fold lesions. *Ear Nose Throat J* 1988; **67:** 357–62.
46. Lumpkin SMM, Bishop SG, Bennett S. Comparison of surgical techniques in the treatment of laryngeal polypoid degeneration. *Ann Otol Rhinol Laryngol* 1987; **96:** 254–7.
47. Mahieu HF, Dikkers FG. Indirect microlaryngostroboscopic surgery. *Arch Otolaryngol Head Neck Surg* 1992; **118:** 21–4.
48. Matsuo K, Kamimura M, Hirano M. Polypoid vocal folds. A ten year review of 191 patients. *Auris Nasus Larynx* 1983; **10:** S37–45.
49. Moesgaard Nielsen V, Højslet PE. Topical treatment of Reinke's oedema with beclomethasone dipropionate (BDP) inhalation aerosol. *J Laryngol Otol* 1987; **101:** 921–4.
50. Morrison MD, Nichol H, Rammage LA. Diagnostic criteria in functional dysphonia. *Laryngoscope* 1986; **94:** 1–8.
51. Morrison MD, Rammage LA, Belisle GM, Pullan CB, Nichol H. Muscular tension dysphonia. *J Otolaryngol* 1983; **12:** 302–6.
52. Moulin G, Cognat T, Delaye J, Ferrier E, Wagschal D. Amylose disseminée primitive familiale (nouvelle forme clinique?). *Ann Dermatol Venereol* 1988; **115:** 565–70.
53. Myerson MC. Smoker's larynx, a clinical pathological entity. *Ann Otol Rhinol Laryngol* 1950; **59:** 541–6.
54. Painter C. The incidence of voice disorders. *Eur Arch Otorhinolaryngol* 1990; **247:** 197–8.
55. Parnes SM. Asbestos and cancer of the larynx: is there a relationship? *Laryngoscope* 1990; **100:** 254–61.
56. Peppard RC, Bless DM, Milenkovic P. Comparison of young adult singers and nonsingers with vocal nodules. *J Voice* 1988; **2:** 250–60.
57. Remacle M, Degols JC, Delos M, Marbaix E, Lawson G. Exudative lesions of the Reinke space – proposition for an anatomopathological classification. In: Kleinsasser O, Glanz H, Olofsson J, eds. *Advances in Laryngology in Europe.* Amsterdam: Elsevier, 1997: 22–5.
58. Remacle M, Dujardin JM, Lawson G. Treatment of vocal fold immobility by glutaraldehyde-cross-linked collagen injection: long-term results. *Ann Otol Rhinol Laryngol* 1995; **104:** 437–41.
59. Riess F, Wendler J. Katamnestische Erhebungen bei Patienten mit Stimmlippenknötchen und -polypen. *HNO Prax* 1976; **2:** 111–16.
60. Righi PD, Wilson KM, Gluckman JL. Thyroplasty using a silicone elastomer implant. *Otolaryngol Clin North Am* 1995; **28:** 309–16.
61. Sataloff RT. Editorial: Surgery for the voice? *Clin Otolaryngol* 1989; **14:** 185–8.
62. Savic D. Characteristiques morphologiques et histopathologiques de l'oedeme chronique des cordes vocales. *JFORL J Fr Otorhinolaryngol Audiophonol Chir Maxillofac* 1976; **25:** 19–20.
63. Sellars SL. Benign tumours of the larynx. *S Afr Med J* 1979; **56:** 943–6.
64. Shindo ML, Hanson DG. Geriatric voice and laryngeal dysfunction. *Otolaryngol Clin North Am* 1990; **23:** 1035–44.
65. Strong MS, Vaughan CW. Vocal cord nodules and polyps – the role of surgical treatment. *Laryngoscope* 1971; **81:** 911–23.

66. Talbot AR. Laryngeal amyloidosis. *J Laryngol Otol* 1990; **104:** 147–9.
67. Tillmann B, Rudert H. Licht- und elektronenmikroskopische Untersuchungen zum Reinkeödem. *HNO* 1982; **30:** 280–4.
68. Toohill RJ. The psychosomatic aspects of children with vocal nodules. *Arch Otolaryngol* 1975; **101:** 591–5.
69. Tsai SP, Waddell LC, Gilstrap EL, Ransdell JD, Ross CE. Mortality among maintenance employees potentially exposed to asbestos in a refinery and petrochemical plant. *Am J Ind Med* 1996; **29:** 89–98.
70. Tsuzuki T, Fukuda H, Fujioka T. Response of the human larynx to silicone. *Am J Otolaryngol* 1991; **12:** 288–91.
71. Varvares MA, Montgomery WW, Hillman RE. Teflon granuloma of the larynx: etiology, pathophysiology, and management. *Ann Otol Rhinol Laryngol* 1995; **104:** 511–15.
72. Von Leden H. Vocal nodules in children. *Ear Nose Throat J* 1985; **64:** 473–80.
73. Wendler J, Seidner W. Ergebnisse operativer Behandlung von Knötchen und Polypen der Stimmlippen bei Erwachsenen. *Folia Phoniatr (Basel)* 1971; **23:** 429–39.
74. Wenig BM, Heffner DK, Oertel YC, Johnson FB. Teflonomas of the larynx and neck. *Hum Pathol* 1990; **21:** 617–23.
75. Yates A, Dedo HH. Carbon dioxide laser enucleation of polypoid vocal cords. *Laryngoscope* 1984; **94:** 731–6.

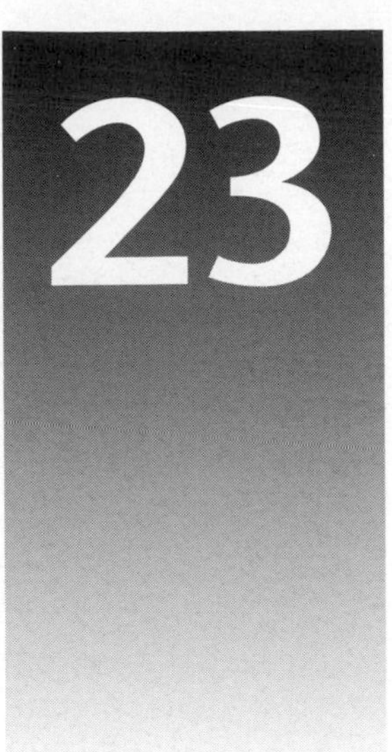

Cysts, pseudocysts and laryngoceles

C Gaelyn Garrett, Mark C Courey and Robert H Ossoff

A variety of benign lesions originate in the larynx. These include both neoplastic and non-neoplastic lesions. This chapter will focus on non-neoplastic cysts and laryngoceles. Understanding the origin of these lesions is predicated on a detailed knowledge of the macroscopic and microscopic anatomy of the larynx and surrounding structures. Please refer to previous chapters for review.

Saccular cysts

The saccule and the ventricle develop as secondary outpouchings of the laryngeal lumen beginning in the latter part of the second month of gestation. They are not derivatives of the visceral pharyngeal pouches. The normal lining of the laryngeal saccule is a pseudostratified, ciliated, columnar epithelium. Mucous glands are located within its submucosa to provide lubrication for the vocal folds.

Saccular cysts occur secondary to a narrowing of the saccular lumen located at the anterior end of the laryngeal ventricle. They are differentiated from air-filled laryngoceles by their lack of communication with the endolarynx. Both congenital and acquired types are described. The congenital type results from complete atresia of the proximal end of the saccule. Holinger *et al.* further subclassified congenital saccular cysts into anterior and lateral varieties based on their location.[9] Anterior congenital saccular cysts are more commonly seen with short saccules and present as a bulge between the true and false vocal folds. Lateral congenital saccular cysts, more commonly seen with longer saccules, present as fullness of the false vocal fold extending to the aryepiglottic fold.

Acquired saccular cysts result from obstruction of the saccular lumen, frequently by a supraglottic carcinoma. Other causes include focal inflammation and trauma. Saccular cysts are lined with normal respiratory epithelium as described above and are submucosal with normal mucosa overlying.

In infants and children, saccular cysts more commonly produce obstructive symptoms such as inspiratory stridor and dyspnea than in adults (Fig 23.1). As the cyst enlarges, voice changes may be noted with a weakened cry in infants. Feeding difficulties may be present. Adults more commonly present with dysphonia. Examination of the larynx reveals the typical submucosal fullness of the false vocal fold with or without involvement of the aryepiglottic fold. Large saccular cysts may extend through the thyrohyoid membrane to produce cervical fullness. Like laryngoceles, both congenital and acquired saccular cysts

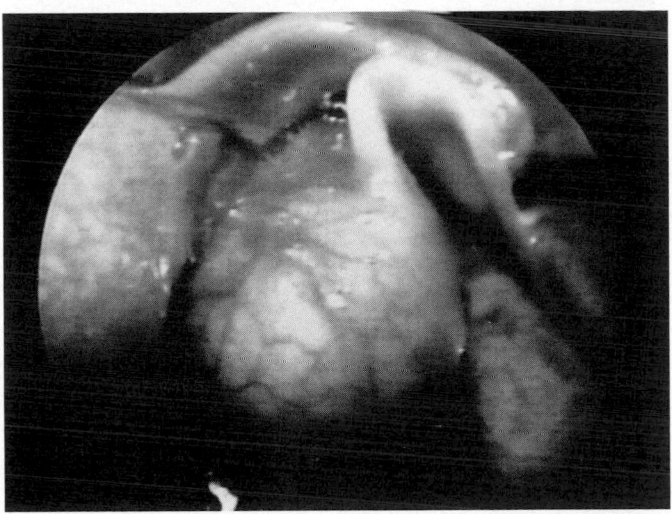

Figure 23.1 *Photograph of a saccular cyst involving the left aryepiglottic fold in an infant. This child presented with acute respiratory distress requiring emergency direct microlaryngoscopy and excision of the lesion.*

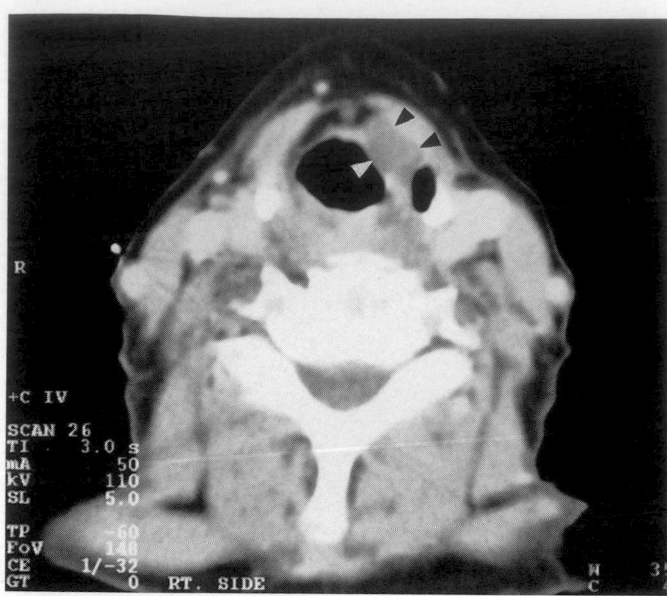

Figure 23.2 *CT scan image of a patient showing a left saccular cyst (arrows).*

may be secondarily infected to produce a laryngopyocele – a potentially life-threatening complication with acute airway obstruction. Imaging studies such as computerized tomography (CT) or magnetic resonance imaging (MRI) scans are helpful to verify and localize the pathology (Fig 23.2).

Both external and endoscopic approaches have been advocated for the treatment of symptomatic saccular cysts. Most authors favor the endoscopic approach initially, especially for the smaller anterior saccular cysts. The actual endoscopic techniques described range from simple needle aspiration[9] to marsupialization to complete excision.[8] Recurrences are common with incomplete excision and therefore more common with an endoscopic approach. In a 1992 series reported by Civantos and Holinger, 17 patients (all < 6 years old) with a diagnosis of saccular cyst underwent an average of six endoscopic procedures each.[3] Those with lateral saccular cysts had more recurrences. Three patients required an external approach for complete excision. Of the 17 patients, 11 underwent planned tracheotomy, generally at the first procedure for airway protection. All were eventually decannulated although three patients later developed subglottic stenosis related to the tracheotomy. Ward *et al.* proposed an external lateral cervical approach for lateral saccular cysts recurring after one or two endoscopic attempts.[17] None of their four pediatric patients required tracheotomy.

Hogikyan and Bastian reviewed their experience with seven adults treated for symptomatic saccular cysts.[8] They describe their technique of complete endoscopic excision using the CO_2 laser at 1.5–2.0 W in a continuous superpulse mode. In some cases the dissection extended beyond the endolarynx through the thyrohyoid membrane. Care was taken to avoid injury to branches of the superior laryngeal vessels and nerve. They conclude that both small cysts and most large lateral cysts can be completely excised via an endoscopic approach, avoiding an external incision and complications related to tracheotomy.

Laryngoceles

A laryngocele is an abnormal dilation of the laryngeal saccule that, unlike the saccular cyst, maintains a communication with the laryngeal lumen. Thus, it is air-filled in the noninfected state. Three subtypes are recognized depending on their location relative to the thyrohyoid membrane. An internal laryngocele is confined to the interior of the thyroid cartilage, involving the false vocal fold and aryepiglottic fold. An external laryngocele extends superiorly with the tract penetrating the thyrohyoid membrane at the point where the superior laryngeal vessels and nerve enter the larynx to cause soft swelling in the neck only. The interior portion of the saccule remains of normal size. A third type, the mixed or combined laryngocele, has features of both the internal and external laryngocele.

Clinically, laryngoceles become apparent when dilated temporarily with air or mucopus when infected. DeSanto considered saccular cysts and laryngoceles part of a spectrum of conditions related to an enlarged saccule.[6] A laryngocele could progress to a saccular cyst and a saccular cyst could progress to a laryngopyocele. Certainly, there is overlap in the clinical pathophysiology of these lesions. Laryngoceles and saccular cysts are both uncommon lesions of the larynx. Stell and Maran determined the incidence of laryngocele to be one per 2.5 million people based on a review of the literature.[16] The mixed type appears to be the most common type of laryngocele.

The etiology of laryngoceles is variable. Laryngoceles are much less common in infants and newborns than in adults. The congenital type is probably related to a congenital abnormality of the saccule. Acquired laryngoceles are more common and may be related to a congenitally large saccule that becomes symptomatic later in life due to various factors. A common notion is that laryngoceles develop in those people whose activities result in prolonged elevated intralaryngeal pressure. A study of 94 wind instrument band members in 1966 revealed that 56% had laryngoceles on neck radiographs taken during Valsalva maneuver.[10] Laryngoceles have also developed following acute periods of elevated intraglottic pressure such as during the labor of childbirth.[2]

Laryngoceles may only cause symptoms when distended with air or if they become temporarily occluded, resulting in a mucus-filled cavity or a laryngopyocele if secondarily infected. In infants and children, symptoms may include intermittent hoarseness and respi-

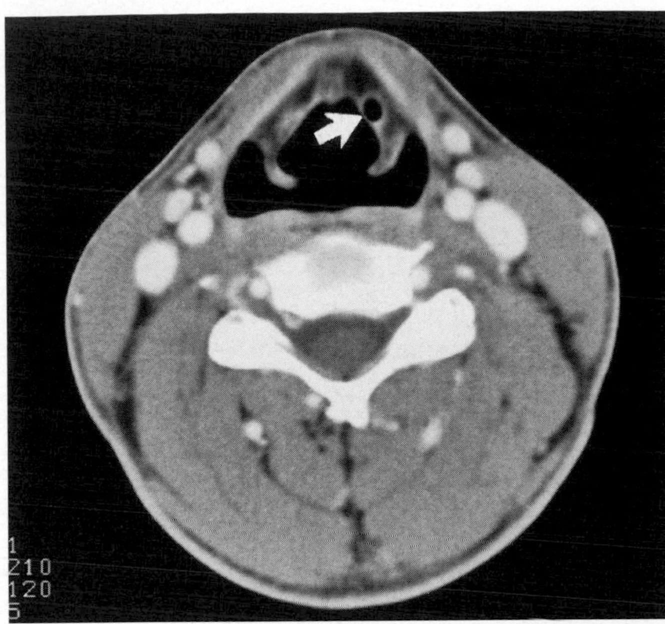

Figure 23.3 *CT scan image of a patient with the incidental finding of a small left internal laryngocele (arrow).*

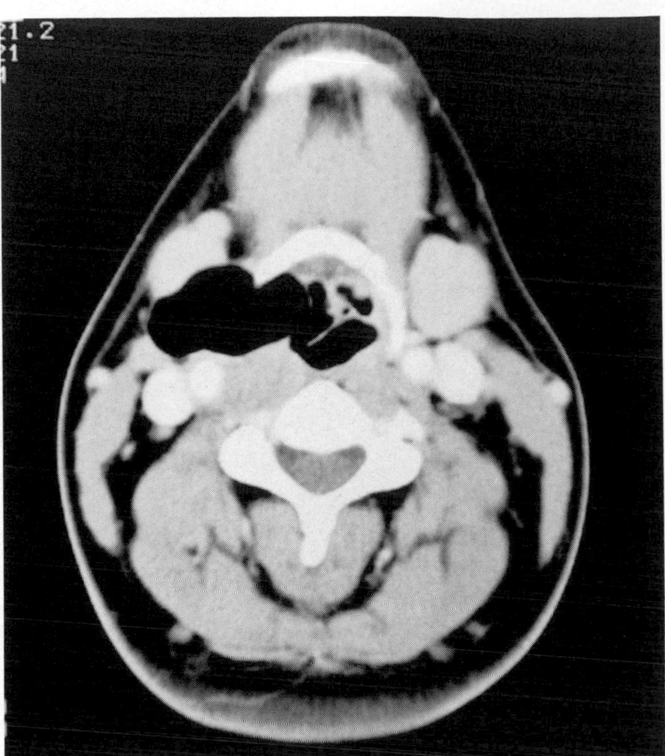

Figure 23.4 *CT scan image of a patient with a large mixed laryngocele. The patient complained of occasional throat fullness and fullness in the submandibular region with swallowing. Indirect laryngoscopy confirmed involvement of the aryepiglottic fold.*

ratory distress that worsens with crying. Adults may complain of dysphonia, cough or fullness in the throat with swallowing. With external or mixed laryngoceles, fullness in the upper neck may be seen on Valsalva maneuver. This fullness is usually decompressible. Evaluation by laryngoscopy reveals unilateral submucosal swelling of the supraglottic larynx. Radiographic evaluation may include plain radiographs as well as CT scanning (Figs 23.3 and 23.4).

The importance of CT scanning is highlighted by the known association of acquired laryngoceles with laryngeal malignancy. This association was first described in 1944 by Schall.[15] The question of whether the presence of a laryngocele predisposes to the development of carcinoma remains unanswered; however, most evidence supports the theory that a laryngocele may develop secondary to a carcinoma that obstructs the laryngeal ventricle and not vice versa.[11,13] Regardless of the true causal relationship, patients with unilateral laryngocele should be evaluated for occult malignancy of the laryngeal ventricle. Any soft tissue mass adjacent to a laryngocele should be further evaluated with direct laryngoscopy and biopsy before proceeding with definitive treatment of the laryngocele.

The treatment of laryngocele is surgical and is usually reserved for symptomatic patients. Like treatment of saccular cysts, that for laryngoceles may include both endoscopic and external approaches. The classic approach has been external via a transverse incision at the level of the thyrohyoid membrane. With the strap muscles retracted anteriorly, the sac of the laryngocele is identified and followed to the thyrohyoid membrane. The sac can then be traced into the larynx where the neck of the sac is suture ligated. The question of planned tracheotomy should be addressed preoperatively. Extensive dissection within the larynx may result in swelling significant enough to cause airway compromise in the postoperative period.

Other laryngeal cysts

Cysts also occur within the larynx unrelated to the laryngeal saccule. These include ductal or mucous retention cysts, squamous inclusion cysts and pseudocysts. They may be found in the ventricle, vallecula, epiglottis, false vocal fold and true vocal fold. The terminology may be confusing when reviewing the literature as there are no standard definitions for these lesions and the pathophysiology is not completely understood for the various histopathologies.

Supraglottic ductal cysts and inclusion cysts

Ductal cysts or mucous retention cysts usually refer to acquired cysts that result from obstruction of the mucous glands in the supraglottis and subglottis. They are most common in the ventricle and false vocal fold but may also be found on the laryngeal or lingual surfaces of the epiglottis.

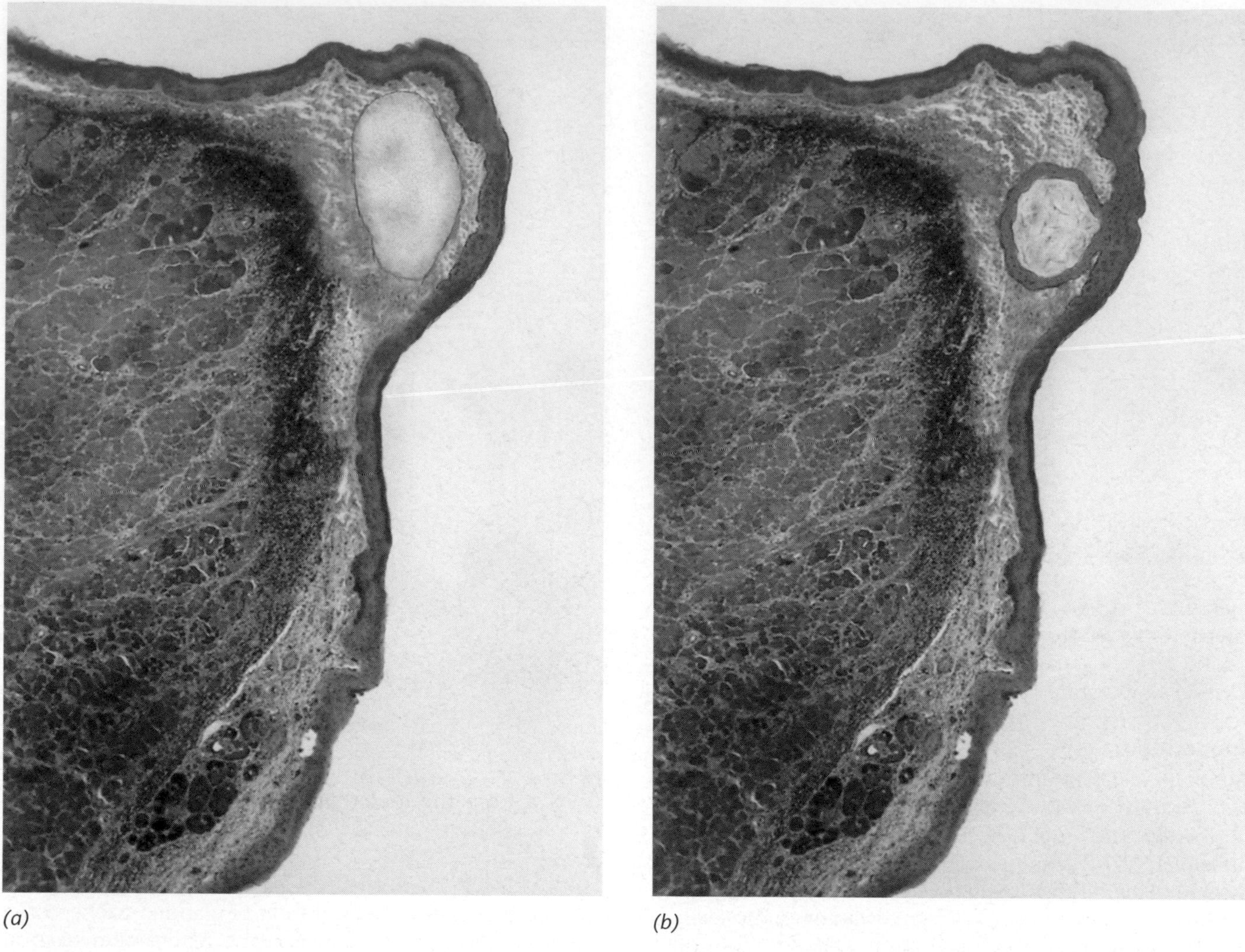

Figure 23.5 *Photomicrograph of a human vocal fold in coronal section with an artist's rendering of (a) a mucous retention cyst and (b) a squamous inclusion cyst resulting from invagination of the mucosal cover into the SLLP.*

Squamous inclusion cysts may also be found in the supraglottis. These cysts are thought to result from ductal narrowing of mucous glands caused by squamous metaplasia of the duct epithelium. The obstruction is due either to complete narrowing from the metaplastic process or from sloughing of squamous debris blocking the lumen. The resulting cyst may be columnar cell-lined or squamous cell-lined depending on the extent of squamous metaplasia.[11]

Symptomatic cysts of the supraglottis are usually treated endoscopically with either marsupialization or complete excision. The CO_2 laser often facilitates the dissection. Recurrences are uncommon with this treatment.

Intracordal vocal fold cysts and pseudocysts

Intracordal vocal fold cysts should be considered separately from other laryngeal cysts relative to pathogenesis and treatment. They, along with vocal fold polyps and nodules, represent a non-neoplastic response of the lamina propria to injury. Both mucous retention, or ductal cysts and squamous inclusion cysts may be found in the true vocal fold within the superficial layer of the lamina propria (SLLP).

Mucous glands are normally absent within the true vocal folds. Therefore, mucus-filled intracordal cysts with a low columnar or cuboidal epithelial lining probably arise from obstruction of a gland within the adjacent supraglottis or subglottis. The obstructed cyst may then migrate into the SLLP of the true vocal fold (Fig 23.5a).

Squamous inclusion, or epidermoid, cysts of the true vocal fold also occur. The pathogenesis of these cysts is speculative and there are theories involving both congenital and acquired factors.[12] One theory suggests that epidermoid cysts result from an invagination of the vocal fold epithelium into the SLLP. This process has been associated with congenital or acquired sulcus vocalis, a furrow along the vibrating edge of the vocal fold where the mucosal cover (epithelium and SLLP) is tethered to the vocal ligament (intermediate and deep layers of the lamina propria). Studies have demonstrated that hyperphonation causes disruption of the basement membrane zone (BMZ) at its junction with the SLLP.[7] This injury is intuitively more likely in the presence of sulcus vocalis where there is tethering of the mucosal cover. The healing process may result in the formation of a new basement membrane over the previous sulcus, creating a squamous-lined sac within the SLLP. The sac would then progress to form an inclusion cyst filled with sloughed squamous debris. This type of lesion has been referred to as a pseudocyst (Fig 23.5b).

Recent immunohistochemical analysis of benign vocal fold lesions has aided our understanding of the vocal fold's response to trauma.[4] Nodules and polyps follow distinct patterns of injury with regards to changes in the BMZ and fibronectin arrangement. Fibronectin is a glycoprotein involved in tissue response to injury and should therefore be a good marker for localizing tissue injury. Nodules have a thickened BMZ and a disordered and more dense fibronectin pattern throughout the lamina propria. Polyps have a more normal BMZ width and the fibronectin is clustered around the neovasculature. Cysts, however, have more variability in the responses seen. The BMZ may be normal or slightly thickened and the fibronectin shows a more normal distribution within the lamina propria. This pattern was seen in both mucous retention cysts and squamous inclusion cysts. With polyps, nodules and cysts, the overlying epithelium is usually uninvolved with the pathologic process.

Clinically, both mucous retention cysts and squamous inclusion cysts have similar presentations. Patients will usually complain of intermittent or chronic vocal difficulties. Professional voice users may notice increased vocal fatigue or a loss of their upper vocal range. Laryngeal examination may reveal fullness of the mid-vocal fold or a discrete lesion interfering with glottic closure. Cysts located more on the superior aspect of the vocal fold may not be apparent on indirect laryngoscopy. With laryngeal videostroboscopy (LVS), however, the mucosal wave is noted to be decreased or absent due to the interruption of the normal vibratory pattern. Intracordal cysts are noted to fluctuate in size correlating with the amount of vocal use. The effect on the mucosal wave may also vary with the condition of the cyst.

Management of vocal fold cysts, like nodules and polyps, should address the source of the offending injury. The most common contributing factor is vocal abuse or misuse. Patient education is extremely important to maximize successful treatment outcome. Patients should be counseled in vocal hygiene with a goal of watery thin mucus lubrication of the vocal folds. Behavioral modifications with speech therapy and singing therapy, if appropriate, are necessary to delay the need for surgical excision or prevent recurrences following excision.

Surgical treatment for benign vocal fold lesions has evolved from the once advocated vocal fold stripping to more delicate microlaryngeal dissection within the SLLP. The goal is restoration of the normal layered architecture of the vocal fold mucosa. Most laryngologists use some variation of a microflap technique which preserves the uninvolved overlying mucosal cover and underlying vocal ligament.[1,5,14] Adequate exposure of the entire endolarynx is essential. Various laryngoscopes are available to allow microsuspension laryngoscopy in most patients. Inadequate exposure is a contraindication for proceeding with surgery until the appropriate instrumentation is available. Regardless of the specific technique used, injury to the vocal ligament should be avoided as this has a high risk of permanent loss of normal vibration and permanent dysphonia. The CO_2 laser does not offer any advantage over cold knife techniques and there is some concern that the laser may cause more scarring via thermal injury to surrounding normal tissue.

The microflap technique begins with an incision on the superior aspect of the true vocal fold. The position of the incision is surgeon-dependent and may vary with type and location of the lesion. A laterally placed incision enables the surgeon to more easily identify and preserve the vocal ligament away from the lesion but usually requires more dissection than a more medially placed incision. The medial incision is appropriate for smaller lesions and for lesions located on the medial vibrating edge without evidence of vocal ligament involvement. Microlaryngeal elevators are used to separate and isolate the cyst from the underlying vocal ligament and overlying mucosal cover. Care should be taken to remove the entire cyst to minimize the risk of recurrence. Any redundant mucosal cover is excised to allow for coaptation of the wound edges.

Postoperative care is as important as the surgical excision. Patients should be counseled before surgery regarding the rehabilitative phase. Most patients are placed at complete voice rest for periods of several days to 2 weeks. Return to voice use is begun under the guidance of the voice team, including the surgeon and speech language pathologist.

References

1. Bastian RW. Vocal fold microsurgery in singers. *J Voice* 1996; **10:** 389–404.
2. Cavo JW, Lee JC. Laryngocele after childbirth. *Otolaryngol Head Neck Surg* 1993; **109:** 766–8.
3. Civantos FJ, Holinger LD. Laryngoceles and saccular cysts in infants and children. *Arch Otolaryngol Head Neck Surg* 1992; **118:** 296–300.
4. Courey MS, Scott MA, Shohet JA, Ossoff RH. Immunohistochemical characterization of benign laryngeal lesions. *Ann Otol Rhinol Laryngol* 1996; **105:** 525–31.
5. Courey MS, Stone RE, Gardner GM, Ossoff RH. Endoscopic vocal fold microflap: a three-year experience. *Ann Otol Rhinol Laryngol* 1995; **104:** 267–73.
6. DeSanto LW. Laryngocele, laryngeal mucocele, large saccules, and laryngeal saccular cysts: a developmental spectrum. *Laryngoscope* 1974; **84:** 1291–6.

7. Gray SD, Hammond E, Hanson DF. Benign pathologic responses of the larynx. *Ann Otol Rhinol Laryngol* 1995; **104:** 13–18.
8. Hogikyan ND, Bastian RW. Endoscopic CO_2 laser excision of large or recurrent laryngeal saccular cysts in adults. *Laryngoscope* 1997; **107:** 260–5.
9. Holinger LD, Barnes DR, Smid LJ. Laryngocele and saccular cysts. *Ann Otol* 1978; **87:** 675–85.
10. MacFie DA. Asymptomatic laryngoceles in wind instrument bandsmen. *Arch Otolaryngol* 1966; **83:** 270–5.
11. Michaels L. Laryngocele, cysts, heterotopia. In: *Pathology of the Larynx*. Berlin: Springer-Verlag, 1984: 51–7.
12. Monday LA, Bouchayer M, Cornut G, Roch JB. Epidermoid cysts of the vocal cords. *Ann Otol Rhinol Laryngol* 1983; **92:** 124–7.
13. Murray SP, Burgess LPA, Burton DM, Gonzalez C, Wood GS, Zajtchuk JT. Laryngocele associated with squamous carcinoma in a 20-year-old nonsmoker. *Ear Nose Throat J* 1994; **73:** 258–61.
14. Sataloff RT, Spiegel JR, Heuer SR *et al.* Laryngeal mini-microflap: a new technique and reassessment of the microflap saga. *J Voice* 1995; **9:** 198–204.
15. Schall L. Laryngocele associated with cancer of the larynx. *Ann Otol* 1944; **53:** 168–72.
16. Stell PM, Maran AGD. Laryngocoele. *J Laryngol Otol* 1975; **89:** 915–24.
17. Ward RF, Jones J, Arnold JA. Surgical management of congenital saccular cysts of the larynx. *Ann Otol Rhinol Laryngol* 1995; **104:** 707–10.

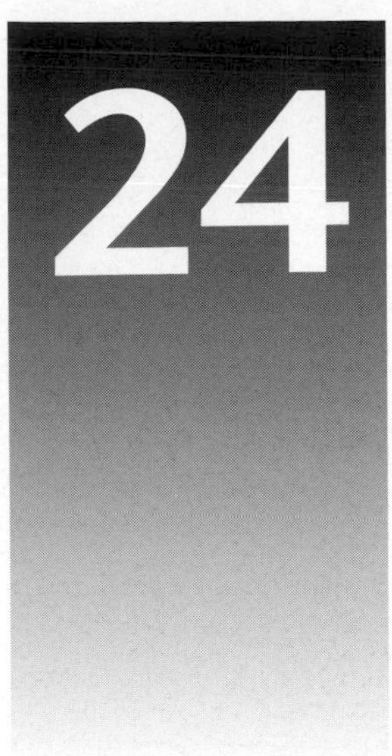

Laryngeal manifestations of acquired immunodeficiency syndrome

Kelvin C Lee and Andrew H Murr

The human immunodeficiency virus and the disease it causes, acquired immunodeficiency syndrome (AIDS), have had an enormous impact on our society through the 1980s and 1990s. What started as curious first reports of clusters of an unusual *Pneumocystis carinii* pneumonia in young gay men in New York and San Francisco in 1981 has progressed into one of the most serious public health problems of the twentieth century.[23,38] No other virus or disease process is as well known to the lay public or has stimulated as much change in social habits throughout the world. The Global AIDS Policy Coalition projected that by the year 2000 the number of people globally infected with HIV since the start of the pandemic would reach as many as 110 million, most of these individuals living in the developing world.[37]

As our understanding of the human immunodeficiency virus (HIV) and its impact on an individual has grown, we have markedly improved our care of patients with AIDS. HIV-infected patients are living longer and, though a cure may be in the distant future, with the advent of protease inhibitors the virus itself may finally be controlled.[5,13] Despite our advances in the identification and treatment of this virus and its related conditions, the number of patients with AIDS continues to increase throughout the world. Though in some places the incidence of new HIV infection has fallen, with their increased life span the prevalence of patients with HIV infection continues to grow.[37] With this growing number of patients 'living with HIV', the importance for all otolaryngologists to understand how to manage this patient population has increased dramatically.

The human immunodeficiency virus

With the massive research effort directed towards AIDS, the etiologic agent was isolated within several years of its first reported cases. We now know that several strains of the human immunodeficiency virus are present throughout the world, with human immunodeficiency virus type one (HIV-1) being the strain most commonly found in the USA and Western Europe. HIV-1 is a retrovirus, which as a family is unique in its ability to convert the single-stranded viral RNA found in the virus into double-stranded DNA which is then incorporated into the host cell genome. HIV-2, a related strain, is thought to be endemic in certain parts of West Africa and causes a very similar infection to HIV-1.[71]

Retroviruses are very simple organisms that are extremely effective in penetrating and surviving in host cells. The virus genome of single-stranded RNA, which codes for only nine known gene products, is encased in the viral protein capsid with several viral enzymes. The viral capsid is contained within a viral lipid bilayer, which contains both viral and host-derived proteins. One of these viral envelope proteins, gp120, has a high affinity for the CD4 membrane receptors. Thus free virions are attracted to cells with CD4 receptors, which they enter and ultimately infect. The cells that have the most CD4 membrane receptors are the CD4 lymphocytes or helper T-lymphocytes. With infection by HIV and the destruction of these cells with viral replication, the numbers of circulating helper T-cells decrease. However, the penetration of the virus into the cell and the incorporation of the newly synthesized viral DNA into the host genome are not usually followed by immediate virus replication. During this latency period the host cell is permanently infected and has impaired function but no detectable levels of virus particle are being produced. What triggers the infected cell to start virus replication is unclear and certain types of host cells may be stimulated by different events. For the helper T-cell or CD4 lymphocyte this includes infection by other DNA viruses such as cytomegalovirus and herpes simplex virus. As the infected host cells become activated and release more free virions, the number of host cells infected by the virus increases. In addition to helper T-lymphocytes, other cells with CD4 membrane receptors become infected, including the cells of the monocyte/macrophage lineage. The number of cells affected is smaller and reflects the smaller number of CD4 receptors found in these cells. The macrophages are important factors in HIV infection in that they are resistant to lysis even with activation of viral replication. They may serve as protected viral reservoirs and may be the means of viral transportation to tissues like the brain. As more and more cells are infected and either impaired by the virus or destroyed, the number of functioning helper T-lymphocytes and later monocytes and macrophages decreases and the patient becomes progressively more vulnerable to infection and neoplasms.[71]

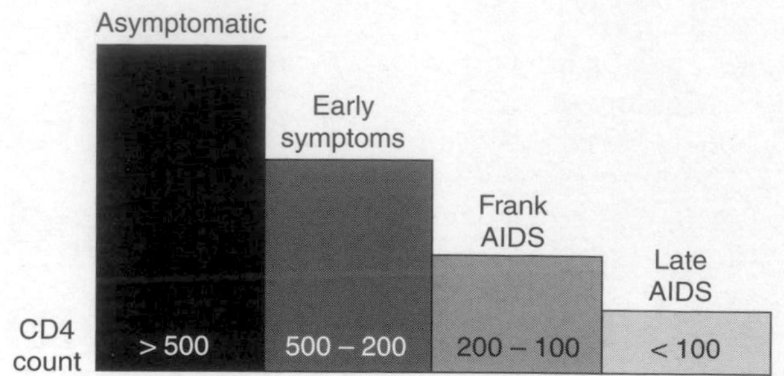

Figure 24.1 *The Walter Reed classification of HIV infection into stages based on CD4 count.[50] These stages are helpful for the clinician to evaluate the relative risk of a patient for the diseases associated with HIV infection.*

Evaluating the HIV-infected patient

As our understanding of HIV infection has improved in the years that followed the first description of an acquired immunodeficiency syndrome, it has been increasingly apparent that it is difficult to categorize all these patients into one neat little group. Patients with HIV infection include a very wide spectrum of individuals, each with a very different risk for the even broader variety of diseases that are associated with HIV. With the widespread use of HIV serologic testing, it has become clear that HIV-infected patients may be completely asymptomatic for many years, often independent of their suspected date of initial infection.[47] Because this syndrome has such variable clinical latency and severity of its manifestations, it is useful to group HIV-infected patients into stages of HIV infection. What we know as AIDS represents only the last stages of HIV infection. The best criteria for grouping patients into stages was found to be the CD4 count.[39,50] The CD4 count is a widely available, relatively inexpensive blood test that correlates with the effect of the virus on the patient's immune system. Using the CD4 count, patients can be grouped into four stages of HIV infection (Fig 24.1).[50] When the CD4 count is over 500 cells/mm^3, most patients are essentially asymptomatic. As the CD4 count drops to 200–500 cells/mm^3, the early manifestations of HIV infection start to appear. As the CD4 count drops below 200 cells/mm^3, the patient becomes vulnerable to many of the processes associated with AIDS. Because of its correlation to clinical disease, the Centers for Disease Control and Prevention in the USA has recently included a CD4 count of 200 cells/mm^3 or less as a defining measure of AIDS. As the CD4 count drops below 100 cells/mm^3, the patient becomes increasingly at risk for the unusual opportunistic infections highlighted in the medical literature.

The ability to divide HIV-infected patients into groups by CD4 count is extremely helpful in determining the aggressiveness of diagnostic evaluation. Though patients may be HIV-infected, if their CD4 count is greater than 500 cells/mm^3, the clinician should expect the types of laryngeal problems found in the general population. As the CD4 count drops down below 500 cells/mm^3, patients become at risk for some of the early manifestations of HIV infection such as laryngeal candidiasis as well as the common laryngeal problems seen in the general population. When the CD4 count falls below 200 cells/mm^3, the unusual infections and neoplasms usually associated with AIDS start to appear. In this group, clinicians should be very aggressive in their evaluation and consider early biopsy for definitive diagnosis. Patients with a CD4 count of below 100 cells/mm^3 should be assumed to have opportunistic infections or neoplasms until proven otherwise. Diagnostic laryngeal endoscopy and biopsy should be performed in this group as soon as possible, to allow for appropriate management. When the CD4 count falls below 50 cells/mm^3, the immune system is so vulnerable that these patients can have several concurrent opportunistic infections or neoplasms. Since in many cases their prognosis is poor even with aggressive medical and surgical therapy, early diagnosis and start of treatment are essential to maximize the therapeutic options available.

Common laryngeal problems found in the HIV-infected patient

Viral infections

Though viral infections of the larynx undoubtedly occur in the general population, they rarely cause significant morbidity or have any long-term impact on the patient. The HIV-infected patient is vulnerable to several very aggressive opportunistic viruses in the late stages of their HIV infection and these organisms can cause a wide range of problems. Of these viruses, cytomegalovirus and herpes simplex have been reported to involve the larynx.

Cytomegalovirus

The cytomegalovirus (CMV) is a virus commonly associated with the manifestations of AIDS and can be a source of significant morbidity for this population of patients. Though serologic evidence of prior infection with this virus is present in 81% of the general population over 35 years of age, the vast majority of those infected remained clinically asymptomatic.[49] CMV is frequently sexually transmitted and in certain HIV-infected populations the number with positive titers for CMV have approached 100%.[12,58] As the HIV disease progresses, the levels of these titers for CMV tend to rise significantly, suggesting reactivation of latent disease. The results of CMV infection usually appear as the patient's CD4 count falls down below 200 cells/mm^3. CMV retinitis is one of most frequent manifestations of this virus, though infections of the gastrointestinal tract, lungs and adrenal glands are also commonly seen.[58]

CMV infections of the upper aerodigestive tract have been reported by a number of authors.[25,31,59,67] Patients usually have a low CD4 count and complain of persistent odynophagia, general malaise and weight loss. When laryngeal involvement is present, patients have cough and hoarseness. On examination of the pharynx or larynx, the virus causes diffuse mucosal inflammation with a central necrotic ulcer. On occasion the swelling can present as a granulomatous mass-like lesion over the arytenoids.[67] These lesions are not very bulky but can cause airway obstruction as the disease progresses. A case of CMV necrotizing tracheitis presenting with emergency airway obstruction has also been reported.[25] Because CMV can frequently be isolated from sputum and mucosal swabs of the throat, definitive diagnosis relies on tissue biopsies and the identification of intranuclear and cytoplasmic inclusions typical of CMV in the sampled tissues. Thus direct laryngoscopy and biopsy are essential for diagnosis.

For invasive CMV infections, intravenous ganciclovir has been traditionally the mainstay of therapy. The cases of laryngeal CMV in the medical literature appeared to respond well to this agent.[67] In the treatment of CMV retinitis, foscarnet has also been effective in preventing progression of infection without some of the toxicity associated with ganciclovir. Combination therapy may be helpful in improving outcome and preventing the emergence of resistant organisms. There is no clear role for surgical intervention, though in cases with prolific granulation tissue, laser excision of the excess tissue can improve the laryngeal airway while antiviral therapy is being given.

In addition to mucosal lesions, CMV is thought to be responsible for at least some cases of idiopathic vocal cord paralysis in HIV-infected patients. Peripheral neuropathies are common in HIV-infected patients as a group. In one patient with idiopathic vocal cord paralysis who died of *Pneumocystis carinii* pneumonia, autopsy results revealed evidence of recurrent laryngeal nerve infection with CMV.[61] Unfortunately the only way to definitively diagnose this cause of vocal cord paralysis would be recurrent laryngeal nerve biopsy or autopsy; thus the rate of occurrence of CMV-related laryngeal paralysis remains difficult to estimate.

Herpes simplex virus

The herpes simplex virus (HSV) is another opportunistic virus that commonly afflicts HIV-infected patients. Like CMV, HSV has a high prevalence in the HIV-infected population overall, with reactivation of the latent virus as the patient's immune system weakens. The most common manifestations of the viral infection involve painful ulcerations of the genital and perioral regions. Involvement of the larynx and esophagus is rare, yet when present, it can cause persistent hoarseness, odynophagia and dysphagia. Biopsy of the lesion with cultures is needed to establish the diagnosis. In most cases infections are treated with intravenous acyclovir.

Bacterial infections

Because of their vulnerable immune systems, these patients have more frequent and more severe bacterial infections than the general population. In addition to the deterioration of the humoral immune system, HIV-infected patients develop impaired chemotaxis and degranulation of their neutrophils which make them very vulnerable to bacterial infections.[16] As long as the patient's CD4 count is above 200 cells/mm^3, the usual pathogens that cause laryngeal and pharyngeal infections are present. Studies of sinusitis and bacteremia in HIV-infected patients suggest an increased vulnerability to staphylococcal and *Pseudomonas* infections.[21,43] Empirical antibiotic therapy should include adequate coverage for these pathogens. Frequently these patients take longer to respond to antibiotic therapy and are more prone to complications than non-HIV-infected patients. As the CD4 count falls below 100 cells/mm^3, more unusual pathogens may be present. From the history and appearance on examination, it may be difficult to determine whether the infection is bacterial, mycotic, mycobacterial or even viral. If patients do not respond to empirical antibiotic therapy, direct laryngoscopy with biopsy for culture and histopathology should be performed to identify the pathogenic organism.

Epiglottitis in adults has become more common in the general population as well as in HIV-infected patients. This diagnosis should be considered in all patients with severe odynophagia and significant dysphagia combined with fevers and malaise. In the HIV-infected patient, the symptoms seem more severe and the progression of infection more rapid with the majority requiring airway intervention. The organisms isolated from epiglottic cultures have included *Streptococcus viridans*, *Streptococcus pneumoniae* and *Staphylococcus aureus*.[55] Candidal epiglottitis has also been reported in HIV-infected patients. Because of this variability of organisms, it is vital to perform throat or, if possible, epiglottic cultures, as well as blood cultures in this group of patients. Definitive therapy includes empiric wide-spectrum intravenous antibiotics and airway protection or observation. At San Francisco General Hospital we frequently give systemic steroids to these patients to reduce soft tissue swelling of the airway unless the patient has an ongoing opportunistic infection. Additional complications, related to the use of systemic steroids in these already immunocompromised patients, have been exceedingly rare. The hospital courses are typically prolonged with slower response to medical therapy, more complications and longer periods of need for airway protection.[55]

Mycobacterial infections

Early in the AIDS epidemic the most common mycobacterium associated with HIV infection was *Mycobacterium avium-intracellulare* now known as *Mycobacterium avium* complex (MAC). These infections with MAC occurred in the last stages of AIDS and usually manifested themselves as a multisystem infection often with mycobacteremia. More recently, it has become clear that HIV-infected patients are also very vulnerable to *Mycobacterium tuberculosis* infection even when their CD4 count is still relatively high.

The patient's primary defense against mycobacterial infection relies on the macrophages and the T-lymphocytes. After initial exposure and ingestion of mycobacteria, macrophages can process the mycobacterial antigens and present them to T-lymphocytes for processing. The T-lymphocytes then release lymphokines that stimulate additional lymphocytes and macrophages to specifically attack the mycobacteria. With infection of the CD4 lymphocytes and macrophages by HIV, these important mechanisms of defense falter and patients become infected with mycobacteria or reactivation of latent infection occurs.[4] In these patients, the risk of reactivation of latent disease for *M. tuberculosis* has been calculated to be 8–10% per year.[51]

Though pulmonary disease remains the most common manifestation, 50–67% of the HIV-infected persons will have extrapulmonary disease, mainly of the lymph nodes or bone marrow.[26] The larynx has been historically recognized as a common extrapulmonary site of tuberculous infection, but almost exclusively in patients with very advanced pulmonary disease or with disseminated disease. More recently, a number of HIV-infected patients have been reported with either primary laryngeal tuberculosis or laryngeal tuberculosis with asymptomatic pulmonary disease. These patients complain primarily of persistent hoarseness and on laryngeal examination have swelling and frequently an exophytic mass of the larynx.[46] Skin testing using PPD for tuberculosis is still useful when appropriate controls are used to rule out anergy. For the HIV-infected patient, a >5 mm skin reaction should be considered a positive test. These patients continue to respond to PPD skin testing even in the later phases of their HIV infection. Some cross-reactivity of the PPD is seen with atypical mycobacterial infections in most cases resulting in a partial response.[34] Definitive diagnosis requires biopsy and culture of the causative organism. Though the classic caseating granulomas with a few acid-fast organisms may suggest *M. tuberculosis*, histopathology alone cannot rule out an atypical mycobacterial infection. Histopathology of tissue infected with *M. avium* complex typically reveals necrotic debris with numerous acid-fast organisms, many more than seen with tuberculosis. This differentiation is important because atypical mycobacterium is frequently resistant to antituberculous medications.[34] In addition, with the increasing incidence of resistant strains of *M. tuberculosis*, culture sensitivities are very helpful in optimizing the prolonged therapy needed for control of this mycobacterium. The medical therapy for extrapulmonary and pulmonary tuberculosis is identical and will lead to complete resolution of the laryngeal lesions in almost every case. There is no role for surgery in these patients aside from diagnostic biopsy.[34]

Fungal infections

In the general population, fungal infections of the larynx are relatively rare and frequently associated with certain predisposing factors.[8,9,17,18,60] HIV-infected persons are more susceptible to fungal infections and increasing numbers of cases involving *Candida*, *Aspergillus*, *Cryptococcus*, *Coccidioides*, *Blastomyces* and *Histoplasma* have been reported.[68] The majority of these cases have had either concurrent pulmonary or systemic infections.

Candida

Candida albicans is the most common fungal organism to afflict those with HIV. Oral mucosal candidiasis is one of the earliest and most frequent manifestations of HIV infection, occurring even when the CD4 count is well over 500 cells/mm^3.[15] As the CD4 count falls below 200 cells/mm^3, patients become even more susceptible to opportunistic infections and these fungal infections often become more extensive and harder to treat. When patients with a low CD4 count and oral candidiasis complain of persistent odynophagia, dysphagia and voice changes, the clinician should suspect extension of the mycotic infection to the larynx and/or esophagus. Patients with esophageal candidiasis report a more severe and deeper substernal pain than seen with pharyngeal infection and the diagnosis can readily be made with radiographic swallow studies with contrast.

Laryngeal lesions can be easily visualized with either indirect laryngoscopy or fiberoptic examination. Though the pseudomembranous type of lesion is the most common seen involving the larynx, atrophic or hypertrophic lesions can occur.[15] The pseudomembranous lesions are the white plaque-like lesions classically associated with oral candidal infections. Atrophic lesions can be more difficult to visualize because they are flat hyperemic lesions, which appear like erythroplakia or telangiectasia. The hypertrophic lesions are thickened plaques, often with some white coloration, and can appear like a neoplastic process. All of these types of candidal lesions rapidly respond to oral antifungal therapy. Empirical antifungal therapy for laryngeal candidiasis can be started without biopsy. Though ketoconazole is effective for candidal infections, because of changes in the gastric physiology in many HIV-infected patients, fluconazole is better absorbed and better tolerated. If the patient does not respond to empiric antifungal therapy, direct laryngoscopy and biopsy are indicated to confirm the diagnosis. Cultures for mycotic as well as mycobacterial organisms should be sent along with specimens for histopathologic examination. These studies will help to rule out other possible etiologies such as other fungal organisms and laryngeal neoplasms. Occasionally candidal infections in this patient population will require more intensive medical therapy such as intravenous amphotericin B to control the infection. Even after apparent control of infection, relapses are frequent and long-term prophylaxis for *Candida* is often essential in the overall management of the patient's symptoms. There is no established therapeutic role for surgery.

Aspergillus

Invasive *Aspergillus* infections have been a well recognized problem in immunocompromised patients. In HIV-infected patients with CD4 counts of less than 50/mm^3, increasing numbers of cases, usually involving multiple sites, have been reported.[36] The majority of cases have involved either the lungs or the paranasal sinuses. Several cases of invasive *Aspergillus* of the larynx have been also been reported.[17,28,36,66] These patients present with hoarseness as their chief complaint and on examination are found to have an ulcerated hypertrophic mucosal lesion of the vocal cords. In one case, the size of the lesion caused significant airway obstruction.[53] Tissue diagnosis is essential because the culture identification of the organism does not imply that invasive *Aspergillus* is present. Only tissue examination and histopathologic proof of invasion can make the diagnosis of invasive aspergillosis. The overall prognosis of patients with HIV-associated invasive *Aspergillus* is very poor. Despite aggressive medical therapy, the mean survival for these patients ranges between 2 and 4 months.[36] The mainstay of therapy has traditionally been intravenous amphotericin B, though a recent study has shown that oral itraconazole may be as effective without the associated side effects.[14] The role of surgical debulking of this fungal infection prior to medical therapy with either itraconazole or amphotericin B remains unclear and requires additional investigation. Currently at San Francisco General Hospital, patients have the majority of the infected tissue excised but without sacrifice of major nerves or other structures. Postoperative wound irrigation with amphotericin B has also been used with some apparent success. The most important factor in the management of these patients is the time to diagnosis. The experience with invasive *Aspergillus* of the paranasal sinuses has highlighted the need for early endoscopy and biopsy of these lesions to maximize any benefit of medical therapy. With earlier diagnosis and initiation of medical therapy and possible surgical therapy, the prognosis of this infection should improve.

Cryptococcus

Cryptococcus neoformans is a well known fungal pathogen with a worldwide distribution and an association with avian habitats. In the general population, cryptococcal infection primarily presents as a pulmonary process. In the HIV-infected patient, these fungal infections have become notorious for an extrapulmonary extension, cryptococcal meningitis. The laryngeal manifestations of cryptococcal infection can result from this central nervous system involvement or direct invasion of the laryngeal mucosa. The symptoms of cryptococcal meningitis include fever, malaise, headache, nausea and vomiting, but the classic bacterial meningitis symptoms of photophobia and neck meningeal signs occur in only 25% of cases.[32] This central nervous system infection can result in cranial neuropathy, such as unilateral or bilateral vocal cord paralysis. In the majority of cases, with treatment of the CNS infection the cranial neuropathies will resolve.

Rare direct laryngeal invasion by *Cryptococcus* has been reported in both the general population and a patient with HIV. In the HIV-infected patient, pulmonary *Cryptococcus* had been previously diagnosed and treated. These patients usually present with chronic hoarseness and on examination have an erythematous mass lesion of the vocal cords.[10] Direct laryngoscopy with biopsy for histopathology and fungal culture is needed to establish the diagnosis. If the diagnosis of extrapulmonary *Cryptococcus* is made, careful evaluation for pulmonary and CNS concurrent infection is essential. The mainstay of therapy for *Cryptococcus* remains intravenous amphotericin B. Medical therapy is very effective in controlling these infections, but because of a high recurrence rate in the HIV-infected patient, long-term maintenance therapy with fluconazole is recommended.

Histoplasma, Coccidioides and Blastomyces

As the HIV epidemic has expanded, an increasing number of laryngeal infections by fungal organisms endemic to certain regions of the world have been reported. Cases of laryngeal histoplasmosis, coccidioidomycosis and blastomycosis have been described, but the majority of these patients have presented with concurrent systemic fungemia and pulmonary symptoms.[20,24,56,69] In almost every case the CD4 count has fallen below 100 cells/mm^3 before these fungal infections develop. The clinical presentation frequently includes a very aggressive course with invasion by the fungal organism of the patient's tissue similar to that found with invasive aspergillosis. The treatment usually includes the antifungal agent appropriate for the organism involved. There is no clear role for surgical debulking of the infected tissue, except for diagnosis. These patients have a poor prognosis overall and often other opportunistic infections or neoplasm complicate the clinical course.

As the incidence of AIDS continues to rise in these areas with endemic fungi, the local otolaryngologist needs to be aware of the possibility of fungal laryngeal infections and be aggressive in performing diagnostic procedures and biopsies in patients at risk.

AIDS-related malignancies of the larynx

It is intriguing to consider that HIV is related to several different types of malignancy that can affect the larynx. Whether the association is secondary to immunodeficiency, specifically cell-mediated immunodeficiency, or secondary to direct viral effect is still unclear. Nevertheless, it is interesting to note that just over a decade ago it was somewhat unusual to associate viral infection with subsequent malignancy in humans. Today, it seems rather logical and the HIV-associated tumors of the larynx are excellent examples of the role of viruses in the development of malignant tumors. Kaposi's sarcoma, squamous cell carcinoma, and malignant lymphoma of the larynx are all known to be associated with HIV infection.[54,57,62]

Kaposi's sarcoma

Kaposi's sarcoma (KS) is the most commonly reported HIV-associated malignancy of the larynx.[44,65,66] In the pre-AIDS era, KS was exceedingly rarely reported as involving the laryngeal structures. In fact a literature review by Abramson and Simons in 1970 identified only 13 cases of laryngeal KS.[2] With the dissemination of AIDS in the early 1980s, however, came a greater number of reported cases of KS. In 1986, the presence of KS was included as an AIDS-defining diagnosis.[44]

KS itself seems to present in several distinct forms. The classic form of KS occurs in white males of Mediterranean or Jewish origin in the 50–70 year old age group. The clinical course is indolent and the prognosis is good. An endemic form of KS has been reported in Africa occurring in young adults and children. This form involves a greater propensity toward dissemination and can affect the spleen, gastrointestinal tract and the lymphatic system. It is more aggressive than classic KS. Finally, there is the epidemic form of KS most commonly associated with homosexual or bisexual males with AIDS, or involving patients who are immunosuppressed due to organ transplantation. This type of KS is often multicentric with involvement of many different organ systems, but especially involving the skin, the entire gastrointestinal tract and the respiratory tract. This is the type of Kaposi's sarcoma that typically can involve the oropharynx and larynx.[22]

Several clinical series have reported the involvement of KS of the larynx. Abemayor and Calcaterra in 1983 noted that of 45 unselected patients with AIDS, 40% had disease related to the head and neck and one patient was reported as having KS of the epiglottis.[1] In 1986, Zibrak reported two cases of laryngeal KS in a group of 61 patients with AIDS. Of the 61 patients, 25 had some form of KS.[70] Stafford *et al.* in 1989 found that of 84 AIDS patients with KS, the head and neck were involved in 56 and the larynx was involved in one patient.[63] Tami and Sharma[65] and Levy and Tansek[35] each separately described one patient with laryngeal KS.[57] Schiff *et al.*[57] described two patients with laryngeal KS and Friedman *et al.*[19] described six patients with laryngeal KS. By far, the largest reported series of laryngeal KS was that of Mochloulis *et al.*, who in 1996 described 17 patients with laryngeal KS.[44]

The presentation of patients with laryngeal KS is what one would expect from most tumors of the larynx. The larynx, however, is usually involved some time after cutaneous or gastrointestinal KS has been firmly established. Symptoms include dyspnea as the most common presenting symptom, closely followed by nonproductive cough, fever, hoarseness and dysphagia. Hemoptysis is possible but quite rare. The site of involvement of laryngeal KS is most commonly the supraglottic larynx alone or in combination with the glottic larynx in 65% of patients. Glottic involvement, alone or in combination with other sites, was found in 29% of patients. Subglottic involvement was found in only one patient or 6%.[44]

The best strategy for diagnosing laryngeal KS is controversial.[19,44] Because KS occurs almost always secondary to quite clinically apparent skin or gastrointestinal involvement, and because its characteristic appearance is that of a violaceous lesion with an irregular surface, the diagnosis is often readily suspected simply upon visual inspection of both the patient's skin and larynx. In fact the differential diagnosis is limited to differentiating KS from bacillary angiomatosis. With this in mind, in the largest clinical series of laryngeal KS the authors warn that 'we would not recommend biopsy of suspected laryngeal Kaposi's sarcoma'.[44] This was due to the potential for life-threatening bleeding from the lesion. On the other hand, most of the case reports generated in the American literature depended on confirmatory biopsy to clinch the diagnosis.[6,19,35,57,65,70] At least one report, that of Tami and Sharma, accomplished a biopsy after a tracheotomy had been placed to secure the airway.[65] The need for histopathologic proof of the neoplasm is often related to the morbidity of the planned treatment, if any is planned. The histologic picture of KS consists of spindle-shaped cells with a large number of vascular channels accompanied by an inflammatory infiltrate. Immunohistochemical staining can be positive for factor VIII antigen.[64]

Treatment for laryngeal KS and KS in general remains controversial. Asymptomatic skin lesions or oropharyngeal lesions do not necessarily require any specific treatment.[64] The neoplasms will continue to grow slowly and in most cases treatment is initiated only when the KS becomes problematic. However, because of the potential for future emergent airway obstruction in laryngeal KS, most clinicians feel that some form of therapy is probably in the patient's best interest. Low-dose radiation ranging from 600 Gy to 2000 Gy appears to offer the best control of symptomatic laryngeal KS.[44] Systemic chemotherapy has been widely described as having efficacy in controlling KS. Etoposide, liposomal doxorubicin, paclitaxel and bleomycin seem to have the highest response rates. Vinblastine, vincristine and interferon-α have also been used with some success.[33] Intralesional injection of vinblastine has been reported in two separate recent papers with regard to laryngeal KS but has a much longer track record with regard to cutaneous KS.[19,29,65] The technique involves the use of 0.2 mg/ml vinblastine sulfate solution injected directly into the symptomatic lesion with a 27 gauge needle. Using this technique, Friedman *et al.* reported a 62% complete regression rate.[19] Finally, endolaryngeal surgical approaches with a CO_2 laser in the form of laser epiglottectomy were reported by Schiff *et al.* to control the airway symptoms from laryngeal KS, but, as expected, this local treatment will have no effect on the KS present at other sites.[57]

Finally, with regard to the etiology of AIDS-related KS, it is noteworthy that recent work has linked a specific herpes virus to the development of KS in the epidemic form.[11,42,44] This virus has been termed herpes simplex 8 or Kaposi's sarcoma associated herpes virus (KSHV). It is theorized that an interplay between KSHV and HIV is required for the immune alteration that leads to the ability to develop Kaposi's sarcoma.[42] Furthermore, it is also hypothesized that the ability to obtain herpes virus DNA from bronchial washings in patients with bronchopulmonary KS may eventually lead to a non-biopsy form of definitive diagnosis for KS in the respiratory tract.[44]

Squamous cell carcinoma

Squamous cell carcinoma is another type of malignancy that can affect the larynx in close association with HIV infection and AIDS.[52,66] Roland *et al.*, in 1993, reported a series of five HIV-infected patients afflicted with squamous cell carcinoma of the larynx, all under the age of 46 and with relatively modest risk factors. Four patients had transglottic tumors and one had a supraglottic tumor. Two of five patients were also infected by human papillomavirus (HPV).[54] Human papillomavirus, especially types 6 and 11, has long been known to be the cause of recurrent respiratory papillomatosis and linked with squamous cell carcinoma. The incidence of squamous cell carcinoma arising from sites of HPV infection is usually quoted as being between 2% and 10%.[48] Authors have described a potential subgroup of squamous cell carcinoma victims in the age group below 45 years and with few, if any, risk factors.[41] These patients do not have a significant history of tobacco and alcohol use and the clinical behavior of the tumors is unusually aggressive. Several clinicians have suggested that a viral etiology may link these individuals. The behavior of the HIV-related laryngeal squamous cell carcinoma has also been described as quite aggressive and experienced clinicians have recommended combined surgery and radiation therapy to attempt to control the disease. Several other individual case reports are scattered throughout the literature postulating an association between HIV and laryngeal squamous cell carcinoma.[3,45] However, the most convincing evidence of such a link lies with reports of the association between HIV, HPV and anogenital squamous cell carcinoma, which is histopathologically similar to laryngeal squamous cell carcinoma.[7,40] Further study is needed to fully understand the relationship of these viruses and the neoplasms they seem to promote.

Non-Hodgkin's lymphoma

Although exceedingly rare, non-Hodgkin's lymphoma (NHL) primary to the larynx has been reported in one case report by Smith *et al.* found in the literature.[62] Nevertheless, non-Hodgkin's lymphoma of other sites is quite commonly found in the HIV-infected population with AIDS. When these tumors appear in the head and neck, their rapidly enlarging size can cause airway obstruction by extrinsic pressure on the larynx or compromise of the recurrent laryngeal nerves. The AIDS-afflicted population differs from other groups with this diagnosis in that AIDS patients have a higher preponderance of the NHL aggressive subtypes. About 40% of AIDS NHLs can be categorized as Burkitt's lymphoma, 30% can be categorized as immunoblastic lymphoma, and 30% can be categorized as large cell lymphoma. Epstein–Barr virus has been identified in many of these lymphomas, approaching nearly 50% of lymphomas in some studies. Furthermore, Kaposi's sarcoma-related herpes virus has also been found to be associated with certain types of body cavity lymphomas. Again, it is postulated that HIV causes an immune suppression that allows the above viruses to participate in the pathogenesis of non-Hodgkin's lymphoma.[30] The diagnosis of non-Hodgkin's lymphoma requires direct endoscopy and biopsy for histopathologic examination. The management of these aggressive lymphomas usually includes combination chemotherapy. Though relatively successful for this tumor in the general population, HIV-infected patients in general have a limited response to this regimen. In one large study of HIV-infected patients with NHL, a median survival of 5.5 months was reported when treated with chemotherapy.[27] Their clinical course on chemotherapy is frequently complicated by opportunistic infections.

Conclusions

Infection by HIV places patients at risk for an overwhelming number of infections and neoplasms of the larynx, many not frequently seen in the general population. However, the risk of these unusual processes changes dramatically with the patient's stage of HIV disease. As the number of patients with HIV infection grows throughout the world, the clinician should become familiar with these infections and neoplasms and when the patient is at greatest risk for a particular disease. In general, the aggressiveness of the evaluation of laryngeal processes should reflect the risk for opportunistic infections and neoplasms. For many of these diseases that are difficult to treat, earlier diagnosis may markedly improve the prognosis of a patient's course.

References

1. Abemayor E, Calcaterra TC. Kaposi's sarcoma and community-acquired immune deficiency syndrome. *Arch Otolaryngol* 1983; **109:** 536–42.
2. Abramson AL, Simons RL. Kaposi's sarcoma of the head and neck. *Arch Otolaryngol* 1970; **92:** 505–8.
3. Alhashimi MM, Krasnow SH, Johnston Early A, Cohen MH. Squamous cell carcinoma of the epiglottis in a homosexual man at risk for AIDS. *JAMA* 1985; **253:** 2366.
4. Barnes PF, Le HQ, Davidson PT. Tuberculosis in patients with HIV infection. *Med Clin North Am* 1993; **77:** 1369–90.
5. Bartlett JG. Protease inhibitors for HIV infection. *Ann Intern Med* 1996; **124:** 1086–8.
6. Beitler AJ, Ptaszynski K, Karpel JP. Upper airway obstruction in a woman with AIDS-related laryngeal Kaposi's sarcoma. *Chest* 1996; **109:** 836–7.
7. Biggar RJ, Rabkin CS. The epidemiology of AIDS-related neoplasms. *Hematol Oncol Clin North Am* 1996; **10:** 997–1010.
8. Boyle JO, Coulthard SW, Mandel RM. Laryngeal involvement in disseminated coccidioidomycosis. *Arch Otolaryngol Head Neck Surg* 1991; **117:** 433–8.
9. Bradsher RW. Histoplasmosis and blastomycosis. *Clin Infect Dis* 1996; **22:** S102–11.
10. Browning DG, Schwartz DA, Jurado RL. Cryptococcosis of the larynx in a patient with AIDS: an unusual cause of fungal laryngitis. *South Med J* 1992; **85:** 762–4.
11. Chang Y, Cesarman E, Pessin MS *et al.* Identification of herpesvirus-like DNA sequences in AIDS-associated Kaposi's sarcoma. *Science* 1994; **266:** 1865–9.
12. Collier AC, Meyers JD, Corey L, Murphy VL, Roberts PL, Handsfield HH. Cytomegalovirus infections in homosexual men. Relationship to sexual practices, antibody to human immunodeficiency virus, and cell-mediated immunity. *Am J Med* 1987; **82:** 593–601.
13. D'Aquila RT, Hughes MD, Jonson VA *et al.* Nepvirapine, zidovudine, and didanosine compared with zidovudine and didanosine in patients with HIV-1 infection. A randomized, double-blind, placebo-controlled trial. National Institute of Allergy and Infectious Disease AIDS Clinical Trials Group Protocol 241 Investigators. *Ann Intern Med* 1996; **124:** 1019–30.
14. Denning DW, Lee JY, Hostetler JS *et al.* NIAID mycoses study group multicenter trial of oral itraconazole therapy for invasive aspergillosis. *Am J Med* 1994; **97:** 135–44.
15. Dichtel WJ. Oral manifestations of human immunodeficiency virus infection. *Otolaryngol Clin North Am* 1992; **25:** 1211–26.
16. Dropulic LK, Leslie JM, Eldred LJ, Zenilman J, Sears CL. Clinical manifestations and risk factors of *Pseudomonas aeruginosa* infection in patients with AIDS. *J Infect Dis* 1995; **171:** 930–7.
17. Ferlito A. Primary aspergillosis of the larynx. *J Laryngol Otol* 1974; **88:** 1257–63.
18. Fletcher SM, Prussin AJ. Histoplasmosis of the larynx treated with ketoconazole: a case report. *Otolaryngol Head Neck Surg* 1990; **103:** 813–16.
19. Friedman M, Venkatesan TK, Caldarelli DD. Intralesional vinblastine for treating AIDS-associated Kaposi's sarcoma of the oropharynx and larynx. *Ann Otol Rhinol Laryngol* 1996; **105:** 272–4.
20. Gerber ME, Rosdeutscher JD, Seiden AM, Tami TA. Histoplasmosis: the otolaryngologist's perspective. *Laryngoscope* 1995; **105:** 919–23.
21. Godofsky EW, Zinreich J, Armstrong M, Leslie JM, Weikel CS. Sinusitis in HIV-infected patients: a clinical and radiographic review. *Am J Med* 1992; **93:** 163–70.
22. Goldberg AN. Kaposi's sarcoma of the head and neck in acquired immunodeficiency syndrome. *Am J Otolaryngol* 1993; **14:** 5–14.
23. Gottlieb MS, Schroff R, Schanker HM *et al. Pneumocystis carinii* pneumonia and mucosal candidiasis in previously healthy homosexual men: evidence of a new acquired cellular immunodeficiency. *N Engl J Med* 1981; **305:** 1425–31.
24. Hajjeh RA. Disseminated histoplasmosis in persons infected with human immunodeficiency virus. *Clin Infect Dis* 1995; **21:** S108–10.
25. Imoto EM, Stein RM, Shellito JE, Curtis JL. Central airway obstruction due to cytomegalovirus-induced necrotizing tracheitis in a patient with AIDS. *Am Rev Respir Dis* 1990; **142:** 884–6.
26. Johnson MP, Chaisson RE. Tuberculosis and HIV disease. *AIDS Clin Rev* 1993; **94:** 73–93.
27. Kaplan LD, Abrams DI, Feigal E *et al.* AIDS associated non-Hodgkin's lymphoma in San Francisco. *JAMA* 1989; **261:** 719–21.
28. Kingdom TT, Lee KC. Invasive aspergillosis of the larynx in AIDS. *Otolaryngol Head Neck Surg* 1996; **115:** 135–7.
29. Klein E, Schwartz RA, Laor Y, Milgrom H, Burgess GH, Holtermann OA. Treatment of Kaposi's sarcoma with vinblastine. *Cancer* 1980; **45:** 427–31.
30. Knowles DM. Etiology and pathogenesis of AIDS-related non-Hodgkin's lymphoma. *Hematol Oncol Clin North Am* 1996; **10:** 1081–109.
31. Lalwani AK, Snyderman NL. Pharyngeal ulceration in AIDS patients secondary to cytomegalovirus infection. *Ann Otol Rhinol Laryngol* 1991; **100:** 484–7.
32. Lee BL, Tauber MG. Cryptococcosis. In: Cohen PT, Sande MA, Volberding PA, eds. *AIDS Knowledge Base*, 2nd edn. Boston: Little Brown, 1994; **6.8:** 1–3.
33. Lee FC, Mitsuyasu RT. Chemotherapy of AIDS-related Kaposi's sarcoma. *Hematol Oncol Clin North Am* 1996; **10:** 1051–68.
34. Lee KC, Schecter G. Tuberculous infections of the head and neck. *Ear Nose Throat J* 1995; **74:** 395–9.
35. Levy FE, Tansek KM. AIDS-associated Kaposi's sarcoma of the larynx. *Ear Nose Throat J* 1990; **69:** 182–4.
36. Lorthollary O, Meyohas MC, Dupont B *et al.* Invasive aspergillosis in patients with acquired immunodeficiency syndrome: report of 33 cases. French Cooperative Study Group on Aspergillosis in AIDS. *Am J Med* 1993; **95:** 177–87.
37. Mann J, Tarantola D. The global AIDS pandemic. Toward a new vision of health. *Infect Dis Clin North Am* 1995; **9:** 275–85.
38. Masur H, Michelis MA, Greene JB *et al.* An outbreak of community-acquired *Pneumocystis carinii* pneumonia:

initial manifestations of cellular immune dysfunction. *N Engl J Med* 1981; **305:** 1431–8.

39. Masur H, Ognibene FP, Yarchoan R *et al.* CD4 counts as a predictor of opportunistic pneumonias in human immunodeficiency virus (HIV) infection. *Ann Intern Med* 1989; **111:** 223–31.
40. Melbye M, Rabkin CS, Frisch M, Biggar RJ. Changing patterns of anal cancer incidence in the United States, 1940–1989. *Am J Epidemiol* 1994; **139:** 772–80.
41. Mendez P Jr, Maves MD, Panje WR. Squamous cell carcinoma of the head and neck in patients under 40 years of age. *Arch Otolaryngol* 1985; **111:** 762–4.
42. Miles SA. Pathogenesis of AIDS-related Kaposi's sarcoma. Evidence of a viral etiology. *Hematol Oncol Clin North Am* 1996; **10:** 1011–21.
43. Milgrim LM, Rubin JS, Rosenstreich DL, Small CB. Sinusitis in human immunodeficiency virus infection: typical and atypical organisms. *J Otolaryngol* 1994; **23:** 450–3.
44. Mochloulis G, Irving RM, Grant HR, Miller RF. Laryngeal Kaposi's sarcoma in patients with AIDS. *J Laryngol Otol* 1996; **110:** 1034–7.
45. Muñoz A, Gómez-Ansón B, Abad L, González-Spínola J. Squamous cell carcinoma of the larynx in a 29-year old man with AIDS. *AJR Am J Roentgenol* 1994; **162:** 232.
46. Nasti G, Tavio M, Rizzardini G *et al.* Primary tuberculosis of the larynx in a patient infected with human immunodeficiency virus. *Clin Infect Dis* 1996; **23:** 183–4.
47. Pantaleo G, Menzo S, Vaccarezza M *et al.* Studies in subjects with long-term nonprogressive human immunodeficiency virus infection. *N Engl J Med* 1995; **332:** 209–16.
48. Pransky SM, Kang DR. Tumors of the larynx, trachea, and bronchi. In: Bluestone CD, Stool SE, Kenna MA, eds. *Pediatric Otolarynglogy*, Vol 2, 2nd edn. Philadelphia: Saunders, 1996: 1402–5.
49. Quinnan GV Jr, Masur H, Rook AH *et al.* Herpes-virus infections in the acquired immunodeficiency syndrome. *JAMA* 1984; **252:** 72–7.
50. Redfield RR, Wright CD, Tramont EC. The Walter Reed staging classification for HTLV-III/LAV infection. *N Engl J Med* 1986; **314:** 131–2.
51. Reider HL, Cauthen GM, Kelly GD, Bloch AB, Snider DE Jr. Tuberculosis in the United States. *JAMA* 1989; **262:** 385–9.
52. Remick SC. Non-AIDS-defining cancers. *Hematol Oncol Clin North Am* 1996; **10:** 1203–13.
53. Richardson BE, Morrison VA, Gapany M. Invasive aspergillosis of the larynx: case report and review of the literature. *Otolaryngol Head Neck Surg* 1996; **114:** 471–3.
54. Roland JT Jr, Rothstein SG, Khushbakhat RM, Perksy MS. Squamous cell carcinoma in HIV-positive patients under age 45. *Laryngoscope* 1993; **103:** 509–11.
55. Rothstein SG, Persky MS, Edelman BA, Gittleman PE, Stroschein M. Epiglottitis in AIDS patients. *Laryngoscope* 1989; **99:** 389–92.
56. Sarosi GA, Davies SF. Endemic mycosis complicating human immunodeficiency virus infection. *West J Med* 1996; **164:** 335–40.
57. Schiff NF, Annino DJ, Woo P, Shapshay SM. Kaposi's sarcoma of the larynx. *Ann Otol Rhinol Laryngol* 1997; **106:** 563–7.
58. Schooley RT. Cytomegalovirus in the setting of infection with human immunodeficiency virus. *Rev Infect Dis* 1990; **12:** S811–19.
59. Seigel RJ, Browning D, Schwartz DA, Hudgins PA. Cytomegaloviral laryngitis and probable malignant lymphoma of the larynx in a patient with acquired immunodeficiency syndrome. *Arch Pathol Lab Med* 1992; **116:** 539–41.
60. Selkin SG. Laryngeal candidiasis and ketoconazole. *Otolaryngol Head Neck Surg* 1985; **93:** 661–3.
61. Small PM, McPhaul LW, Sooy CD, Wofsy CB, Jacobson MA. Cytomegalovirus infection of the laryngeal nerve presenting as hoarseness in patients with acquired immunodeficiency syndrome. *Am J Med* 1989; **86:** 108–10.
62. Smith MS, Browne JD, Teot LA. A case of primary laryngeal T-cell lymphoma in a patient with acquired immunodeficiency syndrome. *Am J Otolaryngol* 1996; **17:** 332–4.
63. Stafford ND, Herdman RC, Forster S, Munro AJ. Kaposi's sarcoma of the head and neck in patients with AIDS. *J Laryngol Otol* 1989; **103:** 379–82.
64. Swift PS. The role of radiation therapy in the management of HIV-related Kaposi's sarcoma. *Hematol Oncol Clin North Am* 1996; **10:** 1069–80.
65. Tami TA, Sharma PK. Intralesional vinblastine therapy for Kaposi's sarcoma of the epiglottis. *Otolaryngol Head Neck Surg* 1995; **113:** 283–5.
66. Tami TA, Ferlito A, Rinaldo A, Lee KC, Singh B. Laryngeal pathology in the acquired immunodeficiency syndrome: diagnostic and therapeutic dilemmas. *Ann Otol Rhinol Laryngol* 1999; **108:** 214–20.
67. Tinelli M, Castelnuovo P, Panigazzi A, D'Andrea F, Caprioglio S. Mass lesions of the larynx due to cytomegalovirus infection in a patient infected with the human immunodeficiency virus. *Clin Infect Dis* 1995; **20:** 726–7.
68. Vrabec DP. Fungal infections of the larynx. *Otolaryngol Clin North Am* 1993; **26:** 1091–114.
69. Wheat J. Endemic mycoses in AIDS: a clinical review. *Clin Microbiol Rev* 1995; **8:** 146–59.
70. Zibrak JD, Silvestri RC, Costello P *et al.* Bronchoscopic and radiologic features of Kaposi's sarcoma involving the respiratory system. *Chest* 1986; **90:** 476–9.
71. Zurlo JJ. The human immunodeficiency virus: basic concepts of infection and host response. *Otolaryngol Clin North Am* 1992; **25:** 1159–81.

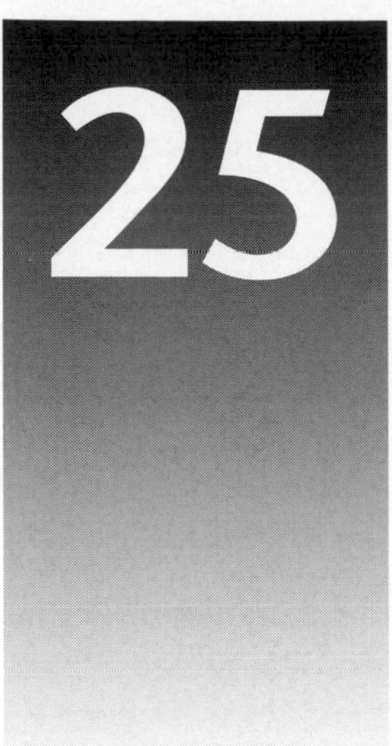

Endocrine disorders of the larynx

Jean Abitbol and Patrick Abitbol

Overview of hormones

Hormones come from the Greek *hormao* which means 'to arouse'. These molecules have the property to stimulate a response in a distant organ via the bloodstream.

We will first describe the hormones and glands, secondly the evolution of the human voice through the hormonal impact from infancy to old age and finally the pathological aspect of endocrine diseases on voice.

The beginning of endocrinology started with voice!

In 400 BC, Aristotle described the effect of castration on the songbird.[8] Galen was the first to describe and to name the thyroid gland. It was only 1500 years later that Leonardo da Vinci started the study of the numerous endocrine organs.

De Humani Corporis Fabrica,[69] published in 1543, provided the first precise book on human anatomy and endocrine glands.

Hormones are the conductors of our body. The mediators between the central nervous system and the glands are the SCN (suprachiasmatic nuclei) and the hypothalamus with its indispensable partner, the pituitary gland. Hence any information treated will have a wide range of responses adapted to physical and psychologic stimuli.[36]

Glands, hormones, transport, action, feedback regulation, receptors, effectors, messenger RNA and genes are the fundamental parameters of the endocrine system. One more thing is involved: time.

The pulse (or the frequency) of emission of hormones is as important as the amplitude (or quantity) produced. The whole process keeps a constant balance in its imbalance.

Endocrinology is the study of the relationship between two cells via a molecule: the hormone. This molecule stimulates, via the bloodstream, a response in a distant organ. The methods of communication by messenger molecules from one cell to another are:

- autocrine (molecule which has an impact on the cell where it has been synthesized);
- paracrine (molecule which has an impact on the adjacent cells to the cell which has synthesized the molecule); and
- pherocrine or endocrine (molecule goes to the bloodstream without any excretory channel).

All hormonal activity needs a target organ or target cells with specific receptors. Its action is limited in time, with a starting point and an end point triggered by a particular signal. The ultimate signal is the one going to the nucleus of the secreting cell to create the specific molecule. Any deviation from this rule will result in endocrine pathologies.

Hormonal actions are 'sensed' at some level to permit a 'normal' level of the hormone impact. Let's take the analogy of Lynn D Loriaux from Oregon University: the home heating system. How does it work in order to keep the temperature at the same level? A home heating system must have a fuel source of energy, a furnace to burn the fuel and heat the house and a thermostat to keep the temperature of the house stable. The thermostat will give orders if any imbalance appears. Sometimes, things get complicated: people open the window, keep going in and

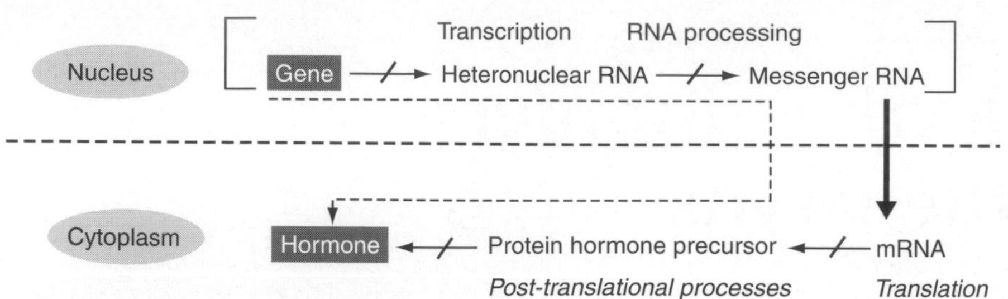

Figure 25.1 *How a hormone is produced from the DNA point of view.*

out. The thermostat keeps working. The furnace will burn more or less fuel depending upon these parameters. Most endocrine systems function in the same way. For example, calcemia, or the plasma calcium level, is strictly regulated. If it decreases, parathormone is secreted to increase it. As the concentration of calcium in plasma comes back to the level expected, the parathormone secretion is reduced and stopped. This is the negative feedback effect. The temperature is the calcium level. The thermostat is the parathyroid. The parathyroid switches on and synthesizes the parathormone. The parathormone is the furnace. The fuel consists of bone cells such as osteoclasts and osteocytes. These cells, triggered by the furnace (the parathormone), will give out calcium. The correct calcemia is reached. The bloodstream through the parathyroid informs that everything is stable and that there is no need to continue the synthesis of the parathormone. Feedback systems are inherently rhythmic. There is a fluctuation around the calcemia, and to make things more complicated, there is a basal fluctuation within strict limits around this independent variable. To go back to our house example, the thermostat turns the heat down every night and up every day within the limits set by the owner.

The endocrine rhythms have been named for a period of duration: circhoral for an hour, circadian for a day, circatrigantan for a month. We know that there is a circadian rhythm of plasma cortisol concentration at 3 a.m. and 8 a.m. The luteinizing hormone (LH) spike is almost a circatrigantan rhythm.

Principles of hormonal action

Genome

The primary function of the genome is to produce the specific protein. The hormones act as the commander.

The genome for a haploid eukaryotic cell consists of approximately 100 000 genes. The action of the hormone is mediated by specific receptors: either on the membrane of the cell, or/and on the nucleus. The expression of genes depends on the organ or the tissue which is involved: in the liver, around 15% of genes may be expressed, in the cerebellum 50–75%.[19]

The mechanism to produce a mature hormone is complex:[16]

- firstly, the gene transfers the information to the heteronuclear RNA via the process of transcription (Fig 25.1);
- secondly, via RNA processing, the heteronuclear RNA becomes a messenger RNA or mRNA; mRNA then travels to the cytoplasm (Fig 25.2);

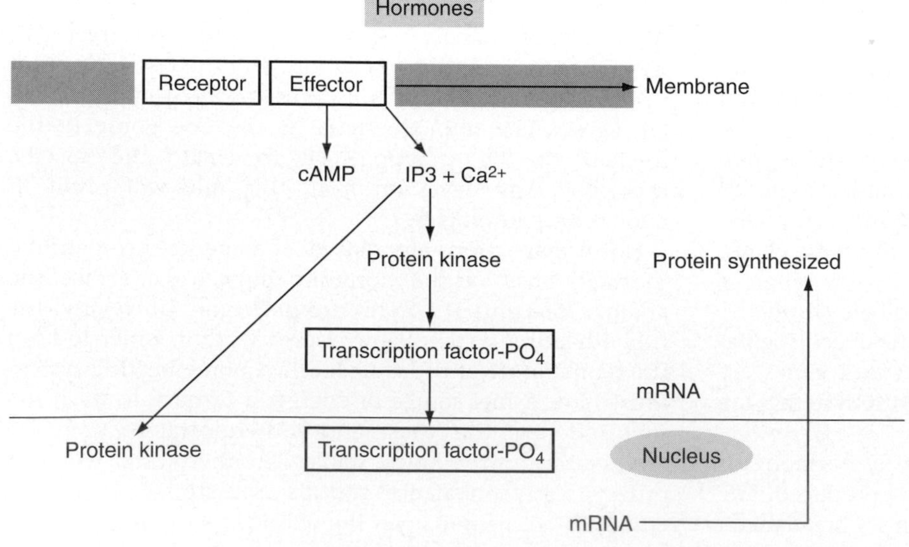

Figure 25.2 *How the hormone goes inside the cell and how it reacts.*

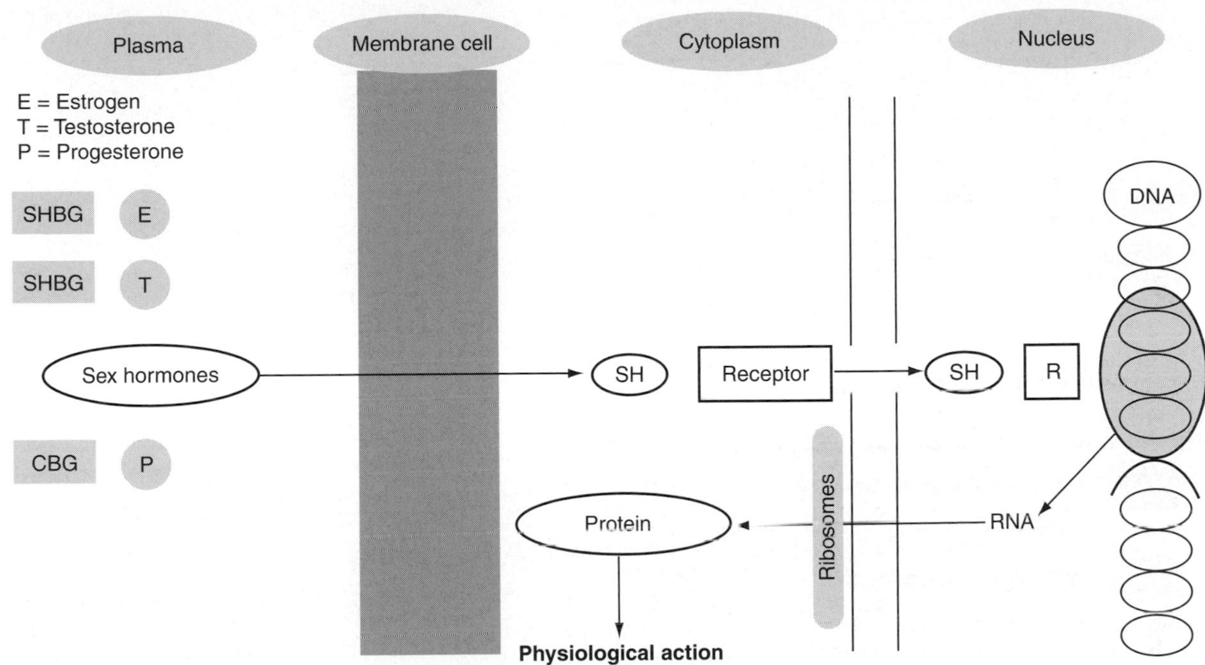

Figure 25.3 *Hormonal impact on the DNA, which will synthesize the protein.*

- thirdly, with the help of ribosomes and the endoplasmic reticulum, a translation from mRNA results in a protein human precursor; and
- fourthly, by the post translation processes, the protein hormone precursor becomes the mature protein hormone. This last step is done in the Golgi apparatus (Figs 25.3 and 25.4).

The ultimate basic element is the gene which is the unit of DNA specific for each being.

Membrane receptors

Hormones like LH, follicle-stimulating hormone (FSH), thyroid-stimulating hormone (TSH), growth factor (GF)

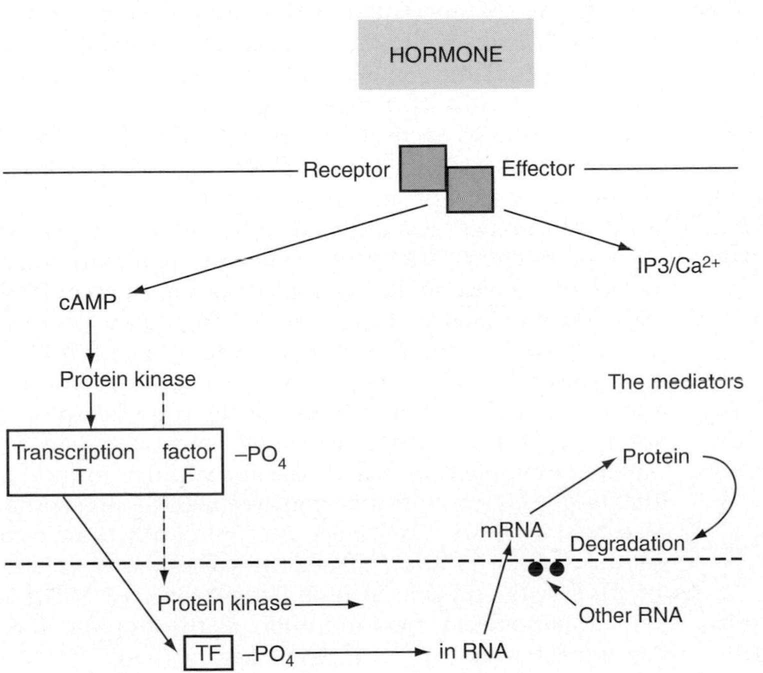

Figure 25.4 *Receptors and effectors of hormones.*

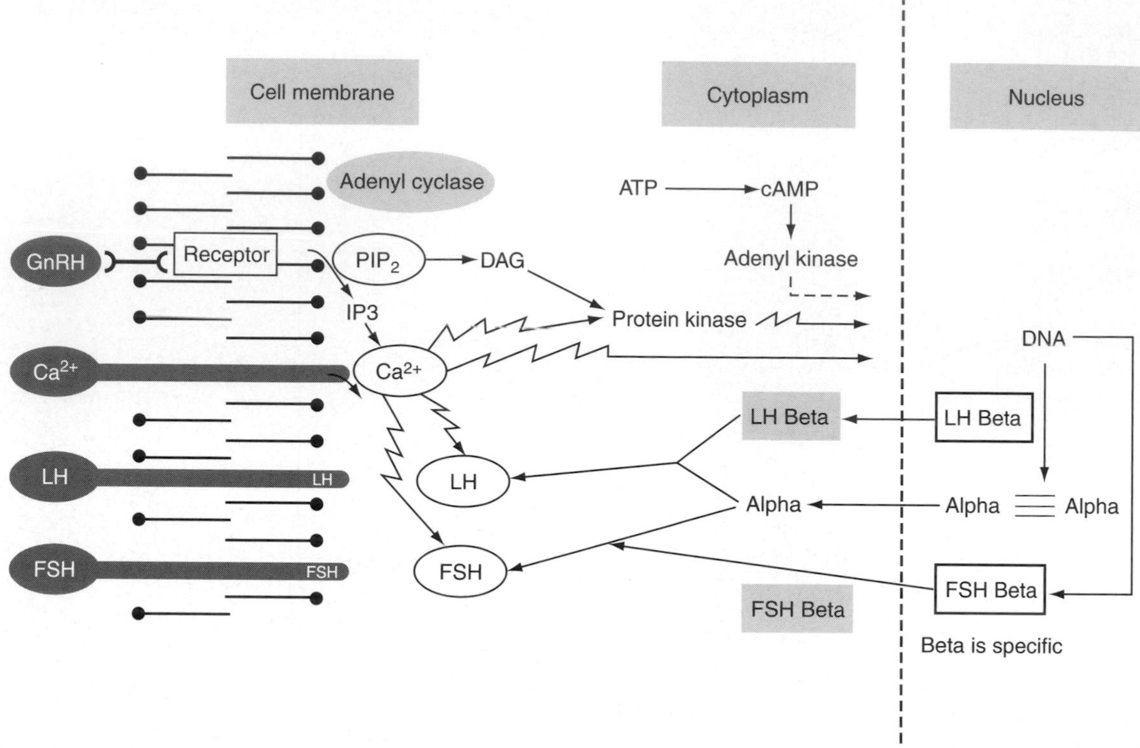

Figure 25.5 *Mechanism of action of GnRH and FSH.*

and insulin, that act on membrane receptors, are not liposoluble.

How do the membrane receptors work? There are three types of action. Type I deals with insulin and growth factors; types II and III deal with peptides, neurotransmitter units, the intramembranous structures and prostaglandins. Growth factors and insulin act like a thyroxine kinase and stimulate the phosphorylation of proteins on tyrosine residues (they act only with a transmembrane segment). The second type binds to receptors with seven transmembrane segments. They are coupled with effector molecules by the globulin proteins. They act on the second messenger cAMP or IP3, which stimulates the phosphorylation of proteins via protein kinases. The third type includes ligand-gated ion channels. Ions activate protein serine-threonine kinases, which stimulate the phosphorylation of proteins. Ion fluxes may induce membrane depolarization, i.e. a non-phosphorylation mediated action (Fig 25.5).[16]

How does a hormone act on a gene?

The hormone stimulates its specific receptor. There follows a complex biochemical chain leading to the formation of an mRNA via the transcription factor-PO_4.[28]

Why is this concept of receptors so crucial in the cycle of hormone life?

Let us take insulin and TSH as examples. TSH binds to its specific receptor on thyroid cells via globulin proteins. Effector is activated and causes a rise in cAMP, which leads to the formation of T3 and T4. There is then a negative feedback due to T3 and T4 that decreases the secretion of TSH. In Graves' diseases, an antibody blocks the TSH receptor and mimics the TSH action leading to the release of T3 and T4. The negative feedback then stops TSH secretion.[56]

Insulin binds to its specific receptor and stimulates directly the tyrosine kinase. It increases glucose metabolism and decreases the blood sugar level. There are two known types of antibodies, anti-R1 and anti-R2, that block the receptors. Anti-R1 increases glucose; anti-R2 decreases glucose. Anti-R2 activates insulin production by a negative feedback action due to the low blood sugar level. Anti-R1 stops insulin secretion (Fig 25.6).

Apart from these two examples, a cross-reactivity may be seen in receptors. There are structural similarities that reflect the evolution of the molecules for thousands of years. This similarity is the result of an affinity between low-specificity receptors, e.g. between insulin and insulin-like growth factor I (IGF-I), which may lead to hyperandrogenism with insulin resistance if the ovary receptor is for IGF-I. It may give a masculine voice with obesity. Another example is an IGF-II receptor sensitive to insulin that may lead to a dramatic hypoglycemia. IGF-I is synthesized mainly in the liver under the control of GH secreted by the anterior pituitary gland. IGF-I acts as a stimulator of cell growth and is located on chromosome 12. IGF-II is on chromosome 11, next to insulin. Corticotrophin, TSH, LH and FSH stimulate local production of IGF-I.

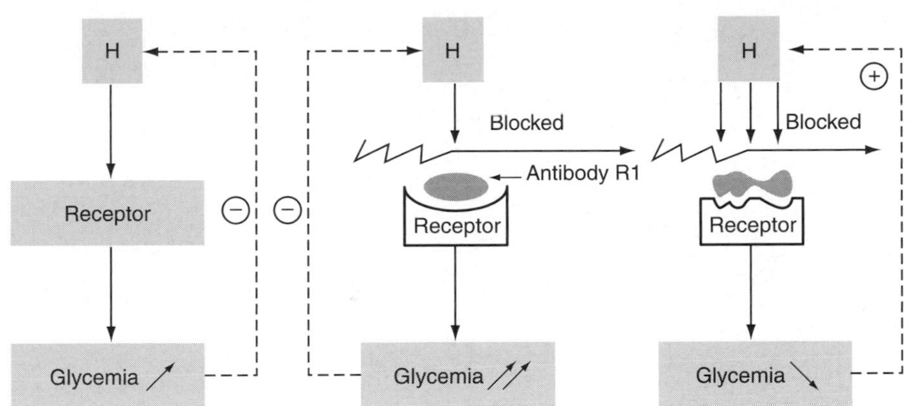

Figure 25.6 *Hormones and impact on glycemia.*

Nuclear receptors

In order to act directly on the nucleus, hormones must be liposoluble. They can then go directly through the membrane of the cell. Examples are steroid hormones, thyroid hormones and active vitamin metabolites such as retinoids, vitamin A metabolites and vitamin D. These hormones go through the cell membrane and activate directly the intracellular receptors in the nucleus.

From then on, the hormone–gene journey is the same as for membrane receptors.

Endocrine glands

The pituitary gland is located in the sella turcica inside the sphenoid bone. It is divided into two parts: the anterior part or adenohypophysis, which secretes FSH, LH, adrenocorticotrophic hormone (ACTH), GH, and the posterior part which is a transmitter and a reserve for neurohormones.

The pineal gland, located at the junction of the cerebrum, the brainstem and the cerebellum, is fixed on the roof of the third ventricle. It is an appendage of the brain and secretes melatonin.

The thyroid gland is located in front of the trachea between the second and the fifth cartilage rings. It secretes the thyroxine hormones: T3, T4.

The parathyroids, located at the posterior face of the thyroid gland, are four in number. They secrete parathormone.

The adrenal gland with the adrenal cortex and the adrenal medulla is located above the kidney. The adrenal cortex secretes mineralocorticoids, glucocorticoids and androgens. The adrenal medulla, like the paraganglia, secretes catecholamines (epinephrine and norepinephrine) and dopamines.

The thymus is located in the upper part of the thorax, at the posterior face of the sternum. It secretes the hormone thymine.

The pancreas secretes glucagon and insulin.

The testicles secrete androgens and 25% of the total daily production of 17β-estradiol (the remainder being derived by conversion of both testicular and adrenal androgens in peripheral tissues). The ovaries secrete estrogens (E), progesterone (P), and the androgen dehydroepiandrosterone (DHEA).

Ganglia of the parasympathetic system secrete catecholamines (epinephrine and norepinephrine) and dopamines.

The endocrine organs without glands are:

- the cerebrum (endorphins): the suprachiasmatic nucleus (SCN), the gyrus, the hypothalamus, the posterior part of the hypophysis (endorphins, catecholamines, dopamines and cytokines);
- the epithelium of the digestive tract: the gastric epithelium (gastrin, secretin);
- the kidney: (renin–angiotensin); and
- the placenta and heart also secrete renin–angiotensin.

Two families of hormones: lipid-soluble and water-soluble

All these hormones can be separated into two big families: lipid-soluble and water-soluble.

The lipid-soluble hormones

The lipid-soluble hormones, because of their structure, enter passively into the cells by virtue of miscibility with the lipid components of the membrane. These hormones interact with cytosol or/and nuclear receptors. They interact with specific gene regulatory sequences. The interaction leads to a hormone action mediated by new protein synthesis. The lipid-soluble hormones are steroids (estrogens, progesterone, androgens, aldosterone), triiodothyronine (T3) and tetraiodothyronine or thyroxine (T4).

Whereas water-soluble hormones, such as insulin, can be transported in plasma in the native state, lipid-soluble hormones must first be 'solubilized' by non-covalent binding proteins. For example:

- testosterone, estrogens, or dehydrotestosterone, circulate as complexes bound to sex-hormone-binding globulin (SHBG);

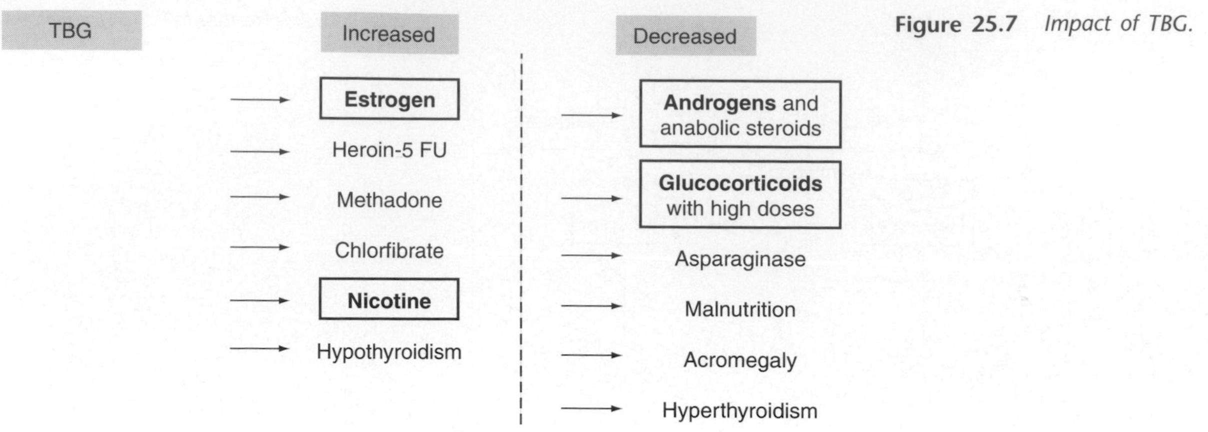

Figure 25.7 *Impact of TBG.*

- cortisol, progesterone and aldosterone circulate as complexes bound to cortisol-binding-globulin (CBG); and
- thyroxine and triiodothyronine circulate bound to thyroxine-binding-globulin (TBG).

The metabolic clearance works in relay with the binding protein and serves as a reservoir to defend the circulating free and biologically active concentration, in addition to permitting vascular transport in an aqueous medium (Fig 25.7).

The water-soluble hormones

The water-soluble hormones are glycoproteins (e.g. LH, FSH, TSH), the catecholamines and dopamines. By themselves, water-soluble hormones are excluded from the interior of the cell. They must interact with cell surface or 'membrane-bound' receptors. They then interact with a second messenger and finally with the nucleus.

The second messengers are not single entities but represent a cascade of events set in motion by a hormone–receptor interaction. This leads to an alteration in the concentration of molecular species, which interact with 'hormone-responsive' elements via gene regulatory elements (GRE). The best understood of the second messengers is the adenyl cyclase system. The hormonal receptor is linked to adenyl cyclase and hence leads to cAMP production.

The hormonal receptor is linked to the enzyme by two globulin proteins: one can suppress and the other can enhance adenyl cyclase activity. So cAMP alone can mediate more than one hormonal response in a given cell. cAMP regulates the 'activation', via phosphorylation, of enzymes in the kinase family that, in turn, catalyze the activation of a cAMP response element binding protein (CREB). CREB is the effector of hormonal action in this second messenger system. Other second messengers depend on the modulation of guanylate cyclase, tyrosine kinase, phosphatidylinositol turnover, calcium flux and ion channel activity (Fig 25.8).

As an example of water-soluble hormones, let see how FSH and LH interact in cells:

- the action of FSH, and LH is specific to the ovary and the testis;
- FSH has a predominant role in maturation of the gonads and regulation of gametogenesis;
- LH regulates steroidogenesis;
- FSH, in the ovary, stimulates the growth of developing follicles beyond the early antral stage. FSH is responsible for the recruitment of a cohort of follicles in each reproductive cycle;[30,39]
- estradiol synergizes with FSH both by stimulating proliferation of the granulosa cells of the ovary and by amplifying the responsiveness of the granulosa cells to FSH;
- the ultimate number of follicles that reach the preovulatory stage depends on the level of continued FSH export;
- FSH stimulates the appearance of LH receptors on both granulosa and theca cells;
- LH is then responsible for theca cell production of androgens from cholesterol;
- FSH then controls aromatization of these androgen precursors to estrogens in the granulosa cells;[45]
- LH plays a major role in the steroid production of the corpus luteum which synthesizes progesterone from the cholesterol precursors that are now available to the granulosa cells owing to the invasion of new vascular channels which appear at the rupture of follicle following ovulation and create the corpus luteum.

In the testis, FSH is required for the development of the seminiferous tubules and for initiation of spermatogenesis at puberty.[9] The spermatogenesis requires high levels of intratesticular androgen that are sustained by LH secretion.

Receptors of FSH and androgen are located on Sertoli cells. FSH in the testis induces the maturation of the Leydig cells, the enhancement of the androgen response to LH, the increase in the numbers of LH receptors, the stimulation of production of androgen-binding protein, and the induction of aromatase activity.[41,66]

LH interacts only with its own specific high-affinity receptors located only on the Leydig cells and controls

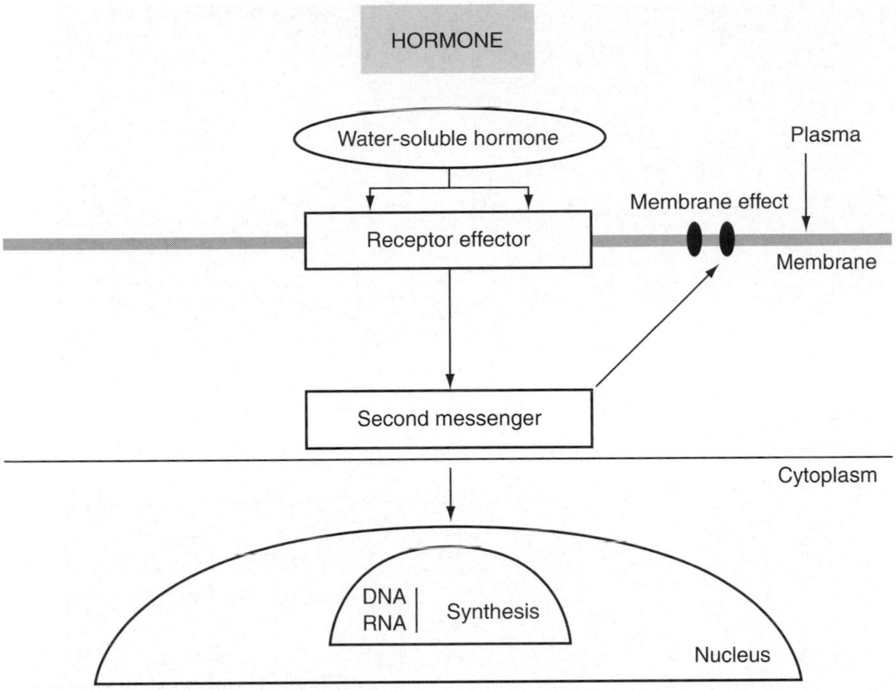

Figure 25.8 *Action of water-soluble hormone.*

testosterone. Pulsatile testosterone secretion follows pulses of LH secretion in normal men.

The larynx as a hormonal target

The larynx is a hormonal target. The sexual maturing or voice mutation is under the control of sex hormones. The voice is changed by the hypothalamus–pituitary axis through its endocrine impact and, during everyday life, because of the hormones of the cerebrum. Emotional stress and the psyche may also provide the hormonal trigger to induce a change in voice production. The voice is at the meeting point of the psyche and the hormonal world, the two great conductors of our being.

The common denominators of endocrine effects on the laryngeal structure are:

- The extravascular spaces: edema, secondary to fluid retention in the extravascular space, in the muscle, the epithelium and Reinke's space. The thickening and the increase in weight on the vocal cords gives a low voice and may cause a dysphonia.
- The epithelium and changes in glandular secretions. Glandular cells are located specifically on the epithelium of all the laryngeal mucous membrane except on the vocal fold which itself is covered by stratified epithelium. Lack of hydration causes a severe dysphonia (Fig 25.9).
- The muscles. The striated muscles of the larynx and the strap muscles may be weak and atrophied or made stronger and hypertrophied in endocrine diseases involving lack of or hyperproduction of testosterone. It must be noted that similar effects may be induced by voice training (muscular hypertrophy) or vows of silence (muscular atrophy).
- The framework: the cartilages of the larynx may be modified (as in acromegaly).
- The neuromuscular transmission. The latent period of response to a stimulus may vary, depending on calcemia, hypothyroidism, epinephrine, the state of the CNS and innervating fibers and vascular conditions.
- Specific laryngeal sensitivities. Cytokines and allergic responses also have an impact on the laryngeal epithelium.

The neuromuscular, neurovascular and neuroreceptor junctions may be sensitive to catecholamines, to temperature, to humidity, and to hydration.

The larynx and sex hormones

Breaking of the voice

Puberty is a hormonal earthquake. Hormones play a new music with the hypothalamus–pituitary axis as the conductor. It gives the adult score and asks the organism to tune its elements. This is to allow the adult music to start in harmony. That period of harmonic tune-up can last from 2 to 5 years between the ages of 12 and 17. Testicles in the male, ovaries in the female, and in both sexes, the adrenal cortex and the thyroid gland, all play a major role during that period of life.

Androgens are the most important hormones responsible for the passage of the boy-child voice to a man's voice, and their impact is irreversible: the Adam's apple appears, the cords lengthen and become rounded, the epithelium thickens

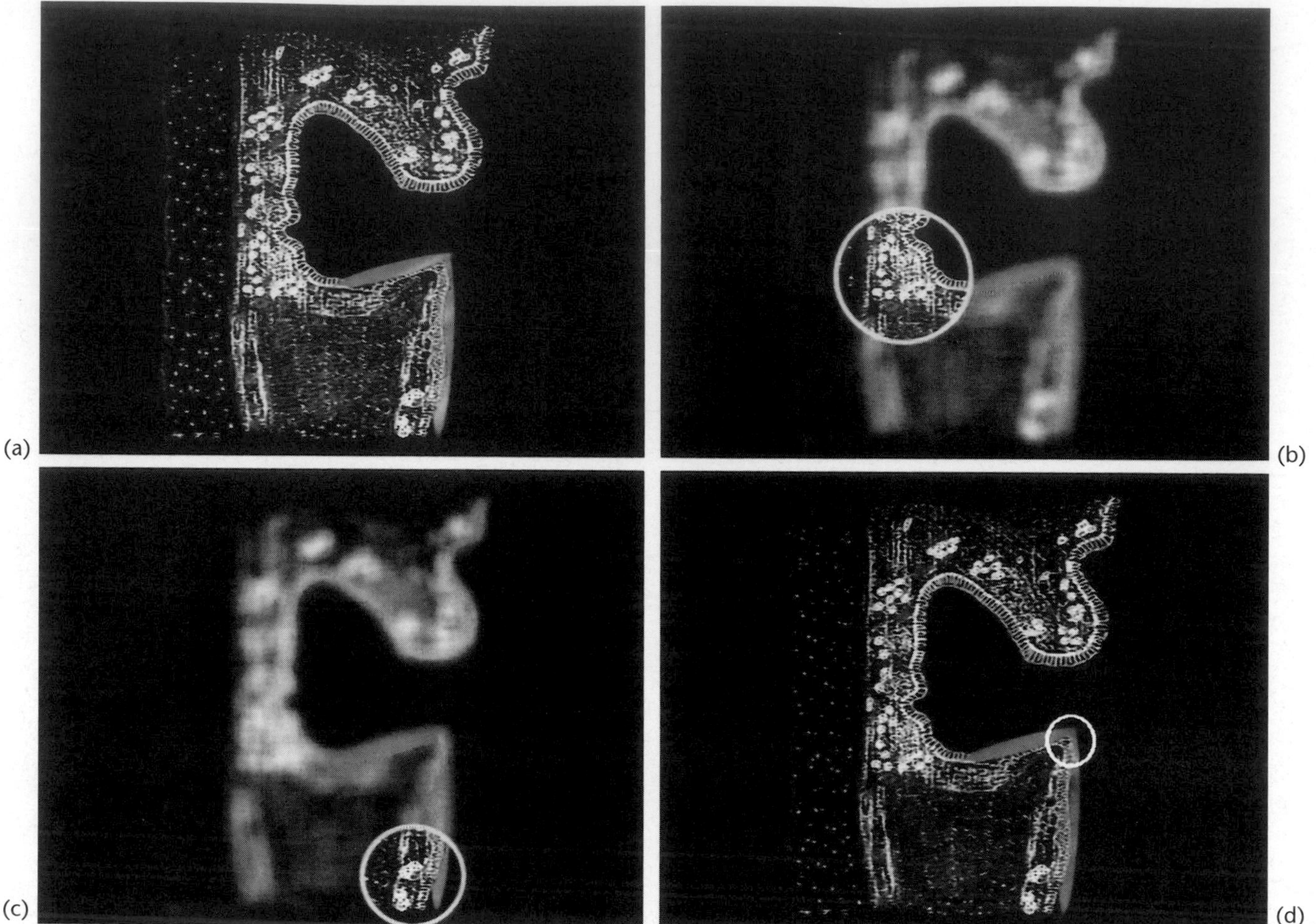

Figure 25.9 *Sagittal slide of the laryngeal structure showing the false vocal fold, the ventricle and the vocal fold. (a) General view. (b) Glandular cells at the ventricle. (c) Glandular cells under the vocal fold; (d) no glandular cells of the free edge of the vocal fold.*

with the formation of three distinct layers, the laryngeal mucus becomes more viscous, the arytenoids become bigger, the thyroarytenoid ligaments become thicker and more powerful, the anterior cricothyroid muscle broadens, becomes more resistant, and its contraction will permit a head voice. (The closure of the cricothyroid space induces a forward tip of the thyroid cartilage. The anterior commissure is thus brought downwards and backwards, thereby shifting the glottic plane from the horizontal. The horizontal projection of the cord is therefore shortened, leading to the production of a high note.) The muscular strength needed for this action is such that it is almost only reserved to men.

Disorders in breaking of the voice result from multifactorial parameters: hormonal mismatch, the psyche, the environment and other factors (diet, social life).

Two examples follow:

- A male adolescent's yodeling voice may be caused by an imbalance between a still childish glottis and an adult thoracoabdominal structure that is providing the driving wind power (sometimes pushing too hard and sometimes not hard enough).
- A male adolescent who keeps a childish voice without yodeling is speaking with a head voice. This is usually due to a psychological problem of a refusal to grow up.

In females, the breaking of the voice is much less apparent, but the female register is not a child's: it is three tones lower, and its spectrograph shows 5–12 formants, as opposed to the child's, with 3–6 formants.

Does voice have a sex? Is it chromosomal or hormonal?

The voice changes with the advancing years, with the scars of life, with its physical envelope and with the emotional world, but the essential element that remains is that voice has a sex and depends on these three principal actors: testosterone, estrogens and progesterone.

In the ancient Greek civilization, the worship of the athlete for his body and of the sirens' voice for the emotional side was recognized by the gods Apollo and Orpheus. In the seventh century BC, Pythagoras rationalized the pitch of a note. He demonstrated the relationship between the length of a string and its tonality. Thus a string narrow at its midpoint gives an octave, at two-thirds of its length, a fifth and at three-quarters of its length, a fourth. But this note, is it male, female or hermaphrodite?

The castrato: a pure example of the impact of a sex hormone on voice

In the fifteenth century the Roman Catholic Church wanted to have high-pitched voices, feminine voices, in the chapel choirs, but without any women. The ecclesiastical world followed scrupulously the maxim of St Paul, 'mulliers in ecclesiae taceant' or 'women should not be heard in the Church'. Castration, to keep the beauty of the female voice, was the eccentricity of the Church at that time, for whom voice was more important than virility. To allow the castrato to have a feminine voice, the castration had to be performed before any sign of puberty, before any secretion of testosterone. Even at this time, the importance of the definitive and indelible hormonal influence of testosterone had been recognized. The castrato has a powerful crystalline voice with an exceptional register. It is an ambiguous voice. The voice comes from a body born XY, but one that has never been clothed by testosterone, and hence this voice does not have a male print.

Let us see in detail the mechanism of the castrato voice. The castrato has the external skeletal envelope of a male (XY) with a vocal lung capacity of 3.5–5 liters. He also possesses the muscular abdominal and pelvic girdle necessary to sustain a male voice. The castrato's resonating chambers are defined by a male-type bony architecture. However, the vocalis muscle is highly sensitive to the impact of male hormones and in particular to the lack of androgens. It therefore keeps its childish characteristics. The quality of the voice is therefore defined by cords having kept a childish texture and being made to vibrate in a female register by the power of a man in a male skeletal environment. However, this is not the whole story. Follow me step by step: as in any musical instrument, there must exist a harmony between the two cords vibrating one against the other, the power of the pulmonary bellows producing the sound energy, and the resonating chambers that allow the amplification and the coloring of the voice. This harmony is especially wafer-thin in the creation of an operatic castrato voice. This is why during the Renaissance, many were called, but few chosen.

The castrato had a voice (according to written reports and to the one and only wax cylinder recording made) with a register of three to four octaves, could hold a note for some 120 seconds and could work his voice for up to 8 hours per day.

Sex hormones

What are the principal effects caused by our three main players, estrogens, progesterone and androgens?

Estrogens

Estrogens are present in women and, at a very low level, in men. They have a hypertrophic and proliferative effect on mucosa. They reduce the desquamating effect of the superficial layers and cause differentiation and complete maturation of the fat cells. The degree of cytoplasmic acidophilia and of nuclear pyknosis, as noted in gynecological cervical smears or in smears from the vocal cords, is a measure of this maturating effect. Estrogens have no effect on striated muscles. Their effects on cerebral tissue are well known. Amongst other things, they are supposed to reduce the risk of contracting Alzheimer's disease.

Progesterone

As its name implies, this hormone promotes gestation and thus is only present in adult women with ovulatory cycles. The effects of progesterone can only be felt if there has previously been an estrogenic impregnation of the tissues.[33,41] Apparently, this is the only known case of hormonal harmony in the human organism, where the impact of estrogens is a prerequisite to allow the action of progesterone to take place, as only estrogens will trigger the possibility of action and of growth in the receptor sites of progesterone. It has an antiproliferative effect on mucosa and accelerates desquamation.

Hence, there is no satisfactory cellular differentiation. On cervical and vocal cord smears, one can observe basophil cells, and, because of the desquamation, an infolding of the cellular edges. Furthermore, one can also observe a drying-out of the mucosa with a reduction in secretions of the glandular epithelium. It has a diuretic effect by its action on sodium metabolism, which is opposed to that of aldosterone. Estrogens increase capillary permeability and allow the through passage of intracapillary fluids to the interstitial space. Progesterone decreases, and even inhibits, capillary permeability, thus trapping the extracellular fluid out of the capillaries and causing tissue congestion. This congestion is quite apparent in the breasts, in the lower abdominal and pelvic tissues as well as in the vocal cords, where it causes premenstrual dysphonia.

Some synthetic progesterones, such as the derivatives of nortestosterone, have an androgenic effect caused by active metabolites. They have a masculine effect on the female voice. They must be never prescribed in voice professionals. That we shall consider at a later stage.

Androgens

Testosterone is the essential male hormone, secreted by the testis. In women, androgens are secreted principally by the adrenal cortex and the derivatives of aldosterone, but also by the theca interna of the ovaries. Studies have shown that androgens cause an increase in the female libido. Furthermore, there is a masculinizing action when the concentration of testosterone is greater than 150 µg/dl. If

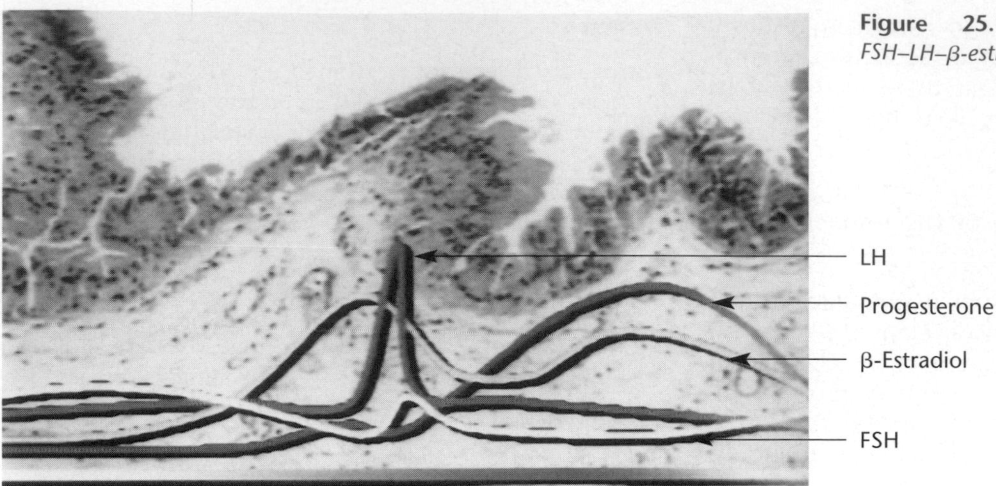

Figure 25.10 *Menstrual cycle display of FSH–LH–β-estradiol–progesterone.*

androgens are essential for male sexuality, they cause in women an often irreversible masculinizing effect at doses greater than 200 μg/dl. Man is the only primate with adrenal glands that secrete an important amount of dehydroandrostenedione (DHA) that is converted to androstenedione. In skin, these androgens cause acne, seborrhea and hirsutism. In mucosa, they cause a loss of hydration with a reduction in glandular secretions. In muscles, they cause a hypertrophy of striated muscles with a reduction in the fat cells in skeletal muscles. There is also a reduction in the whole fatty mass.

Anabolic steroids can have an irreversible effect due to the increase in volume and power of the muscular mass. In high doses, they also lead to the development of definitive masculine vocal characteristics.

Puberty

The passage from childhood to adulthood occurs when the secondary sexual characteristics appear as well as the physical and physiologic changes that are peculiar to each sex. The hypothalamohypophyseal axis and its testicular or ovarian response determine and influence the physical, psychic and emotional sexuality of the person. In the Western world, the average age of puberty is around 8–13 years for the girl and 9–14 years for the boy. In the girl, estrogens and progesterone will produce a woman's voice, and in the boy, testosterone will produce a man's voice. This means a third lower than a child's voice for the woman and an octave lower for the man. The pulmonary capacity, the cardiovascular apparatus, the level of hemoglobin and the striated muscle mass all increase in man.

The changes in males are considered in detail in the section above on the breaking of the voice.

In females, there is little development of the thyroid cartilage or of the cricothyroid membrane. The vocal muscle thickens slightly, but remains very supple and quite narrow. The squamous mucosa also differentiates into three quite distinct layers on the free edge of the cords. The sub- and supraglottic glandular mucosa becomes hormone-dependent to estrogens and progesterone. The ovaries start to work. The first menstrual cycles appear, at first rather irregularly and then regularly. The hormonal rhythm harmonizes the body of the adolescent girl. The conductor is the hypothalamohypophyseal axis by the action of FSH and LH on the ovary. The musical partition, or lunar rhythm of the cycle of life starts, and will carry on for the next 40 years. During the menstrual cycle, we can distinguish the follicular and the luteal phases, linked together by ovulation (Fig 25.10).[30] During the follicular phase, the secretion of estrogens increases progressively, activated by FSH between day 4 and day 8, and reaching a peak on day 13 of the cycle. LH reaches its peak on day 14, leading to ovulation. The ovule is snapped up by the Fallopian tube. The luteal phase allows the creation of a new endocrine gland, the corpus luteum, which secretes progesterone and estrogens.

The exocervical squamous mucosa has three layers: the lamina propria, and the chorion with a basal and a parabasal membrane. The junction between the different cells is relatively large in the first part of the cycle and less so in the second phase. This intercellular space is therefore hormone-dependent. Its importance in the human voice has been emphasized in the paragraph on progesterone.

The endocervix has a glandular ciliated epithelium with serous and mucous glands, which is also spectacularly hormone-dependent. Estrogens produce a fluid mucus and progesterone produces a thick mucus. At menopause, there is atrophy of the mucosa of the uterine cervix with a relative conservation of the glandular secretions as long as there is continued secretion of estrogens. The presence of androgens causes a thickening of the cervical mucosa, a loss of its suppleness and of its sheen, as well as a drying out of the seromucous glands.

In the ovary, estrogens are secreted by the cells of the granulosa and of the theca interna. Progesterone is secreted by the corpus luteum, which disappears at menopause. Testosterone and its derivatives are produced

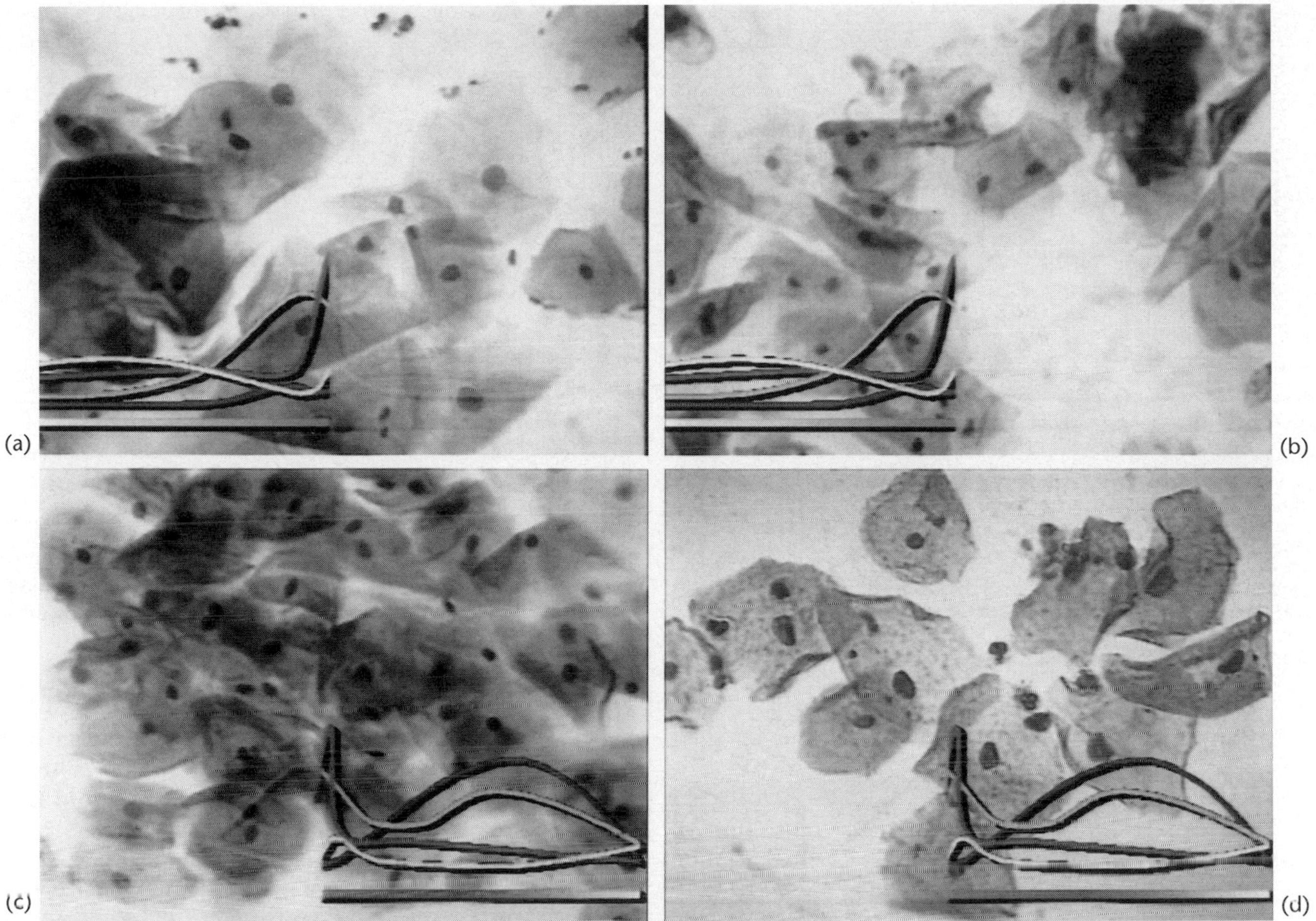

Figure 25.11 *Parallelism of smear test between vocal fold (a,c) and cervix (b,d).*

by the cells of the theca interna and transported to the cells of the granulosa, where they are changed to estradiol.[20] At menopause, and this is even more apparent since the ovaries have practically stopped producing estrogens, the androgen derivatives are changed to estrones in the fatty cells by the cytochrome P450. Thus, the development of a masculine voice at menopause varies with each individual case and depends on each woman's hormonal profile.

The female voice

The premenstrual voice syndrome

Estrogens cause an important thickening of the endometrial mucosa and an increase in the secretions of the endocervical glandular cells.[43] A similar hormonal effect is noted with the laryngeal mucosa, with an increased secretion of the glandular cells above and below the vocal cords. Thus, in some patients, the estrogen–progesterone influence also modifies the structure of the laryngeal mucosa just before ovulation, and the tone of the voice can be slightly altered by the presence of mucus on the vocal cords. This increase in the production of mucus, although quite important, does not usually bother the speaking or the singing voice.

Before the periods, the vocal symptoms are much more pronounced.[4] Morphologically and functionally, the cervix, distal part of the uterus, is independent of the endometrium. Just before ovulation, there is a slight edema. In fact, the cervix acts like a real hormonal trigger in response to estrogens and progesterone at the level of its epithelium, its chorion, and of its squamous and glandular cells.

Progesterone increases the viscosity of the secretions of the glandular cells, the acidity level, but decreases their volume, causing a relative dryness.

In a study carried out with Professor Jean De Brux, in 1986, we demonstrated a surprising correlation between cervical and vocal cord smears (Fig 25.11).[4,5,63]

During the premenstrual period, the dryness of the vocal cords, the increase in the acidity level, often worsened by an esophageal reflux common at this time, the reduced tonicity of the vocal muscle, the edema of the vocal cords and the venous dilatation of the microvarices all combine to cause the premenstrual syndrome.

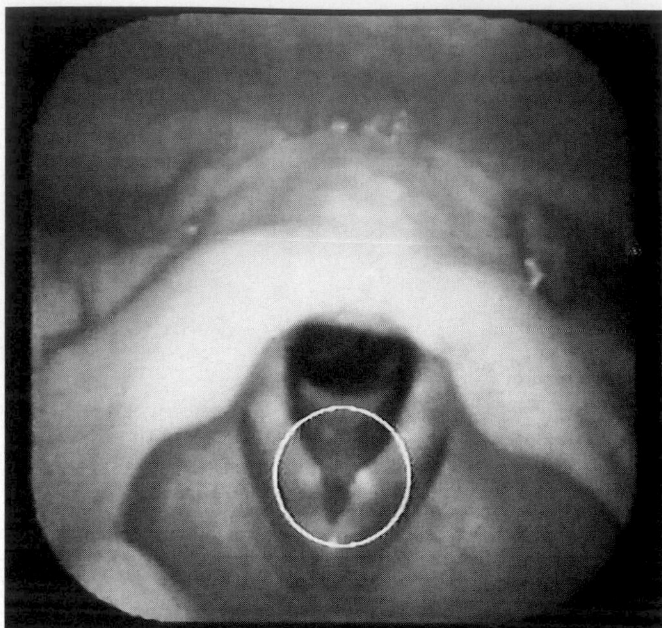

Figure 25.12 *Kissing nodules.*

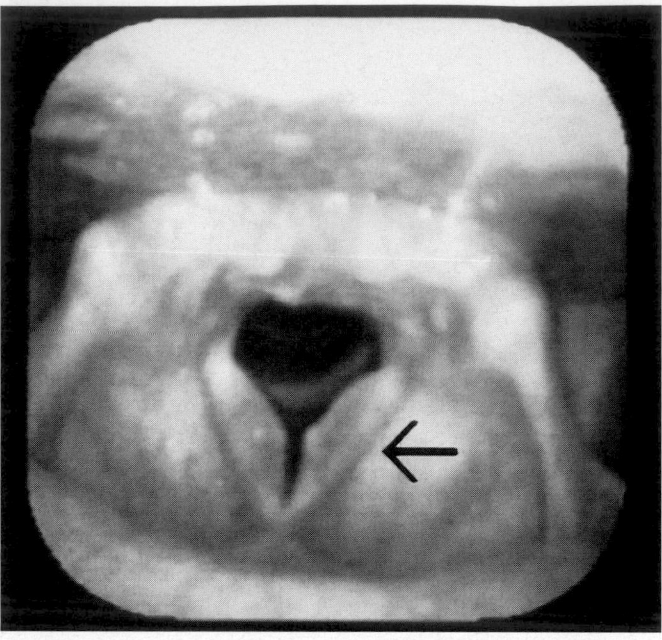

Figure 25.13 *Polypoid cord.*

The clinical signs of the premenstrual syndrome are:[1,34]

- voice fatigue;
- a narrow register, with a loss of high tones and of pianissimo in singers. The low tones are rarely affected;
- a loss of vocal power; and
- a loss of certain high harmonics, with a more metallic and husky voice.

The above signs are frequently associated with other well known signs such as increased nervousness, irritability, pelvic pains, a bloated sensation and asthenia.[29,31]

Dynamic vocal exploration by televideolaryngoscopy and spectrography shows:

- congested vocal cords;
- frequent microvarices on the superior surface of both cords;
- edema of the posterior third of the cords and of the cricoarytenoid joint;
- a less supple epithelium, with a vibration of decreased amplitude, and a vibratory asymmetry quite visible on stroboscopy;
- a lowering of the muscular tone;
- a diminished power of contraction of the vocal muscle;
- a narrow register; and
- vocal cord nodules (Fig 25.12). These nodules are bilateral and symmetrical and are usually almost asymptomatic. They are located on the middle third of the cords and lead to a lowering of the register by about two to three tones, giving a 'blues' voice.

Stroboscopy reveals asymmetric cordal vibrations, with a lack of synchronism and a low amplitude.[24,48,49,51]

Let us remember that the singers of the Opera of La Scala di Milano used to have 'grace days'. They were not asked to sing during the premenstrual period and while menstruating, but they were still paid.

The premenstrual voice syndrome may be explained by the impact of estrogens and progesterone on the vocal musculo–mucosal complex and the resultant rheological, vascular, hydration, secretory and energetic effects.[47] The involvement of aldosterone has often been raised, but is controversial.[46,52] Progesterone and estrogens have a synergistic effect.[50] Attempted explanations of the rheological effects on tissues have included the progesterone/aldosterone ratio and the progesterone/estrogen ratio, but there is no definitive answer as yet. Objectively, one can note:

- a loss of tone in all striated muscles (the vocal muscles, the abdominal muscular belt and the intercostal muscles resulting in reduced pulmonary puff);
- edema in the interstitial tissues and in Reinke's space. This edema is normally reversible, but less so in smokers, who, after some years, develop Reinke's edema or pseudomyxoma (Fig 25.13) that leads to a male voice due to vocal cord thickening. It may occur in women from the age of 35, but never after the menopause. A woman who has not suffered from pseudomyxoma before her menopause will never suffer from it;
- a dilatation of the microvarices that may be complicated by small ruptures leading to a hematoma. This explains why vocal professionals should abstain from taking aspirin at this time (Fig 25.14); and
- a relaxation of the cardia muscles constituting the angle of Hiss, leading to occasional episodes of gastro-

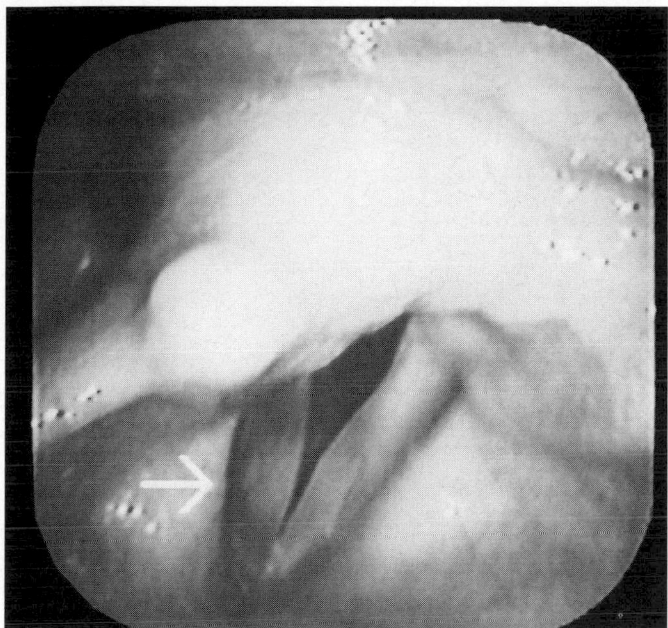

Figure 25.14 *Slight hemorrhage of the right vocal fold, 2 days before menses.*

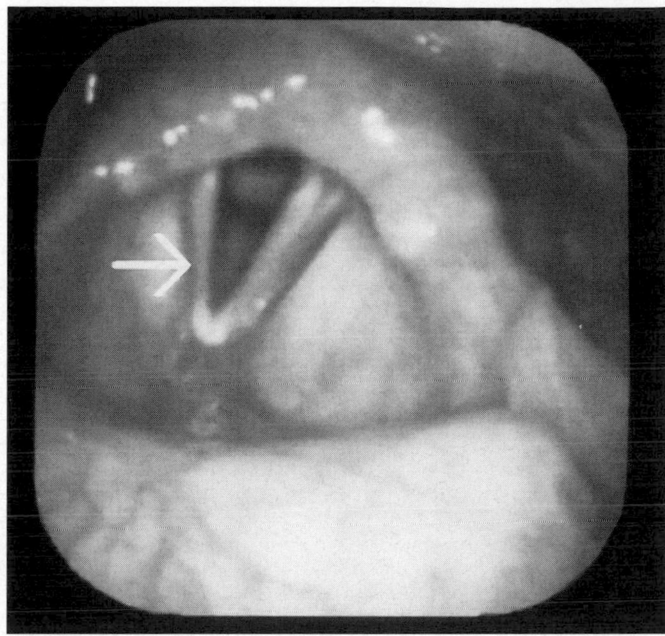

Figure 25.15 *Atrophy of the right vocal fold.*

esophageal reflux. This acid reflux may cause a posterior laryngitis with edema of the posterior third of the vocal cords and a reduced mobility of the edematous cricoarytenoid joints.

The respiratory, pulmonary and nasopharyngeal mucosa is also subject to allergic inflammatory effects. During the premenstrual period, a tenfold increase in allergenic response is noted in 2% of patients.

Hence, the estrogen–progesterone effect leads to a thickening of the laryngeal mucus, frequent throat clearing and a reduction of hydration of the free edges of the cords. Vocal lubrication is reduced and vocal fatigue becomes apparent after about 25–30 minutes of phonation.

The menopausal voice syndrome

In menopause, the hormonal climate is greatly modified and results in changes in the voice.[2,3] We are witnessing the hormonal earthquake of the 50-year-old woman. The periods become irregular and vary in quantity as the progesterone impregnation is reduced at premenopause. At menopause, the disappearance of ovarian follicles leads to the definitive end of menstruation and of progesterone secretion.[6,7] The hypothalamohypophyseal axis is greatly disturbed and there is an increase in FSH and LH secretions to stimulate the ovary. The ovary becomes a curious endocrine organ, as its secretions change, consisting not only of estrogens but also of male hormones. Henceforth, androgens are free to act.[15,17]

The effects of androgens are multiple.[26,32,38] They act on the cerebral cortex, especially on the left hemisphere, on the genital organs (uterus, ovaries, breasts), on sebaceous glands, on striated muscles, and hence on the vocal muscles. This has been demonstrated by the study of smears of the vocal cords and cervical smears, where there is a striking parallelism: there is a relative mucosal atrophy but there is also a muscular atrophy that worsens with age and with diminished use of the voice (Fig 25.15). Glandular cells in the sub- and supracordal mucosa become rarer. Hence there is reduced hydration of the free edges of the cords.[13] There is a dryness during phonation, leading rapidly to vocal fatigue and to dysphonia.

The clinical signs of the menopausal voice syndrome are:

- a lowering of vocal intensity;
- a vocal fatigue;
- a narrow register with a loss of high tones; and
- a loss of melody in the spoken and the speaking voice ('I have lost the color of my voice').

The evolution of the vocal syndrome is very progressive and is specially noticed in voice professionals: first by popular singers, opera singers and comedians, then by barristers, hostesses and finally by school teachers. This imperceptible vocal evolution is noticed in sharp tones and in pianissimos. Many women consult much more because they are worried than because of objective vocal symptoms. These voice professionals act as if the hormonal earthquake caused by the menopause destabilizes the whole of their emotional and vocal self.

There are direct vocal signs, but also indirect signs affecting all the psychologic makeup that can be so fragile at this particular time of a woman's life. The vocal smears as well as the cervical smears show a mucosal subatrophy with basophils and an important reduction of glandular cells.

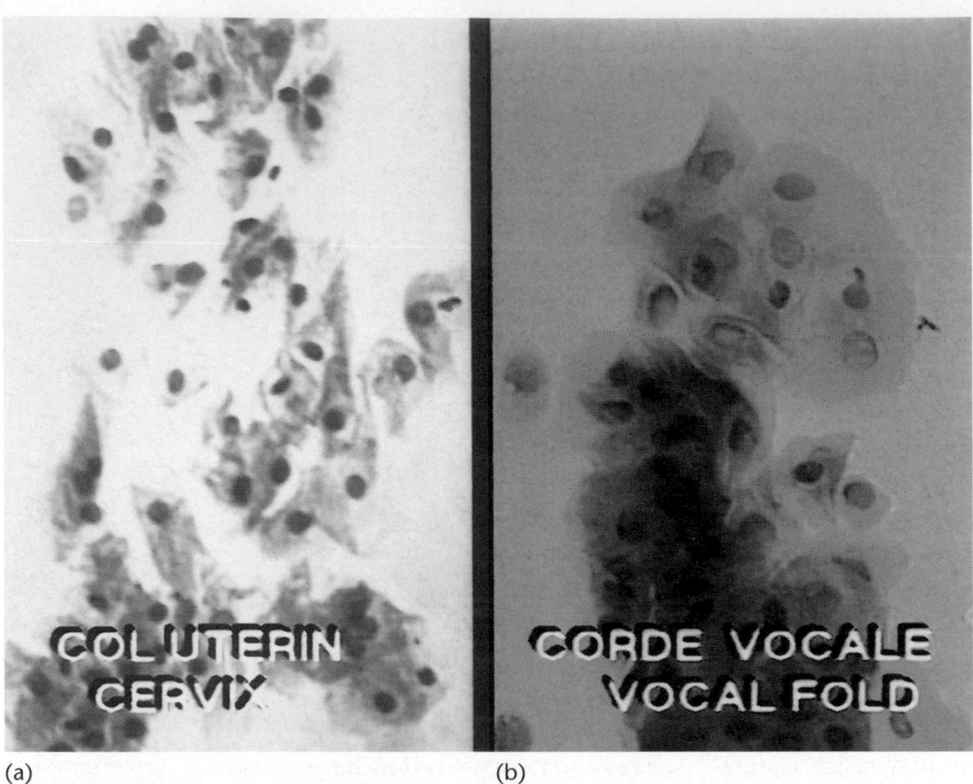

(a) (b)

Figure 25.16 *Smear test at menopause: (a) cervix; (b) vocal fold.*

The following signs are noted:

- during dynamic vocal exploration, acoustically, a slight loss of speed in staccato tones and, at the extreme ranges of the register, a loss of intensity, a narrow register and a loss of formants in the high tones (hardly noticeable in the day-to-day spoken voice), and, anatomically, less supple vocal cords, with a thinner mucosa and a reduced vibratory amplitude; and
- a vocal fold cytology in accordance with the cervical smear and showing a subatrophic mucosa with basophils and a reduction in glandular cells in the mucosa of the ventricular band (Fig 25.16).

In some patients, the following signs are also observed:

- the start of a unilateral muscular atrophy;
- a bilateral muscular atrophy;
- a thinning of the vocal cord mucosa with a reduction in amplitude during phonation and an asymmetry between the right and left cords noted during stroboscopy;
- the mucosa loses its pearly white appearance and becomes dull with, sometimes, some microvarices becoming visible at premenopause;
- the cricoarytenoid joints move normally, but this diminishes after the age of 65 years, with a loss of the suppleness of the ligaments and some arthrosis; and
- the electrolaryngogram is less strong and is irregular, bearing witness to the reduced resistance of the interglottic vibrations.

The spectroacoustic analysis of the voice shows:

- a 20–30% power reduction in the calling voice, the projected voice and the singing voice;
- a narrow register with the loss of some frequencies. This seems to vary with individual cases. The vocal athletes such as singers and comedians may find that two or three tones are altered, but for them, this may be of dramatic importance; and
- the timbre appears to be flat and colorless as some harmonics have been lost.

The author considers menopausal patients to fit two broad types: the 'Modigliani' type, rather thin, with little adipose tissue, and the 'Rubens' type, with a rounded figure. What is the importance of this difference?

Since 1976, it has been shown that estrogen synthesis can take place in fatty cells in men and in women.[21] The relation between obesity and the increase in estrone secretion with reference to the subject's age has also been proved. In patients of equal weight, there is a greater secretion at menopause. Cytochrome P450 is responsible for this biosynthesis of estrone from androgens in the fat cells,[35,40,60,72] and the gene involved is *cyp19* (Fig 25.17). At equal body weight, transcription of P450 aromatase in fat cells increases with age. Hence androstenedione and other androgen derivatives are transformed to estrogens in lipocytes. More recently, it has been shown that this transformation not only took place in the lipocytes, but also in the cells of the stroma in contact with, and surrounding, the fat cells. These cells can therefore be

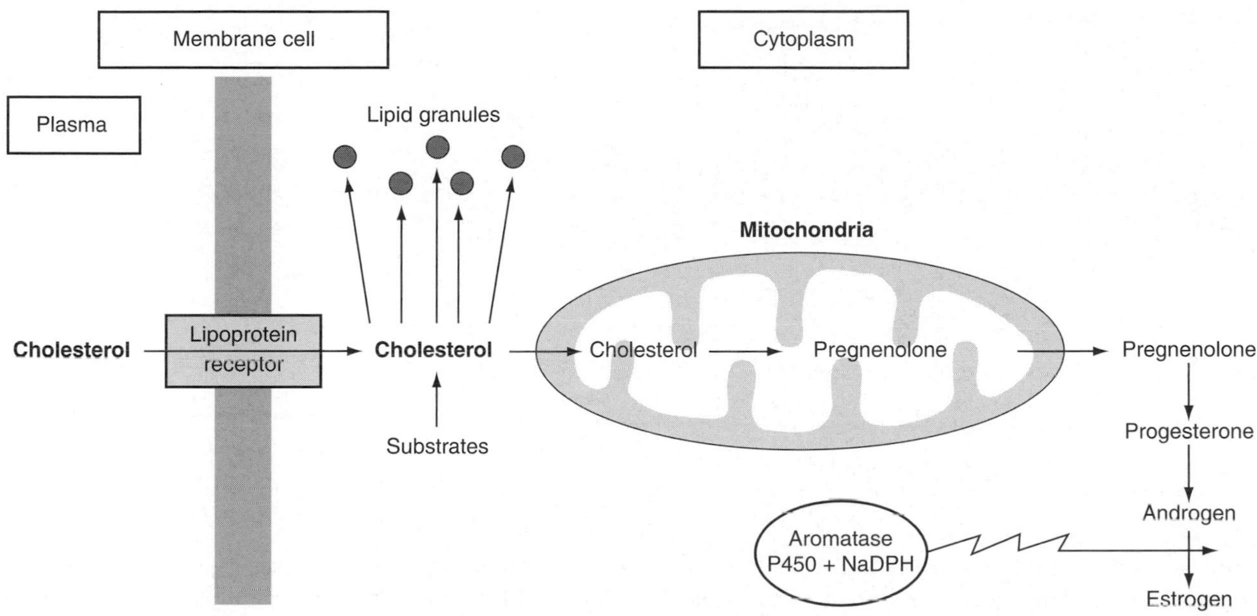

Figure 25.17 *The journey of the cholesterol from the plasma to mitochondria and transformation into sex hormone.*

considered to be 'prelipocytes'. It should be mentioned that this action is increased by glucocorticoids.[21,25,37]

Hence, the major site for estrogen synthesis in the menopausal woman is the lipocyte and the same applies for the obese man.[14,53,55,57,61,64] It seems to be why an obese tenor has a low testosterone level, as the testosterone is trapped by the adipose tissues and undergoes transformation. By contrast, the deep bass with a slim body has a higher testosterone level, as there is no mass of adipose tissue to lead to estrone metabolism.[59] As we grow older, the lean muscle mass diminishes and the fat mass increases, with a new body cell distribution. Glucocorticoids help the increase in the fat mass, thus showing that great care must be taken when prescribing steroids to a menopausal patient.[23]

Estrone is an estrogen with a weaker action on the target organs than estradiol. Its synthesis in the fat cells is multifactorial. It is stimulated by glucocorticoids, by cAMP and its derivatives but is inhibited by many growth factors.

What role does insulin play in all this? The lipocytes possess a cellular membrane with insulin-specific receptors that allow glucose entry into the cells, thus allowing oxidation and lipogenesis. Maintenance of this property allows the absorption of glucose by the specific receptors of these cells. In the middle of the membranes of striated muscle cells, there is a loss of the insulin response with a reduction of insulin receptors. These muscle cells become insulin resistant, insulin secretion increases by the feedback mechanism, resulting in hyperinsulinism. This secondary hyperinsulinism allows fat cells to increase their glucose uptake, as they still have their insulin-specific receptors. There is an increase in the number of fat cells, the obese patient becomes even fatter and the muscle cells become even leaner. Glucocorticoids accelerate this process by causing amyotrophy of the muscle cells and increasing the mass of fat cells, thus contributing to the secondary hyperinsulinism. Fat cells are privileged target organs for glucocorticoids.

An obese menopausal woman possesses important possibilities for the transformation of androgens to estrones and estrone sulfate. Hormone replacement therapy therefore needs careful control, as one needs to watch the risk of a secondary hyperestrogenemia. As the fat cell mass increases, the level of endogenous estrogens also increases. If the hormone replacement dose stays high, it may result in a classical hyperestrogenemia syndrome (tense feeling in the breasts, flatulence, edema, irritability). Each case must be given individual attention.

The 'Rubens' type is certainly much less dependent on hormone replacement therapy than the 'Modigliani' type, but needs closer attention.

The 'Modigliani' patient has little adipose mass, and hence androgens are only slightly transformed to estrones or estrone sulfate, if at all.[67,68,70,71] The androgenic action is strong and is often triggered rapidly. In these cases, we feel that hormonal replacement therapy for voice professionals is essential.[27]

Sex hormonal medication and voice disorders

Anabolic steroids may result in a masculine voice. We do see virilization of the voice after androgenic treatment in women for mammary cancer, and for menstrual or climacteric complaints.

In some athletes for East Europe, anabolic medication was given for muscular performances and asthenia. The tragedy for these women was that these drugs were given

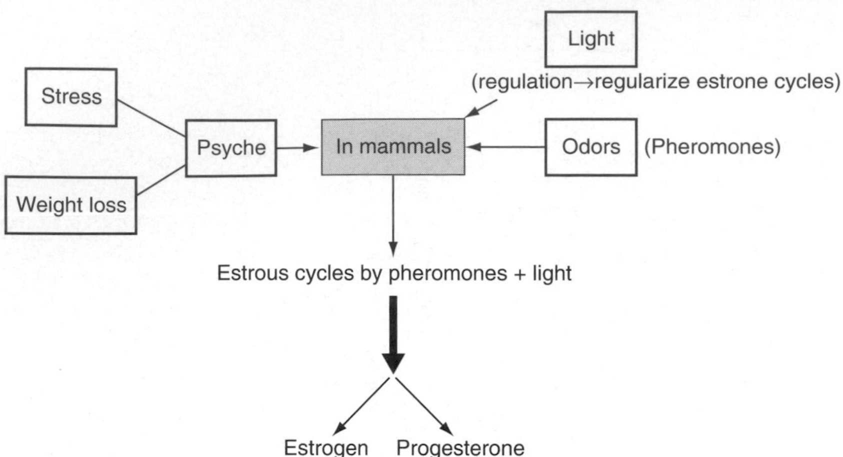

Figure 25.18 *SCN with the suprahypothalamic system.*

around the immediate postpubertal period. Their voices became deeper and hardly came back to normal. These facts point out the importance of anabolic steroids and the impact of male hormones on the voice during the evolution of the human being within the two pillars of the life clock:

- puberty and menopause in women; and
- puberty and andropause in men.

Vocal parameters are disturbed after 2–4 months on androgen drugs. The pitch drops by three to six tones, the register narrows from 2.5 octaves to 1.5 and attaining high notes becomes very difficult.[32]

The therapy is first to stop all androgenic hormones. Unfortunately, most of the vocal changes are usually irreversible. Surgery of the laryngeal framework or endoscopic laser surgery may return the voice to a feminine range.

Current contraceptive pills do not affect the voice. Some of the 'old pills', about 20 years ago, contained synthetic progesterone components with androgenic side effects. They must never be prescribed. Virilization of the female voice with one of the first-generation pills was first reported by Zilstroff in 1965.[73]

Occidental women

In the 1970s, a lot of women wanted to smoke like men, to have their hair cut like men, to dress like men, and, to have a deep voice like men. In the late 1990s, they have become more feminine, but they still have a masculine voice if they smoke. More than before, there are career women: business women, lawyers or journalists. Most of them know how to keep their femininity, but some of them are 'guys in skirts'. These women are often hyperkinetic and have a strained voice production. They were named by Leo Van Gelder and Bergstein in 1970 as being of 'androgenic gestagenic' type.[10]

These women have a tendency to virilization symptoms such as hirsutism, acne, hypomenorrhea. They can be identified by a low estrogen production and are of 'estrogenic type' or still an 'estrogenic gestagenic type'.

This speculative and clinical classification of endocrine-gynecologic types into three different profiles may call to mind the three registers soprano, mezzo-soprano and alto. We have found that androgen levels are higher in altos than in sopranos and that serum calcium levels are more stable in altos than in sopranos. Aldosterone, progesterone and estrogen levels stay reasonably level. The female hormone harmony function is shown in Fig 25.18 with all parameters.

Laryngopathia gravidarum

In our experience, 15% of women have a vocal change during the last 5 months of pregnancy, almost always associated with a rhinitis. In a 1942 study, Schemer had about 20% of women with voice changes during the last trimester of pregnancy.[11]

Intersexuality and voice disorders

Turner's syndrome and Klinefelter's syndrome are the typical examples of intersexuality and voice disorders. Some groups of hermaphrodites have both ovaries and testicles, but this is exceptional. The voice is then under the sole control of the testosterone level, as above 200 µg/dl, the voice is masculine.

The speaking voice may be transformed artificially in transsexuality or homosexuality.

Thyroid disorders

Mechanisms of thyroid hormone action

The thyroid gland has a lot of physiologic effects on fetal growth, obesity and the basic metabolic rate. There are two main impacts: on the cellular differentiation and development, and effects on metabolism reaction.

The syndrome of cretinism in humans demonstrates the thyroid hormone impact during development. But more than that, it suggests that there is an effect during developmental windows in a multifactorial way with other hormones.

During childhood, the thyroid plays a crucial role during puberty. It influences the register of the voice and influences the growth parameters. In adulthood, it will affect the metabolic parameters and its action is measured by the basal metabolic rate. It is increased in hyperthyroidism and decreased in hypothyroidism.

The innervation is provided by the sympathetic and parasympathetic nervous systems. The adrenergic nerve, the sympathetic fibers, come from the superior cervical ganglia. The acetylcholinesterase-positive fibers, the parasympathetic fibers, come from the jugular ganglia. Both the cholinergic and the adrenergic fibers are around the blood vessels, between the thyroid follicles.

This close association between the thyroid follicles, the thyroid vessels (with their laryngeal branches) and the sympathetic and parasympathetic systems probably explains the direct effect of psychoemotional stress on T3 and T4 production. The author has noted thyroid swellings that come and go at times of stress and in some premenstrual syndromes.

Hyperthyroidism

Hyperthyroidism, of which Graves' disease is the most common kind, is due to overproduction of thyroid hormone. It is considered to be of autoimmune etiology and its main symptoms are a goiter and an ophthalmopathy. If the ophthalmic manifestations such as exophthalmus, extraocular muscle hypertrophy, orbital edema and an exposed cornea are serious, this infiltrative ophthalmopathy is independent of the thyroid hormone level in the plasma. Voice disorders are poorly defined and are especially due to muscular hyperstimulation by the elevated levels of thyroxine. There is an increase in the respiratory rate, and a reduction in vital capacity. Anxiety is increased and the voice becomes hoarse and tremulous. The vocal folds look hypervascularized and hyperkinetic.[44] There is also a problem with frequent esophageal reflux associated with gastric hypermotility, that causes a posterior edema of the cords, with a chronic cough and dysphonia.

Hyperthyroidism is very frequently associated with a hypervascular thyroid. In such cases, it has been the author's observation that the vocal folds look hypoxic. This could be explained by a 'laryngeal artery steal syndrome'. The bloodstream is kidnapped by the goiter. The vocal fold muscles are weak and a vocal fatigue occurs. Examination of the vocal folds shows a glottic chink during phonation with a loss of amplitude in the vibrations of the epithelium, resulting in a hoarse and breathy voice. A high pitch is very hard to maintain, low pitches are weak but possible. Similar observations have been made after total thyroidectomies where the laryngeal arteries have been ligated (personal observations).

Hypothyroidism

Hypothyroidism is due to lack of production of thyroxine. If congenital and untreated, it will lead to cretinism and a small larynx. The voice is hoarse and the hearing is decreased. The speech is slow, hesitant and movements are clumsy. The exploration of the larynx shows cramps of the vocal folds and muscle stiffness. The vocal folds are rarely hypertrophied, but the epithelium is dry and has a narrow amplitude during vibrations. There is a mucinous edema.

The cricoarytenoid joint is stiff and pain may appear during speaking. The vocal folds are pale and in some patients, there may be an edema of Reinke's space.

There is a voice fatigue and a weak intensity. The register is narrow and confined to low tones. The maximum phonation time is reduced.

Respiration is altered with dyspnea and shortness of breath, nasal congestion, and low oxygen saturation, which is worsened by sleep apnea. Sleep apnea is unavoidable because of enlargement of the tongue, hypertrophy of oropharyngeal muscles with interstitial edema and muscle fiber enlargement, respiratory muscle weakness and depression of the respiratory center.

Hypophyseal disorders

Growth hormone

Growth hormone insufficiency

The body appearance is abnormal. The bones are small. There is a protuberant forehead, with very small hands and feet, and a small skull. The skin is thin. Some males may have a microphallus. The striated muscles are small and slim. However, the fat/muscle-mass ratio and the weight/height ratio tend to be normal during prepuberty.

The voice in childhood and in male adults is rather peculiar. The resonance cavities are abnormal. The sinus cavities and the nasal fossae are small. Dental eruption is delayed and permanent teeth are irregularly positioned. Bone aging is also very delayed. The lungs are also small.

The thyroid cartilage stays childish for a long time. The epithelium is thin and the amplitude of vibrations during phonation is not wide.

The vocal fold muscle is thin and short. The voice has a high pitch (thin epithelium and slim and short thyroarytenoid muscle) and the intensity is satisfactory. The register is correct. In males, we observe a childish vocal spectrum, whilst in women, there is an almost normal female spectrum. However, both show a lack of harmonics with childhood formants.

Growth hormone excess

Hypersomatotropism and acromegaly. Connective tissue grows in the entire body as a result of excess GH secretion. The disease is very easy to recognize through the skin and connective tissue transformation: there is facial tissue swelling and acromegaly, a fat, wet, handshake, an important hypertrophy of distal bones (hands and feet), a gigantism in all the skeleton (coastal bones, inferior and superior maxillary, frontal bone protuberance, vertebral bones, joints).

The skin is hairy in women, with abundant sweating because of sebaceous gland hypertrophy.

There is an important androgen-like effect except on striated muscles and gonadal development at puberty. Cartilage growth is prolonged. The body proportions are eunuch-like. The liver, kidneys, thyroid gland and other internal organs are all increased in size. There is often a thickening of the cardiac ventricular wall and septum, which results in hypertension.

The vocal tract presents abnormalities.

The resonance cavities

- The skin of the face and the lips are thickened.
- The sinus cavity increases. There is often a prognathism.
- The soft palate and uvula are enlarged and thickened.
- The nasal and oropharyngeal tissues are very thick and less flexible.

The laryngeal anomalies (observations based on personal patients)

- The epiglottis is huge.
- The thyroid cartilage is increased and soppy.
- The mobility of the cricoarytenoid joint is impaired.
- The vocal folds have a very thick epithelium with a normal vibration, and a long thyroarytenoid muscle.

The respiratory functions

The respiratory functions are weak.[54] The voice is deep, of low intensity and narrow register, but the harmonics and formants are satisfactory.

Gonadotrophic disorders

Gonadotrophic adenoma

In men

A lack of LH secretion (because of a physical compression of the cells by the adenoma so that the hormones are not able to go in bloodstream), will result in a lack of testosterone. This leads to a decreased libido with asthenia. Intensity of the voice is weak, the register becomes narrow, the pitch does not change, the voice has fewer harmonics and the timbre is insipid.

In women

The voice does not change, but there is an indirect consequence on the voice, a reduced muscular tone in the vocal fold, resulting from the impact of other hormones such as ACTH or TSH.

Hypergonadotrophic disorders

In men

High FSH levels are almost always associated with testicular failure. Hypoandrogenous symptoms appear such as gynecomastia, defects of spermatogenesis and a falsetto voice.

The testicular gland is smaller than a normal one by some 40%. Klinefelter's syndrome XXY is the most common etiology. This genetic disease is associated with structural abnormalities: long bones, excessive growth, very high levels of FSH and LH.

The testosterone/estradiol ratio is elevated. The testicle is an important secretor of estradiol.

- The larynx is lengthened, with long, thin cords. The arytenoids are less mobile.
- The voice has a narrow register. It lacks timbre as well as power.

Similar symptoms are observed in mosaic patients 46XY/XXY and also in 46XX males in morphotype.

Noonan's syndrome is very rare. Here, LH and FSH levels are high and the testicular secretion is low. There is mental retardation and cryptorchidism. It is an autosomal dominant syndrome 46XY. As there is a similarity in physical profile with Turner's syndrome with webbed neck, short stature, it is also known as the male Turner's syndrome. Voice is affected because of a depressed nasal bridge, a high arched palate, dental malocclusion, pectus excavatum and hypotonia. It is a female voice, with vocal atonia, a narrow register and a shift of the register in the high tones.

Infection with the mumps virus may lead to testicular failure. Usually, it is a failure of spermatogenesis, but sometimes the testosterone producing Leydig cells may also be damaged. There is lack of testosterone and the voice is like a pseudo 'castrato'.

These symptoms may also appear in males with diminished blood flow to the testicles, with bilateral testicular torsion, chemotherapy, or irradiation before puberty.

After puberty, the voice lacks strength, but the register stays male.

The most severe testicular deficiency is due to a pathology of both testicles. Exceptionally, it may be due to a problem with gonadotrophins, receptors, or antibodies.

In women

The FSH level is greater than twice normal during the follicular phase. There is a hypoestrogenic syndrome with amenorrhea. When these symptoms appear before 40 years of age, it is an early menopause or a premature ovarian failure.

LH is also high. There is no progesterone, and a very low level of estrogens.

- The vocal symptoms are similar those of menopause, but more dramatic.
- The pathognomic signs are: hot flushes with insomnia, vaginal dryness.
- In these women, menopause appears before menarche!
- It may be observed after irradiation or chemotherapy.
- Autoimmune diseases may be involved. Antibodies to

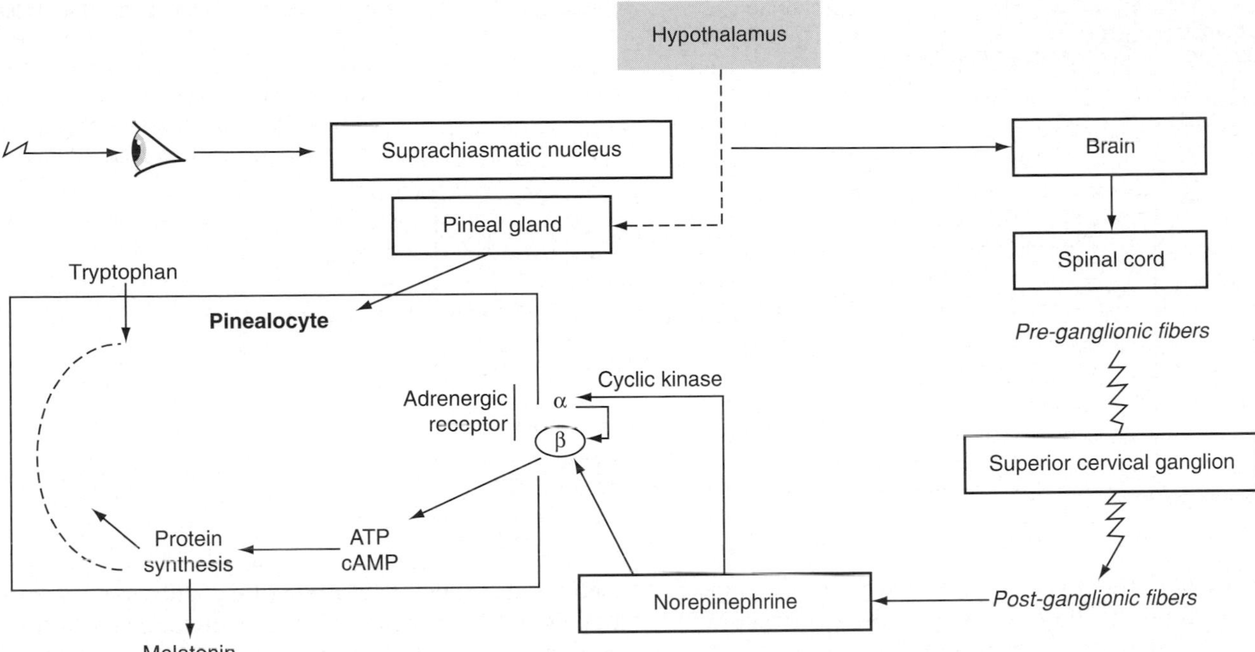

Figure 25.19 *The conductor: hypothalamus.*

both the FSH receptors and the LH receptors have been found in patients during suffering from lupus erythematosus.[57]

Hypogonadotrophic disorders

In men

Lack of testosterone with low or normal levels of FSH and LH indicate abnormal hypothalamic function resulting in alterations in quantity and rhythm of the GnRH production. The voice is less powerful, more high pitched and weak, just like a senile voice. This is due to a paring down of the bulk of the vocal muscle, giving the high voice, and a thinning of the epithelium causing a loss of vibratory amplitude and hence of vocal power.

In women

These patients usually suffer from insomnia, a chronic illness or too much emotional stress, indulge in excessive physical exercise like athletes, or have lost or put on too much weight. Basically, they have suffered from a major physical or mental upheaval. The harmony of these hypothalamic secretions with the environment is fundamental and may be destabilized by external or internal aggressions: for example, stage fright may induce in a voice professional many responses, some positive and some negative. She may lose her vocal timbre because of an epinephrine-induced vasoconstriction; she may become amenorrheic through inhibition of FSH and LH secretion; she may also give a once in a lifetime performance because of the doping effect of endorphines from her own hypothalamus.

In the polycystic ovarian syndrome (PCOS), androgen excess is the typical sign with amenorrhea or oligomenorrhea usually starting at adolescence. This leads to an irreversible masculinization of the voice.[65]

Hypothalamus

Disorders of the hypothalamus affect the larynx via the pituitary gland (Figs 25.19 and 25.20).

Pineal gland

The pineal gland is an endocrine gland in mammals whilst in fish, it is photoreceptive. The natural history of pineal gland through evolution explains the photoreceptive cells in pinealocyte.

The main role of this gland is to organize the body rhythms and the light–dark cycles by inducing the secretion of pineal hormone melatonin. Melatonin is also secreted by the retina and the gut.

Melatonin is secreted by the influences of the SCN, the clock of our body synchronized with the retina. It is synthesized during the dark phase of the day. It effects the CNS and most of these actions come from that target. Melatonin influences the GnRH secretion.

It has an effect on the quality of the voice at different times of the day and night.

Parathyroid disorders

Hypoparathyroidism causes hypocalcemia. It stops or slows down the calcification of the larynx and may cause

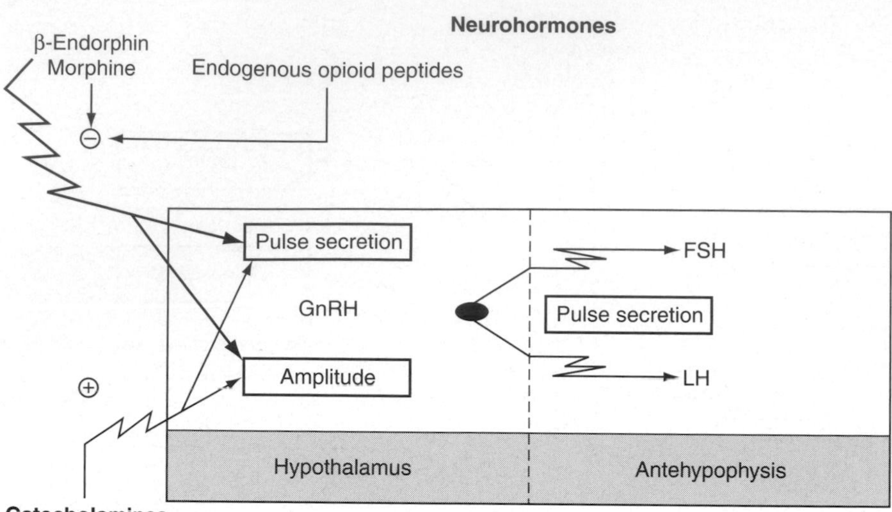

Figure 25.20 *Impact of the neurohormones. Gonadotropin-releasing hormone (GnRH), or LHRH (luteinizing hormone releasing hormone), is a decapeptide produced by the hypothalamic gland or, more precisely, hypothalamic neurons.*

osteomalacia. The hypocalcemia may cause muscle cramps, hyperexcitability and spasmodic contractions. It may lead to lethal complications such as laryngospasm or a heart attack.

Voice fatigue, hoarseness, stridor and, rarely, aphonia are observed. Stridor, arrhythmia and muscle fatigue with spastic muscle contraction are signs of hypocalcemia. It may lead to paresthesia, circumoral tingling and, ultimately, tetany. Chvostek's sign will help for the diagnosis of a stridor and hoarseness, such as Trousseau's sign (a compression of the vessels of the upper arm gives a tetanic state). Videolaryngoscopy shows the development of a vocal fold tetany when the subject is asked to hold an 'aaa'. In emotional stress, these symptoms are increased because the patient 'consumes' more and more calcium when stressed, and also because of less blood supply due to the vasoconstriction.

In artists and voice professionals, these signs must be looked for to avoid and prevent such accidents before going on stage by giving calcium therapy and parasympathetic therapy.

Hyperparathyroidism causes hypercalcemia, with gastrointestinal, renal, musculoskeletal and central nervous systems disorders. Weakness and hyporeflexia are observed, such as dysphonia with aphonia.[65]

Adrenal disorders

Addison's disease is a deficiency of the adrenal cortex with hypoproduction of cortisol and aldosterone. Weakness, muscular adynamia, a weak larynx and dysphonia are observed.[42]

The adrenal cortex gland controls the tonus of striated muscles by controlling the supply of energy to the muscle cells.

In hyperproduction of adrenal cortex hormones, the voice is stronger, the male voice is powerful with a wide register, and the female voice is more often a contralto with a powerful musculature. The child with signs of virilization, also called 'Hercules child', is observed in cases of hyperproduction of hormones of the adrenal cortex.

In adrenal insufficiency, the subject is weak, always tired, the muscular toxins cannot be eliminated. The voice is normal for 10 minutes and then, suddenly, it breaks, with a husky voice leading to aphonia. The vocal folds move for a few minutes and then stop, almost like an intermittent claudication. The vocal fold muscles soon become pathologic, showing the importance of the energy necessary to run these muscles, especially the posticus or posterior cricoarytenoid muscles. Shouting and singing become almost impossible and the register becomes very narrow. It is easier for the patient to speak in a reclined position than in a standing position.

These symptoms demonstrate that epinephrine is the antidote to muscle fatigue. Frequently, there is also an associated hypothyroidism.

Diabetes mellitus

Diabetes mellitus is the disease resulting from a disorder of the endocrine part of the pancreas. More than 10 million people in the USA and 14 million in Europe are diabetic. This pathology is a defect in the metabolic pathways of glucose.

Coronary artery disease and eye problems such as diabetic retinopathy with microaneurysms, conjunctival and iridial hemorrhages resulting in glycogen deposits, depigmentation and neovascularization, are the most dramatic complications. Neural pathology may present as an acute or chronic peripheral neuropathy, involving the limbs as well as the cranial nerves in the head and neck. The autonomic nervous system may also be concerned.

As far as voice disturbance is concerned, involvement of the spinal cervical nerves is the most commonly observed mononeuropathy. It causes vocal fatigue because of pain, sensory loss, weakness of the cervical muscles as well as because of an alteration of sympathetic and parasympathetic function. Exceptionally, attack of the third, fifth, sixth, seventh, eighth, and twelfth cranial nerves have been described.[18,22] The vagus nerve is rarely involved, but may cause a vocal fold dysfunction such as a paresis or a paralysis.

The dysphonia can be associated with dysphagia and food inhalation. This vocal fold paralysis may be seen with a peripheral lesion of the vagus nerve or a nuclear or supranuclear disease.[58] In a case of vocal fold paralysis or paresis, a test of carbohydrate metabolism must be done to rule out diabetes. Indeed, apart from neuropathy, diabetes may also give capillary pathology and a poor oxygenation of the vocal fold muscles, with 'cramps of the larynx' and a very important vocal fatigue.

Voice disorders may also occur because of a hearing loss caused by diabetes. So, in these patients, when there is a dysphonia, an audiogram should always be carried out. In infective laryngitis with reflux, the role of diabetes is critically important. Healing may be a problem if this patient is not treated with very particular attention.

Conclusions

This chapter would not be complete if mention was not made of an article in *Nature* on 16 February 1995. Shaywitz *et al.*[62] showed that in man, the cerebral projection of speech was not only on the left hemisphere but also on the right side, the side of emotions.

The vocal imprint is characteristic to each individual. It reveals the individual's personality and translates his/her emotions. The voice evolves with age and is hormone-dependent in women. Castrato and the changes in a woman's voice bear witness to the importance of the hormonal impact.

The human voice is movement, sex, charming and sensual. It evolves with age, the scars of life, its joys and its emotions.[12]

The voice is in the space–time continuum and our conscience controls it. Nevertheless, the human voice remains intangible.

Acknowledgment

The author wishes to thank Dr Serge Maurice for his efforts on revising the manuscript.

References

1. Abitbol J. Vocal cord hemorrhages in voice professionals. *J Voice* 1988; **2:** 261–6.
2. Abitbol J. *The Female Voice.* [Movie of 27 min]. San Diego: Singular Pubishing Group, 1996.
3. Abitbol J, Abitbol P. *The Feminine Voice and the Cycle of Life.* [Movie of 24 min]. San Diego: Singular Publishing Group, 1998.
4. Abitbol J, Abitbol P, Abitbol B. Sex hormones and the female voice. *J Voice* 1999; **13:** 424–46.
5. Abitbol J, De Brux JK, Millaud G, Felgeres A. Does a hormonal vocal cord cycle exist in women? Study of vocal premenstrual syndrome in voice performers by videostroboscopy-glottography and cytology on 38 women. *J Voice* 1989; **3:** 157–62.
6. Adashi EY. The climacteric ovary: an androgen-producing gland. In: Adashi EY, Rock JA, Rosenwabs Z, eds. *Reproductive Endocrinology, Surgery, and Technology*, Vol. 2. New York: Lippincott-Raven, 1996: 1745–57.
7. Applegarth LD. Emotional implications. In: Adashi EY, Rock JA, Rosenwabs Z, eds. *Reproductive Endocrinology, Surgery, and Technology*, Vol. 2. New York: Lippincott-Raven, 1996: 1953–68.
8. Aristotle. *Historia Animalium.* Book 9. Vol. 4. In: Rambaud J. *Thèses de l'Ecole de Médicine de Paris*, 1853.
9. Bremner WJ, Matsumoto AM, Sussman AM, Paulsen CA. Follicle-stimulating hormone and human spermatogenesis. *J Clin Invest* 1981; **68:** 1044–52.
10. Brodnitz FS. Hormones in the human voice. *Bull N Y Acad Med* 1971; **47:** 183–91.
11. Brodnitz FS. Panel discussion I. In: Lawrence VL, Weinberg B, eds. *Transcripts of the Eighth Symposium on Care of the Professional Voice.* New York: The Voice Foundation, 1979: 69–72.
12. Brodnitz FS. Menstrual cycle and voice quality. *Arch Otolaryngol* 1979; **105:** 300.
13. Buchsbaum HJ. *The Menopause.* New York: Springer-Verlag, 1987.
14. Bulun SE, Mahendroo MS, Simpson ER. Aromatase gene expression in adipose tissue: relationship to breast cancer. *J Steroid Biochem Mol Biol* 1994; **49:** 319–26.
15. Chang RJ, Judd HL. The ovary after menopause. *Clin Obstet Gynecol* 1981; **24:** 181–9.
16. Chin WW. Hormonal regulation of gene expression. In: De Groot LJ, ed. *Endocrinology.* Philadelphia: Saunders, 1995: 6–16.
17. Chodzko-Zajko WJ, Ringer RL. Physiological aspects of aging. *J Voice* 1987; **1:** 18–26.
18. Clements RS Jr. Diabetic neuropathy: new concepts of its etiology. *Diabetes* 1979; **28:** 608–11.
19. Darnell J, Lodish H, Baltimore D. *Molecular Cell Biology.* New York: Scientific American Books, 1990.
20. De Kretser DM, Kerr JB. The cytology of the testis. In: Knobil E, Neill J, eds. *The Physiology of Reproduction.* New York: Raven, 1988: 837–932.
21. Edman CD, MacDonald PC. The role of extraglandular estrogens in women in health and disease. In: James VHT, Serio M, Giusti G, eds. *The Endocrine Function of the Human Ovary.* New York: Academic Press, 1976: 135–40.
22. Ellenberg M. Diabetic neuropathy: clinical aspects. *Metabolism* 1976; **25:** 1627–55.
23. Emperaire JC. *Gynécologie Endocrinienne du Praticien*, 5th edn. Paris: Editions Frison-Roche, 1995.
24. Endicott J, Halbreich U, Schacht S, Nee J. Premenstrual changes and affective disorders. *Psychosom Med* 1981; **43:** 519–29.
25. Evans DJ, Hoffmann RG, Kalkhoff RK, Kissebah AH. Relationship of androgenic activity to body fat topography, fat cell morphology, and metabolic aberrations in premenopausal women. *J Clin Endocrinol Metab* 1983; **57:** 304–10.
26. Fedor-Feyberg P. The influence of estrogens on the

well-being and mental performances in climacteric and post-menopausal women. *Acta Obstet Gynecol Scand* 1979; **64**: 1–6.
27. Gambrell RD Jr. The menopause: benefits and risks of estrogen-progestogen replacement therapy. *Fertil Steril* 1982; **37**: 457–74.
28. Gammelhoft S, Kahn CR. Hormone signaling via membrane receptors. In: De Groot LJ, ed. *Endocrinology*. Philadelphia: Saunders, 1995: 49–57.
29. Gates GA, Montalbo PJ. The effects of low dose beta blockade on performance anxiety in singers. *J Voice* 1987; **1**: 105–8.
30. Gougeon A. Dynamics of follicular growth in the human: a model from preliminary results. *Hum Reprod* 1986; **1**: 81–7.
31. Gramming P, Sundbert J, Ternstrom S, Leanderson R, Perkins W. Relationship between changes in voice pitch and loudness. *J Voice* 1988; **2**: 118–26.
32. Grodin JM, Siiteri PK, MacDonald PC. Source of estrogen production in postmenopausal women. *J Clin Endocrinol Metab* 1973; **36**: 207–14.
33. Grossman A, Kruseman ACN, Perry L *et al.* New hypothalamic hormone, corticotropin-releasing factor, specifically stimulates the release of adrenocorticotropic hormone and cortisol in man. *Lancet* 1982; **1**: 921–2.
34. Hammarbäck S, Damber JE, Bäckstrom T. Relationship between symptom severity and hormone changes in women with premenstrual syndrome. *J Clin Endocrinol Metab* 1989; **68**: 125–30.
35. Harada N. A unique aromatase (P-450arom) mRNA formed by alternative use of tissue-specific exons 1 in human skin fibroblasts. *Biochem Biophys Res Commun* 1992; **189**: 1001–7.
36. Harris GW. Neural control of the pituitary gland. *Physiol Rev* 1948; **28**: 139–79.
37. Hauner H, Schmid P, Pfeiffer EF. Glucocorticoids and insulin promote the differentiation of human adipocyte precursor cells into fat cells. *J Clin Endocrinol Metab* 1987; **64**: 832–5.
38. Hemsell DL, Grodin JM, Brenner PF, Siiteri PK, MacDonald PC. Plasma precursors of estrogens II. Correlations of the extent of conversion of plasma androstenedione to estrone with age. *J Clin Endocrinol Metab* 1974; **38**: 476–9.
39. Hodgen GD. The dominant ovarian follicle. *Fertil Steril* 1982; **38**: 281–300.
40. Inkster SE, Brodie AMH. Expression of aromatase cytochrome P-450 in premenopausal and postmenopausal human ovaries: an immunocytochemical study. *J Clin Endocrinol Metab* 1991; **73**: 717–26.
41. Kerr JB, Sharpe RM. Follicle-stimulating hormone induction of Leydig cell maturation. *Endocrinology* 1985; **116**: 2592–604.
42. Luchsinger R, Arnold G. *Voice – Speech – Language. Clinical Communicalogy: its Physiology and Pathology.* Belmont: Wadworth Publishing, 1965.
43. MacDonald PC, Dombroski RA, Casey ML. Recurrent secretion of progesterone in large amounts: an endocrine/metabolic disorder unique to young women? *Endocr Rev* 1991; **12**: 372–401.
44. Malinsky M, Chevrie Muller, Cerceau N. Etude clinique et electrophyiologique des altérations de la voix au cours des thyrotoxicoses. *Ann Endocrinol (Paris)* 1977; **38**: 171–2.
45. McNatty KP, Makris A, DeGrazia C, Osathanondh R, Ryan KJ. The production of progesterone, androgens, and estrogens by granulosa cells, thecal tissue, and stromal tissue from human ovaries in vitro. *J Clin Endocrinol Metab* 1979; **49**: 687–99.
46. Meisfelt RL. The structure and function of steroid receptor proteins. *Crit Rev Biochem Mol Biol* 1989; **24**: 101–17.
47. Montagnani CF, Arena B, Maffulli N. Estradiol and progesterone during exercise in healthy untrained women. *Med Sci Sports Exerc* 1992; **24**: 764–8.
48. Mortota JF. Issues in the diagnosis and research of premenstrual syndrome. *Clin Obstet Gynecol* 1992; **35**: 587–98.
49. Mortola JF. The premenstrual syndrome. In: Adashi EY, Rock JA, Rosenwabs Z, eds. *Reproductive Endocrinology, Surgery, and Technology*, Vol. 2. New York: Lippincott-Raven, 1996: 1635–47.
50. Mortola JF, Girton L, Fischer U. Successful treatment of severe premenstrual syndrome by combined use of gonadotrophin-releasing hormone agonist and estrogen/progestin. *J Clin Endocrinol Metab* 1991; **72**: 252A–F.
51. Mortola JF, Girton L, Beck L, Yen SSC. Diagnosis of premenstrual syndrome by simple, prospective, and reliable instrument: the calendar of premenstrual experiences. *Obstet Gynecol* 1990; **76**: 302–7.
52. Munday M, Brush MG, Taylor RW. Progesterone and aldosterone levels in the premenstrual tension syndrome. *J Endocrinol* 1977; **73**: 21P–22P.
53. Nagamani M, Hannigan EV, Dinh TV, Stuart CA. Hyperinsulinemia and stromal luteinization of the ovaries in postmenopausal women with endometrial cancer. *J Clin Endocrinol Metab* 1988; **67**: 144–8.
54. Neill JD. Prolactin secretion and its control. In: Knobil E, Neill JD, eds. *The Physiology of Reproduction*. New York: Raven Press, 1988: 1379–90.
55. Perel E, Killinger DW. The interconversion and aromatization of androgens by human adipose tissue. *J Steroid Biochem* 1979; **10**: 623–7.
56. Rees Smith BR, McLachlan SM, Furmaniak J. Autoantibodies to the thyrotropin receptor. *Endocr Rev* 1988; **9**: 106–21.
57. Roncari DAK. Hormonal influences on the replication and maturation of adipocyte precursors. *Int J Obes* 1981; **5**: 547–52.
58. Rontal M, Rontal E. Lesions of the vagus nerve: diagnosis, treatment and rehabilitation. *Laryngoscope* 1977; **87**: 72–86.
59. Rubin J, Sataloff RT, Korovin G, Gould WJ. *The Diagnosis and Treatment of Voice Disorders*. New York: Igaku-Shoin Medical Publisher, 1995.
60. Sasano H, Okamoto M, Mason JL *et al.* Immunolocalization of aromatase, 17α-hydroxylase and side-chain-cleavage cytochromes P-450 in the human ovary. *J Reprod Fertil* 1989; **85**: 163–9.
61. Schneider J, Bradlow HL, Strain G, Levin J, Anderson K, Fishman J. Effects of obesity on estradiol metabolism:

decreased formation of nonuterotropic metabolites. *J Clin Endocrinol Metab* 1983; **56**: 973–8.

62. Shaywitz BA, Shaywitz SE, Pugh KR *et al.* Sex differences in the functional organization of the brain for language. *Nature* 1995; **373**: 607–9.
63. Silverman EM, Zimmer CH. Effect of the menstrual cycle on voice quality. *Arch Ortolaryngol* 1978; **104**: 7–10.
64. Strähle U, Boshart M, Klock G, Stewart F, Schütz G. Glucocorticoid- and progesterone-specific effects are determined by differential expression of the respective hormone receptors. *Nature* 1989; **339**: 629–32.
65. Taylor AE, Schneyer A, Sluss P, Crawley WF Jr. Ovarian failure, resistance and activation. In: Adashi EY, Leung CK, eds. *The Ovary*. New York: Raven Press, 1993.
66. Tindall DJ, Miller DA, Means AR. Characterization of androgen receptor in Sertoli cell-enriched testis. *Endocrinology* 1977; **101**: 13–23.
67. Tsai Morris CH, Aquilano DR, Dufau ML. Cellular localization of rat testicular aromatase activity during development. *Endocrinology* 1985; **116**: 38–46.
68. Vermeulen A. The hormonal activity of the postmenopausal ovary. *J Clin Endocrinol Metab* 1976; **42**: 247–53.
69. Vesalius A. *De Humani Corporis Fabrica*. Basel: 1543.
70. Waterman MR, Simpson ER. Regulation of adrenal cytochrome P-450 activity and gene expression. *Rev Toxicol* 1987; **98**: 259–87.
71. Wotiz HH, Davis JW, Lemon HM, Gut M. Studies in steroid metabolism. V. The conversion of testosterone-4-C14 to estrogens by human ovarian tissue. *J Biol Chem* 1956; **222**: 487–91.
72. Ying Zhao, Nichols JE, Buln SE, Mendelson CR, Simpson ER. Aromatase P450 gene expression in human adipose tissue. Role of a Jak/STAT pathway in regulation of adipose-specific promoter. *J Biol Chem* 1995; **270**: 449–57.
73. Zilstroff J. Quoted by: Luchsinger R, Arnold G.[42]

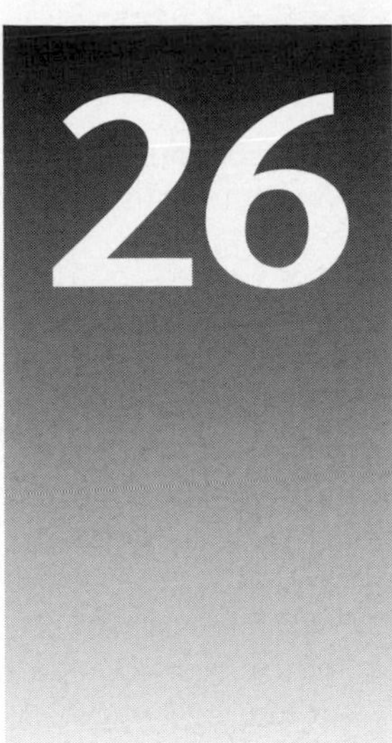

Gastroesophageal reflux and voice disorders

James H Kelly

Although the exact prevalence of gastroesophageal reflux disease (GERD) is not known, a 1976 survey by Nebel and colleagues found that over one-third of the study group reported heartburn on at least a monthly basis and 10% of those surveyed had heartburn on a daily basis.[26,36] Additionally there is a substantial group of patients with esophageal disease who are 'silent' refluxers.[26,36]

Since the late 1960s, GERD in adults has been implicated in a growing number of extraesophageal disorders involving the larynx, pharynx and tracheobronchial tract. These disorders include contact granuloma and ulcer, chronic laryngitis, functional dysphonia, vocal cord nodules, chronic cough, postnasal drip, globus pharynges, laryngeal cancer and asthma, among others.[3,4,6,9,27–29,32,35,37,42,46–48]

In the pediatric age group, in addition to many of the disorders listed above, the spectrum of GERD-related disorders is even more startling and includes laryngospasm, subglottic stenosis, recurrent croup, sudden infant death syndrome (SIDS), otitis media and many more. It is not within the scope of this chapter to cover all disorders; however, excellent articles show the full spectrum of these diseases.[2,3,5,10,13,14,16,27,28,30,45,49] It should be noted that not all investigators recognize this strong association between reflux and laryngeal disease.[11,25,31,43]

Evaluation of this diverse group of GERD-related disorders is further complicated by the findings that at least half the patients with extraesophageal disorders do not have the typical symptoms of heartburn or regurgitation.[9,27,29,42] It seems reasonable, therefore, to identify reflux disease into the categories of GERD and laryngopharyngeal reflux (LPR), a term coined by Koufman,[29]since the symptomatology and pathophysiology appear to be different.

The purpose of this chapter, therefore, is to briefly review normal pharyngoesophageal transit, to review the reflux barriers, to discuss the pathophysiology of GERD/LPR and its relationship to voice disorders and finally to discuss the diagnosis and treatment of GERD/LPR in an otolaryngology setting.

Normal pharyngoesophageal transit

Normal pharyngoesophageal transit begins when the bolus is presented to the pharynx by the posterior motion of the tongue. The transit of the bolus through the pharynx requires the sealing off of the oral cavity and nasopharynx and the opening of the upper esophageal sphincter (UES). Opening of the UES is accomplished by both the relaxation of the tonically contracted cricopharyngeus muscle (CP) and the upward and anterior movement of the larynx, cricoid and hyoid. Additionally, the airway is protected by the aforementioned laryngeal elevation and three other tiers of closure of the laryngeal aperture.[41] Upon entry into the proximal esophagus, the bolus is propelled distally by primary peristalsis (initiated by the swallow) at approximately 2–4 cm/s. The lower esophageal sphincter (LES) then opens to allow the bolus entry into the stomach. Secondary peristalsis (initiated by esophageal distension) then clears the bolus.

It is evident that the UES, esophageal transit and the LES must play important roles in laryngopharyngeal reflux. These will be considered below.

The reflux barriers

With the development of sensitive pH probes, it became evident that transient periods of reflux, particularly after eating, occurred universally. This phenomenon is known as physiological reflux.[20] [Some authors prefer to use the term gastroesophageal reflux (GER) to distinguish this from GERD. This terminology, however, seems unnecessarily confusing, and the term physiological reflux will be used here.]

Since instances of physiological reflux occur frequently, there must obviously be mechanisms to protect the esophageal mucosa from damage during these episodes. These mechanisms are collectively known as reflux barriers and include the UES, esophageal mucosal resistance, acid clearance and salivary buffering, and the LES. These will each be considered separately.

The UES

The tonic contraction of the UES has been well documented both manometrically and electromyographically.[1,21] This tonic contraction prevents aerophagia, protects against reflux and assures orderly progression of the bolus to the stomach. The tone of the UES is decreased by sleep and general anesthesia[17,18,22] and it could be postulated that these conditions would increase the risk of laryngopharyngeal reflux (LPR). While it was originally thought that acid infusion increased UES tone, further studies failed to show increased tone with acid infusion and, more importantly, showed no increase in tone with spontaneous acid reflux even in patients with proven peptic esophagitis.[20] Likewise, while distension of the esophagus using a small balloon increases tone, distensions of long segments of the esophagus, using either long balloons or gas, decrease UES tone.[18] Inspiration increases UES tone (to prevent aerophagia) as does stress.[17,21-23]

Thus, while in most circumstances the UES is an effective barrier to LPR, certain circumstances, mentioned above, can reduce UES tone and make this barrier easier to overcome.[44]

Esophageal mucosal resistance

As with the esophagus, the stomach and the duodenum are exposed to an acid/pepsin environment and need protective mechanisms to prevent cellular damage. In the stomach and duodenum the first line of defense against acid is the pre-epithelial layer consisting of a mucous layer, an unstirred water layer and surface bicarbonate.[28,29,38] The mucous layer acts primarily as a mechanical barrier although it also prevents pepsin from penetrating to the surface of the epithelium. The unstirred water layer and surface bicarbonate ions neutralize hydrogen ions very effectively.[38] These pre-epithelial factors do not seem to be active in the esophagus which must therefore depend on epithelial and post-epithelial factors to protect the esophageal mucosa. Epithelial factors include the cell membrane and intercellular junctional elements. Post-epithelial factors include blood supply and tissue acid buffers. Despite the lack of a pre-epithelial barrier, esophageal epithelium can withstand a direct contact with HCl at pH 2 for several hours without sustaining damage.[38]

A full discussion is beyond the scope of this chapter, but can be obtained in the excellent review by Orlando.[38]

Acid clearance and salivary buffering

Acid clearance and salivary buffering are factors which limit the amount of time acid remains in contact with the esophagus.

During an episode of reflux, the esophagus can clear over 90% of the volume of the reflux by secondary peristalsis. Whilst this reduces the volume of reflux, pH may remain low until swallowing is initiated, bringing saliva with a high bicarbonate concentration into the esophagus by primary peristalsis. This raises the pH and clears the remainder of the reflux.[3,20,29] As will be seen later, deficiencies in these mechanisms can be responsible for esophageal mucosal damage in GERD.

Finally, although these mechanisms are effective in protecting the esophageal mucosa, they offer little or no protection to the upper airway mucosa.

The LES

The LES is the initial and primary barrier to esophageal reflux. Anatomically, the LES consists of an intrinsic sphincter and an extrinsic sphincter. The intrinsic sphincter has been shown to be a thickened ring of smooth muscle in the distal esophagus, measuring approximately 3–4 cm, along with the sling fibers from the stomach.[34,39] The extrinsic sphincter is composed of the crural diaphragm attached to the esophagus by the phreno-esophageal ligament. As with the UES, the LES is tonically contracted.

To be an effective reflux barrier, the LES pressure must adjust to intragastric (and intraabdominal) pressures to maintain a pressure gradient between the stomach and the esophagus. As with the UES, the LES must also open in an appropriate manner to permit the passage of a bolus into the stomach. Both the intrinsic and extrinsic sphincter contribute to this pressure, with the crural diaphragm contributing up to 25% of LES competence.[28] Even with the resection of the intrinsic sphincter, the crural diaphragm can maintain a pressure adequate to prevent reflux.[20] It is likely, then, that in GERD, deficiencies in both the intrinsic and extrinsic sphincter are present.

Pathophysiology of GERD

GERD, according to Katzka and DiMarino,[20] 'must occur in the setting of decreased LES pressure (fixed or transient), with reflux material bathing the esophagus for a prolonged time.' It was formerly thought that patients with GERD universally had decreased LES basal pressure; however, normal LES pressures were observed both in normal subjects with physiologic reflux and patients with mild to moderate reflux. In this setting, reflux was noted to occur during episodes of transient relaxation of the LES, which involved both the intrinsic and extrinsic sphincters. (Transient relaxation is defined as lasting 10–60 seconds and not associated with a swallow or esophageal distension.)[34,39]

Transient relaxations are more common in the postprandial period, particularly after meals that are high in fat content.[34,39] They also tend to occur more in the standing and right decubitus position. Gastric distension also seems to play a role.[34] Not all transient relaxations are associated with reflux, but episodes of reflux associated with transient relaxation are more frequent if there is a hiatal hernia.[34,39]

Transient LES relaxation is now considered the most important factor in GERD. Whilst it would seem logical, it is not known if other factors associated with GERD (such as cigarette smoking and alcohol) are also associated with more frequent transient LES relaxation.

The pathophysiology of esophageal mucosal damage in GERD has also received considerable attention. In addition to the direct effects of the hydrogen ion (acid), pepsin enzymatic damage to cells is an important mechanism in cellular damage.[3,18]

Bile acids also play a role in esophageal mucosal damage. At a pH of 2 bile acids precipitate while at a pH of 7, bile acids are ionized and remain in solution. Between these pH values, a mixture of ionized and precipitated salts exists. Since bile salts must be in a non-polar ionized form to penetrate mucosal cells with resultant damage, therapeutic agents such as H2-blockers and proton pump inhibitors, which increase the pH into this range may be toxic to the epithelial layer.[3,18] It must be noted, however, that extensive experience with these agents have not shown that this mechanism is a clinical problem.[3,39]

Conditions which interfere with salivary buffering, such as xerostomia from radiotherapy would also be expected to influence mucosal damage. Likewise, abnormalities in esophageal peristalsis would also be expected to produce mucosal damage in a selected group of patients.

Although hiatal hernia has been both implicated and exonerated in GERD, recent evidence has shown that the presence of a hiatal hernia both increases the duration of acid exposure and also increases the number of transient episodes of LES relaxation (see above) and is, therefore, much more involved in the pathogenesis of GERD than previously thought.[34]

The relationship of GERD, LPR and voice disorders

Animal studies

Although GERD, by definition, must be present in episodes of LPR, there are differences in pathophysiology and symptomatology that make laryngopharyngeal disorders secondary to reflux unique.

Pathophysiology of LPR

Following their publication of three patients with contact ulcers of the larynx associated with GERD, Cherry and Marguiles applied gastric acid to two dogs daily over a period of 6 weeks and were able to induce vocal cord granulomas in both animals.[4,7] Since this would be equivalent to one episode of LPR daily, this small study suggests the extreme sensitivity of laryngeal mucosa to reflux, even in the absence of prior mucosal damage. In another study, Koufman applied an acid/pepsin mixture to the subglottis of dogs in an area previously denuded of mucosa with a diamond burr. (A group of animals with denuded mucosa and no acid/pepsin was used as a control.) Animals exposed to the acid/pepsin mixture developed non-healing ulceration whereas control animals did not. The animals were only exposed for 3 nonconsecutive days per week.[27] This study suggests that even intermittent non-daily reflux can produce injury, particularly if there is prior mucosal damage. Whilst experimental animal studies are limited, they help to explain some of the clinical studies mentioned below.

Clinical studies

Most clinical studies have focused on the diagnosis of LPR, the association of LPR with laryngopharyngeal signs and symptoms, and therapeutic trials of patients thought to have signs and symptoms related to LPR.

The diagnosis of LPR is difficult. There are a wide variety of tests used in the diagnosis of GERD but most are not applicable to LPR.

Tests used in the diagnosis of GERD include the following:

- barium and acid barium radiography;
- acid perfusion (Bernstein) test;
- esophagoscopy (± biopsy);
- esophageal manometry (± UES manometry);
- scintigraphy;
- single-probe 24-hour pH monitoring; and
- dual-probe 24-hour pH monitoring.

Each of these will be discussed separately.

Barium radiography

Barium radiography has been used for a long time in the diagnosis of esophageal disorders. Strictures, diverticula and tumors are easily demonstrated by this method; however, there is low sensitivity for demonstrating reflux. (Hiatal hernias can be demonstrated, however, and their relationship to GERD is noted above.) By extension, the diagnosis of LPR can seldom be made with barium radiography. The addition of acid barium to this study (an extension of the Bernstein test) has been described by Donner *et al.*[8] This test has proved useful in delineating some causes of noncardiac chest pain, but is not a sensitive indicator of reflux. Barium radiography is most helpful in patients with proven reflux to delineate strictures or esophageal mucosal damage.

The acid perfusion (Bernstein) test

The acid perfusion (Bernstein) test has been used in the past as a test to determine whether the patient's chest pain is due to reflux. Whilst this test has excellent specificity, the sensitivity is poor (36%) and it is therefore not helpful in the diagnosis of reflux.[26]

Esophagoscopy

Esophagoscopy is helpful in delineating strictures and mucosal damage secondary to reflux. It has the additional advantage of being able to sample suspicious areas for Barrett's esophagus, tumors or esophagitis. Since fewer than half of patients with reflux have one of these findings, the sensitivity of this method is poor.

Esophageal manometry

Esophageal manometry is helpful in delineating dysmotility disorders of the esophagus and LES. Dysmotility or hypertensive UES increase the time of acid contact with the esophageal mucosa, making the patient more prone to esophagitis and Barrett's esophagus. Since dysmotility is not universal in GERD/LPR, this test has limited usefulness in the diagnosis of these entities. UES manometry would be a helpful test in determining the integrity of the UES in patients with GERD who might be at risk for LPR. However, whilst strides are being made in the technology and use of UES manometry, there are technical problems that remain to be solved. Except in some centers, therefore, UES manometry has limited usefulness.[21–23]

Scintigraphy

Scintigraphy has been used in determining if refluxed material is aspirated. Results using this method have been disappointing in most patients and the method is not specific or sensitive enough to be helpful in the diagnosis of LPR.[26]

Single-probe 24-hour pH monitoring

This has become the gold standard for the diagnosis of GERD. The probe tube typically contains a manometer for accurate placement (approximately 5 cm above the LES). This test has excellent sensitivity and specificity of 85 and 95%, respectively.[26] In the diagnosis of LPR, however, there are several problems. First, this test cannot determine which episodes of esophageal reflux are also LPR episodes. Secondly, as mentioned above, LPR episodes may be intermittent (not even daily) and thus may be missed on single-probe monitoring. Finally, again as noted above, the mucosa of the laryngopharynx has been shown to be more sensitive to reflux damage and therefore may be a significant factor even in the presence of a normal pH study for the esophagus.[27,29]

Dual-probe 24-hour pH monitoring

This technique has begun to be used by several investigators to overcome the deficiencies of single-probe techniques in the diagnosis of LPR.[15,19,27] In the dual-probe technique, the lower probe is placed 5 cm above the LES (as with the single-probe technique) but there is a proximal probe that is placed either in the hypopharynx, approximately behind the laryngeal introitus or approximately 2 cm below the UES. Either technique will identify patients with LPR that would have been missed with the single-probe technique. The use of these two techniques makes clear the need for standardization. Some investigators have noted a higher incidence of reflux in the standing position in those patients with laryngopharyngeal complaints, but this has not been universally seen. Hypopharyngeal probes have also had some technical problems that have largely been overcome. There has also been concern that a probe through the UES would make a subject prone to LPR by keeping open the UES.[3] Koufman, however, has shown that in normal controls there is no documented reflux.[27] This dual-probe technique is becoming the standard in the investigation of LPR. It should be noted that between 10 and 15% of patients can not tolerate the probe, and a number of patients modify their diet and lifestyle when the probe is in place. This has obvious implications for the sensitivity of this test.

Symptoms and signs of LPR

As has been previously noted, the symptoms of LPR are nonspecific and often vague. Patients may complain of heartburn, regurgitation and chest pain (the most frequent complaints in GERD patients) but most do not. In LPR the most frequently described symptoms relate to the voice as either 'voice problems' or hoarseness. Sore throat, throat pain, nonproductive cough, throat clearing and even postnasal drip appear on most lists of the patient's initial symptoms.

Signs of LPR are likewise nonspecific. Posterior laryngitis, considered the classical laryngeal sign of LPR, is often not present. Laryngeal edema, considered the most frequent sign of LPR, is very observer dependent. Other signs such as vocal cord polyps, nodules, plica ventricularis, leukoplakia and carcinoma are frequently mentioned by clinicians, particularly those with an interest in LPR-related disorders.[27,29]

Thus, according to the large number of articles written on this subject, it could easily be said that any sign or symptom related to the laryngopharynx could be LPR related.

Risk factors for LPR also should be included in this discussion. Alcohol, tobacco, obesity, high-fat diets, eating close to mealtimes, caffeine and numerous drugs are only a few of the risk factors that make a patient prone to LPR (as well as GERD). Again, numerous articles list large numbers of risk factors, making these less helpful in diagnosing LPR.

Therapeutic trials

Because of this nonspecificity of symptoms and signs of LPR and the expense (or unavailability) of dual-probe monitoring, many investigators have advocated therapeutic trials of either alteration of lifestyle, medications or both, to aid in the identification of LPR-related disorders.

Hansen *et al.* have taken a stepwise approach to patients suspected of LPR.[12] The first step is reflux precautions, consisting of avoidance from eating and drinking 3 hours prior to bedtime and elevation of the head of the bed 8–10 inches (3–4 cm). He reports a 51% response rate to these reflux precautions. Of the remaining patients, 54% had good results from 6 weeks of H2-blocker therapy. The remaining 23% of patients were treated with omeprazole (20 mg/day) with an 83% success rate. Overall results were a 96% success rate. Two percent of patients required fundoplication.[12]

The opposite approach is to treat patients with large doses of omeprazole (20 mg twice daily) for 1–3 months with positive results confirming the diagnosis.[29,33] The non-responders underwent an extensive evaluation. Each approach has obvious advantages and disadvantages.

Diagnosis and treatment of LPR-related voice disorders

Diagnosis

Koufman has stated that GERD/LPR is the single most common cause and related cofactor of laryngeal and voice disorders.[29] Even if that estimate is high, it is apparent that a large number of patients presenting to the laryngologist with voice-related problems have GERD/LPR. It behoves the laryngologist, therefore, to have a high index of suspicion in these patients. Sataloff has noted that professional singers are particularly prone to this problem because of their professional lifestyle.[40] These patients must be considered to be at even more risk than the average patient. A careful investigation of risk factors should be undertaken as part of the history or as a patient questionnaire. Patients with severe heartburn or regurgitation should be seen by a gastroenterologist for appropriate diagnostic studies, as mentioned earlier. Patients with no symptoms of GERD should be considered for pH studies, taking into account cost and the availability of these studies. If a therapeutic trial is considered, particularly with attempted modification of lifestyle, the length of treatment, cost and patient compliance must be considered. Therapeutic drug trials should consist of omeprazole 20 mg twice a day for at least 1–3 months, since it has been shown that laryngeal disease does not respond to acid suppressors as rapidly as esophageal disease. H2-blockers may be used as maintenance, but probably do not suppress acid sufficiently in many patients with laryngeal pathology.[24,27,29] Patients who fail the therapeutic trial should be investigated thoroughly in concert with a gastroenterologist.

Treatment

As with the diagnosis of LPR-related disorders, treatment is controversial. Pope has proposed an algorithm for the treatment of GERD, but it does not address patients with primarily or solely laryngopharyngeal symptoms.[39] Other treatment plans differ markedly.

Based on what is known (and not known) about LPR-related voice disorders, each clinician should develop his/her own algorithm that takes into account risk factors, patient compliance, cost and the availability of services (such as dual-probe monitoring). This treatment plan should include consideration of interventions in several areas: lifestyle/dietary modification, pharmacologic therapy and surgical intervention (fundoplication/biopsy).

Any treatment plan should involve careful assessment and reassessment of the patient and, considering the association of LPR and laryngeal cancer by some investigators, prompt selective biopsy of suspicious lesions. Treatment options in each of these areas will be considered below.

Lifestyle/dietary modification

Each patient should be given a list of foods and drinks to be avoided. Inclusive lists have been published in several articles. Counseling should identify risk factors such as smoking, obesity and heavy alcohol use. These areas are hard for the patient to modify and may require professional group or individual therapy of a specialist. A low-fat diet should also be emphasized along with the avoidance of food/drink for 2–3 hours before bedtime. The head of the bed should be elevated 8–10 inches if the patient will tolerate this. It should be emphasized to the patient that these modifications should continue in addition to other therapies.

Pharmacologic therapy

As was noted earlier, there are two main acid suppressive drug classes: H2-antagonists and hydrogen ion pump blockers. The treatment regimens for H2-antagonists consist of either cimetidine 300 mg q.i.d. or ranitidine 150 mg b.i.d. For hydrogen ion pump blockers, omeprazole 20 mg b.i.d. is given. (Some clinicians prefer to start with 20 mg q.d. and increase the dose to b.i.d if there is no response.) Acid suppression should be given for 1–3 months, depending on the response. If there is no response on maximal doses of omeprazole at 3 months, the patient should be reevaluated. If acid reflux is still present, surgical treatment of reflux (fundoplication) should be considered (see below).

If the results of medical therapy are good, maintenance therapy should be considered since there is a high incidence of relapse after discontinuing acid suppression, particularly with patients with LPR.[27,29,39]

The treatment plan for maintenance therapy is also controversial. Chronic acid suppression for periods of up to 5 years, using omeprazole, seems to be safe;[39] however, studies beyond this time period have not been done, since this is a relatively new drug. Recently, cisapride, a prokinetic drug that reduces the duration of acid exposure to the esophagus has been introduced to the treatment regimen. Whilst this drug is useful in both the active treatment of esophageal mucosal damage and the prevention of relapse in GERD,[39] its role in the treatment of LPR has not been defined.

Surgical intervention

The role of surgical treatment of GERD/LPR is still being defined. Laparoscopic fundoplication, which reduces morbidity compared to open procedures, has been successful in the long-term management of those patients who fail medical therapy. This technique is very operator dependent as to efficacy and morbidity and therefore may not be an option in some institutions.

In today's economic climate, the cost of long-term suppressive therapy must also be considered, particularly in young patients who will require many years of therapy. Omeprazole, in a dose of 20 mg b.i.d., costs over US$200.00/month. Cisapride costs approximately US$50.00/month and cimetidine or ranitidine between US$75 and US$95/month.[39] By contrast, the cost of 24-hour ambulatory pH monitoring is approximately US$400. In many patients, H2-blockers do not prevent relapse and are therefore not a choice for a maintenance regimen. Some investigators feel that all LPR patients fit into this category.[27,29] As is mentioned above, there is concern about long-term acid suppression with omeprazole, although it will probably be several more years before this can be adequately assessed. Under these circumstances, it would appear that surgical intervention will begin to play a larger role in the treatment of these patients.

Conclusions

- LPR should be viewed as a separate but related disorder to GERD, and seems to be a cause or a comorbid factor in many patients with voice disorders.
- Long-term dual-probe pH monitoring may well become the 'gold standard' in the evaluation of patients with LPR; however, the test needs to be standardized and is not universally available.
- When dual-probe monitoring is not available or is inconclusive, a therapeutic trial of omeprazole, 20 mg b.i.d. for 1–3 months is reasonable.
- Long-term pharmacologic maintenance therapy is controversial, but seems to require omeprazole in patients with LPR.
- Surgical management may become increasingly important in medical failures, noncompliance with medical therapy, and in the young patient.
- Lifestyle/dietary changes should be utilized in conjunction with any therapy.
- Underlying non-LPR causes of voice disorders (vocal abuse, mucosal damage, etc.) should continue to be addressed.

References

1. Asoh R, Goyal RK. Manometry and electromyography of the upper esophageal sphincter in the opossum. *Gastroenterology* 1978; **74:** 514–20.
2. Bernard F, Dupont C, Viala P. Gastroesophageal reflux and upper airway diseases. *Clin Rev Allergy* 1990; **8:** 403–25.
3. Blaugrund J, Kelly JH. Laryngotracheal manifestations of gastroesophageal reflux disease. *Curr Opin Otolaryngol Head Neck Surg* 1996; **4:** 138–42.
4. Cherry J, Margulies SI. Contact ulcer of the larynx. *Laryngoscope* 1968; **78:** 1937–40.
5. Contencin P, Narcy P. Gastroesophageal reflux in infants and children. *Arch Otolaryngol Head Neck Surg* 1992; **118:** 1028–30.
6. Cote DN, Miller RH. The association of gastroesophageal reflux and otolaryngologic disorders. *Compr Ther* 1995; **21:** 80–4.
7. Delahunty JE, Cherry J. Experimentally produced vocal cord granulomas. *Laryngoscope* 1968; **78:** 1941–7.
8. Donner MW, Silbiger ML, Hookman P, Hendrix TR. Acid barium swallows in the radiographic evaluation of clinical esophagitis. *Radiology* 1966; **87:** 220–5.
9. Fraser AE. Review article: gastro-oesophageal reflux and laryngeal symptoms. *Aliment Pharmacol Ther* 1994; **8:** 265–72.
10. Gomes H, Lallemand P. Infant apnea and gastroesophageal reflux. *Pediatr Radiol* 1992; **22:** 8–11.
11. Hallewell JD, Cole TB. Isolated head and neck symptoms due to hiatus hernia. *Arch Otolaryngol* 1970; **92:** 499–501.
12. Hansen DG, Kamel PL, Kahrilas PJ. Outcomes of antireflux therapy for the treatment of chronic laryngitis. *Ann Otol Rhinol Laryngol* 1995; **104:** 550–5.
13. Hollwarth M, Uray E. Physiology and pathophysiology of the esophagus in childhood. *Prog Pediatr Surg* 1985; **18:** 1–13.
14. Hotaling AJ, Silva AB. Gastroesophageal disease in the pediatric population. *Adv Otolaryngol Head Neck Surg* 1995; **9:** 263–88.
15. Jacob P, Kahrilas PJ, Herzon G. Proximal esophageal pH-metry in patients with 'reflux laryngitis'. *Gastroenterology* 1991; **100:** 305–10.
16. Jindal JR, Milbrath MM, Shaker R, Hogan WJ, Toohill RJ. Gastroesophageal reflux disease as a likely cause of 'idiopathic' subglottic stenosis. *Ann Otol Rhinol Laryngol* 1994; **103:** 186–91.
17. Kahrilas PJ. Functional anatomy and physiology of the esophagus. In: Castell DO, ed. *The Esophagus*, 2nd edn. Boston: Little, Brown, 1995: 1–28.
18. Kahrilas PJ, Dodds WJ, Dent J, Haeberle B, Hogan WS,

Arndorfer RC. Effect of sleep, spontaneous gastroesophageal reflux, and a meal on upper esophageal sphincter pressure in normal human volunteers. *Gastroenterology* 1987; **92:** 466–71.
19. Katz PO. Ambulatory esophageal and hypopharyngeal pH monitoring in patients with hoarseness. *Am J Gastroenterol* 1990; **85:** 38–40.
20. Katzka DA, DiMarino AJ Jr. Pathophysiology of gastroesophageal reflux disease: LES incompetence and esophageal clearance. In: Castell DO, ed. *The Esophagus*, 2nd edn. Boston: Little, Brown, 1995: 443–54.
21. Kelly JH. Use of manometry in the evaluation of dysphagia. *Otolaryngol Head Neck Surg* 1997; **116:** 355–7.
22. Kelly JH, Kuncl RW. Myology of the pharyngoesophageal segment: gross anatomic and histologic characteristics. *Laryngoscope* 1996; **106:** 713–20.
23. Kelly JH, Ravich WJ, Purcell LL, Jones B. Therapy of dysphagia. In: Cummings CW, Frederickson JM, Harper LA, Schuller DE, eds. *Otolaryngology – Head and Neck Surgery*, 2nd edn, Update 1. St Louis: Mosby, 1995: 72–90.
24. Kibblewhite DJ, Morrison MD. A double-blind controlled study of the efficacy of cimetidine in the treatment of the cervical symptoms of gastroesophageal reflux. *J Otolaryngol* 1990; **19:** 103–9.
25. Kjellén G, Brudin L. Gastroesophageal reflux disease and laryngeal symptoms. Is there really a causal relationship? *ORL J Otorhinolaryngol Relat Spec* 1994; **56:** 287–90.
26. Klinkenberg Knol EC, Castell DO. Clinical spectrum and diagnosis of gastroesophageal reflux disease. In: Castell DO, ed. *The Esophagus*, 2nd edn. Boston: Little, Brown, 1995: 435–42.
27. Koufman JA. The otolaryngologic manifestations of gastroesophageal reflux disease (GERD): a clinical investigation of 225 patients using ambulatory 24-hour pH monitoring and an experimental investigation of the role of acid and pepsin in the development of laryngeal injury. *Laryngoscope* 1991; **101(Suppl 53):** 1–78.
28. Koufman JA. Gastroesophageal reflux disease. In: Cummings CW, Frederickson JM, Harper LA, Schuller DE, eds. *Otolaryngology – Head and Neck Surgery*, 2nd edn. St Louis: Mosby, 1993: 2349–67.
29. Koufman JA. Gastroesophageal reflux and voice disorders. In: Rubin JS, Sataloff RT, Korovin GS, Gould WJ, eds. *Diagnosis and Treatment of Voice Disorders*. New York: Igaku-Shoin, 1995: 161–75.
30. Little JP, Matthews BL, Glock MS *et al.* Extraesophageal pediatric reflux: 24 hour double-probe pH monitoring in 222 children. *Ann Otol Rhinol Laryngol Suppl* 1997; **169:** 1–16.
31. Lomasney TL. Hiatus hernia and the respiratory tract. *Ann Thorac Surg* 1977; **24:** 448–50.
32. McNally PR, Maydonovitch CL, Prosek RA, Collette RP, Wong RK. Evaluation of gastroesophageal reflux as a cause of idiopathic hoarseness. *Dig Dis Sci* 1989; **34:** 1900–4.
33. Metz DC, Childs ML, Ruiz C, Weinstein GS. Pilot study of the oral omeprazole test for reflux laryngitis. *Otolaryngol Head Neck Surg* 1997; **116:** 41–6.
34. Mittal RK, Balaban DH. The esophagogastric junction. *N Engl J Med* 1997; **336:** 924–32.
35. Morrison MD. Is chronic gastroesophageal reflux a causative factor in glottic carcinoma? *Otolaryngol Head Neck Surg* 1988; **99:** 370–3.
36. Nebel OT, Fornes MF, Castell DO. Symptomatic gastroesophageal reflux: incidence and precipitating factors. *Am J Dig Dis* 1976; **21:** 953–6.
37. Olson NR. The problem of gastroesophageal reflux. *Otolaryngol Clin North Am* 1986; **19:** 119–33.
38. Orlando RC. Pathophysiology of gastroesophageal reflux disease: esophageal epithelial resistance. In: Castell DO, ed. *The Esophagus*, 2nd edn. Boston: Little, Brown, 1995: 455–68.
39. Pope CE II. Acid reflux disorders. *N Engl J Med* 1994; **331:** 656–60.
40. Sataloff RT. Reflux and other gastroenterologic conditions that may affect the voice. In: Sataloff RT, ed. *Professional Voice: The Science and Art of Clinical Care*. New York: Raven Press, 1991: 179–83.
41. Shaker R. Functional relationship of the larynx and upper GI tract. *Dysphagia* 1993; **8:** 326–30.
42. Traube M. The spectrum of the symptoms and presentations of gastroesophageal reflux disease. *Gastroenterol Clin North Am* 1990; **19:** 609–16.
43. Urschel HC, Paulson DL. Gastroesophageal reflux and hiatal hernia: complications and therapy. *J Thorac Cardiovasc Surg* 1967; **53:** 21–32.
44. Vakil NB, Kahrilas PJ, Dodds WJ, Vanagunas A. Absence of an upper esophageal sphincter response to said reflux. *Am J Gastroenterol* 1989; **84:** 606–13.
45. Waki EY, Madgy DN, Belenky WM, Gower VC. The incidence of gastroesophageal reflux in recurrent croup. *Int J Pediatr Otorhinolaryngol* 1995; **32:** 223–32.
46. Ward PH, Hanson DG. Reflux as an etiologic factor of carcinoma of the larynx. *Laryngoscope* 1988; **98:** 1195–9.
47. Waring JP, Lacayo L, Hunter J, Kata E, Suwak B. Chronic cough and hoarseness in patients with severe gastroesophageal reflux disease. Diagnosis and response to therapy. *Dig Dis Sci* 1995; **40:** 1093–7.
48. Woo P, Noordzij P, Ross JA. Association of esophageal reflux and globus symptom: comparison of laryngoscopy and 24-hour pH manometry. *Otolaryngol Head Neck Surg* 1996; **115:** 502–7.
49. Zalzal GH, Choi SS, Patel KM. The effect of gastroesophageal reflux on laryngotracheal reconstruction. *Arch Otolaryngol Head Neck Surg* 1996; **122:** 297–300.

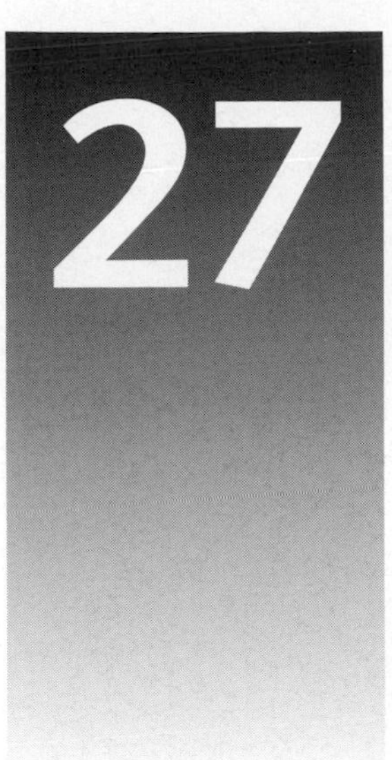

Dysphagia and laryngeal diseases

Abigail Arad-Cohen and Andrew Blitzer

Dysphagia is the subjective symptom of difficulty in swallowing and can be a manifestation of systemic disease or a primary disease of the upper aerodigestive tract at any level. Many disorders produce sensory and/or motor disorder of the oropharynx, hypopharynx, esophagus or larynx, causing dysphagia and/or odynophagia and/or aspiration. Dysphagia can be a manifestation of uncoordination between the various stages of normal swallowing as well as from congenital, inflammatory, infectious or neoplastic conditions. Laryngeal dysfunction from neoplastic or non-neoplastic causes usually presents as dysphonia, or change in quality of voice may present as dysphagia. This chapter deals with dysphagia resulting from diseases involving the larynx and its function, including post-treatment (surgery, irradiation and chemotherapy).

Normal swallowing physiology

Swallowing is produced by a complicated, synchronized system of muscular contractions and relaxation of voluntary and involuntary muscular activity that results in the movement of a bolus of material from the oral cavity, through the pharynx, past the laryngeal inlet, and then into the esophagus. When these events are disordered, aspiration, choking, nasal reflux or regurgitation may occur.

The oral phase of swallowing, which is voluntary, consists of the tongue preparing the bolus for swallowing (Figs 27.1 and 27.2). Food is mixed with saliva and big particles are sorted out to be chewed again. The tongue then compresses the bolus against the palate, shaping it and coating it with mucous, and squeezes the bolus into the oropharynx. The soft palate then elevates, separating

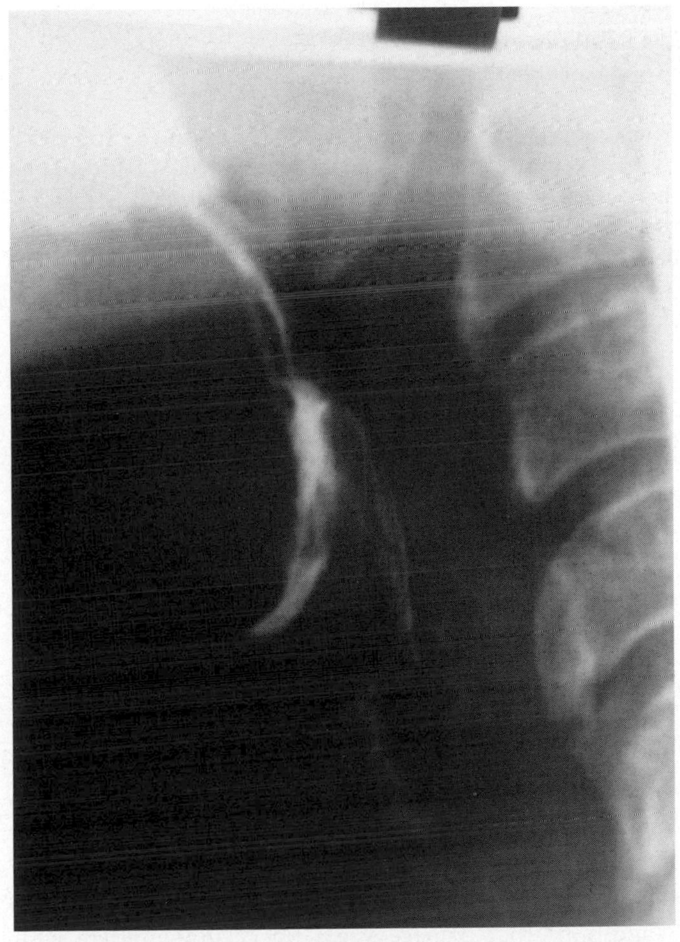

Figure 27.1 *Barium swallow showing the oral phase and early pharyngeal phase of swallowing.*

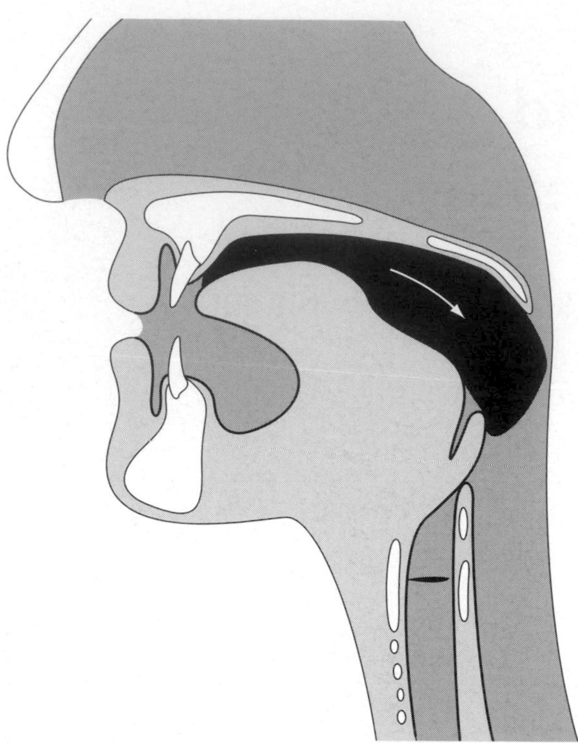

Figure 27.2 *Diagram of swallowing showing the oral phase and early pharyngeal phase of swallowing.*

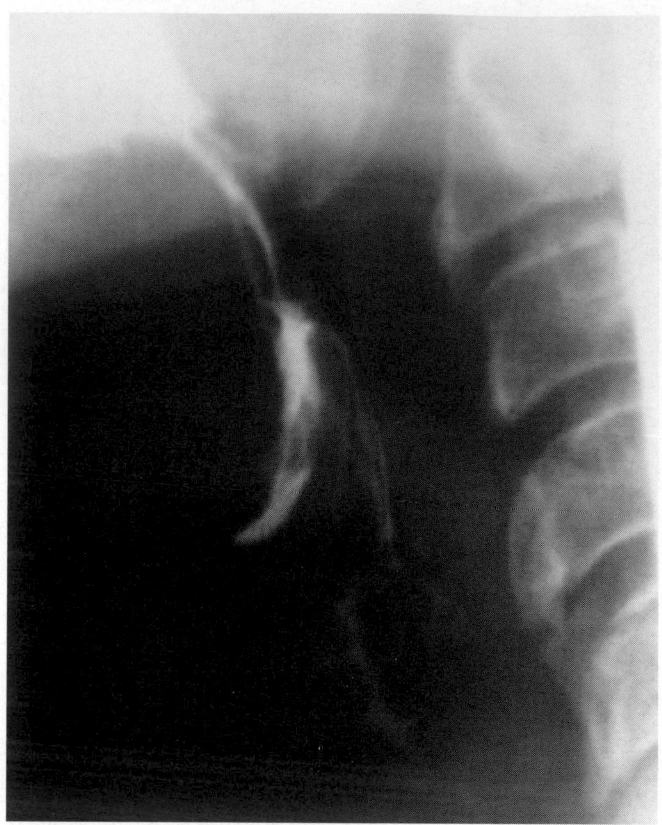

Figure 27.3 *Barium swallow showing the pharyngeal phase of swallowing with closure of the supraglottis by the tipping of the epiglottis and retrodisplacement of the bolus.*

the nasopharynx from the oropharynx, preventing nasal reflux. When the bolus reaches the vallecula, the tongue base moves posteriorly, the epiglottis is tipped posteroinferiorly, and the larynx is raised by the supraglottic musculature. This is the pharyngeal or involuntary phase of swallowing. During this phase, respiration is inhibited. The bolus is diverted posterolaterally, by the epiglottis, away from the airway. The bolus descends into the hypopharynx, with the airway raised and protected by the epiglottis, the aryepiglottic folds, false cords and closure of the true vocal cords (Figs 27.3–27.6).[1,4,14]

The esophageal phase begins when the bolus passes through the upper esophageal sphincter. If the upper esophageal sphincter (the cricopharyngeus muscle) fails to relax and open, or the esophagus fails to contract, swallowing will be impaired and aspiration may occur (Figs 27.7 and 27.8).[40,42]

The nerve fibers supplying the cricopharyngeus arise in the vagal nuclei and pass without synapse to the motor end plates via the vagus nerve. The motor end plates are cholinergically mediated through nicotinic junctions. The tonic contraction is neurogenic, whilst central inhibition is responsible for the relaxation during swallowing.[13] The cricopharyngeus normally exerts a pharyngeal pressure of 15–23 mmHg and must be overcome by the hypopharynx to induce the opening of the upper esophageal sphincter. Conditions that damage vagal fibers and interfere with the relaxation of the cricopharyngeus, such as basilar artery thrombosis, may cause cricopharyngeal spasm or

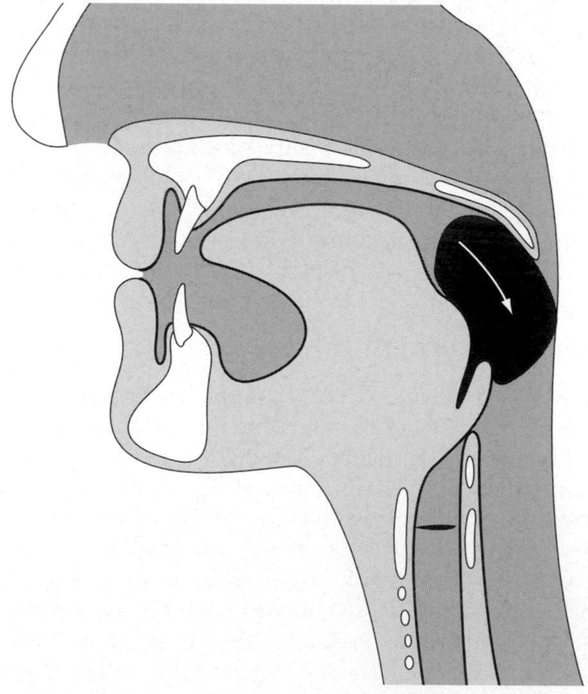

Figure 27.4 *Diagram of swallowing showing the pharyngeal phase of swallowing with closure of the supraglottis by the tipping of the epiglottis and retrodisplacement of the bolus.*

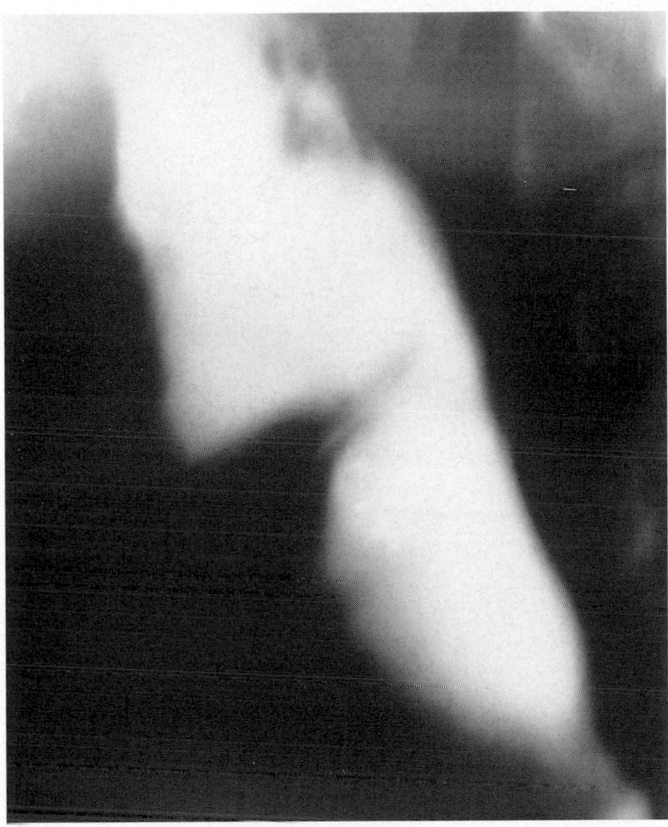

Figure 27.5 *Barium swallow showing the pharyngeal phase and early esophageal phase of swallowing.*

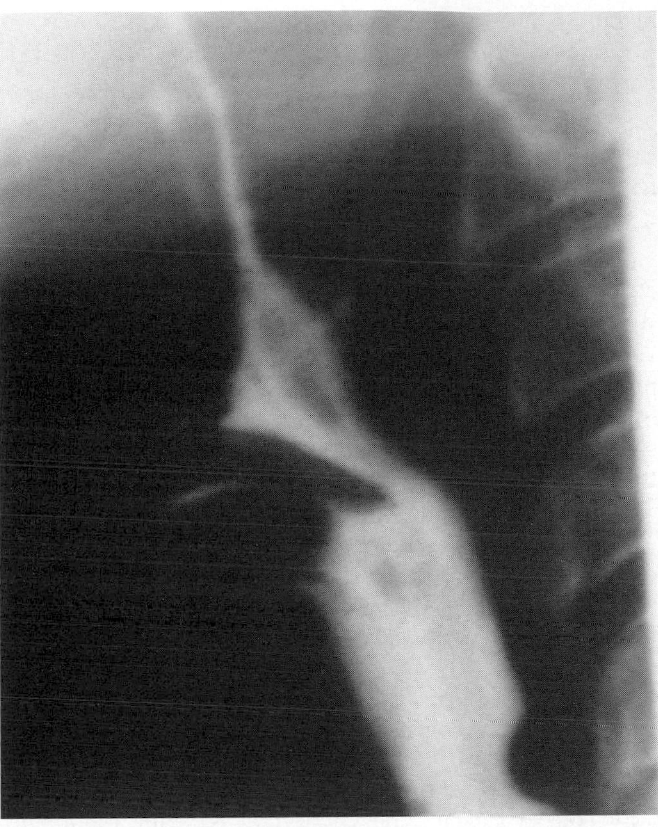

Figure 27.7 *Barium swallow showing the late pharyngeal and esophageal phase of swallowing with complete closure of the supraglottis and an open upper esophageal sphincter.*

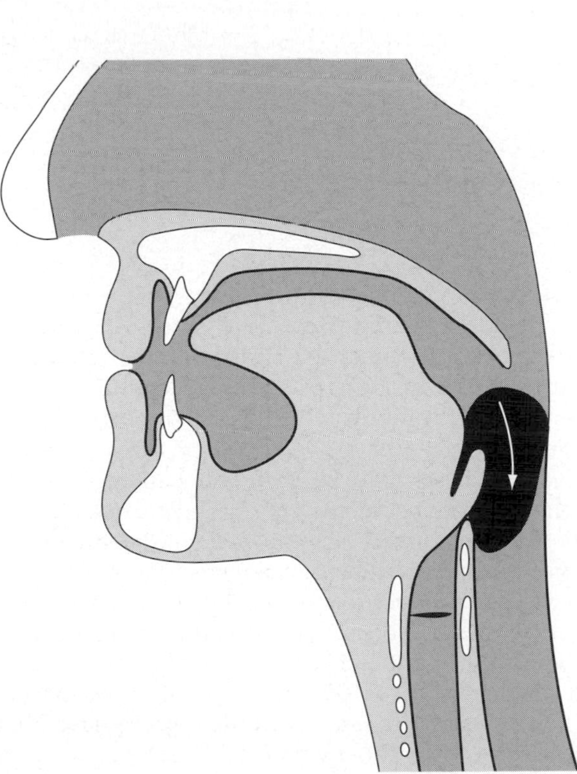

Figure 27.6 *Diagram of swallowing showing the pharyngeal phase and early esophageal phase of swallowing.*

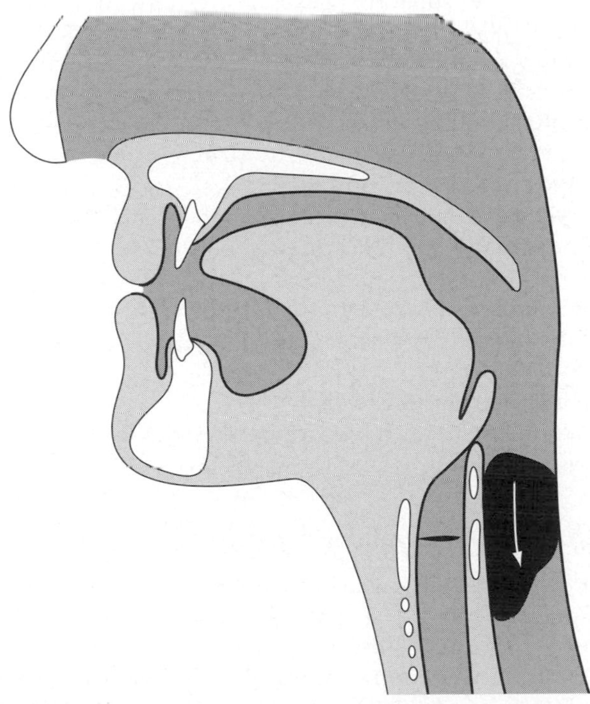

Figure 27.8 *Diagram of swallowing showing the late pharyngeal and esophageal phase of swallowing with complete closure of the supraglottis and an open upper esophageal sphincter.*

achalasia. Neuropathic and myopathic processes may also produce a relative cricopharyngeal achalasia, dyssynchrony and dysphagia.

Laryngo/pharyngo/esophageal interrelationship

The pharynx represents a common cavity for breathing and eating where there is a crossing of air and food/liquid. During the oral phase, food/liquid is ventral to the air stream; during the esophageal phase air occupies the ventral position in the trachea. The crossing of these pathways is the 'weak link' in the chain and takes place in the pharynx. To accomplish a normal, uncomplicated swallow there must be efficient and complete transport of the bolus through the upper esophageal sphincter (UES) and protection of the airway from aspiration.[16,33,34]

During oropharyngeal swallowing three precisely coordinated events occur:

- elevation of the larynx and closure of the airway;
- opening of the UES;
- reflex inhibition of breathing.

In addition to closure of the larynx and opening of the UES, the nasal and oral cavities are closed off, so that the only outlet from the pharynx is the esophagus. Oropharyngeal dysphagia occurs when either effective transport of the bolus and/or protection of the airway is compromised.[33]

The larynx functions as a sphincter to protect the lower airway.[29] The epiglottis flexes posteriorly and caudally during swallowing to deflect the bolus posteriorly and laterally, away from the glottic inlet. The laryngeal sphincter consists of three tiers, which close in a caudad to cephalad direction. The true vocal folds close first, followed in a rapid sequence by closure of the false folds and then the aryepiglottic folds.

Laryngeal penetration or aspiration occurs (Fig 27.9) if one or more of the following happens:

- premature spill from the oral cavity into the pharynx;
- uncoordination between oropharyngeal motility and glottic closure;
- ineffective glottic closure;
- incomplete bolus transport with residue in the pharynx post swallow.[34]

Evaluation of swallowing function

In order to decipher the cause of dysphagia, each phase of swallowing must be evaluated. The evaluation should include a thorough history and physical examination. A fiberoptic laryngoscopy during the swallow can identify any defects in the larynx or pharynx, pooling of secretions in the vallecula or hypopharynx, or a mass lesion that may produce obstruction. A FEES (functional endoscopic evaluation of swallowing) is performed, where

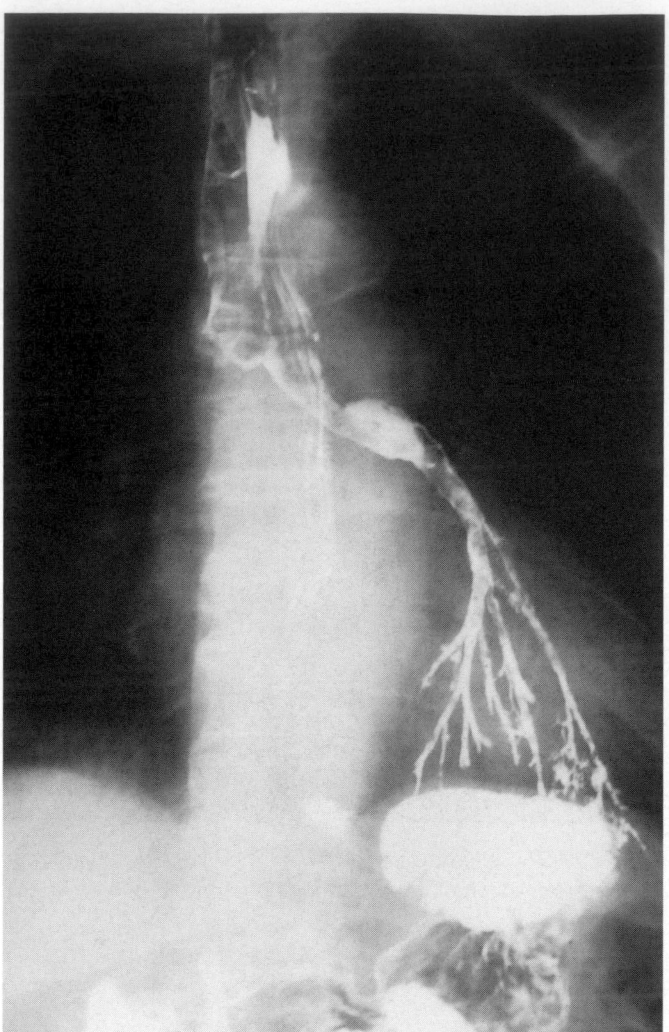

Figure 27.9 *Barium swallow in patient with aspiration showing a bronchogram from aspirated barium.*

a bolus of colored material is given to the patient to swallow while the endoscope is in place. Aberrations of swallowing can be visualized and persistent green material can be found in areas of impaired function. This can be combined with sensory testing (FEEST) with an air-puff stimulus.

Salivary analysis may be useful in patients who have oral phase problems, identifying problems or quantity or composition of saliva.[39] The most definitive analysis is a modified barium swallow or 'cookie swallow' in which a video tape is produced and can be replayed at various speeds to identify subtle changes within the phases of the swallow. The patient is kept in an upright position and given small amounts of barium of different consistencies. This best assesses the oral and pharyngeal phases of the swallow, observing for adynamic areas, relative or true obstructions and dyssynchrony. Assessment of aspiration related to the consistency of the bolus, the position of the patient, and any other associated dysfunction can also be made during this study. The best head position that may benefit planned swallowing therapy can easily be determined during the swallow.[21,22]

Multiple port manometry, in which simultaneous pressure measurement can be taken in the pharynx, cricopharyngeus and esophagus, is a useful way of identifying subtle failures of pressure generation or hyperfunction of the sphincter. Manometry does not, however, yield any information about aspiration. McConnel[24] has shown that the combination of manometry and videofluoroscopy may more accurately diagnose the site of dysfunction.

Ultrasonography has been used to help in assessing the oral phase of swallowing, but cannot be used for the pharyngeal or esophageal phases due to interference of the cervical spine. This study is noninvasive and safe and can be repeated on regular intervals without harm to the patient.[35,36] Radionuclide scans have also been found useful to document aspiration in the evaluation of the patients who have dysphagia. A radioactive bolus, usually composed of ^{99}Tc sulfur colloid, is fed to the patient. The swallow is recorded with a gamma scintillation camera as the bolus passes from the oropharynx to the esophagus. The pharyngeal transit time, clearance rate and degree of aspiration can be easily quantified.[36] CT and MRI scans can be used to detect brainstem or cortical lesions that may be the etiology of a neurologic dysfunction producing dysphagia.

Laryngopharyngeal sensory testing is a new avenue for evaluating the causes of aspiration. The light touch part of the sensory apparatus can be evaluated utilizing a pressure- and duration-controlled puff of air delivered to the anterior wall of the pyriform sinus or aryepiglottic fold (the area innervated by the superior laryngeal nerve). The air puff is delivered from an internal port of a flexible fiberoptic laryngoscope. To determine an individual's sensory pressure threshold, air pressure is varied according to the psychophysical method of limits whilst the duration of the air puff is held constant at 50 milliseconds (ms).[5]

Testing begins by orienting the subject to the supraglottic stimulus with a suprathreshold stream of air for 5 seconds. After a 15 second rest period, presentation of air puffs begins. Six blocks of stimulus administration trials are given in which a threshold is obtained for each block. The mean of the lowest detected pressures from the six blocks is used as that subject's sensory threshold. Both the right and left sides of the pharynx and supraglottic larynx are studied. Sensory decrease and consequent decreased reflexes may lead to aspiration.[5] In the future, sensory nerve grafting in sensory-deficient patients may help to prevent aspiration.[6]

Dysphagia after surgery

Dysphagia in the tracheotomized patient

Tracheostomy is one of the more commonly performed procedures in otolaryngology and head and neck surgery. Currently a tracheostomy is performed for a variety of indications, the most common of these being acute and chronic airway obstruction. Tracheostomy may also be performed in patients who require prolonged ventilatory support. Such patients usually have underlying pulmonary or central nervous system disease. Tracheostomy may also be done to bypass or eliminate the dead space of the upper airway, as in chronic lung patients who have fixed low tidal volume. Tracheostomy is performed by many physicians to aid in the care of patients with chronic aspiration, but, as will be discussed, tracheostomy may cause more problems with aspiration than it solves.[27]

The major swallowing disorder associated with tracheostomy is aspiration. A number of authors reported on post-tracheostomy aspiration. In 1965, Asherson[3] described a patient that was tracheotomized for bilateral vocal fold paralysis who developed such severe aspiration that he eventually underwent total laryngectomy. In 1966, Feldman *et al.*[15] discussed three tracheotomized chronic lung patients who demonstrated severe aspiration. Bonanno[9] studied 43 tracheotomized patients, of whom three developed dysphagia and aspiration, with x-ray evidence of abnormal laryngeal elevation during swallow. Studies by Cameron *et al.*[12] and Bone *et al.*[10] used dye to demonstrate evidence of aspiration in tracheotomized patients. In 1977, Shahvari *et al.*[32] reported the use of a modified tracheostomy tube connected to wall suction that removed between 200 and 600 ml of secretions per day, giving further evidence that tracheostomy can result in significant aspiration.

Tracheostomy has an effect on the second, or pharyngeal stage of swallowing, where the bolus passes through the pharynx, the suprahyoid muscles elevate and move the larynx anteriorly under the tongue base; the epiglottis tilts backward; and the three-tiered laryngeal closure occurs. The peristaltic wave forces the bolus of food into the upper esophagus, the entire process occurring in less than 1 second, while the respiration is reflexly interrupted for only a fraction of the respiratory cycle. The pharyngeal stage of swallowing involves the sensory limbs of the ninth and tenth cranial nerves and the motor limb of the tenth nerve.

The effect of tracheotomy on laryngeal function (Fig 27.10) may be separated into three categories: the mechanical effect on the position of the larynx; the loss of pharyngeal pressure due to leakage around the tube; and the refined neurophysiologic regulation of the intrinsic muscles.

Tracheostomy limits the elevation of the larynx, causing fixation of the trachea to the anterior neck skin,[15] particularly when suturing the trachea to the skin or using a horizontal skin incision and due to the tube itself. The reduced elevation and anterior movement of the larynx may allow food and/or secretions to enter the partially unprotected airway.

Betts[8] felt that external pressure by the tracheostomy cuff led to esophageal obstruction, causing food and secretions to stagnate above the cuff in the proximal esophagus and hypopharynx. These then overflow into the

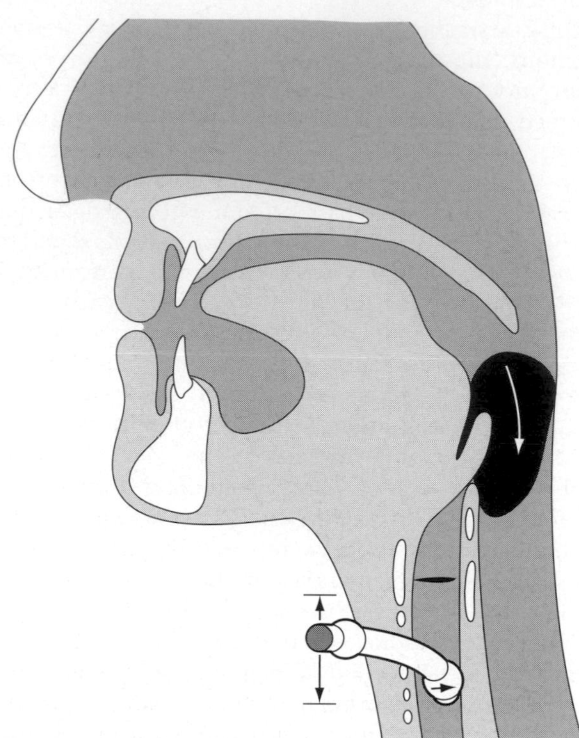

Figure 27.10 *Diagram showing tracheostomy tube in place with cuff inflated. The cuff impinges on the posterior tracheal wall, indenting the esophagus and making swallowing more difficult. The bolus is kept above the upper esophageal sphincter. The tracheostomy tube also limits or prevents the elevation of the larynx further impairing swallowing.*

airway when the cuff is deflated or when the patient inspires forcefully. Feldman *et al.*[15] believed that this stagnated material caused local chondritis of tracheal cartilage, resulting in tracheomalacia, so that there would no longer be a tight cuff-to-trachea seal. This would lead to more secretions and food leaking into the trachea until the physician inflated the cuff with more air, improving the seal temporarily but perpetuating a vicious cycle. He also postulated that long-term diversion of air through a tracheostomy may cause a desensitization of the larynx so that the patient may be unaware of the aspiration, and the protective cough mechanism may be blunted.

Leverment *et al.*[19] suggested that swallowing dysfunction may be due to an increase of intraluminal pressure at the cuff level and at 5 and 10 cm below the pharyngoesophageal junction, which can lead to the above-mentioned condition.

Sasaki and colleagues discussed the effects of tracheotomy in two studies.[11,30] In the first they demonstrated in dogs that chronic upper airway bypass can lead to uncoordinated laryngeal closure that will lead to aspiration. They found that laryngeal respiratory behavior producing phasic inspiratory vocal fold abduction is altered by tracheotomy. Laryngeal protective function by reflex glottic closure may also be altered by tracheotomy. It produces a central dissociation of laryngeal closure reflex, probably by an altered 'sensitivity of the medullary adductor motor neurons to their sensory cues'. The strength of closure is also altered due to weakened and unsustained adductor response to SLN stimulation.

In the second paper they discussed both the neurophysiologic effect of tracheotomy as well as the mechanical effect (reduced elevation). They concluded that:

- phasic abductor activity diminishes as ventilatory resistance decreases;
- the elimination of ventilatory resistance results in cessation of laryngeal abductor activity within 3–5 minutes. This loss persists as long as airway resistance remains low and can be reestablished by increasing ventilatory resistance gradually;
- the longer the duration of reduced resistance, the more difficult it is to reestablish abductor function once it is lost;
- adductor dysfunction may contribute to glottic closure failure, resulting in diminished cough and aspiration;
- reduced elevation of the larynx prevents adequate supraglottic closure during deglutition contributing to aspiration.

Although tracheotomy is commonly used as a procedure to prevent aspiration in patients with CNS or pulmonary disease, it has been shown that it may actually cause more aspiration than it prevents, due to mechanical and neurophysiologic factors. However, in patients with reversible CND or pulmonary disease, a well planned tracheotomy with careful postoperative care can be a short-term aid to aspiration.

Dysphagia after total and partial laryngectomy and laryngopharyngectomy

All laryngectomies have an altered swallowing mechanism as a result of the removal of the larynx. The reported incidence varies from 10 to 58%.[7,28] This incidence may be underestimated since the patient may not be actively complaining about the presence of dysphagia.

During normal swallowing, laryngeal elevation aids in the opening of the pharyngoesophageal (PE) segment. The PE segment develops a negative pressure that is important for bolus passage. After total laryngectomy the patient does not develop this negative pressure and shows an increased propulsive pressure generated by the tongue. The decreased pressure gradient is reflected in an increased pharyngeal transit time (1217 ms versus 835 ms in normal subjects)[4] and a decreased pharyngeal bolus velocity (6.6 cm/s versus 8.7 cm/s in normal subjects). The greatest increase occurs in the hypopharyngeal transit time (1061 ms versus 790 ms). The pressure gradient is changed also in the oropharynx but not to the same degree (658 ms versus 570 ms). The tongue, therefore, is the only significant propulsive force, and any impairment in tongue movement or any obstruction in the neopharynx would affect swallowing.[26]

The high pressure in the pharynx during deglutition after total laryngectomy, which is probably even higher in the immediate postoperative period due to mucosal edema, could help to explain the high incidence of postoperative fistula. Another frequent complication after total laryngectomy is hypopharyngeal stenosis. This creates not only a problem in swallowing but also in speech rehabilitation. The most important determinant for stenosis appears to be the site of the lesion. When a partial pharyngectomy is needed, the chance of stenosis is higher. The morbidity of postoperative stenosis is considerable. The diet must be altered, frequent dilatations are required and there is a decreased ability to produce esophageal speech.

The major problem with deglutition following conservation surgery of the larynx and hypopharynx results from aspiration secondary to glottic insufficiency. The major determinants of aspiration are glottic insufficiency from the excision of all or part of the arytenoid cartilage, excision of part of the tongue base, and failure to control the tumor with previous irradiation. This is true for vertical hemilaryngectomy as well as horizontal supraglottic laryngectomy patients.

Staple and Ogura[37] demonstrated that the three major requirements for adequate swallowing were closing of the glottic chink by the vocal cords (it was not necessary that both cords function but that the remaining cord be able to oppose strongly the fixed or reconstructed cord), apposition of the larynx to the base of the tongue, and a patent esophagus to avoid delay. In conservation surgery of the larynx, it may be necessary to remove or interfere with two of these protective mechanisms.

When the supraglottic structures, including the superior laryngeal (sensory) nerves are surgically removed, the patient no longer has the ability to sense clear fluid passing through the pharynx into the esophagus. Without sensation, attempts to swallow clear liquids can cause aspiration.

In a study by Logemann and Bytell,[22] 25% of supraglottic laryngectomy patients had a problem in the preparatory stage of swallowing. There was difficulty in maintaining a liquid or a thin paste bolus. There was some slowing in oral transit time when compared to normal subjects. Pharyngeal transit time was also slowed and at this stage material fell over the base of the tongue and into the pharynx diffusely rather than in a cohesive bolus in 75–92% of the patients. This occurred more often when a portion of the base of the tongue was included in the surgical resection. Pharyngeal peristalsis was reduced in 25–37% of the patients. Laryngeal closure or constriction was reduced in 50% of the patients, and laryngeal elevation was reduced in 25% of the patients. Aspiration of material into the airway occurred in 50% of patients in this series.

Walther[41] found aspiration to occur in 56% after hypopharyngo-laryngeal resection and in 67% after unilateral oropharyngo-laryngeal resection. As mentioned earlier in this chapter, UES opening does not occur until the pressure gradient is large enough to push the bolus through the collapsed pharyngeal walls (now no longer anatomically held by the hyoid and thyroid cartilages). This pressure gradient can only be generated in the base of the tongue region. After laryngopharyngectomy or laryngectomy with additional lingual defects, the functional obstruction at the pharyngeal outlet can not be overcome by inadequate propulsive forces at the pharyngeal inlet, and considerable swallowing impairment results.

Swallowing disorders after radiotherapy and adjuvant chemotherapy

A study by Lazarus *et al.*[18] examined the nature of swallowing problems seen in patients with diagnosed tumors of the head and neck who were treated primarily with external beam radiation and adjuvant chemotherapy. All subjects underwent videofluorographic examination of their swallowing. Swallowing disorders were observed in both the oral and the pharyngeal stages.

The majority demonstrated clinical pharyngeal-stage swallowing disorders, including delayed triggering of the pharyngeal swallow, reduced posterior motion of the tongue to the posterior pharyngeal wall, reduced laryngeal elevation, and reduced laryngeal closure during the swallow. Reduced posterior movement of the tongue base resulted in tongue base, vallecular, and upper posterior pharyngeal wall residue. Most patients who aspirated did so after the swallow, as this residue slipped into the airway by gravity. Multiple swallows were required to clear pharyngeal residue.

The head and neck cancer patients who received radiotherapy demonstrated reduced coordination and abnormal timing of pharyngeal events, with the pharyngeal events occurring later in the swallow relative to the onset of CPO (cricopharyngeal opening).

Both anterior movement of the posterior pharyngeal wall and posterior movement of the tongue base were late relative to the CPO. This delay most likely contributed to the reduced bolus clearance through the pharynx.

This impairment found in the head and neck cancer patients may have resulted from radiation damage to the cricopharyngeal muscular portion of the sphincter. Late vertical and anterior laryngeal and hyoid motion also contributes to reduced laryngeal vestibule closure during the swallow, resulting in aspiration.

The acute/subacute effects of mucositis probably also have an impact on swallow function. It is not clear to what extent the swallowing problems were related to treatment side effects, such as pain, soreness, mucositis and nausea, or to oropharyngeal motility disorders. Long-term follow-up of swallow function in radiated head and neck cancer patients will elucidate how mucositis affects swallowing. Also, the effects of chemotherapy on oropharyngeal swallowing are unknown at this time.

Dysphagia after laryngotracheal reconstruction

Most cases of mild-to-moderate subglottic stenosis can be successfully treated with laryngotracheal reconstruction. The procedure involves exposure of the cricoid, anterior part of thyroid cartilage and the upper par of the trachea. The cricoid is divided in the midline with extensions based on extent of the stenosis. The cricoid is split posteriorly with care taken not to split the posterior commissure. The cartilage graft is sutured into place.[17] Cricotracheal resection with primary anastomosis is performed in more severe cases, and includes also resection of the stenosed trachea, dissecting it away from the esophagus, and then performing thyrotracheal and lateral cricotracheal anastomosis.[38]

Postsurgical dysphagia may be related to several causes. Dissection around and splitting of the cricoid may interfere with normal cricopharyngeus muscle action due to scarring. There may be some temporary weakness of the vocal cords related to trauma to the recurrent laryngeal nerves. The presence of a tracheotomy at the postsurgical period in some patients may lead to dysphagia, as described previously. In cases of cricotracheal reconstruction, the upper limb of the T-tube must be placed above the vocal cords to prevent permanent scarring resulting from friction of the cords over the tube. These patients may experience aspiration requiring temporary insertion of a nasogastric tube. Cricotracheal resection requires a suprahyoid release, which may contribute to dysphagia and aspiration. At the end of the procedure, the head is maintained in a flexed position by sutures placed from the chin to the chest, contributing also to difficulty in swallowing.

Management

The diagnosis of aspiration is made mainly by clinical observation and then by radiographic studies such as barium swallow and/or cinefluoroscopy. Management should be tailored to the specific cause.

Treatment of the tracheotomized patient includes surgical and nonsurgical considerations. As previously mentioned, use of vertical incision instead of horizontal incision and Bjork flap may lessen the chance of aspiration.[27] After surgery, the tracheotomy cuff should be minimally inflated so as not to compress the posterior wall of the trachea and the esophagus, and should be deflated frequently, preceded by thorough suction through the tube and above the cuff level. Similar suctioning should be performed following oral intake. Other methods of alimentation may be necessary to prevent airway soilage. In severe cases, surgical procedures such as laryngeal closure, laryngotracheal diversion and even total laryngectomy may be needed to solve the problem and are discussed elsewhere in this book.

Surgical treatment of postsurgical glottic incompetence after conservation surgery of the larynx has centered on Teflon injection of the pseudocord scar and reconstruction of a new pseudocord.[31] Arnold[2] and Lewy[20] reported satisfactory results after Teflon injection into an inadequate pseudocord after hemilaryngectomy. Both pointed out that the procedure is limited by the thickness of the scar, but if there is tissue space that will accept the Teflon, it is a good solution.

For glottic incompetence with large tissue loss, the pseudocord must be reconstructed either with cartilage, muscle mucosa or skin, with or without laryngeal stents.

Post-laryngectomy hypopharyngeal stenosis is relatively frequent and the morbidity is considerable. The diet must be altered, and the patient must be restricted to soft foods or liquids. Frequent dilatations are the most common form of therapy. If dilatations are not successful, a surgical option should be considered. Some mild stenoses can be treated with an extraluminal release of a band of scar tissue or even a myotomy. A Z-plasty can be effective with narrow-band strictures. Repairs with a deltopectoral flap are multistage, and myocutaneous flaps are another alternative. Gastric pull-up or bowel interposition may be necessary for severe or very long stenotic segments. A single-stage repair using free microvascular intestinal transfer grafts[25] has also been indicated in patients who do not respond to dilatations and when other intraluminal or extraluminal procedures are not adequate. This can be performed as a patch side graft or as a full luminal graft.

Voluntary swallowing techniques were introduced to improve the patient's ability to protect the airway and eliminate aspiration after supraglottic and other partial laryngectomies. The supraglottic swallow was designed to close the airway in supraglottic laryngectomy patients at the true vocal folds before and during the swallow, thus preventing aspiration during the swallow.[21] In this technique, patients are required to take a breath, hold the breath before and during the swallow, and cough at the end of the swallow before inhaling. The cough is designed to clear any residual material from inside or near the airway entrance. A super-supraglottic swallowing maneuver has been described more recently,[23] which is designed to close the airway at the entrance, i.e. the false vocal folds and the arytenoid to the base of the epiglottis. It includes the same steps as the above, but during the voluntary breath-holding period, the patient is asked to bear down, increasing the effort of closing. This maneuver tilts the arytenoids further forward, towards the base of the epiglottis and pulls in the false vocal folds, generally completely closing the airway entrance above the true vocal folds. This method was used in a group of patients who received high-dose chemotherapy and radiotherapy for tumors of the posterior oral cavity, pharynx and larynx. It not only closes the airway entrance but also elevates the larynx further during the early part of the swallow.

Dysphagia and aspiration can not always be prevented by surgical or nonsurgical means and in certain cases may lead to discontinuation of any oral intake.

Conclusions

This chapter has discussed deglutition problems associated with surgery of the larynx including tracheostomy, total and conservation surgery of the larynx and laryngotracheal reconstruction.

Any laryngeal disease – neoplastic, inflammatory, infectious or congenital as well as nonsurgical treatment for cancer of the head and neck, i.e. irradiation and chemotherapy – might cause dysphagia and/or aspiration.

If these problems are anticipated, recognized, and treated by a team approach of surgeon, nurse, dietitian and voice and swallowing therapist, rehabilitation of swallowing function can be achieved in most cases.

References

1. Ardan GM, Kemp FH. The protection of laryngeal airway during swallowing. *Br J Radiol* 1952; **25:** 406–16.
2. Arnold G. Vocal rehabilitation of paralytic dysphonia. IX. Technique of intracordal injection. *Arch Otolaryngol* 1962; **76:** 358–68.
3. Asherson N. Laryngectomy in the management of dysphagia. *Lancet* 1965; **2:** 1295–6.
4. Atkinson M, Kramer P, Wyman SM, Ingelfinger FJ. The dynamics of swallowing. I. Normal pharyngeal mechanisms. *J Clin Invest* 1957; **36:** 581-8.
5. Aviv JE, Martin JH, Keen MS, Debell M, Blitzer A. Air pulse quantification of supraglottic and pharyngeal sensation: a new technique. *Ann Otol Rhinol Laryngol* 1993; **102:** 777–80.
6. Aviv JE, Mohr JP, Blitzer A, Thomson JE, Close LG. Restoration of laryngopharyngeal sensation by neural anastomosis. *Arch Otolaryngol Head Neck Surg* 1997; **123:** 154–60.
7. Balfe DM, Koehler RE, Setzen M, Weyman PJ, Baron RL, Ogura JH. Barium examination of the esophagus after total laryngectomy. *Radiology* 1982; **143:** 501–8.
8. Betts RH. Posttracheostomy aspiration. *N Engl J Med* 1965; **273:** 155.
9. Bonanno PC. Swallowing dysfunction after tracheotomy. *Ann Surg* 1971; **174:** 29–33.
10. Bone DK, Davis JL, Zuidema GD, Cameron JL. Aspiration pneumonia. Prevention of aspiration in patients with tracheostomies. *Ann Thorac Surg* 1974; **18:** 30–7.
11. Buckwalter JA, Sasaki CT. Effect of tracheotomy on laryngeal function. *Otolaryngol Clin North Am* 1984; **17:** 41–8.
12. Cameron JL, Reynolds J, Zuidema GD. Aspiration in patients with tracheostomies. *Surg Gynecol Obstet* 1973; **136:** 68–70.
13. Christenson J. Innervation and function of the esophagus. In: Stipa S, Belsey RHR, Moraldi A, eds. *Medical and Surgical Problems of the Esophagus*. London: Academic Press, 1981: 14–16.
14. Didio LJA, Anderson MC. *The 'Sphincters' of the Digestive System*. Baltimore: Williams & Wilkins, 1968.
15. Feldman SA, Deal CW, Urquhart W. Disturbance of swallowing after tracheotomy. *Lancet* 1966; **1:** 954–5.
16. Gay T, Randell JK, Spiro J. Oral and laryngeal muscle coordination during swallowing. *Laryngoscope* 1994; **104:** 341–8.
17. Lano CF Jr, Duncavage JA, Reinisch L, Ossoff RH, Courey MS, Netterville JL. Laryngotracheal reconstruction in the adult: a ten year experience. *Ann Otol Rhinol Laryngol* 1998; **107:** 92–7.
18. Lazarus CL, Logemann JA, Pauloski BR *et al*. Swallowing disorders in head and neck cancer patients treated with radiotherapy and adjuvant chemotherapy. *Laryngoscope* 1996; **106:** 1157–66.
19. Leverment NJ, Pearson FG, Rae S. A manometric study of the upper oesophagus in the dog following cuffed tube tracheostomy. *Br J Anaesth* 1976; **48:** 83–9.
20. Lewy RB. Glottic reformation with voice rehabilitation in vocal cord paralysis. *Laryngoscope* 1963; **73:** 547–55.
21. Logemann JA. *Evaluation and Treatment of Swallowing Disorders*. San Diego: College Hill, 1983.
22. Logemann JA, Bytell DE. Swallowing disorders in three types of head and neck surgical patients. *Cancer* 1979; **44:** 1095–105.
23. Logemann JA, Pauloski BR, Rademaker AW, Colangelo LA. Super-supraglottic swallow in irradiated head and neck cancer patients. *Head Neck* 1997; **19:** 536–40.
24. McConnel FMS. Analysis of pressure generation and bolus transit during pharyngeal swallowing. *Laryngoscope* 1988; **98:** 71–8.
25. McConnel FMS, Cerenko D, Mendelsohn MS. Dysphagia after total laryngectomy. *Otolaryngol Clin North Am* 1988; **21:** 721–6.
26. McConnel FMS, Hester TR, Mendelsohn MS, Logemann JA. Manofluorography of deglutition after total laryngopharyngectomy. *Plast Reconstr Surg* 1988; **81:** 346–51.
27. Nash M. Swallowing problems in the tracheotomized patient. *Otolaryngol Clin North Am* 1988; **21:** 701–9.
28. Nayar RC, Sharma VP, Arora MML. A study of the pharynx after laryngectomy. *J Laryngol Otol* 1984; **98:** 807–10.
29. Negus VE. *The Comparative Anatomy and Physiology of the Larynx*. New York: Hafner, 1962.
30. Sasaki CT, Suzuki M, Horiuchi M, Kirchner JA. The effect of tracheostomy on the laryngeal closure reflex. *Laryngoscope* 1977; **87:** 1428–33.
31. Sessions DG, Zill R, Schwartz SL. Deglutition after conservation surgery of the larynx and hypopharynx. *Otolaryngol Head Neck Surg* 1979; **87:** 779–96.
32. Shahvari MBG, Kigin CM, Zimmerman JE. Speaking tracheostomy tube modified for swallowing dysfunction and chronic aspiration. *Anesthesiology* 1977; **46:** 290–1.
33. Shaker R. Oropharyngeal dysphagia: practical approach to diagnosis and management. *Semin Gastrointest Dis* 1992; **3:** 115–28.
34. Shaker R, Dodds WJ, Dantas RO, Hogan WJ, Arndorfer RC. Coordination of deglutitive glottic closure with oropharyngeal swallowing. *Gastroenterology* 1990; **98:** 1478–84.
35. Shawker TH, Sonies B, Stone M, Baum BJ. Real-time ultrasound visualization of tongue movement during swallowing. *JCU J Clin Ultrasound* 1983; **11:** 485–90.
36. Sonies B, Baum BJ. Evaluation of swallowing pathophysiology. *Otolaryngol Clin North Am* 1988; **21:** 637–48.
37. Staple TW, Ogura JH. Cineradiography of the swallowing mechanism following supraglottic subtotal laryngectomy. *J Radiol* 1966; **87:** 226–30.

38. Stern Y, Gerber ME, Walner DL, Cotton RT. Partial cricotracheal resection with primary anastomosis in the pediatric age group. *Ann Otol Rhinol Laryngol* 1997; **106:** 891–6.
39. Stuchell RN, Mandel ID. Salivary gland dysfunction and swallowing disorders. *Otolaryngol Clin North Am* 1988; **21:** 649–61.
40. van Overbeek JJ, Betlem HC. Cricopharyngeal myotomy in pharyngeal paralysis. Cineradiographic and manometric indications. *Ann Otol Rhinol Laryngol* 1979; **88:** 596–602.
41. Walther EK. Dysphagia after pharyngolaryngeal cancer surgery. Part I: pathophysiology of postsurgical deglutition. *Dysphagia* 1995; **10:** 275–8.
42. Yoshida Y. Localization of efferent neurons innervating the pharyngeal constrictor muscles and the cervical esophagus muscle in the cat by means of horseradish peroxidase method. *Neurosci Lett* 1981; **10:** 91–5.

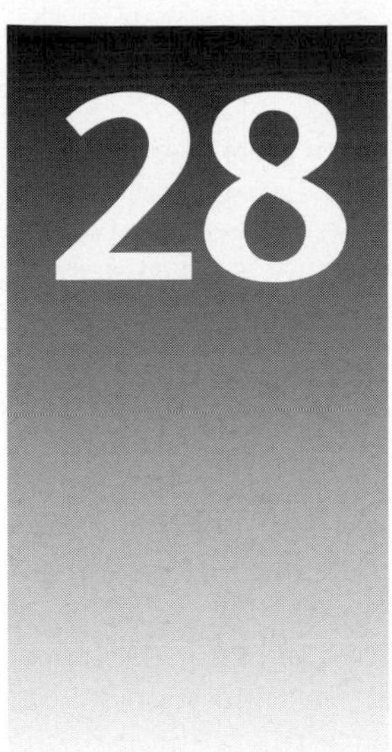

Neurologic disorders of the larynx

Marvin P Fried and Arthur M Lauretano

The complexity of laryngeal function becomes critically apparent when one deals with neurologic dysfunction. In contrast to such entities as inflammatory or neoplastic disease, neurologic disorders are often quite subtle in onset and progression, leading to a broad spectrum of symptoms and findings making diagnosis often difficult and therapy complex. We currently are only at the outset of understanding how the larynx truly functions and the aberrations that can be produced. A limited understanding of laryngeal function is therefore reflected in the history obtained, diagnostic studies performed and therapy offered. Early symptoms of mild dysphonia or cough may frustrate the physician seeking an etiology. The purpose of this chapter is to offer an overview to the complex neurological disorders and the current state of our scientific knowledge.

Pertinent neuroanatomy

The central cortical representation of laryngeal innervation has been demonstrated in the motor cortex in experimental situations.[15] Microstimulation can produce stimulation of a number of laryngeal muscles, producing both abduction and adduction. The complexity of the response reflects the filtration process of neuronal connections from central to peripheral. Unilateral vocal cord dysfunction is not usually affected by lateralized lesions of the cerebral cortex. Descending cortical bulbar fibers descend, decussate and arise at the nucleus ambiguous, the motor nucleus of the tenth cranial nerve. This nucleus is situated in the midportion of the brainstem half way between the floor of the fourth ventricle and the inferior olive.[42] Neural cells of origin of the laryngeal musculature arise in the lower portion of the nucleus ambiguus. The innervation is predominantly unilateral; however, crossing does occur.

The vagus leaves the base of the skull via the jugular foramen in proximity to the ninth and eleventh cranial nerves. The superior laryngeal nerve leaves the vagus at the nodose ganglion. Before entering the larynx, it divides into internal and external branches. The external laryngeal nerve innervates the cricothyroid muscle. The internal laryngeal nerve penetrates the thyrohyoid membrane being distributed to the laryngeal mucosa above the vocal folds with sensory and secretory innervation.

On the left side, the recurrent laryngeal nerve descends into the chest. It loops around the aorta, then, tracking cephalad, it returns to the larynx, being the predominant source of innervation. On the right side, the recurrent nerve arises from the vagus anterior to the subclavian and travels in close relationship to the inferior thyroid artery into the tracheoesophageal groove. On both sides, the nerve enters just posterior to the cricothyroid joint, dividing into anterior and posterior branches. This distribution of these branches is variable; however, the anterior branch usually supplies the lateral cricoarytenoid and thyroarytenoid muscles. The posterior branch supplies the posterior cricoarytenoid and interarytenoid muscles. Sensory and secretory innervation of the laryngeal mucosa inferior to the glottis is carried through the recurrent laryngeal nerve.

The superior and inferior laryngeal nerves both carry sympathetic and parasympathetic fibers, the sympathetic nerves arising from the superior and middle ganglion.[12]

Even more complex is the variety of sensory receptors within the larynx. Chemoreceptors have been identified that produce cardiorespiratory reflexes through the superior laryngeal nerve and then nodose ganglion.[7] Mechanoreceptors make a significant contribution to the regulation of respiration, including upper airway patency. This may play a role in disorders, such as obstructive sleep apnea, and have clearly been demonstrated as being altered in the tracheotomized patient.[1]

Diagnosis

History

Patients who have neurologic dysfunction of the larynx most frequently present, as with other etiologies, with a symptom of hoarseness. This may be isolated or in association with other symptoms related to the underlying cause. The incidence of neurogenic laryngeal disorders is quite variable, spanning the gamut from vocal fold immobility secondary to impingement on the recurrent laryngeal nerves to vocal aberrations related to much rarer primary neurologic disorders, such as myasthenia gravis. Voice disorders are commonly seen in patients with Parkinson's disease, occurring in nearly 90% of these individuals.[36] These disorders are much less common in patients with essential tremor and even less frequently seen in Huntington's disease and cerebellar ataxia.[36]

Associated symptoms should be sought. These include cough and aspiration due to incomplete glottic closure. Aspiration may also be due to sensory deficits within the endolarynx. Other cranial neuropathies and more subtle findings, such as dysarthria, may be present.

The onset of the symptoms is critical, often being related to a surgical procedure or neck trauma in vocal fold paralysis, however, insidious in slowly progressive lower motor neuron neurologic diseases. There are, however, no specific vocal symptoms characteristic of any neurologic disorder.

Office examination

A complete head and neck examination is mandatory, including the cranial nerves. Since multiple neuropathies may coexist, appropriate examination of the extraocular musculature, facial and neck sensation, tongue mobility, gag reflex, neck turning and shoulder mobility is warranted.

Laryngeal examination should begin with a mirror which gives a broad overview of the laryngopharynx. The absence of a gag reflex for this examination should be noted. Telescopic visualization can also be performed, offering greater detail secondary to improved illumination, as well as magnification.

Flexible fiberoptic endoscopy allows vocalization with connected speech and close observation during normal respiration. Laryngeal motion in particular is assessed, evaluating symmetry, as well as the mucosal wave. Localized or diffuse tremor can be observed, as well as paradoxical vocal fold motion.[16]

The use of the flexible endoscope, however, for some neurological diseases, such as spasmodic dysphonia, offers no distinct benefit.[47]

Stroboscopy

In the assessment of unilateral vocal fold immobility, Semon's law governing the position of the vocal cord in motor paralysis has not withstood careful scrutiny.[25] Although the vocal fold may be in or near the midline, its actual position is quite variable, depending on the duration and severity of the motor dysfunction, its location, the degree of arytenoid mobility on the cricoarytenoid joint, vocal fold mass, as well as numerous other factors.[46] The vocal fold may be shortened with anterior rotation of the arytenoid. When comparing configuration of the glottis in patients with either vagal or recurrent laryngeal nerve dysfunction, Woodson could not statistically differentiate between the two. One possible explanation for the variability of vocal fold position was thought to be related to the status of the cricothyroid muscle and its innervation by the superior laryngeal nerve. Koufman *et al.*[26] concluded that the cricothyroid muscle does not predictably influence the position of the vocal fold and unilateral paralysis based on laryngeal electromyography. Moreover, stroboscopy also has found limited utility in the assessment of patients with unilateral vocal fold paralysis. Those patients who have a large glottal gap due to the vocal fold not approximating the midline could not generate an adequate stroboscopic signal for analysis.[17] By contrast, however, laryngeal stroboscopy can help assess subtle differences in motion of the vocal folds, the mucosal wave, as well as tremor or uncoordinated movement. This latter finding often may be the first hint of neurogenic dysfunction and may require evaluation over a period of time, particularly if dysphonia is an early presenting complaint such as in those individuals with amyotrophic lateral sclerosis.

Voice evaluation

The complete evaluation of patients with neurogenic voice dysfunction often will require assessment by a clinical voice laboratory to assess objective voice measures, such as acoustic aerodynamic and electroglottographic parameters. Taken alone, however, they are insufficient in making a definitive diagnosis, but may offer supplementary data, as well as parameters to assess progression or treatment outcome.[32] The interaction with an experienced speech pathologist is critical for this assessment. Examination begins with simply listening to the voice, evaluating phonatory stability, tremor and movement of supporting laryngeal structures.[36] Observation of lingual and palatal movement during vocalization is also critical.

Airflow studies show increase in the mean flow rates, as well as glottal leakage in patients who have a vocal cord paralysis. There is a reduced phonation time and a requirement for frequent inhalations during conversational speech and increased mean airflow rates.[45]

Subglottal air pressure can be correlated with sound pressure level (SPL) of the voice. Both subglottal pressure and vocal SPL should be obtained in compensatory vocal hyperfunction when glottal activity is impaired and will yield elevated subglottic pressures, yet with relatively normal SPL.[19] Ramig and associates have described acoustic analysis in patients with neurologic disease, such as myotonic dystrophy, Huntington's disease, Parkinson's disease and amyotrophic lateral sclerosis. In patients with vocal fold dysfunction, there may be a reduction in phonation time with associated diminution in the dynamic range and in loudness and frequency range. Increases in the signal-to-noise ratio, increase in the aperiodicity, jitter and shimmer also can be found in patients with vocal fold paralysis.[32]

Electroglottography (EGG), which is a noninvasive method of evaluating vocal cord contact during phonation, is also disturbed in neurogenic disease. Although it is of limited clinical value, it has been shown that in vocal fold paralysis, the vocal fold open quotient is increased and the speech quotient is decreased.[28] EGG may be difficult to obtain, particularly in patients with a broad neck with excessive subcutaneous tissue. EGG is most beneficial when evaluating in conjunction with the entire range of other parameters including videostroboscopy.

Electromyography

Assessment of the integrity of the innervation of the laryngeal muscles with electromyography (EMG) has both diagnostic and prognostic relevance.[21,31,34] It finds particular value in the diagnostic assessment of vocal fold paralysis, often differentiating between paralysis and fixation and determining prognosis for recovery.[3,33,35] Monopolar needle examination can differentiate between vocal fold paralysis and cricoarytenoid fixation. EMG of the cricothyroid and thyroarytenoid muscles can differentiate vagal, superior and recurrent laryngeal nerve paralyses. EMG patterns are assessed for spontaneous and evoked activity. The presence of polyphasic and/or joined motor unit potentials indicates reinnervation. Denervation is characterized by spontaneous low-voltage and fibrillation potentials or electrical silence. The presence of evoked giant polyphasic potentials mixed with fibrillation potentials indicates partial denervation and reinnervation. Recruitment patterns during voluntary activity, such as phonation and cough, allow an estimate of the degree of voluntary activity in the muscle being evaluated.[40]

In patients with neurogenic vocal cord paralysis, Parnes and Satya-Murti[31] reported a 90% accuracy rate in predictive value of outcome. EMGs that showed decreased or absent motor unit potentials, fibrillation or positive waves had poor prognosis for return of function whereas those that demonstrated normal motor units or polyphasic potentials had likely return of function.

The difficulty with EMG is the problem of sampling. Location of the electrode in the proper muscle may be problematic; retesting may be difficult since placement of the electrode can be variable. As with other studies, EMG data needs to be taken as one parameter in the battery of tests.[3]

Radiographic studies

Radiographic studies have become critical in the assessment of neurologic laryngeal dysfunction. In the case of unilateral vocal fold paralysis, CT scan from the cranial base to the thorax has become a standard method to assess for a mass lesion that may be impinging on the course of the vagus nerve.[40] However, a limitation of CT is that it may be insensitive to the detection of more cephalic proximal lesions, particularly in the brainstem, basal cistern and skull base.[24]

Jacobs *et al.*[24] offer an algorithm for patients with suspected vagal neuropathies and appropriate diagnostic studies to be performed. They divide the vagus nerve into proximal distal components based on anatomy. They recommend considering the proximal vagus as arising from the brainstem nuclei and the medulla oblongata to distal to the superior laryngeal nerve at the level of the hyoid bone. Often these pathologies, when due to mass lesions, may be associated with neuropathies of cranial nerves IX, XI and XII. Associated clinical findings of an absent or reduced gag reflex, uvular deviation and nasopharyngeal reflux can be found. The cough reflex can also be absent due to involvement of the internal branch of the superior laryngeal nerve. More distal neuropathies can often present as isolated vocal fold dysmotility for neurologic dysfunction that are not due to mass lesions; intracranial MRI is appropriate.

Infants, in particular, should be considered for cranial and cervical radiologic evaluation since central nervous system abnormalities are often associated with vocal fold paralysis and are rarely seen in an otherwise normal infant.[5] Recently, ultrasound has been shown to accurately address the issue of vocal fold mobility in infants and children. The studies of ultrasound reported by Friedman[13] are preliminary, and potential applications are being explored. Benefits include a noninvasive study that is well tolerated and will allow data to be recorded and stored.[13] In adults, color doppler ultrasound imaging has also been shown to be of benefit, particularly when laryngoscopy may be difficult to perform.[30] Doppler imaging may be able to detect vocal fold motion, as well as air flow, and has a potential to differentiate between paresis and paralysis.

Operative endoscopy

In the vast majority of patients, the above diagnostic investigations will be all that is required to assess the manifestations, as well as etiology of laryngeal dysfunction. This is particularly the case when a thorough mirror or office flexible fiberoptic laryngeal examination reveals no mucosal lesions. Occasionally, however, direct endoscopy may be warranted. This should be considered in situations where the subglottis is not adequately visualized, and a suspicion of any mucosal abnormality is noted. At the time, cricoarytenoid joint mobility can be assessed and esophagoscopy can be performed.

Common causes of vocal fold paralysis

Iatrogenic trauma, malignancy and idiopathic causes represent the three most common etiologies of unilateral vocal fold paralysis, each accounting for approximately 30% of cases. Bilateral paralysis, much less common overall, is predominantly related to iatrogenic trauma, with other causes representing a very small fraction of cases.

Iatrogenic

Surgery is one of the most common causes of vocal cord paralysis, in most series accounting for approximately 30% of cases.[27] Surgery of the thyroid is clearly the most common operative procedure leading to vocal cord paralysis, with unilateral paralysis being more frequent; however, in terms of bilateral paralysis, thyroid surgery is by far the most common etiology, with neurologic, nonsurgical trauma and idiopathic being much less common causes. Additional surgical causes of vocal fold paralysis include esophagectomy, lung resection, carotid endarterectomy, neck dissection, mediastinoscopy, cardiac surgery and cervical disc surgery.

Malignant disease

Nearly one-third of vocal fold paralysis is due to malignancy.[14,27] Of these, approximately 50% are due to lung cancer, 20% esophageal, and 10% thyroid.[20,27] Most of these paralyses are unilateral (86% according to Hirano *et al.*[20]). Other causes include temporal bone malignancies, posterior fossa tumors, nasopharyngeal tumors, paragangliomas of the carotid sheath structures, metastatic disease and lymphoma.

Idiopathic

For one-third of vocal fold paralyses (primarily unilateral), a specific cause is never identified. Many of these are presumed to be viral. Some investigators believe the incidence of idiopathic paralysis may be higher but that some patients may have a temporary paralysis that resolves before they seek medical therapy. Prior to considering a paralysis to be idiopathic, a thorough investigation for other causes, especially malignancy, must be undertaken. The cause of vocal fold paralysis should not be considered idiopathic, according to some authorities, until at least 18 months after initial diagnosis.[27]

Nonsurgical trauma

Automobile accidents, skull fractures and penetrating trauma may injur the recurrent laryngeal nerve. Generally, this group has accounted for only about 7% of vocal cord paralyses, and in some studies also includes stretching of the nerve from cardiac or great vessel enlargement and compression of the nerve from endotracheal tube cuffs.

Inflammatory causes

Ninety-five percent of cases in this group are due to pulmonary tuberculosis, either from apical or mediastinal scarring or from mediastinal nodes.[27] Other inflammatory causes include jugular thrombophlebitis, subacute thyroiditis, meningitis, influenza, diphtheria, typhoid fever and granulomatous disease (including TB) of the skull base.[27]

Neurologic causes

Neurologic causes have been reported to account for 1–8% of vocal fold paralysis cases. Cerebrovascular disease and brainstem ischemia, epilepsy, Parkinson's disease, multiple sclerosis, syringobulbia, amyotrophic lateral sclerosis, poliomyelitis, Charcot–Marie–Tooth, Guillain–Barré and head injuries are all potential causes of unilateral or bilateral true vocal fold paralysis. Alcoholic and diabetic neuropathies, as well as vinblastine neuritis, have also been described as etiologies.[27]

Miscellaneous causes

Hemolytic anemia, thrombosis of the subclavian vein, syphilis, collagen diseases, myasthenia gravis and lead and arsenic ingestion have caused a limited number of cases of vocal fold paralysis.[27]

Unusual causes of vocal fold paralysis

Within the categories noted above, there are less frequently sited etiologies for vocal fold paralysis. In some disorders (e.g. Shy–Drager) vocal fold paralysis may be more common and problematic than initially thought. In other disorders, such as myasthenia gravis, the occurrence of vocal fold paralysis is so rare that a careful investigation must be made to identify the underlying cause of the paralysis.

Neuromuscular disorders

Shy–Drager syndrome

Shy–Drager syndrome is a rare, progressive, autonomic failure of the nervous system described by Shy and Drager in 1960.[2] The syndrome is one of several multiple system atrophy syndromes, which also include striatal nigral degeneration and olivopontocerebellar atrophy. Shy–Drager syndrome consists of orthostatic hypotension, urinary and rectal incontinence, loss of sweating, iris atrophy, external ocular palsies, rigidity, tremor, loss of associated movements, impotence, atonic bladder, loss of rectal sphincter tone, fasciculations, wasting of digital muscles, evidence of a neuropathic lesion on EMG suggestive of anterior horn cell involvement and a neuropathic lesion on muscle biopsy. Although not presented as a feature in the initial report of the syndrome, vocal cord paralysis has subsequently been described. The disease most commonly occurs in men, beginning in the sixth decade, and is progressive and irreversible. Average survival time is 7–8 years after onset of orthostatic hypotension and 4 years after the onset of neurologic symptoms. Cause of death is usually aspiration, sleep apnea or cardiac arrhythmia.

Diagnosis is confirmed by the presence of orthostatic hypotension and typical neurologic features, including pyramidal signs (hyperreflexia, dysarthria), extrapyramidal signs (rigidity, mask-like facies), and cerebellar signs. Intellectual or sensory deterioration is rare. Abnormalities of serum catechols may be seen. Head CT and CSF are normal. MRI often reveals areas of decreased density in the posterior putamen. EEG may show diffuse dysrhythmia, slow wave activity, or it may be normal. EMG may suggest peripheral neuropathy.

Vocal cord paralysis in Shy–Drager syndrome is usually bilateral. Paralysis generally occurs in more advanced stages of the disease. These patients may also have disordered central respirations. Vocal cord paralysis may be an initial presenting symptom. Shy–Drager patients with vocal cord paralysis typically exhibit bulbar palsies as well as cerebellar signs. Snoring, stridor, hoarseness and sleep apnea are frequently related to the cord paralysis. Histologically, these patients show marked atrophy of the posterior cricoarytenoid muscles and little atrophy of other laryngeal muscles. Although the muscles show signs of denervation, no loss of motor nuclei can be clearly shown.[18] Loss of small myelinated fibers in motor branches of the recurrent laryngeal nerve has been seen in patients not yet experiencing vocal cord paralysis, whilst patients with paralysis also had loss of large myelinated fibers.[18,22]

Treatment for Shy–Drager is difficult. Dopaminergic drugs for the treatment of parkinsonian symptoms often exacerbate the orthostatic hypotension. Salt, fludrocortisone and Jobst stockings may help with the hypotension, as well as the use of caffeine, indomethacin, ephedrine and dihydroergotamine.[2] The bilateral true vocal cord paralysis often leads to airway obstruction and aspiration, requiring tracheostomy and feeding tube placement. Vocal cord abductor paralysis (VCAP) has been sited as a frequent cause of sudden death at night in patients with Shy–Drager syndrome, even in the absence of voice or swallowing symptoms, indicating a need for early intervention.[23] Thus far, tracheostomy has remained the primary airway treatment for these patients, as opposed to arytenoidectomy, cordotomy and other procedures also used in the treatment of bilateral vocal cord paralysis.[23]

Parkinson's disease

Parkinson's disease (PD) is an idiopathic, progressive neurologic disorder manifested by tremor, bradykinesia, rigidity and postural instability. Pathologically, it is a neurodegenerative disorder characterized by depigmentation of the substantia nigra and by the presence of Lewy bodies. VCAP is rare in Parkinson's disease; this is in contrast to the frequency of VCAP in multiple system atrophy (MSA). Since multiple system atrophy has some parkinsonian features, differentiating the two disorders is sometimes difficult. From a laryngeal perspective, fiberoptic laryngoscopy has confirmed that PD patients exhibit stridor both while awake and asleep; MSA patients are predominantly stridorous when asleep. Histologically, PD patients show no evidence of atrophy of the intrinsic muscles of the larynx, whereas MSA patients characteristically have selective neurogenic atrophy of the posterior cricoarytenoid muscle. Finally, VCAP-related stridor in patients with PD is transiently relieved with haloperidol or methylphenidate, whereas such an effect is not seen with the MSA patients. These findings indicate that VCAP in Parkinson's disease is due to a persistent overactivity of the intrinsic muscles of the larynx. Of note, a high incidence of dysphagia has been seen in Parkinson's disease patients with VCAP.[23,38]

Myasthenia gravis

Myasthenia gravis is an autoimmune disorder resulting from a breakdown in T- and B-cell tolerance to acetylcholine receptor.[10] Patients develop variable muscle weakness exacerbated by exercise. Stridor secondary to vocal fold paralysis is an uncommon presentation of this disorder, and thus diagnosis of myasthenia gravis may be delayed in a patient presenting only with stridor. Careful history-taking may indicate the presence of other bulbar palsies, with symptoms worsening toward the end of the day. A positive response to edrophonium confirms the diagnosis.

Treatment of myasthenia gravis is generally successful, with anticholinesterases being the mainstay of symptomatic treatment. Treatment of the underlying autoimmune disorder consists of steroids, immunosuppressive drugs, and in some cases, thymectomy. Respiratory problems in myasthenia gravis are more commonly related to respiratory muscle paralysis. Patients presenting with stridor due to bilateral vocal fold paralysis often undergo tracheotomy due to delayed diagnosis of the underlying disorder.[10]

Additional central nervous system etiologies

Most laryngeal paralyses relate to a peripheral injury to the laryngeal nerves. However, vocal fold paralysis accompanying central nervous system disorders has been well documented. In addition to the aforementioned central causes, cerebrovascular accidents affecting upper motor neurons and the pyramidal tracts have been noted to cause bilateral vocal fold paralysis. In cases of mild strokes, the larynx may show subtle changes, at times only appearing swollen, at other times producing a frank but intermittent stridor which may be mistaken for asthma. These patients will have intermittent dysphonia as well. Failure to respond to steroids is common among these patients.[43]

Lesions or cerebrovascular accidents (CVAs) involving the lower motor nuclei of the vagus nerve (dorsal and ventral nucleus ambiguus) result in unilateral or bilateral vocal fold paralysis, with findings similar to those seen with a high division of the vagus nerve in the neck. Since there are many cranial nerve nuclei in proximity to the nucleus ambiguus within the brainstem, lesions or CVAs affecting this area tend to produce multiple cranial neuropathies. Thus, these patients typically have problems with deglutition, phonation, articulation and facial expression. In addition to tumors and CVAs, syringomyelia and amyotrophic lateral sclerosis may cause similar lower motor neuron vocal fold paralysis.[43] Patients with bilateral vocal fold paralysis from lower motor neuron lesions typically require tracheotomy.

Arnold–Chiari malformation may have cerebellar and/or brainstem damage secondary to herniation through the abnormally enlarged foramen magnum. Many patients have stridor as a presenting symptom. Many of these patients die from increased intracranial pressure, but also possibly from airway obstruction. These patients have been considered to have bilateral abductor paralysis, although close observation may show some involuntary abduction of the folds.[43]

Herpes vocal cord paralysis

Herpes simplex virus (HSV) has been suspected as the cause of a variety of cranial neuropathies. HSV has been isolated from ganglia of cranial nerves and is also responsible for subsequent demyelination and neural damage. Unilateral vocal cord paralysis has been described in association with HSV infection. Pathogenesis is thought to begin with the reactivation of latent HSV genes within the nerve ganglion, followed by viral replication and centrifugal migration along the nerve. Neural damage may then ensue at the ganglion or within the nerve itself. Use of aciclovir has been reported for a patient with vocal cord paralysis due to HSV; in spite of amelioration of the mucosal lesions, the paralysis did not resolve.[11]

Superior laryngeal nerve paralysis

The superior laryngeal nerve (SLN) originates from the vagus just below the nodose ganglion. The internal branch carries sensory fibers and enters the larynx via the thyrohyoid membrane. The external branch carries motor fibers to the cricothyroid muscle.[4] SLN paralysis or paresis has been classically described as an iatrogenic injury during thyroidectomy. Viral etiologies have been sited in other studies as the most common cause of paralysis of the SLN.[9] Nonsurgical trauma, thyroid lesions, metastatic disease, neuritis and idiopathic causes have all been sited.[4] Clinical manifestations are variable. Loss of high pitch range, poor vocal performance, overall lowered pitch and loss of falsetto may be observed. In singers and professional speakers, such paralysis may lead to muscle tension dysphonia in an attempt to produce a stronger voice. Findings on examination may be subtle, but classic signs are a rotation of the posterior commissure toward the weakened/paralyzed side, with a resultant shortening and bowing of the weakened true vocal fold. The affected fold typically appears lower (more inferior to) the normal side. Steroids and antiviral agents have been used if a viral etiology is suspected. Laryngeal framework surgery has also been used to reproduce the tensing effect of the cricothyroid muscle.

Pulmonary/thoracic etiologies

Cystic fibrosis

Cystic fibrosis (CF) is a hereditary, systemic disorder affecting the glandular structures of the body, particularly the lung.[48] The disease is linked to chromosome 7. The pulmonary artery hypertension and right ventricular hypertrophy characteristic of cor pulmonale can result in pulmonary artery dilation. Vocal cord paralysis, always on the left, has been seen in CF patients. The mechanisms proposed are:

- compression of the left recurrent laryngeal nerve against the ligamentum arteriosum or aortic arch by a dilated pulmonary artery;
- stretching of the nerve (similar to that seen with aortic aneurysms);
- injury due to minor degrees of cardiac rotation seen with cardiac hypertrophy; and
- secondary local factors such as enlarged lymph nodes or calcific aortic plaques in the aortic triangle.

Mitral stenosis, congenital heart disease, atherosclerotic heart disease, primary pulmonary hypertension, recurrent pulmonary embolism and cor pulmonale may all potentially result in a left vocal fold paralysis.[48]

Sarcoidosis

Intrathoracic lymphadenopathy has been reported to occur in 60–90% of patients with sarcoidosis. Seventy-five percent of patients with such nodes have enlargement of the aortopulmonary node group. Surprisingly, there is a paucity of reports in the literature of vocal cord paralysis related to sarcoidosis. Nevertheless, a small number of cases of sarcoidosis have been reported, in which one or both recurrent laryngeal nerves have been paralyzed. A review of the literature by Tobias *et al.* cites compression of the recurrent laryngeal nerve by adenopathy as the potential cause at least for left vocal fold paralysis.[41]

Iatrogenic causes

Radiation therapy

Vocal cord palsy has been described as a delayed and uncommon complication of radiation therapy. In general, the cranial nerves are considered radioresistant to cancericidal radiation doses. Paralysis has been described as a delayed complication in the treatment of nasopharyngeal, glottic and thyroid cancer.[39] Such paralysis may occur years after completion of the radiotherapy. Such paralysis is more often bilateral.

Artificial airway

The laryngeal mask airway (LMA) is considered a safe and convenient method of providing an airway during general anesthesia while avoiding some of the complications of endotracheal intubation. With increasing use, complications have been noted, most of which are attributed to high cuff pressures at the site of placement of the mask. Paralysis from neuropraxia of the recurrent laryngeal nerve has been attributed to LMA use in a small number of cases, due to diffusion of nitrous oxide into the mask and resultant increased cuff pressures.[8] Similar injuries to the hypoglossal nerve have been reported. Although the LMA is considered a preferred alternative to endotracheal intubation in voice professionals, preoperative counseling still needs to address the risk of vocal fold paralysis in these patients.

Endotracheal intubation has also been described as a cause for vocal cord paralysis. The paralysis is thought to occur from compression of the recurrent laryngeal nerve between the cuff of the tube and the thyroid cartilage, with injury typically occurring at the junction of the membranous cord and the vocal process of the arytenoid. Generally, the paralysis is an adductor paralysis from involvement of the anterior branch of the recurrent laryngeal nerve, resulting in a paramedian position of the vocal fold. Hoarseness is common whereas airway distress (even for rare bilateral cases) is reported to be unusual.[6] Cuff pressure may increase during general anesthesia due to diffusion of nitrous oxide into the cuff, causing the paralysis. Care in positioning the cuff below the cords and maintenance of appropriate cuff pressure are critical in preventing this complication. Fortunately, this injury generally results in a temporary paralysis.

Nasogastric tubes

The nasogastric tube can produce a bilateral vocal fold paralysis, at times of sudden onset. Pathophysiology is thought to be paresis of the posterior cricoarytenoid muscles due to ulceration and infection over the posterior lamina of the cricoid in proximity to the tube.[37] Patients requiring prolonged nasogastric tube feeding are at risk. Throat pain is a particularly important symptom in these patients. Odynophagia and otalgia may also be present. Esophagoscopy is necessary to diagnose the ulceration. Tracheotomy is often required for bilateral vocal fold paralysis. The nasogastric tube should be removed and the ulcer cultured. Antibiotic coverage, including anaerobic coverage, should be started parenterally. Steroids have been added in some patients to reduce inflammation. Alternative methods of feeding, including gastrostomy or jejunostomy tubes or hyperalimentation, should be employed. Recovery has been reported to take from 1–2 weeks to as long as 1–2 months (e.g. in diabetic renal transplant patients).[37] In rare cases, scarring can result in permanent fixation of the paralyzed cords.

Anterior cervical spine surgery

The anterior approach to the cervical spine was introduced in 1957 and has become a popular and widely used procedure by orthopedic spine surgeons and neurosurgeons. Various complications from this approach have been described: esophageal perforation, vertebral artery injury, Horner's syndrome, cervical nerve root injury and recurrent laryngeal nerve injury (RLN). RLN injury has the highest incidence of these complications. The right recurrent laryngeal nerve is the more commonly injured nerve. Weisberg studied the anterior cervical approach in cadavers and found the left RLN to be consistently in the tracheoesophageal groove, whereas the right side was more variable.[44] Use of the Cloward retractor in this study did not stretch the left RLN, but resulted in displacement and tension of the right RLN. Other studies have also identified the right RLN as being at more risk during the anterior cervical approach.[29] Some patients have taken up to 12 months to recover nerve function, whereas in others the paralysis remains permanent.

Conclusions

Vocal fold paralysis can disrupt phonation, deglutition and airway and pulmonary function. A thorough understanding of the laryngeal neuroanatomy and knowledge of all potential causes of vocal fold paralysis are essential in the diagnosis and treatment of this disorder. Advances in laryngeal framework surgery and endolaryngeal laser approaches offer increasingly definitive therapy for vocal fold paralysis. The procedure necessitates a more accurate and careful determination of the etiology of a vocal fold paralysis in its subsequent natural history.

References

1. Asher VA, Sasaki CT, Gracco LC. Laryngeal physiology: normal and abnormal. In: Fried MP, ed. *The Larynx. A Multidisciplinary Approach*. St Louis: Mosby, 1996: 45–54.
2. Bawa R, Ramadan H, Wetmore SJ. Bilateral vocal cord paralysis with Shy–Drager syndrome. *Otolaryngol Head Neck Surg* 1993; **109**: 911–14.
3. Beninger MS, Crumley RL, Ford CN *et al*. Evaluation and treatment of the unilateral paralyzed vocal fold. *Otolaryngol Head Neck Surg* 1994; **111**: 497–508.
4. Bevan K, Griffiths MV, Morgan MH. Cricothyroid muscle paralysis: its recognition and diagnosis. *J Laryngol Otol* 1989; **103**: 191–5.
5. Boey HP, Cunningham MJ, Weber AJ. Central nervous system imaging in the evaluation of children with true vocal cord paralysis. *Ann Otol Rhinol Laryngol* 1996; **104**: 76–7.
6. Cavo JW. True vocal cord paralysis following intubation. *Laryngoscope* 1985; **95**: 1352–9.

7. Cooper DM, Lawson W. Laryngeal sensory receptors. In: Blitzer A, Brin MF, Sasaki CT, Fahn S, Harris KS, eds. *Neurologic Disorders of the Larynx*. New York: Thieme, 1992: 12–28.
8. Daya H, Fawcett W, Weir N. Vocal fold palsy after use of the laryngeal mask airway. *J Laryngol Otol* 1996; **110**: 383–4.
9. Dursun G, Sataloff RT, Spiegel JR, Mandel S, Heuer R, Rosen DC. Superior laryngeal nerve paresis and paralysis. *J Voice* 1996; **10**: 206–11.
10. Fairley JW, Hughes M. Acute stridor due to bilateral vocal fold paralysis as a presenting sign of myasthenia gravis. *J Laryngol Otol* 1992; **106**: 737–8.
11. Flowers RH III, Kernodle DS. Vagal mononeuritis caused by herpes simplex virus: association with unilateral vocal cord paralysis. *Am J Med* 1990; **88**: 686–8.
12. Fried MP, Miller SM. Adult laryngeal anatomy. In: Fried MP, ed. *The Larynx. A Multidisciplinary Approach*. St Louis: Mosby, 1996: 33–43.
13. Friedman EM. Role of ultrasound in the assessment of vocal cord function in infants and children. *Ann Otol Rhinol Laryngol* 1997; **106**: 199–209.
14. Furukawa M, Furukawa MK, Ooishi K. Statistical analysis of malignant tumors detected as the cause of vocal cord paralysis. *ORL J Otorhinolaryngol Relat Spec* 1994; **56**: 161–5.
15. Gacek RR, Malmgren LT. Laryngeal motor innervation – central. In: Blitzer A, Brin MF, Sasaki CT, Fahn S, Harris KS, eds. *Neurologic Disorders of the Larynx*. New York: Thieme, 1992: 29–35.
16. Hanson DG. Neuromuscular disorders of the larynx. *Otolaryngol Clin North Am* 1991; **24**: 1035–51.
17. Harris ML, Morrison M. The role of stroboscopy in the management of a patient with a unilateral vocal fold paralysis. *J Laryngol Otol* 1996; **110**: 141–3.
18. Hayashi M, Isozaki E, Oda M, Tanabe H, Kimura J. Loss of large myelinated nerve fibres of the recurrent laryngeal nerve in patients with multiple system atrophy and vocal cord palsy. *J Neurol Neurosurg Psychiatry* 1997; **62**: 234–8.
19. Hillman RE, Holmberg EB, Perkell JS, Walsh M, Vaughan CW. Phonatory function associated with hyperfunctionally related vocal fold lesions. *J Voice* 1990; **4**: 52–63.
20. Hirano M, Tanaka S, Fujita M, Fujita H. Vocal cord paralysis caused by esophageal cancer surgery. *Ann Otol Rhinol Laryngol* 1993; **102**: 182–5.
21. Hiroto I, Hirano M, Tomita H. Electromyographic investigation of human vocal cord paralysis. *Ann Otol* 1968; **77**: 296–304.
22. Isozaki E, Naito A, Horiguchi S, Kawamura R, Hayashida T, Tanabe H. Early diagnosis and stage classification of vocal cord abductor paralysis in patients with multiple system atrophy. *J Neurol Neurosurg Psychiatry* 1996; **60**: 399–402.
23. Isozaki E, Shimizu T, Takamoto K *et al*. Vocal cord abductor paralysis (VCAP) in Parkinson's disease: difference from VCAP in multiple system atrophy. *J Neurol Sci* 1995; **130**: 197–202.
24. Jacobs CJM, Harnsberger HR, Lufkin RB, Osborn AG, Smoker WRK, Parkin JL. Vagal neuropathy: evaluation with CT and MR imaging. *Radiology* 1987; **164**: 97–102.
25. Kirchner JA. Semon's law a century later. *J Laryngol Otol* 1982; **76**: 645–57.
26. Koufman JA, Walker FO, Joharji GM. The cricothyroid muscle does not influence vocal fold position in laryngeal paralysis. *Laryngoscope* 1995; **105**: 368–72.
27. Maran AGD. Vocal cord paralysis. In: Maran AGD, Stell PM, eds. *Clinical Otolaryngology*. Oxford: Blackwell, 1979.
28. Murty GE, Carding PN. Combined glottographic measurement of vocal cord paralysis in the outpatient clinic. *Clin Otolaryngol* 1982; **17**: 3–5.
29. Netterville JL, Koriwchak MJ, Winkle M, Courey MS, Ossoff RH. Vocal fold paralysis following the anterior approach to the cervical spine. *Ann Otol Rhinol Laryngol* 1996; **105**: 85–91.
30. Ooi LLPJ, Chan HS, Soo KC. Color doppler imaging for vocal cord palsy. *Head Neck* 1995; **17**: 20–3.
31. Parnes SM, Satya-Murti S. Predictive value of laryngeal electromyography in patients with vocal cord paralysis of neurogenic origin. *Laryngoscope* 1985; **95**: 1323–6.
32. Ramig LA, Scherer RC, Titze IR, Ringel SP. Acoustic analysis of voices of patients with neurologic disease: rationale and preliminary data. *Ann Otol Rhinol Laryngol* 1988; **97**: 164–72.
33. Rontal E, Rontal M, Silverman B, Kilany PR. The clinical differentiation between vocal cord paralysis and vocal cord fixation using electromyography. *Laryngoscope* 1993; **103**: 133–6.
34. Schaefer SD. Laryngeal electromyography. *Otolaryngol Clin North Am* 1991; **24**: 1053–7.
35. Shindo ML, Woo P. Evaluation and management of unilateral vocal fold paralysis. *American Academy of Otolaryngology – Head and Neck Surgery, Recertification Study Guide*. In press.
36. Smith ME, Ramig LO. Neurological disorders and the voice. In: Gould WJ, Rubia JR, Korovin G, Satoloff R, eds. *Diagnosis and Treatment of Voice Disorders*. New York: Igaku-Shoin, 1995: 203–24.
37. Sofferman RA, Haisch CE, Kirchner JA, Hardin NJ. The nasogastric tube syndrome. *Laryngoscope* 1990; **100**: 962–8.
38. Stacy M, Jankovic J. Differential diagnosis of Parkinson's disease and the Parkinsonism plus syndromes. *Neurol Clin* 1992; **10**: 341–58.
39. Stern Y, Marshak G, Shpitzer T, Segal K, Feinmesser R. Vocal cord palsy: possible late complication of radiotherapy for head and neck cancer. *Ann Otol Rhinol Laryngol* 1995; **104**: 294–6.
40. Terris DJ, Arnstein DP, Nguyen HH. Contemporary evaluation of unilateral vocal cord paralysis. *Otolaryngol Head Neck Surg* 1992; **107**: 84–90.
41. Tobias JK, Santiago SM, Williams AJ. Sarcoidosis as a cause of left recurrent laryngeal nerve palsy. *Arch Otolaryngol Head Neck Surg* 1990; **116**: 971–2.
42. Tyler HR. Neurologic disorders. In: Fried MP, ed. *The Larynx. A Multidisciplinary Approach*. St Louis: Mosby, 1996: 181–5.
43. Ward PH, Hanson DG, Berci G. Observations on central neurologic etiology for laryngeal dysfunction. *Ann Otol* 1981; **90**: 430–41.
44. Weisberg NK, Spengler DM, Netterville JL. Stretch-induced nerve injury as a cause of paralysis secondary to

the anterior cervical approach. *Otolaryngol Head Neck Surg* 1997; **116:** 317–26.

45. Woo P, Cotton R, Brewer O, Cooper J. Functional staging for vocal cord paralysis. *Otolaryngol Head Neck Surg* 1991; **105:** 440–8.
46. Woodson GE. Configuration of the glottis in laryngeal paralysis. I: Clinical study. *Laryngoscope* 1993; **103:** 1227–34.
47. Woodson GE, Zwirner P, Murry T, Swenson M. Use of flexible fiberoptic laryngoscopy to assess patients with spasmodic dysphonia. *J Voice* 1991; **5:** 85–91.
48. Zitsch RP, Reilly JS. Vocal cord paralysis associated with cystic fibrosis. *Ann Otol Rhinol Laryngol* 1987; **96:** 680–3.

Psychology and voice disorders*

Deborah C Rosen, Reinhardt J Heuer and Robert T Sataloff

Although 'voice', the newest subspecialty of otolaryngology, now provides a greatly improved standard of care for *all* patients with voice disorders, most of the advances in this field resulted from interest in and the study of *voice professionals*.

Professional performers are not only demanding, but also remarkably self-analytical. Like athletes, performers have forced health care providers to change our definition of normalcy. Ordinarily, physicians, psychotherapists and other professionals are granted great latitude in the definition of 'normal'. For example, if a microsurgeon injures his or her finger, and the hand surgeon restores 95% of function, the surgeon-patient is likely to be satisfied. If the same result occurs in a world class violinist, that last 5% (or 1%) may mean the difference between renown and obscurity. Traditionally, we have not been trained to recognize, let alone quantify and restore, these degrees of physical perfection. Arts medicine practitioners have learned to do so, including in the field of voice. The process has required advances in scientific knowledge, clinical management, technology for voice assessment, voice therapy, and surgical technique. The drive to expand our knowledge has also led to unprecedented teamwork and interdisciplinary collaboration. As a result, voice care professionals have come to recognize important psychologic problems commonly found in patients with voice disorders. Such problems were routinely ignored in past years. Now they are sought for diligently throughout evaluation and treatment. When identified, they often require intervention by a psychologic professional with special knowledge about voice disorders, as well as by a speech-language pathologist (SLP) and other voice team members.

Arts medicine psychologists specializing in the management of performance anxiety are becoming more common, but there are still very few psychological professionals with extensive experience in diagnosing and treating other psychologic concomitants of voice disorders. It is important for the physician and all other members of the voice care team to recognize the importance of psychologic factors in patients with voice disorders and to be familiar with mental health professionals in various disciplines in order to build a multidisciplinary team, generate appropriate referrals, and coordinate optimal patient care.

Psychiatrists are licensed physicians who have completed medical training, residency in psychiatry, and often additional training. They are qualified not only to establish medical and psychiatric diagnoses and provide therapy, but also to prescribe medications. *Psychologists* make mental health diagnoses, administer psychological tests, and provide therapy. In most locations, they do not prescribe medications, but often work closely with a physician (usually a psychiatrist) who may prescribe and help manage psychotropic medications during the course of psychotherapy. Clinical psychologists have a Masters or Doctoral degree in psychology and may have subspecialty training. Other clinical disciplines (i.e. *social work, nursing, counseling*) license graduate-level practitioners to provide psychotherapy. Laryngologists, phoniatrists and speech-language pathologists are not formally mental health professionals, although all have at least limited training in psychological diagnosis. Specialty definitions vary from country to country. In the USA, laryngologists are responsible for medical diagnosis and treatment, and voice surgery. They also prescribe any medications needed to

*Adapted in part from Sataloff RT. *Professional Voice: Science and Art of Clinical Care*, 2nd edn. San Diego, Calif; Singular Publishing Group, Inc., 1997, with permission.

treat organic voice problems and occasionally take responsibility for prescribing psychoactive medications. Speech-language pathologists are responsible for behavioral therapy for speech, language and swallowing disorders. In many other countries, phoniatrists perform behavioral therapy in addition to making diagnoses. Phoniatrists are physicians. Traditionally, in some countries they have been members of an independent specialty that does not include laryngeal surgery. In other countries, they have been subspecialists of otolaryngology. The European Union has recently determined that in the future, in member countries, phoniatry will be a subspecialty of otolaryngology. Both speech-language pathologists and phoniatrists include at least some psychological assessment and support in their therapeutic paradigms. However, they are not fully trained mental health professionals and must be constantly vigilant to recognize significant psychopathology and recommend appropriate referral for treatment by a psychologist or psychiatrist. Finding a mental health professional familiar with the special needs and problems of voice patients, especially singers and actors, is not easy. Arts medicine psychology is a relatively new field, as voice was in otolaryngology in the early 1980s. Nevertheless, it is usually possible to find a psychological professional who is either knowledgeable or at least interested enough to become knowledgeable. Resources are available in the literature to assist the interested mental health professional,[40] and incorporating such a colleague into the voice care team is extremely beneficial.

Psychology and voice disorders: an overview

Patients seeking medical care for voice disorders come from the general population. Consequently, a normal distribution of comorbid psychopathology can be expected in a laryngology practice. Psychological factors can be causally related to a voice disorder and/or consequences of vocal dysfunction. In practice, they are usually interwoven. The first task of the otolaryngologist treating any patient with a voice complaint is to establish an accurate diagnosis and its etiology. Only as a result of a thorough, comprehensive history and physical examination (including state-of-the-art technology) can the organic and psychologic components of the voice complaint be elucidated. All treatment planning and subsequent intervention depend on this process. However, even minor voice injuries or health problems can be disturbing for many patients and devastating to some professional voice users. In some cases, they even trigger responses that delay the return of normal voice. Such stress, and fear of the evaluation procedures themselves, often heighten the problem and may cloud diagnostic assessment. Some voice disorders are predominantly psychogenic, and psychological assessment may be required to complete a thorough evaluation.

The essential role of the voice in communication of the 'self' creates special potential for psychologic impact. Severe psychological consequences of voice dysfunction are especially common in individuals in whom the voice is pathologically perceived to be the self, such as professional voice users. However, the sensitive clinician will recognize varying degrees of similar reaction among most voice patients who are confronted with voice change or loss.

Our work with professional voice users has provided insight into the special intensification of psychological distress they experience in association with lapses in vocal health. This has proved helpful in treating all patients with voice disorders, and has permitted recognition of psychological problems that may delay recovery following vocal injury or surgery.

In all human beings, self-esteem comprises not only who we believe we are, but also what we have chosen to do as our life's work. A psychological 'double-exposure' exists for performers who experience difficulty separating the two elements. The voice is in, is therefore of, indeed is, the self. Aronson's extensive review of the literature provides an opportunity to examine research that supports the maxim that the 'voice is the mirror of the personality' – both normal and abnormal. Parameters such as voice quality, pitch, loudness, stress pattern, rate, pauses, articulation, vocabulary, syntax and content are described as they reflect life stressors, psychopathology and discrete emotions.[4] Sundberg describes Fonagy's research on the effects of various states of emotion on phonation. These studies revealed specific alterations in articulatory and laryngeal structures and in respiratory muscular activity patterns related to 10 different emotional states.[52] Vogel and Carter include descriptive summaries of the features, symptoms and signs of communication impairment in their text on neurologic and psychiatric disorders.[54] The mind and body are inextricably linked. Thoughts and feelings generate neurochemical transmissions that affect all organ systems. Therefore, not only can disturbances of physical function have profound emotional effects, disturbances of emotion can have profound bodily and artistic effects.

Professional voice users: a special case

It is useful to understand in greater depth the problems experienced by professional voice users who suffer vocal injuries. Most of our observations in this population occur among singers and actors. However, it must be remembered that, although they are the most obvious and demanding professional voice users, many other professionals are classified as professional voice users. These include politicians, attorneys, clergy, teachers, salespeople, broadcasters, shop foremen (who speak over noise), football quarterbacks, secretaries, telephone operators and others. Although we are likely to expect profound emotional reactions to voice problems among singers and actors, many other patients may also demonstrate similar reactions. If we do not recognize these reactions as such, they may be misinterpreted as anger, malingering, or other difficult patient behavior. Some patients are unconsciously afraid that their voices are lost forever and are psychologically unable to make a full effort at vocal recovery after injury or surgery. This blocking of the frightening possibilities by rationalization ('I haven't made a maximum attempt so I don't know yet if my voice will be satisfactory') can result in prolonged or incomplete recovery after technically flawless surgery. It is incumbent upon the laryngologist and other members of the voice team to understand the psychological consequences of voice disturbance and to recognize them not only in extreme cases, but even in their more subtle manifestations.[40]

Typically successful professional voice users (especially actors, singers and politicians) may fall into a personality subtype that is ambitious, driven, perfectionistic and tightly controlled. Externally, they present themselves as confident, competitive and self-assured. Internally, self-esteem, the product of personality development, is often far more fragile. Children and adolescents do the best they can to survive and integrate their life experiences. All psychological defense mechanisms are means to that end. Most of these defenses are not under conscious control. They are a habitual element of the fabric of one's response to life, especially in stressful or psychologically threatening situations.

All psychological adjustment expresses itself through the personality of the patient, and it is essential to focus on the personality style of every performer who seeks psychological help. This can best be done during psychological assessment and evaluation by exploring daily activities, especially those pertaining to the performer's involvement with his/her art, the patient's growth and personality development as an artist, and relationships with people both within and outside his/her performing environment. Each developmental phase carries inherent coping tasks and responsibilities, which can play an important part in the patient's emotional response to vocal dysfunction. Learning about, cherishing and managing our unique, individual psychological vulnerabilities is critical to adaptive psychological function throughout life.

Research into body image theory also provides a theoretical basis for understanding the special impact of stress or injuries to the voice in vocal performers. The body is essential to perception, learning and memory and the body serves as a sensory register and processor of sensory information.[48] Body experience is deeply personal and constitutes a private world typically shared with others only under conditions of closest intimacy. Moreover, the body is an expressive instrument, the medium through which individuality is communicated verbally and nonverbally.[48] It is therefore possible to anticipate direct correspondence between certain physical illness or injury and body and self-image. Among these are psychosomatic conditions and/or body states with high levels of involvement of personality factors. In these cases, body illness or injury may reactivate psychopathologic processes that began in early childhood or induce an emotional disorder such as denial or inappropriately prolonged depression.[48] Psychological reactions to a physical injury are not uniformly disturbing or distressing and do not necessarily result in maladjustment. However, Shontz[48] notes that reactions to body injury are more a function of how much anxiety is generated by the experience than by the actual location, severity, or type of injury itself.

Patients are notoriously adaptive and capable of living with most types of difficulties, injuries, or disabilities if they feel there is a good reason for doing so. If one's life has broad meaning and purpose, any given disorder takes on less significance. When a physical disability or any given body part becomes the main focus of concern or has been the main source of self-esteem in a person's life, that life becomes narrowed and constricted. Patients adapt satisfactorily to a personal medical condition when the problems of living related to the injury cease to be the dominant element in their total psychological life.

A unique closeness exists between one's body and one's identity; this body-self is a central part of self-concept. The interdependence of body image and self-esteem means that distortion of one will affect the other. The cognitive-behavioral model for understanding body image includes the perceptual and affective components, as well as attitudinal ones. From the cognitive perspective, any body image producing dysphoria results from irrational thoughts, unrealistic expectations and faulty explanations.[16] Body-image constructs and their affective and cognitive outcomes relate to personality types and cognitive styles. For example, depressive personality types chronically interpret events in terms of deficiencies and are trapped by habitual self-defeating thoughts. Anxious personality types chronically overestimate risks and become hypervigilant. These types of cognitive errors generate automatic thoughts which intensify body-image-related psychopathology.[40]

It is the task of personality theorists to explain the process of the genesis of the self. There are numerous coherent personality theories, all substantially interrelated. The framework of Karen Horney (1885–1952) is particularly useful in attempting to understand the creative personality and its vulnerabilities. In simplification, she formulated a 'holistic notion of the personality as an individual unit functioning within a social framework and continually interacting with its environment'.[21] In Horney's model, there are three selves. The *actual self* is the sum total of the individual's experience; the *real self* is responsible for harmonious integration; and the *idealized self* sets up unrealistically high expectations which, in the face of disappointment, result in self-hatred and self-alienation.[21] We have chosen Horney's theory as a working model in evolving therapeutic approaches to the special patient population of professional voice users. They are the laryngologist's most demanding consumers of voice care and cling to their physician's explanations with dependency.[39,40]

It may be useful, for theoretical clarity, to divide the experience of vocal injury into several phases. In practice, however, these often overlap or recur and the emotional responses are not entirely linear.

- *The phase of problem recognition.* The patient feels that something is wrong, but may not be able to clearly define the problem, especially if the onset has been gradual or masked by a coexisting illness. Usually, personal 'first aid' measures will be tried, and when they fail, the performer will manifest some level of panic. This is often followed by feelings of guilt when the distress is turned inward against the self, or rage or blame when externalized.
- *The phase of diagnosis.* This may be a protracted period if an injured performer does not have immediate access to a laryngologist experienced in the assessment of vocal injury. He or she may have already consulted with voice teachers, family physicians, allergists, nutritionists, peers, or otolaryngologists and speech-language pathologists without specialized training in caring for professional voice users. There may have been several, possibly contradictory, diagnoses and treatment protocols. The vocal dysfunction persists, and the patient grows more fearful and discouraged. If attempts to perform are continued, they may exacerbate the injury and/or produce embarrassing performances. The fear is of the unknown, but it is intuitively perceived as significant.
- *The phase of treatment: acute/rehabilitative.* Now, fear of the unknown becomes fear of the known, and of its outcome. The performer, now in the sick role, initially feels overwhelmed and powerless. There is frequently a strong component of blame that may be turned inward. 'Why me? Why now?' is the operant, recurrent thought. Vocal rehabilitation is an exquisitely slow, carefully monitored, frustrating process, and many patients become fearful and impatient. Some will meet the criteria for major depression, which will be discussed in additional detail, as will the impact of vocal fold surgery.
- *The phase of acceptance.* When the acute and rehabilitative treatment protocol is complete, the final prognosis is clearer. When there are significant lasting changes in the voice, the patient will experience mourning. Even when there is full return of vocal function, a sense of vulnerability lingers. These individuals are likely to adhere strictly, even ritualistically, to preventive vocal hygiene habits and may be anxious enough to become hypochondriacal.[39–41]

The psychological professional providing care to this special population must be well versed in developmental psychology, experience the world of the performer, and retain an unshakable empathy for the extraordinarily psychologically disorganizing impact of potential vocal jury. It is critical to harken back to one of the earliest lessons taught to all psychotherapists-in-training. That is, the therapist must, through accurate empathy, earn the right to make interpretations and interventions. When this type of insightful and accurate support is available to the professional voice user, the psychotherapist may well be the patient's rudder in the rough seas of diagnosis, treatment and rehabilitation.

Psychogenic voice disorders

Voice disorders are divided into organic and nonorganic etiologies. Various terms have been used interchangeably (but imprecisely) to label observable vocal dysfunction in the presence of emotional factors that cause or perpetuate the symptoms. Aronson argues convincingly for the term psychogenic, which is 'broadly synonymous with functional, but has the advantage of stating positively, based on an exploration of its causes, that the voice disorder is a manifestation of one or more types of psychological disequilibrium, such as anxiety, depression, conversion reaction, or personality disorder, that interfere with normal volitional control over phonation'.[4]

Psychogenic disorders include a variety of discrete presentations. There is disagreement over classification among speech-language pathologists, with some excluding musculoskeletal tension disorders from this heading. Aronson, and Butcher *et al.* conclude that the hypercontraction of extrinsic and intrinsic laryngeal muscles, in response to emotional stress, is the common denominator behind the dysphonia or aphonia in these disorders. In addition, the extent of pathology visible on laryngeal examination is inconsistent with the severity of the abnormal voice. They cite four categories:

- *musculoskeletal tension disorders*: including vocal abuse, vocal nodules, contact ulcers, and ventricular phonation;
- *conversion voice disorders*: including conversion muteness and aphonia, conversion dysphonia, and psychogenic adductor 'spasmodic dysphonia';
- *mutational falsetto (puberphonia)*;
- *child-like speech in adults.*[4,9]

Psychogenic dysphonia often presents as total inability to speak, whispered speech, extremely strained or strangled speech, interrupted speech rhythm, or speech in an abnormal register (such as falsetto in a male). Usually, involuntary vocalizations during laughing and coughing are normal. The vocal folds are often difficult to examine because of supraglottic hyperfunction. There may be apparent bowing of both vocal folds consistent with severe muscular tension dysphonia, creating anterior–posterior 'squeeze' during phonation. Longstanding attempts to produce voice in the presence of this pattern may even result in traumatic lesions associated with vocal abuse patterns, such as vocal fold nodules. Normal abduction and adduction of the vocal folds may be visualized during flexible fiberoptic laryngoscopy by instructing the patient to perform maneuvers that decrease supraglottic load, such as whistling or sniffing. In addition, the singing voice is often more easily produced than the speaking voice in these patients. Tongue protrusion and stabilization during the rigid telescopic portion of the examination will often result in clear voice. The severe muscular tension dysphonia associated with psychogenic dysphonia can often be eliminated by behavioral interventions by the speech-language pathologist, sometimes in one session. In many instances moments of successful voice have been restored during stroboscopic examination.

Electromyography may be helpful in confirming the diagnosis by revealing simultaneous firing of abductors and adductors. Psychogenic dysphonia has been frequently misdiagnosed as spasmodic dysphonia, partially explaining the excellent 'spasmodic dysphonia' cure rates in some series.

Psychogenic voice disorders are not merely the *absence* of observable neurolaryngeal abnormalities. This psychiatric diagnosis cannot be made with accuracy without the *presence* of a psychodynamic formulation based on 'understanding of the personality, motivations, conflicts, and primary as well as secondary gain' associated with the symptoms.[32,40]

Conversion disorders are a special classification of psychogenic symptomatology and reflect loss of voluntary control over striated muscle or the sensory systems as a reflection of stress or psychological conflict. They may occur in any organ system, but the target organ is often symbolically related to the specifics of the unconsciously perceived threat. The term was first used by Freud to describe a defense mechanism that rendered an intolerable wish or drive innocuous by translating its energy into a physical symptom. The presence of an ego-syntonic physical illness offers *primary gain*: relief from the anxiety, depression, or rage by maintaining the emotional conflict in the unconscious. *Secondary gain* often occurs by virtue of the sick role.

Classic descriptions of findings in these patients include indifference to the symptoms, chronic stress, suppressed anger, immaturity and dependency, moderate depression and poor sex role identification.[32,58] Conversion voice disorders also reflect a breakdown in communication with someone of emotional significance in the patient's life; wanting but blocking the verbal expression of anger, fear, or remorse, and significant feelings of shame.[4,40]

Confirmed neurologic disease and psychogenic voice disorders do coexist and are known as somatic compliance.[20,44] Of course, potential organic causes of psychiatric disorders must always be thoroughly ruled out. Insidious onset of depression, personality changes, anxiety, or presumed conversion symptoms may be the first presentation of CNS disease.[14]

The speech-language pathologist's role in treating psychological disturbances in patients with voice disorders

Speech-language pathology is a relatively new profession in the USA. Its roots are in psychology. The original members of the field came primarily from psychology backgrounds. Early interest in the psychological aspects of voicing are evidenced in texts such as *The Voice of Neurosis*.[31] Luchsinger and Arnold present an excellent review of the early literature in their text, *Voice–Speech–Language*.[27] At the present time, speech-language pathologists need to be familiar with models of treatment from the psychological tradition, the medical tradition and the educational tradition. When discussing the speech-language pathologist's role in managing functional voice problems, it must be made clear at the outset that the speech-language pathologist does not work in isolation but as part of a team, including, at a minimum, a laryngologist and speech-language pathologist. Singing instructors, acting instructors, stress specialists, psychologists, neurologists and psychiatrists must be readily available and cognizant of the special needs of voice patients.

Psychology is defined as the study of human behavior, and the speech-language pathologist's role in treating voice-disordered patients is normalizing the patient's speaking and communication behavior. In this sense, all of the activities of speech-language pathologists with voice-disordered patients is 'psychological'. The purpose of this chapter is not to present a full description of the role of the speech-language pathologist but to describe those areas in which the speech-language pathologist must deal with issues not directly related to the physical vocal mechanism. However, a brief overview of the activities engaged in by the speech-language pathologist and the voice patient help set the groundwork for a discussion of psychological issues. A more detailed description has been published elsewhere.[43]

Preparation for treatment

The speech-language pathologist must be aware of, and be able to interpret, the findings of the laryngologist, including strobovideolaryngoscopy. Particular attention should be paid to findings demonstrating muscle tension or lack of glottic closure not associated with organic or physical changes. The perceptions of the laryngologist regarding organic and functional aspects of the patient need to be known.

A case history is taken, reviewing and amplifying the case history reported by the laryngologist. The case history should include but not be limited to the following:

1. Circumstances surrounding the onset, development, and progress of the voice disorder, including:
    - illnesses of the patient
    - recent changes in employment
    - speaking responsibilities associated with the patient's employment
    - effects of the voice disorder on employment
    - employment environment
    - speaking activities outside of employment

- environment in which social speaking activities occur
- effects of the voice disorder on social exchange and social activities
- activities the patient has had to give up because of the voice disorder
- illness or difficulty among family members or friends
- stress factors at work and at home
- methods of dealing with stress.

2. Exploration of the social structure of the patient and environment including:
   - family and living arrangements
   - friends and social gathering places
   - relationships with co-workers and superiors.
3. The patient's response to the voice disorder needs to be explored as follows:
   - what bothers the patient most about the voice disorder?
   - what has the patient done to change voicing and how effective have these attempts been?
   - estimates of the speaking times at work and socially, now and before the voice disorder
   - how does the patient feel about speaking at the present time – stressed, indifferent, depressed, challenged?
4. General health issues should be addressed:
   - chronic illness, including asthma, allergies, diabetes, thyroid dysfunction, chronic fatigue
   - head and neck trauma, including whiplash, concussion, spinal degeneration, temporomandibular joint disease, facial injury
   - surgery
   - high fevers
   - non-vocal symptoms, including swallowing difficulty, pain on speaking or swallowing, numbness, neck stiffness or reduced range of motion, voice quality, speaking rate, movement limitations of the articulators, nasal regurgitation, tremor or shakiness.
5. Medications:
   - prescription medications
   - over-the-counter drugs, including NSAIDs, cough drops, decongestants, antihistamines, mouthwash, vitamins, alcohol, tobacco and caffeine products, and water intake.

Subjective and objective measures of the patient's vocal mechanism and communication skills need to be obtained including the following:

1. Average fundamental frequency and loudness of the patient's conversational voice.
2. Average fundamental frequency, loudness and speaking rate during a selected reading passage, both in normal reading and in the professional voice (if a professional speaker).
3. Acoustic and aerodynamic measures of sustained vowels including:
   - measures of perturbation
   - measures of breathiness and noise
   - measures of vocal breaks and quality change
   - measures of air flow
   - measures of glottic pressure.
4. Preferred breathing patterns for speech:
   - shallow, deep, appropriate for phrase length
   - clavicular, thoracic, abdominal, or mixed
   - coordination with voicing – exhalation initiated before voicing, glottic
   - closure prior to initiation of exhalation, coordinated breath/voicing.
5. Neck and laryngeal use:
   - positioning of the larynx during speech – high, low, inflexible
   - tension in the extralaryngeal muscles, particularly the omohyoid
   - laryngeal/hyoid space – present, reduced
   - positioning of the hyoid – tipped, tense, discomfort on palpation of the cornu.
6. Use of the articulators:
   - oroperipheral examination including lip movements and symmetry, tongue movements and symmetry, palatal sufficiency in non-speech contexts, diadochokinetic rates
   - ability to separate jaw and anterior tongue activity during the production of /l/, /t/, /d/, /n/
   - tongue tension during speech
   - jaw tension and jaw jutting during speech
   - looseness of temporomandibular joint during speech movements.

The speech-language pathologist should be able to develop a plan of behavioral changes. The case history provides an ample sample of the patient's voice use in an interview situation. It is important to note how the patient's voice changes when talking about certain topics and to note evidence of improvement or fatigue as the interview proceeds. It provides data on what speaking activities are most important to the patient and which may need to be addressed initially in therapy. It provides information of the patient's willingness to talk about stressful issues or needs beyond direct focus on voicing and speech skills, which may be important regarding referral to other specialists dealing with stress and emotional or physical health. It establishes an initial rapport, or lack of it, with the clinician that may predict success, or failure, in therapeutic intervention. It also provides the speech-language pathologist with a sample of the patient's communication style and verbosity.

The physical assessment provides the speech-language clinician with objective support for what the clinician has heard and information about how the patient is producing the voice. Since behavioral change instituted during therapy is based on eradication of symptoms of maladaptive voice or communication, to list and evaluate confirmed symptoms at this stage leads to the development of an overall therapeutic plan. Focus should be on the identification of the underlying behavior or behaviors responsible for maintaining the current voice in order to address these underlying behaviors first, which reduces the length of therapy and should predict improvement of voicing.

Therapeutic stage

Information giving is essential at the beginning of therapy and throughout the course of therapy. Patients need to know the reason for the activities in which they are engaging and why these activities are important in changing their current voice problem. Without a thorough understanding of the reasons for changing behavior the probabilities of behavioral change are poor.

The patient needs to know that a voice disorder is not usually caused by a single agent, but is maintained by a combination of physical changes, if present, communication demands on the voice, the patient's skills in producing speech, and the patient's attempts to compensate for vocal changes. The goal in therapy is to initially manage communicative demands, and improve the patient's ability to produce more normal voice. Reassessment of the need for medical/surgical interventions for physical changes is planned with the patient. Reassurance is provided that the goal of therapy is not to change personality or limit communication opportunities, but to return these at least to the level of communication enjoyed prior to the onset of the voice problem.

Patients need to have information regarding their current breathing pattern. It may be insufficient for the demands placed on the patient's voice or a contributor to increased tension in the vocal mechanism. Abdominal breathing is the natural and preferred method of breathing by the body. Abdominal breathing is not a new skill. Patients engage in abdominal breathing when they are relaxed and when they are sleeping.

Patients can be asked to observe or recall the breathing patterns of their pets. They can be asked to observe or recall the breathing patterns of babies engaging in comfort sounds versus painful or paroxysmal crying. They can be asked to observe or recall the breathing of significant others in repose. Their observations can be discussed and used as confirmation of the above information.

Patients need to be informed that predominantly clavicular or thoracic breathing is usually the product of stress, a societal preference toward tight clothing, and/or demands by parents, teachers and society in maintaining a tight tucked-in stomach. All of these factors lead to a reduction of abdominal release during inhalation that leads to restriction in diaphragmatic downward motion and maximal inflation of the lungs.

Patients are taught that taking a deep, high-chest breath increases air pressures in the lungs greatly, triggering a Valsalva response with closure of the glottis and laryngeal and chest muscle tension. The kind of breath the patient takes may influence tension in other parts of the vocal mechanism. High-chest breathing can contribute to a feeling of breathlessness and tightness in the chest. Abdominal breathing produces lesser increases of lung air pressure and removes the tension from the neck and larynx. The patient needs to know what he/she is about to say before he/she inhales the breath to say it, and this concept is discussed and practiced. This simple construct eliminates respiratory/laryngeal incoordination, reduces revisions and struggle during speaking and allows the patient to focus on how he/she is saying something rather than on the content of what is being said. Speech should be a continuous breath event, beginning with inhalation of the appropriate amount of air, through easy transition to exhalation and voicing to the end of the utterance. Instruction and discussion of these matters prior to the initiation of a program of breath-support exercises increases the patient's willingness to change and turns the reluctant patient into an active participant in the process of change. Specific breathing exercises to incorporate abdominal breathing are available in many other publications.

Similarly, the patient needs to know that modification of articulation postures and open, relaxed jaw positioning improve loudness and acuity in noisy environments and can be invaluable in improving communication without effort and fatigue in most speaking circumstances. Tongue tension or pulling the tongue back in the mouth leads to tension in the hyoid and larynx region. These effects can easily be demonstrated and discussed by having the patient tense the tongue or retract the tongue while digitally monitoring tension under the chin and at the sides of the larynx. The same effects can be demonstrated during talking activities. Patients need to learn to explore the feelings associated with tension and extra speaking effort.

Instruction in behavior is provided so that the patient understands that the vocal folds are opened by the flow of air from the lungs and closed due to their own elasticity and Bernoulli's principle. The vocal folds are vibrating much too rapidly to be manipulated by laryngeal effort, and patients need to comprehend that the emotional system and the conscious speech system share control of voicing, which varies with emotional context. The patient needs to know that laryngeal control is primarily automatic and that efforts to produce voice are counterproductive. The quality of the patient's voice during physiologic sound-making, such as laughter, and a gentle cough can predict the quality of sound when extra effort is removed. Humming and sighing are also effective means of demonstrating the effect of reduced effort. Modeling by the clinician of easy, well supported, well resonated voice during these conversations can be a highly effective means of modifying the patient's vocal production in the therapy setting.

Closed, tense jaw articulation and substitution of jaw movement for tongue and lip movements increase tension and fatigue in the face and increase the amount of pulling on the temporomandibular joint capsule. These same methods of speaking reduce lip reading and loudness in noisy speaking situations. Patients learn that in American English only six sounds, /s/, /z/, /ch/, /dz/ and /z/ require closure of the jaw. All other consonants and all vowels can be produced by modifying the position of the lips and tongue with no, or minor, jaw adjustment. Most of speech can be produced with the jaw in a relaxed, partially open neutral position. This can be demonstrated by monitoring tension in the masseter muscle; placing the fingers of both hands in front of the ears and alternately clenching and opening the jaw. The patient will be able to feel the bulking of the masseter during clenching and the stretching of the masseter muscle fibers when the jaw is wide open. The neutral speaking position is identifiable by the absence of muscle bulk or stretched fibers. The patient needs to experience the feeling of relaxation associated with this speaking position. The patient can then be instructed in producing the syllable /la/ by simply lifting the tongue and touching the roof of the mouth behind the upper front teeth and then dropping the tongue to a relaxed position behind, but touching, the lower front teeth. This is extended to other consonants (/ta/, /da/, /na/, /ka/, and /ga/). When the patient is proficient in eliminating jaw tension in these contexts, the effect of lip movement in addition to relaxed jaw and tongue by producing words such as, too, due, coo, load, coat, etc., is practiced. Lip consonants without tensing the jaw are then added. The sounds /f/, /v/, /th/, voiced /th/ need to be monitored for jaw jutting. Open relaxed jaw with improved oral resonance and relaxed tongue can then be practiced in words and phrases. Then the patient can practice in sentences. Practice should initially be done monitoring jaw position and movement with fingers between the posterior molars and with a mirror. As the patient begins to feel comfortable with a relaxed jaw, the tactile monitoring and then the visual monitoring can be eliminated. At this point, the patient should identify phrases and sentences he/she uses frequently, such as, Hello, Put them away, I don't like that behavior, etc., which can be used as frequent daily reminders in their normal speech of more normal oral resonance and speech production. This assists in carry-over. Practice continues with sentences including jaw closure sounds and open vowels, such as, 'He is going', 'Let me have a piece of pie', 'I chose two friends to go with me', etc. The open relaxed jaw can then be extended into question and answer activities, monologue and dialogue.

A pattern of frequent tension checks needs to be established with the cooperation of the client. These need not be elaborate warm-up exercises or cool-down practice. The patient may decide to practice abdominal breathing in the shower, blowing the water away from his/her face, or humming with a relaxed jaw while inhaling the warm steamy air. The patient may be able to stroke the face, jaw or neck at each stop light while driving to or from work or take an easy belly breath followed by a relaxed sigh. The patient may check his/her jaw tension before picking up the telephone to say 'hello'. A brief reminding note can be taped to the inside of the telephone receiver. Abdominal breathing can be practiced leaning over the desk while reading memos or correcting examination papers. A sip of water between tasks can help the patient focus on relaxation of the jaw, throat and can be preceded by a deep abdominal inhalation. The patient can be very creative and very helpful in identifying times when correct vocal behavior can be practiced. Multiple reminders during the busy day can be more effective than a half-hour practice in the isolation of the patient's home, and are more likely to be done.

All these exercises are helpful in aiding the patient to become aware of the subtle nature of tension in the speaking mechanism, but may be overwhelmed by overriding tension not associated directly with speaking behavior in the face and neck. A decision must be made as to whether the speech-language pathologist has the skill to develop a more stringent relaxation regimen or if the patient needs, and is amenable to, a referral to an expert in stress management.

A discussion of relevant and irrelevant talking is necessary, if the patient talks excessively. The patient needs to know that total vocal rest, if extended past a week, can lead to muscle atrophy and an additional voice problem. The concept of vocal naps during the day and the possibility of reducing talking, or more positively, becoming a better listener in noisy environments, should be introduced. The patient is more knowledgeable than the therapist in when and how long these quiet times can be inserted into the daily schedule.

Patients under stress will bring their 'job-voice' home with them. The patient will often complain that family members nag about the use of too loud a voice, of being too demanding, or of using too many directions. A vocal nap during the ride home with an added cool-down protocol can be helpful in providing a positive transition. The patient should be reminded that singing in the car over the noise of traffic and radio and engine noises can be abusive.

The patient needs to know that everyone lip reads in noisy environments. If the patient has been successful in developing open oral resonance and articulation patterns, the ability of the patient's listeners to understand in noisy situations is enhanced. A slower rate of talking is also helpful in improving comprehension. The patient should be instructed in the effective use of light to highlight his/her face during such conversations.

Voice patients under stress often violate the rules of conversation, including rules of relevance, brevity and turn taking. A discussion of these rules may lead to an awareness of inappropriate communication patterns or the revelation of an underlying personality difficulty that may lead to a referral to a psychologic professional. Often persons with difficulty in personal relationships and/or coping with their circumstances can admit to a voice disorder, but not the underlying personal difficulties. The experience of voice therapy, especially supportive rather than prescriptive voice therapy, may lead to the acceptance of a referral to a professional trained in dealing with these underlying difficulties that might have been rejected at initial interview. The combination of an inability to relax following focal voice exercises, an inability to modify communication behaviors, a tendency for the patient to revert to discussions of personal problems rather than focus of the process of communication, all assist the therapist in reinforcing the idea that the patient's problem lies outside the realm of traditional voice therapy. A statement by the therapist such as, 'You have very real problems, but I am not trained to deal with them. I know someone who can help you' can be the beginning of a successful referral.

Finally, the patient needs to know that voice therapy is short term and finite. The goal of therapy is to identify underlying behavioral, emotional and physical factors, modify current vocal behaviors and develop better communication skills. The therapist must be aware that the stressed patient can develop inappropriate dependence upon the therapist. If therapy sessions begin to focus more on the patient's day-to-day personal problems than on voice, the time for referral is long past. Patients need to know that voice therapy usually is successful in only a few sessions, unless there are other problems that maintain the maladaptive vocal behavior. The therapeutic goal in these cases is to identify the underlying problems and make the appropriate referrals. This is a difficult concept for some patients, particularly singers, who are used to taking singing lessons most of their life.

Examples of psychological aspects of voice disorders

Patients often respond to a voice change by struggling to continue to use their voices in their daily jobs. Teachers will continue to teach, preachers continue to preach, and sales personnel continue to sell. The fear of losing their livelihood drives them to modify their speaking techniques, usually applying extra effort, which results in fatigue, pain and progressive voice loss. They will stop doing enjoyable leisure activities that involve talking and begin to feel impoverished both personally and socially. Feelings of self-worth are also diminished. They feel as though they are not doing their job as well as possible and often consider job changes that do not suit their training or skills.

The speech-language pathologist (SLP) can be very helpful in reducing these feelings by focusing on a plan to return the patient to comfortable functioning in the current occupation. If the patient is successful in modifying the effortful and compromised voice using the techniques described above, these reactions subside. It behoves the SLP to develop a therapeutic program that will provide the most rapid return of better voicing. The patient needs to be evaluated for the key elements producing vocal fatigue and vocal quality changes. A program of vocal hygiene that can alleviate environmental and behavioral stresses in the workplace, a program of reasonable vocal rest during the work day, and the initiation of a program which will reinstate the balance between respiratory, voicing and resonance effort in vocal technique are very important. A timetable of when the patient can resume specific activities or when the treatment program will be reviewed to assess alternate treatment options gives the patient something to work toward.

Case 1

Case 1 had been a fifth grade school teacher for 20 years. She denied having any previous voice problems, other than vocal fatigue by the end of the week at the end of the school year. She also assisted her husband, a pediatrician, as his receptionist during evening office hours. However, she now presented with progressive hoarseness. She was diagnosed with vocal fold swelling, gastroesophageal reflux laryngitis, and pinpoint vocal nodules by a laryngologist. She was seen by a speech-language pathologist one month prior to the end of the school year.

Case history revealed important life differences. The previous summer the regular receptionist at her husband's office had taken a maternity leave and she had volunteered her services over the summer months. It was a busy office and she spent many hours on the telephone and talking with patients. Her voice did not feel rested at the beginning of the school year.

Because of her excellent teaching record she had been assigned a student teacher who required a great deal of counseling, typically after school hours. She found herself rushing from school to her husband's office without time to eat. She began eating after office hours, experiencing heartburn and disrupted sleep. Her voice was worse in the morning and even more fatigued after the school day. She was physically tired before the day began. She had been given a prescription for ranitidine (Zantac), but did not believe it was helping her.

She noted that her students, her husband and the patients at her husband's office complained that she was 'yelling at them'. She was very worried about her ability to continue teaching with no voice. She was worried about the status of her marriage. She was frustrated by the fact that she was at least a month behind in school lesson plans and correction of homework papers and tests. She had tried correcting papers at her desk in her husband's office but found the mess intolerable and interfering with her receptionist tasks. She said: 'Now I have to carry three bags of work home, and somehow it never gets done.' She was seriously considering quitting teaching but was ambivalent because she really enjoyed teaching and felt she had a great deal to give both to her students and student teachers. Her principal was urging her to make a decision about teaching the next year and also about taking on another student teacher. She felt that engaging in voice therapy would only complicate her already busy schedule. She stated: 'The harder I try, the worse things seem to get.' She then cried.

Evaluation of her voice revealed a shallow thoracic breathing pattern. She had developed a pattern of taking a quick breath and holding it prior to initiation of voicing, resulting in glottal attack rates of 54% (normal 15%). Her voice was loud, low pitched and rough. She was using a tense jaw, jutting forward during speech. These characteristics were even worse when demonstrating her current teaching voice. She felt her voice was very different in the classroom now than before her voice problems began.

The following therapeutic plan was developed. Direct voice therapy was deferred until July following the end of school and a brief vacation. In the meantime she was urged to continue using the ranitidine and to institute a more rigorous program to control her reflux. The program included the use of liquid antacids following each meal and at bedtime to neutralize the contents of her stomach should she reflux, elevation of the head of her bed to reduce night-time reflux and to promote better sleep, and to try to find time to eat a light meal prior to the onset of office hours. The matter of paper work was discussed. She felt she might be able to combine her counseling sessions with her student teacher with grading activities and also decided she would allow the student teacher to help her with the paper grading. This left her with lesson plans that she felt she accomplished by coming in to work 20 minutes early. She decided to not take a new student teacher in the fall, but to try to teach. Because of this decision she committed herself to six sessions of voice therapy over the summer. A plan was developed to provide those sessions followed by reevaluation by the laryngologist. If the therapy was unsuccessful she could apply for a 3 months leave of absence from teaching.

She returned for therapy in July. She was feeling better physically and was sleeping better. Therapy focused on reducing vocal effort, reestablishing abdominal breathing, reducing glottal stopping, jaw relaxation and open oral resonance for loudness. Classroom teaching materials were used for exercises. She was able to modify her vocal behaviors easily, although she continued to voice concern about her ability to use them in the classroom. A probable set of voice rests during the school day was discussed and cool-down procedures to implement on the trip to the office were planned. At the end of the therapy, review by the laryngologist demonstrated a reduction in the size of the vocal nodules, resolution of vocal swelling and reduced reflux findings. She decided to try teaching but was still worried. A plan was developed to see her for therapeutic review 2 weeks into the school year, then, if needed, mid-fall, at winter break, at spring break and at the end of the school year. If she felt she did not need to come in, she would call and report how her voice was progressing.

At the meeting 2 weeks into the school year, she reported that she was surviving. She was still concerned about whether she was using her voice correctly. Through discussion, she decided she would enlist her students as monitors, particularly for loudness. During the fall, she called to say she was doing well. Her voice was strong and she was much less tired. She reported that her class had taken their role in monitoring her voice very enthusiastically and seriously. Her admission of voice problems and need for help had become an advantage for noise control in her classroom and in student/teacher interactions. She was planning to develop a vocal hygiene section in her curriculum.

At winter break, she attended one session for review. Her glottal attacks were reduced to 8%. She reported her voice was not as fatigued and she was eagerly looking forward to return to teaching after the break. Breath support and oral resonance had improved.

At spring break, she reported her voice was different. She no longer experienced vocal fatigue. She was using a lighter voice in the classroom. Glottal attack remained under 10%. She was sleeping all night. Her reflux appeared to be under control. She stated: 'I now realize that I don't have to take all responsibility for communicating in the classroom. The kids have been very responsive.' She was dismissed from therapy but reminded to contact the therapist if she experienced any problems.

Some patients appear to react to life stresses by overuse of their voices and excessive tension focused in the speaking mechanism. They may consider themselves talkative and congenial persons but actually talk constantly, rapidly, or in an excessively loud voice. They appear to be afraid of silence or afraid that if they give up their turn to talk they will not be able to talk again. They often complain of pain and tension in the neck and jaw or of a feeling of breathlessness. They may seek treatment when their inappropriate speaking patterns lead to benign lesions of the larynx or when some other organic change in the vocal mechanism causes their voice to break down. Modeling slower, softer voicing and turn taking during therapeutic sessions can be very helpful in reducing these vocal faults and providing a more reasonable speaking pattern. The development of relaxation programs for the face and neck to be used frequently during the day is useful. Discussions of the rules of discourse may be helpful.

Some patients bring with them a severe overall body reaction to the stresses of their life. They complain of fatigue, sleeplessness, tension and pain. They are unable to turn off their 'work voice' at home. They complain of lack of time to complete all the activities in which they are engaged. Standard therapeutic procedures often are ineffective because they are unable to distinguish the subtle changes in support, voicing or resonation due to the overriding levels of general tension. They appear to be out of harmony with their body. Focal relaxation of the vocal mechanism is unsuccessful. They usually deny having emotional problems and have difficulty dealing with the daily stress, but continue to return to nonvocal issues during the course of therapy. The SLP can be helpful in allowing these patients to experience a supportive one-on-one relationship as a prelude to referral to a psychologic professional. Often after several sessions with the SLP protesting that, 'We are talking about issues I am not able to help you with, but Dr X can', the patient is receptive to referral. Often referral to a stress manager or professional trained in Feldenkreis or Alexander technique or some other relaxation/body awareness method can be useful. The patient may return to the SLP following resolution of some of these issues. The SLP needs to be careful not to continue the therapeutic relationship so long that the patient becomes dependent on an ineffectual but sympathetic ear.

Case 2

Case 2 presented with a large hemorrhagic cyst on one vocal fold and a reactive lesion directly opposite the cyst on the other vocal fold. She was married and had an adopted son. She was a grade school teacher. She had been forced to take a sabbatical because her voice had deteriorated. On evaluation she presented with a loud, hoarse voice with frequent glottal attacks and frequent aphonic breaks. She was extremely verbal with frequent run-on sentences and sentence revisions. She demonstrated a pattern of taking a rapid, large chest breath followed by holding the breath with her larynx at the end of inhalation. She demonstrated excessive tension in the speech musculature. Her conversational style was repetitious. Interestingly, her teacher's voice was better controlled. She admitted that yelling at a sporting event probably caused the cyst. She was seen prior to surgery. Therapy consisted in promoting a softer, more breathy voice. The combination of being relieved from teaching duties and modifying voicing behaviors was successful in eliminating the reactive lesion. Surgery for the hemorrhagic cyst was planned and carried out successfully. She was able to complete a week of voice rest following the surgery. The following weeks of gradual increased voice use were difficult for her. Therapy focused on reducing glottal attacks, improving breath support and monitoring loudness. Materials included readings and repeated sentences and phrases. Materials from her classroom texts were used in preparation for her return to the classroom. She made excellent progress. However, when therapy moved to monitoring her new skills in general conversation, it became clear that she was unable to recognize her loudness level, control her excessive talking or identify hard glottal attack.

She returned to school and was seen on a limited schedule similar to that used with the previously described patient. She complained of continued vocal fatigue and hoarseness. She developed a pattern of bringing small gifts. She had limited success in developing self-monitoring skills outside of controlled materials or classroom activities. She successfully completed the school year with no return of vocal fold masses. However, her monitoring skills and general levels of tension remained unchanged. The termination of therapy was discussed. She was very anxious about the termination, citing the continued fatigue and difficulties in monitoring her speech outside of the classroom. It was suggested that emotional factors might play a role in her lack of success in changing these behaviors and that she might wish to begin seeing the psychologist associated with the practice. At this point, she admitted to a long history of both physical and verbal abuse, first from her father and then from her husband. It became clear that her failures in therapy led to criticism by the therapist that satisfied her unconscious need for abuse.

Patients with aphonia

There appear to be three categories of patients who have little voicing capability in the absence of structural or neurological etiology. Some patients present with a whispered voice without vocal paralysis, vocal injury or other pathology. Usually the vocal folds appear to be normal. Initial case history may or may not reveal psychological trauma associated with the onset. Nonspeech sounds such as cough, laugh, cry and throat clearing are present and normal. These sounds can be extended gradually into speech. If the patient is ready to give up the aphonic behavior, therapy is relatively brief, usually within one session.

Case 3

Case 3 presented with a loud strained whispered voice. The laryngologist had found no laryngeal pathology. Case history revealed no changes in lifestyle, or environment, at the time of onset. However, the voice problem began about 1 year after her husband's retirement as owner and manager of a large grocery store. The family lived in a small town some distance from any cultural area. She felt the voice loss was related to a bad cold and allergy she had experienced at the time of onset. Normal voice was observed during throat clearing, coughing and laughter. When asked 'what bothered her about her voice loss', she answered, 'I can't talk to my friends!'

Therapy consisted of extending the throat clear from 'ah? hum' to longer and longer hum-m-m-m sounds. She was then able to produce the hum word without the throat clear. The 'hum' was extended into single 'm' words and phrases beginning with 'm' words. At this point, she reverted to whisper. The process was repeated with additional focus on relaxed production. This time she was able to extend to days of the week, counting, short phrases, sentences and, finally, conversation. It is not unusual to have to start at the beginning several times with these patients. She was very relieved and thankful to be able to talk again. During the ensuing conversation, she said: 'Now, maybe he will let me rejoin my bridge club.' When re-questioned about changes in her lifestyle, she admitted that since her husband's retirement her life had changed extensively. She had thought, however, that it was only part of what to expect when one's spouse retired. He had begun to criticize her housekeeping in the same managerial style he used with his employees at the store. He had always done this, but now that he was retired and home it became almost constant. She was resentful because he did not volunteer to help. After about a year, he became more and more concerned with expenses and living on a fixed income. He complained about her extravagance in entertaining her bridge club every other month, even though he continued to golf regularly and he continued to attend his bowling team matches. He finally forbade her to entertain her bridge club and essentially took away her only source of pleasure and enjoyment. It was at this point her voice deteriorated.

The mechanism of conversion reaction was then discussed in terms of the conflict between anger, resentment and frustration versus maintenance of a loving relationship that might suffer irreparable damage if feelings were verbalized. She agreed that this was what had happened. These matters were discussed with her husband and the couple consented to marriage counseling on their return to their local community.

Some patients accrue secondary gain from a voice disorder. Often these patients come to the voice pathologist on the insistence of others. There frequently is a lack of affect surrounding the patient's feeling about his/her voice problem.

Case 4

Case 4 was a very wealthy widowed woman. She was brought to the voice center at the insistence of her unmarried sister who had come to live with her after the death of her husband. Onset of the voice problem had been gradual, beginning with speech within the home. The laryngologist reported normal vocal folds with no evidence of structural or neurologic pathology. The patient demonstrated little concern about her voice problem other than an inconvenience. When asked how her voice interfered with her life, she stated, with a little smile: 'Well, when I am at parties, everyone has to come up to me to converse, and of course, I cannot reprimand or manage the servants, and I can't do the grocery shopping, my sister has to do that.' Although physiologic sounds were present in normal voice, she was unable to extend them into any semblance of speech voicing. She took umbrage at the suggestion of counseling or any emotional etiology for her voice problem and terminated contact. She refused to have her case discussed with her sister. It appeared to be clear that her voice problem would not improve until her sister and friends stopped reinforcing the positive impact of her voice problem.

A second group of aphonic patients present with tense aphonic speech with intermittent squeaky, high-pitched syllables or words. They are often misdiagnosed with spasmodic dysphonia, currently thought to be a neurological disorder. Careful differential diagnosis is important. However, initial evaluation and treatment are similar regardless of initial diagnosis.

These patients may present with a history of emotional disorder or severe stress, reflux, asthma and/or chemical sensitivity resulting in laryngospasm. Strobovideolaryngoscopy usually reveals severe muscle tension with anterior–posterior constriction, elevated laryngeal position, reduced abduction and adduction and, in many cases, evidence of reflux laryngitis. Evaluation of the vocal mechanism finds the larynx held high in the neck. There is tension in the jaw, tongue and extralaryngeal muscles. Breathing is high in the chest with excessive inspiratory effort. Therapy includes Aronson's digital manipulation,[4] yawn-sigh, swallow and gargling activities to lower and relax the larynx. Tongue and jaw must be relaxed, using techniques described previously. Good abdominal breathing must be developed. Therapy needs to be intensive, on a daily basis. Appointments on a weekly basis allow too much time for the tension reactions to re-establish themselves, reducing the effectiveness of therapeutic intervention. Referral to a stress manager or psychologist is sometimes necessary. If voice therapy is successful in establishing normally pitched voice with little evidence of tension, but spasmodic aphonic breaks persist, the patient should be re-evaluated for the presence of spasmodic dysphonia.

Case 5

Case 5 presented with a high-pitched squeaky voice with frequent aphonic breaks. He felt his voice problem was directly related to his work situation. He was a middle manager in a utility. He felt his company was in the process of down-sizing, but instead of firing of employees, the company designated some employees as eligible for up-grade training. The training consisted of EST-like sessions with no bathroom or food breaks and constant berating of the employee. Several of his fellow employees quit. He vowed to fight the system. However, at this point he lost his voice. He was transferred within the company from sales to a computer-intensive position. His voice returned to the presenting squeaky quality. He felt the stress of his treatment at work and resulting stress at home were directly related to his problem. Evaluation revealed high, tense laryngeal position, pain on palpation of the hyoid bone supporting the tongue, and 'chest heave' breathing pattern. He was seen for a period of 3 days. Initially he was unable to maintain a relaxed lowered laryngeal position. He was able to monitor his larynx position digitally and was aware of the mechanism. When his larynx was lowered he produced normally pitched but breathy voice. Cues to make his voice louder improved voice quality but tended to introduce laryngeal tension and lifting of the larynx. Continued therapy, to relax the tongue and jaw and to develop abdominal breathing, were effective in producing normal voice. He refused suggestions for referral to the voice team psychologist. He contacts the therapist on occasion and continues to be symptom-free.

Case 6

Case 6 was a teacher's assistant in a preschool program. She came to school early one day and found the janitor cleaning the floors with a strong disinfectant liquid cleaner. Excessive cleaning fluid had spilled from the container and had spread across the floor. She was unable to breathe and was sent to emergency care, requiring muscle relaxants and oxygen to restore breathing. Her breathing improved but her voice became high-pitched and squeaky. She experienced two other incidents of breathing difficulties associated with the smells in a new store and when buying carpet. She was unable to use commercial cleaning products in her home without experiencing shortness of breath. She was diagnosed with laryngospasm. Strobovideolaryngoscopy revealed severe muscle tension and elevated larynx, but normal laryngeal function. Voice evaluation revealed high laryngeal positioning, extreme tension in the neck and extralaryngeal muscles and a rapid, shallow, thoracic breathing pattern. The patient was convinced that her voice problem was related to 'damage while hospitalized' and was considering suing the hospital.

Gentle digital massage and head and neck relaxation exercises restored her voice to normal. Therapy then focused on reducing fears of breathing and voicing. She was given strategies, including slow, deep, abdominal breathing and jaw and throat relaxation patterns, to counteract the return of the laryngeal spasms. She consented to referral to stress management/psychology. Therapy with the psychologist focused on deep relaxation and hypnotic suggestion to reduce fears and anxiety. She was able to return to work. She still avoided areas with strong smells but was able to utilize her compensation techniques. She has not required hospitalization for breathing difficulties since.

A third group of aphonic patients present with aphonia accompanied with low-pitched, rough, strangled voice quality. Strobovideolaryngoscopy reveals extreme supralaryngeal tension with both anterior/posterior and medial compression of supralaryngeal structures. Often laryngeal examination is discontinued and voice therapy pursued because of the difficulty in viewing the vocal folds beneath the extreme supralaryngeal closure. Emotional trauma is usually present in these cases. Again, these patients are often misdiagnosed as having spasmodic dysphonia. Frequently, the same techniques utilized with whispering patients are helpful in modifying the vocal behavior towards normal. In addition, inhalation speech can be helpful in breaking the supraglottic tension.

Case 7

Case 7 lost her voice following the death of her grandson. Her voice was low, rough, strangled and intermittently aphonic. Voice evaluation demonstrated generalized reduction of movement in the respiratory and articulatory systems with excessive tension in the extralaryngeal musculature. During the history, she described the death of her grandson. Her daughter and son-in-law went out to dinner, leaving their son with her and her husband. During the evening, the child suffered a severe asthma attack and died in her arms despite CPR. During the telling of this story her voice became more and more strangled. The therapist commented that she sounded like she wanted to cry and offered a tissue. At this, she burst into tears and great sobbing. She began to cry in a normal voice: 'I am so angry.' The therapist asked if she was angry because of the death of her grandson. She replied: 'No, I am angry because I have not had a chance to grieve.' Continuing in a normal voice, she related that her husband, daughter and son-in-law were devastated by the death, which left her to make all arrangements for the autopsy, funeral and burial. Her anger was especially directed toward her husband, who did not help, nor give her any expression of sympathy or sensitivity to the depth of her feelings about the death and its aftermath. At the end of this revelation, the therapist gently brought her attention to the fact that her voice had become quite normal. She said: 'Yes, but that's not the problem.' She agreed to and was immediately referred to the voice team psychologist. She was followed periodically by speech therapy. Her voice remained stable. The psychologist reported that her problems with her family were much more extensive than those she had related to the speech-language pathologist.

Case 8

Case 8 was referred from his local speech-language pathologist to be evaluated for possible spasmodic dysphonia. He had been unable to obtain any normal speech after several months of therapy. His therapy had focused on relaxation techniques and breathing.

The patient presented with severe muscle tension and low-pitched rough voice with a predominating whisper. Laryngoscopy could not be completed due to the severe supraglottic constriction. He denied any emotional trauma associated with the onset of his voice problem. His wife, however, felt it might be related to the death of his mother, followed within a month by the death of his father. He was also in the process of beginning retirement. All direct attempts at relaxing his voice, including inhalation speech, were ineffective or caused his voice to become worse. During instructional episodes and general conversation, he produced an occasional normal word or phrase. The therapist decided that direct therapy was not effective and began modeling normal easy voicing in conversation. Normal words and phrases were pointed out, and he was asked to reproduce the same vocal feeling and style in further conversation. Conversation focused on positive experiences and pleasurable activities. Over the course of four sessions, the frequency of normal voice continued to increase. His wife reported episodes of normal voice at home. By the fifth session, his voice was consistently normal except for a reduction in vocal loudness. There was no evidence of spasm. At this point, strobovideolaryngoscopy was completed and was within normal limits. At the next session, the subject of his parent's deaths was broached. He denied that this was a problem that 'a good man should let it bother him. A man should be strong enough to deal with such an inevitable occurrence.' He felt it had been inappropriate of his previous female therapist to focus on that problem and found it difficult to cooperate with her in relaxation and breathing tasks. He was not ready to discuss his reaction. At the next session, he maintained his voicing. He also was able to begin to modify his breathing pattern to increase support and loudness. At the next session, he announced that he felt his voice had returned to normal and terminated therapy. He was seen at 6 months follow-up with the laryngologist and continued to maintain relatively normal voice.

A fourth form of aphonia is voluntary muteness. Voluntary muteness in the absence of severe laryngeal pathology, developmental language delay, or severe hearing loss is very rare. In 35 years of experience with voice patients, this author (RJH) has seen only one such case.

Case 9

Case 9 was a 12-year-old boy. His mother, a loquacious and verbal woman, brought him to the voice center. She was concerned about his preparation for bar mitzvah. She was planning a large ceremony and big party, which she thought he would enjoy. However, he would not talk to her about the event or talk to the cantor or rabbi during training lessons. She had taken him to a psychologist, but he would not talk to her either. He was doing well in school although she did not know how much talking he did there. She reported that his father was a soft spoken man of few words. She felt that voice therapy might be helpful in increasing his loudness and ability to perform at his bar mitzvah.

Strobovideolaryngoscopy demonstrated a normal larynx. However, the laryngologist was unable to get him to vocalize with any strength. The therapist agreed to attempt short-term therapy, but felt that he had found a powerful tool to control his mother.

He reluctantly participated in breathing exercises and better oral resonance. He would practice portions of the readings required at the bar mitzvah service, but only in exchange for a turn at a computer game.

He arrived at the third session more animated than he had ever been before. His teacher had given the class a book report assignment. Each student was to read a book and then report orally to the class about the story from the point of view of one of the characters in the book. The report could only be 5 minutes long. He had chosen *Tom Sawyer* and wanted to report in the guise of that character. He discussed in detail his plans for a costume and asked for help in presenting an already prepared presentation. We worked on appropriate breath support and phrasing, projection and open oral resonance and editing for length. He asked for an additional session to give us more time prior to his presentation. It was hoped that a breakthrough had occurred. He was working as hard as any aspiring actor, reporting that he received an A+ on his presentation. However, when the work resumed on his bar mitzvah readings, the old reluctance returned. He was able to demonstrate his skills if rewarded, but continued to be silent at home. His mother reported that he would at least mumble his readings to the cantor. Plans for a large bar mitzvah were cancelled. His mother was reluctant to re-engage in psychotherapy, and the patient discontinued voice therapy.

Voice problems associated with psychosis

Rarely does the voice of the psychotic patient present as the most relevant symptom. Several studies have been published characterizing the speech of the schizophrenic. These characteristics are considered to be the byproduct of affect, aura and relational disturbances. Speech therapy for those voice characteristics is rarely considered. However, occasionally such a patient will be seen in a voice center.

Case 10

Case 10 had a successful career in a medical subspecialty. However, she aspired to a career in opera. She had taken many lessons, but had been discouraged by her family and teachers to pursue this professionally. She had been highly unsuccessful while auditioning for roles. She came to the voice center to have her singing/speaking voice evaluated. Strobovideolaryngoscopy revealed normal laryngeal structures. She revealed, during history-taking, that her voice was fine at work, because of the lead shielding at the hospital. However, at home, her voice was disrupted and changed in quality, particularly when she was practicing singing and acting and at auditions. When asked why, she reported that 'they' were shooting laser beams at her and shocking her, which disrupted her voice and made her voicing very tense. When asked, 'Who they were?' She replied, 'Certain others who are jealous of my talents and want to thwart my career in singing.' She also reported that the beams 'they' were using burned her and produced changes in her skin color around her neck and shoulders.

When reading a passage, she winced, dodged, and several times cried out in pain. When this behavior was questioned, she reported calmly that 'they' had followed her to the center and were shooting laser beams and using electric shock on her. She was reluctant to work on her speaking voice because the problems of tension that she had were caused by an external force and not by her.

Her evaluation by our singing specialist was similar. She was urged by the entire team to submit to evaluation by a psychiatrist, but would not do so.

Voice problems associated with adolescence

Mutational falsetto is high-falsetto voicing, often with frequent pitch breaks. The voice is thin and high pitched.

Falsetto voice requires a different shaping of the glottis and different breath support than typical voicing. The larynx must ride high in the neck to produce falsetto. It is a normal phenomenon; most males can produce it. It is used frequently in singing by rock and roll singers and developed extensively by classical countertenors, but it is not a preferred means of speech communication. It occurs in some young men following the onset of laryngeal growth associated with adolescence. The techniques described above for use with patients with squeaky voices are useful in this group. Usually, normal voicing is easily achieved during the evaluation and trial therapy sessions. Often the patient has both falsetto and normal voice, but prefers the falsetto for various personal reasons. Most of these patients are nonmuscular young men with little self-confidence. It has often been misdiagnosed as spasmodic dysphonia because of the pitch breaks.

Case 11

Case 11 was a 23-year-old auto body repairman. He was concerned about laryngeal cancer. His girlfriend and parents accompanied him to the voice clinic. Strobovideolaryngoscopy revealed normal larynx and the presence of falsetto voicing. During the voice evaluation, he was asked if he had any other voices. In a normal deep baritone he answered 'Yes.' He used the deep voice around his colleagues at the auto body shop. He used the falsetto voice with his girlfriend, his family and his high school friends. His life was organized around the premise that the two groups of people were never present at the same time. When asked why he needed the dichotomy of voice, he answered that he was afraid his girlfriend and family wouldn't like his other voice. He was asked if he would be willing to try. His girlfriend was brought into the room and he used his deep voice. She, of course, was thrilled. He was relieved, and his voice problem was solved.

Case 12

Case 12 was a 19-year-old college student. He had just completed his freshman year at a religious college. He had attended a choir school during his primary school years and had sung many soprano solos. His best singing occurred just prior to adolescent voice change. He continued to sing soprano although his voice became thin and he had difficulty keeping his voice from cracking following vocal mutation. His speaking voice continued to be high, breathy and characterized by pitch breaks.

When he arrived at college, he enrolled in the religious music department, hoping to continue a career in choral singing. His singing teacher, instead of being impressed by his high voice, referred him to a local speech-language pathologist. He was diagnosed with spasmodic dysphonia, presumably because of the numerous pitch breaks. He was referred for neurological workup and Botox injection. His singing teacher was not convinced of this diagnosis and referred him to our voice center.

Strobovideolaryngoscopy revealed normal larynx with falsetto voice patterning. He was convinced that 'spasmodic dysphonia had destroyed his singing voice'. He was counseled on the effects of adolescent voice change. We explored the large size and angular shape of his larynx, comparing it to the much smaller, rounded larynx of a child. The symptoms of spasmodic dysphonia were described and tapes of spasmodic dysphonic voices were played for him.

Attempts at producing low-pitched normal voice extending from cough and throat-clearing sounds were successful but transition into speech sounds was difficult. He was asked to put his finger across his 'Adam's apple' and tuck his chin down toward his chest. This maneuver made falsetto voicing impossible. Normal low-pitched voicing was achieved and transferred to syllables, words, phrases, questions/answers and monologue. The positioning cues were faded to gentle downward tactile cues. He was engaged in conversation using the 'new' voice for at least 30 minutes. He was asked to use his new voice with other personnel, his family (who had accompanied him to the center), and on the telephone to his singing teacher. His family was relieved that Botox injections would not be necessary. Breath support was practiced in context of his speech. By the end of the evaluation and trial therapy session, he was convinced that he was a baritone and could continue singing in that role. He no longer felt he had spasmodic dysphonia. The singing specialist at the voice center saw him and it was reported that he was able to maintain his speaking voice and begin some singing exercises focusing on lower range extension and breath support. He was asked to call the center the following day to report on continued use of the 'new' voice. During that call, the patient reported that he had retained his lower voice. He was looking forward to returning to college and working with his singing teacher on developing his baritone voice.

Occasionally, males with mutational falsetto demonstrate personal conflicts with their fathers, attachment problems with their mothers, or gender confusion. These patients tend to produce normal voice reluctantly and fail to maintain it, often complaining that such a voice is not appropriate for them. Counseling and referral to a psychological professional to focus on these difficulties is necessary.

Young women do not present with mutational falsetto. Rarely, a young postpubescent girl will present with immature voice. This is characterized by high pitch and melody, inflection, articulation and word choice more reminiscent of a preschool child than a postpubertal young adult. Usually, strong dependent behaviors are described in the history.

Case 13

Case 13 was a 17-year-old high school student who aspired to a career in musical theater. She had been highly successful in obtaining roles as a child in productions of

Annie. She had been thwarted lately in winning any role because of her voice. She was close to tears and appeared to be very depressed. Laryngological examination demonstrated normal structures but muscle tension associated with high pitch. Her voice was very high pitched and immature with a mild lisp and 'r' sound distortions. She was seen in therapy and made progress in controlled contexts. However, she was unable to transfer her more mature voice to home and school environments. She was very unhappy about this and felt that something was blocking her ability to use her more mature voice outside the office. She readily accepted referral to psychologic services. However, because of travel distance she was seen by someone closer to her home.

Summary

In summary, speech-language pathologists provide many services in the context of a team approach to functional voice disorders. The speech-language pathologist must be able to modify disordered voices into functional voices with sufficient stamina to endure the demands of lifestyle and environment. The speech-language pathologist provides a caring and supportive environment that allows patients to explore possible underlying causes. Speech-language pathologists assist in the differential diagnosis of functional from organic disorders. He or she must be able to discern the difference between functional voice patterns and those that require medical/surgical treatment, and to share such insights with the laryngologist responsible for making medical diagnoses. Sensitivity to the fact that the voice is the mirror of emotions and help to identify those emotions are essential. Speech-language pathologists must provide prudent and appropriate referral to other professionals trained in dealing with the psychological and emotional issues. Above all, each speech-language pathologist must be aware of his/her own limitations and develop strong and cooperative relationships with other professionals who care for patients with voice disorders.

The mental health professional's role in treating psychological disturbances in patients with voice disorders

General psychopathologic presentations

Otolaryngologists and all other health care providers involved with patients with voice disorders should recognize significant comorbid psychopathology and should be prepared to consult an appropriate mental health professional. Psychologists and psychiatrists are responsible for psychologic diagnosis and treatment, but it is important to select a mental health professional with advanced understanding of the special problems associated with voice disorders (especially, but not exclusively, in professional voice users). Patterns of voice use may provide clues to the presence of psychopathology, although voice disturbance is certainly not the principal feature of major psychiatric illness. Nevertheless, failure to recognize serious psychopathology in voice patients may result not only in errors in voice diagnosis and failures of therapy, but, more importantly, in serious injury to the patient, sometimes even death.

Although a full depressive syndrome, including melancholia, can occur as a result of loss, it fulfills the criteria for a major depressive episode when the individual becomes preoccupied with feelings of worthlessness and guilt, demonstrates marked psychomotor retardation and other biologic markers and becomes impaired in both social and occupational functioning.[3] Careful listening during the taking of a history will reveal flat affect, including slowed rate of speech, decreased length of utterance, lengthy pauses, decreased pitch variability, monoloudness and frequent use of vocal fry.[8,40,54] William Styron described his speech during his depressive illness as 'slowed to the vocal equivalent of a shuffle'.[51]

Major depression may be part of the patient's past medical history, may be a comorbid illness, or may be a result of the presenting problem. The essential feature is a prominent, persistent dysphoric mood characterized by a loss of pleasure in nearly all activities. Appetite and sleep are disturbed and there may be marked weight gain or loss, hypersomnia, or one of three insomnia patterns. Psychomotor agitation or retardation may be present. Patients may demonstrate distractibility, memory disturbances, and difficulty concentrating. Feelings of worthlessness, helplessness and hopelessness are a classic triad. Suicidal ideation, with or without plan, and/or concomitant psychotic features, may necessitate emergency intervention.

Major affective disorders are classified as unipolar or bipolar. In bipolar disorder, the patient will also experience periods of mania: a recurrent elated state first occurring in young adulthood. (First manic episodes in patients over 50 should alert the clinician to medical or CNS illness, or to the effects of drugs.) The presentation of the illness includes the following major characteristics on a continuum of severity: elevated mood, irritability/hostility, distractibility, inflated self-concept, grandiosity, physical and sexual overactivity, flight of ideas, decreased need for sleep, social intrusiveness, buying sprees, and inappropriate collections of possessions. Manic patients demonstrate impaired social and familial behavior patterns. They are manipulative, alienate family members, and tend to have a very high divorce rate.[3,24] Vocal presentation will manifest flight of ideas (content), rapid-paced, pressured speech, and often increased pitch and volume. There may be dysfluency related to the rate of speech, breathlessness and difficulty in interrupting the language stream. Three major theories, based on neuroanatomy, neuroendocrinology and neuropharmacology, are the most currently promulgated explanations for these disease states, but they are beyond the scope of this chapter.[24,42,56]

Treatment of affective disorders includes psychotherapy. Diagnosis and short-term treatment of reactive depressive states may be performed by the psychologist on the voice team, utilizing individual or group therapy modalities. Longer-term treatment necessitates a referral to a community-based psychotherapist, ideally one whose skills, training and understanding of the medical and artistic components of the illness are well known to the referring laryngologist. The use of psychopharmacologic agents is a risk/benefit decision. When the patient's symptom severity meets the criteria for major affective disorder, the physiological effects of the disease, as well as the potential for self-destructive behavior, must be carefully considered.

Anxiety is an expected response in reaction to any medical diagnosis and the required treatment. However, anxiety disorders are seen with increasing incidence. Vocal presentations of anxiety vary with the continuum of psychiatric symptoms, ranging from depression to agitation and including impairment of concentration. Psychotherapy, including desensitization, cognitive/behavioral techniques, stress management, hypnosis and insight-oriented approaches are helpful. Patients must learn to tolerate their distress and identify factors that precipitate or intensify their symptoms (see Stress management, p.382). Medication may be used to treat underlying depression and decrease the frequency of episodes. However, it leaves the underlying conflict unresolved and negatively affects artistic quality.[39,40,45] Some medical conditions are commonly associated with the presenting symptom of anxiety. These include CNS disease, Cushing's syndrome, hyperthyroidism, hypoglycemia, the consequences of minor head trauma, premenstrual syndrome, and cardiac disease such as mitral valve prolapse and various arrhythmias. Medications prescribed for other conditions may have anxiety as a side effect. These include such drugs as amphetamines, corticosteroids, caffeine, decongestants, cocaine, and the asthma armamentarium.[54]

Although psychotic behavior may be observed with major affective disorders, organic CNS disease or drug toxicity, schizophrenia occurs in only 1–2% of the general population.[53] Its onset is most prominent in mid to late adolescence through the late 20s. Incidence is approximately equal for males and females and schizophrenia has been described in all cultures and socioeconomic classes. This is a group of mental disorders in which massive disruptions in cognition or perception, such as delusions, hallucinations or thought disorders, are present. The fundamental causes of schizophrenia are unknown but the disease involves excessive amounts of neurotransmitters, chiefly dopamine. There is a genetic predisposition. Somatic delusions may present as voice complaints. However, flattening or inappropriateness of affect, a diagnostic characteristic of schizophrenia, will produce voice changes similar to those described for depression and mania. Where hallucinatory material creates fear, characteristics of anxiety and agitation will be audible. Perseveration, repetition and neologisms may be present. The signs and symptoms also include clear indications of deterioration in social or occupational functioning, personal hygiene, changes in behavior and movement, an altered sense of self, and the presence of blunted or inappropriate affect.[3,53,54] The disease is chronic and control requires consistent use of antipsychotic medications for symptom management. Social support in regulating activities of daily living is crucial in maintaining emotional control. Family counseling and support groups offer the opportunity to share experiences and resources in the care of individuals with this difficult disease.

Psychoactive medications

All psychoactive agents have effects that can interfere with vocal tract physiology. Treatment requires frequent, open collaboration between the laryngologist and the biologic psychiatrist. The patient and physicians need to carefully weigh the benefits and side effects of available medications. Patients must be informed of the relative probability of experiencing any known side effect. This is especially critical to the professional voice user and plays an important role in developing a treatment plan when there is no imminent serious psychiatric risk.

Antidepressant medications include compounds from several different classes. Tri- and tetracyclic antidepressants (TCAs) block the reuptake of norepinephrine and serotonin and have secondary effects on pre- and postsynaptic receptors. An H1–H2-receptor blockade has also been demonstrated.[47]

Schatzberg and Cole summarize the side effects of TCAs as:

- anticholinergic (dry mouth and nasal mucosa, constipation, urinary hesitancy, gastroesophageal reflux);
- autonomic (orthostatic hypotension, palpitations, increased cardiac conduction intervals, diaphoresis, hypertension, tremor);
- allergic (skin rashes);
- CNS (stimulation, sedation, delirium, twitching, nausea, speech delay, seizures, extrapyramidal symptoms); and
- other (weight gain, impotence).[47]

These may be dose-related and agent-specific.

Monoamine oxidase inhibitors (MAOIs) are useful in depression that is refractory to tricyclics. The mode of action involves inhibiting monoamine oxidase (MAO) in various organs, especially MAO-A, for which norepinephrine and serotonin are primary substrates. The full restoration of enzyme activity may take 2 weeks after the drug is discontinued.

The side effects of MAOIs may be extremely serious and troublesome. The one most commonly reported is dizziness secondary to orthostatic hypotension. When MAOIs are taken, hypertensive crisis with violent headache and potential cerebrovascular accident, or hyperpyrexic crisis with monoclonus and coma, may be produced by ingesting foods rich in tyramine, or by many medications, including meperidine (Demerol), epinephrine, local anesthetics containing sympathomimetics, decongestants, selective serotonin reuptake inhibitors (SSRIs) and surgical anesthetics. Other side effects include sexual dysfunction, sedation, insomnia, overstimulation, myositis-like reactions, myoclonic twitches, and a small incidence of dry mouth, constipation and urinary hesitancy.[12,47]

A few antidepressants have been developed with different chemical structures and side effect profiles. Trazodone (Desyrel) is pharmacologically complex, and its specific mode of action is not completely clear. It has proved helpful in depression associated with initial insomnia. Three side effects are particularly noteworthy: sedation, acute dizziness with fainting (especially when taken on an empty stomach) and priapism.[33,34,40]

Nefazodone hydrochloride (Serzone) is another antidepressant with an unknown mechanism. Its chemical structure is different from the SSRIs, tri/tetracyclics and MAOIs. It appears to inhibit neuronal reuptake of serotonin and norepinephrine. It has been advertised as useful in depressions characterized by anxiety. Side effects include significant orthostasis, potential activation of mania, and a questionable potential for priapism. Decreased cognitive and motor performance, dry mouth, nausea, dizziness, are also noted as well as other frequently recurring side effects. This drug has notable medication interactions with Hismanal, Halcion, Xanax and Propulsid. It is not recommended for patients with unstable heart disease.[35]

Bupropion (Wellbutrin) was released in 1989. Its biochemical mode of action is not well understood. It is not anticholinergic. The most commonly reported complaint is nausea. However, a potential risk of seizures exists, and the drug is not recommended in patients with a history of seizures, head trauma, or anorexia or bulimia.[12,47]

A smaller group of antidepressant drugs that selectively inhibit the reuptake of serotonin are most likely to be selected as first pharmacological agents. These include fluoxetine (Prozac), sertraline (Zoloft), and paroxetine (Paxil). They appear to be effective in typical episodic depression and for some chronic refractory presentations.[33,47] Major side effects are significant degrees of nausea, sweating, headache, mouth dryness, tremor, nervousness, dizziness, insomnia, somnolence, constipation and sexual dysfunction. There are drug interactions with the concomitant administration of tryptophan, MAOIs, warfarin, cimetidine, phenobarbital and phenytoin.[33–35]

Mood-stabilizing drugs are those that are effective in manic episodes and prevent manic and depressive recurrences in patients with bipolar disorder. These include lithium salts and several anticonvulsants. Lithium is available in multiple formulations, and prescribing is guided by both symptom index and blood levels. Lithium side effects are apparent in diverse organ systems. The most commonly noted is fine tremor, especially noticeable in the fingers. With toxic lithium levels, gross tremulousness, ataxia, dysarthria and confusion or delirium may develop. Some patients describe slowed mentation, measurable memory deficit and impaired creativity. Chronic nausea and diarrhea are usually related to gastrointestinal tract mucosal irritation, but may be signs of toxicity. Some patients gain weight progressively and may demonstrate edema or increased appetite. Lithium therapy affects thyroid function. In some cases it is transitory, but there may be goiter with normal T3 and T4 but elevated TSH levels.[47]

Polyuria and secondary polydipsia are complications of lithium and may progress to diabetes insipidus. In most cases, discontinuing the medication reverses the renal effects. Prescribed thiazide diuretics can double the lithium level and lead to sudden lithium toxicity. NSAIDs decrease lithium excretion. Cardiovascular effects include the rare induction of sick sinus syndrome. The aggravation of psoriasis, allergic skin rashes, and reversible alopecia are associated with lithium therapy, as are teratogenic effects.[47]

Three anticonvulsant compounds appear to act preferentially on the temporal lobe and the limbic system. Carbamazepine (Tegretol) carries a risk of agranulocytosis or aplastic anemia, and is monitored by complete blood counts and symptoms of bone marrow depression. Care must be taken to avoid the numerous drug interactions that accelerate the metabolism of some drugs or raise carbamazepine levels.[47]

Valproic acid (Depakote, Depakene) is especially useful when there is a rapid-cycling pattern. The major side effect is hepatocellular toxicity. Thrombocytopenia and platelet dysfunction have been reported. Sedation is common, and tremor, ataxia, weight gain, alopecia and fetal neural tube defects are all side effects that patients must comprehend.[22,47]

Anxiolytics are the psychotropic drugs most commonly prescribed, usually by nonpsychiatric specialists, for somatic disorders. It behoves the laryngologist to probe for a history of past or current drug therapy in markedly anxious or somatically focused patients with vocal complaints. Benzodiazepines produce effective relief of anxiety but have a high addictive potential that includes physical symptoms of withdrawal, including potential seizures, if the drug is stopped abruptly. It is well to remember that this class of drugs is commonly available on the streets and from colleagues. The most common benzodiazepine side effect is dose-related sedation, followed by dizziness, weakness, ataxia, decreased motor performance, and mild hypotension. Clonazepam (Klonopin) is a benzodiazepine and may produce sedation, ataxia, and malcoordination, as well as (rarely) disinhibition, agitation or a situational anger.[47] Alterations of sensory input, either by CNS stimulants (cocaine, amphetamines and over-the-counter vasoconstrictors) or depressants, are potentially dangerous in a voice professional. The patient who is unaware of these effects should be apprised of them promptly by the laryngologist.[40,46]

Phenobarbital and meprobamate are no longer commonly used as anxiolytics in the USA. Clomipramine (Anafranil) is useful in the anxiety evident in obsessive-compulsive disorder. The side effects are similar to those of the tricyclic antidepressants: dry mouth, hypotension, constipation, tachycardia, sweating, tremor and anorgasmia.[47] Fluoxetine has also proved effective for some patients with obsessive-compulsive disorder, and appears better tolerated.[47]

Hydroxyzine, an antihistamine, is occasionally prescribed for mild anxiety and/or pruritus. It does not produce physical dependence but does potentiate the CNS effects of alcohol, narcotics, CNS depressants and tricyclic antidepressants. Side effects include notable mucous membrane dryness and drowsiness.[47]

Buspirone (Buspar) is not sedating at its usual dosage levels, and it has little addictive potential. Side effects include mild degrees of headache, nausea and dizziness. However, it is poorly tolerated in patients accustomed to the more immediate relief of benzodiazepines.[47]

β-Blockers are used by some clinicians to mask physiologic symptoms of sympathetic arousal in performance anxiety. Their side effects are serious and may include bradycardia, hypotension, weakness, fatigue, clouded sensorium, impotence and bronchospasm. There is controversy regarding their potential to induce depression.[47] Although the problem of upper respiratory tract secretion dryness was diminished and other symptoms of performance anxiety were lessened in two studies,[45] the drugs are potentially dangerous. Moreover, they leave the underlying conflict unresolved and negatively affect artistic quality.[45] Some authors still prefer them, especially in those patients who may be at risk for drug dependency.

Various antipsychotic drugs [haloperidol (Haldol), chlorpromazine HCl (Thorazine), perphenazine (Trilafon), molindone (Moban), loxapine HCl (Loxitane) and clozapine (Clozaril)] have a mode of action that involves dopamine antagonism, probably in the mesolimbic or mesocortical areas. They also have endocrine effects through dopamine receptors in the hypothalamic–pituitary axis.[47] These potent agents have very significant side effects. Sedation, accompanied by fatigue during early dosing and akinesia with chronic administration, is frequently described. Anticholinergic effects include postural hypotension, dry mouth, nasal congestion and constipation. The endocrine system is also affected, with a direct increase in blood prolactin levels. Breast enlargement and galactorrhea are seen in men and women and correlate with impotence and amenorrhea. Weight gain is often excessive and frequently leads to noncompliance. Skin complications such as rash, retinal pigmentation and photosensitivity occur. Rare but serious complications include agranulocytosis, allergic obstructive hepatitis, seizures, and sudden death secondary to ventricular fibrillation.[47] A drug recently marketed which selectively blocks dopamine receptors without blocking receptors in the basal ganglia is risperidone (Risperdal).[33]

Approximately 14% of patients receiving long-term (greater than 7 years) treatment with antipsychotic agents develop tardive dyskinesia ranging from minimal tongue restlessness to incapacitating, disfiguring choreiform and/or athetoid movements, especially of the head, neck and hands. Unfortunately, there is no cure for the condition once it develops, nor are there accurate predictors for which patients will be affected.[47]

The mode of action in neurologic side effects of the neuroleptics is primarily cholinergic–dopaminergic blockade. Dystonia usually involves tonic spasm of the tongue, jaw and neck but may range from mild tongue stiffness to opisthotonos.[47] Pseudoparkinsonism may occur very early in treatment and is evidenced by muscle stiffness, cogwheel rigidity, stooped posture and mask-like facies with loss of salivary control. Pill-rolling tremor is rare. Akathisia, an inner-driven muscular restlessness with rhythmic leg jiggling, hand wringing, and pacing, is extremely unpleasant. Multiple drug regimens are employed to diminish these symptoms.[47]

Neuroleptic malignant syndrome is a potentially fatal complication of these drugs. Patients manifest hyperthermia, severe extrapyramidal signs and autonomic hyperarousal. Neuroleptics also affect temperature regulation generally and can predispose to heat stroke.[47]

Ongoing psychiatric treatment of patients with voice disorders mandates a careful evaluation of current and prior psychoactive drug therapy. In addition, numerous psychoactive substances are used in the medical management of neurologic conditions such as Tourette's syndrome (haloperidol), chronic pain syndromes (carbamazepine), and vertigo (diazepam, clonazepam).

The laryngologist must thus identify symptoms that may be causally related to drug side effects and avoid drug interactions. It is appropriate (with the patient's consent) to consult with the prescribing physician directly to advocate the use of the psychoactive drug least likely to produce adverse effects on the voice while adequately controlling the psychiatric illness.[46]

Eating disorders and substance abuse

The rapport of the laryngologist and voice team may also allow patients to reveal other self-defeating disorders. Among the most common in arts medicine are body dysmorphic (eating) disorders and substance abuse problems. Comprehensive discussion of these subjects is beyond the scope of this chapter but it is important for the laryngologist to recognize such conditions, not only because of their effects on the voice, but also because of their potentially serious general medical and psychiatric implications. In addition to posterior laryngitis and pharyngitis, laryngeal findings associated with bulimia include subepithelial vocal fold hemorrhages, superficial telangiectasia of the vocal fold mucosa and vocal fold scarring.[45]

Bulimia is a disorder associated with self-induced vomiting following episodes of binge eating. It may occur sporadically, or it may be a chronic problem. Vomiting produces signs and symptoms similar to severe chronic reflux as well as thinning of tooth enamel. Bulimia nervosa can be a serious disorder and may be associated with anorexia nervosa. Bulimia may be more prevalent than is commonly realized. It has been estimated to occur in as many as 2–4% of female adolescents and female young adults. Laryngologists must be attentive to the potential for anorexia and exercise addiction in the maintenance of a desirable body appearance in performers.

Appetite suppressants

There is enormous popular interest in the use of appetite suppressants in weight management. Many myths persist about proper weight management approaches in singers and the value and/or risk of weight loss. The availability and popularity of appetite suppressant drugs, and marketing approaches which included making them available in franchised weight loss centers, led many Americans to explore the use of 'Fen-Phen' [phentermine (Ionamine and others) and fenfluramine (Pondomin)]. Another drug that gained popularity is dexfenfluramine hydrochloride (Redux). These medications have limited efficacy in changing metabolism and limiting craving. Many patients took these drugs in combinations that were never approved for concomitant use. Laryngologists and psychologic professionals caring for singers and other performers should be certain to investigate the potential use of these medications, which were voluntarily withdrawn from the market by their manufacturer in 1997 because of a significant correlation with cardiac valve damage and with pulmonary hypertension.

Alcohol, benzodiazepines, stimulants, cocaine and narcotics are notoriously readily available in the performing community and on the streets. Patients who demonstrate signs and symptoms, or who admit that these areas of their lives are out of control, have taken the first step to regaining control, and this should be acknowledged while efficiently arranging treatment for them. The window of opportunity is often remarkably narrow. The physician should establish close ties to excellent treatment facilities where specialized clinicians can offer confidential outpatient management, with inpatient care available when required for safety.[40]

Neurogenic dysphonia

Patients with neurological disease are likely to experience psychiatric symptoms, especially depression and anxiety. These disorders cause physiological changes that may exacerbate or mask the underlying neurological presentation. Metcalfe and colleagues cite the incidence of severe depression and/or anxiety in neurological patients at one-third.[30] Site of lesion affects the incidence, with lesions of the left cerebral hemisphere, basal ganglia, limbic system, thalamus and anterior frontal lobe more likely to produce depression and anxiety.[18] These same structures are important in voice, speech and language production; so, depression and anxiety logically coexist with voice and language disorders resulting from CNS pathology.[2,18] Dystonias and stuttering are also associated with both neurological and psychogenic etiologies, and must be carefully distinguished by the laryngologist before instituting interdisciplinary treatment.[29]

Stress management

Stress pervades virtually all professions in today's fast-moving society. A singer preparing for a series of concerts, a teacher preparing for presentation of lectures, a lawyer anticipating a major trial, a businessperson negotiating an important contract, or a member of any other goal-oriented profession, each must deal with a myriad of demands on our time and talents. In 1971, Brodnitz reported on 2286 cases of all forms of voice disorders and classified 80% of the disorders as attributable to voice abuse or psychogenic factors resulting in vocal dysfunction.[8] However, regardless of the incidence, it is clear that stress-related problems are important and common in professional voice users. Stress may be physical or psychological, and it often involves a combination of both. Either may interfere with performance. Stress represents a special problem for singers, because its physiologic manifestations may interfere with the delicate mechanisms of voice production.[40]

Stress is recognized as a factor in illness and disease and is probably implicated in almost every type of human problem. It is estimated that 50–70% of all physicians' visits involve complaints of stress-related illness.[15] Stress is a psychological experience that has physiological consequences. A brief review of some terminology may be useful. *Stress* is a term that is used broadly. Our working definition is emotional, cognitive and physiological reactions to psychological demands and challenges. The term *stress level* reflects the degree of stress experienced. Stress is not an all-or-none phenomenon. The psychological effects of stress range from mild to severely incapacitating. The term *stress response* refers to the physiologic reaction of an organism to stress. A *stressor* is an external stimulus or internal thought, perception, image, or emotion that creates stress.[19] Two other concepts are important in a contemporary discussion of stress: *coping* and *adaptation*. Lazarus has defined coping as 'the process of managing demands (external or internal) that are appraised as taxing or exceeding the resources of the person'.[26] In the early 1930s, Hans Selye, an endocrinologist, discovered a generalized response to stressors in research animals. He described their responses using the term *general adaptation syndrome*. Selye (cited in Green and Snellenberger[19]) postulated that the physiology of the test animals was trying to adapt to the challenges of noxious stimuli. The process of adaptation to chronic and severe stressors was harmful over time. There were three phases to the observed response: *alarm*, *adaption* and *exhaustion*. These phases were named for physiologic responses during a sequence of events. The alarm phase is the characteristic fight or flight response. If the stressor continued, the animal appeared to adapt. In the adaptation phase, the physiologic responses were less extreme but the animal eventually became more exhausted. In the exhaustion phase, the animal's adaptation energy was spent, physical symptoms occurred, and some animals died.[19]

Stress responses occur in part through the autonomic nervous system. A stressor triggers particular brain centers, which in turn affect target organs through nerve connections. The brain has two primary pathways for the stress response, neuronal and hormonal, and these pathways overlap. The body initiates a stress response through one of three pathways: through sympathetic nervous system efferents which terminate on target organs such as the heart and blood vessels; via the release of epinephrine and norepinephrine from the adrenal medulla; and through the release of various other catecholamines.[19] A full description of the various processes involved is beyond the scope of this chapter. However, stress has numerous physical consequences. Through the autonomic nervous system, it may alter oral and vocal fold secretions, heart rate and gastric acid production. Under acute, anxiety-producing circumstances, such changes are to be expected. When frightened, a normal person's palms become cold and sweaty, the mouth becomes dry, heart rate increases, his or her pupils change size, and stomach acid secretions may increase. These phenomena are objective signs that may be observed by a physician and their symptoms may be recognized by the performer as dry mouth and voice fatigue, heart palpitations and 'heartburn'. More severe, prolonged stress is also commonly associated with increased muscle tension throughout the body (but particularly in the head and neck), headaches, decreased ability to concentrate, and insomnia. Chronic fatigue is also a common symptom. These physiologic alterations may lead not only to altered vocal quality, but also to physical pathology. Increased gastric acid secretion is associated with ulcers, as well as reflux laryngitis and arytenoid irritation. Other gastrointestinal manifestations, such as colitis, irritable bowel syndrome and dysphagia are also described. Chronic stress and tension may cause numerous pain syndromes although headaches, particularly migraines in vulnerable individuals, are most common. Stress is also associated with more serious physical problems such as myocardial infarction, asthma and depression of the immune system.[19,45,50] Thus, the constant pressure under which many performers live may be more than an inconvenience. Stress factors should be recognized, and appropriate modifications should be made to ameliorate them.

Stressors may be physical or psychological, and often involve a combination of both. Either may interfere with performance. There are several situations in which physical stress is common and important. Generalized fatigue is seen frequently in hard-working singers, especially in the frantic few weeks preceding major performances. In order to maintain normal mucosal secretions, a strong immune system to fight infection, and the ability of muscles to recover from heavy use, rest, proper nutrition and hydration are required. When the body is stressed through deprivation of these essentials, illness (such as upper respiratory infection), voice fatigue, hoarseness, and other vocal dysfunctions may supervene.

Lack of physical conditioning undermines the power source of the voice. A person who becomes short of breath while climbing a flight of stairs hardly has the abdominal and respiratory endurance needed to sustain him or her optimally through the rigors of performance. The stress of attempting to perform under such circumstances often results in voice dysfunction.

Over-singing is another common physical stress. As with running, swimming, or any other athletic activity that depends upon sustained, coordinated muscle activity, singing requires conditioning to build up strength and endurance. Rest periods are also essential for muscle recovery. Singers who are accustomed to singing for 1 or 2 hours a day stress their physical voice-producing mechanism severely when they suddenly begin rehearsing for 14 hours daily immediately prior to performance.

Medical treatment of stress depends upon the specific circumstances. When the diagnosis is appropriate but poorly controlled anxiety, the singer can usually be helped by assurance that his or her voice complaint is related to anxiety and not to any physical problem. Under ordinary circumstances, once the singer's mind is put to rest regarding the questions of nodules, vocal fold injury, or other serious problems, his or her training usually allows compensation for vocal manifestations of anxiety, especially when the vocal complaint is minor. Slight alterations in quality or increased vocal fatigue are seen most frequently. These are often associated with lack of sleep, over-singing and dehydration associated with the stress-producing commitment. The singer or actor should be advised to modify these and to consult his or her voice teacher. The voice teacher should ensure that good vocal technique is being used under performance and rehearsal circumstances. Frequently, young singers are not trained sufficiently in how and when to 'mark.' For example, many singers whistle to rest their voices, not realizing that active vocalization and potentially fatiguing vocal fold contact occur when whistling. Technical proficiency and a plan for voice conservation during rehearsals and performances are essential under these circumstances. A manageable stressful situation may become unmanageable if real physical vocal problems develop.

Several additional modalities may be helpful in selected circumstances. Relative voice rest (using the voice only when necessary) may be important not only to voice conservation but also to psychological relaxation. Under stressful circumstances, a singer needs as much peace and quiet as possible, not hectic socializing, parties with heavy voice use in noisy environments and press appearances. The importance of adequate sleep and fluid intake cannot be overemphasized. Local therapy such as steam inhalation and neck muscle massage may be helpful in some people and certainly does no harm. The doctor may be very helpful in alleviating the singer's exogenous stress by conveying 'doctor's orders' directly to theater management. This will save the singer the discomfort of having to personally confront an authority and violate his or her 'show must go on' ethic. A short phone call by the physician can be highly therapeutic.

When stress is chronic and incapacitating, more comprehensive measures are required. If psychological stress manifestations become so severe as to impair performance or necessitate the use of drugs to allow performance, psychotherapy is indicated. The goal of psychotherapeutic approaches to stress-management includes:

- changing external and internal stressors;
- changing affective and cognitive reactions to stressors;
- changing physiologic reactions to stress; and
- changing stress behaviors.

A psychoeducational model is customarily used. Initially, the psychotherapist will assist the patient in identifying and evaluating stressor characteristics. A variety of assessment tools are available for this purpose. Interventions designed to increase a sense of efficacy and personal control are designed. Perceived control over the stressor directly affects stress level and it changes one's experience of the stressor. Laboratory and human research has determined a sense of control to be one of the most potent elements in the modulation of stress responses. Concrete exercises that impose time management are taught and practiced. Patients are urged to identify and expand their network of support as well. Psychological intervention requires evaluation of the patient's cognitive model. Cognitive restructuring exercises as well as classical behavioral conditioning responses are useful, practical tools that patients easily learn and utilize effectively with practice. Cognitive skills include the use of monitored perception, thought, and internal dialogue to regulate emotional and physiological responses. A variety of relaxation techniques are available and are ordinarily taught in the course of stress-management treatment. These include progressive relaxation, hypnosis, autogenic training and imagery and biofeedback training. Underlying all these approaches is the premise that making conscious normally unconscious processes leads to control and self-efficacy.[40]

As with all medical conditions, the best treatment for stress in singers is prevention. Awareness of the conditions that lead to stress and its potential adverse effect on voice production often allows the singer to anticipate and avoid these problems. Stress is inevitable in performance and in life. Performers must learn to recognize it, compensate for it when necessary, and incorporate it into their singing as emotion and excitement – the 'edge'. Stress should be controlled, not pharmacologically eliminated. Used well, stress should be just one more tool of the singer's trade.

Performance anxiety

Psychological stress is intrinsic to vocal performance. For most people, sharing emotions is stressful even in the privacy of home, let alone under spotlights in front of a room full of people. Under ordinary circumstances, during training, a singer or actor learns to recognize his or her customary anxiety about performing, to accept it as part of his or her instrument, and to compensate for it. When psychologic pressures become severe enough to impair or prohibit performance, careful treatment is required. Such occurrences usually are temporary and happen because of a particular situation such as short notice for a critically important performance, a recent family death, etc. Chronic disabling psychological stress in the face of performance is a more serious problem. In its most extreme forms, performance anxiety actually disrupts the skills of performers; in its milder form it lessens the enjoyment of appearing in public.[10]

Virtually all performers have experienced at least some symptoms of hyperarousal during their performance history and all fear their reemergence. Some fortunate people seem to bypass this type of trauma, exhibiting only mild symptoms of nervousness ahead of performance, which disappear the moment they walk on stage.[6] In these individuals, personal physiology works consistently for instead of against them.[10] The human nervous system functions exquisitely for the great majority of our needs, but in performance anxiety it begins to work against the performer in those very circumstances when he or she wants most to do well. Human autonomic arousal continues to be under the sway of primal survival mechanisms, which are the basic lines of defense against physical danger: they prepare the individual to fight or flee in response to the perception of threat.[10] They are essential to our survival in situations of physical danger. However, the dangers that threaten performers are not physical in nature, but the human nervous system cannot differentiate between physical and psychological dangers, producing physiological responses that are the same. When the physical symptoms associated with extreme arousal are enumerated, it is easy to understand why they can be major impediments to skilled performance and may even be disabling. They include rapid heart rate, dry mouth, sweating palms, palpitations, tremor, high blood pressure, restricted breathing, frequency of urination and impaired memory.[10]

This process is cognitive, and Beck and Emery[6] describe the development of cognitive sets using an analogy to photography. The individual scans the relevant environment and then determines which aspect, if any, on which to focus. Cognitive processing reduces the number of dimensions in a situation, sacrifices a great deal of information, and induces distortion into the picture. Certain aspects of the situation are highlighted at the expense of others, the relative magnitudes and prominence of various features are distorted, and there is loss of perspective. In addition, they describe blurring and loss of important detail. These are the decisive influences upon what the individual sees. They describe how the cognitive set influences the picture that is perceived. The existing cognitive sets determine which aspects of the scene will be highlighted, which glossed over, and which excluded. The individual's first impressions of an event provide information that either reinforces or modifies the preexisting cognitive set. The initial impression is critical because it determines whether the situation directly affects the patient's vital interests. It also sets the course of subsequent steps in conceptualization and the total response to a situation.[6] According to the cognitive model, at the same time the individual is evaluating the nature of the threat, he or she is also assessing internal resources for dealing with it and their availability and effectiveness in deflecting potential damage. The balance between potential danger and available coping responses determines the nature and intensity of the patient's stress response. Two major behavioral systems are activated, either separately or together, in response to the threat: those mediated by the sympathetic branch of the autonomic nervous system, 'the fight or flight response', and those related to the parasympathetic branch, 'the freeze or faint' response.[6]

A major feature of performance anxiety is that the actual fear prior to entering the situation appears plausible. A complex web of factors in this situation may aggravate the patient's fears. These may include the relative status of the performer and the evaluator, the performer's skill, his or her confidence in the ability to perform adequately in a given 'threatening situation' and the appraisal of the degree of threat (including the severity of potential damage to one's career and self-esteem). The individual's threshold of automatic defenses that undermine performance and the rigidity of the rules relevant to the performance in question are also factored into the intensity of the response. Unfortunately, the experience of fear increases the likelihood of the undesirable consequences. A vicious cycle is created in which the anticipation of an absolute, extreme, irreversible outcome makes the performer more fearful of the effects and inhibited when entering the situation.[6] Negative evaluation by judges or audiences is the common psychic threat. The individual suffering from performance anxiety believes that he or she is being scrutinized and judged. Components under observation include fluency, artistry, self-assurance and technique.

Although most fears tend to decline with continued exposure and expertise, Caine notes that even highly skilled performers do not always experience lessening of performance anxiety over time.[10] Indeed, she describes a dilemma for the expert performer in which a potentially humiliating and frightening mistake is less and less tolerable. A behavioral feedback loop becomes established. The act of performance becomes the stimulus perceived as a threat. In situations of danger, the individual's physiology primes him or her to become more alert and sensitive to all potential threats in the surrounding environment. Anticipating mistakes increases arousal, which further enhances access to memories of mistakes and feelings of humiliation, which activates more fears and more arousal. This process is linked by catastrophic thoughts, physiologic manifestations of anxiety, and imagery. Unfortunately, this process is often initiated very early in a young performer's training.[10]

A variety of psychotherapeutic treatment approaches to performance anxiety have been described in the literature. The most effective of these are cognitive and behavioral strategies, which assist performers in modulating levels of arousal to more optimal levels. Cognitive therapy addresses the essential mechanism sustaining performance anxiety: the cognitive set a performer brings to the performance situation. The autonomic nervous system is merely responding to the threat as it is perceived, and the intensity of the response correlates to the degree of threat generated by the sufferer's catastrophic expectations and negative self-talk. Cognitive restructuring techniques are extremely effective in producing the necessary adjustments. Monitoring internal self-dialogue comprises the first step in recognizing the dimension of the problem. These excessively self-critical attitudes enhance the probability of mistakes. Homework exercises designed to monitor critical thoughts are assigned. In the second step of cognitive treatment, adaptive, realistic self-statements are substituted. Behaviorally based treatment approaches such as thought-stopping, paired relaxation responses and 'prescribing the symptom' are also utilized. Hypnosis is efficacious, providing relaxation techniques and introducing positive, satisfying and joyful imagery.[40]

Brief psychotherapeutic approaches produce effective outcomes, but some proponents of the psychodynamic approach argue that the underlying conflicts will resurface in some form of symptom substitution. This author's (DCR) clinical approach includes an exploration for secondary gain offered by disabling performance anxiety. The performer's unconscious fear must be addressed for these treatments to remain effective and to avoid eventual symptom substitution. Patients are asked: 'What does this symptom accomplish for you?' The question may sound unsympathetic, and the patient may need to search deeply for the answer. This search requires significant courage. If the patient makes effective use of the treatment strategies, what might be expected of him or her? Where might success lead? Is he or she ready to go on to the next phase in a performance career, or does it remain safer to be immobilized? Which problem is honestly more terrifying: the symptom of performance anxiety or the possibility of success? What would be the consequences of resolving the immobilizing performance anxiety? The patient is asked to imagine a life in which the problem is no longer present. This exploration is often conducted using the relaxation and enhanced perception available in hypnosis.[40] Most of these questions are painful ones to answer. For some performers, success beckons with one hand and signals caution with the other. Eloise Ristad describes this with extraordinarily pragmatic wisdom:[37]

> *The part of us that holds back knows that change involves challenges-losses as well as gains. Change always means dying a little; leaving behind something old and tattered and no longer useful to us even though comfortably familiar.*

A successful psychotherapeutic response to disabling performance anxiety requires a thorough explanation of the personal meaning of the symptom to the patient as well as an extensive and exciting repertoire of strategies for effecting personal change.

Reactive responses

Reaction to illness is the major source of psychiatric disturbance in patients with significant voice dysfunction. Loss of communicative function is an experience of alienation that threatens human self-definition and independence. Catastrophic fears of loss of productivity, economic and social status and, in professional voice users, creative artistry, contribute to rising anxiety. Anxiety is known to worsen existing communication disorders, and the disturbances in memory, concentration and synaptic transmission secondary to depression may intensify other voice symptoms and interfere with rehabilitation.

The self-concept is an essential construct of Carl Rodgers' theories of counseling. Rodgers described self-concept as composed of perceptions of the characteristics of the self and the relationships of the self to various aspects of life, as well as the values attached to the perceptions. Rodgers suggested that equilibrium requires that patients' self-concepts be congruent with their life experiences. It follows, then, that it is not the disability *per se* that psychologically influences the person, but rather the subjective meaning and feelings attached to the disability. According to Rodgers, the two major psychologic defenses which operate to maintain consistent self-concept are denial and distortion.[38]

Families of patients are affected as well. They are often confused about the diagnosis and poorly prepared to support the patient's coping responses. The resulting stress may negatively influence family dynamics and intensify the patient's depressive illness[59] As the voice-injured patient experiences the process of grieving, the psychologist may assume a more prominent role in his or her care. Essentially, the voice-injured patient goes through a grieving process similar to patients who mourn other losses such as the death of a loved one. In some cases, especially among voice professionals, the patients actually mourn the loss of their self as they perceive it. The psychologist is responsible for facilitating the tasks of mourning and monitoring the individual's formal mental status for clinically significant changes.[39–41] There are a number of models for tracking this process. The most easily understood is that of Worden,[57] as adapted by the author (DCR). Initially, the task is to *accept the reality of the loss*. The need for and distress of this is vestigial during the phase of diagnosis, is held consciously in abeyance during the acute and rehabilitative phases of treatment, but is reinforced with accumulating data measuring vocal function. As the reality becomes undeniable, the mourner must be helped to express the full range of grieving affect. The rate of accomplishing this is variable and individual. Generally, it will occur in the style with which the person usually copes with crisis and may be florid or tightly constricted. All responses must be invited and normalized. The psychologist facilitates the process and stays particularly attuned to unacceptable, split-off responses or the failure to move through any particular response.

As attempts to deny the loss take place and fail, the mourner gradually encounters the next task: *beginning to live and cope in a world in which the lost object is absent.* This is the psychoanalytic process of *decathexsis*, requiring the withdrawal of life energies from the other and the reinvesting of them in the self. For some professional voice users, this may be a temporary state as they make adjustments required by their rehabilitation demands. In other cases, the need for change will be lasting; change in fach, change in repertoire, need for amplification, altered performance schedule or, occasionally, change in career.[39–41]

As the patient so injured seeks to heal his or her life, another task looms. Known as *recathexis*, it involves *reinvesting life energies in other relationships, interests, talents, and life goals.* The individual is assisted in redefining and revaluing the self as apart from the voice. The voice is then seen as the *product* of the self, rather than as equivalent to the self. For many performers this is painfully difficult.[39–41,57] Rosen and Sataloff have described in detail research applying the various theoretical models of grief resolution to the perception of vocal injury in professional voice users.[39]

The surgical experience

When vocal fold surgery is indicated, many individuals will demonstrate hospital-related phobias or self-destructive responses to pain. Adamson *et al.* describe the importance of understanding how the patient's occupational identity will be affected by surgical intervention.[1] Vocal fold surgery impacts on the major mode of communication that all human beings utilize; the impact is extraordinarily anxiety-producing in professional voice users. Even temporary periods of absolute voice restriction may induce feelings of insecurity, helplessness and dissociation from the verbal world. Carpenter details the value of an early therapy session to focus on the fears, fantasies, misconceptions and regression that frequently accompany a decision to undergo surgery.[11]

A proper surgical discussion highlights vocal fold surgery as *elective*. The patient chooses surgery as the only remaining means to regaining the previously 'normal' voice, or to a different but desirable voice. Responsible care includes a thorough preoperative and written discussion of the limits and complications of surgery, with recognition by the surgeon that anxiety affects both understanding and retention of information about undesirable outcomes. Personality psychopathology or unrealistic expectations of the impact of surgery on their lives are elements for which surgical candidates can be screened.[28,36,48] Recognizing such problems preoperatively allows preoperative counseling and obviates many postoperative difficulties.

Although a thorough discussion is outside the scope of this chapter, surgically treated voice patients include those undergoing laryngectomy, with or without a voice prosthesis. The laryngectomized individual must make major psychological and social adjustments. These include not only those adjustments related to a diagnosis of cancer, but also to a sudden disability: loss of voice. With the improvement in prognosis, research has begun to focus on the individual's quality of life after the laryngectomy. There is wide variability in the quality of preoperative and postoperative psychological support reported by patients during each phase of care. Special psychological issues in professional voice users diagnosed with laryngeal cancer are discussed in detail in other works.[40] Providing this support is a crucial role for the voice team's psychologist.[7,17,49]

Role of the psychological professional

Both psychology and psychiatry specialize in attending to emotional needs and problems. Psychiatrists, as physicians, focus on the neurological and biological causes and treatment of psychopathology. Psychologists have advanced graduate training in psychological function and therapy. They concern themselves with cognitive processes such as thinking, behavior and memory; the experiencing and expression of emotions; significant inner conflict, characteristic modes of defense in coping with stress; and personality style and perception of self and others, including their expression in interpersonal behavior. Other mental health professionals also provide psychotherapy to performers. In the authors' practice, clinical psychologists serve as members of the voice team. They work directly with some patients and offer consultation to the physician and other professionals.

Assessment of patients is done throughout the physician's history-taking and physical examinations, as well as in a formal psychiatric interview when appropriate in our center. Personality assessment, screening for or evaluating known psychopathology, and assessing potential surgical candidates is performed. Occasionally, psychometric instruments are added to the diagnostic interview. Confidentiality of content is extended to the treatment team to maximize interdisciplinary care. Because of their special interest in voicing parameters, the voice team psychologists are especially attuned to the therapeutic use of their own voices for intensifying rapport and pacing/leading the patient's emotional state during interventions.[5,13,23,25,55]

Psychotherapeutic treatment is offered on a short-term, diagnosis-related basis. Treatment is designed to identify and alleviate emotional distress and to increase the individual's resources for adaptive functioning. Individual psychotherapeutic approaches include brief insight-oriented therapies, cognitive/behavioral techniques, Gestalt interventions, stress-management skill building and clinical hypnosis.

After any indicated acute intervention is provided, and in patients whose coping repertoire is clearly adequate to the stressors, a psychoeducational model is used. The therapy session focuses on a prospective discussion of personal, inherent life stressors and predictable illnesses. Stress management skills are taught and audiotapes provided. These offer portable skills and supplemental sessions may be scheduled by mutual decision during appointments at the center for medical examinations and speech or singing voice therapy. A group therapy model, facilitated by the psychologist, has also been used to provide a forum for discussion of patient responses during the various phases of treatment. Participants benefit from the perspective and progress of other patients, the opportunity to decrease their experience of isolation and the sharing of resources.

Long-term psychodynamic psychotherapy, chronic psychiatric conditions, and patients requiring psychopharmacologic management are referred to consultant mental health professionals with special interest and insight in voice-related psychological problems. The voice team's psychologists also serve in a liaison role when patients already in treatment come to our center for voice care. In addition, the psychologist participates in professional education activities in the medical practice. These include writing, lecturing and serving as a preceptor for visiting professionals. Specially trained psychologists have proven to be an invaluable addition to the voice team, and close collaboration with team members has proven to be valuable and stimulating for psychologists interested in the care of professional voice users.

Conclusions

Psychophysiological research informs our treatment and maximizes the benefits of medical interreactions in every specialty. This is the rightful role of the arts medicine psychologist: to possess mastery of the knowledge bases of psychology and medicine and also an experiential understanding of the performing arts so that he or she may stand in alliance with the injured performer on the journey to explore, understand and modify the psychological impact of performance-related injuries. The speech-language pathologist must understand the psychological factors that may cause, or be caused by, voice disorders. The SLP must also recognize his/her limits as a psychotherapist and know when to refer to and collaborate with a mental health professional while maintaining responsibility for voice modification and some degree of psychological support. The laryngologist must recognize the need for therapy in individual patients, accurately diagnose the presence of organic and functional disorders, select and coordinate the therapy team, and retain overall responsibility for the therapeutic process and the patient's outcome. Those who are privileged to care for that uniquely human capability – the voice – quickly come to understand the essential role of psychologic awareness in our treatment failures and successes.

References

1. Adamson JD, Hersuberg D, Shane F. The psychic significance of parts of the body in surgery. In: Howells JG, ed. *Modern Perspectives in the Psychiatric Aspects of Surgery*. New York: Brunner Mazel, 1976: 20–45.
2. Alexander MP, LoVerme SR Jr. Aphasia after left hemispheric intracerebral hemorrhage. *Neurology* 1980; **30:** 1193–202.
3. American Psychiatric Association. *Diagnostic and Statistical Manual of Mental Disorders III-R*. Washington, DC: American Psychiatric Association, 1987: 206–10.
4. Aronson A. *Clinical Voice Disorders*, 3rd edn. New York: Thieme Medical Publishers, 1900: 117–45, 314–15.
5. Bady SL. The voice as curative factor in psychotherapy. *Psychoanal Rev* 1985; **72:** 479–90.
6. Beck A, Emery G. *Anxiety Disorders and Phobias: a Cognitive Perspective*. New York: Basic Books, 1985: 38–50, 151.
7. Berkowitz JF, Lucente FE. Counseling before laryngectomy. *Laryngoscope* 1985; **95:** 1332–6.
8. Brodnitz FS. Hormones and the human voice. *Bull N Y Acad Med* 1971; **47:** 183–91.
9. Butcher P, Elias A, Raven R. *Psychogenic Voice Disorders and Cognitive-Behavior Therapy*. San Diego: Singular Publishing Group, 1993: 3–22.
10. Caine JB. Understanding and treating performance anxiety from a cognitive-behavior therapy perspective. *NATS J* 1991; **47:** 27–51.
11. Carpenter B. Psychological aspects of vocal fold surgery. In: Gould WJ, Sataloff RT, Spiegel JR, eds. *Voice Surgery*. St Louis: Mosby, 1993: 339–43.
12. Cole JO, Bodkin JA. Antidepressant drug side effects. *J Clin Psychiatry* 1990; **51:** S21–6.
13. Crasilneck HB, Hall J. *Clinical Hypnosis: Principles and Applications*, 2nd edn. Orlando: Grune and Stratton, 1985: 60–1.
14. Cummings JL, Benson DF, Houlihan JP, Gosenfield LF. Mutism: loss of neocortical and limbic vocalization. *J Nerv Ment Dis* 1983; **171:** 255–9.
15. Everly GS. *A Clinical Guide to the Treatment of the Human Stress Response*. New York: Plenum Press, 1989: 40–3.
16. Freedman R. Cognitive behavioral perspectives on body image change. In: Cash TF, Pruzinsky T, eds. *Body Images: Development Deviance and Change*. New York: Guilford Press, 1990: 273–95.
17. Gardner WH. Adjustment problems of laryngectomized women. *Arch Otolaryngol* 1966; **83:** 31–42.
18. Gianotti G. Emotional behavior and hemispheric side of lesion. *Cortex* 1972; **8:** 41–55.
19. Green J, Snellenberger R. *The Dynamics of Health and Wellness. A Biopsychosocial Approach*. Fort Worth: Holt, Reinhardt and Winston, 1991: 61–4, 92, 98, 101–36.
20. Hartman DE, Daily WW, Morin KN. A case of superior laryngeal nerve paresis and psychogenic dysphonia. *J Speech Hear Disord* 1989; **54:** 526–9.
21. Horney K. Cited by: Meissner W. Theories of personality. In: Nicholi A, ed. *The New Harvard Guide to Psychiatry*. Cambridge, MA: Harvard University Press, 1988: 177–99.
22. Janitec P, Davis J, Prescorn F, Ab S. *Principles and Practice of Psychopharmacology*. Baltimore: Williams & Wilkins, 1993: 164–84, 230–89, 433–9.
23. King M, Novick L, Citrenbaum C. *Irresistible Communication*. Philadelphia: Saunders, 1983: 21, 22, 115–27.
24. Klerman G. Depression and related disorders of mood. In: Nicholi A, ed. *The New Harvard Guide to Psychiatry*. Cambridge, MA: Harvard University Press, 1988: 309–36.
25. Lankton S. *Practical Magic: a Translation of Neuro-Linguistic Programming into Clinical Psycho-Therapy*. Cupertino: Meta Publications, 1980: 174.
26. Lazarus RS, Folkman S. *Stress Appraisal and Coping*. New York: Springer-Verlag, 1984: 283.
27. Luchsinger R, Arnold E. *Voice–Speech–Language – Clinical Communicology: Its Physiology and Pathology*. Belmont: Wadsworth, 1965.
28. Macgregor FC. Patient dissatisfaction with results of technically satisfactory surgery. *Aesthetic Plast Surg* 1981; **5:** 27–32.
29. Mahr G, Leith W. Psychogenic stuttering of adult onset. *J Speech Hear Res* 1992; **35:** 283–6.
30. Metcalfe R, Firth D, Pollock S, Creed F. Psychiatric morbidity and illness behaviour in female neurological in-patients. *J Neurol Neurosurg Psychiatry* 1988; **51:** 1387–90.
31. Moses PJ. *The Voice of Neurosis*. New York: Grune and Stratton, 1954.
32. Nemiah J. Psychoneurotic disorders. In: Nicholi A, ed. *The New Harvard Guide to Psychiatry*. Cambridge, MA: Harvard University Press, 1988: 234–58.
33. *Physician's Desk Reference*. Oradell: Medical Economics Data, 1994: 2000–3, 2267–70.
34. *Physician's Desk Reference*. Oradell: Medical Economics Data, 1996: B20.
35. *Physician's Desk Reference*. Oradell: Medical Economics Data, 1997: 1615, 1878, 2239.
36. Ray CJ, Fitzgibbon G. The socially mediated reduction of stress in surgical patients. In: Oborne DJ, Grunberg M, Eisner JR, eds. *Research and Psychology in Medicine*. Vol. 2. Oxford: Pergamon Press, 1979: 521–7.
37. Ristad E. *A Soprano on Her Head: Right Side Up Reflections on Life and Other Performances*. Moah: Real People Press, 1982: 154, 155.
38. Rodgers CA. A theory of personality and interpersonal relationships as developed in a client centered framework. In: Koch S, ed. *Psychology: a Study of a Science*. New York: McGraw-Hill, 1959: 184–256.
39. Rosen DC, Sataloff RT. Psychological aspects of voice disorders. In: Gould WJ, Rubin J, Korovin G, Sataloff RT, eds. *Diagnosis and Treatment of Voice Disorders*. New York: Igaku-Shoin Medical Publishers, 1993: 491–501.
40. Rosen DC, Sataloff RT. *Psychology of Voice Disorders*. San Diego: Singular Publishing Group, 1997.

41. Rosen DC, Sataloff RT, Evans H, Hawkshaw M. Self-esteem in singers: singing healthy, singing hurt. *NATS J* 1993; **49:** 32–5.
42. Ross E, Rush A. Diagnosis and neuroanatomical correlates of depression in brain-damaged patients: implications for a neurology of depression. *Arch Gen Psychiatry* 1981; **38:** 1344–54.
43. Rulnick RK, Heuer RJ, Perez KS, Emerich KA, Sataloff RT. Voice therapy. In: Sataloff RT, ed. *Professional Voice: the Science and Art of Clinical Care,* 2nd edn. San Diego: Singular Publishing Group, 1997: 699–720.
44. Sapir S, Aronson AE. Coexisting psychogenic and neurogenic dysphonia: a source of diagnostic confusion. *Br J Disord Commun* 1987; **22:** 73–80.
45. Sataloff RT. Stress, anxiety and psychogenic dysphonia. In: Sataloff RT, ed. *Professional Voice: the Science and Art of Clinical Care.* New York: Raven Press, 1991: 195–200.
46. Sataloff RT, Lawrence VL, Hawkshaw M, Rosen DC. Medications and their effects on the voice. In: Benninger MS, Jacobson BH, Johnson AF, eds. *Vocal Arts Medicine: the Care and Prevention of Professional Voice Disorders.* New York: Thieme Medical, 1994: 216–25.
47. Schatzberg A, Cole J. *Manual of Clinical Psychopharmacology,* 2nd edn. Washington, DC: APA Press, 1991: 40, 50, 55, 58, 66, 68, 69, 72–7, 110–25, 158–65, 169–77, 185–227, 313–48.
48. Shontz F. Body image and physical disability. In: Cash T, Pruzinsky T, eds. *Body Images: Development, Deviance and Change.* New York: The Guilford Press, 1990: 149–69.
49. Stam H, Koopmans J, Mathieson C. The psychological impact of a laryngectomy: a comprehensive assessment. *J Psychosoc Oncol* 1991; **9:** 37–58.
50. Stroudmire A. *Psychological Factors Affecting Medication Conditions.* Washington, DC: American Psychiatric Press, 1995: 187–92.
51. Styron W. *Darkness Visible: a Memoir of Madness.* New York: Random House, 1990.
52. Sundberg J. *The Science of the Singing Voice.* DeKalb: Northern Illinois University Press, 1985: 146–56.
53. Tsuang M, Faraone S, Day M. Schizophrenic disorders. In: Nicholi A, ed. *The New Harvard Guide to Psychiatry.* Cambridge, MA: Harvard University Press, 1988: 259–95.
54. Vogel D, Carter J. *The Effects of Drugs on Communication Disorders.* San Diego: Singular Publishing Group, 1995: 31–143.
55. Watkins J. *Hypnotherapeutic Techniques.* New York: Irvington Publishers, 1987: 114.
56. Weissman MM. The psychological treatment of depression. Evidence for the efficacy of psychotherapy alone, in comparison with, and in combination with pharmacotherapy. *Arch Gen Psychiatry* 1979; **38:** 1261–9.
57. Worden W. *Grief Counseling and Grief Therapy.* New York: Springer-Verlag, 1982: 7–18.
58. Ziegler FS, Imboden JB. Contemporary conversion reactions: II conceptual model. *Arch Gen Psychiatry* 1962; **6:** 279–87.
59. Zraick RI, Boone DR. Spouse attitudes toward the person with aphasia. *J Speech Hear Res* 1991; **34:** 123–8.

Spasmodic dysphonia: evaluation and management with botulinum toxin

Andrew Blitzer and Mitchell F Brin

Spasmodic dysphonia, a focal laryngeal dystonia, is a chronic neurologic disorder of central motor processing characterized by action-induced spasms of the muscles controlling the vocal folds. The vocal folds are normal at rest, but with an action-induced, task-specific movement, inappropriate muscle contraction occurs, typically causing dysphonia during speaking.

Spasmodic dysphonia ('spastic dysphonia'), historically, was considered a disorder of uncertain origin. For many, it was thought to have a psychogenic etiology, since many patients often have sensory tricks (such as yawning or laughing when beginning to speak) to ameliorate the abnormal voice production. In addition, stress made the symptoms worse, and relaxation, alcohol or tranquilizers often made the symptoms better. Many of the patients can laugh and sing normally, but they almost universally have difficulty speaking on the telephone.[5,6,10]

Marsden and Sheehy[24] in 1982 first noticed that:

> *all evidence points to the conclusion that blepharospasm and oromandibular dystonia seen in Meige disease is another manifestation of adult-onset torsion dystonia, [and] since dysphonia may occur in the same syndrome, it is quite likely that dysphonia itself may be the sole manifestation of dystonia.*

In 1984, our group recognized that the characteristics of 'spastic dysphonia' were similar to the dysphonia found in some patients with generalized and multifocal dystonia. Both the clinical examination and EMG characteristics led us to the conclusion that most cases of dysphonia clinically diagnosed as 'spastic dysphonia' are focal forms of cranial dystonia.[6,8] Other focal forms include blepharospasm, torticollis, oromandibular dystonia and occupational writer's cramp. We found that laryngeal dystonia may present focally or in association with other dystonic movements.[10] Neuropathologic studies of the brains of dystonic patients have shown lesions in the region of the basal ganglia (putamen, head of the caudate and the upper brainstem).[25,33]

The classification of primary dystonia (idiopathic) includes patients in whom there is no evidence by history, examination or laboratory studies showing a secondary cause for the dystonic symptoms, with the exception of trauma. Therefore, there must be a normal perinatal and early developmental history, no prior history of neurologic illness or exposure to drugs known to cause acquired dystonia (e.g. phenothiazine). There also must be normal intellectual, pyramidal, cerebellar and secondary examinations and diagnostic studies.[5,10,24]

The dystonic symptoms generally start in one site. Spread to other regions is seen in childhood-onset dystonia, whilst the disorder tends to remain focal in the adult-onset type. In our series, 16% of patients with primary laryngeal involvement develop spread of the disorder to another body part. This data suggests that patients should be advised of possible spread to another part and they should be examined and followed on a regular basis for signs of other dystonic involvement.[5,10] The family history is also important, and in our series of over 900 patients, 12% of the patients with primary laryngeal dystonia had a family history of dystonia.[10] Recently, the autosomal dominant (non-dopa-responsive) idiopathic torsion dystonia DTY1 gene was identified on chromosome 9q34.[19,28]

The majority of patients with laryngeal dystonia have the adductor type. In our series of over 900 patients, 87% had the adductor type characterized by a strain-strangled voice that is harsh. They often have a tremor, inappropriate pitch or pitch breaks, breathiness and glottal fry. The stroboscopic examination shows hyperadduction at the glottal or supraglottal level. The most extreme cases may have sphincteric closure of the arytenoids and epiglottis. Aronson *et al.*[3] and Ludlow *et al.*[20] have described the tremor in spasmodic dysphonia to be similar to that of essential tremor. Blitzer *et al.*[8] studied spasmodic dysphonia patients electromyographically and found that 25% had an irregular tremor of 4–8 Hz on phonation, with no resting tremor. An additional 6% had a regular tremor similar to that of essential tremor.

The abductor type of laryngeal dystonia was found in 13% of our patient series.[7] This group had spasms of the posterior cricoarytenoid muscles producing a breathy, effortful hypophonic voice with vocal arrests causing aphonic or whispered segments of speech. In the abductor patients, the laryngostroboscopic examination showed synchronous and untimely abduction of the true vocal folds, causing an extremely wide, open glottic chink. The abductor spasms are triggered by consonant sounds, particularly when they are in the initial position in words. For instance, having a patient say 'taxi' or 'Harry's hat' will lead to a breathy break in sound production. Several of our patients have a true mixed adductor-abductor type in which the patients produce a mixture of breathy breaks with tight, harsh sounds. Sometimes this is seen with compensatory strategies, but when one form is treated with botulinum toxin, the other gets worse. This necessitates both adductor and abductor muscles be treated. Cannito and Johnson[11] proposed that both adductor and abductor abnormalities are present in all spasmodic dysphonia patients, but the symptomatic presentation depends upon whether there is more adductor or abductor activity. Some spasmodic dysphonia patients utilize compensatory strategies. Some of the adductor spasmodic dysphonia patients will present with a hypophonic or aphonic voice to prevent the adductor spasms and broken speech patterns. The abductor spasmodic dysphonia patients may begin to speak with their vocal folds tightly contracted in an attempt to overcome the breathy dysphonia simulating the adductor presentation.

We[17] have also described 12 patients who have stridor based on dystonic paradoxical vocal fold motion, which we have termed adductor breathing dystonia. These patients have normal laryngeal movements for other functions (cough, speaking, swallowing) do not develop hypoxia, and the stridor disappears upon falling asleep.

Patient evaluation

All of the patients have a detailed head and neck examination with particular attention to spasms, tremor, or motor dysfunction. Fiberoptic laryngoscopy and stroboscopy are performed in all patients to observe the glottal function for /i/ and connected speech segments to observe disruptions, spasms, breathy breaks and tremor. Indirect laryngoscopy cannot display the vocal phenomenology due to the anterior traction of the tongue and the inability of the patient to produce connected speech segments.[5,7,10]

All of the patients should have a detailed neurologic examination since dystonia is a brainstem disorder. This should include examining the patient performing postures and tasks that may bring out signs of dystonia, tremor and other neurologic phenomena. Since dystonic symptoms may be related to another underlying neurologic disorder (i.e. multiple sclerosis, Wilson's disease, etc.) the examination should evaluate for the etiology of the symptoms. A speech pathologist should also examine the spasmodic dysphonia patient with acoustic and aerodynamic measures to evaluate for tremor, fundamental frequency, pitch and amplitude perturbations, harshness, fluency breaks and breathiness.[10]

Laryngeal electromyography is often performed in spasmodic dysphonia patients to evaluate tremor and areas of muscle hyperactivity. In our initial study, 17% of the spasmodic dysphonia patients tested showed enlarged potentials, 4% had small potentials, and 6% had reduced numbers of motor unit potentials. Polyphasic potentials were found in 11% of the patients (perhaps showing evidence of a denervation and reinnervation process) and 2% had evidence of pseudomyotonic discharges. A more consistent finding was that, when the EMG signal and voice spectrogram were placed on the same time line, a greater than normal delay in onset of sound production was found.[8]

Koufman[18] found that spectral analysis was particularly helpful in comparing the characteristics of spasmodic dysphonia and muscle tension dysphonia (MTD). He found that voice breaks were usually present in spasmodic dysphonia but not in MTD. Spasmodic dysphonia patients also had well-defined formants, whereas the MTD patients did not, and the MTD patients had excessive high-frequency spectral noise that was minimal in spasmodic dysphonia patients. Shipp *et al.*[31] found that there were abnormally high subglottic pressures in patients who have adductor spasmodic dysphonia.

Therapy

Patients with greater involvement than focal dystonia (segmental, multifocal and generalized) are usually treated with pharmacotherapy. This usually begins with an anticholinergic, benzodiazepine, or baclofen.[1] The choice of drug to initiate usually depends upon the age of the patient, prior exposure to medications, and other concurrent medications or medical problems. Dosage is initially low, and gradually increased as tolerated. Sometimes combinations of low-dose medication are better tolerated than high doses of a single agent. Anticholinergics are the drugs most often used, helping 50% of children and 40% of adults with dystonia. Difficulty with concentration, cognitive impairment, dry mouth and blurred vision are the major side effects of these drugs. Baclofen has also been found useful in many patients.[9]

Surgery has also played a role in the management of spasmodic dysphonia. Dedo[12] first reported a method of providing local therapy, based on his theory that weakening the vocal cords would eliminate sustained contractions. He designed a treatment to impair one vocal cord to theoretically make the bilateral spasms impossible. He found initially that lidocaine blockade of one recurrent laryngeal nerve (RLN) could provide temporary improvement in speech fluency. Based on this observation, Dedo advocated RLN section as a method of providing permanent cessation of the vocal spasms. Dedo in a large series reports only 15% failure after time, and suggests that these cases of failure may be corrected with a laser thinning of the vocal folds.[13]

The initial very promising results of RLN section did not stand up with time in many patients. Aronson and DeSanto[2] reviewed the Mayo Clinic series and critically evaluated the voices of the patients treated with RLN section. They found that by 3 years, only 36% of the spasmodic dysphonia patients continued to have improvement, and that only one of 33 patients continued to have a normal voice. They also found that of the 64% that failed at 3 years, 48% had a worse voice than before the surgery. Ludlow *et al.*[21] theorized that the RLN section failures were due to an ingrowth of new motor nerve fibers into the stump of the sectioned RLN. Based on this premise, Netterville *et al.*[27] proposed an RLN avulsion technique of a large portion of the remaining RLN.

Tucker[32] proposed a different approach to the spasms and tension of the vocal folds in spasmodic dysphonia. He suggested a laryngeal framework procedure, in which the anterior commissure is retrodisplaced, shortening the anterior–posterior dimension of the vocal folds. This technique fails in many cases due to the way the muscle stretch receptors work, and it may leave the patient with a poor voice. Genack *et al.*[16] found in an animal model that a laser could be used to perform a myectomy to reduce the tension of the muscle spasm in spasmodic dysphonia and thereby relieve the symptoms. Lastly, Friedman *et al.*[15] described the use of an implantable nerve stimulator to counter the excessive contracture of the muscles. The initial report revealed technical difficulties and a small sample size.

Botulinum toxin therapy

In April 1984, I [AB] first treated a patient who had spasmodic dysphonia with intramuscular injections of botulinum toxin (BTX). He had Meige syndrome and his blepharospasm had been successfully managed with BTX. He was given small doses unilaterally until a fluent voice pattern was produced. Other authors initially reported similarly good results with BTX injections for spasmodic dysphonia.[23,26] Since this time our group has treated over 900 patients with laryngeal dystonia with excellent results and minimal side effects.

BTX is a potent neurotoxin produced by the bacterium *Clostridium botulinum*. There are seven serologically different toxins produced, of which type A is presently used therapeutically. It was first developed by Alan Scott[30] in San Francisco as a therapeutic modality for the management of strabismus, and then for blepharospasm. BTX type A acts as a zinc-dependent metalloprotease which specifically cleaves the SNAP-25 target protein, causing an inhibition of synaptic acetylcholine vesicle exocytosis from the nerve ending, thereby preventing synaptic transmission.[4] The result of BTX injection is a dose-related muscle weakness that can be used to manage hyperfunctional muscle activity in focal dystonia, spasticity, gastrointestinal achalasia, hyperfunctional facial lines, tremor and many other conditions.

The laryngeal injection technique that we have described for the adductor type of spasmodic dysphonia[5] uses a monopolar hollow-bore Teflon-coated electromyography needle which is connected to an EMG machine. The patient is generally placed in a supine position with the neck extended. The needle is curved slightly to allow a more anterior placement, and is then placed through the neck skin and cricothyroid membrane into the thyroarytenoid muscle under EMG guidance. The patient is asked to phonate, and when the needle is in a very electrically active area of the muscle, the toxin is injected. The patient is also instructed to try not to cough or swallow when the needle is in the airway or in the thyroarytenoid muscle. The patient who has an uncontrollable cough or gag is given 0.3 ml of 1% lidocaine injected through the cricothyroid membrane into the subglottic airway. This usually causes the patient to cough, which sprays the anesthetic agent over the vocal fold mucosa. The anesthetic is not given routinely because it may diminish the EMG interference pattern, making identification of the most active place in the muscle more difficult.

The BTX-A that we have used is obtained from Allergan, Inc. in Irvine, CA. It is sent as frozen lyophilized toxin and is reconstituted with normal saline (without preservative) to a final concentration of 2.5 units per 0.1 ml. Further dilutions are performed by adding additional saline to the syringe, keeping a uniform volume of 0.1 ml. Our dose range for the 13-year period was 0.005–30 U with an average of 3.09 ±3.1. With our theory of exacerbating the dystonic symptoms on the functional vocal cord after unilateral weakness, and our goal of minimizing dose, we began bilateral dosing in most patients. Our current average starting dose is 1 U per thyroarytenoid muscle. The doses are then modified to the patient's response. Some patients have staggered doses, others have unilateral small doses, and still others have mini-doses bilaterally, which are given more frequently. These other strategies developed to try to maximize the patient's good voice. The breathy period can be minimized, but often more frequent dosing is needed. The average onset of effect was 2.4 days, with the peak effect at 9.0 days. The duration of benefit in the entire group was 15.1 weeks. The patients' initial rating averaged 52.4% function with a final result after injection of 89.7% function with an average improvement of 37.3%.

The adverse effects from the adductor laryngeal Botox injections included mild breathiness in 35% of patients and mild choking on fluids in 15% of patients. Less than 1% had local pain or sore throat related to the injection, slight blood-tinged sputum, itch, or rash.

We have also treated spasmodic dysphonia patients who failed RLN section and those who had an anterior commissure release (Tucker procedure). Although many of these patients had benefit from the injection, their voices were never as good as those patients who did not have surgery.

Ford *et al.*[14] reported an indirect laryngoscopic technique for injecting toxin into the vocal folds. They reported that the technique has the advantage of being 'familiar to the otolaryngologist and requires no special (EMG) equipment or training'. The onset of the response to toxin appears delayed (9.1 days) as compared to the percutaneous EMG technique, but the degree of benefit and the duration of efficacy appear to be comparable. Another technique was described by Rhew *et al.*[29] in which the toxin is injected through a needle placed within the operative channel of a flexible fiberoptic laryngoscope.

Based on the benefit seen in adductor spasmodic dysphonia patients, who were treated with BTX-A, we attempted to reduce the symptomatic adductor breathing spasms with similar doses. Patients received between 0.625 and 3.75 U in each thyroarytenoid muscle, depending on the severity of the spasms. These patients showed a significant symptomatic improvement and an improvement of their flow–volume loops. One of the limitations in benefit is that most of these patients also had diaphragmatic dysfunction on testing. These patients often needed concomitant systemic therapy. The mean duration of benefit in this group was 14 weeks. Half the patients injected had a breathy voice lasting 1–2 weeks.

Based on the good results we found in treating the adductor spasmodic dysphonia group, we began to inject abductor spasmodic dysphonia patients in 1989. Since that time we have treated 154 abductor patients with improvement in most. The injections are also performed percutaneously in a previously described technique.[7] In brief, the larynx is rotated away from the side of the intended injection. The hollow-bore EMG needle is then placed posterior to the posterior edge of the thyroid lamina, and advanced through the inferior constrictor muscle until reaching the cricoid cartilage. It is then moved out slightly under EMG guidance to the optimum position in the posterior cricoarytenoid muscle (PCA). The patient is asked to sniff, which maximally activates the PCA muscle, and the BTX-A is injected. An alternative technique may be used, particularly in young individuals with soft cartilage. A small amount of 1% lidocaine is injected into the subglottic airway, after which the EMG needle is placed through the cricothyroid membrane just above the cricoid cartilage anteriorly. The needle is advanced in this plane, and then directed laterally until engaging the rostrum of the cricoid cartilage. The needle is then pushed through the cartilage until there is a burst of EMG signal when the needle enters the PCA muscle. Again, the patient is asked to sniff to make sure that the needle is in an active place within the PCA muscle, and then the BTX is injected. In the older patient, this technique is difficult due to calcification of the cricoid cartilage.

I [AB] generally start with an injection of 3.75 units of BTX in 0.15 ml to weaken or paralyze one PCA muscle. In one of five of our abductor spasmodic dysphonia patients, weakening or paralyzing just one PCA muscle produces significant voice improvement. The others need both PCAs injected. Conservative doses of 0.675–2.5 units in 0.1 ml are given into the contralateral PCA, if the voice is not improved at 3 weeks from the first injection. The toxin dose for the second or third treatment is based on the amount of residual function of the previously injected PCA, the degree of persistent vocal disability, and whether the patient has had any respiratory symptoms. No further injections are given if there has been any stridor or if the glottic chink appears very narrow on examination. To date none of our 130 treated abductor patients have needed to be intubated or tracheotomized related to the BTX treatment. The patients who have been injected, but still have breathy breaks may need additional modalities used to help control their symptoms. About 15% of our patients have been given small doses of systemic agents such as Klonopin, Ativan or baclofen. This combination of toxin and systemic agent has improved the vocalization for many of the patients.

Some of the patients have had added benefit from bilateral cricothyroid injections, based on the observations of Ludlow *et al.*[22] who found abnormal cricothyroid activity in many abductor spasmodic dysphonia patients. Additionally, 12 of our patients had benefit from a type 1 thyroplasty performed to limit the abduction of one vocal fold.

Analysis of our entire abductor spasmodic dysphonia group found 30% with tremor and 30% had segmental cranial or axial dystonia, with many having respiratory muscle involvement. These factors made the degree of improvement less than in the adductor spasmodic dysphonia group overall. The average onset of effect of the toxin in the abductor group was 4.1 days with the peak effect at 10 days. The duration of benefit was on average 10.5 weeks, somewhat shorter than in the adductor group.

The adverse effects of BTX injection in the abductor spasmodic dysphonia group include four patients who developed exertional wheezing/stridor when going up stairs or jogging, and 10 patients who reported mild dysphagia to solids. The dysphagia is probably related to some of the toxin diffusing into the inferior constrictor muscle. These side effects have been transient, usually resolving within 1 week.

Our 12-year experience of more than 900 patients with spasmodic dysphonia (laryngeal dystonia) shows that until there is a treatment directed toward the central nervous system, local injections of BTX provide a safe and effective means of controlling patient symptoms. There is a learning curve in obtaining consistently good responses with small doses and few side effects, as noted by our continued downward trend in dosing and our ever-increasing benefit ratio.

References

1. Adler CH. Botulinum toxin. A therapy in dystonia. *Hosp Pract (Off Ed)* 1991; **26:** 35, 38, 41–2.
2. Aronson AE, DeSanto LW. Adductor spastic dysphonia: three years after recurrent laryngeal nerve resection. *Laryngoscope* 1983; **93:** 1–8.
3. Aronson AE, Brown JR, Litin EM, Pearson JS. Spastic dysphonia. II. Comparison with essential (voice) tremor and other neurologic and psychogenic dysphonias. *J Speech Hear Disord* 1968; **33:** 219–31.
4. Binz T, Blasi J, Yamasaki S *et al.* Proteolysis of SNAP-25 by types E and A botulinal neurotoxins. *J Biol Chem* 1994; **269:** 1617–20.
5. Blitzer A, Brin MF. Laryngeal dystonia: a series with botulinum toxin therapy. *Ann Otol Rhinol Laryngol* 1991; **100:** 85–9.
6. Blitzer A, Brin MF, Fahn S, Lovelace RE. Clinical and laboratory characteristics of focal laryngeal dystonia: study of 110 cases. *Laryngoscope* 1988; **98:** 636–40.
7. Blitzer A, Brin MF, Stewart C, Aviv JE, Fahn S. Abductor laryngeal dystonia: a series treated with botulinum toxin. *Laryngoscope* 1992; **102:** 163–7.
8. Blitzer A, Lovelace RE, Brin MF, Fahn S, Fink ME. Electromyographic findings in focal laryngeal dystonia (spastic dysphonia). *Ann Otol Rhinol Laryngol* 1985; **94:** 591–4.
9. Brin MF, Blitzer A, Stewart C, Fahn S. Treatment of spasmodic dysphonia (laryngeal dystonia) with injections of botulinum toxin: review and technical aspects. In: Blitzer A, Brin MF, Sasaki CT, Fahn S, Harris K, eds. *Neurological Disorders of the Larynx*. New York: Thieme, 1992: 214–29.
10. Brin MF, Fahn S, Blitzer A, Ramig LO, Stewart C. Movement disorders of the larynx. In: Blitzer A, Brin MF, Sasaki CT, Fahn S, Harris K, eds. *Neurological Disorders of the Larynx*. New York: Thieme, 1992: 240–8.
11. Cannito MP, Johnson P. Spastic dysphonia: a continuum disorder. *J Commun Disord* 1981; **14:** 215–23.
12. Dedo HH. Recurrent laryngeal nerve section for spastic dysphonia. *Ann Otol* 1976; **85:** 451–9.
13. Dedo HH, Behlau MS. Recurrent laryngeal nerve section for spastic dysphonia: 5–14 year preliminary results in the first 300 patients. *Ann Otol Rhinol Laryngol* 1991; **100:** 274–9.
14. Ford CN, Bless DM, Lowery JD. Indirect laryngoscopic approach for injection of botulinum toxin in spasmodic dysphonia. *Otolaryngol Head Neck Surg* 1990; **103:** 752–8.
15. Friedman M, Toriumi DM, Grybauskas VT, Applebaum EL. Implantation of a recurrent laryngeal nerve stimulator for the treatment of spastic dysphonia. *Ann Otol Rhinol Laryngol* 1989; **98:** 130–4.
16. Genack SH, Woo P, Cotton RH, Goyette D. Partial thyroarytenoid myectomy: an animal study investigating a proposed new treatment for adductor spasmodic dysphonia. *Otolaryngol Head Neck Surg* 1993; **108:** 256–64.
17. Grillone G, Blitzer A, Brin MF. Treatment of adductor breathing dystonia with botulinum toxin. *Laryngoscope* 1994; **104:** 30–3.
18. Koufman JA. A classification of laryngeal dystonias. *Visible Voice* 1992; **1:** 1–2.
19. Kramer PL, de Leon D, Ozelius L *et al.* Dystonia gene in Ashkenazi Jewish population is located on chromosome 9q32-34. *Ann Neurol* 1990; **27:** 114–20.
20. Ludlow CL, Naunton RF, Bassich CJ. Procedures for the selection of spastic dysphonia patients for recurrent laryngeal nerve section. *Otolaryngol Head Neck Surg* 1984; **92:** 24–31.
21. Ludlow CL, Naunton RF, Fujita M, Sedory SE. Spasmodic dysphonia: botulinum toxin injection after recurrent nerve surgery. *Otolaryngol Head Neck Surg* 1990; **102:** 122–31.
22. Ludlow CL, Naunton RF, Terada S, Anderson BJ. Successful treatment of selected cases of abductor spasmodic dysphonia using botulinum toxin injection. *Otolaryngol Head Neck Surg* 1991; **104:** 849–55.
23. Ludlow CL, Naunton RF, Sedory SE, Schulz GM, Hallett M. Effects of botulinum toxin injections on speech in adductor spasmodic dysphonia. *Neurology* 1988; **38:** 1220–5.
24. Marsden CD, Sheehy MP. Spastic dysphonia, Meige disease and torsion dystonia. *Neurology* 1982; **32:** 1202–3.
25. Marsden CD, Obeso JA, Zarranz JJ, Lang AE. The anatomical basis of symptomatic hemidystonia. *Brain* 1985; **108:** 463–83.
26. Miller RH, Woodson GE, Jankovic J. Botulinum toxin injection of the vocal fold for spasmodic dysphonia. A preliminary report. *Arch Otolaryngol Head Neck Surg* 1987; **113:** 603–5.
27. Netterville JL, Stone RE, Rainey C, Zealear DL, Ossoff RH. Recurrent laryngeal nerve avulsion for the treatment of spastic dysphonia. *Ann Otol Rhinol Laryngol* 1991; **100:** 10–14.
28. Ozelius LJ, Hewett JW, Page CE *et al.* The early-onset torsion dystonia gene (DTY1) encodes an ATP-binding protein. *Nat Genet* 1997; **17:** 40–8.
29. Rhew K, Fiedler DA, Ludlow CL. Technique for injection of botulinum toxin through the flexible nasolaryngoscope. *Otolaryngol Head Neck Surg* 1994; **111:** 787–94.
30. Scott AB. Botulinum toxin injection of eye muscles to correct strabismus. *Trans Am Ophthalmol Soc* 1981; **79:** 734–70.
31. Shipp T, Izdebski K, Shutte HK, Morrissey P. Subglottal air pressure in spastic dysphonia speech. *Folia Phoniatr (Basel)* 1988; **40:** 105–10.
32. Tucker HM. Laryngeal framework surgery in the management of spasmodic dysphonia. Preliminary report. *Ann Otol Rhinol Laryngol* 1989; **98:** 52–4.
33. Zweign RM, Hedreen JC, Jankel WR, Casanova MF, Whitehouse PJ. Pathology in brainstem regions of individuals with primary dystonia. *Neurology* 1988; **38:** 702–6.

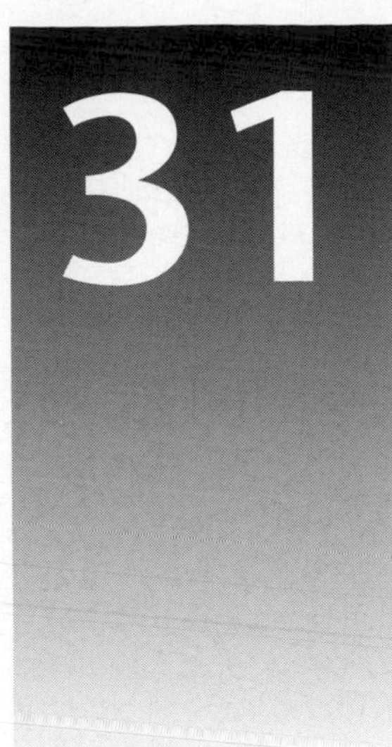

Laryngeal stenosis

J Gershon Spector

Definition

The larynx is located at the pivotal point in the aerodigestive system. The cricoid cartilage is the only complete ring and surrounds the narrowest lumen in the airway system. The larynx has three major functions in humans:

- a conduit for gaseous respiration;
- sphincteric mechanism for airway protection during deglutition; and
- phonation or voice production.

Mucociliary transport is also an important variable in airway cleansing and when inadequate can further compromise and restrict laryngeal function.

Laryngeal stenosis can be described as a partial or total obstruction of the airway through the laryngeal lumen.[2] Although formerly laryngeal stenosis was caused by generalized diseases such as diphtheria, syphilis, tuberculosis, cancers or lye burns, today prolonged tracheal intubation and external trauma account for the majority of acute and chronic laryngeal injuries. Because of the protected anatomy of the larynx below the mandible and above the sternum, iatrogenic laryngeal injuries are rare. However, persistent urban and vehicular violence contributes to the higher incidence of laryngeal injuries.

Laryngeal stenosis is generally subdivided into acute and chronic states. Acute stenosis injuries are further subdivided into soft tissue injuries and open or closed laryngeal soft tissue injuries with fracture or dislocation of the outer cartilaginous framework (compound injuries). Chronic laryngeal stenosis is subdivided by the anatomic site of the stenosis, e.g. supraglottic, glottic, subglottic or combined. These areas differ in their external cartilaginous skeletal support, epithelial lining, mobility, transluminal pressure changes, and luminal deformability to intrinsic and extrinsic physical forces. Compliance, elasticity and resilience (deformability) depend on the anatomic and physiologic characteristics of each luminal laryngeal area. In addition to the stenotic location, the composition, length and thickness of the stenosis are of paramount importance in the therapeutic decision analysis and outcome evaluation. Congenital and disease-based stenosis can be classified as subsets within this classification system for chronic stenosis.

Pathophysiology

Sphincteric properties

The laryngeal inlet acts as a sphincter to protect the airway. Closure of the laryngeal sphincter allows an increase in the intrathoracic pressure to develop. Furthermore, closure of the glottis allows for increased intra-abdominal pressure to develop in order to aid in defecation, micturition and parturition.

Prior to the second year of life, the epiglottis and supraglottis are located in the naso- or oropharynx.[50] On swallowing foods or liquids, the airway and food passages are separated at the level of the nasopharynx. On a structural and anatomic basis this separation prevents aspiration in neonates. With increasing age the larynx descends lower into the neck and the trachea becomes more intrathoracically located. For example, at birth the tracheal carina is at the level of the sternal notch and almost 80% is located in the neck. With increasing age the trachea descends into the thoracic cage so that by the age of 50 years only four tracheal rings are located at the level of the sternal notch. Therefore, with increasing age the food and airway passages develop a common lumen (oropharynx and hypopharynx). This maturation increases the risk of aspiration while at the same time it enriches our lives with a mature and recognizable phonatory function partly due to the vibratory and resonance properties of the hypopharynx and larynx.[82]

During swallowing the adult airway is protected by two mechanisms:

- mechanical properties; and
- proprioceptive reflexes.

The mechanical factors include the elevation of the larynx to bring the pharyngoesophageal lumen towards the bolus of food. The laryngeal inlet is covered by the epiglottis and by the base of the tongue to protect the airway. The epiglottic tilt and cartilaginous shape direct the food bolus sideways towards the esophagus via the pyriform fossae. At the same time there are reflexes mediated via the glossopharyngeal nerve in the hypopharynx and superior laryngeal nerves in the supraglottis. As a result of central inhibition, the airflow is arrested by closure of both the supraglottic and glottic sphincters, e.g. the false cords and true cords are squeezed in adduction to occlude the airway. The closed vocal cords have a flat cephalic surface and a dome-shaped inferior surface. The flat upper surface acts as a shelf to trap food and secretions. The dome-shaped undersurface allows for expiratory plosive forces (air) to clear the glottis during abduction. The latter reflexes are mediated by the internal branches of the superior laryngeal nerves as stimuli are carried centrally (CNS).[33,81]

Phonatory properties of the glottis will be discussed in other sections of this text.

Endoluminal airway

The airway can be conceived as a flexible cylinder. The airway circumference is related to the radius of the cross-section of the airway lumen. This relationship is numerical (circumference, C is equal to 2 times π radius; $C = 2\pi r$). The luminal surface area is the key feature in the adequacy of respiration and is related to the square of the radius (surface area equals π times the radius squared; $SA = \pi r^2$). Thus small changes in the luminal circumference and diameter produce large changes in luminal surface area.

The resistance to airflow by a stenotic segment is proportional to the length of the stenosis and inversely proportional to the fourth power of the radius of the stenotic cross-sectional surface area. The Bernoulli effect states that the work done by a cylindrical flow system is equal to the potential energy, kinetic energy and resistance of the system (Work = Potential Energy + Kinetic Energy + Resistance). The kinetic energy is related to the mass (air) and the square of the velocity of flow within the system (Kinetic Energy = $1/2MV^2$). Velocity of flow is directly related to the mass of air and inversely related to the diameter or surface area of the system ($SA=M/V$). A special derivation of the kinetic equation assumes that the mass of air does not change during respiration. Thus, the airflow velocity is directly related to the surface area (diameter or radius) of the cylinder lumen. This is called the Venturi equation ($AV = AV$; Area 1 × Velocity 1 = Area 2 × Velocity 2). Therefore, as the diameter or surface area of the lumen decreases, the airflow or velocity of flow for the same amount of air must increase. Furthermore, in a non-distensible cylinder (rigid fibrosis) the peripheral resistance and turbulent flow must also increase inversely with luminal surface area. Distensible or flexible luminal walls will reduce the resistance and turbulence of the airflow. In addition, increased resistance and turbulence may further decrease gaseous exchange and increase noise (wheezing) in the system during increased exertion of breathing.[81]

Hypoventilation

The nose is the preferred airway to the lungs. The neonate is an obligatory nasal breather. In adults, mouth breathing is employed when ventilatory demands exceed the nasal airway capacity. Ordinarily, nasal airway maximal capacity during inspiration is 1.5–2.1 l/s. The peak nasal flow resistance varies from 0.5 to 2.5 cmH_2O at 5 l/s. The larynx is primarily a valve interposed in the airway to prevent aspiration. Subglottic pressures during phonation are usually 6–10 cmH_2O. During vigorous breathing or singing, the pressure may rise to 40 cmH_2O and the airflow may range from 100 to 300 ml/s.[82]

Significant laryngeal stenosis presents a picture quite different from chronic obstructive pulmonary disease. Laryngeal obstruction is characterized by increased ventilatory effort to maintain normal alveolar ventilation while exhaustion develops. In exhausted patients death occurs in minutes (neonates) or hours (adults) after the onset of

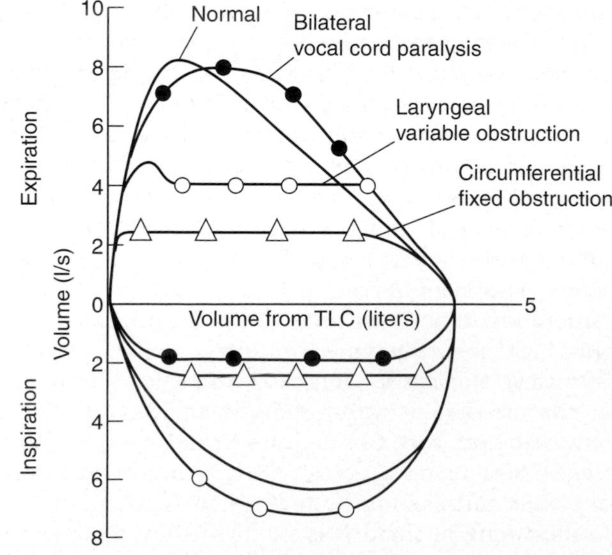

Figure 31.1 *Composite flow–volume loop studies from some characteristic types of laryngeal obstruction.*

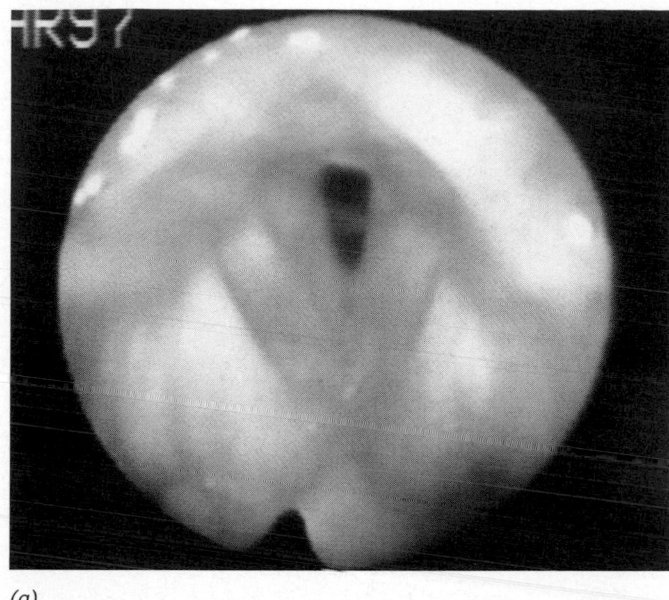

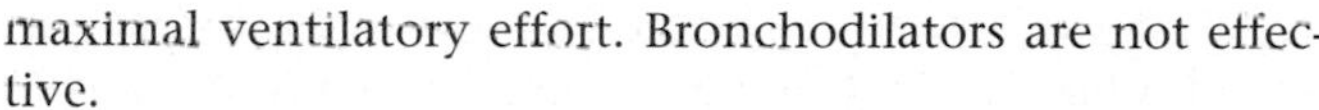

(a)

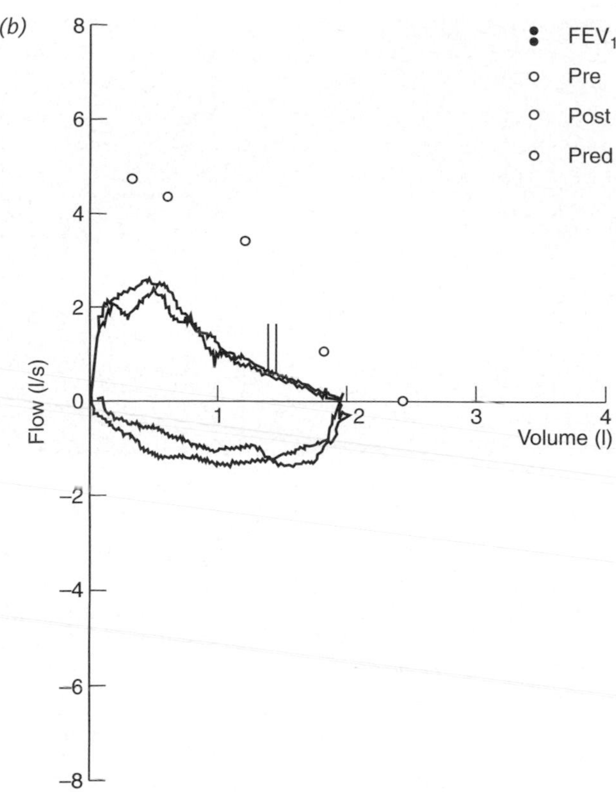

Figure 31.2 *(a) Soft subglottic stenosis following prolonged intubation 3 months prior to treatment. (b) Flow–volume loop study in the same patient. Note that the expiratory phase is reduced as compared to the inspiratory phase.*

maximal ventilatory effort. Bronchodilators are not effective.

The laryngeal narrowing can be acute or chronic. Acute obstructions are tolerated less well and may precipitate death on instrumentation. Those chronic obstructions that are at equilibrium hemodynamically and respirationally are better tolerated. The latter are amenable to instrumentation. In addition, the airway obstruction may be either rigid (fixed) or soft (distensible). Soft or flexible stenoses are better tolerated since these (edema, granuloma, membranes, spasticity of muscles, muscle tone loss) are displaceable without loss of the external cartilaginous framework support. Rigid stenoses result from intraluminal fibrosis, through-and-through tissue scarring (involving the cartilaginous framework) or external compression (invasive carcinomas, thyroid compression, comminuted compound laryngeal fractures, certain subglottic stenoses) and are not well tolerated by instrumentation. These require an airway (tracheotomy) below the obstruction prior to manipulation of the defect.

In addition to the size and nature of the stenosis, the location of the stenosis is also important. Generally, laryngotracheal stenoses are categorized physiologically as intrathoracic or extrathoracic obstructions. A flow–volume loop study may be of great diagnostic value (Fig 31.1). Wheezing, not to be confused with asthma, is common. Limitation of airflow during inspiration and expiration signifies a fixed obstruction of the entire larynx (supraglottic to subglottic regions). Limitation of airflow during expiration is a sign of subglottic stenosis that is variable, such as congenital subglottic stenoses, carcinoma with subglottic extension, subglottic hemangiomas or papillomata (Fig 31.2). Limitation during inspiration is more consistent with glottic or supraglottic obstruction such as laryngomalacia, epiglottitis, supraglottic carcinoma, or traumatic subluxation of the epiglottis.[82]

Extrathoracic soft or malacic obstructions will, on ventilation tests, give poor results on the forced inspiratory volume in one second (FIV_1) and produce inspiratory stridor. The peak inspiratory flow rate (PIFR) is reduced greater than the forced expiratory volume in one second (FEV_1). On the other hand, intrathoracic variable obstructions (tracheomalacia) produce lower volumes on the FEV_1 than on the FIV_1 due to the collapsing airway resulting from the negative intrathoracic pressure forces. In the latter instance, therefore, the cough reflex is reduced. The intrathoracic airway is smaller during expiration and the narrowing produces the typical expiratory wheezing.[82]

On flow–volume loop studies, fixed circumferential lesions of the laryngeal lumen will show a reduction in the peak flow rates in both inspiration and expiration, giving the characteristic plateau effect (Fig 31.3). Thus the FIV_1 and FEV_1 have decreased values. These are usually chronic diseases and may be well compensated, e.g. postdiphtheritic obstructions without vocal cord paresis. They do not produce symptoms until the cross-sectional area of the lumen is less than 50% of normal. Fixed extrathoracic laryngeal stenoses, because they are not malleable, produce a reduced flow in both expiration and inspiration (plateau effect or flattened flow–loop study) and the FEV_1/PEFR (Empey index) will increase. Significant obstructions will have an Empey index of >10.

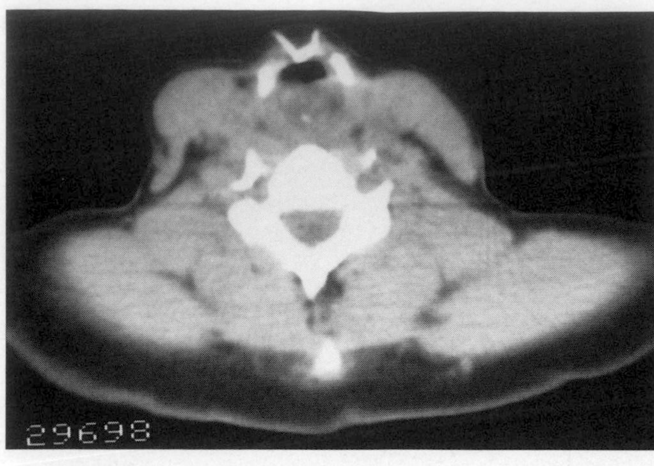

(a)

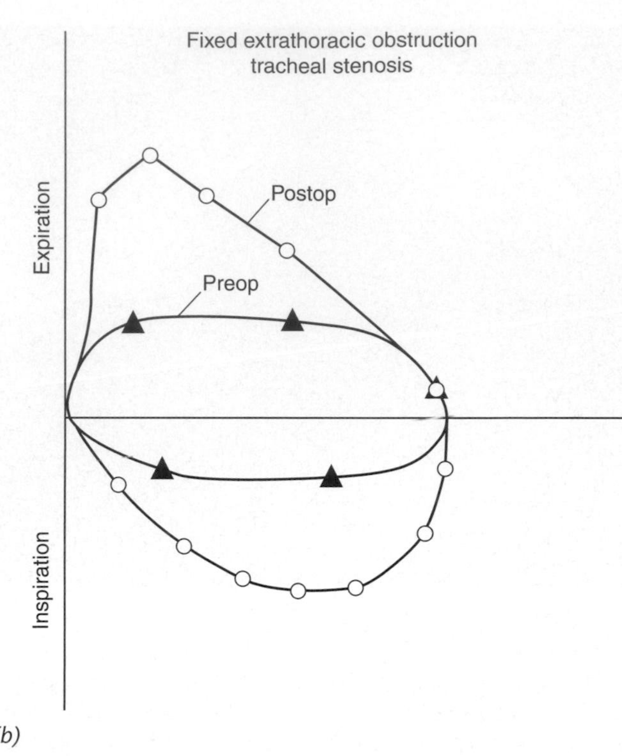

(b)

Figure 31.3 *(a) Subglottic and upper tracheal obstruction following blunt neck trauma which was corrected with a hyoid myocartilaginous transpositional graft. (b) Flow–volume loop study in the same patient prior to surgical correction (notice the flattened plateau effect). After repair there is expansion of the curve in both inspiration and expiration.*

The increased airflow resistance and problems with mucous clearance will further aggravate these symptoms to produce a greater obstruction physiologically than measured by conventional computer tomographic airway assessment measurements. As a general rule, laryngeal obstructions which allow an inspiratory flow rate of >1.5 l/s can be tolerated without the need of a tracheotomy.[26,83]

Generally, fixed intrathoracic obstructions (tracheal stenosis) and variable extrathoracic obstructions (laryngeal webs) tend to be benign. Variable intrathoracic obstructions (bronchogenic carcinomas) include a high proportion of malignancies. Fixed extrathoracic obstructions can be benign (laryngeal cicatricial stenosis) or malignant (invasive stage IV laryngeal carcinomas). Therefore, spirographic data alone are not suitable for definitive clinical diagnosis. Laryngoscopy and bronchoscopy are mandatory for clinical and tissue diagnosis. The combination of scar tissue, soft granulation tissues and framework injuries make differential diagnosis difficult, on spirographic criteria. Functional ventilation studies in combination with endoscopy and radiology are mandatory additions to the history and physical examination for proper diagnosis. In certain types of stenosis, the configuration of the narrowing will give rise to noises that can be analyzed. These can define the location and nature of the stenosis. Laryngeal webs classically lend themselves to noise analysis studies.[33,80,81]

Circulation

Laryngeal obstructions lead to alveolar hypoventilation. The cardinal feature of alveolar hypoventilation is an abnormally high $P\text{CO}_2$ (hypercapnia) which is often accompanied by a drop in the $P\text{O}_2$ (hypoxia). In patients with normal lungs, the main causes are CNS abnormalities in the respiratory drive, stiffness of the chest wall, or obstructive upper airway disease (laryngeal or tracheal stenosis). In chronic cases of upper airway obstruction the CNS is unresponsive and has a diminished sensitivity to CO_2. The resting arterial CO_2 ($P\text{aCO}_2$) may be variable. The bicarbonate level (HCO_3^-) is higher in the blood and cerebrospinal fluid due to renal adaptation to respiratory acidosis (compensatory metabolic acidosis). The arterial O_2 levels are reduced. The situation of an elevated $P\text{aCO}_2$, depressed $P\text{aO}_2$, elevated serum HCO_3^- and reduced serum pH cause CNS depression to respiratory drive and constitute a danger to life since they promote further hypoxia. Eventually these hemodynamic abnormalities culminate in cor pulmonale. The right side of the heart workload is increased by a constriction of the pulmonary vascular bed (increased vascular resistance). In the severe acute phase of the disease (traumatic laryngeal stenosis), both the pulmonary and systemic arterial pressures may be elevated. This would produce an increased cardiac output. The resulting arterial circulation is characterized by three biochemical changes:

- arterial hypoxia (low $P\text{aO}_2$, hypoxemia);
- retention of CO_2 (high $P\text{aCO}_2$, hypercapnia);
- lower pH (respiratory acidosis).

Occasionally metabolic acidosis follows as a compensatory measure. The latter further depresses the serum pH by retention of lactic acid and carbonic acid ($H_2CO_3^-$) by the

Table 31.1 Classification of laryngeal stenosis

Developmental

- Primary
  - Agenesis or aplasia
  - Atresia
  - Congenital subglottic stenosis
  - Laryngeal webs
  - Clefts
  - Laryngomalacia
- Secondary
- Laryngeal
    - Laryngocele
    - Cysts
    - Ventricular prolapse
    - Vocal cord paralysis
  - Esophageal
    - Megaesophagus
    - Tracheoesophageal fistulae
    - Esophageal atresia or stenosis
  - Laryngeal masses
    - Teratoma
    - Cystic hygroma
    - Meconium or fecal aspiration
    - Myxedema
    - Ectopic thyroid
    - Subglottic hemangioma

Inflammations

- Primary
  - Bacterial
    - Epiglottitis
    - Laryngotracheal
    - Diphtheria
    - Laryngitis
  - Granulomatous
    - TBC (human, avian)
    - Scleroma
    - Sarcoid
    - Leprosy
  - Luetic laryngitis
    - Acquired
    - Congenital
  - Fungal
    - Histoplasmosis
    - Actinomycosis
- Secondary
  - Thyroiditis
  - Neoplastic chondritis
  - Radiation chondritis
  - Post-traumatic sepsis
  - Postsurgical sepsis

Traumatic

- External trauma
  - Blunt neck injuries
  - Penetrating neck injuries
    - Low velocity – knife
    - High velocity – bullets
  - Postoperative
  - Complex comminuted injuries
    - Neck injuries
    - Neurologic and muscular injuries
    - Vascular injuries
    - CNS injuries
- Internal trauma
  - Post-intubation
  - Post-tracheotomy
  - Cuff injuries
  - Foreign bodies
  - Chemical injuries
  - Physical (thermal) injuries
  - Postoperative

Neoplastic

- Laryngeal
  - Benign
    - Papillomata
    - Chondroma
    - Fibromas
    - Neurofibroma
    - Chemodectomas
    - Hemangiomata
  - Malignant
    - Epithelial
      - Squamous cell carcinoma
      - Adenocarcinoma
      - Adenoid cystic carcinoma
    - Neuroendocrine
      - Typical carcinoid
      - Atypical carcinoid
      - Small cell neuroendocrine carcinoma
    - Skeletal muscle
      - Rhabdomyosarcoma
      - Fibromyosarcoma
    - Cartilage – chondrosarcoma
    - Vascular
      - Kaposi sarcoma
      - Hemangiopericytoma
- Extralaryngeal malignant tumors
  - Invasive thyroid adenocarcinoma
  - Tracheal carcinoma
    - Squamous cell carcinoma
    - Adenocystic carcinoma
  - Esophageal carcinoma
  - Hypopharyngeal carcinoma
  - Metastatic tumors to the larynx
  - Lymphoma and Hodgkin's –
  - Hemopoietic tumors

Neuromuscular deficits

- Bilateral vocal cord paralysis
- Postoperative neuromuscular deficits
- CNS injuries
- Shy–Drager syndrome

Idiopathic and miscellaneous

- Amyloid
- Lipoid proteinosis
- Angioneurotic edema
- Relapsing polychondritis
- Rheumatoid arthritis; lupus erythematosus
- Wegener's granulomatosis
- Eosinophilic granulomatosis
- Immobile cilia syndrome
- Obesity – Pickwickian syndrome
- Secretional obstruction
  - Cystic fibrosis
  - Postradiation
  - Diabetes mellitus
  - Autonomic deficit syndromes
- Epidermolysis bullosa
- Pemphigoid
- Gastroesophageal reflux

kidneys. (At the same time the respiratory tidal volume is reduced.)[82]

Other circulatory problems are related to the action of cardiovascular reflexes. Baroreceptors in the aortic arch and carotid bifurcation are affected by vagal stimulation from the superior laryngeal and recurrent laryngeal nerves. Stimulation of the vagus nerve (intubation, endoscopy) will cause a reduction of the heart rate. This reflex can be enhanced by morphine and reduced by atropine.[82]

Mucociliary flow

The true vocal cords are covered by stratified squamous epithelium. The remainder of the larynx has a ciliated columnar epithelium with goblet cells and minor salivary gland covering. Trauma, fibrosis and inflammation damage the respiratory epithelium and paralyze ciliary motility in the adjacent nontraumatic areas. This prevents mucociliary transport in a greater region than the damaged area of the larynx. The mucous secretions are arrested below the damaged area. They may accumulate and further reduce the airway diameter. The only way to traverse this mucous obstructive area (stenotic site and paretic region) is by plosive expiratory coughing. The cough is considered a backup system for the mucosal transport in the airway. Thus coughing in patients with laryngeal stenosis is a common clinical finding.[82]

Mucosal regeneration can occur even in stenotic laryngeal segments. The rate of regeneration varies from 1 mm/day to 1 mm/week. The ability to transport mucus is rather good when at least part of the luminal circumference of the stenotic site has functioning ciliated epithelium. Thus scattered islands of respiratory epithelium may be adequate to promote mucus transport. The mucous blanket is pulled over the denuded areas by the ciliary motility in the adjacent areas.[82]

The mucous blanket in the respiratory tract has two components, which differ in their viscosity and elasticity. A soluble low-viscosity and elasticity layer (with low resistance) lies on top of the beating cilia. This layer acts as a conveyor belt, which is moved by the synchronized beating cilia. On top of this mucous conveyor belt lies another mucous layer, which is of high viscosity and elasticity. The main function of the uppermost mucous layer is to trap particulate material and debris that gain entrance into the lower airway system. Thus small gaps and defects in the respiratory epithelium can be traversed by the mucous blanket due to the cross-linked macromolecules that hold the mucous together as the cilia pull the entire mucous blanket over the denuded areas. If the mucosal defect is larger and it is not possible to traverse the injured site, then pooling of secretions occurs below the stenotic site.

Classification

The etiologic classification of laryngeal stenosis is presented in Table 31.1. Although not totally comprehensive, this classification represents a basis on which to formulate a differential diagnosis. This classification should be distinguished from the various therapeutic classifications that have been formulated for specific common causes of laryngeal stenosis, e.g. subglottic stenosis, postintubation stenosis, traumatic stenosis, etc. Many of the disease entities will not be covered in this chapter since they will be discussed elsewhere in the text. The main focus in this chapter will be on the common congenital and traumatic stenotic lesions of the larynx.

Congenital malformations

Congenital malformations that lead to laryngeal stenosis may be divided into two pathologic subgroups, e.g. primary and secondary. Primary or intrinsic laryngeal malformations are caused by maldevelopment of the larynx itself. Secondary malformations are due to extralaryngeal malformations that interfere with the laryngeal airway. It should be remembered that approximately 50% of laryngeal malformations are associated with other organ anomalies (heart, eyes, neck, anus, vertebral bodies and reproductive organs).[36] The most common congenital malformations that lead to laryngeal airway compromise are laryngomalacia, bilateral vocal cord paralysis, subglottic stenosis and laryngeal webs.

Laryngeal webs

Laryngeal webs occur due to incomplete canalization of the epithelial lamina at the stage of luminal development.[4] The solid cellular epithelial plug that occludes the rudimentary lumen at 12 weeks *in utero* fails to recanalize from the laryngeal ventricles, true cords and false vocal folds. This may be a failure in apoptosis or cellular vacuolization, which leads to incomplete luminal development and to partial obstruction. Neonates may present from birth with a weak, unusual or absent cry and varying degrees of stridor, respiratory distress and airway obstruction. When laryngeal atresia is present, the baby may make violent attempts at ineffective respiration. Asphyxia occurs rapidly if a tracheotomy is not performed. Older children will present with repeated attacks of stridor or croup, especially following laryngotracheal bronchitis or laryngitis. They also tend to have an abnormal and weak cry. Respiratory distress, cyanosis, recurrent croup and weak cry are the cardinal presenting features of laryngeal webs.

Most webs are thin and transparent posteriorly. The webs tend to be thicker anteriorly at the anterior commissure. The webs occur anteriorly and extend backwards towards the posterior commissure between the two vocal cords to varying degrees of thickness and luminal occlusion. The upper surface is flat and the posterior edge is

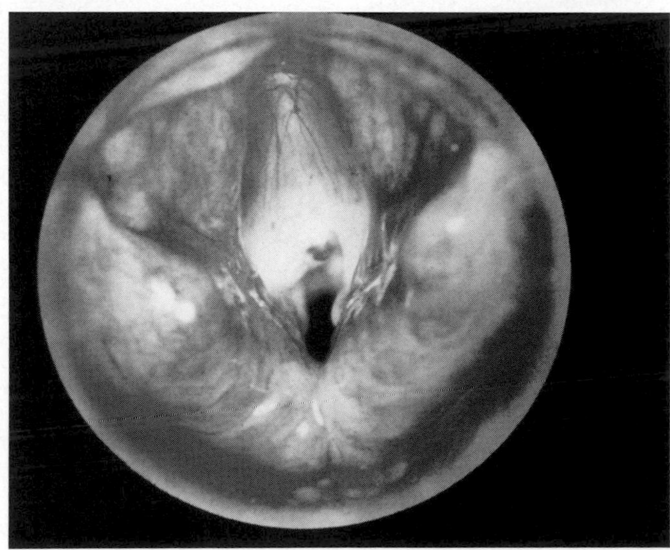

Figure 31.4 *Congenital thick laryngeal web which involves the anterior subglottic area. This is a combined glottic–subglottic stenosis.*

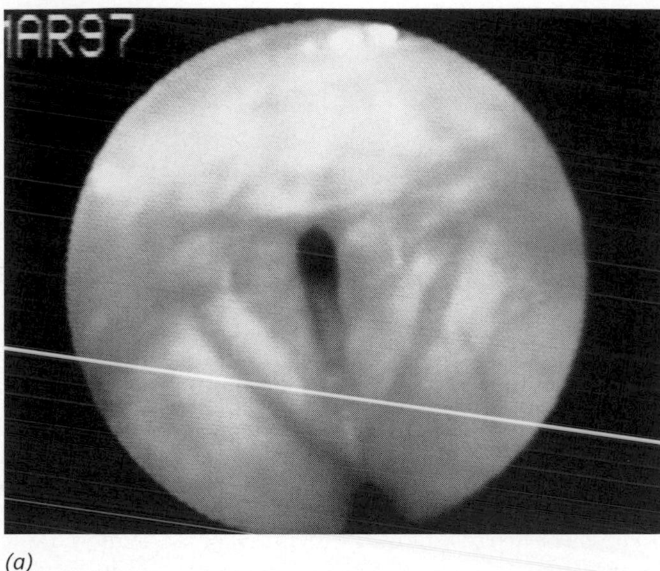

(a)

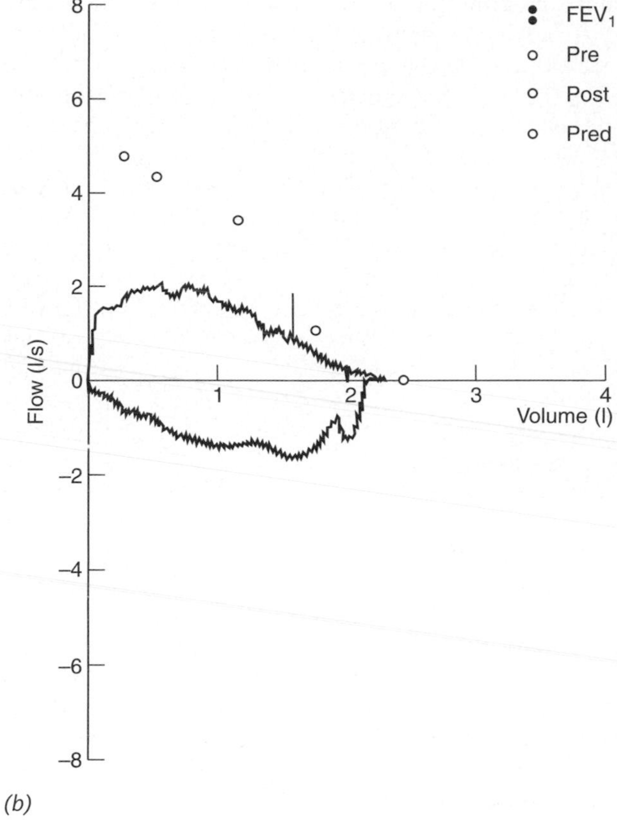

(b)

Figure 31.5 *(a) Subglottic stenosis with intact laryngeal skeleton. (b) Flow–volume loop study in the same patient denoting the plateau effect. There is a reduction of expiratory flow greater than the inspiratory flow.*

concave. The undersurface is convex. The upper surface is covered with squamous epithelium and the under surface with respiratory epithelium mucosa. In between there is a fibrous layer. Benjamin classifies congenital webs by their location, e.g. glottic, subglottic, interarytenoid and supraglottic.[4] Supraglottic webs are extremely rare. Subglottic webs can occur with or without subglottic stenosis and cricoid cartilage involvement. Interarytenoid webs are the most difficult to treat and, when associated with subglottic stenosis, usually require a preliminary tracheotomy. Glottic webs may be associated (frequently) with subglottic airway reduction (Fig 31.4).

Subglottic stenosis

Subglottic stenosis can be classified as soft tissue stenosis or combined cricoid cartilage malformation (hard stenosis).[91] *Soft tissue subglottic stenosis* is due to swelling or hypertrophy of mucous glands, fibrous tissue proliferation, thickened conus elasticus and hypertrophied submucosa (Fig 31.5). The cricoid cartilage development is normal. *Hard stenosis* is due to malformations of the cricoid cartilage.[45] This may be due to cartilage malformation, congenital small ring, overgrowth circumferentially of the cricoid cartilage, inward luminal thickening, or incomplete canalization (associated with laryngeal webs). Cricoid cartilage agenesis may be complete or partial. These may be associated with a small cricoid ring, annular malformations, or failure of luminal canalization. The cricoid may have an abnormal shape, producing a large anterior or posterior lamina, elliptical shape or flattened shape. Incomplete cricoid cartilaginous rings may produce partial, occult (submucosal) or complete laryngeal clefts. The most common laryngeal atresia is developed by membranous and/or cartilaginous stenosis at the cricotracheal junction.[90] An improper subluxation of the first tracheal ring under a malformed inferior border of the cricoid cartilage produces the classic *long* subglottic hard stenosis, e.g. the trapped first tracheal ring.

There have been various systems developed for grading the degree of subglottic stenosis.[14] Prior to 1984, a subjective system (grades 1–4) was based on the cross-sectional area of the stenotic site (lumen) and was correlated successfully with prognosis for therapeutic recovery.[85] The stenotic grade was correlated with luminal reduction as follows:

- grade 1, < 70%;
- grade II, 70–90%;
- grade III, > 90%; and
- grade IV, no visible lumen.

In 1986, Grundfast *et al.* proposed a classification based on the stenotic segment length, cross-sectional diameter and consistency (hard or soft stenosis). This system

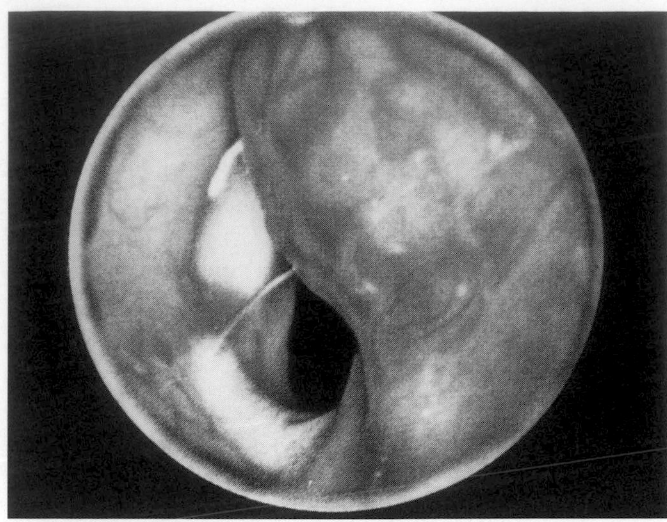

Figure 31.6 *Internal laryngocele.*

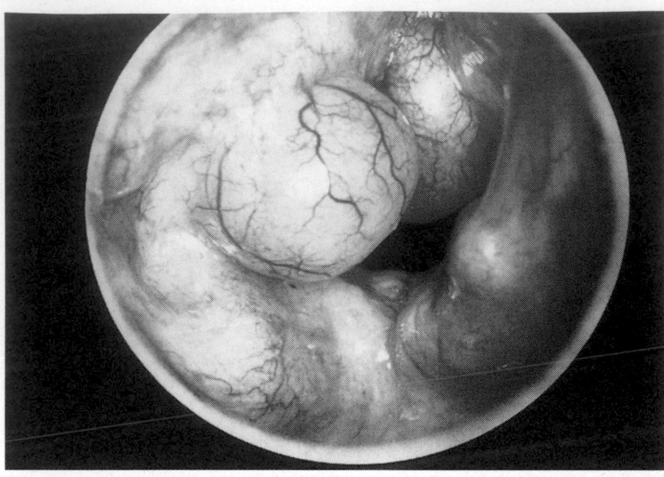

Figure 31.7 *Internal laryngocele and a saccular cyst causing glottic intermittent obstruction.*

required radiographic and endoscopic measurements.[40] In 1988, the American Society of Pediatric ORL agreed to adapt the FLECS classification system (FLECS is an acronym for *F*unction, *L*umen, *E*xtent, *C*onsistency and *S*ite of *S*tenosis.) This system has proved to be complete but too cumbersome for routine use. Cotton *et al.* proposed a simplified classification based on the outer diameter of the endotracheal tubes (standardized sizes) that can pass the obstruction site.[16] The standardized tube sizes are precisely measured and can be converted to standard circumferential and cross-sectional areas. However, the latter classification, though facile for clinicians, is not adequate for data reporting and analysis.

Laryngoceles

Laryngoceles represent a dilatation of the ventricular saccule.[82] They may be filled with air or secretions (mucus or pus). If the laryngocele is dilated with air, there is a communication with the mucosal surface of the laryngeal ventricle. Internal laryngoceles are confined to the larynx and manifest as a bulge in the false vocal fold or aryepiglottic fold (Fig 31.6). External laryngoceles present as masses which extend superiorly above the rim of the thyroid lamina. They produce a bulge in the thyrohyoid membrane. Characteristically they follow the lateral rim of the epiglottic cartilage and are medial to the superior laryngeal neurovascular bundle. The combined laryngoceles have both an internal and external saccular dilatation. Since the lining of the laryngoceles is respiratory epithelium with goblet cells and secretory glands, the lumen is filled with secretions in those laryngoceles that do not communicate with the laryngeal ventricle. These can become infected to produce laryngopyoceles. It should be remembered that 12–18% of glottic carcinomas are associated with laryngoceles. Laryngoceles may be associated with certain professions in which high intralaryngeal pressures are created, e.g. wind or brass instrument players. Occasionally the redundant ventricular mucosa and laryngeal saccule may eviscerate into the laryngeal lumen to produce a ventricular prolapse (Fig 31.7). This may produce intermittent stridor. However, prolapsed mucosa, if not septic, rarely causes airway incompetence.

Laryngomalacia

Laryngomalacia may cause intermittent inspiratory stridor and reduced inspiratory airflow (Fig 31.8). This is a sequela of an omega-shaped epiglottis which is associated with a diffuse absence, deformity or flaccidity of the supraglottic cartilaginous and/or ligamentous framework. The flaccidity of the epiglottis and supraglottic soft tissues

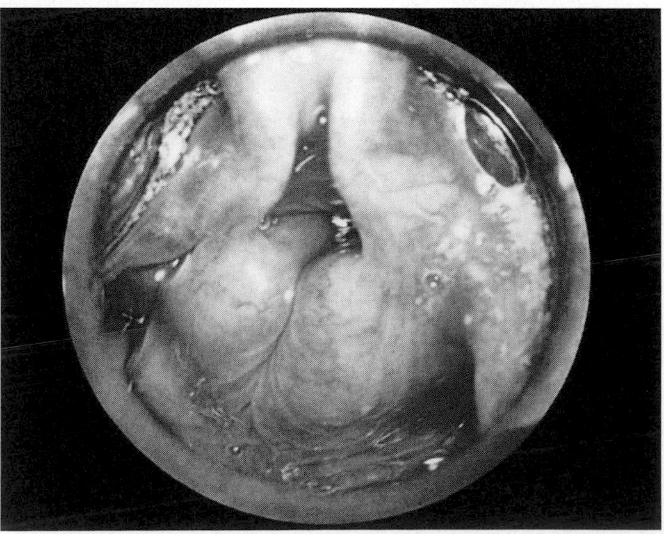

Figure 31.8 *Laryngomalacia in a neonate during inspiration causing inspiratory stridor.*

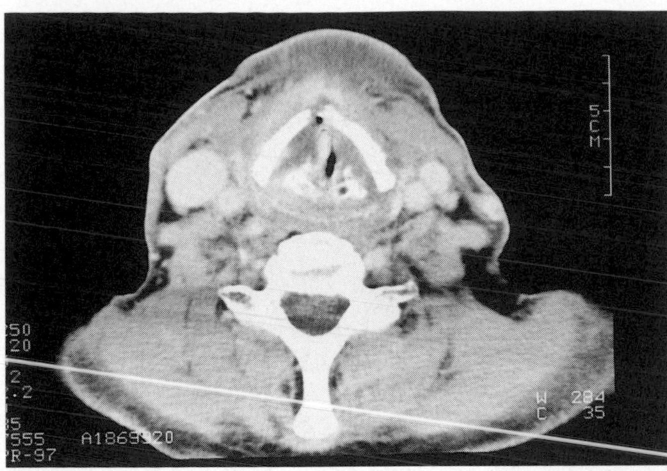

Figure 31.9 *Subglottic extension of squamous cell carcinoma with laryngeal skeletal invasion producing laryngeal airway compromise.*

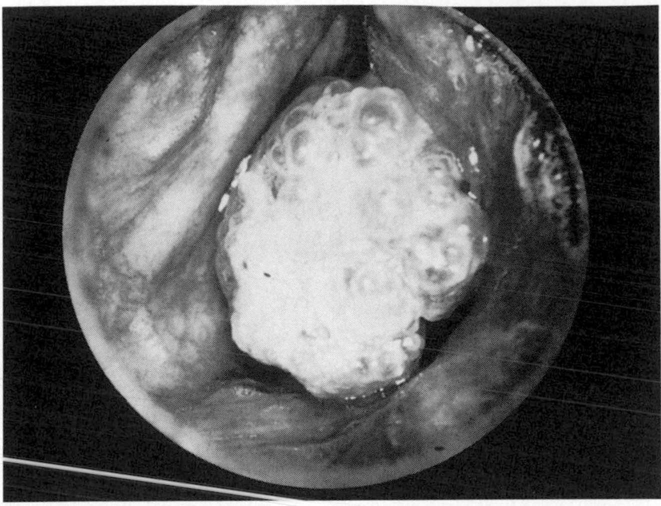

Figure 31.10 *Laryngeal viral papillomata causing obstruction and airway compromise.*

collapses on inspiration. On inspiration, due to the Bernoulli effect of the in-rushing air, the soft tissues are sucked into the endolaryngeal lumen to produce the characteristic inspiratory stridor. The soft tissue mass in the lumen decreases the inspiratory airflow (decreased FIV_1). The expiratory outflow of air is not affected. Thus major obstructions are rare.

Acquired stenosis

The vast majority of acquired laryngeal stenoses are due to endoluminal trauma (intubation or endoscopic procedures), external laryngeal trauma (blunt or penetrating), inflammatory disease (acute epiglottitis, laryngotracheal bronchitis) or bilateral vocal cord paralysis (usually postoperative – thyroid, cardiovascular, pulmonary or CNS procedures). Other common causes include:

- a high proportion of malignancies of the larynx or hypopharynx (squamous cell carcinomas) (Fig 31.9);
- postradiation therapy edema;
- granulomatous disease (TBC, Lues); and
- general systemic diseases – rheumatoid arthritis, lupus erythematosus, relapsing polychondritis, aspirations due to varying causes, angioneurotic edema, chemical inhalations, burn injuries (inhalation of hot gases), etc. (Fig 31.10).

Most of the acquired diseases which can cause laryngostenosis will be covered elsewhere in this text. The main focus of this section will deal with three issues: post-intubation injuries, external laryngeal trauma and post-tracheotomy airway compromise.

Post-intubation stenosis

It is estimated that the incidence of significant laryngotracheal stenoses following intubation is between 0.9 and 8.3%. In the early 1960s and 1970s, the incidence was higher (12–20%). The most common site of injury is the subglottic region in children and the posterior commissure area of adult larynges. Since MacEwen introduced the oral tracheal tube in 1880 there have been proponents who claimed that prolonged oral tracheal intubation produces minimal risks and opponents who noted a significant incidence of serious complications. The latter group suggests that tracheotomy leads eventually to fewer laryngeal complications. Fearon *et al.* noted that in 504 tracheotomies in children there were no major complications as opposed to 11 laryngotracheal complications in 72 prolonged oral tracheal intubations (8 hours or longer).[29] Previously, Baron and Kahlmoos described the complications of prolonged intubation in children.[3]

Holinger noted that the narrowest diameter of the infantile larynx is at the glottis where the anteroposterior diameter is 7 mm and the posterior glottic commissure width is 4 mm. The surface area is 14 mm^2. One millimeter of edema reduces the surface area to 65% (9 mm^2). This will produce serious obstruction symptoms in children but not adults. Furthermore, subglottic submucosa has a loose areolar tissue and respiratory epithelium. These produce swelling, edema and ulceration with even the slightest endoluminal foreign body trauma. Since the subglottic area is surrounded by a complete cartilaginous ring of the cricoid cartilage, outward expansion of swollen tissue is prevented. The resultant effect is endoluminal constriction and airway compromise.[46]

A number of factors have been described as predisposing to laryngeal stenosis in intubated patients.[29] The *duration* of intubation correlates with the risk of significant laryngeal injury. There appears to be no absolutely safe time limit. Significant injuries have been observed after 8 hours of intubation in adults and 1 week in neonates. Whited reported prospectively that almost all patients who were examined endoscopically after

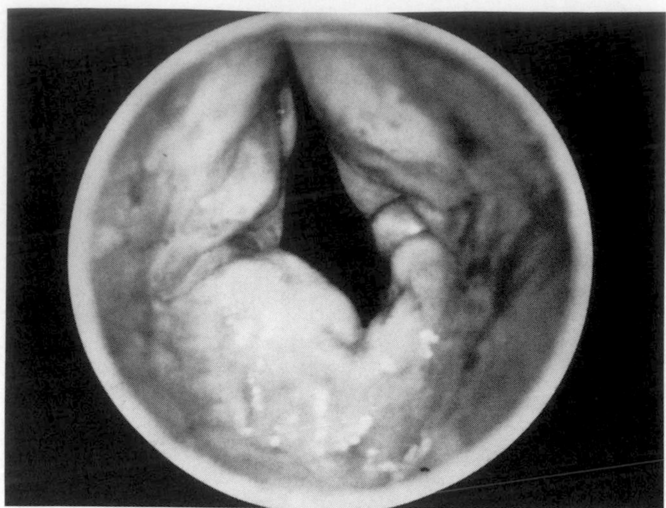

Figure 31.11 *Prolonged intubation of >2 weeks with assisted ventilation. Note extensive true and false vocal cord edema, necrosis of the left arytenoid cartilage, and posterior glottic stenosis.*

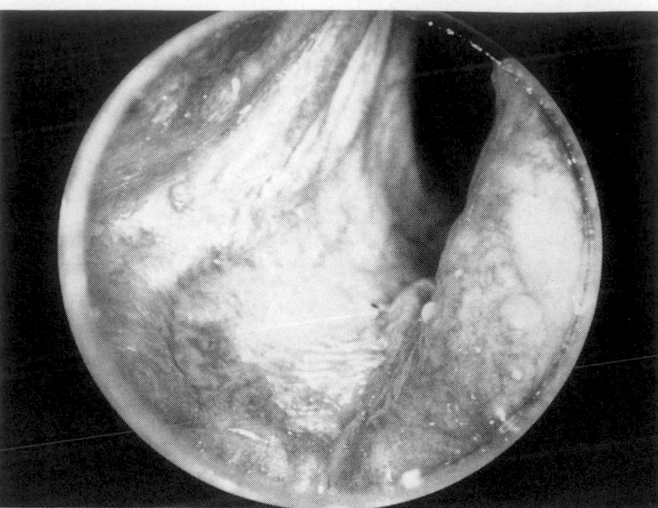

Figure 31.12 *Following prolonged intubation there was necrosis of the vocal process of the arytenoid and posterior glottic scarring that included the mucosa and interarytenoid muscle.*

prolonged intubation had superficial ulcerations and erythema of the laryngeal mucosa.[94] In 200 patients, following prolonged intubation, the overall incidence of laryngeal stenosis was 6%. Posterior glottic stenosis occurred after 5–10 days of intubation (4%) and increased to 14% after 10–24 days of intubation. Even in expert hands, injury cannot be avoided and there is a limit for long-term intubation. Generally, the limits for prolonged intubation are evident after 7 days and are clearly manifested after 10 days of intubation. Conversion to a tracheotomy following 7–10 days of intubation was advocated.

Others have noted that 63% of patients intubated in a critical care setting had early injuries of the larynx; however, only 10% developed long-term stenosis. Nevertheless, most studies suggest that the vast majority of intubations result in injuries, but only a few are of significance. Donnelly, in an autopsy study, described the histopathology of endolaryngeal intubation trauma in 99 adults.[20] The brunt of the trauma was on the vocal processes of the arytenoid cartilages, the subglottic mucosa, the cricoid lamina and the interarytenoid area. The degree of injury was related to the length of time of intubation. Intubations of 12 hours or less produced shallow ulcers, loss of epithelium and compression of mucosal capillary beds. Between 12 and 48 hours there were deep ulcers with stromal necrosis. After 48 hours of intubation there were vocal process ulcers, deeper and broader subglottic ulceration and exposed inner perichondrium. After 96 hours of intubation there was excavation of the laryngeal cartilages and after 120 hours there was cartilage necrosis (Fig 31.11). Reparative intubation granulomas or late reparative vocal process of arytenoid phenomena require at a minimum perichondrial ulceration. Gould and Howard did a similar study in neonates.[37]

Earlier damage occurs within hours of intubation, leading to ulcerations of the vocal process of the arytenoids, vocal cord rims and subglottic epithelium. There is earlier cartilage ulceration of the arytenoids, cricoid lamina and thyroid cartilages. In a prospective study of 3 years' duration on 289 newborns weighing <1500 g at birth that were intubated, Nicklaus *et al.* noted that 2.4% developed subglottic stenosis.[68] Generally, prolonged neonatal intubation produces stenosis in 0.25–8.0% of the patients. Laryngeal injuries following prolonged intubation can be quantified according to site of the lesion in the following sequence of probabilities: subglottic, 70%; supraglottic, 5–10%; glottic, 5–10%; and tracheal, 5%. Hawkins *et al.* documented that 15 of 16 neonates intubated for longer than 6 days showed ulcerative lesions in the subglottic area.[42] In addition, they described the occurrence of posterior glottic post-intubation injuries, e.g. between the arytenoid cartilages. There were two forms of posterior glottic narrowing. One was due to posterior glottic synechiae or bands which bridge between the two vocal processes of the arytenoids (superficial variant). The second was scarring that involved the entire posterior commissure including the underlying interarytenoid muscle with/without cartilage damage (Fig 31.12). In most cases the anterior commissure was spared. Bogdasarian *et al.* described four degrees of glottic injury:

- interarytenoid synechiae;
- scarring in posterior commissure involving the interarytenoid muscle with mobile joints;
- fixation of one cricoarytenoid joint; and
- fixation of both cricoarytenoid joints.[7]

Cohen described the 'pseudolaryngeal paralysis' due to cricoarytenoid joint fixation by scar following prolonged

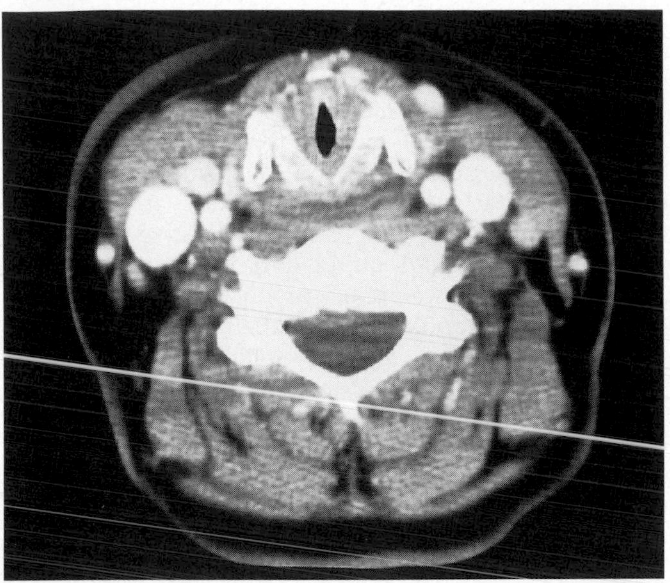

(a)

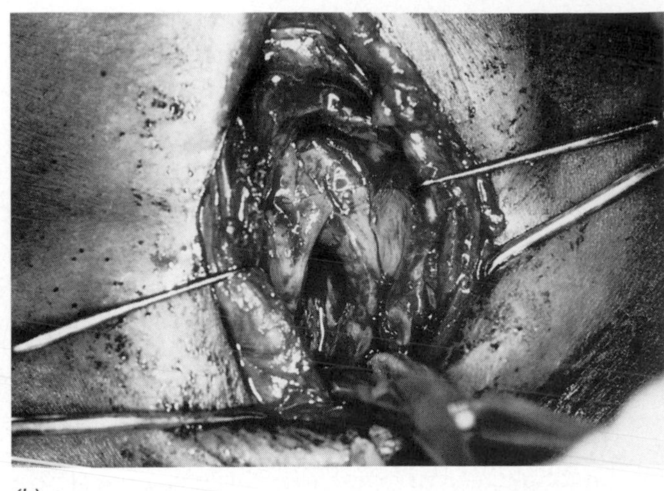

(b)

Figure 31.13 *Prolonged intubation causing glottic and subglottic stenosis with necrosis of the laryngeal skeleton. (a) CT scan demonstrates subglottic stenosis with destruction of the anterior cricoid cartilage. (b) At exploration in the same patient a partial midline thyrotomy demonstrated a combined glottic–subglottic stenosis, necrosis of the anterior cricoid ring, granulation tissue and edema.*

intubation.[10] There were no true paralyses of the vocal cords after lysis of the scar. Some have labelled this syndrome as the 'stiff larynx' since vocal cord mobility is diminished.

Endotracheal tube size is a second variable which predisposes to laryngeal stenosis. Way and Sooy noted in monkeys that increasing the endotracheal tube by one size (larger) from a proper fit produced noticeable mucosal damage in the larynx.[92] Oversized tubes produce early mucosal damage and underlying cartilage ulceration and necrosis. Generally it is recommended that a small air leak be present following intubation and that ventilation be at <20 cmH_2O. Cuffed tubes that are inflated further increase the endoluminal tube size. Inflation of the tube cuff to internal pressures above 20–30 cmH_2O will occlude the mucosal and submucosal circulation in the subglottic region. This will cause devascularization with ischemic necrosis of the soft tissues and cartilages of the trachea and cricoid. The latter will predispose to subglottic stenosis. The intermittent reduction of the pressure in the cuff, the use of a double cuff, or the use of low-pressure cuffs will ameliorate the risk (Fig 31.13). However, one should remember that the interface between the cuffs in a double cuff tube will create shearing forces which could produce subglottic stenosis.[12]

Repeated intubation or *traumatic* intubation predisposes to early mucosal and cartilaginous damage, especially if the tube size is large. The aseptic mucosal injury due to compression with a large tube is further damaged by mechanical trauma, leading to greater laryngeal damage. Today, the endotracheal tubes are standardized with a known outer and inner diameter size. These sizes can be correlated with known neonatal or adult endoluminal surface area dimensions. Therefore, the proper tube matched to the patient age is possible by standardized tables (for example see Eckenhoff[24]). Other intubation injuries include subluxation of the arytenoid cartilage, cricoarytenoid joint trauma, laryngeal hematoma, mucosal lacerations and vocal cord paralysis. Two prospective studies indicate that the risk of the above-mentioned complications is 6%. Arytenoid cartilage subluxation was found in one case per 1000 patients. It is important to be able to differentiate post-subluxation arytenoid fixation from vocal cord paralysis, which can be achieved by direct endoscopy and arytenoid manipulation or laryngeal EMG studies. Kuriloff *et al.* noted that with cricothyrotomy (electively done in 48 patients) there was a 52% incidence of airway complications, most commonly subglottic stenosis.[49] Brantigan and Grow reported on 655 patients with elective cricothyrotomy and prolonged intubation.[8] The complication rate was 6%; much less than tracheotomy. However, others reversed this opinion and advocated tracheotomy when laryngotracheal injury was expected.[67] Today cricothyrotomy is used mainly as an emergency access to the airway. Then it should be converted to a regular tracheotomy within 12–24 hours. Cricothyrotomy is not advocated for prolonged intubation since it causes cricoid cartilage necrosis and circumferential high subglottic stenosis.

Shearing forces between the endotracheal tube and patient are of paramount importance in laryngeal stenosis. This is especially true with incapacitated or obtunded patients. The pneumatic action of the respirator, which acts on a fixed endotracheal tube, causes a relative motion between the tube and the incapacitated patient's larynx. In alert, restless patients, persistent motion and swallowing produce similar forces between the moving larynx and the fixed endotracheal tube. These produce friction and continuous trauma to the laryngeal mucosa. Adequate sedation may be required in the restless patient to avoid further laryngeal damage. Couraud *et al.* noted that 95% of laryngeal and tracheal stenoses (strictures) in 300 patients treated by the thoracic service were due to resuscitation injuries.[17] Since 1978 they treated 181 laryngotracheal injuries of which 80 cases (44%) were laryngeal injuries. These injuries resulted in stenoses in various laryngeal areas and frequently involved more than one area, as well as trachea. The implication of these findings is that shearing forces can produce more extensive damage to different laryngeal areas, including the glottis, supraglottis and subglottis, in addition to the cervical trachea. Lanza *et al.* reported that in 52 patients with head injuries, the early complication rate with endotracheal tube intubation was 61%.[51] The complication rate with tracheotomy was 20%. Prolonged intubation and the use of respiratory assistance were major sources of complications (P = 0.008). Some have advocated that to avoid complications one should:

- change the position of the inflatable tube cuff;
- use two interchangeable cuffs;
- use a soft, low-pressure, malleable cuff;
- inflate the cuff with enough air pressure (or saline) to allow the respirator to work;
- increase humidification in the inspired air;
- have the patient bronchoscoped (fiberoptic endoscope) before decannulation; and
- suspect delayed stenosis with dyspnea, wheezing, coughing, stridor or cyanosis.

Symptoms may be delayed from 1 week to 10 months.

Prolonged ventilatory-assisted respiration in neonates is the most common cause of acquired subglottic stenosis.[11] Nevertheless, because of the subglottic structure and composition of the neonatal larynx, prolonged intubation is tolerated better in neonates and children than in adults. There is a relatively higher hydration and decreased rigidity in the neonatal cartilages. The cartilages have greater resilience in infants due to the composition of the cartilaginous matrix. Neonates and premature children have greater cellularity and a gel-like matrix with a high fluid content. With development, the cartilaginous matrix becomes less hydrated, more fibrous and more rigid. Eventually in the adult it may calcify. However, extremely premature children (<1000 g) tolerate intubation less well, since the larynges are too small for the smallest endotracheal tubes. Therefore, the very low birth weight neonates (1000 g) have a higher incidence of subglottic stenosis following prolonged intubation.[5,68,84]

The presence of *infection* is acknowledged as a major factor predisposing to laryngeal stenosis. Preexisting infection of the tracheobronchial tree prior to intubation, especially, predisposes to mucosal and submucosal necrosis and chondritis. In addition, following prolonged intubation, tracheotomy predisposes to both laryngeal and tracheal stenosis. McGovern *et al.* noted an increased incidence of laryngeal stenosis (twofold increase) when post-intubation tracheotomy was performed.[57] They hypothesize that minor intubation injuries are aggravated by tracheotomy. To test this hypothesis, Sasaki *et al.* performed experiments on 12 dogs to demonstrate that the magnitude of scar tissue produced in the larynx is related to the amount of the inflammatory response.[74] Subglottic mucosal injuries following tracheotomy resulted from $>10^5$ bacteria per gram of tissue. This led to mucosal ulceration and underlying chondritis. The mechanism of contamination is by mucociliary flow rather than by lymphovascular invasion. The upward movement of the mucociliary flow away from the tracheotomy site damages the subglottic area by contamination. The use of systemic antibiotics (pre- and postoperatively) and meticulous stomal care limit the amount of injury. Needless to say, the size of the bacterial inoculum and duration of exposure are contributing factors to major injury. The combination of aseptic mucosal and submucosal injuries, combined with bacterial invasion, result in underlying chondritis which leads to subglottic stenosis. The most common organisms isolated in humans are *Pseudomonas aeruginosa* and *Staphylococcus aureus*.

Most cuffed endotracheal tubes accumulate secretions above the cuff. This pooling serves as a culture medium for bacterial contamination. In addition, many patients have nasogastric tubes, gastroesophageal reflux, reflex gastric or esophageal regurgitation which further contaminate the airway system by a chemical (acid) injury. Furthermore, all endoluminal tubes have micropores in the walls of the tube (Portex, polyvinyl chloride, Silastic, etc.). On prolonged exposure to contamination, bacteria or fungi can grow in the walls of the tube. These are not susceptible to antibiotics or stomal care. They present a constant source of infection. The only way to control this problem is by replacing the endoluminal tubes on a regular basis. The use of soft tubes that mold at body temperature is less irritating to the luminal surface. All tubes used should be disposable. Sterilization with ethylene oxide provides toxic residues and contamination in the tube wall pores. In general, nasogastric tubes that are rigid can cause esophageal and laryngopharyngeal mucosal injury. When combined with an endotracheal tube, these may cause esophageal fistulae, reflux or pressure necrosis.

The presence of simultaneous *systemic illnesses* or injuries also influences the development of laryngeal stenosis following prolonged intubation. Clearly most patients who require prolonged intubation have other associated injuries or traumas, which need to be addressed. These increase laryngeal susceptibility to injury and in many cases reduce the therapeutic response. Dwyer *et al.* noted that general debility, chronic illness, anemia, neutropenia, in addition to dietary deficiencies, predispose to laryngeal trauma at intubation.[23] Today we can add the immunosuppression therapies, cardiothoracic procedures, hypoxemic states, immunocompromised states and a vast variety of chronic illnesses. It is well known that dehydration leads to friability of the endoluminal mucosa of the larynx, diminishes mucous secretion, arrests the movement of the mucociliary blanket, and promotes local contamination by stasis of debris and crusting. Renal malfunction and cardiac disease can lead to persistent airway edema and poor circulation. Drug reactions and angioneurotic edema will lower resistance to infection. For example, intubation in the face of acute epiglottitis (*Haemophilus influenzae*) predisposes to a greater complication rate than in an uninfected larynx. The inflammatory exudate can extend from the base of the tongue to the pre-epiglottic space to involve the deep spaces of the larynx and intrinsic musculature. The presence of chronic infectious diseases (TBC, Lues, diphtheria) may predispose to greater damage following intubation. The same can be said for chronic inflammations such as Wagner's granulomatosis, sarcoid, lupus erythematosus, pemphigoid, polychondritis and epidermolysis bullosa. In many patients with severe head injuries, who require prolonged ventilation support, the use of tracheotomy is more efficient than intubation. The latter will be associated with sepsis and laryngeal trauma to a greater extent than cervical tracheotomy (P<0.008).[51] Studies have shown that diabetes mellitus and hypotensive episodes produce avascular necrosis of the subglottic area in prolonged-intubation patients. Especially true is the higher incidence of cuff injuries following chronic debilitating disease. Prolonged intubation following obstructive laryngoesophageal carcinoma and postradiation edema predisposes to laryngotracheal chondritis. The latter may be associated with sloughing of major portions of the airway system.

Traumatic stenosis

External trauma to the larynx is generally subdivided into blunt trauma and penetrating injuries. Blunt trauma is by far the most common. Nevertheless, the use of firearms and knives in our city streets has increased the incidence of visceral penetrating injuries. A classification for laryngeal stenoses following external trauma is presented in Table 31.2. This essentially takes into consideration the site and extent of the stenosis, but does not consider the severity, depth, or associated injuries (e.g. vocal cord paralysis). Thus supplemental descriptive terms must be used to augment this classification.

The incidence of laryngeal stenosis is estimated to be one case per 14 500–42 500 emergency room visits. Recently there has been a significant decline in injuries associated with motor vehicles and an increase in penetrating injuries (knife wounds or gunshots).[41,75] Older patients have been considered at a higher risk from blunt injury, sustaining comminuted laryngeal skeletal fractures, because of the increased laryngeal cartilage calcification. However, the vast majority of laryngeal traumatic injuries occur in young adults. Although women have been considered more vulnerable to laryngeal injuries, because of their longer and more slender necks, there are relatively few women with laryngeal fractures.

Table 31.2 Surgical classification of acquired laryngeal stenosis

Hypopharynx	Glottic
Anterior	Anterior
Posterior	Posterior
Circumferential	Circumferential
Combined	Combined
	Subglottic
Larynx	High
Supraglottic	Low
Anterior – base epiglottis	Combined
Posterior – A–E folds and interarytenoid	**Tracheal**
Circumferential	Incomplete
Combined	Complete
	Short segment
	Long segment

The larynx, because it is anteriorly located and prominent in the neck, is susceptible to both blunt trauma and penetrating injury. The risk is greater when the neck is hyperextended (car accidents), because the mandible and sternum do not provide protection. Furthermore, the larynx tolerates lateral blunt trauma better than anterior trauma. Laryngeal lateral mobility due to ligamentous and muscle attachments as opposed to anterior–posterior fixation to the trachea and hyoid provides lateral elasticity and recoil against trauma from the sides. Anterior injuries to the larynx compress it against the cervical spine. This causes spreading of the thyroid alae and subsequently fractures the thyroid cartilage in the midline (Fig 31.14). Usually calcified areas fracture first. In younger

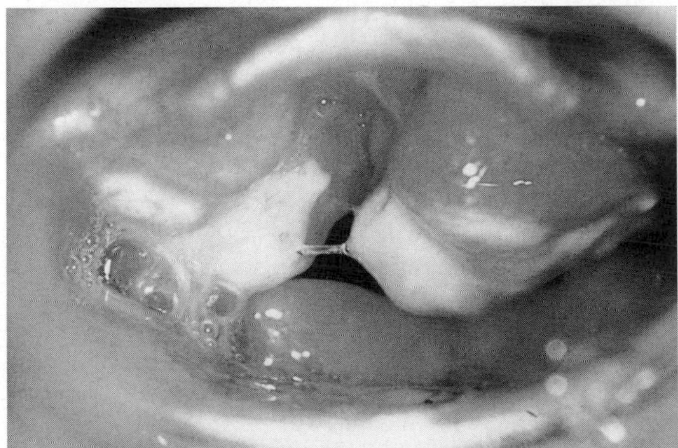

Figure 31.14 *Acute blunt laryngeal trauma resulting in a foreshortened anteroposterior glottic diameter, bilateral vocal cord edema, supraglottic hematomata and a pharyngeal hematoma. The right arytenoid cartilage is dislocated.*

patients the elasticity of the laryngeal cartilage causes a post-traumatic snapback on recoil to produces more characteristic, soft tissue damage rather than fractures, avulsions or separations. These tear the mucosa by stretching and compression, to produce extensive hematomata. Because in children the larynx is more pliable and less protrusive anteriorly, the blunt trauma force is dissipated over a wider area and is greatly absorbed by the neck tissues. This produces more soft tissue injury than skeletal fractures. In older patients, composite lesions of the laryngotracheal skeleton are more common following significant anterior trauma and constitute over 90% of the injuries. Melvin *et al.* showed that compression of laryngeal specimens against a flat surface caused thyroid cartilage damage first, followed by cricoid fractures.[60] In the female larynx, being less prominent and more elastic, simultaneous thyroid and cricoid cartilage fractures were more common. Thus, thyroid fractures or combined fractures with the cricoid are more common than solitary cricoid cartilage fractures. Cricoid fractures are more commonly associated with cricotracheal injuries (85% of the time), leading to dislocation, separation or avulsion. Furthermore, cricotracheal separation is not uncommon in closed injuries from ropes or wires. Slender wire or rope may produce unique injuries in the laryngotracheal complex.[39] These wires and ropes enter the path of least resistance. Below the cricoid they cause laryngotracheal separation. Above the cricoid they enter the cricothyroid membrane, causing cricothyroid separation, dislocation of the arytenoids and recurrent laryngeal nerve palsy. Between the hyoid and thyroid the injury will separate the two structures at the thyrohyoid membrane, causing damage to the superior laryngeal nerves and fracture of the hyoid.[30]

Laryngeal injuries are often associated with other types of trauma. The cervical spine must be evaluated for fractures or dislocations. Manipulation must be avoided, lest the physician produces spinal compression in unstable injuries. Displacement of the larynx can produce laryngotracheal separation, pharyngoesophageal laceration fistulae, and superior and recurrent laryngeal nerve palsies. Other injuries to be expected are to the central nervous system, major blood vessels, nerves in the neck, facial skeletal fractures (most commonly, the mandible) and lung or chest injuries (fractured ribs leading to pneumothorax).

Acute blunt laryngeal injuries are usually classified according to the site of injury and severity of the injury. More commonly the laryngeal stenotic site is not specific (glottic, supraglottic, subglottic) but a combination of injuries (laryngotracheal separation, glottic–subglottic stenosis). Shaefer has subdivided acute trauma into four categories:

- group 1 includes minor trauma, endolaryngeal hematoma and mucosal lacerations;
- group 2 has edema, hematoma, and mucous membrane disruption;
- group 3 has severe edema, mucosal tears, exposed cartilage and cord immobility; and
- group 4 includes avulsed soft tissue and fracture comminution of the laryngeal cartilages.[75]

These can be classified as minor injuries and major injuries. Minor injuries usually do not require surgical treatment or airway intubation. They usually are treated with antibiotics, steroids, humidification, voice rest, dietary and reflux measures, and bed rest. Laryngeal edema and hematoma form quickly after trauma, reaching peak swelling at 3–4 hours. If tracheotomy is not needed after the first post-traumatic day, it can probably be avoided. Most mild injuries involve the soft tissues. Generally edema and hematoma form on the true vocal cords, aryepiglottic folds, false cords and arytenoids. Occasionally there are associated superficial mucosal lacerations, which may be allowed to heal spontaneously. Major injuries cause massive edema and hematoma, as well as large and deep lacerations of the mucosa and underlying muscles. These may expose the underlying cartilage or be associated with comminuted displaced cartilage fragments. In more severe injuries, there is partial laryngeal cartilage framework destruction, vocal cord transection and nerve damage. Finally, the latter injuries may produce combined laryngotracheal damage. Major injuries require airway control (usually tracheotomy) and surgical reconstruction.[75]

The site of stenosis may be supraglottic, glottic, subglottic or a combination of these sites.

Supraglottic stenosis may be anterior, posterior or circumferential. Posterior stenosis is almost always secondary to post-intubation or prolonged-intubation trauma causing interarytenoid scarring (see above). Anterior stenosis is mostly due to anterior blunt trauma where the hyoid is fractured, the thyroid cartilage is flattened and widened (or fractured) to decrease the thyroid prominence, and the base of the epiglottis is avulsed and rotated posteriorly into the lumen of the airway. Generally, there is disruption of the thyrohyoid membrane and thyroepiglottic ligaments. Epiglottic displacement posteriorly is due to avulsion of the epiglottis from the petiole above the anterior commissure area. Thus tears in the false cords, aryepiglottic folds, hypopharyngeal walls and laryngeal ventricles are common. The latter may produce circumferential stenosis with avulsion and dislocation of the arytenoid cartilages. Circumferential stenosis involving the superior hypopharynx and supraglottic area, but sparing the arytenoids, can occur following subtotal supraglottic laryngectomies (Fig 31.15).

Glottic stenosis can be anterior, posterior or circumferential stenosis. Posterior stenosis is almost always related to prolonged intubation. It may be associated with arytenoid cartilage dislocation, vocal cord paralysis, post-intubation granulomas and interarytenoid webs. In the older literature, posterior stenosis was uniquely associated with bronchopulmonary tuberculosis. Characteristically, TBC produced posterior scars of the glottis and epiglottic

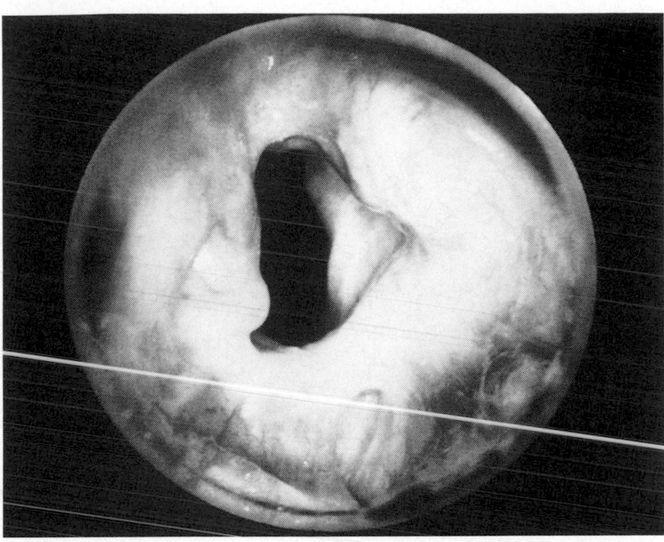

Figure 31.15 *Circumferential supraglottic stenosis following subtotal supraglottic laryngectomy with postoperative radiation (6600 cGy) for squamous cell carcinoma.*

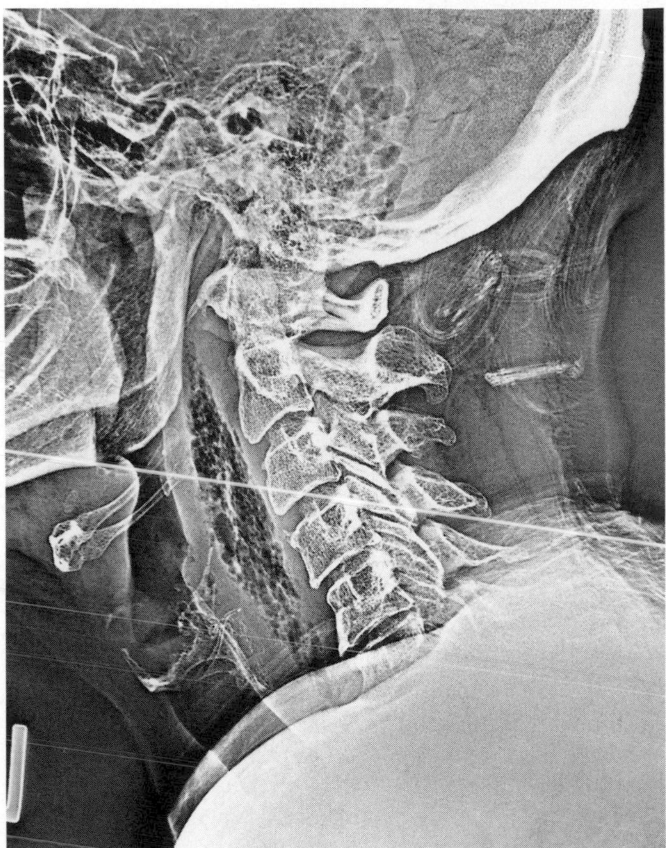

Figure 31.16 *Blunt neck trauma causing laryngeal fracture and pyriform-hypopharyngeal tear. Note the convex shape of the anterior neck, subcutaneous edema and retropharyngeal air. The retropharyngeal space is widened.*

granulomas. Isolated posterior laryngeal fractures are rare. They cause interarytenoid disruptions, lacerations of the thyroarytenoid muscles, dislocation or avulsion of the arytenoid cartilages from the cricoarytenoid joints and compression damage to the recurrent laryngeal nerves. Anterior glottic stenosis is more common following improper or extensive endoscopic surgery of the anterior commissure as well as blunt trauma. Blunt trauma produces midline vertical fractures of the thyroid lamina (cartilage) with lacerations of the anterior vocal cords, false cords, base of the epiglottis and aryepiglottic folds. The larynx becomes foreshortened in the anteroposterior axis, the thyroid protuberance (Adam's apple) collapses, the laryngeal lumen becomes more horizontal and vocal cord mobility is affected. The anterior neck becomes convex with subcutaneous blood or air (Fig 31.16). In the older literature, anterior webs and stenosis were associated with luetic gumma (a major differential diagnostic finding from TBC). Circumferential stenosis is associated with massive laryngeal trauma and comminution of the thyroid cartilages. Occasionally the lateral laryngeal walls fracture with displacement of the thyroid alae into the pyriform sinus or hypopharynx to produce massive lacerations and fistulae. These are usually associated with arytenoid and epiglottic base avulsions and a flattened anteroposterior axis of the larynx. In the older literature, complete glottic stenosis was associated, with or without vocal cord paralysis, with diphtheria. Massive glottic trauma will usually produce cricoid fractures and subglottic stenosis in association with glottic stenosis.

Subglottic stenosis is usually congenital, post-intubation or post-tracheotomy. Isolated subglottic stenosis following blunt trauma is rare. Generally, subglottic stenosis is subdivided into high stenosis, e.g. transglottic injuries, or low stenosis, e.g. laryngotracheal injuries. High stenosis usually results from thyroid cartilage and cricoid cartilage fractures. The anterior cricoid arch is usually fractured in two or more locations near the midline. The cricoid prominence is lost with displacement of fragments posteriorly to occlude the lumen (with edema and hematoma). The cricothyroid membrane is lacerated and the cricotracheal attachment is separated. The posterior cricoid rostrum is rarely fractured but the cricoarytenoid joints may be damaged or avulsed. Most low subglottic injuries involve the laryngotracheal attachment. These are the so-called 'clothesline injuries'. These injuries are due to excessive forces applied anteriorly to a hyperextended exposed neck and hyperinflated airway (breath-holding). Frequently they are associated with one or both recurrent laryngeal nerve transections or avulsions. Occasionally the inferior hypopharynx at a level below the cricopharyngeus muscle or the esophagus is lacerated to produce fistulae. The trachea may retract substernally and the larynx moves upwards. However, the continuity of the visceral fascia connective tissue may maintain an airway for a certain period of time. It is important to make a proper diagnosis and avoid instrumentation so as not to throw the patient into respiratory distress or obstruction. Gentle intubation in the operating room with tracheotomy standby is the procedure of choice in maintaining an airway prior to surgical correction. Another cause of subglottic stenosis is prolonged use of a cricothyrotomy for airway control, which can produce subglottic stenosis and chondritis of the cricoid arch.

Penetrating laryngeal injuries can cause damage to vessels and nerves in the central or lateral cervical visceral compartment. Penetrating injuries of the neck can be divided into high- or low-velocity injuries.[52,86] Most recently the use of high-velocity bullets has predominated. Mostly these injuries are multiple in the head and neck region, resulting in severe impact damage. Large defects of the larynx may be incompatible with life unless an airway is established quickly. Consequently, smaller neck wounds are salvaged routinely. It is the amount of kinetic energy released on impact that determines the degree of damage. Thus, small-caliber, high-velocity bullets produce more damage than slower and heavier bullets. Bullets that travel long distances dissipate their velocity and energy to produce low velocity and more circumscribed damage. The mortality of penetrating neck wounds is between 3 and 6%. In 50% of these, death is due to damage to the cervical spine or carotid vessels. McInnis *et al.* advocated early exploration (100 patients) of the neck.[58] Over 50% of the patients had unsuspected associated injuries. Nevertheless, laryngotracheal injuries do not constitute the most frequent wartime injuries and causes of death.[62] Generally, the algorithm for high-velocity injuries requires immediate airway exploration, followed by the control of bleeding, maintenance of the cardiovascular tone and stabilization of central neurologic damage, prior to the exploration of the neck and reconstitution of the airway.

Post-tracheotomy stenosis

The incidence of tracheotomy procedures have increased. Tracheotomy is used primarily to alleviate airway obstruction, airway toilet for clearance of secretions, with assisted ventilation and for control of the airway in severely debilitated patients. The incidence of low subglottic stenosis has increased due to the combined use of prolonged intubation and tracheotomy. Verougstraebe and Plisnier, considering post-tracheotomy stenosis, divided and classified the lesions as suprastomal, stomal, intermediate and distal stenoses. Montgomery classified the lesions based on location and pathophysiology of the injury. This classification has four subgroups: above tracheotomy site, at the tracheotomy site, below tracheotomy site and distal to the tracheotomy site. In general, more than 90% of post-traumatic laryngotracheal stenoses are due to obstructions caused by intubation or tracheotomy injuries. Furthermore, more than 90% of the stenoses are in the stomal and suprastomal areas. Meyer and Flemming classified stenosis as functional stenosis (laryngo- or tracheomalacia), cicatricial stenosis (partial loss of substance) and postresection or post-traumatic defects

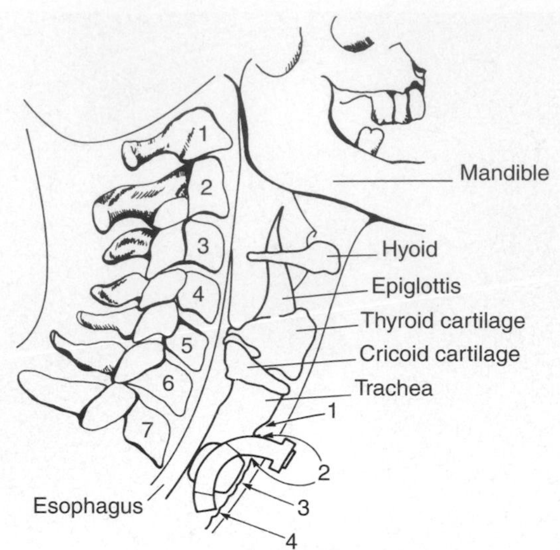

Figure 31.17 *Schematic representation of four types of stenosis that can occur following tracheotomy. These are: 1, suprastomal stenosis; 2, stomal stenosis; 3, cuff stenosis; and 4, cannular tip distal stenosis.*

(total loss of substance). The latter classification is based on two concepts: the length and location of the stenosis and the thickness of the wall or lumen that is lost. Tracheotomy can produce four types of stenosis: suprastomal, stomal, infrastomal (cuff injuries) and distal stenosis (cannular tip stenosis) (Fig 31.17). For the purposes of this chapter, the suprastomal stenosis is of major concern. The other injuries produce stenosis mainly in the trachea. Suprastomal stenosis is caused by hurried improper tracheotomies, large-caliber tracheotomy tube, highly placed tracheal incisions, or significant cartilage damage during the procedure. The first tracheal ring is inserted under the cricoid cartilage and the first tracheal interspace is between the first and second tracheal rings. Thus a high tracheotomy in the first interspace will cause the first or second tracheal cartilage to impinge on the subglottic area (Fig 31.18). Occasionally the tracheal ring will buckle in when a large cannula is inserted to occlude the airway. This cartilaginous fracture (superior stomal lip) will lead to a loss of the anterior wall support during extubation. Care should be taken not to place a sharp tracheal hook on the cricoid or first tracheal ring and to avoid cartilage laceration during upward mobilization of the trachea. The external sharp trauma to the cartilage with fracturing causes the tissues to devascularize and form granulation tissue, granulomas and cartilage necrosis. As the tracheal cuff lies inferior to the tracheotomy site, secretion accumulations and superficial sepsis on top of the cuff (occluding the airway and preventing the action of the mucociliary blanket) will further damage the devitalized and traumatized tracheotomy site. The pathogens are usually *Pseudomonas*, enteric organisms or *Staphylococcus aureus*. In addition, the curved shape of the tracheotomy tube will produce pressure and shearing forces (ventila-

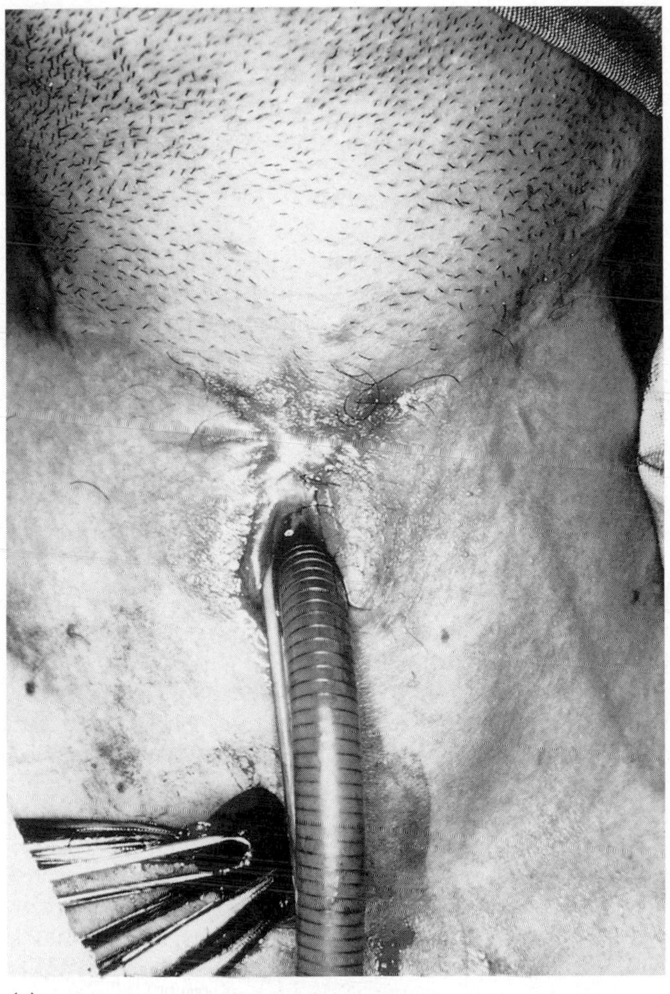

(a)

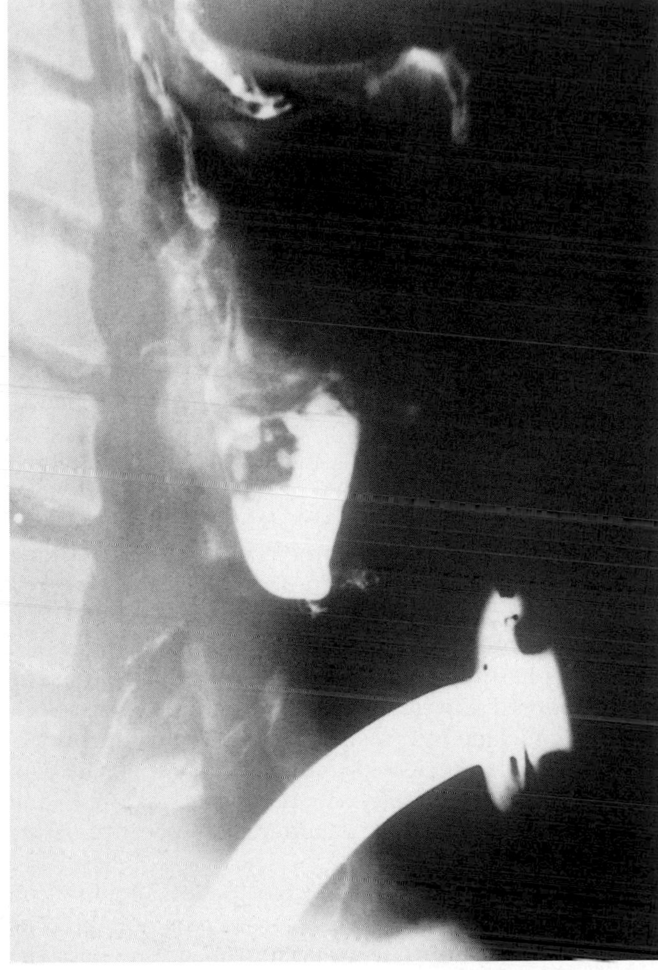

(b)

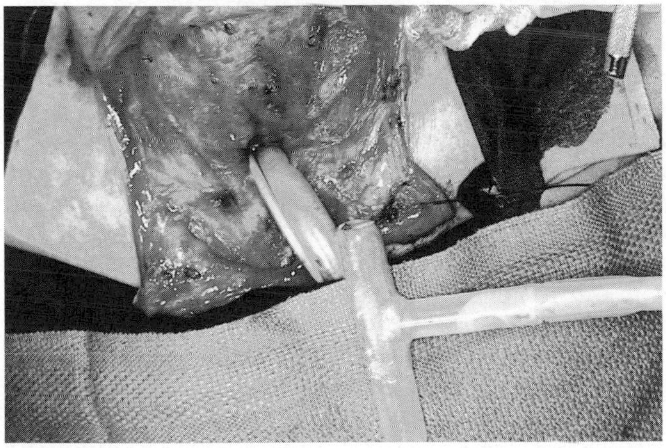

(c)

Figure 31.18 *(a) Combined glottic and subglottic stenosis following a high tracheotomy performed in an emergency room because of penetrating neck and chest wounds due to ballistic injury. (b) An aspirated barium swallow contrast study demonstrates total subglottic stenosis. (c) During a second stage of the reconstruction a mucosally lined upper limb of a Montgomery T-tube is inserted through the lowered tracheotomy site for internal stenting and epithelialization.*

tion) on the anterior cricoid ring and inferior tracheostomy lip (second tracheal ring) in high tracheotomies. Since many patients have systemic disease (hypertension, diabetes mellitus, collagen vascular disease, CNS trauma), wound repair may be hampered. Overinflated cuffs may cause vascular compromise of the luminal surface mucosa and submucosa and increase cricoid ring ischemic necrosis, cartilage slough and soft tissue loss. Tracheotomy is more dangerous in premature infants, causing a 50% complication rate. In full term infants there is a 24% complication rate.[47] Furthermore, repeated insertions and replacement of tracheotomy tubes aggravate the situation and produce subglottic stenosis because of physical trauma and introduced sepsis. Ulceration, granulomas, cartilage collapse, extensive cellulite and edema are signs of infection and tissue damage. These should alert the clinician to the potential for subglottic stenosis. Generally, a higher incidence of stenosis is reported with an H-type incision than with a circumferential incision in the intercartilaginous spaces.

Clinical presentation

The cardinal feature of laryngeal stenosis is dyspnea associated with noisy breathing. Other signs include hoarseness, pain and tenderness, hemoptysis, dysphagia, subcutaneous emphysema, respiratory distress, neck hematoma, flattening of the neck profile and flattening of the laryngeal prominence. Supraglottic stenosis produces inspiratory stridor. Glottic and transglottic stenoses each produce inspiratory and expiratory stridor. Subglottic and tracheal stenoses produce expiratory stridor, wheezing or snorting. Patients manifest slow, deep breathing in order to decrease the work of respiration. In the acute phase, the breathing is rapid and shallow. The voice produced is weak, breathy or absent. Other associated signs include intercostal, epigastric and supraclavicular retractions, increased heart rate and exhaustion. These may lead to asphyxia. The onset, duration and degree of the obstruction determine the severity of the symptoms.

The tidal volume is increased, but the lung volume and forced expiratory volume (FEV_1) remain normal. The patient may demonstrate wheezing or stridor over the larynx on auscultation. Occasionally sonorous rhonchi or low-pitched whistling may occur in the subglottic area due to retention of secretions (more common during inspiration). The expiratory phase of respiration may be prolonged to >4–6 seconds. These findings do not improve with medication (bronchodilators).

The patient will complain of a sensation of breathlessness, which is aggravated by activity. These reflexes are mediated by muscle receptors in the larynx and chest wall. Chemoreceptors of the carotid and aortic bodies monitor CO_2, O_2 and pH via the glossopharyngeal or vagus afferent nerves that travel to the CNS respiratory centers (in the posterior fossa) and then on to higher consciousness centers in the cortex. The maximum breathing capacity is reduced and the respiratory rate is less than 10/min. Most patients will have a persistent cough, which may be short and weak. With secretions in the subglottic area, the cough may be associated with periods of asphyxia. Foreign bodies may be associated with an expiratory tracheal clap as well as a dry and persistent clearing of the throat (a brassy, dry and unproductive cough). Laryngeal tumors may produce a cough with hemoptysis or tissue expectoration (necrotic tumor). Patients may exhibit a fever when associated with pulmonary aspiration or infection (pneumonia). This persistent cough will lead to generalized chest wall and abdominal muscle pain. In chronic disease there may be cyanosis in the skin and nail beds due to reduced oxygenated hemoglobin in the dermal subpapillary venous plexus. The severity and duration of the obstructions determine the symptom complex at presentation. Endoscopic examination may reveal intralaryngeal damage (massive edema, mucosal tears, exposed subluxed cartilage in the lumen, and loss of vocal cord function).

The hypoxemia interferes with cellular metabolic function, especially in the CNS. The carotid and aortic bodies are major chemoreceptors that perceive changes in $Pa{O_2}$. Changes in alveolar O_2 ($PA{O_2}$ 50 mmHg or less), changes in arterial $Pa{O_2}$, and less than 70% hemoglobin saturation are stimulatory. These cause an increase in the respiratory rate and heart rate, a higher systolic blood pressure, an elevated peripheral and pulmonary vascular resistance (peripheral vasoconstriction), elevated adrenal cortical activity, and an elevated CNS respiratory drive.

Sudden obstructions are associated with rapid hypoxemia, unconsciousness, and respiratory or vascular collapse. Death may follow in minutes. In the meantime, dyspnea, hyperpnea, tachycardia, hypertension and neurologic symptoms occur. Neurologic symptoms include headaches, restlessness, mental confusion, disorientation, depression, irritability, muscle weakness, nausea, vomiting and incoordination.

Chronic obstructions may produce similar symptoms of a milder variety that are compensated by the slow progression of the disease. However, a sudden strain on the system (exercise or O_2 therapy) can provoke rapid deterioration. The symptoms may include an elevated blood flow rate, polycythemia, mild hypercapnia and mild acidosis. The elevated CO_2 level is a direct CNS respiratory stimulant that causes an increased respiratory rate, headaches, irritability, confusion, tingling sensations, weakness, lassitude, decreased reflexes, muscle tremors and eventually convulsions, CO_2 narcosis and coma. Coma is caused by a fall in CSF pH (acidosis) due to hydrogen ion accumulation, which is secondary to the respiratory acidosis. In these chronic states the sole respiratory drive is the hypoxemic effect on the peripheral chemoreceptors. Thus O_2 therapy may be detrimental due to physiologic denervation of these organs. The use of O_2 will lead to apnea and CO_2 narcosis. In these states, the CNS is particularly sensitive to narcotics or sedatives. These drugs are prohibited and not included in the therapeutic regimen.

Laryngeal airway obstructions present with various clinical signs. These are divided into laryngeal, neck and soft tissue, and generalized signs. Fixation of the larynx or upward motion during respiration or swallowing denotes paralaryngeal disease. Laryngeal tactile fremitus denotes subglottic or tracheal obstruction. The larynx may be flattened with no landmarks to denote anterior blunt injury. The area of the anterior neck may be covered by a hematoma, ecchymosis or constriction due to rope or wire injury. The laryngeal cartilages may be splayed out laterally and the crepitation on laryngeal side-to-side motion may be absent. There may be subcutaneous emphysema as denoted by tissue crepitation. This indicates a ruptured viscus. Endoscopic examination of the laryngeal lumen may show foreshortening of the anterioposterior diameter, edema, hematomata, laryngeal fractures, arytenoid dislocation and avulsions, and a narrowed airway. Generally, tumors, webs, sepsis, and granulomatous disease are self-evident. Subglottic stenosis may be difficult to differentiate and quantify. The latter needs a radiologic evaluation as well as endoscopy.

The generalized observation denotes a prolongation of the forced vital capacity (>6 seconds), increased functional residual capacity, increased airway resistance and a decreased FEV_1 during the first phase of expiration. Mild symptoms occur with a cross-sectional area reduction of the lumen of 50%. Serious symptoms occur when the laryngeal glottic cross-sectional diameter is reduced to 2 mm or less. The latter produces dyspnea on exertion and stridor. The suprasternal notch is deepened on inspiration. Persistent venous distensions in the neck veins are signs of increased venous pressure secondary to chronic coughing, increased respiratory effort or cor pulmonale. The Valsalva or Mueller maneuver does not produce bulging or retraction in the supraclavicular and suprasternal notches. The neck muscles are tight, denoting secondary muscle fixation to facilitate troubled breathing. The patient's neck is usually extended and accessory muscles of respiration are fixed to facilitate breathing.

Many patients have pre-existing disease such as cardiac, pulmonary and neurologic deficits. The most common causes for laryngotracheal stenosis are due to prolonged intubation following cardiac, pulmonary and neurologic procedures. It is of paramount importance to obtain full information of the presenting conditions prior to attempting the correction of laryngeal stenosis. Cardiac disease (CAD), asthma, chronic obstructive pulmonary disease (COPD), hypertension, diabetes mellitus, atherosclerotic cerebrovascular disease are the usual coexisting problems. Furthermore, the pharmacologic history of the medication taken by the patient should be obtained. A thorough history and physical examination, radiographic studies (see below), pulmonary function test, arterial gases and flow–volume loop studies should be part of all preoperative evaluations. The flow–volume loop study should differentiate between a fixed upper airway obstruction and either a variable intrathoracic or extrathoracic obstruction. A high degree of suspicion is required to rule out COPD and bronchial asthma. Furthermore, patients should refrain from smoking for at least 2 weeks prior to surgical correction.

Radiology and endoscopy

In addition to a complete history, physical examination and laboratory tests, radiologic studies and endoscopy are required for complete stenosis evaluation.

Radiologic tests are required to reveal the location, extent and composition of the stenosis. Once the airway is established, the neck is splinted to protect the cervical spine (if necessary) and a physical examination is completed; the larynx is examined with a mirror or flexible laryngoscope. Although overpenetrated lateral soft tissue neck radiographs and xeroradiograms demonstrate the tracheal air column well, the computerized tomographic (CT) scan is the radiologic procedure of choice.[2,28,81,82,93] The key feature is to delineate the site, composition, type and extent of the stenosis. Particularly important is determination of soft tissue and mucosal cicatricial stenosis from injuries of the cartilaginous framework. In addition, the stenotic length and laryngeal regions involved should be delineated. CT scans in the coronal plane allow for precise delineation of the stenosis, its composition and length. Fluoroscopy may be used to delineate dynamic functional obstructions (laryngomalacia, vocal cord paralysis). Contrast laryngograms are rarely needed. They carry significant risk in the presence of a compromised airway and poor pulmonary toilet. Esophageal contrast studies are employed in suspected aspiration, esophageal or hypopharyngeal tears or fistulae, and with concomitant penetrating injuries.

Endoscopy, with or without a preceding tracheotomy, is reserved for laryngeal assessment prior to definitive therapy.[63] The flexible fiberoptic laryngoscope has facilitated evaluation and decreased the risk of pre- and postoperative manipulation of the traumatic area. The endoscopy is generally under topical or local anesthesia with general anesthesia as standby. As a primary goal, it is important to delineate the superior border of the stenosis as it is related to the cardinal anatomic landmarks such as the vocal cords, arytenoid cartilages, cricoid cartilage, epiglottis, base of tongue and tracheotomy orifice. The inferior border is delineated by the preceding radiologic studies and at exploration or tracheotomy. Endoscopy can also be performed in a retrograde manner via the tracheotomy site to delineate the inferior border of the stenosis. Occasionally, rigid bronchoscopy can be used for emergency treatment in laryngeal trauma (laryngotracheal separation). The bronchoscopy can be insinuated past the obstruction, the distal airway suctioned, and ventilation maintained. Then a careful tracheotomy under sterile conditions is performed over the rigid bronchoscope. A biopsy may also be taken at the same time. Rigid endoscopy usually provides a better view of the obstruction than flexible endoscopic evaluation. Examination with a flexible bronchoscope passed through the endotracheal tube, or tracheotomy site, will allow for the evaluation and suctioning of the lower airway.

Management

For a historical review of treatments for laryngeal stenosis, the reader is referred to references 2, 69, 81 and 82.

General principles of repair in acute stenosis

When examined carefully, the issues involved in laryngeal stenosis are in fact extensive and complex. The severity, extent and composition of the stenosing lesions affect the prognosis and determine the methods of therapeutic intervention. Therefore, prevention of stenosis from improper or prolonged intubation, tracheotomy or neck trauma is of paramount importance. On the other hand, the diagnosis and extent of the injury determination are critical in therapeutic option selection. The clinician must also be patient and be prepared for multiple-stage procedures in order to eventually achieve a desired result. Most laryngeal injuries are mild acute blunt traumas or superficial intubation mucosal injuries that can be managed conservatively. The role of medical versus surgical management is based in many instances on the clinician's experience. In general, acute traumatic stenoses are divided into four categories based on the severity of the laryngeal defect. These are mild injuries that can be treated medically, moderate injuries that require a tracheotomy and repair, severe injuries that require a tracheotomy and exploration, and compound injuries that require tracheotomy, open exploration and stenting.

Mild stenosis – medical management

Mild stenoses commonly involve the soft tissues only and develop from blunt neck trauma or traumatic intubations. They manifest as edema, hematomata, ecchymosis or superficial lacerations of the mucosa. These injuries are aggravated by prolonged nasogastric tube intubation, prolonged airway intubation, acid gastric reflux or postradiation laryngeal mucositis. Occasionally undisplaced, non-comminuted uncomplicated laryngeal fractures can be observed without surgical intervention. However, care must be taken to rule out major cartilaginous injuries or associated problems of sepsis (chondritis) by a computed tomographic study.

These mild stenoses are managed conservatively by observation, vital sign monitoring and medications. Depending upon the findings within the endolaryngeal lumen on fiberoptic flexible laryngoscopy, it may be necessary to support the patient and place the larynx at rest. The medical treatment should include bedrest with the head elevated (to avoid reflux or aspiration), voice rest, humidification (mask) of the breathed air, brief antibiotic prophylaxis, and careful dietary management (avoid coughing). There should be a minimum of 24 hours of close observation. The use of corticosteroids (prednisone) is a debatable issue. Steroids have been recommended to reduce endolaryngeal edema. However, there have been no prospective randomized studies to document their benefit. Nevertheless, when steroids are used they should be started immediately after the traumatic event (within hours) to be considered beneficial. Antacids are used to reduce reflux gastric acidity. For the same reason racemic epinephrine nebulizers are used to cause vasoconstriction, reduce edema and decrease bleeding within the laryngeal mucosa. Studies have shown that edema and hematoma form quickly in the larynx and reach their peak swelling within 3–4 hours after the trauma. Thus, to be effective, medication must be given as soon as possible. On the other hand, if a patient is without respiratory distress after 24 hours of observation, the likelihood of airway compromise and the need for a tracheotomy are significantly reduced in the immediate post-traumatic period.

Moderate soft tissue stenosis – tracheotomy

Intermediate soft tissue stenoses generally require control of the airway and medical management. Some injuries occlude the airway by massive hematoma, edema or soft tissue mucosal lacerations but do not disrupt the cartilaginous framework or neuromuscular function of the larynx. Such stenoses are generally due to blunt neck trauma, undisplaced fractures or prolonged intubations. Exploration of the larynx or endoluminal intubation in such cases is unnecessary and may promote further injury. Therefore, a tracheotomy to control the airway and place the larynx at rest is used in conjunction with the aforementioned medications as the treatment of choice. Once the edema and hematoma have subsided, the soft tissue injury can be assessed further and appropriate measures instituted. The main issues raised in these types of injuries are the need for early repair and stenting. A stent should be used as an internal fixation device to prevent luminal scarring and stenosis and to maintain endolaryngeal configuration. As a general rule, disruption of the anterior commissure (true and false cords), or massive soft tissue loss in the lumen in acute injuries require stenting. The more mucosa that is saved, approximated and carefully closed to prevent submucosa, muscle or cartilage exposure the less the need for stenting. The use of stenting in chronic stenosis or staged resections of cicatrization causing luminal cross-sectional loss is discussed below. However, prolonged stenting in acute injuries should be avoided whenever possible. Stenting produces its own set of problems with tissue erosion, sepsis and progressive cicatrization.

There is controversy surrounding the indications for surgery, timing of the surgery and the type of procedure to perform. The indications for surgery range from establishing an airway to open repair of laryngeal skeletal injuries. The tracheotomy should be done under local anesthesia. Once the airway is established, radiographic studies (CT or MRI) are performed to establish the severity, composition and location of the injury. Then rigid endoscopy is performed to delineate the cephalic border of the injury site and assess the resultant endolaryngeal function (arytenoid dislocation, recurrent nerve paralysis, etc.). In selected patients with edema, hematoma, minor mucosal lacerations, without cartilage exposure or dislocation, and without damage to vital areas (anterior commissure, interarytenoid space, arytenoid dislocation), no further therapy is necessary. Single undisplaced paramedian thyroid laminar fractures are not repaired. On the other hand, comminuted fractures, inner perichondrial exposure, cartilage dislocations, massive soft tissue loss or lacerations, functional deficits and vital anatomic area damage require repair.

Severe stenosis – exploration

Severe laryngeal stenoses, requiring tracheotomy under local anesthesia and explorative repair, are subdivided into two groups of reconstructions, e.g. open repairs and open repairs with stenting. Surgical exploration is recommended within 24 hours of injury.[76] Early adequate evaluation and treatment of endolaryngeal injuries are essential to preserve the phonatory or sphincteric laryngeal functions and the avoidance of stenosis. The main goals for surgery are to restore normal laryngeal skeletal stability, provide an epithelial-lined internal covering and restore neuromuscular and sensory function. As a general rule, open explorations are required when: the airway obstruction requires tracheotomy, there is progressive subcutaneous emphysema, there is fracture and dislocation of the cartilaginous framework, there are massive endolaryngeal lacerations, and there are extensive mucosal disruptions or tissue loss.[53] Traditionally, the larynx is opened through a median vertical thyrotomy incision. The exploration is similar for both blunt and penetrating injuries. However, large penetrating anterior cervical skin lacerations that are communicating with open laryngeal fractures may serve as a means by which to explore, expose and repair deeper structures in the neck and larynx.

Large mucosal lacerations, exposed cartilage, displaced (but not comminuted) large thyroid laminal fractures, false vocal fold lacerations, minor anterior commissure lacerations, and free vocal cord margin lacerations can all be repaired without stenting. Other traumatic lesions that can be repaired without stenting include single anterior or angulated thyroid laminar fractures, single paramedian displaced laminar fractures, multiple undisplaced thyroid or cricoid fractures and disruptions of the cricoarytenoid points. In general, when a fracture can be stabilized, the mucosal or epithelial covering can be repaired, and the lining is adequate to cover all the exposed denuded surfaces, then stenting is not required. Non-stenting repairs require meticulous closure of all the mucosal lacerations with 6-0 absorbable sutures with the knots inverted and cartilage fragments stabilized with 5-0 braided stainless steel wires or miniplates. Meticulous perichondrial closure is achieved with 4-0 proline (Dexon) sutures. The anterior vocal folds are stabilized and lengthened with 4-0 submucosal chromic gut sutures to the outer perichondrium or Broyles' ligament. Such anterior commissure repairs are possible if there is adequate mucosal coverage, otherwise an anterior Silastic keel is required in order to avoid anterior web formation.[70]

Severe combined stenosis – stenting

Stenting is required where there is disruption of the anterior commissure or unstable comminuted laryngeal skeletal fractures with dislocation and massive soft tissue loss (Fig 31.19). Stents can also be used to stabilize skin and mucosal free grafts in denuded areas of the larynx and to prevent web formation across the denuded adjacent raw surfaces. Disruption of the anterior commissure requires a stent to preserve the scaphoid shape of this site. Loss of the anterior one-third of the thyroid lamina (usually associated with base of the epiglottis dislocation and false vocal fold lacerations) requires stenting to maintain the anteroposterior vocal fold length and preserve the anteroposterior glottic diameter which is essential for good voice production. The most common use for stenting is in comminuted unstable skeletal fractures that are associated with massive mucosal wounds and soft tissue loss. Stenting prevents endolaryngeal adhesions or webs and stabilized the endolaryngeal skeleton.

A variety of stents are available. Generally, stenting is a compromise between achieving stability of the cartilaginous skeleton and mucosal coverage and the inherent endolaryngeal injuries and infections promoted by the foreign body in the laryngeal lumen.[87] The properties of the stent should include the following seven parameters:

- The stent should be soft and tolerable to avoid further mucosal injury;
- The stent should be long enough to reach from the supraglottis to the undersurface of the first tracheal ring;
- The stent should be stabilized in the laryngeal lumen to avoid motion or shearing forces;
- The stent should reconfigure the endolaryngeal lumen;
- The stent should be made from nonirritating, nontoxic and inert materials;
- The stent should be left in place a minimum amount of time (usually 10–14 days); and
- The stent should serve as a carrier for skin, mucosa or other grafts.

Ideally, the stent should be rigid enough to maintain the internal support of the airway, yet flexible enough not to damage the mucosal or soft tissue repairs. The stent should move with the larynx during respiration or swallowing. It should be easy to place and remove. Generally, anterior commissure injuries may require only a Teflon keel.[65] The latter should be long enough to prevent anterior web formation, but avoid interarytenoid ulceration or trauma. Keels tend to produce less trauma since they produce fewer contact points with laryngeal mucosa.[59,64] Transglottic or subglottic injuries are usually stented with Montgomery silicone fitted stents, finger cots, configured Portex endotracheal modified tubes or other stents. Subglottic and tracheal injuries are corrected with T-tube prostheses, which incorporate a tracheotomy site into the stented area. Generally, we prefer the use of a low tracheotomy and a separate stent above it, rather than a combined T-tube (Fig 31.20). However, the former is not always possible.

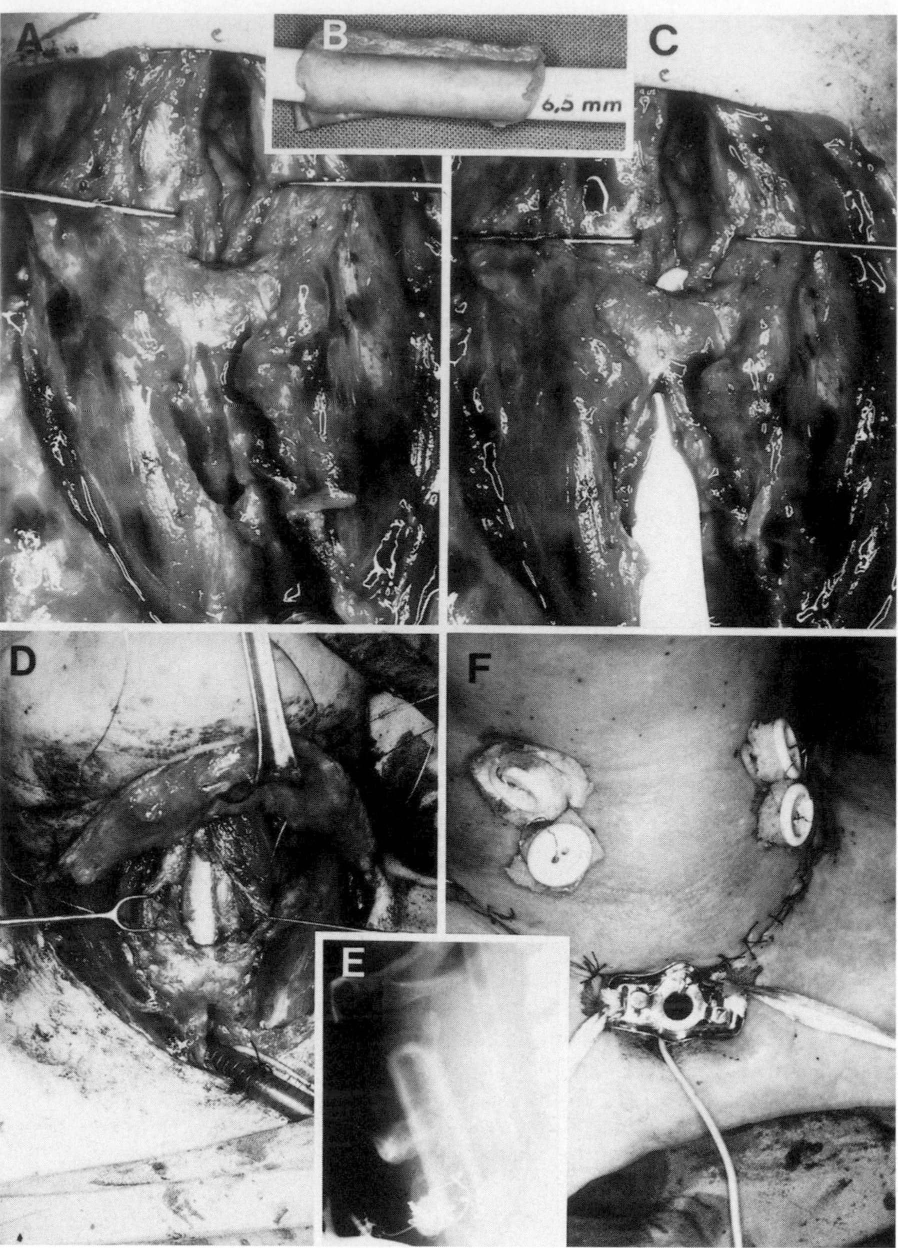

Figure 31.19 *Combined laryngotracheal stenosis with an intact cricoid arch following anterior blunt neck injury. (a) Exploration of the stenosis through a midline thyrotomy incision and tracheotomy. (b) A skin-lined 6.5 mm endotracheal tube stent. (c) Placement of stent under the cricoid into the glottic, subglottic and upper tracheal area. (d) Stent in place prior to wound closure. (e) Confirmation of stent location by a lateral soft tissue radiograph. (f) Wound closed and stent held in place with two stenting wire sutures.*

Unlike blunt trauma that tends to produce more extensive soft tissue injuries and inapparent collateral trauma, penetrating laryngeal injuries tend to be more demarcated. Stab wounds are well defined whereas gunshot injuries are associated with more massive damage and other associated injuries (esophageal tears, spinal cord damage, pneumothorax, tracheal lacerations, recurrent laryngeal nerve injuries, pharyngeal lacerations, thyroid trauma and great vessel damage). Many of these associated complications can lead to death. Great vessel lacerations and tracheoesophageal damage, especially, should be repaired as soon as possible. With respect to the aerodigestive system, a preliminary tracheotomy is required. The trachea is repaired with extraluminal minimal tension sutures. This may require tracheal mobilization from the adjacent soft tissue and laryngeal release. The cervical esophageal repair should be a two-layer closure in the transverse plane. The use of muscle [sternocleidomastoid (SCM), strap muscles, etc.] cervical fascia to be inserted between the trachea and esophagus, or other pedicle flaps to buttress the repair may be required. Adequate drainage (anteriorly so as not to cross the major vessels) or controlled end-to-side esophagostomy may be needed to avoid complications (tracheo-esophageal fistulae, mediastinitis, wound infections with slough, carotid artery rupture). In extremely rare occasions with massive life-threatening injuries, a laryngectomy and esophageal repair may be required in order to control the bleeding, the airway and fistulous infection.

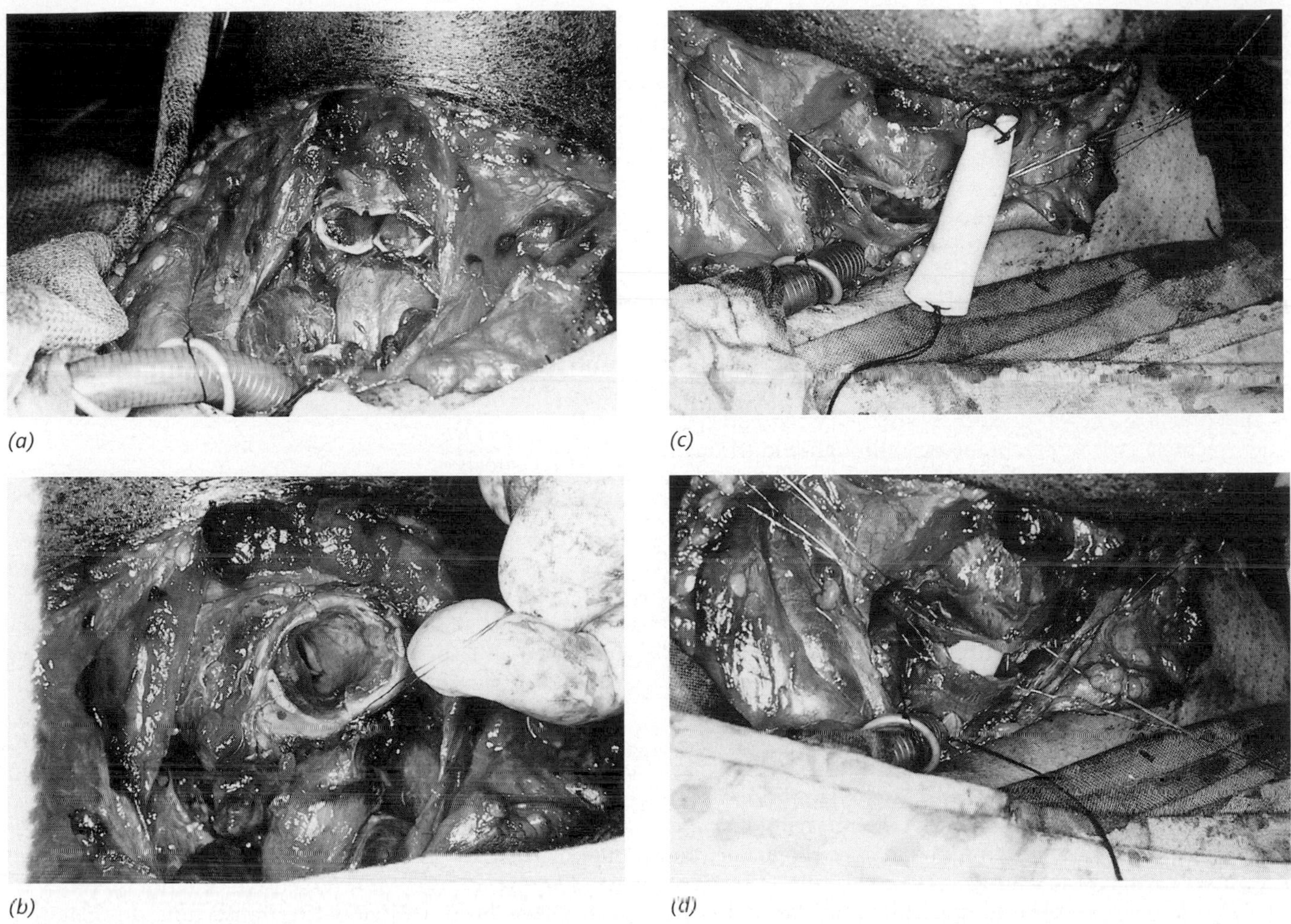

Figure 31.20 *Laryngotracheal separation with crush injury of the subglottis and upper trachea. (a) Note the crush injury of the subglottis and upper trachea. The mediastinally retracted lower trachea is intubated. (b) The upper tracheal crush injury is reconstructed with extraluminal 4-0 braided wire sutures. Note that the esophagus is intact and the right recurrent laryngeal nerve is not severed. The left recurrent laryngeal nerve was crushed during the injury. (c) The tracheotomy site has been lowered and 27 gauge stainless steel extraluminal sutures are placed laterally and anteriorly to reconstruct the airway. Posteriorly, Vicryl 2-0 sutures are used extraluminally. A silicone stent with the luminal ends closed is pre-measured and aligned to reconstitute the lumen. (d) Stent in place and the airway is reconstituted. Note that if there was no crush injury a stent would not be required. Since there was adequate mucosal coverage no grafting was necessary.*

Specific laryngeal repairs – chronic stenosis

The initial evaluation should include a detailed history, physical examination, indirect and flexible direct laryngoscopy. The latter should evaluate the status of the airway, vocal cord mobility and location of the stenotic segment. Pulmonary function tests combined with volume–flow loop studies provide valuable data in determining the functional airway. Videolaryngoscopy and simultaneous tape recordings of the voice will establish the degree of vocal abnormality and can be used for comparison with postoperative results. Computed tomographic scans in the high resolution mode (2 mm cuts) and occasionally magnetic resonance films of the larynx and cervical trachea will delineate the location, site and composition of the stenosis. Then, following a tracheotomy (if necessary), direct microscopic laryngoscopy (with or without lasers) is performed to confirm the location, composition and severity of the stenosis. Laser excision of granulation tissue (CO_2 or KTP), granulomas or foreign debris prior to institution of definitive therapy is mandatory since it will allow a more accurate repair.[22] It is best to wait until all granulation tissue is replaced by scar or epithelium prior to institution of definitive open procedures. Generally, about 25% of the circumference or half (one side) of the larynx is treated with laser removal of granulation tissue at one sitting. It is best to stage the procedures. Previously placed stents and keels are removed in order to evaluate the airway and reduce the sepsis.

Supraglottic stenosis

Supraglottic stenoses can be anterior, posterior or circumferential. *Anterior stenosis* is most commonly due to blunt anterior cervical trauma, which causes subluxation into the lumen of the base (petiole) of the epiglottis. This is associated with false cord laceration, anterior commissure injury and anterior vocal cord lacerations. These injuries may be associated with glottic injuries and a foreshortened anteroposterior glottic chink. Webs in this area can be resected endoscopically with a laser. The base of the epiglottis can be resected or sutured forward through the thyroid ala and fixed to the outer perichondrium near the thyroid notch with Dexon or Vicryl sutures (2-0). If there is mucosal loss, a Teflon keel is inserted endoscopically and secured with percutaneous through-and-through sutures. When there is extensive soft tissue or mucosal loss, an open midline thyrotomy or midline pharyngotomy may be necessary to reattach or resect the base of the epiglottis, repair the false cord tissue deficits, reconstruct the anterior commissure and lengthen the anteroposterior glottic lumen. Generally, a Teflon keel or stent is inserted. Stents are used to reconstruct the lumen and, more importantly, as mucosal or skin graft carriers. Early removal of the stent or keel (14 days) is advocated.

Posterior supraglottic scars, webs or stenoses are most often seen following prolonged intubations. The scar may span the corniculate cartilages or muscular processes of the arytenoids and obliterate the interarytenoid space. They may also cause limitation of movement of the arytenoid cartilages (pseudovocal cord paralysis) because of scarring. The posterior glottic chink will be narrowed and arytenoid abduction will be limited. Occasionally, the stenosis may extend to the aryepiglottic folds to further narrow the supraglottic lumen. Thin webs and scars can be released endoscopically with a CO_2 laser to the depth of the interarytenoideus muscle and absorbable 4-0 sutures can be placed endoscopically on the mucosal edges to resurface this area with epithelium. If the scar is deeper and involves the interarytenoideus muscle and cricoid rostrum, an open procedure is advocated. Following a midline thyrotomy, the posterior glottic interarytenoid mucosa is elevated. The scar and occasionally the fibrotic muscle are resected then the area is resurfaced with mucosa. The latter is a V-Y advancement repair (similar to pulling down a window shade) where the mucosa from the postcricoid region or aryepiglottic folds is advanced as a sliding flap to cover the denuded raw surfaces. Suturing is done with 4-0 to 6-0 mild chromic gut sutures or Dexon with the knots inverted extraluminally. Stenting is generally not required unless there is a need for skin or mucosal grafting to the posterior supraglottis.

Circumferential supraglottic stenosis most often is associated with conservation laryngeal surgical procedures (partial laryngopharyngectomy and subtotal supraglottic laryngectomy), caustic ingestions (lye), or massive trauma. The main issue is loss of soft tissue substance followed by cicatricial scarring. Following conservation surgery, the resection may be redone with removal of the scar, elevation of the larynx and direct resuturing to the base of the tongue. The other stenoses may be treated by partial laser-staged excisions with secondary epithelialization, supraglottic laryngectomy or reconstruction with vascularized flaps (radial forearm free flap; latissimus dorsi, pectoralis major, or platysmal myocutaneous flaps). Care must be taken to preserve the superior laryngeal neurovascular bundles. A cricopharyngeal myotomy is performed as an adjunct procedure to facilitate swallowing. The use of a vascularized flap facilitates healing, reduces the complications significantly and corrects the problem in a single-stage procedure.

Glottic stenosis

Glottic stenosis may be anterior, posterior or complete. A subset of glottic stenoses includes vocal cord deformities, unilateral or bilateral vocal cord paralyses, dislocated arytenoids and post-traumatic granulomas. *Anterior* glottic stenosis most often is due to congenital webs or malformations, anterior blunt neck injuries or aggressive endoscopic surgical resections. The anterior commissure is usually involved with cicatricial webs of varying degrees of thicknesses. Small webs, which are less than 3 mm in width and do not produce airway or voice problems, can be left undisturbed. These usually are secondary to congenital malformations, endoscopic anterior commissure manipulations or conservation surgery (frontolateral hemilaryngectomy). More extensive anterior stenoses or webs have been treated with transection. In children, dilatation with a rigid bronchoscope will occasionally lyse the anterior thin web. In adults, webs between the anterior and middle of the vocal cords have been corrected by microlaryngeal lysis of the adhesions with laser or microscissors. If adequate mucosa is present, it can be elevated and returned to cover the denuded lysed area. We have used a drop of fibrin glue or serum to make the mucosa adhere to the free edges of the vocal cords. More extensive and thicker webs will require an endoscopically placed Teflon keel to prevent anterior web formation. The keel must not impinge on the posterior commissure epithelium, in order to avoid posterior glottic scarring. The keel is removed after 2–3 weeks. Anterior comminuted fractures of the glottis foreshorten the anteroposterior diameter of the glottic airway, lacerate the vocal cords, disrupt Broyles' ligament and are often associated with anterior cartilaginous fractures with or without dislocation. Occasionally, the petiole of the epiglottis is sheared and displaced posteriorly. More rarely, the anterior arch of the cricoid cartilage is fractured. In such cases, following mucosal repair, lengthening of the anterior vocal cords and increasing the anteroposterior glottic length requires the use of an indwelling laryngeal stent. Generally, there is a deficit of soft tissue and mucosa. Thus anterior commissure grafting may be required. Furthermore, if the fractures are comminuted and cartilage is missing, a bone or cartilage graft interposition may be needed to stabilize the external cartilaginous framework. Most routinely we use a hyoid interposition bone graft which is attached to the infrahyoid strap muscles. The graft is placed on a cervical fascial graft, which overlies the stent. The fascia is readily obtained from the sternomastoid muscles. Other interpositional grafts used were nasal septal cartilage, rib cartilage, clavicle, iliac crest, auricular cartilage (in children), and manubrial periosteal–osseous grafts.[1,9,13,32,35,55,66,88] The skeletal grafts are fixed with extraluminal 4-0 braided wire or miniplates. In more severe traumas, an epiglottic pull-down procedure can resurface the anterior larynx. In the latter case, the anteroposterior diameter is foreshortened and the lateral glottic airway is widened, producing a poor quality voice. The epiglottis and its endoluminal mucosal covering can resurface the glottis, subglottis and upper first tracheal ring area in a single-stage procedure. It is more commonly used following oncologic frontolateral or anterior commissure resections. Care must be taken to preserve the lateral superior neurovascular sensory bundles when freeing the epiglottis from the surrounding tissues.

Posterior glottic stenosis most commonly occurs following prolonged endotracheal intubations. In the past the most common causes were tuberculosis and diphtheria. Care must be taken to diagnose cricoarytenoid joint function and vocal cord mobility. Scarring may cause a picture of pseudoparalysis where in fact the vocal cords and cricoarytenoid joints are functional. Both trauma and recurrent nerve paralysis are required to produce joint arthrodesis in dogs.[61] The laryngeal cicatrization is at the level of the vocal processes of the arytenoid. Often there is a dimple or sinus tract posterior to the web, which denotes the true level of the posterior glottic chink. The severity of the stenosis is directly related to the severity of the trauma. Stenosis may involve the mucosa and submucosa, and interarytenoid muscle. When extremely severe there is necrosis of the cricoid cartilage rostrum with loss of the cephalic cartilaginous support. The latter may manifest as a deeper interarytenoid notching. Superficial scarring can be corrected with microlaryngeal laser web excision. Care is taken to protect the perichondrium on the vocal processes of the arytenoid and the subglottis. The posterior dimple or sinus tract can be used as a landmark to denote the true level of the posterior glottic aperture. After opening the scar, the cricoarytenoid joints are palpated for mobility. The anesthesia and paralysis are lightened to denote vocal cord mobility. This technique can be repeated if webs reform. These procedures are successful because the frequent arytenoid motion during phonation and deglutition tend to limit restenosis. In more severe stenosis involving loss of mucosa, interarytenoid muscle fibrosis and cricoid or arytenoid cartilage necrosis, an open midline thyrotomy procedure is required. The posterior defect may need mucosal flap advancement with a V-Y window-shade technique or stenting with mucosal or skin grafts to resurface the inadequate epithelial coverage. A posterior cricoid cartilage rostrum graft interposition may be required with cartilage loss.[73]

Complete glottic stenosis is rare and most often seen following severe trauma, diphtheria and caustic ingestions. Generally, there is a dimple or a sinus tract to delineate the approximate location of the lumen. These techniques require tracheotomy under local anesthesia, an open exploratory midline thyrotomy and mucosal coverage. There is extensive soft tissue or mucosal loss. Usually the subglottis is also affected. These repairs almost always require stenting and mucosal grafts. Some prefer the use of split-thickness skin or dermis whilst others use advancement mucosal flaps from the pyriform sinus and aryepiglottic folds or free buccal mucosal grafts. Some graft the entire area whereas others graft one side of the larynx and allow the contralateral side to reepithelialize on its own. In extremely severe cases with thick stenosis, but functional arytenoids, some authors have advocated hemilaryngectomy procedures or other conservation surgical resections. Nevertheless, it is better to reconstitute the airway without resection as the initial therapeutic option. In complete stenosis with laryngeal framework cartilage loss, cartilage interposition anteriorly and posteriorly is possible.[73] The free cartilaginous grafts are fixed with miniplates and covered with mucosa.[73]

Subglottic stenosis

The composition of the subglottic stenotic segment can be *soft* (soft tissues scarring) or *hard* (soft tissue and cartilaginous skeletal damage). The location can be *high* (involving the glottis) or *low* (involving the first tracheal ring). In traumatic lesions, subglottic stenosis is generally associated with glottic or anterior commissure injuries. The most common causes for subglottic stenosis are congenital, traumatic (surgical or external blunt trauma) or post-intubation. Subglottic stenosis is a frequent problem with long-term cricothyrotomy procedures and cannulation. Studies have shown that subglottic stenosis is associated with stenting and tracheotomy because of a higher incidence of local bacterial contamination.

The multiple treatment methods for acquired subglottic stenosis indicate the lack of a single reliable operative approach. The goal of the reconstruction is to provide a stable airway and normal voice. In order to achieve this, it is necessary to provide a sturdy external supportive cartilaginous framework, to preserve the neurovascular structures and provide an epithelial covering for the lumen. Depending on the severity of the stenosis, the treatments have ranged in a progressive scale of severity from observation with or without dilatation, partial endoscopic laser resections with dilatation or stenting, cricoid-splitting techniques to laryngotracheal resections and reanastomosis.

Soft tissue subglottic stenosis has been treated with repeated dilatations and scar excisions. Thin narrow stenosis can be dilated repeatedly (six times or more) to eventually achieve a competent lumen. Thicker stenoses are partially resected with lasers under microscopic control in a multistage procedure. These may be augmented by stenting and grafting of the subglottic area. McGee *et al.* studied the CO_2 laser for treatment of subglottic stenosis in dogs without the use of stents, antibiotics or steroids.[56] At 3 weeks there was tissue edema and a patent airway. Later, granulation tissue and collagen deposition restenosed the subglottis. The use of stents and epithelial coverage with a suitable graft was advocated. Healy *et al.*, using a similar canine model, noted that in severe 80% stenosis the use of stents, antibiotics and steroids correlated with a greater success following excisions with the carbon dioxide laser.[43] Soft stents were more successful than hard stents. Some have stated that the use of systemic steroids could be detrimental. Toohill *et al.*, in a series of canine experiments, noted that both segmental scar resections and total scar resections produced restenosis.[88] However, total scar resection produced more granulation and scar that later developed progression of the stenosis. Thus segmental resection by itself was not beneficial, but total scar resection was actually harmful. Strong *et al.* used partial resection with stenting to correct subglottic stenosis with success in 15 of 20 patients.[85] However, Kaufman *et al.* noted rapid granulation tissue formation and rapid restenosis followed the use of stents.[48] Many authors have advocated the use of systemic or intralesional steroid injections to avoid granulation tissue formation. The latter may be augmented by serial dilatations. Holinger reported success with repeated sequential resections of scar and avoidance of tracheotomy.[44] Dedo and Sooy developed the micro-trapdoor mucosal flap.[19] The preservation of the overlying mucosa and resection of the underlying scar tissue enabled them to decannulate 17 of 19 patients. The success was related to the preservation of the mucosal covering in the subglottic area. Simpson *et al.* reported on 60 patients and noted that endoscopic partial techniques were most successful.[79] They noted that the predisposing causes of failure were associated with preceding infection, tracheotomy, circumferential scarring, scar tissue width greater than 1 cm in vertical dimension and combined glottic fibrosis (especially the posterior glottic chink and interarytenoid area). Today we employ a combination of these techniques. We prefer to have the scar matured without granulation tissue. Whenever possible we try to avoid tracheotomy. Anesthesia under Venturi jet flow ventilation or endotracheal intubation is used. Segmental scar excision is performed with a CO_2 laser under microlaryngoscopy. Mucosal flaps are created and preserved. These procedures are repeated until an adequate lumen is established. In combined glottic–subglottic stenosis we use an open exploration technique via midline thyrotomy with or without mucosal grafting and short-term stenting (2 weeks).

For severe *combined stenosis* (hard stenosis) the reconstructive techniques used with soft stenosis are combined with two extralaryngeal skeletal methods, e.g. interpositional grafts for cricoid expansion or cricotracheal resections with anastomosis. There are a variety of techniques available, which attests to the fact that no procedure is fully reliable. Furthermore, a second procedure may be necessary in approximately 50% of the most severe stenoses. Generally, prosthetic devices have met with little success. We have abandoned their use in subglottic expansion techniques. All patients in this group of severe stenosis require a preliminary tracheotomy for airway control. The tracheotomy should be sufficiently low in the neck in order to bypass the area of obstruction (fourth or fifth tracheal ring if possible in children and third or fourth tracheal ring in adults). The subglottic repair requires an open exploratory procedure via a transverse incision in the larynx, including the thyrohyoid and cricothyroid membranes, thyroid lamina and cricoid cartilage. In selective cases only the cricoid cartilage and cricothyroid membrane need to be opened, whilst the thyroid lamina may be left intact. The scar tissue is identified and removed, but the mucosa is left intact. Stenosis following external trauma may be confined to the cricoid arch area but may be circumferential within the lumen. After intubation, subglottic scarring is likely to be submucosal and predominantly posterior (or circumferential). In most instances the resultant mucosal and soft tissue defect, after scar removal, is significant with bare areas of cartilage exposure. These areas should be covered by autologous tissue. Most commonly very thin (18×10^{-3} inch) hairless skin grafts, buccal mucosa, dermal grafts, nasal septal mucosa, sinus mucosa, or vaginal mucosal grafts have proved to be successful. These are sutured around suitable soft or molded stents, which are placed endoluminally and secured with through-and-through sutures to the soft tissue of the neck or overlying skin. In low-lying stenosis, a Montgomery silicone T-tube is most useful. Other stents include Teflon (Conley, Knight), Portex (polyvinyl chloride), molded endotracheal tubes, silicone (Montgomery) and acrylic stents. The closure of the external laryngeal skeleton will generally require materials that will maintain structural integrity and expand the luminal cross-sectional area.

It is best to use materials that can be incorporated into the reconstruction. For these reasons, synthetic prostheses or preserved autographs and homografts have not been successful. It is important to avoid graft rejection and poor incorporation of the grafted material into the host tissues. These will lead to leakage, infection and proliferative granulation tissue formation. Chondritis with restenosis, scar contraction, visceral erosion and great vessel rupture with subsequent life-threatening hemorrhage are some of the major complications. Autologous cartilage and bone grafts have better success and are widely used today. Looper, in 1938, first proposed the use of hyoid interpositional grafts that were sandwiched between fascia and interposed between anterior cricoid ring deficits.[55] Finnegan *et al.* used the hyoid attached to the strap muscles as a pedicled vascular composite graft.[32] We use the latter method frequently. Lofgren *et al.* used composite mucosal and cortical bone grafts in a multistage procedure in dogs.[54] Others have used full cartilage grafts from the auricle, nasal septum, rib (costal cartilage), and composite bone grafts from the sternum (with periosteum), iliac crest, split calvarium and myoperiosteal grafts. It has been known that vascularized periosteum can lead to osteoneogenesis. The degree of osteogenesis varies with the site of transplantation, e.g. more bone is formed within a muscle or bone bed than in subcutaneous tissue. Fonkalsrud and Plested use periosteal reconstruction of the tracheobronchial tree in dogs.[34] They noted that delayed vascularized grafts were more successful. Tovi and Gittot used sternomastoid clavicular periosteal reconstructions and demonstrated adequate tissue rigidity and osteoneogenesis in laryngeal and tracheal defects.[89] Blair used intercostal pedicled grafts in the tracheobronchial tree.[6] Friedman *et al.* used sternomastoid muscle and manubrial periosteal flaps in canines and man.[35] They noted rapid healing, vascularization, rapid epithelialization, minimal granulation tissue formation, and facile utility due to its conformation to the defect site. The use of composite grafts has been beneficial and useful for more than 70 years.

There have been numerous additions to the laryngotracheoplastic procedures in order to expand the external cartilaginous framework. Rethi and later Grahne divided the posterior lamina of the cricoid in pediatric patients, excised necrotic cartilage, and grafted and stented for 4 months.[38,73] Crysdale and Platt (after Rethi) performed both anterior and posterior divisions of the cricoid cartilage with cartilage interpositions. These techniques have been shown to have favorable long-term results and firmly established the concept of cricoid framework expansion by anterior and posterior division of the cartilage with long-term stenting.[18] Evans and Todd developed a stairstep division of the anterior cricoid and trachea for framework expansion.[27] Cotton interposed costal cartilage grafts in both the anterior and posterior cricoid lamina in order to maintain an expanded cartilaginous outer framework.[13] Later Cotton and Evans described the four quadrant cricoid divisions with/without stenting.[15] These divisions include an anterior, posterior and two lateral cricoid cartilage divisions. The two lateral divisions allow for lateral expansion in severely stenotic subglottic lesions. The reported decannulation rate was 76% in severely stenosed cases. Single-stage procedures may be augmented by cartilage grafts. In single-stage laryngotracheal reconstructions with stenting, the decannulation rate was 83%. Others have described the castellated anterior incision,[27] refined cartilaginous carving techniques with various composite grafts and myocutaneous grafts (platysma, strap muscles, latissimus dorsi, etc.) or free flap reconstructions.

In *combined severe low subglottic stenosis* favorable results have been obtained by partial resection of the cricoid and/or first tracheal ring and primary reanastomosis. Tracheal and subglottic stenoses that are associated with a normal glottis can be treated by partial cricoid resection and cricotracheal anastomosis.[72] A tracheal mucosal flap can be created to line the posterior cricoid lamina.[39] The anastomotic tension must not exceed 124 g/cm^2.[69] If the subglottic stenosis is associated with total cricoid destruction (chondritis), an inferior cricotracheal resection is performed and a tracheothyroid or anterior tracheohyoid anastomosis can be performed. This can be combined with long-term stenting, perichondrial grafts and periosteal flaps in the posterior resection bed. The arytenoids and recurrent nerves need to be preserved. In cases where there is subglottic stenosis associated with laryngeal stenosis and bilateral vocal cord paralysis, the use of a Rethi procedure with/without arytenoidectomy and long-term stenting with grafting is advocated. There are a great variety of methods and individual modifications that are required to be tailor-made for specific individual injuries. Personal long-term experience with surgical techniques is mandatory. As a general rule, most conservative approaches should be tried first in order to obtain an adequate mucosally lined lumen, a sturdy outer framework and functional neuromuscular activity.

Post-tracheotomy stenosis

We have used computed tomography to delineate pediatric subglottic stenosis and tracheal stenosis as mucosal defects, supporting cartilaginous defects and combined stenosis.[28] From a surgical point of view it appears that the following parameters are important:

- the length of the stenosis;
- the location of the defect;
- the thickness of the defects (mucosa, submucosa, cartilaginous framework or combined);
- the age of the patient (older patients can undergo smaller tracheal resections and newborns tolerate intubation longer); and
- the nature of the injury.

Generally, cuff injuries are annular; suprastomal and cannular tip injuries involve the anterior wall; stomal injuries involve the anterior and lateral walls; and intubation injuries involve mostly the posterior mucosa and submucosa. The incidence of laryngotracheal stenosis, based on the location of the lesion, decreases as one moves inferiorly away from the larynx. The most common lesions, listed in a decreasing order of incidence are laryngotracheal, subglottic, suprastomal, stomal, infrastomal (high) tracheal, and infrastomal (low) retrosternal.

Suprastomal stenosis is a result of buckling in of the anterior cartilaginous tracheal wall (superior stomal lip) or cricoid cartilage with fracture or loss of anterior wall support. This can be corrected by composite resection of the necrotic cartilage, with hyoid bone interposition and stenting with mucosa or skin.

Stomal stenosis is caused by sepsis, a tight-fitting tracheal cannula and excessive excision of anterior tracheal cartilage. These break the cartilaginous spring and cause buckling in of the free edges of the transected tracheal cartilage and loss of the lateral cartilaginous support. Nevertheless, the major cause of stenosis is infection complicated by granulation tissue formation and focal chondritis. This infection leads to loss of anterior wall support, which may not be recognized until after decannulation (the cannula acts as a temporary stent). In the presence of cartilaginous damage (surgical resection and vascular compromise), sepsis produces chondritis and, eventually, combined stenosis. This defect is usually corrected by removal of necrotic tissue, granulation tissue or granuloma, and mucosal stenting within a T-tube.

Infrastomal stenosis is a result of prolonged periods of pressure necrosis by the tracheotomy tube or cuff. Shearing forces by the cuff (associated usually with assisted respiration) produce mucosal inflammation, vascular stasis, chondritis and delayed stenosis. Most injuries are associated with infection resulting from dependent pooling of secretions in the inferior sulcus (where the cuff meets the trachea). The damage is circumferential. Granulation tissue and granulomas are common. As a rule, there is delayed stenosis (occurring 2–3 weeks after extubation). These are corrected with resection of the stenosis and end-to-end tracheal anastomosis without stenting.

Distal tracheostenosis occurs secondary to the improper curvature of the tracheotomy tube. The distal anterior lip of a convex metal tube will impinge on the anterior tracheal wall, producing pressure and shearing forces. The mucosa is denuded, the vasculature is compromised, and the cartilage is exposed. This cartilage becomes infected. Granulation tissues or granulomas form, leading to chondritis and anterior tracheal wall collapse. The anterior tracheal wall lesions lie in the substernal trachea. This defect is corrected with external extraluminal anterior wall support and intraluminal laser excision of the stenosis, scar or granuloma.

Results

The documentation of successful reconstruction of laryngeal stenosis varies in the literature. For complete analysis there should be:

- videolaryngoscopy documentation of the airway;
- flow–loop studies to demonstrate dynamic respiratory function tests;
- voice analysis to document the phonatory quality;
- modified barium swallow to demonstrate the presence of unsuspected or silent mucous aspiration;
- high-resolution computed tomograms to denote extralaryngeal cartilaginous skeletal grafted cartilage or bone integrity; and
- tracheal extubation to denote voluntary and unassisted respiration.

Needless to say, most studies do not include all these parameters. Generally, the ability to have unassisted breathing without aspiration and a reasonable quality of voice are used empirically as a sign of successful reconstruction.

A second issue of importance is the long-term management of the postoperative patient in whom a tracheotomy or stent is in place. This is especially true in the pediatric population. It is important to communicate with the referring physician and caretaker with regard to tracheotomy care, humidification, cannular care and clean wound care. It is especially important to clean the cannula, remove inspissated secretions and crusts, maintain antibiotic coverage and be aware of the subtle signs of airway compromise and complications. The development of stridor, granulation tissue in the stomal area and peristomal or cutaneous cellulitis require early intervention to avoid restenosis. These assessments may be difficult for the general practitioner or pediatrician. Frequent communication with the outpatient caretaker, to the optimal benefit of the patient, is important in long-term care. Specific written communication, with telephone or computer follow-up in a language that can be understood, is important. In our institution, a nurse trained in airway management (as well as a social worker) follows up on all tracheotomy and laryngeal reconstructed patients to make sure that careful attention to details, such as humidification, suctioning, cannula changing, evidence of excessive trauma or sepsis and clean wound care (sterile gloves should be used to manage tracheotomy and wound care), is maintained. With the advent of managed care, in the USA, many patients are discharged early and managed as outpatients at local facilities. It is difficult to obtain appropriate nursing care in such locations. It therefore behoves the reconstruction team to keep close watch during the postoperative care period.

The third issue to be addressed in the analysis of results is the evaluation of the emotional and psychologic aspects of this patient population. It is important to define and discuss openly the surgeon's and patient's expectations and priorities. Incongruity between these expectations may affect the final outcome of the repair. Alteration of appearance, communication function and airway use may have devastating effects on the patient and create mental changes of the body image. These may lead to decreased ability to cope. The resultant effects may limit the emotional expression, reduce the intellect and self-worth and impact unfavorably on the sociocultural interactions or expectations of the patient (relationships and interactions with others). The head and neck area plays an important role in defining body image. Distortion of this area can affect our self-image and our dealings with other people. Postoperatively patients undergo various stages of adaptation which include shock, withdrawal, denial, acknowledgement (facing up to reality) and reconstruction (rebuilding the damaged body image). The last two phases denote that the patient has started reintegration and self-responsibility in the recovery process. Dropkin *et al.* noted that the pivotal period is 4–6 days postoperatively.[21] Patients not exhibiting self-care after 1 week of treatment may need assistance with their adjustment in their body image integration. This is especially true in the postoperative adjustment to a new tracheotomy. An interesting observation is that patients who were able to integrate their new tracheotomy state developed significant fear and anxiety during decannulation procedures. A great deal of emotional distress occurs when patients were not able to integrate the give-and-take relationship between voice production and airway patency as related to aspiration. There was a lack of congruence between the surgeon's and patient's expectations. Coping effectiveness is therefore a critical factor in the recovery outcome and quality of survival. Decreased ability in coping with stress and irrational beliefs are major issues that need to be addressed openly by clinicians and health care professionals.

It is generally agreed that in short incomplete stenosis of the larynx, endoscopic staged resections with lasers or knife without tracheotomy produce the best results. Almost 100% function can be achieved endoscopically in supraglottic partial anterior stenosis. Posterior and circumferential stenosis of the supraglottis repaired with open techniques generally achieves approximately 100% decannulation but the voice quality and silent aspiration (if the superior laryngeal nerves are damaged) may become a problem. For example, almost 20–30% of supraglottic laryngectomies have some form of minor silent aspiration. Glottic partial anterior webs and stenosis can be handled endoscopically with single or multistage laser resection with uniformly good results in all cases. However, total glottic stenoses have successful decannulation in the range of 60–94% and posterior glottic stenoses are decannulated in 86–93% of the cases after open procedures. Long-term stenting seems to have slightly better decannulation rates than short-term stenting but with a poorer voice quality. In combined glottic–subglottic stenosis the successful decannulation rate is 77–98%. The use of mucosal or skin grafts over extraskeletal bone or cartilage grafts has been reported to have a rate of successful decannulation in children of 76–84% and in adults of 83–100%. Usually multistage procedures are indicated for successful outcome. Treatment of subglottic stenosis (grades 3 and 4) with endoscopic laser excision without stenting or reconstruction has a success rate of 0–50%, especially if the stenoses are circumferential, greater than 1 cm in thickness, involve the glottis or trachea and include the posterior subglottic wall. Some have used laser radial incisions and dilatation in such cases with a success rate of 58%. In acute traumatic subglottic stenosis, the use of skin grafts, stents and external skeletal support has produced a success rate of 77–93%. However the voice quality was poor (adequate voice in 49% of cases). In low stenoses involving the subglottis and trachea, the rate of successful decannulation following cricoid resection with end-to-end anastomosis to the trachea is in the 80–88% range. However, if the glottis is also stenosed, the rate of successful decannulation drops to the 50–60% range. The success rate with grafting and long-term stenting rather than resection in similar lesions is in the 81–86% range. However, if the glottis is totally involved and the arytenoids are fibrosed or paralyzed, the decannulation rate decreases to 60–65%.[1,6,9,13,15,18,19,21,22,25,27,31,32,34,35,38,44,48,54,55,66,71,72,77–79,88,89]

Complications

Complications of laryngeal reconstruction can be divided into early and delayed problems.

Early complications

The most common early complication is pooling of secretions with resultant pulmonary atelectasis. Occasionally this follows intraoperative aspiration of blood or other secretions or the introduction of a long tracheotomy tube that is inserted into one right mainstem bronchus. The latter causes atelectasis in the opposite lung as a result of poor ventilation.

Laryngeal edema can result from endotracheal intubation or surgery, a long stent that compresses the subglottis or glottis, or the use of laryngotracheal procedures. The edema is treated with steroids (inhaled topical steroids) and racemic epinephrine within the perioperative period.

Apnea may follow surgery when air or O_2 is used following tracheotomy. Since in patients with chronic upper airway obstruction, CO_2 is the main respiratory drive, O_2 therapy physiologically denervates the chemoreceptor respiratory drive.

Hypotension may result from a decrease in CO_2 retention following tracheotomy. CO_2 mediates (via the CNS) increased cardiac output, high blood flow, increased peripheral resistance and hypertension.

Hemorrhage can occur during or immediately after surgery as a result of damage to the anterior jugular vein, the inferior thyroid veins, the innominate artery, the internal jugular veins, and the aortic arch and its branches. Delayed bleeding is usually secondary to bleeding of the thyroid isthmus, which is not adequately sutured at the time of surgery.

Injury to the recurrent laryngeal nerves is a major concern, especially with post-traumatic cicatricial combined laryngeal tracheal stenosis.

Pneumothorax and pneumomediastinum are major concerns, since patients in respiratory distress may have a high-rising pleura, which can be perforated during surgery. These may be manifested by shock, subcutaneous emphysema and deteriorating respiratory functions. An underwater seal chest tube is required.

A tracheoesophageal fistula is an unusual complication that may result from improper surgical technique, necrosis secondary to an excessively large tracheotomy tube or stent, or inadvertent laceration.

Subcutaneous emphysema can occur from air leakage around a tracheotomy tube that is packed too tightly. However, one must suspect the most dreaded complication of this kind of surgery: separation of the suture line or partial laryngotracheal separation. This is most often caused by excessive tension on the suture line or damage to the tracheal or laryngeal blood supply (avascular necrosis). In the immediate postoperative period it signifies a surgical error. This complication requires immediate reoperation with repair, insertion of a T-tube or tracheotomy. The repair is usually delayed until there is reduction of the inflammation and the beginning of fibrosis. Following stenting or surgical repair, delayed surgery is performed for late stenosis.

Delayed complications

Pneumonia is a delayed complication that occurs at the end of the first postoperative week. It is associated with poor tracheal toilet, atelectasis, the use of contaminated suction tips, or poor sterile techniques (nosocomial infection).

Aerophagia (air swallowing) can cause abdominal distension, pulmonary atelectasis, diaphragmatic elevation and respiratory distress. It is most common in young children. The treatment is to decompress the stomach with a nasogastric tube and adjust the tracheotomy tube to one that is slightly smaller.

A disturbing but common problem is tracheal tube dislocation into the anterior mediastinum, resulting in respiratory distress and occasionally death. Our policy is not to change the tracheotomy tube until the stoma is mature (lined with skin) and to suture the initial tracheotomy tube to the cervical skin.

Delayed respiratory distress can occur secondarily to inspissated secretions obstructing the tracheal tube lumen, tracheal crusting (tracheitis sicca), bleeding, granulation tissue (tip granuloma), an overinflated soft tracheal cuff, or improper tracheal tube curvature (occlusion along the anterior tracheal wall).

Dysphagia, usually temporary, is a result of postoperative pain, aspiration, vagal nerve paralysis, or the use of a large tracheal tube with esophageal compression by a tracheal cuff.

Difficulty in decannulation can occur after prolonged tracheal intubation. It is best treated by a gradual decrease in tracheal tube size to a no. 4 tube and the progressive plugging of the tube until it is tolerated for 12 hours or more.

A persistent tracheocutaneous fistula implies that the tract is lined by skin. This situation requires surgical closure a few weeks following decannulation. Occasionally these tracts have intratracheal inflammation and granulomas, which must be removed before closure.

A worrisome complication is persistent granulation tissue in the larynx lumen or at the anastomotic suture line, which may lead to partial stenosis. This complication is handled endoscopically with minimal trauma and the CO_2 laser. Cutaneous cellulitis or laryngeal chondritis require systemic intravenous antibiotics. Nebulized steroids are given as well as systemic steroids, for a period of 2 weeks. The stenosis is handled conservatively by rigid endoscopic dilatation. Mature restenosis requires resection. This is usually delayed for 4–6 months following the original procedure. This time period allows for more rigid fibrosis and decreases the incidence of inflammation of the laryngeal walls. The key feature is to make the initial resection or reconstruction work by eliminating tension, maintaining careful tissue approximation, using extraluminal absorbable synthetic polymeric sutures, removing all devitalized tissues and conserving as much viable tissue as possible during the initial definitive procedure.

References

1. Alonso WA, Bridger GP, Youngblood J, Delahunty JE, Bordley JE. Cricoid arch transplantation: long term follow-up. *Laryngoscope* 1971; **81**: 1968–70.
2. Arjmand EM, Spector GJ. Airway control and laryngotracheal stenosis. In: Ballanger JJ, Snow JB Jr, eds. *Otolaryngology Head and Neck Surgery*, 15th edn. Baltimore: Williams & Wilkins, 1996: 466–97.
3. Baron SH, Kahlmoos HW. Laryngeal sequelae of endotracheal anesthesia. *Ann Otol* 1951; **60**: 767–76.
4. Benjamin B. Congenital laryngeal webs. *Ann Otol Rhinol Laryngol* 1983; **92**: 317–26.
5. Bergstrom J, Moberg A, Orell SR. On the pathogenesis of laryngeal injuries following prolonged intubation. *Acta Otolaryngol (Stockh)* 1962; **55**: 342–6.
6. Blair E. Study of the viable intercostal pedicle graft in tracheobronchial surgery. *J Thorac Surg* 1958; **36**: 869–78.
7. Bogdasarian RS, Olson NR. Posterior glottic laryngeal stenosis. *Otolaryngol Head Neck Surg* 1980; **88**: 765–72.
8. Brantigan CO, Grow JB. Cricothyrotomy: elective use in respiratory problems requiring tracheotomy. *J Thorac Cardiovasc Surg* 1976; **71**: 79–83.
9. Caputo V, Consiglion V. The use of the patients own auricular cartilage to repair deficiency of the tracheal wall. *J Thorac Cardiovasc Surg* 1961; **41**: 574–95.
10. Cohen SR. Pseudolaryngeal paralysis: a postintubation complication. *Ann Otol* 1981; **90**: 483–8.
11. Connor GH, Maisels MJ. Orotracheal intubation in the newborn. *Laryngoscope* 1977; **87**: 87–91.
12. Cooper JD, Grillo HC. The evolution of tracheal injury due to ventilatory assistance through cuffed tubes: a pathologic study. *Ann Surg* 1969; **169**: 334–48.
13. Cotton R. Management of subglottic stenosis in infancy and childhood. Review of a consecutive series of cases managed by surgical reconstruction. *Ann Otol* 1978; **87**: 649–57.
14. Cotton RT. Pediatric laryngotracheal stenosis. *J Pediatr Surg* 1984; **19**: 699–704.
15. Cotton RT, Evans JN. Laryngotracheal reconstruction in children. Five-year follow-up. *Ann Otol* 1981; **90**: 516–20.
16. Cotton RT, Gray SD, Miller RP. Update of the Cincinnati experience in pediatric laryngotractual reconstruction. *Laryngoscope* 1989; **99**: 1111–16.
17. Couraud L, Brichon PY, Velly JF. The surgical treatment of inflammatory and fibrous laryngotracheal stenosis. *Eur J Cardiothorac Surg* 1988; **2**: 410–15.
18. Crysdale WS, Platt LJ. Division of the posterior cricoid plate in young children with subglottic stenosis. *Laryngoscope* 1976; **86**: 1451–8.

19. Dedo HH, Sooy CD. Endoscopic laser repair of posterior glottic, subglottic and tracheal stenosis by division or micro trap door flap. *Laryngoscope* 1983; **94:** 445–50.
20. Donnelly WH. Histopathology of endotracheal intubation. An autopsy study of 99 cases. *Arch Pathol* 1969; **88:** 511–20.
21. Dropkin MJ, Scott DW. Body image reintegration and coping effectiveness after head and neck surgery. *J Soc Otolaryngol Head Neck Nurs* 1983; **2:** 7–16.
22. Duncavage JA, Ossoff RH, Toohill RJ. Carbon dioxide laser management of laryngeal stenosis. *Ann Otol Rhinol Laryngol* 1985; **94:** 565–9.
23. Dwyer CS, Kronenberg S, Saklad M. The endotracheal tube: a consideration of its traumatic effects with a suggestion for the modification thereof. *Anesthesiology* 1949; **10:** 714–22.
24. Eckenhoff JE. Some anatomic considerations of the infant larynx influencing endotracheal anesthesia. *Anesthesiology* 1951; **12:** 401–10.
25. Eliachar I, Roberts JK, Welker KB, Tucker HM. Advantages of the rotary door flap in laryngotracheal reconstruction: is skeletal support necessary? *Ann Otol Rhinol Laryngol* 1989; **98:** 37–40.
26. Engstrom H, Grimby G, Soderholm B. Dynamic spirometry in patients with tracheal stenosis. *Acta Med Scand* 1964; **176:** 329–34.
27. Evans JNG, Todd GB. Laryngotracheoplasty. *J Laryngol Otol* 1974; **88:** 589–97.
28. Faw K, Muntz H, Seigel M, Spector GJ. Computed tomography in the evaluation of acquired stenosis in the neonate. *Laryngoscope* 1982; **92:** 100–5.
29. Fearon B, MacDonald RE, Smith C, Mitchell D. Airway problems in children following prolonged endotracheal intubation. *Ann Otol* 1967; **81:** 976–86.
30. Feliciano DV, Bitondo CG, Mattox KL *et al.* Combined tracheoesophageal injuries. *Am J Surg* 1985; **150:** 710–15.
31. Figi FA. The etiology and treatment of cicatricial stenosis of the larynx and trachea. *South Med J* 1947; **40:** 17–26.
32. Finnegan DA, Wong ML, Kashima HK. Hyoid autograft repair of chronic subglottic stenosis. *Ann Otol* 1975; **84:** 643–9.
33. Fishman AP. *Pulmonary Diseases and Disorders.* Vol. 1. New York: McGraw-Hill, 1980.
34. Fonkalsrud EW, Plested WG. Tracheobronchial reconstruction with autologous periosteum. *J Thorac Cardiovasc Surg* 1966; **52:** 666–74.
35. Friedman M, Grybauskas V, Toriumi DM, Skolnik E, Chilis T. Sternomastoid myoperiosteal flap for reconstruction of the subglottic larynx. *Ann Otol Rhinol Laryngol* 1987; **96:** 163–9.
36. Gay I, Feinmesser R, Cohen T. Laryngeal web, congenital heart disease and low stature. A syndrome? *Arch Otolaryngol* 1981; **107:** 510–12.
37. Gould SJ, Howard S. The histopathology of the larynx in the neonate following endotracheal intubation. *J Pathol* 1985; **146:** 301–11.
38. Grahne B. Operative treatment of severe chronic traumatic laryngeal stenosis in infants up to three years old. *Acta Otolaryngol (Stockh)* 1971; **72:** 134–7.
39. Grillo HC. Primary reconstruction of airway after resection of subglottic laryngeal and upper tracheal stenosis. *Ann Thorac Surg* 1982; **33:** 3–18.
40. Grundfast KM, Morris MS, Bernsley C. Subglottic stenosis: retrospective analysis and proposal for standard reporting system. *Ann Otol Rhinol Laryngol* 1987; **96:** 101–5.
41. Gussack GS, Jurkovick GJ, Luterman A. Laryngotracheal trauma. A protocol approach to a rare injury. *Laryngoscope* 1986; **96:** 660–5.
42. Hawkins DB. Pathogenesis of subglottic stenosis from endotracheal intubation. *Ann Otol Rhinol Laryngol* 1987; **96:** 116–21.
43. Healy GB. Experimental model for the endoscopic correction of subglottic stenosis with clinical application. *Laryngoscope* 1982; **92:** 1103–15.
44. Holinger LD. Treatment of severe subglottic stenosis without tracheotomy: a preliminary report. *Ann Otol* 1982; **91:** 407–12.
45. Holinger LD, Oppenheimer RW. Congenital subglottic stenosis: the elliptical cricoid cartilage. *Ann Otol Rhinol Laryngol* 1989; **98:** 702–6.
46. Holinger P, Johnston K. Factors responsible for laryngeal obstruction in infants. *JAMA* 1950; **143:** 1229–30.
47. Kenna MA, Reilly JS, Stool SE. Tracheotomy in the preterm infant. *Ann Otol Rhinol Laryngol* 1987; **96:** 68–70.
48. Koufman JA, Thompson JN, Kohut RI. Endoscopic management of subglottic stenosis with one CO_2 surgical laser. *Otolaryngol Head Neck Surg* 1981; **89:** 215–20.
49. Kuriloff DB, Setzen M, Portnoy W, Gadaleta D. Laryngotracheal injury following cricothyrotomy. *Laryngoscope* 1989; **99:** 125–30.
50. Laitman JT. The evolution and development of the human upper respiratory tract. In: Ruben RJ, Van De Water TR, Rubel EW, eds. *Biology of Change in Otolaryngology.* Amsterdam: Elsevier Science, 1986: 105–13.
51. Lanza DC, Parnes SM, Koltai PJ, Fortune JB. Early complications of airway management in head injured patients. *Laryngoscope* 1990; **100:** 958–68.
52. LeMay SR Jr. Penetrating wounds of the larynx and cervical trachea. *Arch Otolaryngol* 1971; **94:** 558–65.
53. Leopold DA. Laryngeal trauma: a historical comparison of treatment methods. *Arch Otolaryngol* 1983; **109:** 106–11.
54. Lofgren LA, Lindholm CE, Jansson B. The autogenous mucosal cyst procedure. Experimental reconstructive surgery of the airway with a new composite graft technique. *Acta Otolaryngol (Stockh)* 1985; **99:** 179–92.
55. Looper EA. The use of the hyoid bone as a stent in laryngeal stenosis. *Arch Otolaryngol* 1938; **28:** 106–11.
56. McGee KC, Nagle JW, Toohill RJ. CO_2 laser repair of subglottic and upper tracheal stenosis. *Otolaryngol Head Neck Surg* 1981; **89:** 91–5.
57. McGovern FH, Fitz-Hugh GS, Edgemon LJ. The hazards of endotracheal intubation. *Ann Otol* 1971; **80:** 556–64.
58. McInnes WD, Cruz AB, Aust JB. Penetrating injuries to the neck. *Am J Surg* 1945; **130:** 416–20.
59. McNaught RC. Surgical correction of anterior web of the larynx. *Laryngoscope* 1950; **60:** 264–72.
60. Melvin JW, Snyder RG, Travis LW *et al.* Response of

human larynx to blunt loading. *Proc 17th Stapp Car Crash Conf* 1973: 101–14.
61. Miller DW, Spector GJ. Surgical obliteration and silastic arthroplasty of the canine cricoarytenoid joint. *Laryngoscope* 1977; **87**: 2049–55.
62. Miller LH. Laryngealtracheal trauma in combat casualties. *Ann Otol* 1970; **79**: 1088–90.
63. Montgomery WW. Endoscopy and surgery of the larynx and trachea. *Radiol Clin North Am* 1978; **16**: 219–26.
64. Montgomery WW, Gamble JE. Anterior glottic stenosis: experimental and clinical management. *Arch Otolaryngol* 1970; **92**: 560–7.
65. Montgomery WW, Montgomery SK. Manual for use of Montgomery laryngeal, tracheal and esophageal prosthesis: update 1990. *Ann Otol Rhinol Laryngol* 1990; **99**: 223–48.
66. Morganstern KM. Composite auricular graft in laryngeal reconstruction. *Laryngoscope* 1972; **82**: 844–7.
67. Murphy D, MacLeon L, Dobell A. Tracheal stenosis as a complication of tracheotomy. *Ann Thorac Surg* 1966; **2**: 44–8.
68. Nicklaus PJ, Crysdale WS, Conley S, White AK, Sendi K, Forte V. Evaluation of neonatal subglottic stenosis: a 3-year prospective study. *Laryngoscope* 1990; **100**: 1185–90.
69. Ogura JH, Spector GJ. Reconstructive surgery of the larynx and laryngeal part of the pharynx: experimental aspects and their clinical application. In: Hinchcliffe R, Harrison D, eds. *Scientific Foundations of Otolaryngology*. Chicago: Year Book, 1976: 894–919.
70. Olson NR. Wound healing by primary intention in the larynx. *Otolaryngol Clin North Am* 1979; **12**: 735–40.
71. Olson NR. Skin grafting of the larynx. *Otolaryngol Head Neck Surg* 1991; **104**: 503–8.
72. Pearson FG, Cooper JD, Neleus JM, Vaunestrand AWP. Primary tracheal anastomosis after resection of the cricoid cartilage with preservation of recurrent laryngeal nerves. *J Thorac Cardiovasc Surg* 1975; **70**: 806–15.
73. Rethi A. An operation for cicatricial stenosis of the larynx. *J Laryngol Otol* 1956; **70**: 283–93.
74. Sasaki CT, Horiuchi M, Koss N. Tracheostomy-related subglottic stenosis: bacteriologic pathogenesis. *Laryngoscope* 1979; **89**: 857–65.
75. Schaefer SD. Treatment of acute external laryngeal injuries. *Arch Otolaryngol Head Neck Surg* 1991; **117**: 635–9.
76. Schaefer SD, Close LC. Acute management of laryngeal trauma. *Ann Otol Rhinol Laryngol* 1989; **98**: 98–104.
77. Schuller DE. Longterm stenting for laryngotracheal stenosis. *Ann Otol* 1980; **89**: 515–20.
78. Schuller DE. Reconstruction of the larynx and trachea. *Arch Otolaryngol Head Neck Surg* 1988; **114**: 278–86.
79. Simpson GT, Strong MS, Healy GB, Shapshay SM, Vaughan CW. Predictive factors of success or failure in the endoscopic management of laryngeal and tracheal stenosis. *Ann Otol* 1982; **91**: 384–8.
80. Slawinski EB, Jamieson DG. Studies of respiratory stridor in young children: acoustical analyses and tests of a theoretical model. *Int J Pediatr Otolaryngol* 1990; **19**: 205–22.
81. Spector JG. Respiratory insufficiency and tracheotomy. Tracheostenosis and airway control. In: Ballanger JJ, ed. *Diseases of the Nose, Throat and Ear*, 14th edn. Philadelphia: Lea & Febiger, 1984: 530–69.
82. Spector JG, Anderson K. Tracheostenosis. In: Cummings CW, Fredrickson JM, Harker LA, Krause CJ, Schuller DE, eds. *Otolaryngology Head and Neck Surgery*. St Louis: Mosby, 1986: 2433–59.
83. Strauss HJ, Scheel W, Bartel M. Comparative cinematographic, endoscopic and functional studies in the preoperative estimation of the severity of tracheal stenoses. *Z Erkr Atmungsorgane* 1989; **172**: 130–42.
84. Striker TW, Stool S, Downes JJ. Prolonged nasotracheal intubation in infants and children. *Arch Otolaryngol* 1967; **85**: 210–13.
85. Strong MS, Healey GB, Vaughan CW, Fried MP, Shapshay S. Endoscopic management of laryngeal stenosis. *Otolaryngol Clin North Am* 1979; **12**: 797–805.
86. Sulek M, Miller RH, Mattox KL. The management of gunshot and stab injuries of the trachea. *Arch Otolaryngol* 1983; **109**: 56–9.
87. Thomas GK, Stevens MH. Stenting in experimental laryngeal injuries. *Arch Otolaryngol* 1975; **101**: 217–21.
88. Toohill RJ. Composite nasal septal graft in the management of advanced laryngotracheal stenosis. *Laryngoscope* 1981; **91**: 233–7.
89. Tovi F, Gittot A. Sternocleidomastoid myoperiosteal flap for repair of laryngeal and tracheal wall defects. *Head Neck Surg* 1983; **5**: 447–51.
90. Tucker GF Jr. Laryngeal development and congenital lesions. *Ann Otol Suppl* 1980; **89**: 142–5.
91. Tucker GF, Ossoff RH, Newman AN, Holinger LD. Histopathology of congenital subglottic stenosis. *Laryngoscope* 1979; **89**: 866–77.
92. Way WL, Sooy FA. Histopathologic changes produced by endotracheal intubation. *Ann Otol* 1965; **74**: 799–805.
93. Wenig BL, Schild JA, Mafee MF. Epiglottic laryngoplasty for repair of blunt laryngotracheal trauma. *Ann Otol Rhinol Laryngol* 1990; **99**: 709–13.
94. Whited RE. A prospective study of laryngotracheal sequelae in long term intubation. *Laryngoscope* 1984; **94**: 367–77.

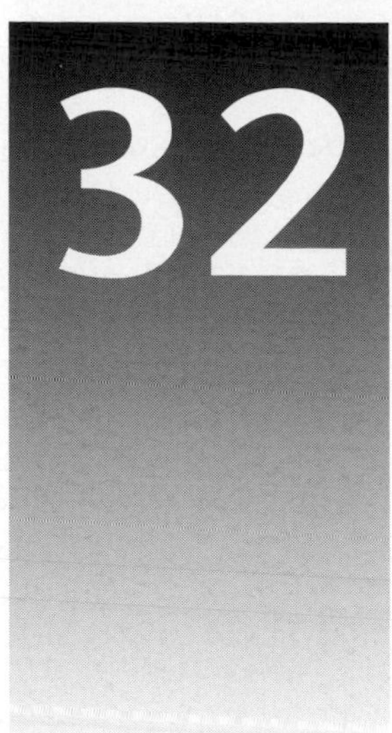

Management of vocal pathology in the voice professional

Charles W Vaughan

Vocal pathology is here defined as degradation of vocal quality. The change may be obvious to all, or only to the voice professional, or perhaps only a possibility.[2] A voice professional is anyone who derives income from vocal communication. Since the level of this income usually depends on how well the audience likes what it hears, the audience is a critical factor in managing vocal pathology in the voice professional.

Management principles

Respect the professional's concerns

Every professional cares for the tools of his/her trade and is far more sensitive to the nuances than are most others. For the voice professional, the tool that provides income and nourishes spirit is 'the voice', often referred to in just such an impersonal term. It is an instrument, no more, no less, entrusted to the care of the professional, and the professional is a better judge of its condition than is the physician. If 'the voice' concerns the vocalist so that help is sought, it is important and worthy of serious management by the physician.

Respect the professional as a person

Typically, the voice professional is an 'artist' in the finest sense of the word, able to understand, distill and communicate ideas, a process that requires sensitivity and intelligence. And those who do this before an audience must like people, and be likable. Contrary to popular belief, they are neither unstable nor unreasonable; typically, they are a pleasure to care for.

Understand the professional's audience

Audiences differ in their makeup and requirements. The audience of an American football team quarterback is his team-mates, who require that his shouted commands, regardless of vocal purity, be heard and understood. By contrast, the audience of an operatic tenor is intolerant of the slightest quality imperfection. The presentation must be 'bel canto' from start to finish.

Although audience expectations may differ, each audience is consistent in its demand that the voice professional provides, at minimum, that which it expects. The voice must be recognized as that of the performer, with quality that is standard for the performer, and the material must be known. Whilst more than expected may be appreciated, less is never accepted, or excused.

Therapy must satisfy the expectations of the professional's audience. If the professional's audience likes rock 'n' roll, the professional does not benefit from therapy biased otherwise. This should go without saying; unfortunately, the following anecdote is not uncommon: removal of vocal nodules resulted in a brilliant coloratura, but ruined the image and career of a ballad singer known for her warm, sexy voice.

Audience satisfaction is the fundamental need of the voice professional. Management of the professional's vocal pathology must be directed at satisfying this need.

Build confidence

Confidence is critical to any athletic endeavor, but particularly for vocal performance. Because it is through the nuances of voicing that we most commonly express emotion, audiences are quick to discover uncertainty and become discomfited by it. An uncertain performance satisfies no-one.

Building confidence starts with the performer's contact with the physician, who also must be professional, effective and confident. Most voice professionals have had sufficient prior experience to judge a physician's competence and to develop bias about management of their own vocal pathology. They know the things the physician should inquire about, the examinations that should be made, and the remedies most likely to be effective.

The patient must have confidence in the treatment. Respect the patient's biases about treatment and, whenever possible, prescribe that which has worked for the patient previously. If the voice professional has confidence in a physician at home, telephone that physician and discuss the findings and the plan for management. Do this in the presence of the patient.

Do no harm

This precept is fundamental to all of medicine, but in the voice professional the concept of harm requires some unique consideration. It is common belief that voice use can further harm vocal folds if the folds are already 'sick'. Certainly nodules, even submucosal hemorrhage, occur in vocalists who perform while suffering an upper respiratory infection. However, these pathologies do not 'ruin the voice'; they are treatable and reversible. More serious by far, but frequently not treatable or reversible, is the damage to the reputation of the professional who either cancels or insists that the 'show must go on' even though audience expectations cannot be met. The unreliable performer exposes the producer to financial risk and finds that jobs are no longer offered; the vocalists whose sick vocal folds cannot provide the audience with what it expects, finds that audiences are cruel. An announcement that the performer is not well, but will do his/her best, alerts the audience for signs of trouble, and any failure is quickly noted, not forgiven and widely reported. The decision to cancel or to perform cannot be made lightly.

A major decision: to perform or to cancel?

Huge sums of money often are at risk, and many other than the performer (the producer, the director, members of the cast, etc.) are affected by and have a legitimate interest in what is going on. Whilst the physician is responsible only to the performer, it is in the performer's best interest if everyone is kept informed. Debilitating illness, exudative laryngitis, and vocal fold hemorrhage present no decision difficulty. The performance is cancelled. Prompt and official (written or personal phone call) notification is given to all who need it. However, when the illness presents a more subtle pathology, every effort should be made to allow the performance. The final decision can await the outcome of this effort.

Lastly, understand that there is little research to support this chapter

It reflects the experience from years of practice and of talking things over with respected colleagues, ... and some SWAG (Scientific, wild A, guess).

Management of specific pathologies

Three categories of pathology – acute, chronic and things we cannot change – are discussed.

Acute vocal pathology

What we are concerned about here is any vocal quality degradation (obvious to all, noted only by the professional, or potential) of recent onset that may affect an imminent performance. Typically, there is some relatively minor glottic inflammation and treatment is pretty standard, no matter what the cause. Voice rest, humidification of the respiratory mucous membrane and emotional support are its essential elements.

Voice rest means: no talking, no singing, no whispering; write notes. This is difficult and nonprofessionals usually cannot do it. The professional understands and willingly conforms, but often needs help in the form of written or verbal communication to the producer/director/co-workers that voice rest has been ordered.

Humidification of the respiratory mucous membrane aids clearance of secretions, or drainage, which is still the most important factor in managing infection. Humidification is improved by avoiding diuretics, including alcohol and anything with caffeine and anticholinergics (most 'cold' medications and antihistamines), by increasing water consumption (drink a minimum of eight 10 oz glasses per day), and inhaling air moistened beyond its saturation point. Although steam kettles and other vaporizers can be used, the simplest and most effective 'tool' is a bathroom with a shower, decent lighting, and a comfortable chair. Closing off the room and running the shower increases humidity to the desired level and the patient spends as much time as possible in this environment, reading, relaxing, silently rehearsing, whatever, but all the while improving drainage, and not talking.

Emotional support means establishing confidence in the performer that everything that should be done, is being done. Establishing confidence is the most important element of the treatment (see above), and often the most difficult because development of a confident relationship between patient and physician takes time. A quick mirror examination of the folds and a prescription for steroids is insufficient. It might even be necessary that the physician be present during the performance – time consuming, but fun! On the other hand, if the performer is only nervous but otherwise in good health, clearly state so.

Medications

Medications to relieve discomfort, to reduce edema, to relieve anxiety, to increase humidification, or to control infection have potential for doing more harm than good. Analgesics and anti-inflammatory agents artificially relieve discomfort and swelling and allow further use of, and injury to, tissue that should be allowed to rest and undergo the orderly process of healing. Analgesics that contain salicylates (aspirin and many 'cold' tablets) inactivate platelet aggregation and increase the risk for cordal hemorrhage. Antihistamines and vasoconstricting decongestants decrease secretions and drainage. Steroids can inhibit vocal 'warm-up'. Chemical sedatives and tranquilizers calm the nervous patient, but when the 'adrenaline flow' is missing, the performance is dead, without pleasure for the audience or the professional. Antibiotics have no effect on viral agents, which are the usual etiology for upper respiratory infection, but they can cause allergic reactions and permit overgrowth of fungi and resistant bacteria.

Why then use medication? The patient wants it. The show must go on at all costs, there is no understudy, and everything that can be done must be done. And in selected patients, some agents are useful.

Medication is prescribed only for a specific, short-term illness. The patient must realize that its purpose is to allow only this singular and uniquely important performance to take place. Medication must not be used routinely to relieve the symptoms of daily vocal abuse, lest permanent damage result. [Of course, all rules have exceptions. If gastroesophageal reflux disease (GERD) is thought to contribute to the acute inflammation of the folds, long-term therapy is appropriate, including omeprazole, 20 mg, PO, q.d.][1]

Prescribe only that which the patient has used previously without difficulty. Prior to an important performance is not the time to risk occurrence of deleterious side effects. Many professionals, singers especially, have experience with a variety of medications, often including ancient formulae passed on from one generation to another but generally unknown to the modern physician. (See the appendix at the end of this chapter for a listing and discussion of their ingredients.) Furthermore, many carry and freely use antibiotics, steroids and many other medications obtained in countries that do not require prescription. Some are OK, but many are dangerous. In the face of unshakable faith in nostrums believed to have worked successfully in the past, it is best to comply if the request is for something harmless, or can be made so.

When everything must be done, we do the following:

- Constant exposure of the respiratory membranes to water-saturated air (see above). Pungent additives are popular, as are a variety of sprays, but act only as placebo.
- Absolute vocal rest until show time and minimal vocal warm-up. No 'trying out the voice'.
- Dexamethasone, 10 mg PO, or IM (this dose is prepackaged in a sterile syringe), at least 1 hour prior to performance. Dexamethasone has a half-life of 36 hours and the dose need not – should not – be repeated.
- Assume GERD and treat empirically.
- Reevaluate the patient, including visual observation of the vocal folds, as needed, and 30 minutes prior to the performance.
- If mild edema persists, oxymetazoline hydrochloride (Afrin†®) 0.05% is sprayed onto the vocal folds by means of one or two oral inhalations. This provides prompt decongestion of glottic mucosa, lasting one to several hours – if decongestion is possible. Revealing the identity of this medication is dangerous. Afrin® is available without prescription and can be misused. Other bronchodilators (isoetharine, isoproterenol, etc.) can be similarly used and misused.
- Continue humidification as much as possible. A small, wet towel may be carried on stage to moisten inspired air.
- Encourage modification of the performance so that it is less demanding physically. As an extreme example, a soprano lead, having completely lost her voice in the second act, completed the opera by mouthing the words as another soprano sang them from the chorus!
- Following the performance, vocal rest and humidification are continued. Post-theater partying must be avoided.

Other medications

The patient may have used and request one or more of the following; they are provided with caution, if at all.

Antibiotics

Antibiotics do not rapidly affect the course of an infection. They are given only if the Gram stain and WBC are consistent with bacterial infection, or if the patient insists on an antibiotic, or if the patient is well into a course of self-treatment. Ideally, antibiotic selection is based on culture and sensitivity, but usually this is impractical. If the patient is not already on one, selection is based on local knowledge of 'what is going around'.

Antihistamines

All antihistamines have anticholinergic activity which decreases secretions, dries the mouth and inhibits drainage. These effects are the exact opposite of what is wanted. Antihistamines should not be used.

Decongestant sprays

- Diphenhydramine hydrochloride (Benadryl®), 2% in saline dispensed in an atomizer, has vasoconstricting action that shrinks swollen vocal cord mucous membranes. Diphenhydramine also acts as a topical anesthetic and can interfere with control of subglottic pressure.

- Beclomethasone dipropionate (Beclovent®, Vanceril®), two oral inhalations, three to four times a day. Each metered dose provides 24 μg beclomethasone dipropionate and each canister provides at least 200 doses. At the recommended schedule, several days are required before the medication reaches effective levels; thus, it is not suitable for emergency measures. With chronic use, *Candida albicans* infection in the mouth, pharynx and larynx is common.

Injectables

- Vitamin B12, 1000 μg, IM once or twice weekly. The only known indications for B12 (sprue, pernicious anemia and perhaps neural conductivity) are unrelated to vocal fold inflammation. On the other hand, it is a harmless placebo.
- ACTH, 40 units, IM. This hormone stimulates the functioning adrenal cortex to produce and secrete adrenal cortical hormones. The package insert for Acthar®, Armour Pharmaceuticals, states that the hormone has 'limited therapeutic value in those conditions responsive to corticosteroid therapy; in such cases, corticosteroid therapy is considered to be the treatment of choice'.

Expectorants

Iodinated glycerol (Organidin), 60 mg, q.i.d. has the lowest amount of iodine of the various similar products available and is the least prone to side effects of iodism: dermatitis, gastrointestinal irritation, parotitis and lithium toxicity if on lithium.

Nerves

Sedatives [barbiturates and tranquilizers, including propranolol hydrochloride (Inderol®)] should not be given, no matter how reasonable the request may seem, nor should alcohol be condoned. The effect of a sedative carries through the next day and interferes with the nervous tension necessary for an exciting performance. Given the peripatetic lifestyle of many professionals, a vicious cycle of sedative–stimulant–sedative is easily established, hard to break, and best avoided.

Chronic vocal degradation

Chronic vocal degradation is any prolonged degradation of vocal quality. It may be obvious to all or perceived only by the performer or coach. Management varies according to cause, but rarely is it simple because:

- Cause and effect are interactive. Physical change in the vocal tract produces compensatory change in vocal effort, typically greater; greater effort typically produces physical change in the vocal tract. Both cause and effect must be managed.
- The relationship between cause and effect is not always clear. Whilst a singer complaining of mild difficulty during register shifts may be found to have vocal nodules, there are many singers with vocal nodules who have no voice difficulty. And of course, there are many perfect vocal folds, but very few great voices!
- There are a lot of causes.

Management of chronic vocal pathology in the professional should be attempted only by those skilled in attending to both cause and effect of vocal problems, usually a team. The team includes laryngologist, voice scientist, representatives from other medical specialties as needed, particularly pulmonary, allergy and endocrinology, and a voice therapist skilled in training vocal effort. The therapist may be a teacher of singing, a speech therapist, a voice scientist, even a physician (a phoniatrist in Europe). The background is unimportant as long as the therapist is effective in teaching vocal support appropriate to the vocal task. A coach may also be useful to guide the choice of roles and material suitable for the performer, and their presentation.

Treatment limited to excision of a vocal fold nodule discovered in a patient with a complaint of vocal fatigue may have appeal to the casual surgeon, but success is uncertain unless true cause and effect are discovered and treated. A list of some of the many excellent symposia, articles and books detailing how to go about this is appended.

Things we can't change

The well known, bad voice

A voice becomes well known because it has somehow affected a large number of people, usually in some positive way. They get to know its owner and to like the voice, no matter what its quality. Since vocal quality defies definition, other than it is liked, or not, it follows that any voice that is liked cannot be bad (no matter how bad). Any voice that is liked can only be good and should not be changed. The problem is that many of these voices are the products of tobacco, alcohol and vocal abuse rarely relieved by vocal training. At times they become useless, lost entirely or too hoarse to be serviceable. When this happens, the treatment goal is restoration of the usual voice of that unique individual. Any infection is treated and an attempt is made to limit further abuse by prescribing voice rest, no alcohol, no smoking and voice therapy. Infection is treated.

No matter how tempting, the polyp, nodules, Reinke's edema, whatever, should be left alone if they contribute to the known image of the voice. There are always exceptions, but any decision to alter the image must be the patient's, entirely.

The aging voice

The vocal tract changes with age. The infant larynx is small, flexible and quite resilient; during childhood the larynx lowers its position in the neck and during puberty it changes shape and enlarges rapidly. About age 20, the thyroid cartilage begins to ossify and become less flexible; fine motor control begins to deteriorate after age 25; muscle mass and strength increase through age 50, then slowly decrease. Mucous secretion diminishes. There are well known vocal characteristics associated with these changes: the infant voice penetrates and is untiring, a mark of puberty is unstable control of voicing, and a weak vocal cackle defines the very old. Less known, but important to the professional, are other results of maturational changes in flexibility, mass and motor control. The coloratura may have 'lost her voice' in her early 20s because, with ossification, her thyroid cartilage has lost its flexibility. Wagnerian opera cannot be sung until the vocal folds have developed sufficient mass. Fine motor control, essential for voice 'support', the exquisite balance of subglottic pressure, glottic resistance, and airflow that is just right for healthy and bel canto voicing, eventually becomes lost.

Not uncommonly, vocal deterioration is found to be the result of unhealthy vocal habits rather than aging, *per se*. Surprisingly common is abuse of the speaking voice of otherwise well-trained singers. In such instances, vocal health is restored by further training. Vocal training may also allow postponement of the inevitable deterioration due to aging. Although some deterioration is obvious in most voices after 60 years of age, some singers have performed professionally well into their 80s! Because we do not hear ourselves as others hear us, an expert listener and teacher usually is essential for guiding the development and maintenance of proper vocal support.

Lifestyle, overwork, emotional problems and disease also may take their toll. Frequent travel, often across time zones, late meals of unusual foods and strange beds make for difficult living conditions. Gastroesophageal reflux that inflames the larynx is common.[1] The vocal folds also thicken and the vocal pitch lowers with hyperthyroidism and antihypertensive medication and with steroids taken for contraception or to counteract the symptoms of menopause. Temporal mandibular joint abnormalities may produce neck muscle tension and alter laryngeal control. Any pathology that reduces lung vital capacity affects 'support', and diabetic neuropathy frequently involves laryngeal motor nerves. Many of these conditions can be ameliorated. For those that cannot, the professional should receive informed advice on which to base realistic plans.

Limits

Every system, no matter how skilled or efficient, has limited ability to endure stress, beyond which it will break down. All athletes understand this. A baseball pitcher pitches no more often than every third day, and grand opera conforms to a similar rotation. Although some voices are tougher than others, skilled vocalists know their limits, and generally do not wish to exceed them. Pressure to do so, however, often is great. Money provides its force and is difficult to resist. Because of it, singers attempt roles such as *Evita*, with daily performances plus biweekly matinees, despite the fact that no matter how tough or skilled, none has been able to endure such stress for the full run of that show. There are many other examples. Students have a lifestyle all their own, often exceeding reasonable limits. They enthusiastically prepare their voice lessons, sing in the church choir and the opera workshop, and to support themselves they wait tables and do 'gigs'. They are friendly, enjoy social contact and partying. Because they are young, they are somewhat resilient and bounce back – but not always. They are frequent visitors to the laryngologist. In every instance, therapy consists of authoritatively prescribing limits. Documentation of these limits is often needed for producers, directors, teachers, whatever.

Surgery

Surgery under general, endotracheal anesthesia, and particularly laryngeal surgery, threatens the voice professional's future as a performer.[3] The fear this generates must be sensitively managed. Consent must be truly 'informed'. Helpful in this are:

- reviewing with the patient the videostroboscopy tape of the lesion;
- illustrating vocal fold anatomy and physiology and the effect of the lesion on both;
- demonstrating the surgical microscope and instruments used during laryngeal surgery;
- video tapes (non-gory) of similar procedures, the endotracheal tube and its safe placement between the arytenoids during surgery; and
- fully discussing all concerns, expressed and unexpressed.

Finally, uncover any misconceptions by requesting that the patient reviews what has been learned, and corrects those replies that are incorrect.

Capped teeth are common in the voice professional and are threatened by use of laryngoscope holders of the Lewy/Kleinsasser type, which are levers that fulcrum on the teeth. Teeth are best protected by use of a true suspension system, such as the 'BU Suspension' (Pilling) for holding the laryngoscope. Work only with an anesthesiologist who shares the patient's concerns, will take the time to address them, and whose ego will not be damaged if the surgeon decides to do the intubation.

Appendix

Medications occasionally requested but not recommended

Most are contraindicated. Use should be limited to those who insist and should be discouraged in all others.

Modern and popular

Decongestant sprays

- Diphenhydramine hydrochloride (Benadryl), 2% in saline dispensed in an atomizer. When sprayed onto the vocal folds, this decongests swollen vocal fold mucosa, but diphenhydramine also acts as a topical anesthetic and interferes with kinesthetic control of subglottic pressure.
- Beclomethasone dipropionate (Beclovent, Vanceril) for oral inhalation. Each method dose provides 24 µg of beclomethasone dipropionate and each canister provides at least 200 metered doses. At the recommended schedule of two inhalations three to four times a day, several days are required before the medication reaches effective levels; therefore, it is not suitable for emergency measures. With chronic use *Candida albicans* infection in the mouth, pharynx and larynx is common.

Injectables

- Vitamin B12, 1000 µg, IM once or twice weekly. The only known indications for B12 (sprue, pernicious anemia and perhaps neural conductivity) are unrelated to vocal fold inflammation.
- ACTH, 40 units, IM. This hormone stimulates the functioning adrenal cortex to produce and secrete the adrenal cortical hormones. To quote the package insert for Acthar, Armour Pharmaceuticals, the hormone has, 'limited therapeutic value in those conditions responsive to corticosteroid therapy; in such case, corticosteroid therapy is considered to be the treatment of choice'.

Ancient formulations

These have generally been abandoned, but are occasionally encountered. Many represent witchcraft rather than science; indeed, most contain irritants, caustics, or astringents.

Inhalants

A teaspoonful of one of the following is added to a pint of steaming water. A cone is placed over the mouth of the vessel and through this, the patient inhales the vapors for 5 minutes, repeating every 2 hours or less often as needed.

'Friar's balsam' – tincturae benzoini compositae 4.0 ml

To this may be added:

- Mentholis 0.2 g;
- Tincture eucalypti in alcohol 4.0 ml; and
- a few drops of chloroform.

More pungent is the following:

- Olei pini sylvestris 8.0 ml;
- Tincturae benzoini compositae 30.0 ml;
- Magnesi carbonatis levis 4.0 g;
- Aquae rosae 30.0 ml; and
- Glycerinum to 90.0 ml.

'Dry' inhalants

These vaporize when poured onto the hand or into a handkerchief and inhaled directly. Typically, they contain chloroform and an admonition that not more than three teaspoonfuls be used on any single occasion!

- Chloroform 7.0 ml;
- Spirits vini rectificati 7.0 ml.

To the chloroform may be added menthol or iodine and ether, or oil of pine:

- Mentholis 1.0 g
- Chloroform 15.0 ml
- Tincturae iodi 4.0 ml
- Spiritus aetheris sulph compositi 4.0 ml
- Spiritus chloroformi 8.0 ml
- Olei sanitas 30.0 ml
- Guaiacol 8.0 ml
- Terebeni 8.0 ml
- Mentholis 1.0 g
- Olei pini pumilionis 1.0 ml
- Chloroformi 8.0 ml
- Spiritus vini rectificati 30.0 ml

Gargles, washes and sprays

Some formulations mimic normal saline:

- Sodii bicarbonatis 0.32 g
- Sodii biboratis 0.32 g
- Sodii chloridi 0.32 g
- Sucrosi 0.32 g

Others contain caustics, astringents and volatile agents, i.e. phenol, menthol, camphor, silver nitrate and oils. Typical are compound carbolic solutions:

- Sodii bicarbonatis 0.2 g
- Sodii biratis 0.2 g
- Phenolis 0.06 g
- Sucrosi 0.32 g

Oily sprays may contain menthol:

- Mentholis 0.32–2.0 g
- Paraffini liquidi (BP) to 30.0 ml
- Chloretoni (chlorbgutolis) 0.3 g
- Camphorae 0.3 g
- Mentholis 0.15 g
- Olei pini pumilii 0.3 ml
- Paraffini liquidi 30.0 ml

Aspirin may be gargled:

- Acidi acetyl-salicylici 0.65 g
- Pulv. tragacanthae co. 0.65 g
- Aquae 30.0 ml

Astringents may be gargled:

- Aluminis 4.0 g
- Acidi tannici 5.3 g
- Aquae destillatae to 300.0 ml
- Boracis 8.0 g
- Glycerini 8.0 ml

- Tincture myrrhae 8.0 ml
- Aquae destillatae to 180.0 ml

Solutions for topical applications usually contain caustics:

Mandl solution:
- Iodi puri 0.4 g
- Potassi iodidi 1.3 g
- Olei menthae piperitae 0.3 ml
- Glycerini 30.0 ml

Argyrol (Protargolum):
- Argyrol (or Protargolum) 3.0 g
- Aquae destillatae 30.0 ml

None of the above medications is recommended.

References

1. Koufman JA. The otolaryngologic manifestations of gastroesophageal reflux disease (GERD): a clinical investigation of 225 patients using ambulatory 24-hour pH monitoring and an experimental investigation of the role of acid and pepsin in the development of laryngeal injury. *Laryngoscope* 1991; **101(Suppl 53)**: 1–78.
2. Sataloff RT. *Professional Voice, the Science and Art of Clinical Care.* New York: Raven Press, 1991.
3. Vaughan CW. Vocal fold exposure in phonosurgery. *J Voice* 1993; **7**: 189–194.

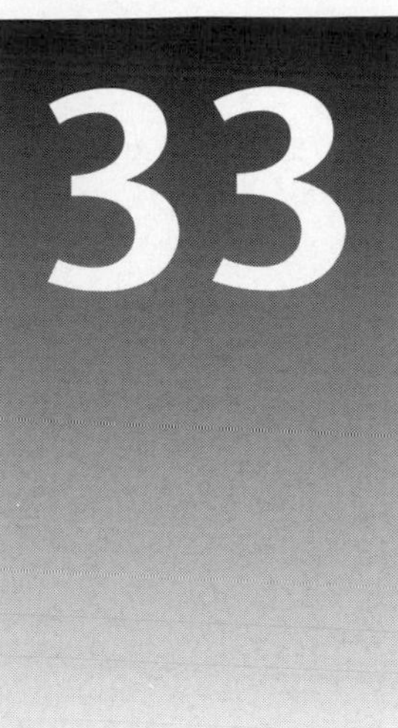

Laryngeal framework surgery

Hans F Mahieu

Phonosurgery is defined by the International Association of Phonosurgeons as any type of surgery that is performed with the aim to improve, or change, voice or speech. This means that the goal of phonosurgery is to restore function rather than to restore normal anatomy.

Modern phonosurgery is therefore based on concepts of physiology of phonation and laryngeal biomechanics and is a functional type of surgery by definition. The delicate structure of the vocal folds and the vulnerable mechanism of phonation, which is susceptible to even minor damage of the vocal fold's epithelium or lamina propria, can sometimes make direct microlaryngeal surgical treatment of the vocal folds a hazardous intervention with regard to the vocal outcome. Of course direct microlaryngoscopic interventions very often cannot be avoided, but in a considerable number of cases restoration of function can be achieved, without jeopardizing the vocal fold's integrity and function, by using an external surgical approach.

By changing the shape or position of some of the laryngeal cartilages and thus providing biomechanical compensation for the phonatory dysfunction, some types of dysphonia can be corrected without touching the vocal folds themselves. These so-called laryngeal framework surgical procedures are performed under local anesthesia to enable voice monitoring during the surgical procedure in order to fine-tune the voice and obtain the best functional result. Laryngeal framework surgery consists of a group of surgical procedures that present a fine example of how correction of voice disorders can be obtained without necessarily reestablishing normal laryngeal anatomy.

Some types of laryngeal framework surgery had already been suggested decades ago, for example, by Payr,[39] who in 1915 described an anterior pedicled transverse, U-shaped

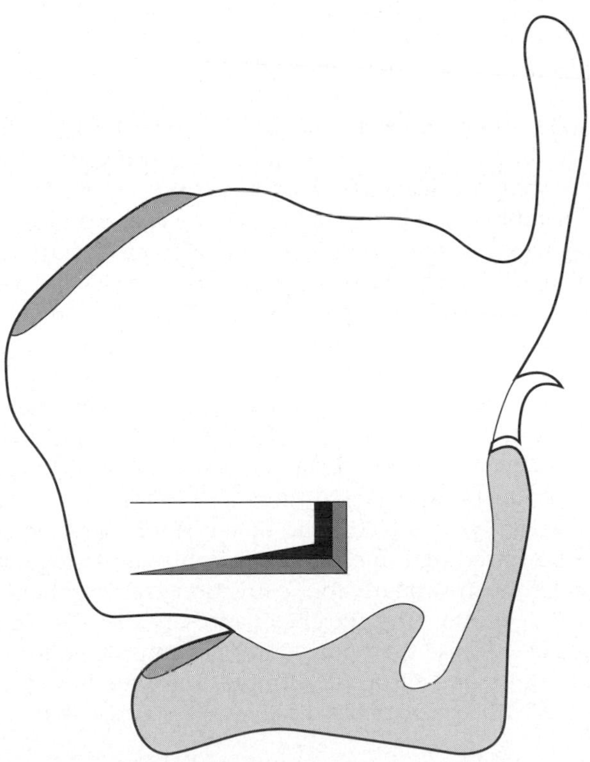

Figure 33.1 *Vocal fold medialization according to Payr.*[39]

cartilage flap, designed in the thyroid ala, which was depressed inward to medialize the vocal fold (Fig 33.1). The effect was, however, limited, probably because the anterior pedicle restricted adequate medialization and fixation of the cartilage in the desired position proved difficult and uncertain.[51] Others, like Seiffert in 1942[51] and Meurman[34] in 1944, proposed the paraglottic implantation of a rib cartilage graft to medialize the vocal fold. Despite all these efforts, the concept remained fragmentary until Isshiki *et al.*,[22] in 1974, presented his innovative ideas for correcting several types of dysphonia by indirect means using laryngeal framework surgical techniques, which he termed thyroplasties. Over the years, Isshiki and colleagues[18–22] have molded these thyroplasties into the versatile set of phonosurgical techniques that is available to us today and which has enabled us to achieve such good results in the treatment of many different types of dysphonia. Although quite a discussion has been going on concerning the correct nomenclature of the different laryngeal framework surgical procedures, the original phrases as coined by Isshiki will be used in this chapter as a tribute to his contribution in this field.

Two different categories of laryngeal framework surgeries can be distinguished:

- procedures with the objective to correct incomplete glottis closure by medialization of one or both vocal folds; and
- procedures with the objective to adjust the tension of one or both vocal folds.

The most frequent indication for correction of glottis closure using a laryngeal framework surgical technique is undoubtedly glottic insufficiency resulting from vocal fold palsy.

In 1911, Brunings[7] was the first to report successful phonosurgical correction of glottic insufficiency in patients suffering from vocal fold paralysis, using intracordal paraffin injections. This technique was abandoned because some patients developed paraffinomas, but the stage was set for other investigators, using several other substances, to inject into the vocal folds. Arnold[1] advocated the use of another alloplastic material, Teflon (polytetrafluoroethylene), in 1962, and this substance is still in use today, although many complications have been reported.[26,38,42,59] More recently, the biomaterial bovine collagen and autologous fat have achieved favorable attention from several authors.[6,11,12,35,40,41,53]

Until recently, this technique of vocal fold augmentation using intracordal injections of soluble substance was the preferred treatment for correction of dysphonia caused by glottic insufficiency and its use is still widespread, because such procedures are considered to be effective, quick and apparently simple. They are, however, associated with considerable disadvantages and risks:

- The mass, volume, and stiffness of the injected vocal fold are influenced by the injected substances. Such changes in vocal fold mass, volume, and stiffness interfere with the vibratory properties of the vocal fold, which can result in a poor voice.
- Distribution of the injected substance is difficult to control. The substance will spread according to the path of least resistance, rather than to the area requiring augmentation.
- The use of injectable substances, especially Teflon, is generally considered contraindicated in a mobile vocal fold, because of the risk of subsequent vocal fold fixation as a result of local tissue reaction.
- Bilateral use of injectable substances is considered contraindicated, because of the risk of airway compromise.
- The treatment is irreversible. Over-injection is difficult to correct and generally requires partial resection of the vocal fold, resulting in severe dysphonia.
- If performed under general anesthesia, as many endolaryngeal injection procedures are, voice monitoring during the procedure is not possible. Consequently it is difficult to estimate the proper amount of substance to be injected.
- Some materials (collagen, fat) are subject to partial absorption so that initial overcorrection is required and repeated injections may be necessary. Other materials (silicone, Teflon) are known to have a tendency to migrate, which may also lead to repeated injections.[11]
- Often vocal fold palsy is associated with a vertical level difference of both vocal folds, although this is not always easily detected on laryngeal examination. Such a level of difference usually can not be corrected by vocal fold injection.
- Last but not least, as already mentioned, a considerable number of complications and local tissue reactions attributable to the injected substances have been published, especially regarding the use of Teflon.[26,38,42,59] The injection of autologous fat and collagen seems to present fewer complications.[6,11,12,35,40,41,53]

These disadvantages do not hold true for laryngeal framework surgical procedures, of which only a few complications have been reported[8,36,61] and which can also be used bilaterally and in case of mobile vocal folds. Therefore, these procedures are presently used by many phonosurgeons as the first choice of treatment for correction of incomplete glottis closure, leaving only a few indications for intracordal injection of soluble substances.

Indications for adjustment of vocal fold tension are various. Too lax vocal folds may result in a weak, hoarse and usually low-pitched voice. Too tense vocal folds may result in a strained, breathy and usually high-pitched voice. Diminished and asymmetrical vocal fold tension, as may accompany vocal fold palsy, may contribute to the breathy voice quality and can result in diplophonia. These and certain pitch-related dysphonias may be eligible for surgical correction of vocal fold tension.

By and large there are five categories of patients who

may benefit from phonosurgical correction of vocal fold tension:

- Patients who are undergoing correction of incomplete glottis closure by means of medialization laryngeal framework surgery and in whom additional correction of vocal fold tension may contribute to a further improvement of the voice.
- Patients who request an elevation of the vocal pitch. The major indications for raising the vocal pitch are androphonia following hormonal medication and gender dysphonia in male-to-female transsexual patients. Voice therapy is the mainstay for gender dysphonias, but additional phonosurgical intervention can be required to raise the habitual vocal pitch.[32] Although vocal pitch is not the only factor in identifying the gender of a speaker, it is generally regarded as the predominant one. Other factors include patterns of intonation, quality of resonance, articulation characteristics, conversational topics and type of vocabulary.[5,37]
- Patients with lax vocal folds, as may be the result of superior laryngeal nerve palsy, extreme flaccid vocal folds resulting from presbyphonia in elderly patients and in some cases following laryngeal trauma.
- Patients with stiff vocal fold(s) due to congenital vocal fold disorders, some cases of sulcus vocalis (after unsatisfactory microlaryngeal surgery) and exceptional cases following laryngeal trauma. In such cases a combination of surgical reduction of vocal fold tension and slight medialization can improve the voice.
- Patients requesting a lowering of the vocal pitch. Although rare, cases of voice therapy-resistant mutational dysphonia and some cases of congenital vocal fold hypoplasia can benefit from surgical reduction of vocal fold tension.

Several surgical procedures have been described to elevate the vocal pitch. First, Donald in 1982 described the creation of a web in the anterior commissure through a laryngofissure.[10] Others, like Waar[67] and Wendler (personal communication), create such webs endoscopically. The general idea of this procedure is that the length over which the vocal fold can vibrate is reduced. By reducing the vibratory length of the vocal fold, the pitch will rise. However, it proves difficult to control the length over which the vocal folds will form a web. Furthermore, all laryngologists are familiar with the negative side effects such as hoarseness and breathiness, which can occur in patients with a laryngeal web.

Furthermore, mass reduction of the vocal folds by CO_2 laser vaporization,[19,56] corticosteroid injection[19] and longitudinal incisions in the vocal fold to induce scarring and consequently increased stiffness in the vocal fold[20,23] have been described as methods to raise the vocal fold pitch. Clearly all these procedures will have more or less severe negative consequences on voice quality. In most cases vocal pitch elevation can safely be achieved by a laryngeal framework surgical technique which mimics the activity of the cricothyroid muscles, thus providing a more physiologic approach to the problem of androphonia or gender dysphonia.

The only reasonably documented method to decrease vocal pitch consists of the laryngeal framework surgical procedures developed by Isshiki.[19,55] Reduction of the anterior–posterior dimension of the thyroid ala is a procedure which enables regulated reduction of vocal fold tension and consequently vocal pitch with voice monitoring during surgery.

No phonosurgical techniques other than laryngeal framework surgical procedures have been described to correct vocal fold tension associated with vocal fold palsy, presbyphonia, or increased vocal fold stiffness. Laryngeal framework surgical techniques constitute a versatile set of phonosurgical procedures enabling the surgeon to treat a large scope of phonatory disorders. They have, therefore, since the late 1980s and early 1990s, rapidly gained popularity as the treatment of first choice for dysphonias resulting from incomplete glottis closure or inadequate vocal fold tension.[3,14,24,25,30–33,36,62]

Sometimes a single modality laryngeal framework surgical technique sufficiently improves the voice, but often a better voice can be obtained by combining different techniques in a single-stage intervention.[27,54] Voice monitoring and functional fiberoptic endolaryngeal monitoring are essential during the surgical procedure, not only to determine the required degree of medialization or change of vocal fold tension, but also to decide whether a combination of laryngeal framework surgical procedures is required. Consequently laryngeal framework surgical techniques must always be performed under local anesthesia.

Good results have been obtained, undoubtedly thanks to the functional monitoring during surgery, which enables a tailored approach to the individually required correction. This clearly requires a more than superficial knowledge of laryngeal biomechanics and phonatory physiology from the surgeon involved in phonosurgery.

This chapter focuses primarily on the surgical aspect of patients requiring correction of incomplete glottis closure or correction of vocal fold tension by means of laryngeal framework surgery. This does not imply that there is no place for voice and speech therapy in these categories of patients, but more often than not they have been treated extensively with voice and speech therapy, often without sufficient voice improvement, before they are presented for laryngeal framework surgical correction. The need for additional speech therapy is therefore judged in each individual case and is not included routinely.

Basic concepts

Voice production essentially is the process of generating vibrating air, which is perceived as sound. The vibrating air is generated by the periodic opening and closing of the glottis with a frequency equaling the fundamental

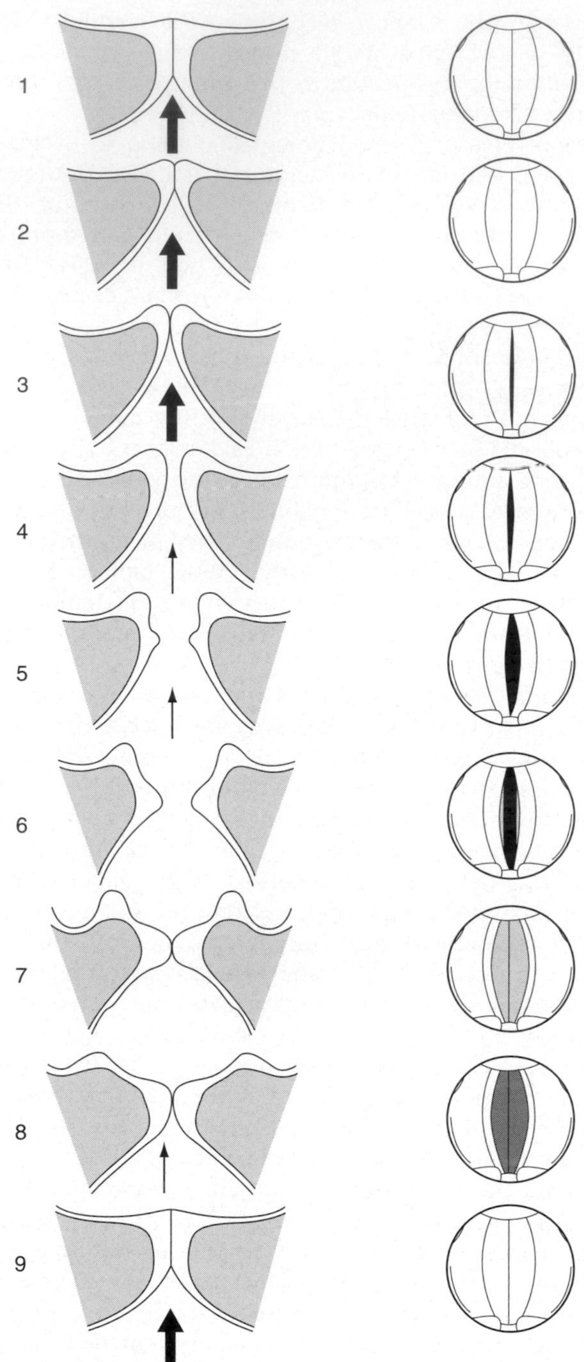

Figure 33.2 *Vocal fold motion during phonation and corresponding stroboscopic image (adapted from Schonharl[46] and Hirano[16]). Aerodynamic force schematically represented by arrow.*

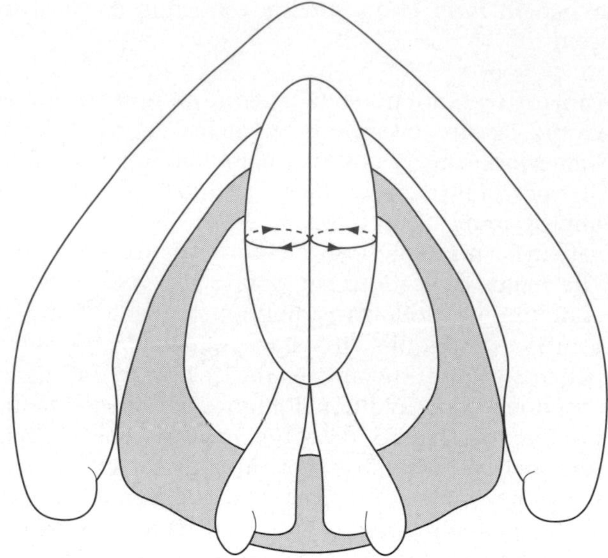

Figure 33.3 *Representation of glottic cycle during phonation.*

frequency of the produced phonation. The basic tone produced there is further modified by the configuration of the vocal tract. The periodic opening and closing of the glottis (Fig 33.2) is regulated by a complex interaction of aerodynamic and myoelastic forces, which are still not fully understood.[15,16,45–47,49,64–66] For the understanding required here, it will suffice to simplify this process of phonation and focus on the basic requirements for the production of voice. In order to phonate, the vocal folds have to adduct and thus close the glottis during the expiration of air from the lungs. This results in an increase of airway resistance and consequently in an increase of subglottic pressure. The rising subglottic pressure will result in a cranial displacement of the free edge of both vocal folds and will cause the vocal folds' free edges to separate in the midline, thus slightly opening the glottis. The opened glottis will allow the passage of a small puff of air and the subglottic pressure will drop. As a result of the drop of subglottic pressure, the myoelastic forces of the vocal folds and the Bernoulli effect caused by the passing puff of air, the vocal fold edges approximate again and the glottis closes, completing the glottic cycle (Fig 33.3). This cycle is repeated periodically and thus the oscillating vocal folds essentially cut the passing expiratory airflow into glottal pulses. The intraglottal and transglottal pressures are changing periodically as well and are extremely important in the maintenance of vocal fold oscillation.[44,58]

The frequency of the glottic cycle obviously determines the frequency of the glottal pulses and thus also the fundamental frequency of the phonation. This fundamental frequency is perceived as the vocal pitch. The fundamental frequency of the glottic cycle is determined by the tension, the mass (especially the vocal folds' cover and transitional layer) and the length of the vocal folds and is largely regulated by the interaction between the cricothyroid muscles and the medial part of the thyroarytenoid muscles. These muscles act as agonist–antagonist pairs; the former to lengthen the vocal folds, and the latter to shorten them. This mechanism is supported by the other intrinsic laryngeal muscles that counterbalance the forces applied to the arytenoid and assist in increasing the tension of the vocal folds. Contraction of the cricothyroid muscles results in an anterior approximation

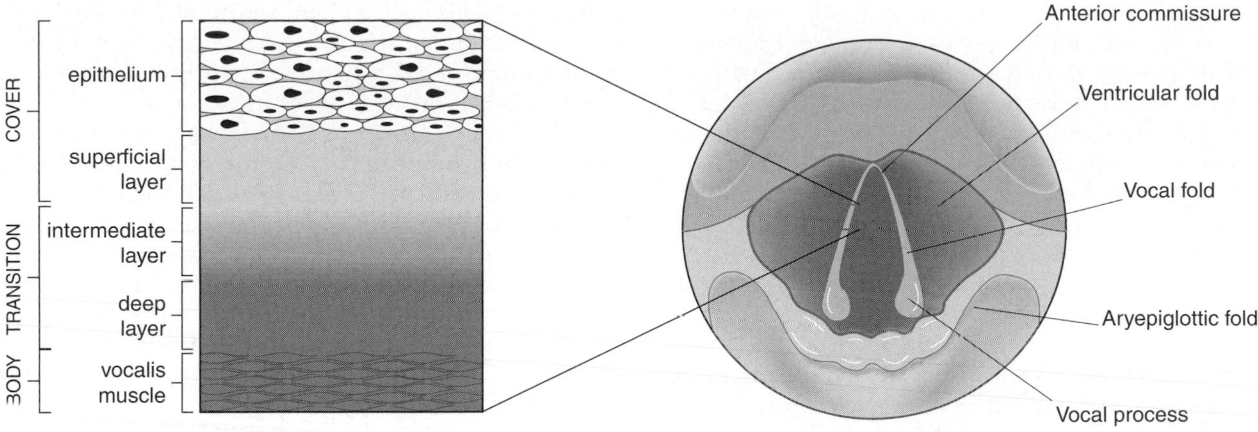

Figure 33.4 *Schematic presentation of the layered structure of the vocal fold. Cover formed by epithelium and the superficial layer (pliable) of the lamina propria, also known as Reinke's space, consisting of amorphous substance and loosely connective tissue. Transition formed by the intermediate layer (elastic) of the lamina propria (largely consisting of elastic fibers) and the deep layer (moderately stiff) of the lamina propria (largely consisting of collagenous fibers). Body formed by vocalis muscle (stiff).*

of the cricoid and thyroid cartilages and consequently the anterior commissure is displaced anteriorly and caudally. As a result of this displacement the vocal folds are elongated. By elongating the vocal folds, the cricothyroid muscles also stretch the vocal folds, thus increasing the tension and thinning and stiffening the vocal folds (body as well as cover), consequently reducing their vibratory mass. The effect of increasing the tension, thinning the vocal folds and reducing the vibratory mass surpasses the effect of the vocal fold elongation and the net result is a rise in fundamental frequency and consequently in vocal pitch. Contraction of the vocalis muscle results in a shortening, thickening and slackening (cover only) of the vocal folds, leading to a lower vocal pitch. The role of subglottic pressure in pitch regulation is an important but complicated issue, and is beyond the description required in this chapter.

There are several prerequisites for proper functioning of the process of phonation:

- The vocal folds have to be able to adduct sufficiently to achieve dynamic glottic closure in phonation. Inability to adduct the vocal folds sufficiently will lead to escape of subglottic air without it having been modulated into periodic puffs of air, also causing high airflow rates and turbulence. This is perceived as a weak and breathy phonation, acoustically characterized by noisy components in the higher frequency domains of the spectrogram.[44,52] One of the obvious consequences of insufficient glottic closure is a reduction of the maximal duration of phonation because of the lack of sufficient subglottic air volume to sustain the phonation. In extreme cases this may lead to hyperventilation during phonation. Furthermore, an insufficient glottic closure will interfere with the subglottic and transglottic pressure buildup, thus hampering the maintenance of oscillation of the vocal folds.
- The delicate layered structure of the vocal folds has to be intact. The vocal fold consists of the epithelium and the superficial layer of the lamina propria acting as the cover, the intermediate and deep layers of the lamina propria acting as a transitional layer and the vocalis muscle as the body (Fig 33.4).[15] This layered structure and especially the loose connection of the cover to the transitional layer allows relatively free mobility of this cover. Fibrosis or edema of the cover or the transitional layer will interfere with the mobility of the cover and will increase the cover's stiffness, consequently interfering with the vocal folds' oscillation and the opening and closing of the glottis. This can result in insufficient glottal closure, in aperiodicity of the glottal cycle, or in asymmetrical vibration of both vocal folds. The resulting voice can have different characteristics, varying from rough and unstable to harsh and breathy and sometimes diplophonia.
- Adjustment of vocal fold tension has to be adequate and balanced. Different intensities of phonation and different vocal pitches require different vocal fold tensions. Regulation of vocal fold tension is especially important to regulate the airflow resistance and consequently the subglottic and transglottic pressures. A too high tension or stiffness of the vocal fold will hamper the vocal fold oscillation, while a too low tension will not sufficiently counterbalance the subglottic pressure buildup. Furthermore, imbalance of the tension of both vocal folds will lead to asymmetrical vibration of both vocal folds and consequently to aperiodicity of the glottal cycle. Acoustically, the resulting voices are characterized by a high jitter rate (perturbation of fundamental frequency) and/or a high shimmer rate (perturbation in amplitude equaling intensity). In extreme cases the frequency of vibration of both vocal folds can differ, leading to diplophonia.

The pathophysiological phenomenon of incomplete glottis closure and inadequate tension are important causes of dysphonia and are preferably corrected without interfering with the delicate structure of the vocal folds. It is clear that laryngeal framework surgical procedures for correction of incomplete glottis closure as well as for correction of vocal fold tension can play an important role in the treatment of many types of dysphonia.

The advantages of the laryngeal framework surgical techniques over alternative procedures concerning the above mentioned aspects are:

- The affected vocal fold is not negatively influenced by inadvertent mass, volume, or stiffness changes.
- Direct control can be obtained over the degree of medialization or tension correction.
- A vertical level difference of both vocal folds in vocal fold palsy can be corrected adequately.
- Most procedures are reversible or correctable in the unlikely event of overcorrection.
- Some of the procedures can be performed without interfering with vocal fold mobility and can therefore also be performed bilaterally.
- The procedures are performed under local anesthesia, so that fine tuning of the voice is possible during the operation and several combinations of techniques can be tested during the operation to achieve the best voice result.
- The voice results have proved to remain stable with only very few exceptions, so that the need for revision procedures is rare.
- Few complications have been reported following laryngeal framework surgeries and those that have been reported were immediately related to the surgical procedure and could be adequately corrected, so that this was usually not detrimental to ultimate voice improvement.[8,32,36,61]

The only obvious disadvantages of laryngeal framework surgery are the elaborateness of the procedures and the fact that clinical observation of 1 day is advised in all but the simplest procedures.

Assessment of laryngeal and vocal function

Laryngeal assessment

Without any doubt the most useful diagnostic tool for assessment of laryngeal function during phonation is videolaryngostroboscopy. Although this assessment method only shows a virtual slow-motion image of the vibrating vocal folds, it enables a good evaluation of the glottis closure and is very helpful in the diagnosis of vocal fold tension dysbalance. In the present day and age it is unthinkable to make proper indications for phonosurgical procedures, without performing videolaryngostroboscopy.[4,17,28,29,57,68,69]

If there is doubt about the cause of an immobile vocal fold, of course adequate diagnostic procedures are to be performed. This will include laryngeal electromyography and, depending on the EMG results, imaging of the neck, mediastinum or skull base, and occasionally endoscopic examination in general anaesthesia.

If the history also reveals dysphagia, it is wise to first evaluate the dysphagic problems before contemplating laryngeal framework surgery. This can include videofluoroscopy, esophageal and hypopharyngeal manometry, 24 hours of pH monitoring and occasionally endoscopic examination. If there are also dysphagic problems requiring surgical treatment, these are best treated before laryngeal framework surgery, because if laryngeal framework surgery is performed first, later endotracheal intubation can annihilate the obtained voice result.

During the surgical procedure laryngeal assessment is performed with a flexible endoscope and a camera, allowing the surgeon to monitor the endolaryngeal consequences of his manipulations with the laryngeal framework. This laryngeal monitoring, in combination with the monitoring of the voice during the surgical intervention, enables the surgeon to obtain the best functional result. Videolaryngostroboscopic assessment of the endolaryngeal situation during surgery can be helpful, but is technically difficult to perform due to the triggering mechanism of the stroboscope, which either interferes with the surgical field or is inadvertently triggered by the noise in the operating theater.

Voice assessment

The best diagnostic tool for voice assessment is still the clinician's ear. Other voice assessment methods may be more objective, but are certainly less sensitive and can only characterize a few of the factors that determine the quality of voice. Therefore the clinician's judgement of the voice remains very important, at the time of the preoperative assessment but even more so during laryngeal framework surgery. This certainly holds true for the individual patient, but does not allow objective assessment of the functional result of phonosurgical procedures. Many different objective voice assessment methods have been proposed for this purpose.

My preferred voice evaluation method is the phonetogram, or voice range profile (VRP), registered according to the guidelines of the European Union of Phoniatricians[50] with a microphone-to-mouth distance of 30 cm. The VRP is a graphical representation of vocal capabilities concerning the fundamental frequency range and the dynamic range determined on several vocal pitches.[48] The advantages of the VRP over acoustical voice assessment are first of all that the VRP contains information on vocal capacity in circumstances other than normal loudness only, whereas acoustical voice analysis is usually performed for normal vocal intensity and habitual vocal pitch only. In normal day-to-day life, the dysphonic patient, however, encounters most problems in making him/herself heard or understood in noisy surroundings, where he/she has to raise the vocal inten-

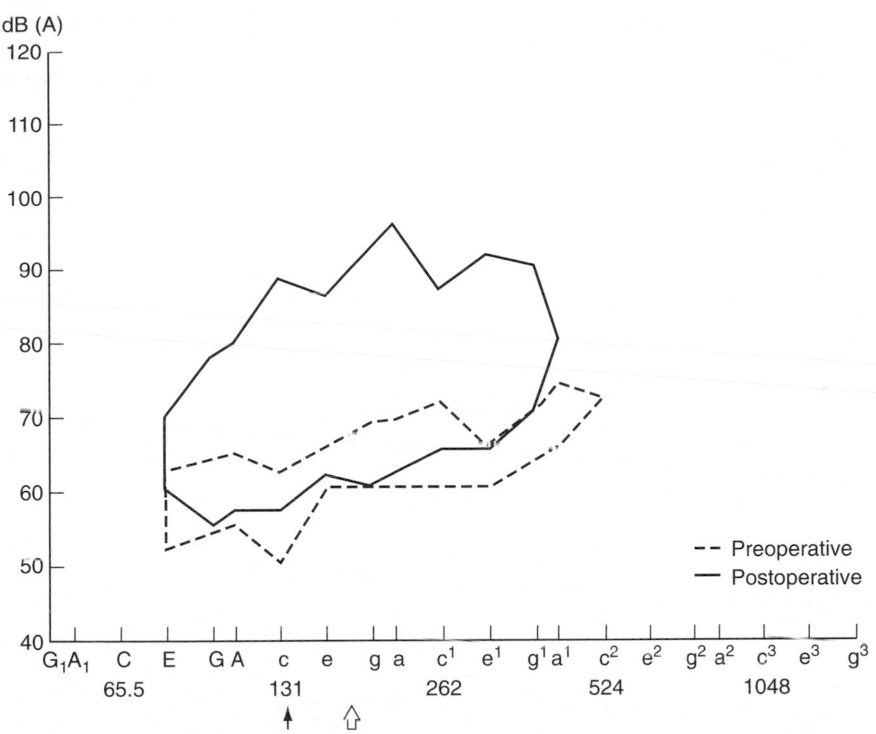

Figure 33.5 *An example of a VRP before and after medialization laryngeal framework surgery of a 43-year-old male. Preoperatively the habitual pitch of the voice was 180 Hz. The preoperative VRP showed a maximal dynamic range of 12 dB, a dynamic range at the level of the habitual pitch of 7 dB, a maximal vocal intensity of 74 dB and a melodic range of 33 semitones. Three months after a combination of thyroplasty type 1 and arytenoid adduction, the habitual pitch was 131 Hz. The postoperative VRP showed a maximal dynamic range of 33 dB, a dynamic range at the level of the habitual pitch of 30 dB, a maximal vocal intensity of 95 dB and a melodic range of 30 semitones.*

⇧ = mean F_0 preoperatively (180 Hz)

▲ = mean F_0 postoperatively (131 Hz)

sity. Furthermore, a VRP presents an easily interpretable and quick overview of the vocal capacity, somewhat resembling the audiogram in audiology, with which every laryngologist is familiar.

Figure 33.5 is an example of a VRP before and after medialization laryngeal framework surgery of a 43-year-old male with a severe dysphonia for 2 years, caused by an immobile right hemilarynx following excision of a glomus tumor and consequently an insufficient glottis closure. Apart from the fact that the voice before correction of the insufficient glottis closure was weak and breathy, the habitual pitch of the voice (180 Hz) was too high for a male. The maximal phonation time was 6 seconds. The VRP before medialization laryngeal framework surgery showed a marked restriction in the dynamic range and maximal vocal intensity. Three months after thyroplasty type 1 the voice was sonorous and stable, with a habitual pitch of 131 Hz, which is considered to be within the normal male range. The maximal phonation time had increased to 26 seconds. The postoperative VRP showed an almost normal vocal capacity for an untrained male voice.

In addition, the maximal phonation time of the sustained vowel /a/ is a very simple and effective method to obtain some information concerning vocal fold efficiency. Although clearly other factors beside vocal efficiency (e.g. pulmonary condition) will have influence on the maximal phonation time, it is an effective tool, which can be used in the office to determine the gain obtained in vocal fold efficiency in the same subject. This is especially helpful in the patients undergoing medialization laryngeal framework surgery.

Determination of the habitual pitch of the speaking voice is obviously important in patients with pitch-related dysphonias. Furthermore, in combination with the VRP it shows which part of the voice profile is most important for the speaking voice. The mean vocal pitch (MVP) is determined during spontaneous speech by means of electroglottography (Glottal Frequency Analyzer – Teltec type GFA 06, Sweden).

From the above-mentioned voice assessment methods the following objective voice parameters can be derived:

- maximal phonation time (Phon Time) in seconds of a sustained vowel /a/ (best of three efforts);
- maximal dynamic intensity range (Dyn Range) in decibels obtained from the VRP (Fig 33.6a);
- dynamic intensity range at the mean habitual pitch of the speaking voice (Dyn Range MVP) in decibels obtained from the VRP (Fig 33.6b);
- maximal vocal intensity (Max Int) in decibels obtained from the VRP (Fig 33.6c);
- melodic range (Mel Range) in semitones obtained from the VRP (Fig 33.6d);
- mean habitual pitch of the voice during speech (MVP).

These voice parameters have been used for the evaluation of the results of laryngeal framework surgery.

During laryngeal framework surgical intervention, voice monitoring is usually performed by the surgeon's ear. Sometimes, however, it can be helpful to perform another type of voice monitoring as well. Recent developments in computerized voice assessment programs presently allow for very quick acoustical voice assessment, almost resembling

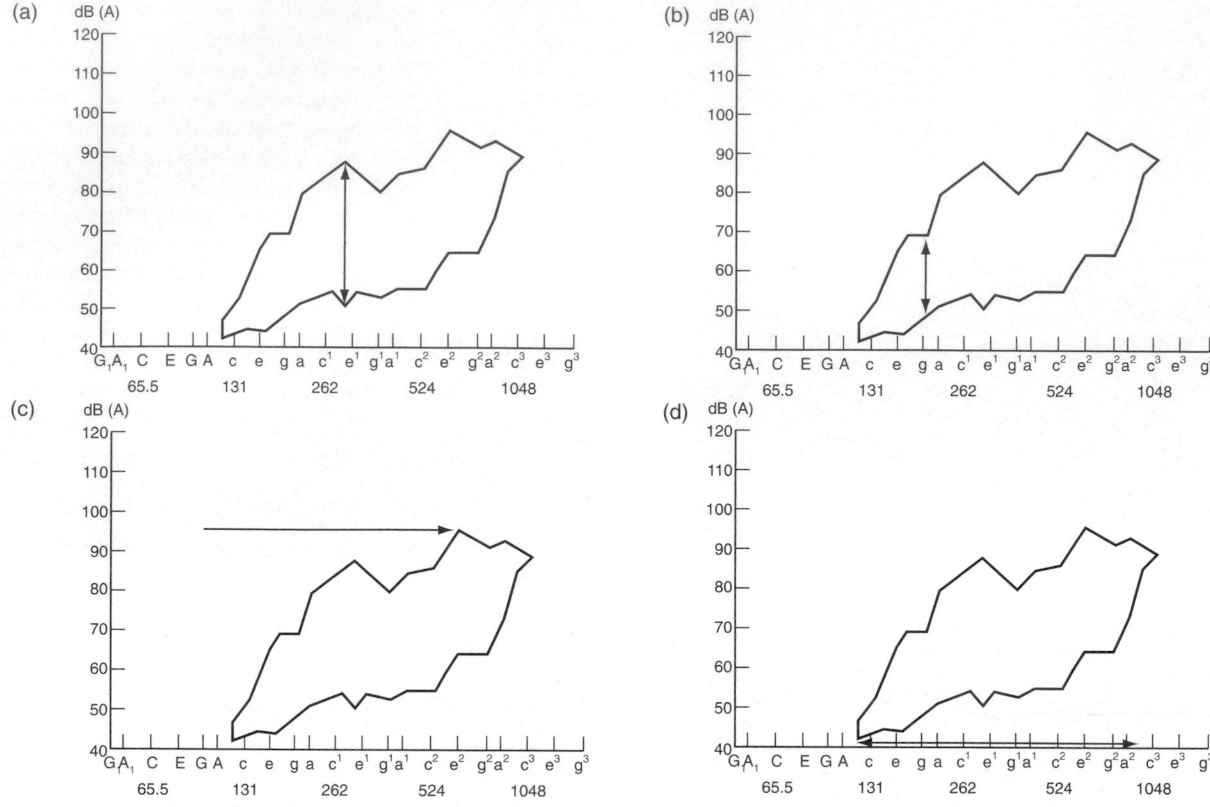

Figure 33.6 *Voice range profile. Vertical axis: vocal intensity in decibels. Horizontal axis: vocal pitch (fundamental frequency) in Herz and in musical notes. (a) Determination of maximal dynamic range (dB). (b) Determination of dynamic range at the level of the habitual speaking pitch (dB). (c) Determination of the maximal vocal intensity (dB). (d) Determination of the melodic range (semitones).*

online voice monitoring. This can be used during the laryngeal framework surgical procedure to assist the surgeon in deciding upon the optimal degree of vocal fold medialization or correction of vocal fold tension. Several aspects of the voice can thus be taken into consideration.

Figure 33.7 depicts a voice sample of a sustained vowel /a/ of a female patient with a breathy and weak voice as a result of long-standing unilateral vocal fold paralysis. The signal is presented on a time scale without further analysis. The upper trace demonstrates the situation at the beginning of the surgical intervention, with a marked lack of periodicity in the signal. First a thyroplasty type 1 was performed, which resulted in a much stronger but still breathy voice. The voice sample on the middle trace following the thyroplasty type 1 shows more regularity, but is not a perfect voice tracing. Because of a slight persisting glottis insufficiency posteriorly and a less than optimal voice, it was decided to expand the procedure with an additional arytenoid adduction. The lower trace shows the voice result obtained perioperatively following the arytenoid adduction, demonstrating a nice periodic signal.

Figure 33.8 shows an example of voice spectra of sustained phonations of the vowel /a/ of a female patient undergoing arytenoid adduction for a severe glottic insufficiency 4 years following resection of a glomus tumor with a unilateral vagal nerve palsy. The upper trace at the

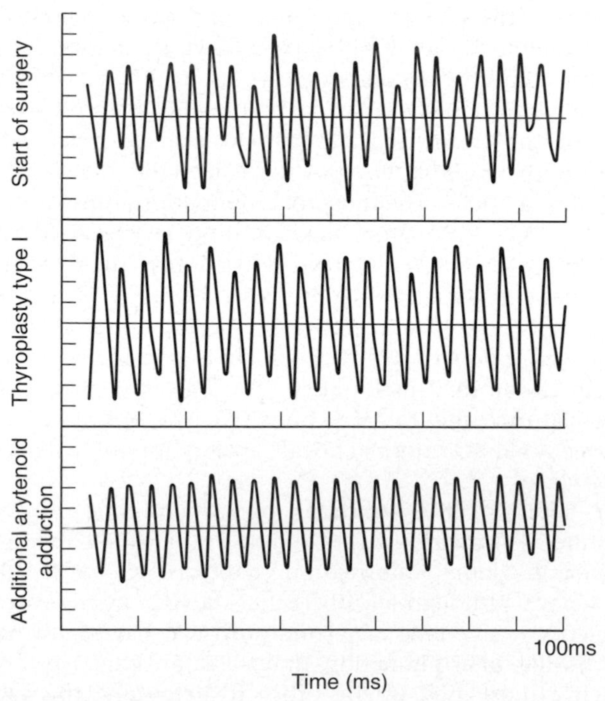

Figure 33.7 *Time signal of voice recorded during laryngeal framework surgery.*

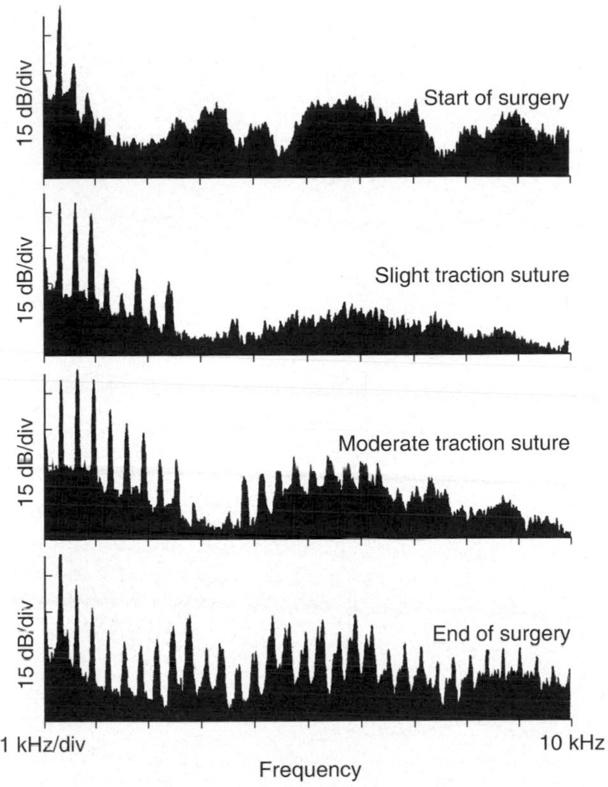

Figure 33.8 *Voice spectra recorded during arytenoid adduction.*

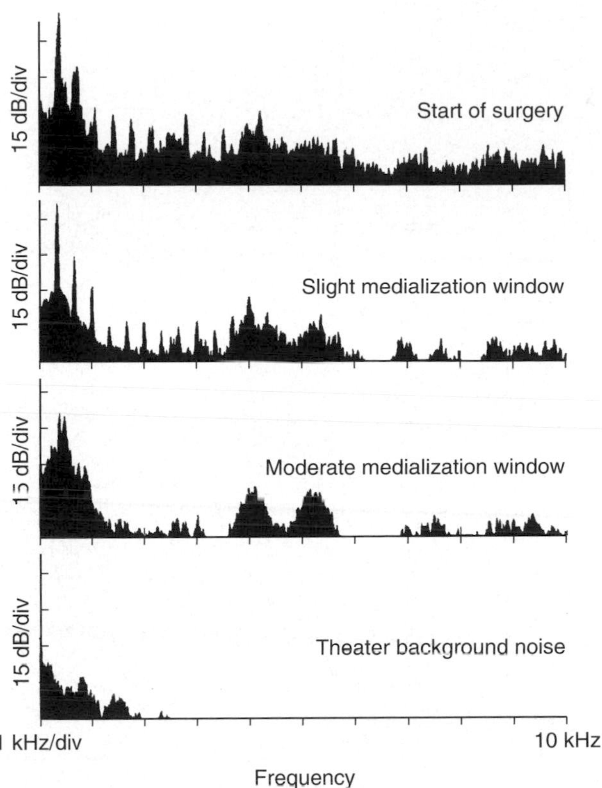

Figure 33.9 *Voice spectra recorded during thyroplasty type 1.*

beginning of the surgery shows a lot of noise, especially in the higher frequency regions, as is often observed in breathy voices with incomplete glottis closure. Furthermore, this signal shows a lack of harmonics. The second and third traces were made with, respectively, little and moderate traction on the arytenoid sutures. Gradually more harmonics appear in the spectra and the noise level diminishes. The lower trace represents the situation at the end of the procedure, demonstrating a rich spectrum with a favorable harmonics-to-noise ratio.

Figure 33.9 shows an example of voice spectra of sustained phonations of the vowel /a/ of a female patient undergoing thyroplasty type 1 for a moderate glottic insufficiency 1 year following penetrating neck injury with a unilateral recurrent laryngeal nerve (RLN) palsy. The upper trace at the beginning of the surgery shows some noise and a poor harmonics-to-noise ratio. The second trace following the creation and slight medialization of the cartilage window shows a marked reduction of the noise and an improved signal-to-noise ratio. The third trace shows the situation with slightly more medialization by means of a Silastic wedge. The harmonics in this signal have disappeared and the fundamental is not clearly distinguishable. This situation represents an overcorrection and was associated with a pressed rough voice quality. The wedge was removed and the cartilage window was fixed with sutures in the position of the second voice trace. The last trace demonstrates the background noise in the operating theater.

This possibility of voice analysis during surgery can be very helpful, especially in those cases where minor changes in the position of the cartilage window have a major impact on the voice result and in cases requiring subtle voice changes.

Classification of laryngeal framework surgery

A classification of laryngeal framework surgery (Fig 33.10a–h) as proposed by Isshiki and some brief characteristics of the procedure and the indications is given below.

Surgery of the thyroid cartilage, the so-called thyroplasties

- Thyroplasty type 1, designed for medialization of the vocal fold and vocal fold augmentation, by means of impression of a cartilage window cut in the thyroid ala. Especially effective in the anterior part of the vocal fold. Indicated for correction of moderate incomplete glottis closure in vocal fold palsy and cases of incomplete glottis closure with mobile vocal folds, such as vocal fold atrophy or presbyphonia. Can be used bilaterally. The most widely used thyroplasty, either as a single procedure or in combination with other types of laryngeal framework surgery.

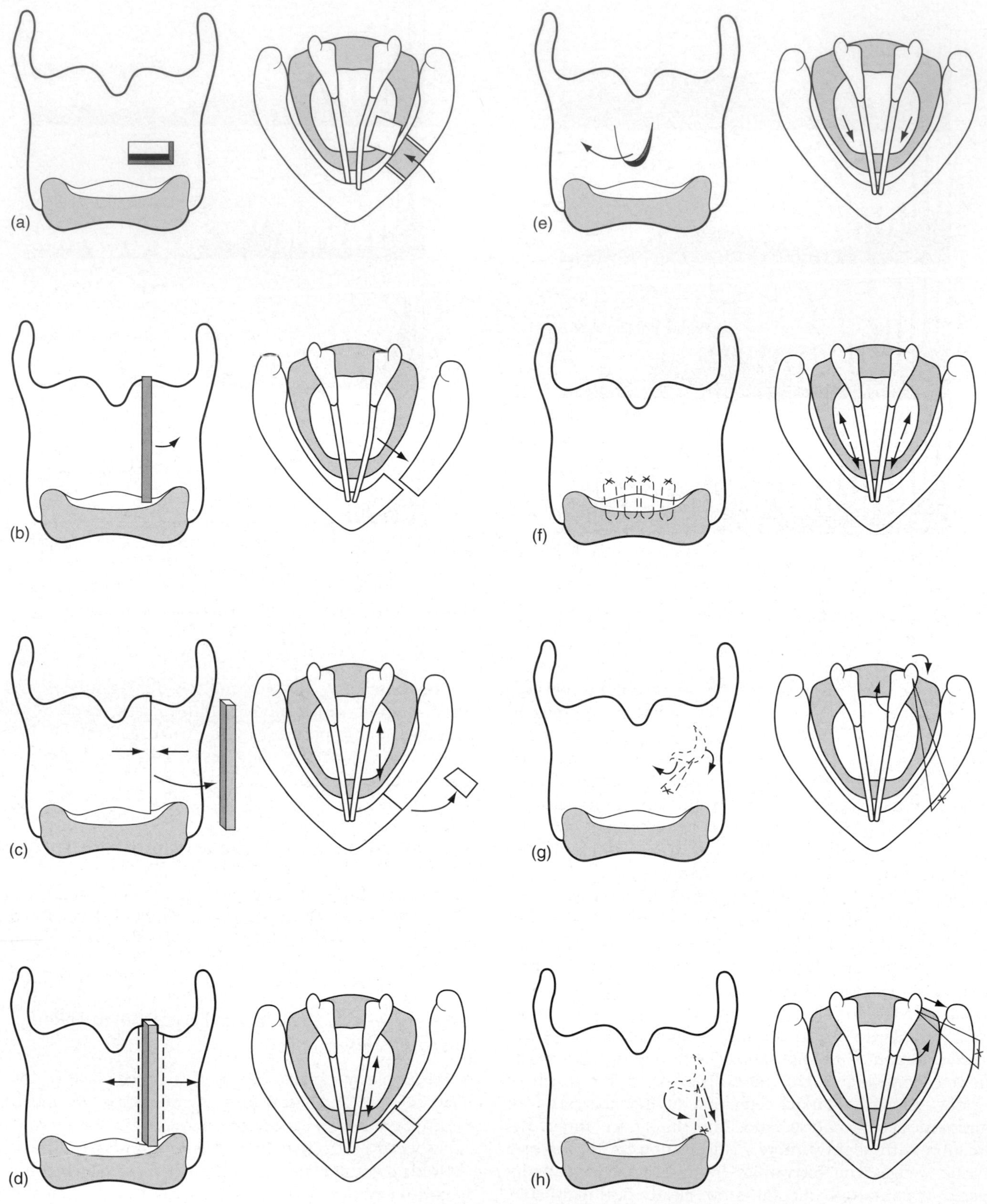

Figure 33.10 *Classification of laryngeal framework surgery: (a) thyroplasty type 1; (b) thyroplasty type 2; (c) thyroplasty type 3; (d) thyroplasty type 4; (e) anterior commissure advancement thyroplasty; (f) cricothyroid approximation; (g) arytenoid adduction; (h) arytenoid abduction.*

- Thyroplasty type 2, designed for lateralization of the vocal fold by means of lateralizing part of the thyroid ala, unilaterally or bilaterally, by making a vertical incision on the thyroid ala and interposing the anterior segment beneath the posterolateral segment. Seldom-used type of thyroplasty, using an anterior midline modification with interposition of a strip of cartilage, suggested in the treatment of spasmodic dysphonia recently. Will not be further discussed in this chapter.
- Thyroplasty type 3, designed for reduction of vocal fold tension by means of reducing the anterior–posterior dimensions of the thyroid ala. Main indications include voice therapy-resistant mutational dysphonia, vocal fold atrophy or hypoplasia and otherwise stiffened vocal folds. Occasionally used type of thyroplasty. If used for atrophy or hypoplasia, then more often than not in combination with thyroplasty type 1. Can be used bilaterally and in mobile vocal folds.
- Thyroplasty type 4, designed for increasing vocal fold tension by increasing the anterior–posterior dimensions of the thyroid ala. Seldom-used type of thyroplasty, suggested as alternative procedure for pitch-raising surgery. Will not be further discussed.
- Anterior commissure advancement thyroplasty, designed for increasing vocal fold tension by displacing a thyroid cartilage flap attached to the anterior commissure anteriorly. Occasionally used thyroplasty, especially used following failed other pitch-raising surgeries in gender dysphonia.

Surgery involving the cricoid and thyroid cartilage

Cricothyroid approximation, designed for increasing vocal fold tension by simulating the position of cricoid and thyroid during falsetto phonation, mimicking contraction of the cricothyroid muscles, is used for correction of lax vocal folds, occasionally in cases of laryngeal palsy. It is often used in combination with thyroplasty type 1 and also for pitch-raising surgery in cases of androphonia or transsexual gender dysphonia.

Surgery involving the arytenoid cartilage

- Arytenoid adduction, designed for vocal fold medialization and correction of vocal fold level difference, by means of sutures attached to the muscular process of the arytenoid mimicking the action of the lateral cricoarytenoid muscle. Indicated for correction of severe incomplete glottis closure in cases of vocal fold palsy. Especially effective for closure of dorsal glottal gap. Can only be used unilaterally and is often used in combination with thyroplasty type 1.
- Arytenoid abduction, designed for vocal fold lateralization, by means of sutures pulling arytenoid laterally. Indicated for correction of airway compromise. Will not be further discussed in this chapter.

Combinations of above-mentioned laryngeal framework surgical procedures

Often combinations of above-mentioned laryngeal framework surgical procedures are used for the best result.

Surgical techniques

The laryngeal framework surgical procedures are performed following an intramuscular premedication of atropine sulfate (0.5 mg) and morphine (10 mg).

At surgery the patient is placed in the supine position with the head extended in such a way that the patient is comfortable and can maintain that position for 1–2 hours. If necessary, rolled sheets can be placed beneath the shoulders. An intravenous drip with saline 0.9% is started to enable the administration of medication intravenously if so required. Vital signs are monitored throughout the procedure by means of pulse oximetry and heart-rate monitoring. Drapes are positioned over a bar placed 10 cm above the patient's chin, leaving the nose and mouth free for access of the fiberoptic endoscope, which is used during several stages of the procedure to monitor the endolaryngeal situation. The surgeon can have a view of the endolaryngeal situation on the video monitor during the procedure. The changes in quality of the voice are, however, the most important assessment parameters during the surgery.

Topographical landmarks consisting of the thyroid notch, the lower border of the thyroid cartilage and the cricoid cartilage are marked with ink on the skin.

Local anesthesia is obtained with infiltration of 10–20 ml of 1% lidocaine hydrochloride with 0.001% epinephrine.

Prophylactic antibiotic treatment is started at the beginning of the surgery and is continued for 5 days postoperatively. Postoperative voice rest ranges from 2 to 4 days, depending upon the laryngoscopic findings. Occasionally steroid administration is added in cases of exceptional postoperative endolaryngeal swelling or codeine medication in cases of excessive coughing.

Postoperative voice therapy, if indicated, in my opinion should start no sooner than 2 months following surgery. The instability of the voice associated with reactive postoperative swelling and readaption of the laryngeal system to the new situation should not be burdened too soon with intensive voice therapeutic training.

Correction of incomplete glottis closure

Thyroplasty type 1

The procedure of thyroplasty type 1 is based on the concept that medial displacement of a cartilage window cut in the thyroid ala, at the level of the vocal fold, will medialize this vocal fold.

The skin incision is made horizontally, in a skin crease, on the anterior portion of the neck at the lower margin

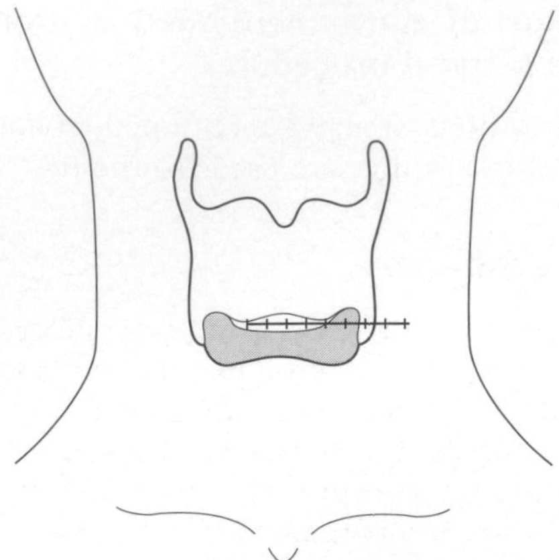

Figure 33.11 *Skin incision for thyroplasty type 1.*

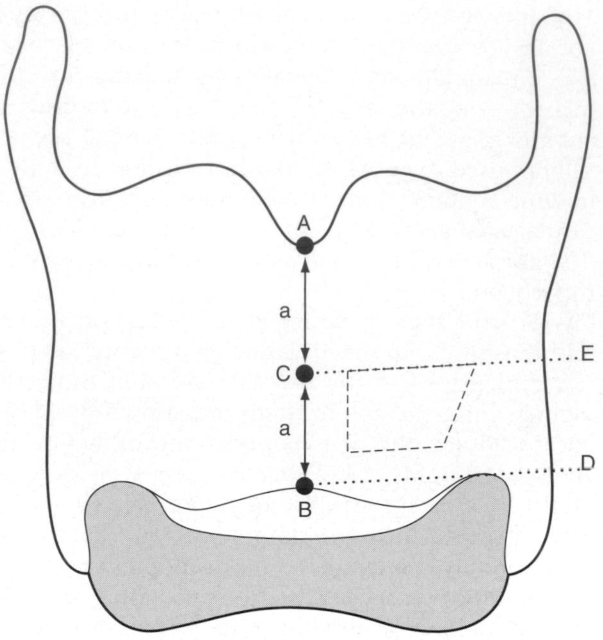

Figure 33.12 *Landmarks for design of cartilage window of thyroplasty type 1: A, thyroid notch; B, midpoint lower margin thyroid ala; C, midpoint between A and B, coinciding with anterior commissure; D, line along upper parts of lower margin of thyroid ala; E, line parallel to D, through C, coinciding with level vocal fold.*

of the thyroid cartilage extending from 1 cm paramedial on the unaffected side to 1 cm lateral from the posterior margin of the thyroid cartilage on the affected side (Fig 33.11). The incision should be sufficiently large to enable extension of the surgery to an arytenoid adduction or cricothyroid approximation. Subplatysmal flaps are elevated to obtain sufficient exposure of the thyroid ala. The strap muscles overlying the thyroid cartilage are retracted laterally and their medial aspects are cut for a better exposure. Stay sutures are placed through the cut ends of these muscles, to allow for repair at the end of the procedure.

The cartilage of the thyroid ala is exposed on the affected side.

The surgical landmarks (Fig 33.12) for the thyroplasty type 1 procedure are:

- the thyroid notch (A);
- the midline point (B) of the lower margin of the thyroid ala;
- the midway point (C) between the two former landmarks (determined with a caliper), which coincides with the position of the anterior commissure;
- the lower margin of the thyroid ala on the involved side; and
- a horizontal line (E) drawn from the point marking the anterior commissure in the posterior direction; this line marks the level of the vocal fold and is running parallel to an imaginary straight line (D) along the lower margin of the thyroid ala.

All these landmarks are marked with electrocautery applied to the caliper. At the level of the vocal fold a cartilage 'window' is designed, adjusted to the individual dimensions (approximately 5 × 8–10 mm in females, 6 × 10–12 mm in males). In order to design the correct position of this cartilage window, it is important to take notice of the lower thyroid ala margin when designing the line representing the level of the vocal fold. This line representing the level of the vocal fold coincides with the upper limit of the cartilage window. A vertical line 4–5 mm paramedial marks the anterior limit of the cartilage window. A horizontal line just above the lower thyroid ala margin marks the lower limit of the cartilage window. The posterior limit of the cartilage window is 10 (female) to 12 mm (male) superiorly and 8 (female) to 10 mm (male) inferiorly from the anterior limit.

The reason for the smaller dimension of the cartilage window inferiorly is that the upper margin of the cricoid cartilage is ascending posteriorly, medial to the inner thyroid cartilage surface (Fig 33.13). This can interfere with medialization of the cartilage window if it is designed too much posteriorly, because the lower posterior part of the cartilage window will be pressed against the lateral surface of the cricoid cartilage.

In order to prepare the cartilage window, the overlying perichondrium is incised, elevated and removed. The cartilage window is then cut either with a knife blade no. 15 or 11 in young or female patients, or, in cases of cartilage calcification, with a fine cutting drill. If a drill is required, the corners of the cartilage window are first marked with the drill. In highly calcified larynges it can be helpful to first drill multiple small holes along the lines of the designed window, and later connect these holes in order to cut the cartilage.

The cartilage window incisions are now completed over the entire cartilage thickness, taking care to preserve the inner perichondrium. The last attachments are freed with a small Rosen dissector or freer. The inner perichondrium

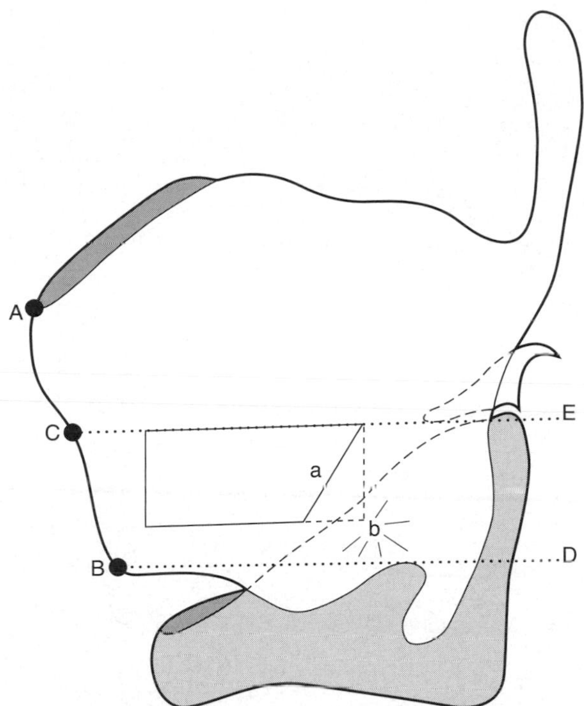

Figure 33.13 *Design of cartilage window of thyroplasty type 1. (a) Correctly designed cartilage window; (b) cartilage window too long in lower posterior corner. Medialization of window impeded by cricoid cartilage.*

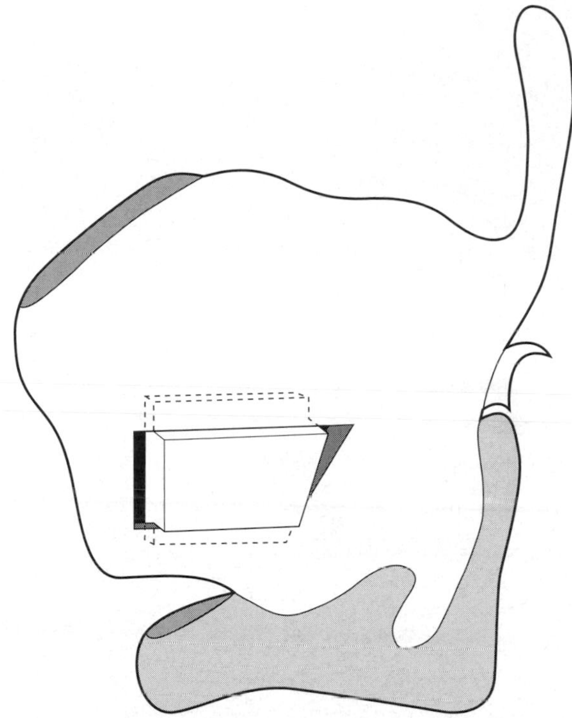

Figure 33.14 *Thyroplasty type 1. Medialization of cartilage window by means of Silastic wedge. Wedge is self-retaining, kept in position by flanges medial to thyroid cartilage. Suitable for more than moderate medialization (3–5 mm).*

around the window is then carefully elevated from the inner cartilage surface in order to enable medialization of the cartilage window. The cartilage window is depressed inward to various depths during phonation to decide the optimal degree of vocal fold medialization under fiberoptic and voice monitoring. More medialization is often required posteriorly and inferiorly than superiorly and anteriorly. Care should be especially taken not to overcorrect anteriorly. Prior to testing the voice the surgeon has to make sure that the head and neck are in a neutral position. It is advisable to let the patient phonate at different intensities and frequencies and to include a short phrase of connected speech in order to get a better impression of the obtained result. For fixation of the cartilage window in the optimal position, either a small Silastic (or other material) wedge (Fig 33.14), or plug (Fig 33.15), or sutures (Fig 33.16) can be used, depending upon the required degree of medialization. The wedge or plug can be modeled according to the requirements. Sometimes a posterior extension is added in an effort to correct a posterior insufficient closure. Personally, I prefer to perform an additional arytenoid adduction in such cases, rather than try to insert a wedge with a very large posterior extension. Usually a snug-fitting wedge, requiring no further fixation, is considered the best option.

Overcorrection at the subglottic, glottic, or supraglottic level is recognized by a pressed and hyperkinetic, rough, voice quality and sometimes at laryngoscopy a protruding

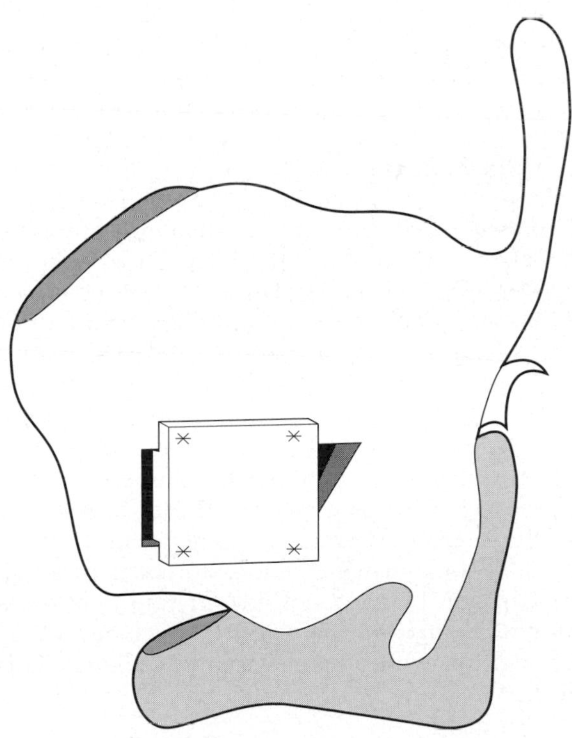

Figure 33.15 *Thyroplasty type 1. Medialization of cartilage window by means of Silastic plug. Plug is kept in position by sutures. Suitable for moderate medialization (2–4 mm).*

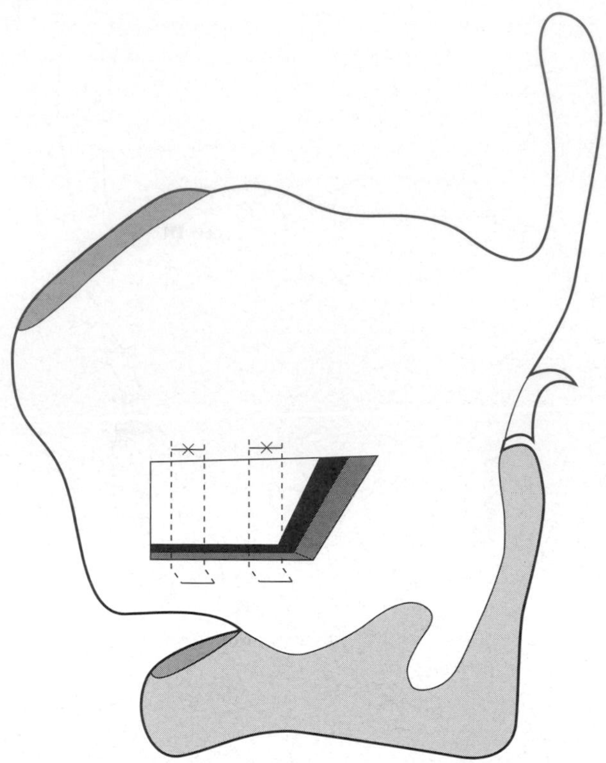

Figure 33.16 *Thyroplasty type 1. Medialization of cartilage window by means of sutures. Suitable for slight medialization (1–2 mm).*

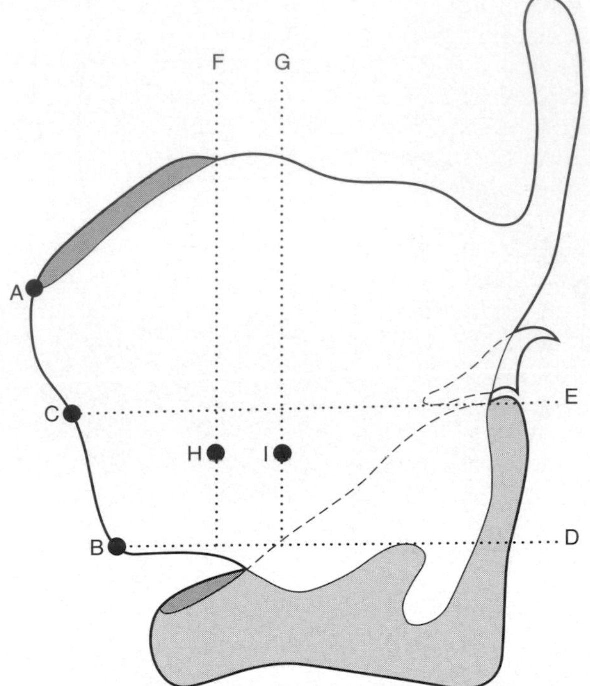

Figure 33.17 *Landmarks for design of arytenoid adduction sutures: A, thyroid notch; B, midpoint lower margin thyroid ala; C, midpoint between A and B, coinciding with anterior commissure; D, line along upper parts of lower margin of thyroid ala; E, line parallel to D, through C, coinciding with level of vocal fold; F, vertical line at junction anterior and middle third of thyroid ala; G, vertical line at junction anterior and posterior half of thyroid ala; H and I, projected points of exit for arytenoid adduction sutures.*

ventricular fold can then be seen. When in doubt whether the optimal degree of medialization has been achieved, the silicon wedge should be removed and remodeled. If the result is not satisfactory, an additional arytenoid adduction should be considered.

Contrary to the recently advocated procedure of removing the cartilage window in order to more directly influence the shape and position of the vocal fold by using differently shaped silicon implants,[8,36,43,61] I personally prefer to leave the cartilage window *in situ*, as a buttress against endolaryngeal extrusion of the silicon implant.

Because thyroplasty type 1 does not interfere with vocal fold mobility, it can be used bilaterally, if necessary, in cases with incomplete glottis closure and mobile vocal folds. The medialization achieved by this procedure is more outspoken in the anterior part of the vocal fold.

Before the surgery is terminated, cricoid and thyroid cartilages are approximated anteriorly to test if vocal fold tension correction by means of cricothyroid approximation will further improve the voice. If this is indeed the case, an additional cricothyroid approximation will be performed.

Arytenoid adduction

The procedure of arytenoid adduction is based on the concept that the vocal fold can be medialized by placing sutures through the muscular process of the arytenoid and pulling these sutures in the same direction as the lateral cricoarytenoid muscle and the vocalis muscle would exert traction on the muscular process.

The skin incision and flap preparation is the same as described for thyroplasty type 1.

The surgical landmarks (Fig 33.17) for the arytenoid adduction are:

- the lower margin of the thyroid ala on the involved side;
- a horizontal line (E) drawn from the point marking the anterior commissure in the posterior direction; this line marks the level of the vocal fold and is running parallel to an imaginary straight line (D) along the lower margin of the thyroid ala (also see landmarks for thyroplasty type 1);
- the posterior margin of the thyroid ala;
- the upper horn of the thyroid ala;
- the lower horn of the thyroid ala;
- the cricothyroid joint;
- the posterolateral surface of the cricoid cartilage;
- the cricoarytenoid joint;
- the muscular process of the arytenoid cartilage;

- a vertical line (F) at the junction of the anterior and middle third of the thyroid ala;
- a vertical line (G) at the junction of the anterior and the posterior half of the thyroid ala; and
- points of exit (H and I) for the sutures along the two vertical lines, located below the line marking the level of the vocal fold.

Following exposure of the thyroid ala cartilage, the posterior margin is exposed over its entire length, elevating and sectioning the thyropharyngeal musculature. Elevation of the perichondrium is continued around the posterior margin to the inner surface of the thyroid cartilage. For a good exposure of the arytenoid region, the cricothyroid joint is dislocated, and the superior horn of the thyroid cartilage may be sectioned (sometimes it is easier not to dislocate the cricothyroid joint and section the upper horn of the thyroid cartilage, but to resect a part of the posterior thyroid ala margin to achieve access to the arytenoid area).

While dislocating the cricothyroid joint and later while locating and approaching the muscular process of the arytenoid, efforts should be made to preserve the RLN, which runs just posteriorly of the cricothyroid joint and enters the larynx between the cricothyroid joint and the cricoarytenoid joint. Although in most cases in which arytenoid adduction is indicated, the underlying cause of the dysphonia will be a recurrent nerve palsy, very often a subclinical reinnervation has taken place, which is insufficient to restore laryngeal mobility but which may provide the musculature with sufficient tonicity to positively influence voice quality.

Following the dislocation of the cricothyroid joint and the resection of the upper thyroid horn, the posterior thyroid margin can be rotated anteromedially, thus exposing the arytenoid region (occasionally in males partial resection of the posterior part of the thyroid ala is required for a better exposure). The arytenoid cartilage can then be palpated through the surrounding musculature. The line on the thyroid ala representing the level of the vocal fold will point in the direction of the muscular process of the arytenoid, which is approximately on the same level as the vocal fold. The cricoarytenoid joint is approached following the posterolateral surface of the cricoid cartilage upward from the dislocated cricothyroid joint. The articular facet of the cricoarytenoid joint is located on the superior lateral ridge of the cricoid plate, approximately 1 cm (females) to 1.5 cm (males) cranially from the cricothyroid joint. During this part of the procedure, it is essential to stay on the solid cricoid cartilage surface in order to prevent entering the piriform sinus, which overlies the muscular process. The cricoarytenoid joint is opened slightly for a sure identification and to exclude cricoarytenoid joint fixation. Observance of the white, glistening articular facet ensures unmistakable identification. Care should be taken not to open the joint too widely to avoid later dislocation.

It can be difficult to grasp the muscular process and the arytenoid joint surface, including some surrounding muscular tissue, with a suture. Therefore two or three sutures are passed, of which the first one is often used to guide the following sutures, taking a larger bite of tissue. Gore-Tex® 5-0 or nylon 4-0 sutures are used for this purpose. Which of the sutures has the best grip on the arytenoid can be tested under fiberoptic control. This suture is tied around the muscular process and is then passed anteriorly in the general direction of the lateral cricoarytenoid and thyroarytenoid muscles, which will result in rotation of the vocal process medially, thus medializing the vocal fold. One end of the suture is brought out in this direction using a straight needle passing through the thyroid ala at the level of the most anterior designed vertical line at the junction of the anterior and middle third of the thyroid ala (F). The other end is brought out at the level of the vertical line at the junction of the anterior and the posterior half of the thyroid ala (G). At this stage it is important to determine whether there is a level difference between both vocal fold processes, which has to be corrected. If there is no important level difference, then the sutures can best be brought out approximately 2–3 mm below the line marking the vocal fold level (E). If a correction of the vocal fold level is required, the suture should be passed lower if the vocal process should be tilted upward, and vice versa.

In cases of calcification it may be necessary to use a cutting drill to pierce the thyroid ala, drilling at the above-mentioned points in a posterior direction. (In the case of a combination of thyroplasty type 1 and arytenoid adduction, the sutures can be attached to the cartilage window; if the combination was anticipated, holes can be drilled in the designed cartilage window for this purpose before actually cutting the window.) In calcified larynges it can be helpful to pass a hollow needle from anterior through the drilled holes in the direction of the arytenoid and then guide the suture through the posterior end of the hollow needle in the anterior direction, in order to get the suture through the holes.

Again under phonatory control, in order to decide the optimal degree of traction, the suture is tied on the outer surface of the thyroid ala. Usually only mild and subtle traction is required. Care should be taken not to pull too hard. In most cases only one suture is required to achieve a good result and the other sutures can then be removed. Before removing these sutures, the voice is tested while they are being pulled in different directions. Occasionally additional traction in the caudal direction will further improve the voice because of additional correction of the level of the vocal process or in cases of slight overcorrection by the first suture.

Overcorrection is recognized by the pressed and hyperkinetic, sometimes breathy, voice quality and the endoscopic laryngeal image. Because arytenoid adduction restricts laryngeal mobility, it can only be used unilaterally. The medialization achieved with this procedure is more outspoken than can be obtained by means of a thyroplasty type 1, but the arytenoid adduction is technically more demanding. The medialization is noticeable

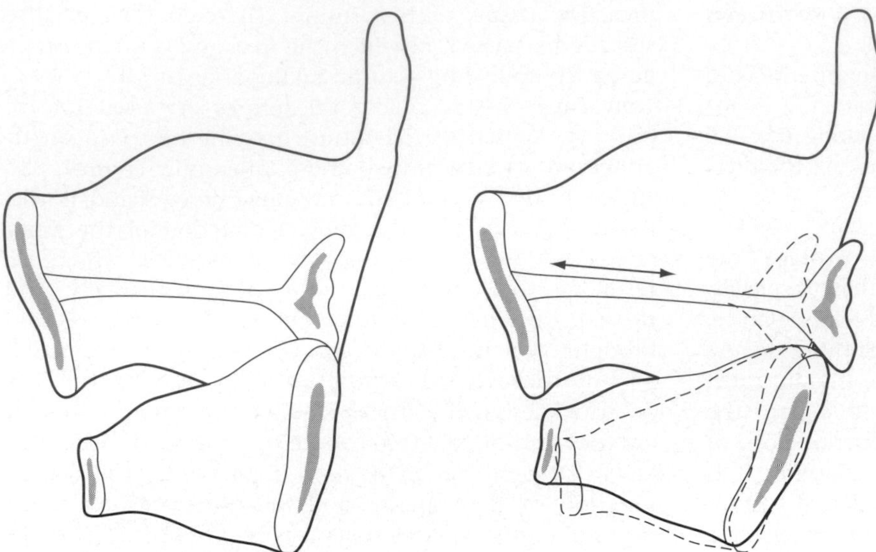

Figure 33.18 *Cricothyroid approximation. Left: resting position. Right: position after cricothyroid approximation, mimicking contraction of cricothyroid muscles as in falsetto phonation, increasing vocal fold tension.*

over the entire length of the vocal fold, but can be insufficient in the anterior part of the vocal fold, as is often the case in vocal fold atrophy. If the result is not satisfactory, an additional thyroplasty type 1 should be considered.

Before the surgery is terminated, cricoid and thyroid cartilages are approximated anteriorly to test if vocal fold tension correction by means of cricothyroid approximation will further improve the voice. If this is indeed the case, an additional cricothyroid approximation will be performed.

Adjustment of vocal fold tension

Cricothyroid approximation

The cricothyroid approximation (Fig 33.18) procedure is based on the concept that approximation of cricoid and thyroid cartilages anteriorly, mimicking their position in falsetto phonation, will result in an increase of tension of both vocal folds.

The skin incision is made horizontally, in a skin crease, on the anterior portion of the neck at the lower margin of the thyroid cartilage extending 2–3 cm bilaterally from the midline. Subplatysmal flaps are elevated to obtain sufficient exposure of the anterior aspect of the thyroid and cricoid cartilages. The strap muscles overlying the thyroid and cricoid cartilages are retracted laterally.

The surgical landmarks (Fig 33.19) for the cricothyroid approximation procedure are:

- the thyroid notch (A);
- the lower margin of the thyroid cartilage anteriorly (B);
- the midway point (C) between the two former landmarks (determined with a caliper), which coincides with the position of the anterior commissure; and
- the cricoid cartilage.

Cricothyroid approximation mimics the function of the cricothyroid muscles, thus stretching the vocal folds and increasing the tension.

Four (or two for unilateral cricothyroid approximation) thick (1-0 or 2-0), double-armored, non-absorbable (Gore-Tex®) sutures are used. Both ends of the sutures are passed through the cricoid just above the lower margin and are advanced along the inner cricoid surface and directed upwards. To reduce the chances of the sutures pulling through, part of the cricothyroid muscle can be included in the suture, or a bolster can be used (2 mm thick Gore-Tex® sheet). The needles are withdrawn at the upper

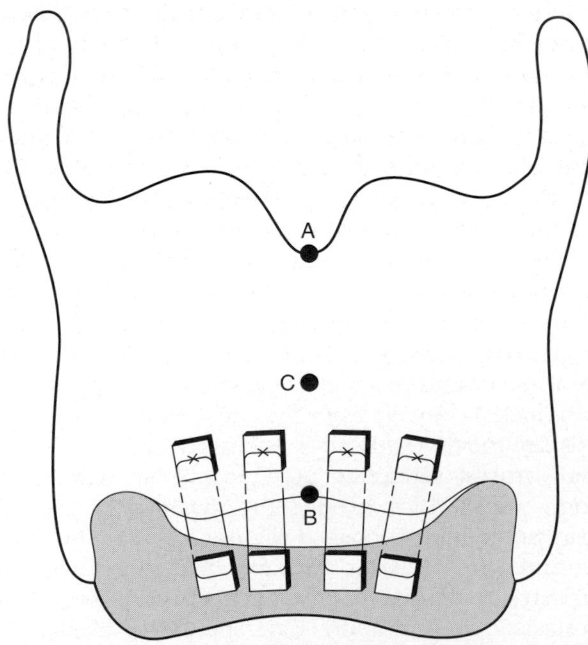

Figure 33.19 *Cricothyroid approximation. Sutures tied over bolsters.*

margin of the cricoid cartilage and then reinserted just behind the lower edge of the thyroid cartilage. They are directed along the inner surface of the thyroid cartilage and directed outward through the middle lower third part of the ala, slightly below the level of the vocal folds. The thyroid cartilage can be difficult to pierce because of calcification. Sometimes a drill is necessary to drill holes.

The voice is tested while the sutures are being pulled, thus approximating cricoid and thyroid cartilages and stretching the vocal folds. In the case of pitch-raising surgery, overcorrection is required up to the point that the vocal folds are so tensed that they can no longer vibrate and the patient is virtually aphonic. The voice will return within the first 2 weeks and thus a pitch rise of more than one octave can be obtained. In the case of correction of vocal fold tension for lax vocal folds or in combination with a medialization type of laryngeal framework surgery, overcorrection is not required.

If the result is satisfactory, the sutures are tied as mattress sutures on the outer surface of the thyroid ala. It is advisable to tie the sutures over a small bolster (2 mm thick Gore-Tex® sheet) to disperse the force on the cartilage. It is, furthermore, wise to have the assistant pushing the cricoid upwards, while tying the sutures, so that the first suture will not pull through the cartilage.

During the whole procedure care should be taken not to enter the airway, which is close to the inner perichondrium of both the cricoid and the lower anterior part of the thyroid cartilage. Perforation of the airway should be suspected if the patient coughs and fiberoptic control is advisable in all cases.

Anterior commissure advancement thyroplasty

The anterior commissure advancement thyroplasty is based on the concept that displacement of the anterior commissure anteriorly will result in an increase of tension of both vocal folds.

The skin incision is made horizontally, in a skin crease, on the anterior portion of the neck a few millimeters above the lower margin of the thyroid cartilage extending 2 cm bilaterally from the midline. Subplatysmal flaps are elevated to obtain sufficient exposure of the anterior aspect of the thyroid cartilage. The strap muscles overlying the thyroid cartilage are retracted laterally.

Surgical landmarks (Fig 33.20) for the anterior commissure advancement are:

- the thyroid notch (A);
- the lower margin of the thyroid cartilage anteriorly (B); and
- the midway point (C) between the two former landmarks (determined with a caliper), which coincides with the position of the anterior commissure.

A superior based cartilage flap is designed with its lower end 2 mm above the lower margin. It extends superiorly about 4 mm above the level of the anterior commissure.

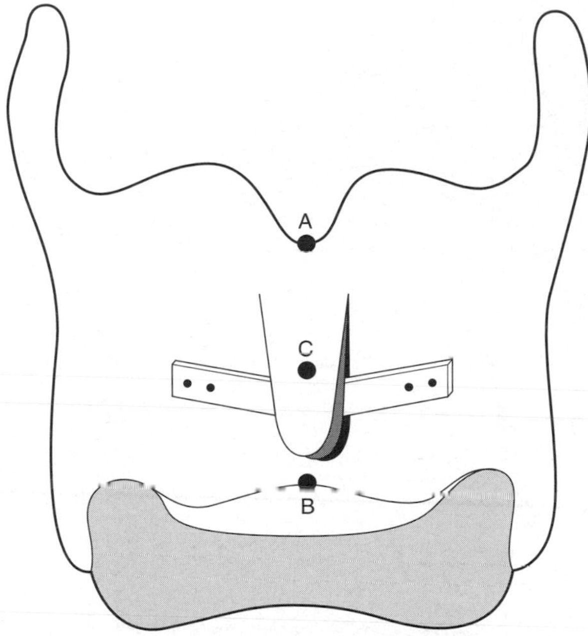

Figure 33.20 *Anterior commissure advancement. Anterior view. Metal shim projecting superior-based cartilage flap. A, Thyroid notch; B, midpoint lower margin of thyroid ala; C, midpoint between A and B, coinciding with anterior commissure.*

Both vertical limbs of the designed flap are approximately 3–4 mm from the midline.

After having incised the external perichondrium, the cartilage flap is cut with a knife blade no. 15 or 11, or with a drill in the case of calcification.

The inner perichondrium of the lower part of the flap is carefully detached with a freer until the flap can be pulled anteriorly, but care should be taken not to detach Broyle's ligament at the anterior commissure insertion.

The flap can be fixed in the anterior position by interposition of a shim, thus stretching the vocal folds (Fig 33.21).

Thyroplasty type 3

Thyroplasty type 3 is based on the concept that a change in the anterior–posterior (A-P) dimension of the thyroid ala will result in a change of vocal fold tension. Excision of a vertical strip of thyroid cartilage will result in a reduction of the A-P dimension of the thyroid ala and consequently in a reduction of the vocal fold tension.

The skin incision is made horizontally, in a skin crease, on the anterior portion of the neck a few mm above the lower margin of the thyroid cartilage extending 2–3 cm bilaterally from the midline. Subplatysmal flaps are elevated to obtain sufficient exposure of the anterior aspect of the thyroid cartilage. The strap muscles overlying the thyroid cartilage are retracted laterally and their medial aspects are cut for a better exposure. Stay sutures are placed through

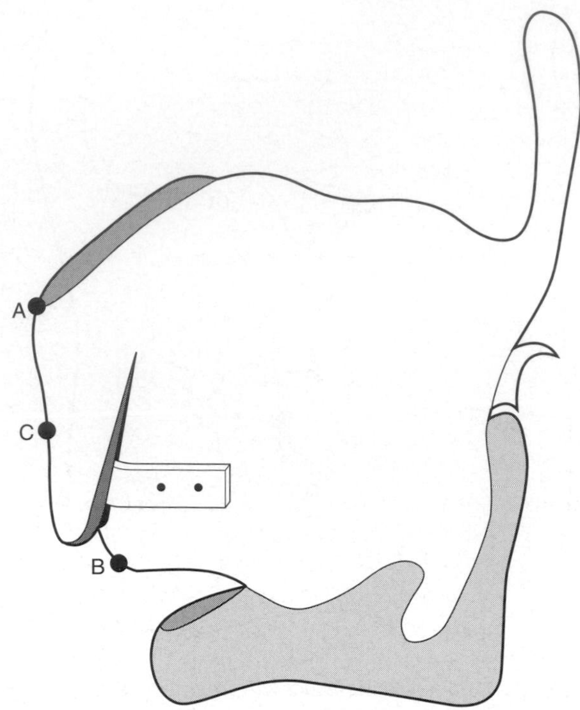

Figure 33.21 *Anterior commissure advancement. Lateral view. Metal shim projecting superior-based cartilage flap. A, Thyroid notch; B, midpoint lower margin of thyroid ala; C, midpoint between A and B, coinciding with anterior commissure.*

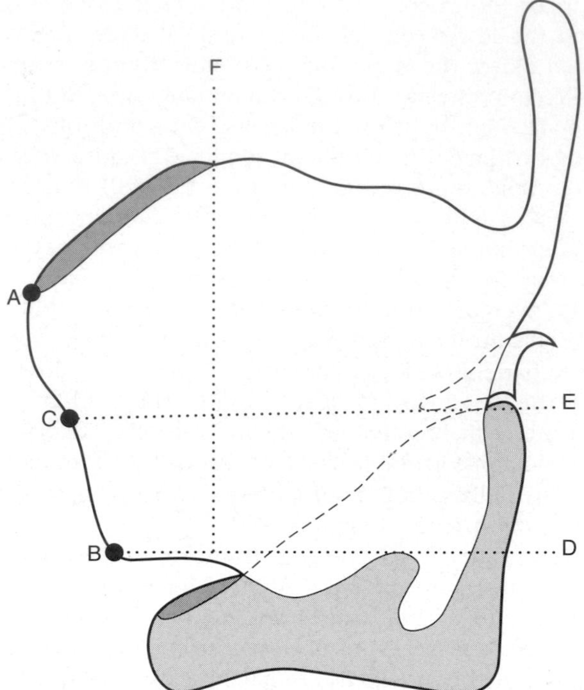

Figure 33.22 *Landmarks for design of thyroplasty type 3. A, Thyroid notch; B, midpoint lower margin thyroid ala; C, midpoint between A and B, coinciding with anterior commissure; D, line along upper parts of lower margin of thyroid ala; E, line parallel to D, through C, coinciding with level of vocal fold; F, vertical line at junction anterior and middle third of thyroid ala.*

the cut ends of these muscles to allow for repair at the end of the procedure. The cartilage of the thyroid ala is exposed on the affected side or bilaterally if indicated.

The surgical landmarks for the thyroplasty type 3 (Fig 33.22) procedure are:

- the thyroid notch (A);
- the lower margin of the thyroid ala on the involved side; and
- a vertical line at the junction of the anterior and middle third of the thyroid ala (F).

The vertical line designed on the thyroid ala one-third from the midline is marked. The outer perichondrium is incised and detached with a freer to expose the cartilage. The cartilage can now be cut with a knife blade no. 15 or 11, or with a drill.

The inner perichondrium is detached on both sides of the incision using a freer.

The anterior and posterior segments can then be overlapped, resulting in shortening of the vocal fold and partial medialization and partial lateralization of the vocal fold. The parts that are medialized or lateralized are dependent upon whether the posterior or the anterior part of the thyroid ala is in the underlay position. The segment can be fixed with mattress sutures (Gore-Tex® or nylon 4-0) in an overlapped position, the anterior part either as underlay or overlay, depending on the effect on the voice.

However, usually the excessive cartilage is excised, after which both segments are approximated with sutures. To determine the dimensions of the segment that is to be removed, the voice is tested and fiberoptic laryngoscopy is performed in the underlay and overlay position. The resection of the determined excess of cartilage is performed rather conservatively, since it is easier to remove another strip of cartilage in cases of undercorrection, than it is to interpose a strip of cartilage in cases of overcorrection. Usually a vertical strip of cartilage of between 2 and 4 mm is removed.

The sutures used for fixation are two mattress sutures and one or two sutures crossing the line of resection, from inside out and vice versa (Gore-Tex® or nylon 4-0). Thus the two cartilage segments are fixed and approximated, but cannot slide over each other (Fig 33.23).

This procedure can be performed unilaterally or bilaterally and can be combined with a thyroplasty type 1 for medialization, which can better control the degree of medialization than the underlay or overlay position of the thyroid segments.

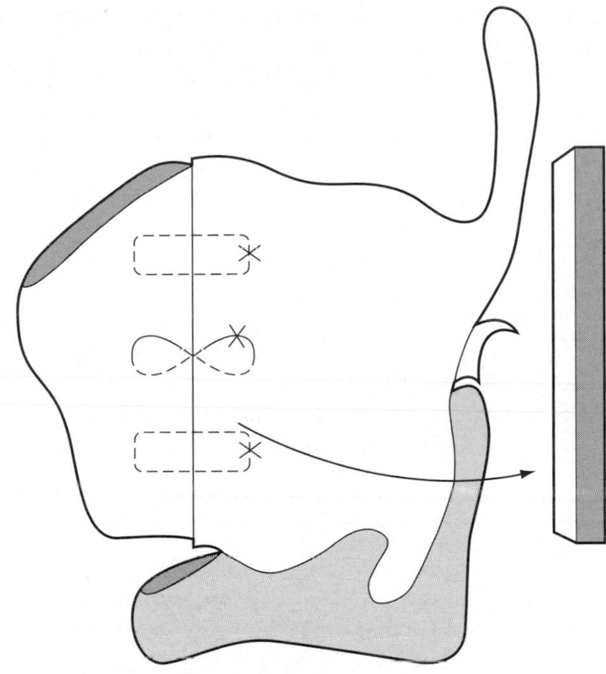

Figure 33.23 *Thyroplasty type 3. Excision of a strip of cartilage along the junction of the anterior and middle third of the thyroid ala. Sutures approximating anterior and posterior segment of the thyroid ala.*

Combinations of laryngeal framework surgery

In cases with a unilateral vocal fold immobility and incomplete glottis closure, a thyroplasty type 1 is usually performed first, because it is the simplest technique. Only if the glottal gap is extremely large or if there is a marked vertical level difference between both vocal folds, will the procedure start with an arytenoid adduction. If this 'single modality' framework surgery results in a satisfactory peroperative voice and adequate glottis closure, the procedure is ended. If the peroperative voice improvement is not satisfactory, then the procedure is extended with the addition of another medialization or tension-adjusting framework technique.

The most frequently used combination in medialization laryngeal framework surgery, in my experience, is thyroplasty type 1 and arytenoid adduction (almost 30% of the cases). The effect of a manual cricothyroid approximation (see adjustment of vocal fold tension) is always tested after the required degree of medialization has been achieved, to hear whether increased tension results in a further improvement of voice. If indicated, surgical cricothyroid approximation can then be added (in approximately 10% of the cases).

Medialization laryngeal framework surgery can thus be performed stepwise as a functionally monitored single-stage procedure under local anesthesia using thyroplasty type 1, arytenoid adduction, cricothyroid approximation or combinations of these procedures (Fig 33.24).

Other employed combinations include thyroplasty type 1 and type 3 and occasionally cricothyroid approximation and anterior commissure advancement.

Special considerations and pitfalls in laryngeal framework surgery

Thyroplasty type 1

Local anesthesia versus general anesthesia

Considering the major impact that even minor changes in the position and medialization of the cartilage window

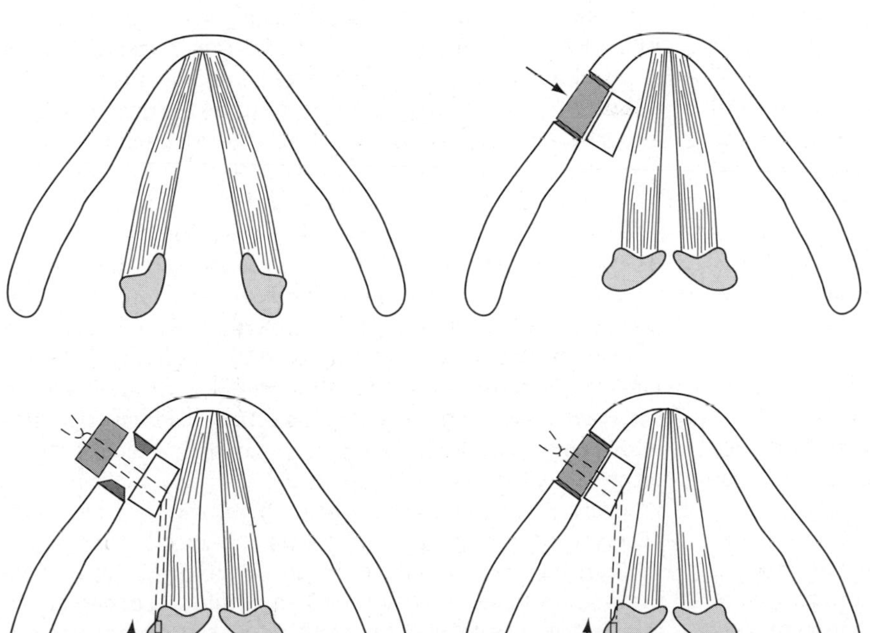

Figure 33.24 *Combination of laryngeal framework surgical techniques.* Upper left*: situation before surgery.* Upper right*: thyroplasty type 1.* Lower left*: additional arytenoid adduction.* Lower right*: additional cricothyroid approximation.*

can have on the voice, voice monitoring during the surgical procedure is considered a sine qua non. General anesthesia is therefore contraindicated and premedication should not be too sedative in order to allow the patient to phonate on request. My personal preference for premedication is 10 mg morphine and 0.5 mg atropine administered intramuscularly 30 minutes prior to surgery. Some surgeons prefer not to administer atropine because the resulting dryness of the mucosa may interfere with voice production. Prevention of laryngospasm and reduction of saliva secretion and consequently reduction of swallowing movements during surgery, which can be obtained by atropine, in my opinion, justify its use.

The above-mentioned considerations hold true for all types of laryngeal framework surgery.

Design of the cartilage window

Two errors which are frequently observed in the design of the cartilage window are:

- a too high projection of the cartilage window, especially in the middle and posterior part of the thyroid ala, resulting in an obliquely designed cartilage window. Usually the anterior landmarks are easily determined, so that the risk of a too high projection of the anterior border of the cartilage window is small. The upper and lower vertical margins of the window should be projected parallel to an imaginary line along the lower border of the thyroid ala. Because the thyroid ala is highly variable in shape and inferior extension, it is not always easy to project an imaginary line along its lower border. Adequate exposure of the lower thyroid ala border can prevent this error. If the cartilage window is made too high, medialization of the window will result in medialization of the ventricular fold instead of the vocal fold. This is recognized by insufficient voice improvement and on fiberoptic laryngeal inspection.
- a too long projection of the cartilage window posteriorly, especially in the posterior lower corner of the window. Because of the position of the cricoid cartilage medially to this area, the medialization of the cartilage window will be impeded posteriorly, resulting in insufficient voice improvement. Resection of the lower posterior corner of the cartilage window will correct this condition.

Endolaryngeal perichondrium

The endolaryngeal perichondrium plays an important role in thyroplasty type 1 and should be preserved as much as possible.

Despite careful preparation, bleeding from the inner perichondrium may occur, which can be difficult to control. Usually this can be managed by application of epinephrine-soaked swabs, or, if this is insufficient, by needle-suction coagulation.

Insufficient elevation of the inner perichondrium from the inner surface of the thyroid ala around the cartilage window will impede medialization of the window, resulting in insufficient voice improvement.

Incision of the inner perichondrium carries the risk of penetration of the laryngeal lumen and can eventually result in dislocation of the cartilage window. If penetration into the airway occurs, this will be at the level of the ventricle because of tears occurring in the inner perichondrium. Should this occur, repair is mandatory. If the airway has been entered and the perichondrium repaired, medialization of the cartilage window should be achieved by means of sutures or a Silastic plug fixed to the thyroid ala, rather than by means of a Silastic wedge, in order to prevent endolaryngeal extrusion.

Fixation of the cartilage window in the optimal position

Usually the Silastic wedge will guarantee sufficient fixation of the cartilage window in the medialized position. Occasionally an additional fixation of the cartilage window and the Silastic plug is required, which can be achieved with nylon 4-0 or Gore-Tex® 5-0 sutures.

Sometimes medialization by means of a Silastic wedge results in overcorrection. Optimal medialization of the cartilage window can then be maintained with sutures or a Silastic plug which is fixed to the thyroid ala with sutures.

Fracture of the thyroid ala cartilage

Fracture of the lower rim of the thyroid ala cartilage can occur if the cartilage window is located near the lower ala border. This can easily occur in female patients because of the smaller dimensions and usually less outspoken calcification of the thyroid cartilage than is encountered in males. Normally fracture of the lower rim does not require repair. Fractures elsewhere can result in instability of the thyroid cartilage and do require repair, for which either nylon or Gore-Tex® sutures can be used.

Edema

In isolated thyroplasty type 1 procedures, endolaryngeal edema occurring during the procedure is rare, but if it occurs it will interfere with voice monitoring. In such a case slight overcorrection is required. It is therefore important to distinguish the voice associated with edema from the voice associated with overcorrection. Edema will result in a rough and unstable voice, whereas overcorrection results in a pressed voice quality.

Severe edema interfering with the airway has not been observed following thyroplasty type 1 only.

Slight vocal fold edema postoperatively is a normal finding and usually requires no treatment. I, however, do not perform thyroplasty type 1 as a day-care treatment, because it is never certain preoperatively whether or not a combination of laryngeal framework surgical procedures will be performed and the potential risk of airway compromise is always present.

Undercorrection and overcorrection

Voice monitoring during the laryngeal framework surgical procedure should be performed in a comfortable and neutral position of the head and neck to prevent under- or overcorrection.

Voice tasks during monitoring should include spoken text as well as sustained vowels at several pitch levels in order to properly judge the obtained result.

Overcorrection can occur when the patient is reluctant to phonate, as can be the case following prolonged periods of severe dysphonia.

Local infection

Prophylactic antibiotics are advisable to prevent local infection. Following this regimen, no serious local infections have been observed following thyroplasty type 1, even in patients who had been previously irradiated to the neck.

Extrusion implant

Endolaryngeal extrusion of the Silastic implant has never been observed in thyroplasty techniques preserving the cartilage window. Several endolaryngeal extrusions have been reported, especially following suboptimal implant placements, following techniques in which the cartilage window is removed.[8,63]

Arytenoid adduction

Local anesthesia versus general anesthesia

Considering the major impact that even minor changes in the position of the arytenoid can have on the voice, voice monitoring is a sine qua non and I, therefore, consider general anesthesia contraindicated (also see comments concerning anesthesia and premedication of thyroplasty type 1).

Exposure of the cricoarytenoid area

Resection of a posterior part of the thyroid ala may be necessary to obtain sufficient exposure of the cricoarytenoid area. This might preclude the necessity to dislocate the cricothyroid joint and sever the superior thyroid horn. On the other hand, resection of the posterior part of the thyroid ala increases the risk of thyroid ala fracture, if used in combination with a thyroplasty 1. Furthermore identification of the cricoarytenoid joint can prove more difficult, without the landmark of the opened cricothyroid joint.

Identification of the cricoarytenoid joint

Identification of the cricoarytenoid joint can be very difficult. The surgeon should always stay on the posterolateral cricoid surface to avoid entering the piriform sinus. Repeated palpation of the muscular process of the arytenoid is required at this stage. The cricothyroid joint is an important surgical landmark, located approximately 1.5 cm caudolaterally from the cricoarytenoid joint.

Personally, I prefer to open the cricoarytenoid joint slightly, for positive identification and visual monitoring of the sutures passing through this joint. Opening the cricothyroid joint too widely will result in posterior instability of the arytenoid. If this occurs, an additional suture can be passed through the arytenoid, which can be fixed to the lower part of the posterior thyroid ala border. This will stabilize the arytenoid joint posteriorly, preventing dislocation anteriorly.

Fixation of the cricoarytenoid joint

Cricoarytenoid joint fixation can be identified by palpation of the arytenoid following exposure of the cricoarytenoid area.

Fixations of the cricoarytenoid joint have to be released before arytenoid adduction can be performed. True ankylosis of the cricoarytenoid joint can make identification almost impossible. In such cases, a 'new joint' has to be created with a drill, to enable adduction of the arytenoid.

Recurrent laryngeal nerve

The recurrent laryngeal nerve is at risk during the approach of the cricoarytenoid joint. Damage to the nerve may increase the dysphonia during the surgery, probably as a result of loss of tonicity that was generated by subclinical or inappropriate innervation (or in cases of joint fixation, even normal innervation!). Therefore, the recurrent laryngeal nerve, passing just posteriorly to the cricothyroid joint, should be preserved whenever possible.

Fractured arytenoid

The arytenoid cartilage can be very fragile and is susceptible to fracture by the sutures being passed through. Including some muscular and capsular tissue in the suture will reduce the risk of fracture. In cases of severe fracture of the arytenoid, the loose fragments have to be removed and the sutures will have to be attached to the surrounding soft tissues.

Undercorrection and overcorrection

Gentle traction on the arytenoid sutures should already result in arytenoid adduction. Failure of adduction can be caused by inappropriately placed sutures, sutures pulled through or unnoticed joint fixation.

Overcorrection can easily occur, especially in the presence of a posterior instability of the cricoarytenoid joint. Overcorrection results in an anterior displacement of the arytenoid and a medial protrusion of the vocal process. Anterior displacement can be corrected by an additional suture that is passed through the arytenoid and is fixed to the posterior thyroid ala border.

Edema

Significant edema of the arytenoid region can be observed during and following arytenoid adduction, especially in cases with ankylosis of the cricoarytenoid joint, requiring special efforts to mobilize the arytenoid. Usually this will not compromise the airway, but occasionally steroid medication has to be administered. Arytenoid adduction as an outpatient procedure is not advisable in any case. Emergency tracheotomies have been reported following day-care surgery.

Edema usually does not develop immediately and therefore normally does not interfere with voice monitoring.

Local infection

Local infection is unlikely if the airway has not been entered. Nevertheless, prophylactic antibiotics are usually administered, because of the frequent combination of arytenoid adduction and thyroplasty 1, which involves the use of an implant.

Cricothyroid approximation

Local anesthesia versus general anesthesia

Considering the major impact that even minor changes in the approximation of cricoid and thyroid can have on the voice, voice monitoring is considered a sine qua non and general anesthesia, contraindicated for most indications of cricothyroid approximation. The possible exception is pitch-raising surgery in male-to-female transsexual patients, in which cases usually a maximal approximation of cricoid and thyroid is required. Therefore, voice monitoring seems to be of slightly less importance. However, also in these cases local anesthesia is preferred to determine the need for additional anterior commissure advancement thyroplasty (see comments concerning anesthesia and premedication of thyroplasty type 1).

Cartilage fracture

Cricothyroid approximation, especially in pitch-raising surgery, results in high tension on the sutures and consequently the risk of cartilage fracture of either cricoid or thyroid cartilage. This can be prevented by dispersing the tension on the mattress sutures, using Silastic or Gore-Tex® bolsters.

Cartilage instability

Cartilage fractures can lead to instability of the cricoid and thyroid cartilages. If necessary, fractures have to be stabilized. Usually the cricothyroid approximation itself will add stability.

The combination of cricothyroid approximation with thyroid notch reduction, as is often indicated in transsexual patients, increases the risk of fracture and instability.

Entering the airway

The airway is in close relationship to the inner surface of the cricoid cartilage. The risk of entering the airway with the sutures is relatively high. Usually this is recognized by a coughing reflex. Nevertheless, it is advisable to perform fiberoptic monitoring.

Local infection

Prophylactic antibiotics are advisable, considering the close relationship of the cricoid and the airway and the tension on the sutures and the bolsters, which increase the risk of local infection.

Anterior commissure advancement thyroplasty

Local anesthesia versus general anesthesia

Considering the major impact that even minor changes in the position of the anterior commissure can have on the voice, voice monitoring is considered a sine qua non and general anesthesia absolutely contraindicated (also see comments concerning anesthesia and premedication of thyroplasty type 1).

Cartilage fracture

Creation of an anterior cartilage window in the thyroid carries the risk of cartilage fracture, since this is the narrowest part of the thyroid.

Combination with thyroid notch correction is contraindicated because of the increased risk of fracture.

Cartilage instability

Cartilage fracture in the anterior part of the thyroid will lead to severe instability and will require repair with sutures or miniplates.

Entering the airway

At and below the level of the anterior commissure the relationship between airway and inner perichondrium is very close, increasing the risk of entering the airway. Usually this is recognized by a coughing reflex. Nevertheless, it is advisable to perform fiberoptic monitoring.

Detachment of Broyle's ligament

In order to advance the anterior commissure cartilage flap, the perichondrium just below the anterior commissure has to be elevated. If this is carried through too high, Broyle's ligament will be detached from the inner thyroid surface. This is recognized by a drop of vocal pitch and a weak voice. Fiberendoscopic evaluation will demonstrate flaccid vocal folds. Repair is then required, suturing the anterior commissure to the thyroid cartilage.

Local infection

Prophylactic antibiotics are advocated, because of the close relationship to the airway and the use of a shim.

Thyroplasty type 3

Local anesthesia versus general anesthesia

Considering the major impact that even minor changes in the A-P dimension of the thyroid cartilage can have on the voice, voice monitoring is considered a sine qua non and general anesthesia absolutely contraindicated (also see comments concerning anesthesia and premedication of thyroplasty type 1).

Cartilage instability

Especially in bilateral thyroplasty type 3 procedures, instability of the thyroid cartilage can occur. Sutures usually are sufficient to stabilize the cartilage pieces but if they are not, then miniplates can be used.

Cartilage fracture

Cartilage fracture can occur, especially when a combination of thyroplasty 3 and thyroplasty 1 is used. This will severely jeopardize the stability of the thyroid cartilage. Repair is mandatory, either with sutures or miniplates.

Entering the airway

The instability of the thyroid cartilage during the surgery, especially in bilateral thyroplasty type 3 cases in combination with thyroplasty type 1, carries the risk of entering the airway at the level of the ventricle, because of tears occurring in the inner perichondrium. Should this occur, repair is mandatory.

Role of voice therapy

Most patients undergoing laryngeal framework surgery have had extensive voice therapy before the surgical procedure. Basic concepts in voice training are therefore known to them, although they often were not able to employ them efficiently, because of the lack of laryngeal function.

In my opinion, preoperative efforts to improve glottic closure by forceful expiration or pushing exercises are of no use and can even be regarded as counterproductive, because the increased subglottic air pressures and increased airflow rates associated with these exercises will negatively influence the glottis closure. Preoperative voice therapy should therefore be restricted to counseling and aimed at prevention of inadequate and counterproductive compensation mechanisms and other negative phonatory habits.

Postoperative voice therapy following correction of glottic closure, if indicated, in my opinion should start no sooner than 2 months following surgery. The instability of the voice associated with reactive postoperative swelling and readaption of the laryngeal system to the new situation should not be burdened too soon with intensive voice therapeutic training.

Voice training in the postoperative period should be focused on retraining adapted counterproductive compensatory phonatory habits. Furthermore, to obtain a well balanced voice quality, exercises with pitch-gliding tones, as well as exercises in the dynamic intensity range, can be performed to regain the optimal flexibility in prosody and accentuation.

Pitch-related dysphonias should primarily be treated by voice therapy. Laryngeal framework surgery is only indicated if voice therapy fails. Following laryngeal framework surgery performed with the primary aim to adjust the vocal pitch, patients are advised to start with voice therapy within a few weeks.

Indications and contraindications for laryngeal framework surgery

In general, the pediatric population is not suitable for laryngeal framework surgery, first of all because the surgery is performed under local anesthesia, which will not be tolerated by children, secondly because the dimensions of the larynx in the younger pediatric population carries the risk of airway compromise, thirdly because extensive laryngeal framework surgery in the growing larynx can interfere with normal outgrowth of the larynx, and last but not least, the changes occurring especially in the male larynx at puberty might alter the degree of the dysphonia. Therefore, usually puberty with its laryngeal changes is awaited before laryngeal framework surgery is contemplated.

In adults the indications for a specific type of laryngeal framework surgery and the timing of these procedures are totally dependent on the etiology and severity of the dysphonia.

Every dysphonia caused by incomplete glottis closure, with the exception of posterior glottic insufficiency with normal vocal fold mobility and incomplete glottis closure caused by a localized vocal fold swelling, can form an indication for medialization with laryngeal framework surgery.

Cases involving bilateral vocal fold immobility are usually not suitable for correction of incomplete glottis closure because of the risk of airway compromise. In cases with mobile vocal folds, arytenoid adduction is normally contraindicated because this procedure will result in vocal fold fixation.

Generally speaking, in cases of vocal fold palsy, thyroplasty type 1 is indicated in anteriorly more outspoken glottis insufficiency, whereas arytenoid adduction is indicated in cases of a more posteriorly located glottis insufficiency. Furthermore, a vertical level difference of both vocal folds, as can often be observed in vocal fold palsy, can be corrected by arytenoid adduction. In patients experiencing repeated aspiration besides dysphonia, the glottic insufficiency is usually best corrected by means of a combination of arytenoid adduction and thyroplasty type 1.

Patients with vocal fold palsy due to mediastinal malignant disease are eligible for medialization laryngeal framework surgery, as long as their general condition permits such an intervention. Otherwise intracordal injection of collagen under local anesthesia can be a good alternative.

Vocal fold atrophy or hypoplasia with or without a vocal fold mobility disorder usually is a good indication for thyroplasty type 1.

In cases of cricoarytenoid joint fixation, an arytenoid adduction procedure can prove very difficult. Therefore it is wise to start with a thyroplasty type 1 procedure in these cases. Despite commonly held beliefs stating otherwise, it is unusual even in long-standing vocal fold palsy to result in cricoarytenoid fixation.[13] In my series I have encountered three patients with a history of long-standing vocal fold palsy, who during surgery proved to have a fixation of the cricoarytenoid joint. In two of these, in retrospect the cause of the vocal fold mobility disorder probably was the cricoarytenoid fixation and not the assumed vocal fold palsy. When cricoarytenoid fixation is suspected, laryngeal EMG is helpful in arriving at the right diagnosis.

Presbyphonia is a good indication for bilateral thyroplasty type 1.

Cases of dysphonia caused by vocal fold fibrosis and incomplete glottis closure can be eligible for a combination of thyroplasty type 1 and type 3. Of course the voice results obtained will be moderate at best and are more directed towards facilitating phonation than obtaining a normal voice quality.

Irradiation or previous partial vocal fold resection for treatment of laryngeal cancer is not an absolute contraindication for laryngeal framework surgery, but the results will be less than obtained for other categories of patients. Furthermore, because of oncologic principles, surgery is not contemplated before the patient has remained free of local disease for at least 2 years.

The major indications for raising the tension of the vocal folds are dysphonias resulting from paralysis of the superior laryngeal nerve or requests to raise the vocal pitch in cases of androphonia following hormonal medication and gender dysphonia in male-to-female transsexual patients.

The indications for reduction of vocal fold tension are restricted to strained, high-pitched voices in congenital hypoplasia or other conditions with stiff vocal folds, e.g. severe sulcus vocalis previously treated by microlaryngeal surgery. In such cases, thyroplasty type 3 is usually combined with thyroplasty type 1. In exceptional cases, voice therapy-resistant mutational dysphonias can be eligible for tension-reducing surgery, resulting in a lower pitch.

Voice therapy is without doubt the mainstay for all vocal pitch disorders, but additional phonosurgical intervention is often required in transsexuals to raise the habitual vocal pitch. Although vocal pitch is not the only factor in identifying the gender of a speaker, it is generally regarded as the predominant one. Other factors include patterns of intonation, quality of resonance, articulation characteristics, conversational topics and type of vocabulary.[5,37]

Timing and planning of laryngeal framework surgery

Timing and planning of laryngeal framework surgery is largely dependent upon:

- the etiology of the dysphonia;
- the degree of dysphonia;
- the time that has passed since the onset of dysphonia;
- the life expectancy of the patient;
- the appearance and mobility of the vocal folds;
- the position of the affected vocal fold;
- the degree of compensation of the contralateral vocal fold;
- other patient-related factors (profession, age, etc.);
- other complaints related to laryngeal dysfunction (aspiration, hyperventilation, etc.); and
- last but not least, the experience of the surgeon.

Timing of laryngeal framework surgery

Etiology is a very important factor in timing, especially if the dysphonia is due to a recurrent laryngeal or vagus nerve paralysis.

In the case of mobile vocal folds, as for instance in severe presbyphonia, there is no reason for delaying the surgery, since there is no chance of spontaneous recovery or compensation.

Laryngeal framework surgical correction of the glottic closure can therefore be planned immediately in all cases of glottic insufficiency with bilateral mobile vocal folds, when voice therapy remains unsuccessful or is not indicated.

In the case of unilateral immobility, the strategy will depend on the cause of the vocal fold immobility.

If, in the case of a paralysis, the continuity of the nerve is intact (e.g. idiopathic paralysis) or believed to be intact, spontaneous recovery of function may be expected up to 1 year following the onset of the paralysis. Therefore it is advisable to plan a surgical treatment no sooner than 1 year following onset, unless other factors prevail.

If the paralysis is a result of a severed nerve without reconstruction (e.g. resection of vagus nerve tumor, resection of the recurrent nerve due to thyroid malignant tumor, etc.), no spontaneous recovery of function can be expected. In these circumstances laryngeal framework surgery can be taken into consideration sooner. If, in such cases, the glottic insufficiency is relatively small it is worthwhile to wait for compensation of the unaffected vocal fold to occur. Voice therapy can be advised during this period, but in my personal opinion, it will not stimulate compensation. If compensation has not been achieved sufficiently within 6 months, surgical treatment can be planned.

If the dysphonia is a result of trauma, it is advisable to wait at least 6 months before framework surgery is contemplated. By that time scar tissue will have settled.

If the glottic insufficiency is a result of a fixed cricoarytenoid joint, there is no reason to postpone surgical treatment. Laryngeal EMG is very helpful to differentiate between laryngeal paralysis and fixation of the cricoarytenoid joint.

In patients with a recurrent laryngeal nerve paralysis as a result of an intrathoracic malignancy, laryngeal framework surgery is usually performed as soon as is convenient for the patient, because of the short life expectancy of these patients. In this category of patients, especially if they are in a poor general condition, vocal fold augmentation by means of intracordal injection can be considered a reasonable alternative. This should, however, be performed under local anesthesia in order to monitor the voice, in which case my personal preference would be a collagen injection.

The degree of dysphonia can influence the timing of laryngeal framework surgery as well. If the degree of dysphonia is very significant, I tend to operate earlier than 1 year following the onset. The patient will, however, have to realize that the performance of an arytenoid adduction will interfere with the chance of spontaneous recovery.

Sometimes patients have other complaints related to the laryngeal dysfunction, such as aspiration as a result of vagal nerve palsy, or hyperventilation as a result of the large airflow during phonation. These factors can form a reason to plan surgery earlier than 1 year following the onset of the palsy. If in cases of severe aspiration other surgical procedures, such as cricopharyngeal myotomy, are contemplated, these should be performed prior to laryngeal framework surgery, because intubation can destroy the results obtained with medialization laryngeal framework surgery. Furthermore, in cases of severe aspiration, arytenoid adduction will be employed more often, because this procedure will aid in the prevention of aspiration.

In selected cases, professional and social factors may urge us to improve the voice sooner as well.

Timing of laryngeal framework surgery for correction of vocal fold tension is less strict than that of medialization framework surgery and it is much more dependent upon the progress obtained with voice therapy. In the case of transsexual gender dysphonia, pitch-raising surgery is often postponed until all gender reassignment surgery has been performed, to reduce the risk of damage of the stretched vocal folds by repeated intubations.

Planning of laryngeal framework surgery

My personal strategy in the planning of medialization laryngeal framework surgery is usually as follows, unless specific factors, as mentioned below, incite me to change my policy.

Usually, in cases of dysphonia with a slight-to-moderate degree of glottic insufficiency, I start with a thyroplasty type 1. If, during the surgery, this is found to result in an insufficient improvement of the voice, an arytenoid adduction is performed additionally. Often, however, a good voice can be obtained by means of a thyroplasty type 1 only. Prior to finishing the surgery the effect of a manual cricothyroid approximation is tested as a rule. If this results in a better voice, the cricoid and thyroid cartilages are approximated permanently with sutures.

The reasons why I prefer this sequence of techniques are:

- Thyroplasty type 1 is a much simpler and less time-consuming procedure than an arytenoid adduction.
- Usually no endolaryngeal edema is observed during a thyroplasty type 1, whereas arytenoid adduction results in a not insignificant edema of the arytenoid region. This may interfere with the voice monitoring during surgery. Even in those cases where a combination of thyroplasty type 1 and arytenoid adduction is considered likely to be required, it seems wise to start with the thyroplasty type 1. Presence of endolaryngeal edema at the time of peroperative voice monitoring should be ruled out by fiberoptic examination of the larynx during surgery. If significant edema or even hematoma is present, overcorrection is required to get a good postoperative voice result.
- Thyroplasty type 1 is a procedure which can more easily be reversed than an arytenoid adduction.
- Swallowing complaints and pain during the first postoperative days are much more often observed following arytenoid adduction than following thyroplasty type 1.

Exceptions of the policy described above can occur:

- In cases with a large glottic insufficiency and/or a level difference between both vocal folds. In such cases an arytenoid adduction alone can be sufficient and I therefore start with this procedure. If, during the surgery, this is found to result in an insufficient improvement of the voice, a thyroplasty type 1 is performed additionally.
- In selected cases of isolated fixation of the

cricoarytenoid joint, an effort can be made to explore the cricoarytenoid joint and fix the arytenoid in a more adducted position. If, however, the fixation of this joint is only part of a more extensive fibrosis, it is much safer to limit the surgery to the simpler procedures, such as thyroplasty type 1 and cricothyroid approximation.

- In cases of normal laryngeal mobility, if medialization is required, it should be achieved without arytenoid adduction.
- In cases with flaccid vocal folds, tension correction by means of cricothyroid approximation seems to be the first choice; if necessary, bilateral thyroplasty type 1 can be added.
- In older patients the medialization required for the best voice result may compromise the airway as a result of a diminished tension of the unaffected vocal fold, associated with older age. This flaccid but otherwise unaffected vocal fold can be adducted passively by the Bernoulli effect during inspiration, resulting in a relative airway obstruction. Therefore, it is wise not to be overzealous in correcting the dysphonia of older patients. The same holds true for patients with poor physical condition, for whom operating time and peroperative stress should be reduced to the minimum. In both patient groups I tend to limit the surgical procedure to a thyroplasty type 1 and perhaps a cricothyroid approximation.
- If the surgeon is not yet experienced in laryngeal framework surgery, it is advisable to limit the procedures to the thyroplasty type 1 and cricothyroid approximation initially, because these procedures are relatively simple. This may not lead to the best obtainable voice result in all cases, but it will definitely improve the voice without much risk.

Results

Materials and methods

Between 1986 and 1997, 213 laryngeal framework surgical techniques were performed by the author, either as combinations or separately as 157 procedures in 150 patients. The patient group consisted of 53 females, 67 males and 30 male-to-female transsexuals. This involved 116 patients who were treated with the intention of correcting the glottis closure and 34 patients who were treated with the intention of correcting the vocal fold tension and consequently the vocal fold pitch.

Voice evaluation was performed in the glottic closure correction as well as the vocal fold tension correction patient categories. The voice evaluation was performed by means of a voice range profile. Assessment was performed preoperatively, between 2 and 6 months postoperatively (short-term results) and more than 1 year postoperatively (long-term results). In addition, the maximal phonation time of the sustained vowel /a/ was recorded in the patients undergoing medialization laryngeal framework surgery. Furthermore, the mean pitch of the voice during normal speech was determined by means of electroglottography (Glottal Frequency Analyzer – Teltec type GFA 06, Sweden) in the glottic closure correction as well as the vocal fold tension correction patient categories.

This resulted in the following objective voice parameters:

- maximal phonation time (Max Phon) in seconds of a sustained vowel /a/ (best of three efforts);
- maximal dynamic intensity range (Dyn Range) in decibels obtained from the phonetogram;
- dynamic intensity range at the mean habitual pitch of the speaking voice (Dyn Range MVP) in decibels obtained from the phonetogram;
- maximal vocal intensity (Max Int) in decibels obtained from the phonetogram;
- melodic range (Mel Range) in semitones obtained from the phonetogram; and
- mean habitual pitch of the voice during speech (MVP).

Results of correction of incomplete glottis closure

The 116 patients who have been treated in our department with the intention of improving the glottis closure, have undergone a total of 181 laryngeal framework surgical techniques in 123 surgical procedures. This patient group consisted of 49 females and 67 males, with a mean age of 49.9 years (range 17–80 years). This involved a single modality laryngeal framework technique in 55% of the procedures (64 thyroplasties type 1; 4 arytenoid adductions) or a combination of laryngeal framework surgical techniques during the same surgical procedure in 45% of the cases (34 thyroplasties type 1 in combination with arytenoid adduction; 6 combinations of thyroplasty type 1 and cricothyroid approximation; 5 combinations of thyroplasty type 1, arytenoid adduction and cricothyroid approximation; 10 other combinations).

None of these patients, who have undergone medialization laryngeal framework surgery, showed a deterioration of the voice. Three patients considered their voice to be unchanged or only marginally improved following the procedure. All three had undergone extensive previous phonosurgical procedures, two of them including Teflon injections. All patients with a dysphonia based on vagus or recurrent nerve paralysis, who had not previously undergone any phonosurgical procedure, obtained a markedly improved voice and were highly satisfied with the result. About one-third of all patients considered their postoperative voice to be absolutely normal, even in demanding circumstances. More than half of the other patients considered their voice to be 'functionally adequate'.

Short-term objective postoperative voice evaluation was obtained in 85 patients following medialization laryngeal framework surgery (Fig 33.25). Thirty-one patients could not be evaluated: seven patients because they were from abroad and the voice assessment performed in the respective referring centers was not consistent; nine patients

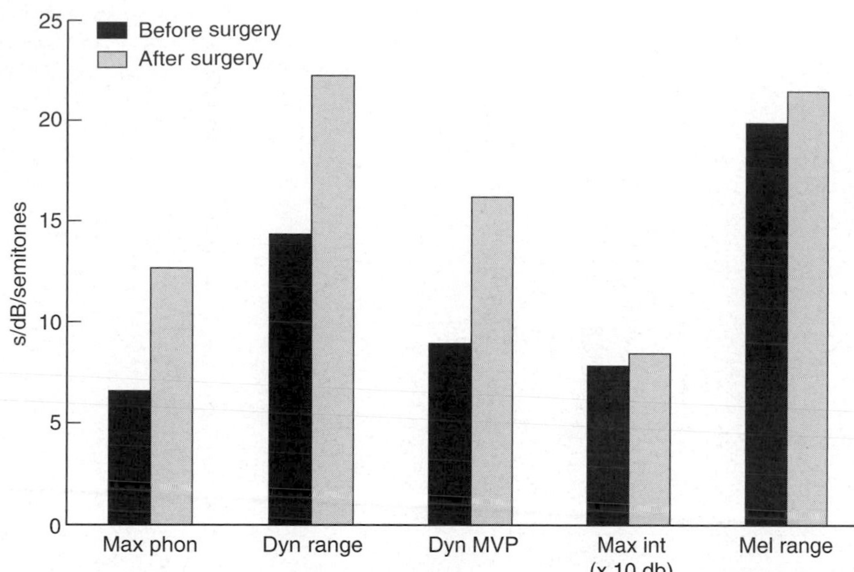

Figure 33.25 *Mean results of medialization laryngeal framework surgery. Overall voice results (n = 85). Max phon, maximal phonation time; Dyn range, maximal dynamic range; Dyn MVP, dynamic range at mean vocal pitch; Max int, maximal vocal intensity; Mel range, melodic range.*

because they had terminal disease (malignant involvement of mediastinum); eight patients because they were unable to produce a VRP. Three patients were lost to follow-up. Four patients still have to return for their first postoperative voice evaluation.

A considerable voice improvement was found in all voice parameters:

- almost doubling of the mean maximal phonation time from 6.6 seconds to 12.7 seconds;
- marked increase of the maximal dynamic range from 14.4 dB to 22.7 dB;
- improvement of the dynamic range at the mean vocal pitch from 9.1 dB to 16.3 dB;
- the maximal vocal intensity improved from 79.6 dB to 85.5 dB; and
- the melodic range demonstrated a slight improvement from 20 to 21.5 semitones.

With the exception of the melodic range results, these improvements are all highly significant (*t*-test $P < 0.001$).

A differentiation of the preoperative voice assessment on the basis of laryngeal framework surgical techniques used (Fig 33.26) shows, as could have been expected, that the most extensive surgery has been performed in the patient group with the worst preoperative voice. This difference is significant (*t*-test $P < 0.05$) for the comparison of the thyroplasty type 1 only group and the combination of thyroplasty type 1 and arytenoid adduction group. In the postoperative voice assessment (Fig 33.27), it is remarkable that the maximal phonation time is only slightly improved following thyroplasty type 1 (mean gain 4.8 seconds) and much more improved following combinations including arytenoid adduction and thyroplasty type 1 (mean gain 8.4 seconds). This difference is, however, not statistically significant. Another point of interest is the slight deteri-

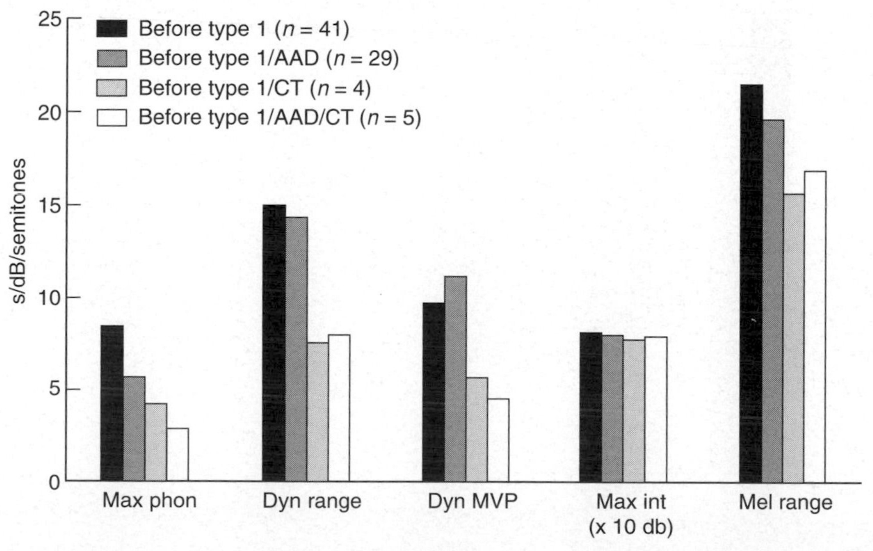

Figure 33.26 *Mean preoperative voice parameters, differentiated according to type of surgery performed. Abbreviations as in Fig 33.25.*

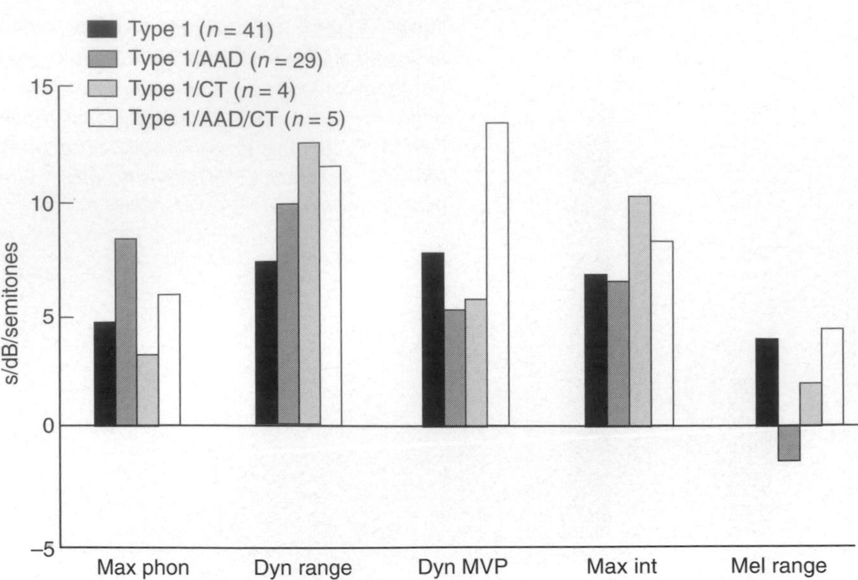

Figure 33.27 *Mean voice gain following surgery, differentiated according to type of surgery performed. Abbreviations as in Fig 33.25.*

oration of the melodic range following procedures including arytenoid adduction (mean loss of 1.6 semitones), whereas the melodic range is clearly improved following thyroplasty type 1 only (mean improvement of 3.6 semitones). This difference is statistically significant (*t*-test P <0.05).

The mean vocal pitch (Fig 33.28) did not change significantly either following thyroplasty type 1 only or following a combination of thyroplasty type 1 and arytenoid adduction. The overall mean pitch of the male group was 122 Hz preoperatively and 121.7 Hz postoperatively. For the female patients this was 188.2 Hz preoperatively and 185.9 Hz postoperatively. These values are within the normal habitual speaking voice range.

A differentiation of the preoperative voice assessment on the basis of initial diagnosis (Fig 33.29) showed a tendency of the voice in vagal nerve palsy to be slightly better preoperatively than recurrent laryngeal nerve (RLN) palsy for the parameters: dynamic range, dynamic range at the level of the mean vocal pitch, the maximal intensity and the melodic range. This proved to be a significant difference for the dynamic range at the level of the mean vocal pitch (P <0.05). There was no significant difference between the other diagnosis groups: hemilaryngeal mobility disorder of unknown origin (ECI), vagal nerve palsy and the miscellaneous group.

Postoperatively (Fig 33.30) the voice gain was significantly less in the miscellaneous diagnosis group than in the other diagnosis groups, for all voice parameters (P <0.05), with the exception of the melodic range (also the difference between vagal nerve palsy and miscellaneous in the dynamic range parameter was not significant). The differences in voice gain between the other diagnosis groups were not significant.

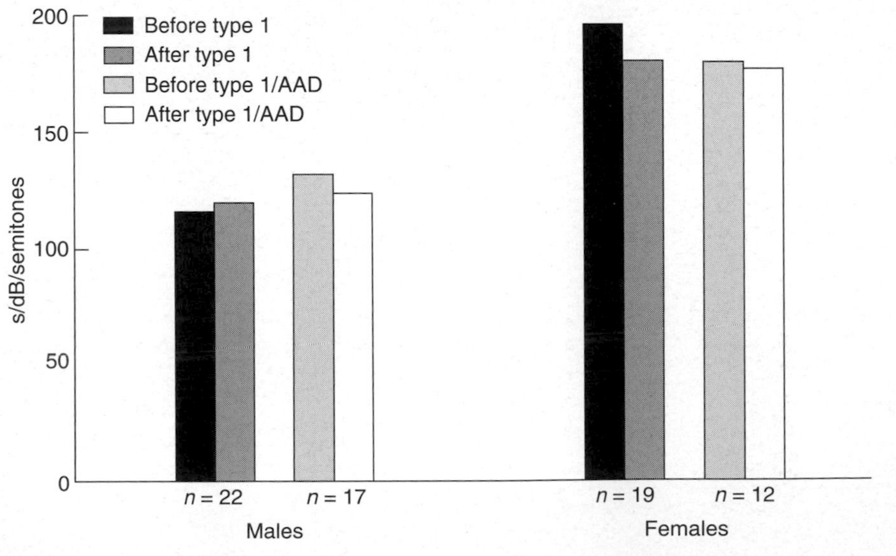

Figure 33.28 *Mean vocal pitch before and after medialization laryngeal framework surgery. Abbreviations as in Fig 33.25.*

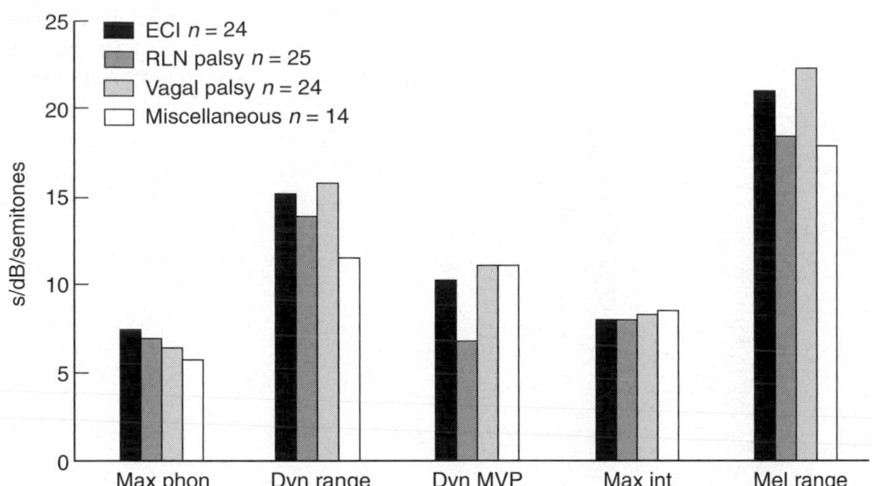

Figure 33.29 *Mean preoperative voice parameters, before medialization laryngeal framework surgery, differentiated according to diagnosis group. ECI, hemilaryngeal mobility disorder of unknown origin; RLN palsy, recurrent laryngeal nerve palsy; Vagal palsy, vagal nerve palsy; Miscellaneous, other causes of incomplete glottis closure. Other abbreviations as in Fig 33.25.*

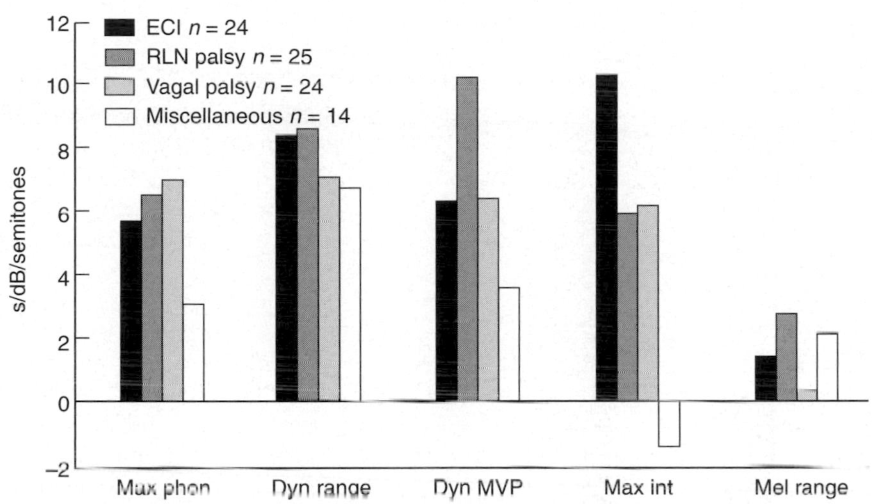

Figure 33.30 *Mean voice gain, following medialization laryngeal framework surgery, differentiated according to diagnosis group. Abbreviations as in Figs 33.25 and 33.29.*

In all diagnosis groups with the exception of the miscellaneous group, voice results were significantly better for all voice parameters following surgery, with the exception of the melodic range. The only significant voice improvement in the miscellaneous group was for the dynamic range. The maximal intensity in the miscellaneous group was even less postoperatively than preoperatively.

Obviously the best results were obtained in patients with dysphonia caused by a 'simple' hemilaryngeal mobility disorder (RLN palsy, vagal palsy or hemilaryngeal mobility disorder without known cause). Worst results were obtained in patients in the miscellaneous group, which contains patients who had previously undergone intracordal Teflon injections, patients with laryngeal fibrosis following laryngeal trauma or surgery, congenital laryngeal disorders, or patients who had undergone radiotherapy to the neck and larynx.

In 33 patients long-term voice evaluation was also obtained (Fig 33.31). It is interesting to notice that the voice results have remained stable or sometimes even slightly improved after a year as compared to the voice evaluation a few months postoperatively. The short-term and long-term results are not significantly different. Differentiated according to the type of laryngeal framework surgery performed (Figs 33.32 and 33.33), there is no difference in long-term results between thyroplasty type 1 only and a combination of thyroplasty type 1 and arytenoid adduction.

Revision medialization laryngeal framework surgery or collagen injection

Four patients had previously undergone medialization laryngeal framework surgery elsewhere (three of which had been performed under general anesthesia) with unsatisfactory results, six patients initially treated in our department required revision laryngeal framework procedure to optimize the result, and seven others required an additional intracordal injection of collagen in local anesthesia to obtain the optimal result.

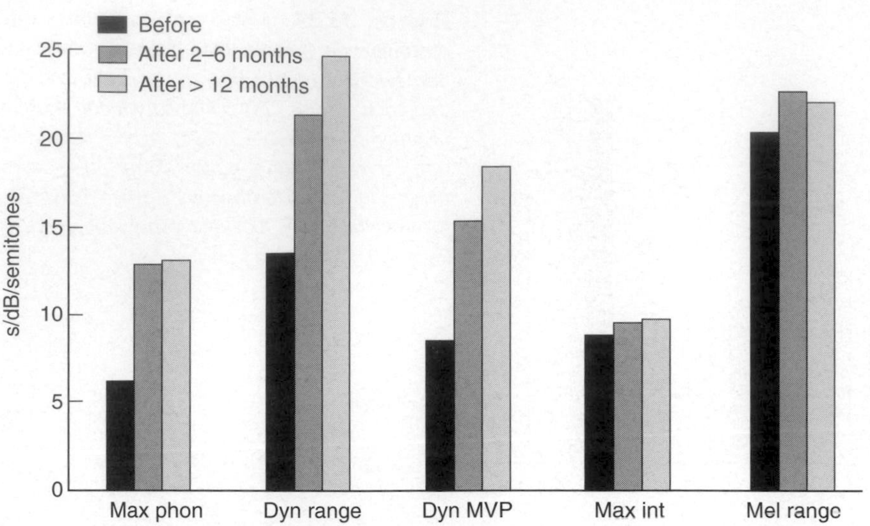

Figure 33.31 *Mean long-term voice results, following medialization laryngeal framework surgery (n=33). Abbreviations as in Fig 33.25.*

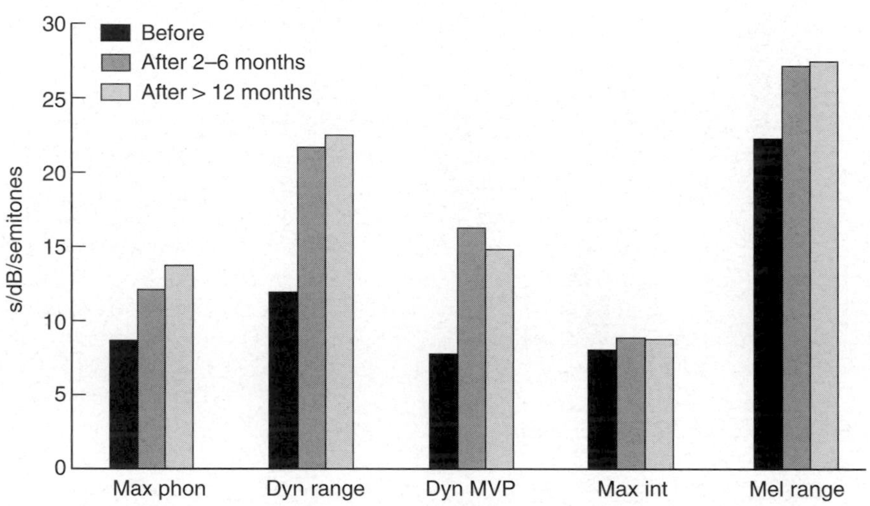

Figure 33.32 *Mean long-term voice results, following thyroplasty type 1 (n=15). Abbreviations as in Fig 33.25.*

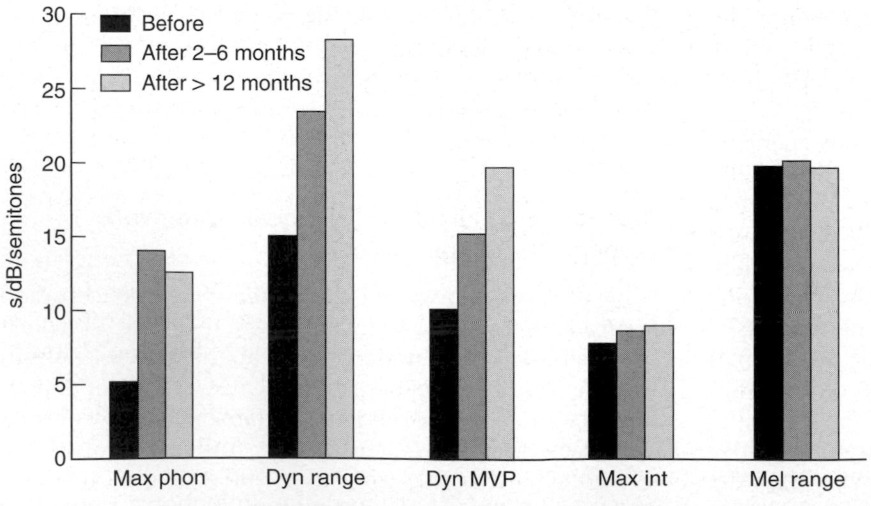

Figure 33.33 *Mean long-term voice results, following combination of thyroplasty type 1 and arytenoid adduction (n=14). Abbreviations as in Fig 33.25.*

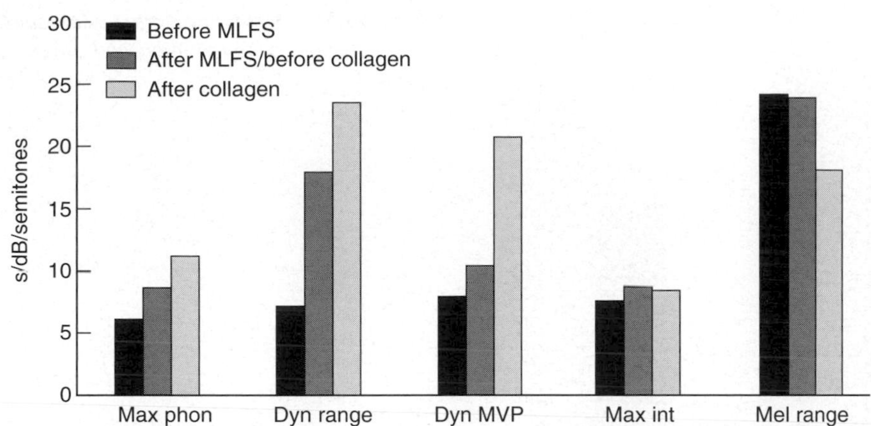

Figure 33.34 *Mean voice results after medialization laryngeal framework surgery (MLFS) and additional intracordal collagen injection (n=7). Abbreviations as in Fig 33.25.*

Of the six patients who were initially treated in our department and required revision framework surgery to optimize the result, only one reintervention was performed to correct initial overcorrection of a thyroplasty type 1. Following the revision thyroplasty type 1 in this case, the voice remained satisfactory and the slight dyspnea on effort dissolved.

In two patients thyroplasty type 1 was initially performed, with improved but not optimal voice results. Secondary arytenoid adduction resulted in a near normal voice in both.

Two patients initially had good voice results following thyroplasty type 1, but again lost their voices following intubation for other surgical procedures. Revision thyroplasty type 1 in combination with arytenoid adduction improved the voice in both, although the initially obtained result was never again achieved.

In one patient during a combination of thyroplasty type 1 and arytenoid adduction, the usually performed routine manual cricothyroid approximation, performed to check whether correction of vocal fold tension will further improve the voice, was inadvertently not performed. Postoperatively this female patient, on videolaryngostroboscopy, demonstrated a reasonable correction of the glottis closure but an insufficient tension of vocal fold, resulting in an unstable low-pitched and rather weak voice. Additional cricothyroid approximation was performed secondarily with an excellent voice result.

In seven cases additional intracordal collagen injections were performed a few months following laryngeal framework surgery. All intracordal collagen injections were performed under local anesthesia and functional laryngostroboscopic control. In five of the seven cases this involved patients who belonged to the miscellaneous diagnosis group: two patients after blunt laryngeal trauma, one patient after previous Teflon injection and two patients after extensive endolaryngeal surgery for bilateral sulcus vocalis. Of the two patients with hemilaryngeal mobility disorders, one patient had a bilateral glomus tumor. Although thyroplasty type 1 was not sufficient to fully correct his incomplete glottis closure, it was deemed unwise to perform an arytenoid adduction because of its irreversibility. This would carry a risk for airway obstruction in the future should the mobility of contralateral vocal fold also be affected by the glomus tumor on the contralateral side. Following thyroplasty type 1, the voice was much better but not sufficient for the patient's needs, who had a voice-demanding profession. It was therefore decided to augment the vocal fold with a minimal amount of collagen. The airway was not compromised and the voice markedly improved.

Although the voices of all seven patients had improved following the medialization laryngeal framework surgery, a further improvement was obtained by the additional collagen injections for all parameters except maximal intensity and melodic range (Fig 33.34). Only the improvement in the dynamic range at the level of the mean vocal pitch was significant ($P < 0.05$).

Results of correction of vocal fold tension

Thirty-two laryngeal framework surgical procedures have been performed by the author with the objective of raising the vocal pitch in 31 patients. This involved one case of androphonia in a young female patient and 30 male-to-female transsexuals. The mean age was 38.3 years (range 19–70). All these patients underwent a cricothyroid approximation and two of them also underwent anterior commissure advancement thyroplasty. One patient later also underwent additional scarification and mass reduction of the vocal folds. Five patients had already undergone anterior web creation elsewhere in an effort to raise the vocal pitch prior to laryngeal framework surgery.

There is a tendency among transsexual patients not to show up for postoperative voice assessment. Twenty-four patients could be assessed objectively between 2 and 6 months postoperatively (Figs 33.35 and 33.36).

Four of the other seven patients have communicated by telephone that they were satisfied with the voice result, but were unable or unwilling to come for postoperative voice assessment. Breathiness and diplophonia were often

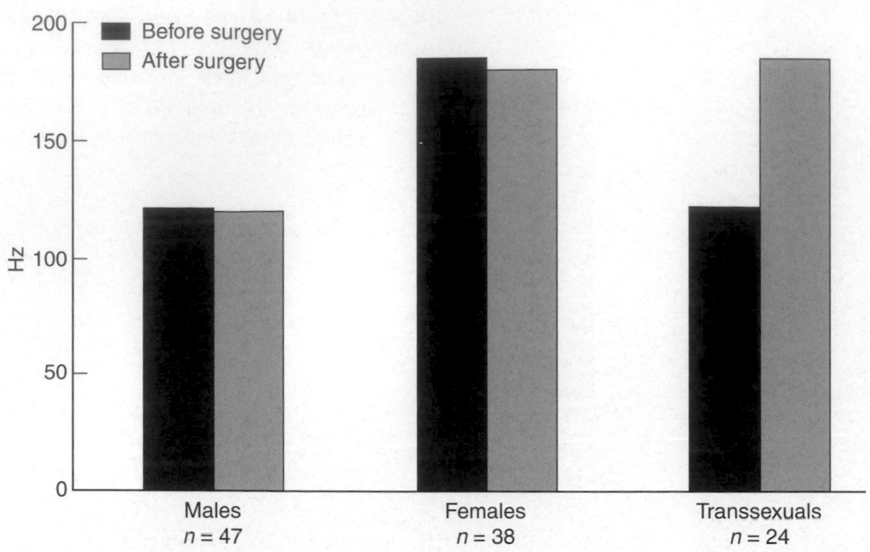

Figure 33.35 *Mean vocal pitch after laryngeal framework surgery. Abbreviations as in Fig 33.25.*

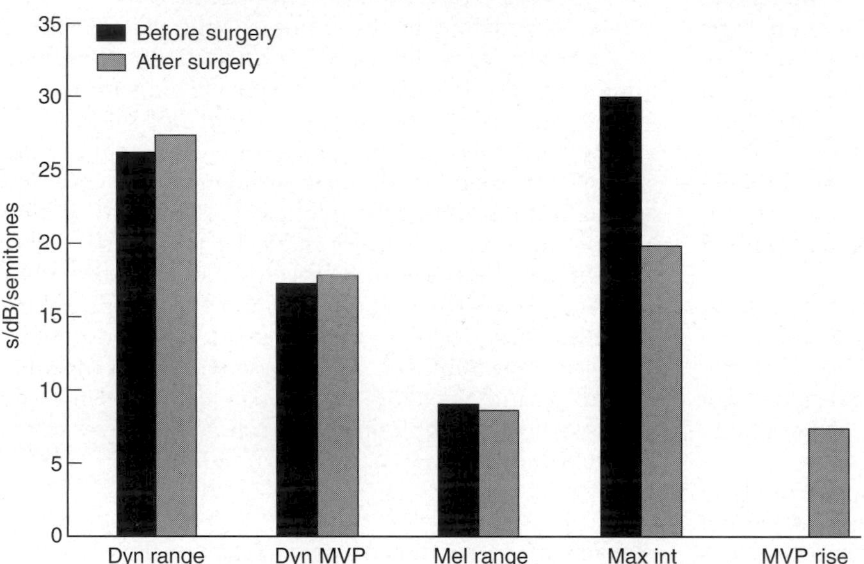

Figure 33.36 *Mean voice results after pitch-raising surgery (n=24). Abbreviations as in Fig 33.25.*

present during the first few weeks postoperatively, but normalized spontaneously within 2 months.

Figure 33.35 shows the mean vocal pitch of the male and female patients before and after medialization laryngeal framework surgery as compared to the transsexual patients before and after pitch-raising surgery. Before surgery the mean vocal pitch of the transsexuals equals the mean vocal pitch of the males and after surgery it equals that of the female patients.

Preoperatively 21 out of 24 transsexual patients had a mean pitch of the speaking voice within the normal male range (98–131 Hz). The mean preoperative pitch was 123.7 Hz. Postoperatively 16 of the 24 patients had achieved a mean pitch within the normal female range (174–262 Hz). The mean postoperative pitch was 186.9 Hz. One patient had no pitch rise after cricothyroid approximation but refused further treatment. One patient only had a minor pitch raise of two semitones.

The overall mean pitch rise of the speaking voice was almost eight semitones. Although the melodic range was almost invariably diminished postoperatively (more than ten semitones mean loss of melodic range), there were no complaints of monotonous voices. The other voice parameters such as maximal dynamic intensity range (preoperatively 26.3 dB; postoperatively 27.3 dB), dynamic intensity range at the mean pitch of the speaking voice (preoperatively 17.0 dB; postoperatively 17.6 dB) and the maximal vocal intensity (preoperatively 89.6 dB; postoperatively 87.8 dB), did not change significantly due to the surgery, signifying no gross loss of overall voice quality.

Most patients were satisfied with the result and considered their voices as 'normal female voices'. Three patients were not satisfied with the result. One had a rise of five semitones on postoperative voice assessment and was almost within the range of the normal female speaking pitch, but did not appreciate this voice as a 'normal female voice'.

Two transsexual patients undergoing vocal pitch-raising surgery demonstrated a drop of pitch after initial successful rise following cricothyroid approximation (one of these procedures was performed elsewhere); both underwent an anterior commissure advancement thyroplasty resulting in an adequate pitch rise, which was, however, short-lived in one of them.

In two female patients a cricothyroid approximation was performed to correct a superior laryngeal nerve paralysis (one unilaterally, one bilaterally). Both demonstrated a slightly higher pitch and a stronger voice postoperatively.

The indication for reduction of vocal fold tension is rare and has occurred only five times, usually in combination with an indication for correction of glottis closure. All dysphonias were the result of a combination of congenital vocal fold hypoplasia and sulcus vocalis, resulting in weak and high-pitched voices. Three patients had undergone previous microlaryngoscopic correction of vocal fold mucosal lesions, including vocal fold sulcus.

Once a thyroplasty type 3 was performed bilaterally and four times a unilateral combination of thyroplasty type 3 and thyroplasty type 1 was required. In one of these an additional thyroplasty type 1 was performed contralaterally. In all cases the mean pitch dropped a few semitones and the glottis closure improved.

Complications

Complications observed as a result of medialization laryngeal framework surgical procedures in my series were minor:

- Two patients developed a local infection, which was successfully treated with antibiotics in both cases. Since that period antibiotics were routinely administered perioperatively on a prophylactic basis.
- One patient developed transient stridor because of edema, which was successfully treated with steroid medication.
- In one male patient in whom a resection of the posterior thyroid ala was performed to facilitate approach of the cricoarytenoid joint during a combined procedure of thyroplasty type 1 and arytenoid adduction, a fracture of the remainder of the posterior thyroid ala occurred without further consequences. The fracture was stabilized with sutures.
- In one elderly female patient, a slight dyspnea on exertion resulted because of overcorrection of a thyroplasty type 1. During the procedure the patient was afraid to phonate and thus monitoring of the voice was not optimal, resulting in the overcorrection, which was not noticed at the time of surgery. Revision surgery was performed 4 months later, successfully correcting the degree of medialization of the cartilage window, with preservation of the achieved voice improvement.
- One patient required reintervention because of local bleeding 1 day postoperatively.
- No extrusions of silicone implants or cartilage windows were observed.
- No airway compromise requiring tracheotomy has been observed.

Complications of laryngeal framework surgery to correct vocal fold tension consisted of:

- Three patients with an anterior fracture of the cricoid cartilage. Since silicone or Gore-Tex® bolsters to disperse the pressure of the sutures on the cartilage have been used for the cricoid, no more fractures of the cricoid have been observed.
- One patient with an anterior fracture of the thyroid cartilage, despite the use of silicone bolsters, which apparently were too weak to withstand the pressure of the suture. Since that time Gore-Tex® bolsters have been used. All fractures resulted from sutures pulling through the cartilage during maximal cricothyroid approximation in transsexual patients. Two patients were young transsexual patients with non-calcified laryngeal cartilages; the other two patients were older than 60 years, with extremely calcified but fragile laryngeal cartilages. All fractures were repaired at the time of initial surgery, without further sequelae. Two of these patients had a good vocal pitch rise, in the other two the results were less satisfactory. In one of these patients eventually a satisfactory result was obtained following anterior commissure advancement as a second-stage procedure.
- One patient developed a wound infection after cricothyroid approximation, despite prophylactic antibiotic treatment, necessitating surgical removal of the silicone bolsters. The further recovery was uneventful.
- No other complications were observed.

Discussion

Some reports in the literature suggested that the long-term results, e.g. 1 year following thyroplasty type 1 with medialization of the cartilage window, are not as good as the immediate and short-term results. Some patients were reported[43] to have experienced a deterioration of the voice after some months, which was attributed to resorption of the cartilage window and consequently a loss of vocal fold medialization. It was therefore advised to remove the cartilage window and medialize the inner perichondrium and the endolaryngeal soft tissues with an implant. Following this policy, however, the first reports of endolaryngeal extrusion of the implants[8,63] started to appear, which had never been observed previously when the cartilage window remained *in situ* and was medialized. In one series reported by Cotter and coworkers in 1995 an extrusion rate of even more than 8% within the first 5 months was found, following removal of the cartilage window.[8] Tucker *et al.*[63] reported an endolaryngeal extrusion rate of 7% within the first 15 months following surgery. In my own series, in which 117 thyroplasty type 1 procedures were performed, either separately or in combination with other procedures, no extrusions of implants have been observed. In all of these patients the cartilage window was preserved and medialized. I have personally observed only one extrusion, which occurred in a patient who had been operated elsewhere and in whom the cartilage window had also been removed. Isshiki (personal communication), who also still preserves and medializes the cartilage window, has never observed an endolaryngeal extrusion of the implant either. However, not all surgeons who remove the cartilage window have observed extrusions. Netterville *et al.*[36] did not encounter any endolaryngeal extrusion of an implant in 116 procedures. Neither have they observed any airway compromise other than mild edema.

The need for removing the cartilage window in my opinion remains questionable. The long-term functional results of my patients following thyroplasty type 1 showed no deterioration of voice over time, as had been found by some authors and was attributed to absorption of the cartilage window.[43] The longest patient in follow-up is now more than 10 years postoperative still with an excellent voice. I therefore consider medialization of the cartilage window a reliable procedure and I regard preservation of the cartilage window as an effective buttress against implant extrusion.

Another point of discussion in the literature concerns the airway compromise following laryngeal framework surgery. Tucker *et al.*[63] mention postoperative airway compromise requiring tracheotomy in 10% of the patients following thyroplasty type 1. In all cases this was caused by hematoma development. Cotter *et al.*[8] have seen no airway compromise following thyroplasty type 1. They explain the difference between the results reported by Tucker and their own by the technique used to remove the cartilage window. Tucker uses an oscillating saw, whereas Cotter and coworkers use a diamond drill.

I personally think that Tucker's policy to routinely add a nerve muscle pedicle reinnervation procedure to the thyroplasty type 1 might have added to his reported high incidence of airway compromise. In order to perform the nerve muscle pedicle procedure, the inner perichondrium has be incised, thus increasing the risk of endolaryngeal hematoma development. Furthermore, it is not clear from either the report of Tucker and coworkers or from Cotter and coworkers whether wound drainage is performed routinely, as is the case in my patients. I have observed one incident of mild postoperative airway compromise due to edema, which reacted favorably to corticosteroid administration. No tracheotomy was required. One other patient was slightly overcorrected, resulting in a slight dyspnea on exertion, which was corrected by revision surgery. One of my other patients was a marathon runner. He underwent a thyroplasty type 1 in combination with an arytenoid adduction without any restriction of his airway.

Mild endolaryngeal hematoma is a normal postoperative finding, especially following combination laryngeal framework surgery, but this invariably resolves within a few days. Nevertheless, it seems wise to keep patients admitted for one or two days following all but the simplest (isolated cricothyroid approximation) procedures.

There is controversy in the literature concerning the effectiveness of arytenoid adduction as a technique to correct glottis closure and improve the dysphonia. Woodson and Murray[70] suggested that arytenoid adduction is not an effective procedure in patients following long-standing paralysis and that they obtained poor functional results, especially in this patient group. However, their overall functional success rate is also less than would be expected. Their description of the postoperative glottic configuration in these patients suggests that many of them also had a marked fold atrophy beside the large glottal gap, which in my experience can best be treated by a combination of arytenoid adduction and thyroplasty type 1. Even in patients with a vocal fold paralysis for more than 20 years I have successfully performed combinations of arytenoid adduction and thyroplasty type 1 with excellent functional results.

Bielamowicz *et al.*[2] compared the results of thyroplasty type 1 with those obtained with arytenoid adduction and found no differences between the two techniques, suggesting an equal effectiveness.

The results obtained in my own series with arytenoid adduction, usually performed in combination with thyroplasty type 1 as presented above, prove the effectiveness of this combined procedure in the correction of glottis closure. Especially, the improvement of the maximal phonation time in the combination of the arytenoid adduction and thyroplasty type 1 group as compared to the thyroplasty type 1 only group is suggestive of the improved efficiency of phonation, which can be obtained with this combined procedure, at the slight cost of a minor reduction in melodic range. These results are in accordance with reports by Slavit and Maragos[54] who also found the combination of arytenoid adduction and thyroplasty type 1 to be very effective.

Despite the reported complications, the authors of these reports invariably conclude that laryngeal framework surgery is the treatment of choice for most patients with incomplete glottis closure resulting from vocal fold palsy. The results presented above support the notion that the group of patients with vocal fold palsy will benefit most from laryngeal framework surgery, but that also in other categories of dysphonic patients reasonable results can be obtained.

As already mentioned, Tucker[60] has suggested a reinnervation procedure (nerve muscle pedicle technique) in addition to medialization laryngeal framework surgery to restore vocal fold tension. Preoperative laryngeal EMG studies have, however, taught us that most of the 'unilateral laryngeal palsy' patients do not have a lack of innervation of the laryngeal musculature, but they have an inappropriate reinnervation leading to synkinesis, tension dysbalance and sometimes even a tendency towards paradoxical laryngeal mobility. Since hyperinnervation of an, albeit subclinical, innervated muscle is physiologically impossible, the effectiveness of such additional reinnervation procedures is questionable.

Reinnervation by transfer of the ansa cervicalis as proposed by Crumley[9] as an alternative to medialization laryngeal framework surgery is feasible because the path of the subclinical innervation is sectioned to enable anastomosis between the ansa cervicalis and the RLN stump. However, this will not lead to restoration of mobility but only to restoration of tonicity, which seems to be indicated only in a selected group of patients. Furthermore, the result of the reinnervation has to be awaited for several months, whereas medialization laryngeal framework surgery produces immediate results and can be fine-tuned functionally.

Conclusions

Laryngeal framework surgery offers a safe and usually effective method to improve incomplete glottis closure and adjust vocal fold tension.

Thyroplasty type 1, especially, has become the first treatment of choice for many phonosurgeons. The reasons for this popularity have been outlined and are supported by the results presented above. We should, however, always keep in mind that we are dealing with surgery aimed at improvement of phonatory function and that sometimes, minor changes of the laryngeal framework can result in major changes of the voice. Therefore the most important factor determining success of these procedures is the monitoring of the phonatory function during the surgery. That is why these procedures should only be undertaken under local anesthesia. Furthermore, the surgeon who is performing this type of surgery should be able to manage the different techniques described above, so that the surgery can be tailored to the individual patient's situation, which will often require a combination of techniques to obtain the best result. In this respect the importance of adjustment of vocal fold tension in addition to vocal fold medialization is often underestimated.

References

1. Arnold GE. Vocal rehabilitation of paralytic dysphonia. *Arch Otolaryngol* 1962; **76**: 358–68.
2. Bielamowicz S, Berke GS, Gerratt BR. A comparison of type 1 thyroplasty and arytenoid adduction. *J Voice* 1995; **9**: 466–72.
3. Blaugrund SM. Laryngeal framework surgery. In: Ford CM, Bless DM, eds. *Phonosurgery: Assessment and Management of Voice Disorders*. New York: Raven Press, 1991: 183–99.
4. Bouchayer M, Cornut G. Microsurgical treatment of benign vocal fold lesions: indications, technique, results. *Folia Phoniatr (Basel)* 1992; **44**: 155–84.
5. Brally RC, Bull GL, Gore CH, Edgerton MT. Evaluation of vocal pitch in male transsexuals. *J Commun Disord* 1978; **2**: 443–9.
6. Brandenburg JH, Kirkham W, Koschkee D. Vocal cord augmentation with autogenous fat. *Laryngoscope* 1992; **102**: 495–500.
7. Brunings W. Ueber eine neue Behandlungsmethode der Rekurrenslaemung. *Verh Vereins Dtsch Laryngol* 1911; **18**: 93–151.
8. Cotter CS, Avidano MA, Crary MA, Cassisi NJ, Gorham MM. Laryngeal complications after type 1 thyroplasty. *Otolaryngol Head Neck Surg* 1995; **113**: 671–3.
9. Crumley RL. Update: ansa cervicalis to recurrent laryngeal nerve anastomosis for unilateral laryngeal paralysis. *Laryngoscope* 1991; **101**: 384–7.
10. Donald PJ. Voice change surgery in the transsexual. *Head Neck Surg* 1982; **4**: 433–7.
11. Ford CN. Laryngeal injection techniques. In: Ford CM, Bless DM, eds. *Phonosurgery Assessment and Management of Voice Disorders*. New York: Raven Press, 1991: 123–41.
12. Ford CN, Bless DM, Loftus JM. Role of injectable collagen in the treatment of glottic insufficiency a study of 119 patients. *Ann Otol Rhinol Laryngol* 1992; **101**: 237–47.
13. Gacek M, Gacek RR. Cricoarytenoid joint mobility after chronic vocal cord paralysis. *Laryngoscope* 1996; **106**: 1528–30.
14. Harries ML. Laryngeal framework surgery (thyroplasty). *J Laryngol Otol* 1997; **111**: 103–5.
15. Hirano M. Morphological structure of the vocal cord as a vibrator and its variations. *Folia Phoniatr (Basel)* 1974; **26**: 89–94.
16. Hirano M. *Clinical Examination of the Voice*. New York: Springer-Verlag, 1981.
17. Hirano M, Bless DM. *Videostroboscopic Examination of the Larynx*. San Diego: Singular Press, 1993.
18. Isshiki N. Recent advances in phonosurgery. *Folia Phoniatr (Basel)* 1980; **32**: 119–54.
19. Isshiki N. *Phonosurgery, Theory and Practice*. New York: Springer-Verlag, 1989.
20. Isshiki N, Taira T, Tanabe M. Surgical alteration of the vocal pitch. *J Otolaryngol* 1983; **12**: 335–40.
21. Isshiki N, Tanabe M, Sawada M. Arytenoid adduction for unilateral vocal cord paralysis. *Arch Otolaryngol* 1978; **140**: 555–8.
22. Isshiki N, Morita H, Okamura H, Hiramoto M. Thyroplasty as a new phonosurgical technique. *Acta Otolaryngol (Stockh)* 1974; **78**: 451–7.
23. Kokawa N. A new surgical procedure for dysphonia due to androgenic or anabolic hormones. *J Jpn Bronchoesophageal Soc* 1977; **28**: 323–32.
24. Koufman JA. Laryngoplasty for vocal cord medialization: an alternative to Teflon. *Laryngoscope* 1986; **96**: 726–31.
25. Koufman JA, Isaacson G. Laryngoplastic phonosurgery. *Otolaryngol Clin North Am* 1991; **24**: 1151–77.
26. Lewy RB. Teflon injection in the vocal cord complications, errors and precautions. *Ann Otol Rhinol Laryngol* 1983; **92**: 473–4.
27. Mahieu HF. Laryngeal framework surgery – a tailored approach to voice improvement. In: Pais Clemente M, ed. *Voice Update*. Amsterdam: Elsevier, 1996: 147–57.
28. Mahieu HF, Dikkers FG. Indirect microlaryngostrobo-

scopic surgery. *Arch Otolaryngol Head Neck Surg* 1992; **118:** 21–4.

29. Mahieu HF, Dikkers FG. Stroboscopy and phonosurgery. *Arch Otolaryngol Head Neck Surg* 1992; **118:** 1003–5.
30. Mahieu HF, Herrmann IF. Erfahrungen mit der Thyreoplastik nach Isshiki. *Arch Otorhinolaryngol* 1988; **245:** 108–10.
31. Mahieu HF, Schutte HK. New surgical techniques for voice improvement. *Arch Otorhinolaryngol* 1989; **246:** 397–402.
32. Mahieu HF, Norbart T, Snel F. Laryngeal framework surgery for voice improvement. *Rev Laryngol Otol Rhinol (Bord)* 1996; **177:** 189–97.
33. Mahieu HF, Norbart T, Wong Chung RP. Laryngeal framework surgery. In: Kleinsasser O, Glanz H, Olofsson J, eds. *Advances in Laryngology in Europe*. Amsterdam: Elsevier, 1997: 426–32.
34. Meurman Y. Mediofixation der Stimmlippe bei ihrer vollständigen Lähmung. *Arch Ohren Nasen Kehlkopfheilkde* 1944; **154:** 296–304.
35. Mikaelian DO, Lowrey LD, Sataloff RT. Lipoinjection for unilateral vocal fold paralysis. *Laryngoscope* 1991; **101:** 465–8.
36. Netterville JL, Stone RE, Luken ES, Civantos FJ, Ossoff RH. Silastic medialization and arytenoid adduction: the Vanderbilt experience. A review of 116 phonosurgical procedures. *Ann Otol Rhinol Laryngol* 1993; **102:** 413–24.
37. Oates JM, Dacakis G. Speech pathology considerations in the management of transsexualism: a review. *Br J Disord Commun* 1983; **18:** 139–51.
38. Ossoff RH, Koriwchak MJ, Netterville JL, Duncavage JA. Difficulties in endoscopic removal of Teflon granulomas of the vocal fold. *Ann Otol Rhinol Laryngol* 1993; **102:** 405–12.
39. Payr E. Plastik am Schildknorpel zur Behebung der Folgen einseitiger Stimmbandlähmung. *Dtsch Med Wochenschr* 1915; **41:** 1264–70.
40. Remacle M, Dujardin JM, Lawson G. Treatment of vocal fold immobility by glutaraldehyde cross-linked collagen injection. Long term results. *Ann Otol Rhinol Laryngol* 1995; **104:** 437–41.
41. Remacle M, Marbaix E, Hamoir M, Bertrand B, van den Eeckhaut J. Correction of glottic insufficiency by collagen injection. *Ann Otol Rhinol Laryngol* 1990; **99:** 438–44.
42. Rubin HJ. Misadventures with injectable polytef (Teflon). *Arch Otolaryngol* 1975; **101:** 114–16.
43. Sasaki CT, Driscoll BP, Gracco C, Eisen R. The fate of medialized cartilage in thyroplasty type 1. *Arch Otolaryngol Head Neck Surg* 1994; **120:** 1398–9.
44. Scherer RC. Physiology of phonation a review of basic mechanics. In: Ford CN, Bless D, eds. *Phonosurgery Assessment and Surgical Management of Voice Disorders*. New York: Raven Press, 1991: 112–23.
45. Scherer RC. Laryngeal function during phonation. In: Rubin JS, Sataloff RT, Korovin GS, Gould WJ, eds. *Diagnosis and Treatment of Voice Disorders*. Tokyo: Igaku-Shoin, 1995: 86–104.
46. Schonharl E. *Die Stroboscopie in der Praktischen Laryngologie*. Stuttgart: Thieme, 1960.
47. Schutte HK. *Efficiency of Voice Production*. Thesis, Gröningen University, 1980.
48. Schutte HK. Phonetogram-voice range profile assessment of voice capacities and its clinical value. In: Pais Clemente M, ed. *Voice Update*. Amsterdam: Elsevier, 1996: 23–8.
49. Schutte HK, Miller DG. Rezonanzspiele der Gesangstimme in ihren Beziehungen zu supra- und subglottalen Druckverlaufen; Konsequenzen fur die Stimmbildungstheorie. *Folia Phoniatr (Basel)* 1988; **40:** 65–73.
50. Schutte HK, Seidner W. Recommendations by the Union of European Phoniatricians (UEP) standardizing voice area measurement/phonetography. *Folia Phoniatr (Basel)* 1983; **35:** 286–8.
51. Seiffert A. Operative Wiederherstellung des Glottisschlusses bei einseitiger Recurrenslähmung und Stimmbanddefekten. *Arch Ohren Nasen Kehlkopfheilkde* 1942; **152:** 366–8.
52. Shadle CH, Barney AM, Thomas DW. An investigation into the acoustic and aerodynamics of the larynx. In: Gauffin J, Hammarberg B, eds. *Vocal Fold Physiology: Acoustic, Perceptual and Physiological Aspects of Voice Mechanics*. San Diego: Singular Press, 1991: 73–80.
53. Shaw GY, Szewczyk MA, Searle J, Woodroof J. Autologous fat injection into the vocal folds: technical considerations and long-term follow-up. *Laryngoscope* 1997; **107:** 177–86.
54. Slavit DH, Maragos NE. Arytenoid adduction and thyroplasty type 1 in the treatment of aphonia. *J Voice* 1994; **8:** 84–91.
55. Slavit DH, Maragos NE, Lipton RJ. Physiologic assessment of Isshiki type 3 thyroplasty. *Laryngoscope* 1990; **100:** 844–8.
56. Tanabe M, Haji T, Honjo I, Isshiki N. Surgical treatment for androphonia (an experimental study). *Folia Phoniatr (Basel)* 1985; **37:** 15–21.
57. Thompson DM, Maragos NE, Edwards BW. The study of vocal fold vibratory patterns in patients with unilateral vocal fold paralysis before and after type 1 thyroplasty with or without arytenoid adduction. *Laryngoscope* 1995; **105:** 481–6.
58. Titze IR. *Principles of Voice Production*. Englewood Cliffs: Prentice-Hall, 1994.
59. Tucker HM. Complications after surgical management of the paralyzed larynx. *Laryngoscope* 1983; **93:** 295–8.
60. Tucker HM. Simultaneous medialization and reinnervation for unilateral vocal fold paralysis. *Oper Techn Otolaryngol Head Neck Surg* 1993; **4:** 83–5.
61. Tucker HM. Complications of laryngeal framework surgery for phonation disorders. *Oper Techn Otolaryngol Head Neck Surg* 1993; **4:** 232–5.
62. Tucker HM. New voices for old. *J Voice* 1995; **9:** 111–17.
63. Tucker HM, Wanamaker J, Trott M, Hicks D. Complications of laryngeal framework surgery. *Laryngoscope* 1993; **103:** 525–8.
64. Van den Berg JW. Myoelastic-aerodynamic theory of voice production. *J Speech Hear Res* 1958; **1:** 227–44.
65. Van den Berg JW, Tan TS. Results of experiments with human larynges. *Pract Otorhinolaryngol (Basel)* 1959; **21:** 425–50.

66. Van den Berg JW, Zantema JF, Doornenbal P Jr. On the air resistance and Bernoulli effect of the human larynx. *J Acoust Soc Am* 1959; **29:** 626–31.
67. Waar CH. Stemveranderingen bij transsexuelen door operatie. *Logoped Foniatr* 1986; **58:** 135–7.
68. Woo P. Quantification of videostroboscopic findings – measurements of the glottic cycle. *Laryngoscope* 1996; **106:** S791–827.
69. Woo P, Casper J, Colton R, Brewer D. Aerodynamic and stroboscopic findings before and after microlaryngeal phonosurgery. *J Voice* 1994; **8:** 186–94.
70. Woodson GE, Murray T. Glottic configuration after arytenoid adduction. *Laryngoscope* 1994; **104:** 965–9.

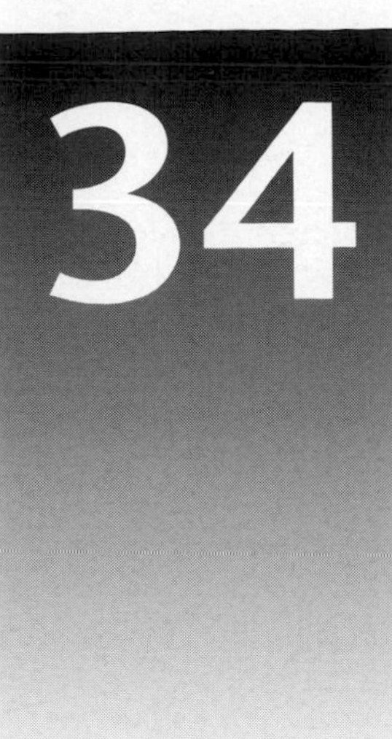

Benign laryngeal neoplasms

Jonas T Johnson and Clark A Rosen

The larynx is a histologically complex organ with epithelium covering fibrous and muscle tissue attached to a cartilage framework. The overwhelming majority of laryngeal neoplasia is malignant. Squamous cell carcinoma, the most common laryngeal neoplasm, is widely attributed to the effects of environmental mutagens (e.g. tobacco).

Less than 10% of laryngeal neoplasia is benign. The laryngeal papilloma accounts for over 95% of these lesions.[35] Laryngeal papillomas are attributed to an acquired viral infection and are classically identified based upon the characteristic surface appearance (Fig 34.1). By contrast, all other benign laryngeal neoplasia can be classified as either uncommon or distinctly rare. These lesions may be suspected based upon their submucosal location, slow growth, relative paucity of symptoms, and, in some cases, characteristic appearance employing either CT or MRI. Excision of benign neoplasms of the larynx is, under most circumstances, curative and, under certain conditions, may be successfully and safely carried out employing endoscopic techniques.

Laryngeal papilloma

Papilloma represents the most common neoplasm of the larynx.[3] Papillomatosis of the larynx airway has plagued both patients and physicians for many years. Despite being a rare affliction, the significant morbidity and mortality that laryngotracheal papillomatosis (LTP) produces on each affected patient has resulted in a multitude of research and potential treatments.

Clinical presentation

LTP tends to present during two age groups, young children (6 months to 5 years) and young adults (18–30 years). The symptoms of LTP at presentation in children is usually hoarseness or airway difficulties. Adult-onset LTP presents with persistent hoarseness, (frequently following an upper respiratory infection or oral-tracheal

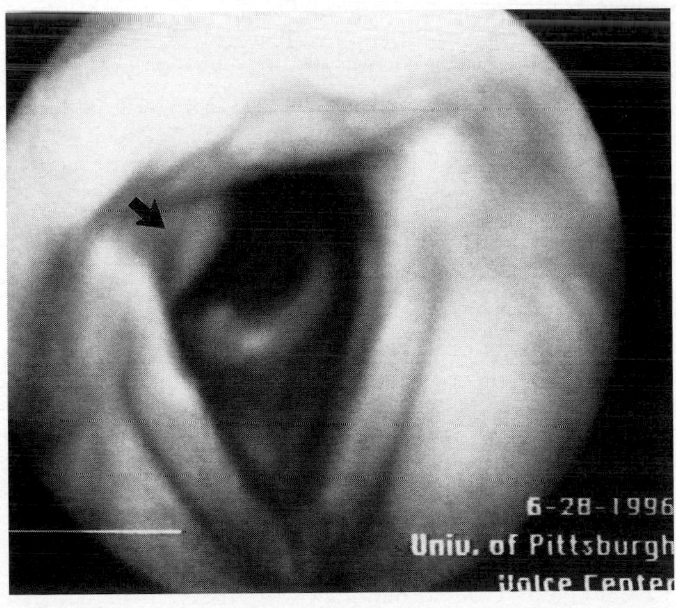

Figure 34.1 *This patient presents with multiple laryngeal papillomas. The appearance of these papillomas is characteristic of this condition.*

intubation) or cough or globus sensation. The severity and clinical course in both pediatric and adult LTP is highly variable and unpredictable. Most common is a recurrent papillary growth following surgical removal.

Papilloma growths may occur throughout the aerodigestive tract, the vocal folds being the most common location. Kashima *et al.* found that LTP tends to occur at the junction of respiratory epithelium with squamous epithelium.[27] LTP is frequently seen in the laryngeal ventricles and can spread distally into the tracheal–bronchial tree, especially when a tracheotomy is present.

Etiology

The etiology of papilloma disease of the larynx for many decades was unknown, despite an early recognition that LTP may be caused by a virus. Ullmann in 1923 proposed that LTP was caused by a virus.[48] He prepared a sterile, cell-free extract from a laryngeal papilloma, injected it into his arm, and developed a skin wart. Despite this creative and insightful work, the etiologic agent of LTP was not soundly proved until 1982.[34] The cause of LTP has been found to be an infection of a human papilloma virus (HPV).

The viral particles of HPV were discovered in a cutaneous wart in 1949 and in a genital wart in 1969. HPV is a double-stranded DNA virus belonging to the papovavirus family. These viruses have a circular, closed DNA that is protected by an icosahedral capsid. At least 54 known types of HPV have been distinguished by DNA hybridization techniques. LTP is most commonly associated with the HPV types 6 and 11. Each type has a greater than 50% difference between genomes. Infection also causes condyloma of the genital tract, predisposition to cervical carcinoma and cutaneous warts.

The application of Southern's transfer technology (Southern blot) is used to detect the HPV genome within laryngeal papilloma tissues. The testing techniques for DNA content of HPV have improved in sensitivity, specificity and ease of methodology. This has allowed for multiple studies of LTP involving typing and clinical correlation. Four subtypes of HPV-6 have been found, HPV-6c, 6d, 6e and 6f. These viruses and HPV-11 share 85% genome patterns and are responsible for the majority of LTPs. At present, it appears that HPV types and subtypes do not correlate with clinical outcomes.[37]

Steinberg *et al.* provided a significant breakthrough in the quest to understand the LTP disease process when they reported the identification of HPV DNA in biopsy samples of patients with a history of LTP.[45] These biopsies were from either uninvolved sites of the larynx in patients with active LTP or normal appearing tissue in patients in remission. This explains the highly variable natural course of LTP and the occurrence of recurrent LTP following long periods of disease-free intervals.

Histology

Epithelial cells infected by HPV undergo transformation and, as the transformed cells proliferate, a wart-like lesion develops. The virus is found within the nuclei of superficial epithelial cells. The typical laryngeal papilloma has a thickened spinous layer within the epithelium. Papillomata appear as projections of keratinized stratified squamous epithelium overlying a fibrovascular core upon microscopic examination. The basal zone of the epithelium is often hyperplastic. Koilocytes, which appear as vacuolated cells with clean cytoplasm, are commonly seen.[31]

Transmission

Recent virologic advances in HPV detection have been coupled with long-standing clinical suspicion that LTP may be related to maternal genital warts. The pertinent issues at hand are:

- Does maternal HPV infection cause LTP?
- What is the mechanism of transmission of the virus from mother to child?
- Would delivery by cesarean section prevent LTP?

In 1956, Hajek reported a case of LTP in a child whose mother had extensive genital condyloma.[40] Cook *et al.* published a retrospective chart review of the HPV status of the mothers of nine children with LTP.[7] Five of these mothers were found to have active condyloma disease at the time of birth. Subsequent studies with larger numbers have substantiated that more than half the mothers of children with LTP have a history of condyloma during pregnancy. Strong *et al.* reported 18 of their 36 LTP patients had mothers with active genital PV disease at the time of birth.[47] Hallden and Majmudar reported a 54% rate of a positive maternal history for genital warts among their 44 children with LTP.[11] Fortunately, a low number of children with mothers that have condyloma at birth develop LTP. Shah *et al.* calculated that the risk of developing juvenile LTP from an infected mother is one in several hundred.[40] Thus there is a connection between maternal HPV disease and an increased risk of children developing LTP.

Initially the presumed method of disease transmission was direct contact in the birth canal. This was supported by a report that the foreskin of 4% of newborn boys harbored HPV. By contrast, a case of a young girl with condyloma and an intact hymen, whose mother had genital HPV, has been reported.[30] In this case, the same HPV type was found in the mother's and daughter's cervix and the cord blood. A well-documented case of a child with LTP that was born by cesarean section with intact membranes puts significant question to the birth canal theory of perinatal transmission.[40]

Transmission of a virus from the maternal lower genital tract to the fetus may occur by an ascending infection reaching the fetus while in the uterus. Transplacental intrauterine transmission also may occur if the infection is blood-borne. Several recent studies have been published using sensitive HPV-probe technology in a prospective manner testing mother and neonate for evidence of HPV.[11,44] These studies strongly suggest an *in utero* transmission of the HPV from mother to fetus. Thus, elective cesarean section for delivery of babies of mothers with active or latent HPV is not recommended.

Treatment

A plethora of treatment modalities have been used over the years for LTP. Medical therapy for LTP in the past has included hormones, escharotics, podophyllin, celandine, antibiotics, magnesium and corticosteroids.[18] The latter was injected intralaryngeally without success. The possibility of a vaccine has been entertained for many years. A bovine papilloma vaccine, autogenous vaccine, attenuated human papilloma virus and the smallpox vaccine have all been tried to treat LTP without success.[42,46] Recently, anecdotal success has been reported using the mumps vaccine injected into the laryngeal papilloma tissue, but no clinical studies have been published to date.

Surgical therapy for LTP has also tried multiple approaches without significant success. Repeated removal with forceps earlier and now with the laser has been shown to be effective temporarily for symptoms of the voice and airway problems.[47] However, surgical removal to date is only a temporizing therapy that frequently results in scar formation to the laryngeal structures.[36]

Tracheotomy has also been a frequent surgery for both airway establishment and in hope of 'putting the larynx at rest'. It has been established that the presence of a tracheotomy may worsen a patient's disease. Present recommendations are to avoid this procedure if possible.[4]

Thermal cautery, diathermy and radiation have been used in the treatment of LTP, usually with initial success but with ultimate failures and serious complications.[47] Electrocautery and diathermy have resulted in serious scar, whilst radiation has been linked with the malignant transformation of LTP.

Interferon (IFN) was first used to treat LTP in 1981 by Haglund *et al.* in Sweden.[13] The known actions of interferons are antiviral, antineoplastic and immunomodulating. This includes induction of enzymes within cells that block viral replication of RNA and DNA, alteration of cell membranes to make them less susceptible to viral penetration, and selective inhibition of growth and proliferation of neoplastic cells. The mechanisms used by IFN to produce the above changes are unknown. IFN can be given either by intramuscular or subcutaneous injection.

Kashima and colleagues performed a prospective, randomized crossover trial using IFN for LTP.[26,29] Six patients in the original observation group developed a complete response following the crossover to IFN treatment. A total of eight of the 57 patients in the study had a complete response from 6 months of IFN treatment. No complete responses were achieved during either of the observational periods. The overall trend was that following discontinuation of IFN therapy a relatively rapid return of disease of increased severity occurred.

The most recent follow-up of this study was published by Leventhal *et al.* in 1991.[29] This provided a median follow-up of 4 years on 60 of the original 66 patients. After the above year of treatment and observation (6 months of each), the patients were treated with IFN as recommended by their physicians. During the long follow-up, 22 of the 60 (37%) patients achieved a complete response at one point during the study. Unfortunately, seven patients relapsed following the complete response (two while on IFN and five while off IFN). Worse results were seen in the partial response category. The recidivism rate for complete and partial responses was 53% over the 4 years of follow-up. The final recommendations from this study were that for patients with severe LTP a 6-month trial of IFN should be given. If no response is achieved, then IFN should be stopped. However, if a partial response occurs, then continued IFN treatment is justified.

Healy *et al.* published their results of a large, randomized, multicenter trial of IFN for LTP in 1988.[16] At 1 year and beyond, they found no significant differences in the outcome measures between the IFN + surgery group and the surgery alone group.

Crockett *et al.* provided a detailed report of the Iowa study group's experience with side effects of IFN therapy.[8] Out of these 26 patients, two experienced neurotoxic side effects. These consisted of seizures following therapy. One patient had self-limiting seizures that were probably associated with the febrile response to IFN. The second patient had a series of petit and grand mal seizures that required anti-seizure medication prior to restarting IFN treatment. Mild alopecia was also reported to have occurred in several patients in most of the studies. Healy found no evidence of growth disturbances from IFN with long-term follow-up.[15]

There is very good evidence that IFN will cause a significant reduction in disease in most patients. In addition, IFN causes maintenance of reduced disease with constant use. However, the curative ability of IFN has not been clearly shown to be present.

Photodynamic therapy (PDT) is an experimental treatment for LTP. This treatment consists of an intravenous injection of an agent that has the ability to localize within abnormal tissue and then be activated with a specialized light source (laser).

The largest clinical experience with PDT for LTP was reported in 1992 by Abramson *et al.*[1] This is a series of 33 patients with severe LTP, all treated with one or two courses of PDT. Thirty patients were available for analysis with an average follow-up of 1 year. Three patients had a complete response with a follow-up of 22, 23 and 27 months, respectively. The average growth rates were statistically improved following PDT. A 50% decreased average growth rate of the LTP disease was observed ($P = 0.004$).

Patients with the worst disease had the best overall response. Adult-onset disease appeared to be more responsive to PDT than the juvenile-onset disease. The mean time between procedures to reestablish an airway improved from 52 days prior to PDT to 100 days following PDT.

The side effects of PDT include the post-treatment photosensitivity reactions of mild erythema, inflammation, pruritus and ocular discomfort. Almost a quarter of the patients had some skin blistering. Photosensitivity occurred for an average of 9 weeks with a range of 4–17 weeks. These were described as a sunburn and only occurred in locations that were exposed to sun and light, e.g. the face and dorsum of the hands. Compliance with the photosensitivity precautions was noted to be the worst in the active, young male patients. Most adults returned to work in 2 weeks and the children received home tutoring for 4–8 weeks after PDT.

The results of PDT are still preliminary but encouraging. Many questions still persist regarding this therapy. Long-term follow-up, toxic effects, different photosensitizing agents and different light sources and delivery methods are all important issues that are presently unknown regarding photodynamic therapy.[41]

Recent studies have shown promise for the treatment of LTP using peroral administration of indole-3-carbinol (I3C). I3C is a chemical found in high concentrations of cruciferous vegetables. I3C has been shown to alter estrogen degradation, resulting in different concentrations of various estrogen metabolites. The estrogen changes induced by I3C have been found to stop HPV-infected cell culture growth and to reduce HPV infection in an animal model.

Preliminary results of an open-label, prospective clinical trial found a 33% complete response and 33% partial response in patients with LTP.[39] I3C is available as a nutritional supplemental. Clinical experience of 3 years has shown no significant side effects or toxicity using I3C for LTP.[39] A double-blind, crossover study using I3C for LTP is pending.

Other experimental treatments for LTP include aciclovir, retinoic acid and ribavirin. A clinical trial for the latter is in progress.

Chondroma

Laryngeal chondromas are uncommon and are seen most often in the sixth or seventh decade of life. Hoarseness, dysphagia, dyspnea, foreign body sensation, or a neck mass may serve as the presenting symptom. The cricoid cartridge is most commonly involved (Fig 34.2). The occasional chondroma rises from the thyroid cartridge and grows externally. Only on very rare occasions have chondromas been reported from the arytenoid cartridge.

Laryngeal chondromas are most frequent in men with a male:female ratio of 4:1.[12,19,20] The cause of these tumors is unknown.

Histologically, the chondroma is hypocellular with 30–40 cells per high power field. Mitotic activity is not a feature of the benign chondroma.

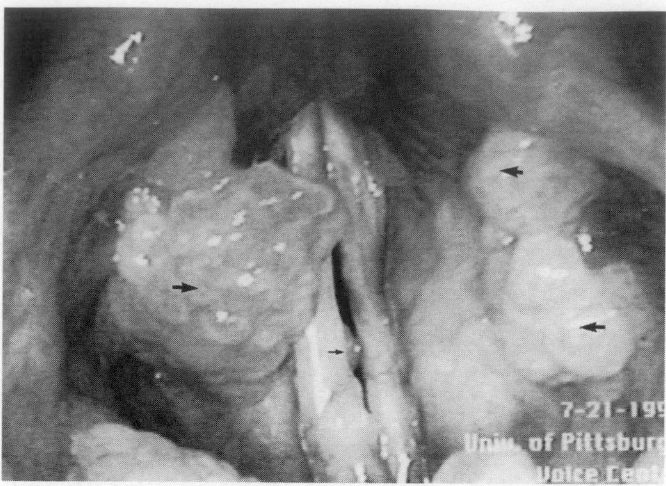

Figure 34.2 *The patient has a cricoid chondroma. Note the submucosal bulging from the posterior right aspect of the larynx.*

Biopsy is difficult because of the soft tissue covering of the laryngeal cartilages and the hard consistency of the lesion, which may resist attempts at biopsy.

The distinction between benign chondroma and a low-grade chondral sarcoma may be pathologically difficult. Establishment of a firm diagnosis may require excision and serial sectioning of the entire lesion. This places a great deal of responsibility upon the clinician faced with treatment planning prior to a firm establishment of a diagnosis. Fortunately, the slow growth of the relatively low-grade chondrosarcoma behaves in a fashion similar to a benign lesion, causing some authors to argue that the treatment should be similar.

Benign chondroma may attain sizes in excess of several centimeters in diameter but they do not metastasize. Excision is curative. Unfortunately, excision may require a total laryngectomy or result in laryngeal dysfunction due to either aspiration or stenosis because of extensive cricoid involvement. Nevertheless, conservative surgical management with local excision designed to preserve the upper airway, whenever possible, is recommended by most authors. A recent report suggests that fine-needle aspiration of cartilaginous tumors may contribute to preoperative establishment of diagnosis.[12]

Paraganglioma

Laryngeal paragangliomas arise from the paraganglia normally located in the larynx.[28] A pair is present in the anterior aspect of the false vocal cord whilst a second pair is found in the subglottic region just superior to the division of the recurrent nerve into its anterior and posterior branches. The superior paraganglia are between 0.1 and 0.3 mm in diameter whereas the inferior paraganglia are between 0.3 and 0.4 mm.

Neoplastic development of a paraganglioma occurs more commonly in women than men by a ratio of 4:1.

These lesions are most commonly recognized in the fourth to sixth decades of life. These are extremely unusual lesions which have been reported in fewer than 70 cases.[10]

Clinical symptomatology is referable to the size and location of the paraganglioma. Hoarseness is the most common symptom.

Functional laryngeal paragangliomas have been reported but are exceedingly rare.[32] Paraneoplastic syndrome is not associated with paraganglioma but may be an indication of an atypical carcinoid tumor, an important clinical distinction. Multiple paragangliomas of the head and neck are frequently encountered in the familial setting.

The laryngeal paraganglioma presents as a submucosal mass. Preoperative imaging with contrast may alert the physician to the highly vascular nature of these lesions. Endoscopic biopsy may result in catastrophic hemorrhage.

Histologically, paragangliomas are characterized by chief and sustentacular cells. Chief cells are polygonal with small nuclei arranged as Zellballen. Paragangliomas are argyrophil-positive and argentaffin-negative. Electron microscopy shows neural secretory granules. Chief cells stain positive for chromogranin and synaptophysin. Paragangliomas are cytokeratin-negative.

The overwhelming majority of laryngeal paragangliomas are benign. The presence of a mitotic activity does not correlate with behavior. The recommended treatment is conservative excision accomplished most commonly through a lateral pharyngotomy approach.

Granular cell tumors

Granular cell tumors are benign lesions. Current opinion is that these are derived from Schwann cells.[6] Granular cell tumors are most commonly seen in the tongue and are extremely rare in the larynx.

Granular cell tumors are submucosal in location. Hoarseness may occur. Stridor and respiratory obstruction is extremely rare. Between 10 and 15% of patients with granular cell tumors may have multifocal involvement under which circumstances the larynx may be involved.

The granular cell tumor may be covered by pseudoepitheliomatous hyperplasia.[5] This observation is the source of histologic error and an erroneous diagnosis of dysplasia or squamous carcinoma may be made.

The tumor is S-100 positive. Malignancy in a granular cell tumor is extremely rare (less than 2%).[9] Simple excision is the treatment for all small tumors which can ordinarily be achieved endoscopically. Larger tumors may require laryngofissure to afford adequate exposure.

Neurilemmoma or benign schwannoma

Neurilemmomas are benign tumors of Schwann cells. The true incidence of laryngeal neurilemmoma and laryngeal neurofibroma is unknown; however, fewer than 100 cases have been reported to date. Rarely, neurilemmomas may be associated with neurofibromatosis type I (von Recklinghausen's disease).[43]

Neurofibroma

Neurofibroma should be distinguished from neurilemmoma because of the association neurofibroma has with neurofibromatosis type I.[43] A small percentage of neurofibromas may transform into malignant tumors. Conversely, neurilemmoma is rarely associated with malignancy. Diagnostic criteria are similar to those used to distinguish these lesions in other regions of the body.

Salivary gland neoplasm

Benign pleomorphic adenoma of the larynx has been reported in fewer than ten cases in the world literature.[2] Most arise from the supraglottic larynx and have been reported as early as adolescence but more commonly in midlife. Histologic diagnosis is uncomplicated. Treatment requires excision.

Oncocytoma

Solitary oncocytomas are extremely rare and only a few cases have been reported in the world literature.[38] Oncocytic hyperplasia, however, may be occasionally encountered in elderly patients.[14] These lesions are most commonly seen in the supraglottic larynx and may be an incidental finding during laryngoscopy. In most cases endoscopic excision can be accomplished and is curative.

Leiomyoma

Fewer than 30 leiomyomas of the larynx have been reported.[23] These lesions arise from smooth muscle and are most common in the supraglottic larynx. Pathologically, leiomyoma are divided into conventional, vascular and epithelioid.

Benign leiomyoma may be distinguished from leiomyosarcoma by the absence of the necrosis, pleomorphism, and significant myotatic activity. Treatment consists of simple endoscopic removal. An external approach may be required for large lesions.

Vascular leiomyoma is more unusual; biopsy or attempted endoscopic removal may be associated with profuse bleeding. Most of the reported epithelioid leiomyomas occur in the gastrointestinal tract. There have been only two documented cases of epithelioid leiomyoma of the larynx.[17,33]

Rhabdomyoma

The most common rhabdomyomas are cardiac in origin. These benign tumors develop from striated muscle. Extracardiac rhabdomyomas may be subclassified into adult and fetal type. The histologic appearance of adult rhabdomyoma is distinctive and usually easily diagnosed on routine histologic section. Electron microscopy, employed in difficult cases, will demonstrate myofilaments, Z-bands and glycogen granules. Complete excision is the treatment of choice.[24,49]

Fetal rhabdomyomas are benign tumors that exhibit immature skeletal muscle differentiation. These typically present before age 10 years; however, as many as 50% of patients may be recognized after 15 years of age.[25] The absence of prominent nuclear atypia is important in distinguishing fetal rhabdomyoma from rhabdomyosarcoma. Excision is the treatment of choice.[21]

Lipoma

Benign lipoma is commonly encountered in a wide variety of locations throughout the body. It is estimated that 13% of lipomas occur in the head and neck.[49] Laryngeal lipomas are exceedingly unusual and, when noted, occur most often in the supraglottic larynx.[22]

Conclusions

With the exception of laryngeal papillomas, benign neoplasms are exceedingly rare when compared to the more commonly encountered malignant lesions of the larynx. Under most circumstances, function-sparing procedures are satisfactory to effect cure. It is essential that the clinician is aware of the wide variety of pathologies that may be encountered. The consulting pathologist must be knowledgeable in these diagnoses to afford the clinician the opportunity to recommend the appropriate therapy when planning treatment. Under many circumstances, excisional biopsy may be accomplished, often using endoscopic techniques, before the final diagnosis is substantiated.

References

1. Abramson AL, Shikowitz MJ, Mullooly VM, Steinberg BM, Amella CA, Rothstein HR. Clinical effects of photodynamic therapy on recurrent laryngeal papillomas. *Arch Otolaryngol Head Neck Surg* 1992; **118**: 25–9.
2. Argat M, Born IA, Maier H, Mohadjer C. Pleomorphic adenoma of the larynx. *Eur Arch Otorhinolaryngol* 1994; **251**: 304–6.
3. Cohen SR, Geller KA, Seltzer S, Thompson JW. Papilloma of the larynx and tracheobronchial tree in children. A retrospective study. *Ann Otol* 1980; **89**: 497–503.
4. Cole RR, Myer CM III, Cotton RT. Tracheotomy in children with recurrent respiratory papillomatosis. *Head Neck* 1989; **11**: 226–30.
5. Compagno J, Hyams VJ, Ste Marie P. Benign granular cell tumors of the larynx: a review of 36 cases with clinicopathologic data. *Ann Otol* 1975; **84**: 308–14.
6. Conley SF, Milbrath MM, Beste DJ. Pediatric laryngeal granular cell tumor. *J Otolaryngol* 1992; **21**: 450–3.
7. Cook TA, Brunschwig J, Butel JS, Cohn AM, Goepfert H, Rawls WE. Laryngeal papilloma: etiologic and therapeutic considerations. *Ann Otol* 1973; **82**: 649–55.
8. Crockett DM, McCabe BF, Lusk RP, Mixon JH. Side effects and toxicity of interferon in the treatment of recurrent respiratory papillomatosis. *Ann Otol Rhinol Laryngol* 1987; **96**: 601–7.
9. Enzinger F, Weiss S. Benign tumors of peripheral nerves. In: *Soft Tissue Tumors*, 2nd edn. St Louis: Mosby, 1988: 719–80.
10. Ferlito A, Milroy CM, Barnes L. Neuroendocrine neoplasms. In: Ferlito A, ed. *Surgical Pathology of Laryngeal Neoplasms*. London: Chapman and Hall, 1996: 173–93.
11. Fletcher JL Jr. Perinatal transmission of human papilloma virus. *Am Fam Physician* 1991; **43**: 143–8.
12. Frober MK, Meschter SC, Brown RE, Garbes AD. Cartilaginous tumors of the larynx. A report of two cases with definitive diagnosis by fine needle aspiration and computer tomography. *Acta Cytol* 1996; **40**: 761–4.
13. Haglund S, Lundquist P, Cantell K, Stander H. Interferon therapy in juvenile laryngeal papillomatosis. *Arch Otolaryngol* 1981; **107**: 327–32.
14. Hartwick RW, Batsakis JG. Non-Warthin's tumor oncocytic lesions. *Ann Otol Rhinol Laryngol* 1990; **99**: 674–7.
15. Healy GB. Personal communication, 1993.
16. Healy GB, Gelber RD, Trowbridge AL, Grundfast KM, Ruben RJ, Price KN. Treatment of recurrent respiratory papillomatosis with human leukocyte interferon. Results of a multicenter randomized clinical trial. *N Engl J Med* 1988; **319**: 401–7.
17. Hellquist HB, Hellqvist H, Vejlens L, Lindholm CE. Epithelioid leiomyoma of the larynx. *Histopathology* 1994; **24**: 155–9.
18. Holinger P, Schild J, Maurizi D. Laryngeal papilloma: review of etiology and therapy. *Laryngoscope* 1968; **78**: 1462–74.
19. Huizenga C, Balogh K. Cartilaginous tumors of the larynx. A clinopathologic study of 10 new cases and a review of the literature. *Cancer* 1970; **26**: 201–10.
20. Hyams VJ, Rabuzzi DD. Cartilaginous tumors of the larynx. *Laryngoscope* 1970; **80**: 755–67.
21. Johansen ECJ, Illum P. Rhabdomyoma of the larynx: a review of the literature with a summary of previously described cases of rhabdomyoma of the larynx and a report of a new case. *J Laryngol Otol* 1995; **109**: 147–53.
22. Jones SR, Myers EN, Barnes L. Benign neoplasms of the larynx. *Otolaryngol Clin North Am* 1984; **17**: 151–78.
23. Kapadia SB, Barnes L. Muscle tissue neoplasms. In: Ferlito A, ed. *Surgical Pathology of Laryngeal Neoplasms*. London: Chapman and Hall, 1996: 321–40.
24. Kapadia SB, Meis JM, Frisman DM, Ellis GL, Heffner DK. Fetal rhabdomyoma of the head and neck: clinicopathologic and immunophenotypic study of 24 cases. *Hum Pathol* 1993; **24**: 754–65.
25. Kapadia SB, Meis JM, Frisman DM, Ellis GL, Heffner DK, Hyams VJ. Adult rhabdomyoma of the head and neck: a clinicopathologic and immunophenotypic study. *Hum Pathol* 1993; **24**: 608–17.
26. Kashima HK, Leventhal BG, Clark K *et al.* Interferon alfa-n1 (Wellferon) in juvenile onset recurrent respiratory papillomatosis: results of a randomized study in twelve collaborative institutions. *Laryngoscope* 1988; **98**: 334–40.

27. Kashima HK, Shah F, Lyles A *et al.* A comparison of risk factors in juvenile-onset and adult-onset recurrent respiratory papillomatosis. *Laryngoscope* 1992; **102:** 9–13.
28. Lawson N, Zak FG. The glomus bodies ('paraganglia') of the human larynx. *Laryngoscope* 1974; **84:** 98–111.
29. Leventhal BG, Kashima HK, Mounts P *et al.* Long-term response of recurrent respiratory papillomatosis to treatment with lymphoblastoid interferon alfa-N1. *N Engl J Med* 1991; **325:** 613–17.
30. Lindeberg H, Elbrxnd O. Laryngeal papillomas: clinical aspects in series of 231 patients. *Clin Otolaryngol* 1989; **14:** 333–42.
31. Meyers C, Frattini MG, Hudson JB, Laimins LA. Biosynthesis of human papillomavirus from a continuous cell line upon epithelial differentiation. *Science* 1992; **257:** 971–3.
32. Milroy CM, Rode J, Moss E. Laryngeal paragangliomas and neuroendocrine carcinomas. *Histopathology* 1991; **18:** 201–9.
33. Mori H, Kumoi T, Hashimoto M, Uematsu K. Leiomyoblastoma of the larynx: report of a case. *Head Neck* 1992; **14:** 148–52.
34. Mounts P, Shah K, Kashima H. Viral etiology of juvenile- and adult-onset squamous papilloma of the larynx. *Proc Natl Acad Sci USA* 1982; **79:** 5425–9.
35. Narozny W, Mikaszewski B, Stankiewicz C. Benign neoplasms of the larynx. *Auris Nasus Larynx* 1995; **22:** 38–42.
36. Ossoff R, Werkhaven J, Dere H. Soft-tissue complications of laser surgery for recurrent respiratory papillomatosis. *Laryngoscope* 1991; **101:** 1162–6.
37. Rimell F, Maisel R, Dayton V. In situ hybridization and laryngeal papillomas. *Ann Otol Rhinol Laryngol* 1992; **101:** 119–26.
38. Robinson AC, Kaberos A, Cox PM, Stearns MP. Oncocytoma of the larynx. *J Laryngol Otol* 1990; **104:** 346–9.
39. Rosen CA, Woodson GE, Thompson JW, Hengesteg AP, Bradlow HL. Preliminary results of the use of indole-3-carbinol for recurrent respiratory papillomatosis. *Otolaryngol Head Neck Surg* 1997; **118:** 810–15.
40. Shah K, Kashima H, Polk BF, Shah F, Abbey H, Abramson AL. Rarity of cesarean delivery in cases of juvenile-onset respiratory papillomatosis. *Obstet Gynecol* 1986; **68:** 795–9.
41. Shikowitz MJ. Comparison of pulsed and continuous wave light in photodynamic therapy of papillomas: an experimental study. *Laryngoscope* 1992; **102:** 300–10.
42. Shipkowitz NL, Holper JC, Worland MC, Holinger PH. Evaluation of an autogenous laryngeal papilloma vaccine. *Laryngoscope* 1967; **77:** 1047–66.
43. Smith BC, Wenig BM. Neurogenic neoplasms including melanoma: In: Ferlito A, ed. *Surgical Pathology of Laryngeal Neoplasms.* London: Chapman and Hall, 1996: 195–255.
44. Smith EM, Johnson SR, Cripe TP, Pignatari S, Turek L. Perinatal vertical transmission of human papillomavirus and subsequent development of respiratory tract papillomatosis. *Ann Otol Rhinol Laryngol* 1991; **100:** 479–83.
45. Steinberg BM, Topp WC, Schneider PS, Abramson AL. Laryngeal papillomavirus infection during clinical remission. *N Engl J Med* 1983; **308:** 1261–4.
46. Stephens CB, Arnold GE, Butchko GM, Hardy CL. Autogenous vaccine treatment of juvenile laryngeal papillomatosis. *Laryngoscope* 1979; **89:** 1689–96.
47. Strong MS, Vaughan CW, Cooperband SR, Healy GB, Clemente MA. Recurrent respiratory papillomatosis: management with the CO_2 laser. *Ann Otol* 1976; **85:** 508–16.
48. Ullmann EV. On the etiology of laryngeal papilloma. *Acta Otolaryngol (Stockh)* 1923; **5:** 317–38.
49. Zbären P, Läng H, Becker M. Rare benign neoplasms of the larynx: rhabdomyoma and lipoma. *ORL J Otorhinolaryngol Relat Spec* 1995; **57:** 351–5.

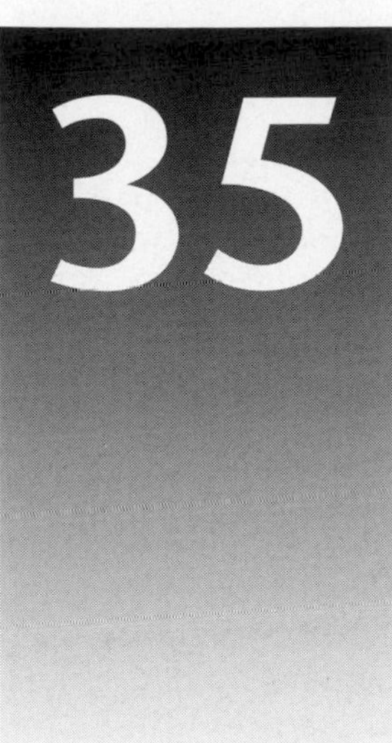

Epidemiology and pathogenesis of laryngeal cancer

Neil Molony, Alessandra Rinaldo, Arnold G D Maran and Alfio Ferlito

The term epidemiology represents the study of the pattern of the disease throughout populations. The term pathogenesis covers risk factors and mechanisms implicated in bringing around the origin of a disease. Patterns of disease in populations will vary due to intrinsic factors (the genetics of a population) and extrinsic factors (environmental factors). The latter will include some under the control of individual subjects, such as smoking and alcohol consumption, and other factors often beyond their control, such as atmospheric pollution.

Laryngeal cancer is a relatively rare disease, but it is the most frequent cancer of the head and neck,[38] apart from skin malignancies[32] and it is also the second most common respiratory cancer after lung cancer.[17] It accounts for roughly 1% of all cancer mortality, amounting to roughly 200 000 deaths annually worldwide.[16] Laryngeal cancer represents 2–5% of all malignancies diagnosed annually worldwide. In the USA, cancer of the larynx accounts for approximately 2% of all cancers and for 25% of all head and neck cancers. In 1990, American cancer statistics reported that approximately 4000 deaths, or nearly 1% of all cancer-related deaths, were due to laryngeal cancer. Each year 12 500 new cases of laryngeal cancer are diagnosed in the USA.[76] Its incidence is increasing over time in much of the world, and this increase is generally attributed to changes in alcohol and tobacco consumption.[17] Important as they are, they are not the only factors involved.

Squamous cell carcinoma represents approximately 85–90% of all malignant laryngeal neoplasms[30] and is the focus of this chapter.

Epidemiological methods

How common a disease is in a population tends to be measured by two indices, incidence and prevalence. Incidence refers to the number of new cases per year per unit of population. This depends on clinicians and pathologists accurately diagnosing the lesion when a patient presents with it and is subjected to biopsy. The accuracy has been measured in the Euro Care study[10] and is close to, but not always equal to, 100%. This refers to First World countries and hence it may not be possible for all countries to give so accurate a figure for incidence of new cases. The second term used is prevalence, how many people have a disease in a unit of population at a given time, irrespective of how long they have had it. Figures for this are less used by cancer registries and are affected by survival, since if many patients live a long time with the lesion this will tend to give it a higher prevalence than a disease of equal incidence which is rapidly fatal. There is a problem of asymptomatic patients with the disease at whatever stage, who would only be picked up by an active screening program. Figures for survival after diagnosis are useful but subject to various confounding factors. The first is lead time bias. By this we mean that if an active screening program identifies a lesion at a very early stage, then subjects identified by this method may appear to live with the cancer far longer than if their diagnosis had been more delayed and they had presented with worse symptoms. A second problem is stage migration. If a pathologist spots tiny signs of cancer in parts of a resected specimen which most other pathologists would have regarded as clear, this automatically increases the T stage of the tumor such that the patient appears to have presented with a more advanced cancer. This could then have the effect of causing an apparent improvement of the survival of that patient by increasing the stage of disease at presentation. This is likely to be a particular problem in specialist centers where the histopathologists are extremely attuned to detecting such lesions and have the experience of dealing with relatively large numbers of such specimens. Crude survival itself needs to be weighted for the age and sex of patients, and their general health; this is termed 'survival analysis' for example by the Kaplan–Meier method.

Clinical studies may broadly be observational, 'let's see what happens', or experimental, 'we think A causes B; let us prove this by means of experiment C'. Epidemiological studies may be conducted in a prospective, cross-sectional or retrospective manner. 'The perfect study' would arguably be a prospective randomized controlled experimental trial of adequate power, regarded as the most effective means of deriving evidence by comparing two corresponding groups. The requirements for conducting a true randomized controlled study are rigorous and have been summarized recently in the 'CONSORT statement'.[3] For a suspected risk factor in carcinogenesis this would involve randomly assigning a large number of subjects to be exposed to, or kept away from, a proposed carcinogen for a considerable period, having eliminated or controlled for all other known or suspected risk factors. This is clearly unethical and also impossible. The next most powerful type of possible study, the strongest that can actually be done, is a non-randomized study conducted in a prospective manner. In this, as an observational study, a cohort of subjects exposed to a suspected risk factor, such as asbestos for cancer of the larynx, are followed forward over a period of time and their health measured. The study is strengthened by having a control group not exposed to the risk factor. These are the most difficult to coordinate and continue, and some subjects will always be lost. This could also be run on a more 'experimental' basis for an epidemiological treatment intervention, such as an anti-smoking campaign or a vaccination; in this, follow-up again needs to be prolonged in order to allow for the natural history of the disease to occur and for a therapeutic effect to take place.

Retrospective studies are easier to accomplish but are of less value than prospective studies. A common technique is the retrospective case-controlled study. To save time, instead of starting with well subjects and seeing if they develop a disease, we can start with people who are already ill and work backwards to attempt to find out why they came to have it. This is done by matching each 'case' with one or more disease-free controls of the same age, socioeconomic status, etc., and looking back in time to see how they differ. This study is weaker, being more open to the effects of chance and bias. Our ill subjects have already selected themselves by becoming ill, and of the 'at risk' group they were presumably the most 'at risk'. How do we know cases or controls are truly random samples? Large numbers are required to overcome the confounding effects of chance. These studies are widely used as a starting point to identify factors that seem to be associated with a particular disease. Association does not imply causation, but is a first step. For example, the Heidelberg study[53] examining exposure to paint and solvents found such exposure to raise the relative risk of developing laryngeal cancer. This can then act as a starting point for future prospective studies, such as identifying particular chemicals in solvents or implementing protective measures. Some prior knowledge of the natural history and of the magnitude of the suspected risk is needed to determine the required duration of a prospective study and the numbers of subjects to be recruited. Inferential statistics can then be used to determine whether or not there was a significant difference in (for our purposes) the incidence of cancer of the larynx between those exposed and those not exposed to the risk factor. In an ideal study, the effect of one variable would be examined in isolation by balancing or eliminating other known risk factors, allowing 'univariate' analysis. In practice this is also impossible for epidemiological studies, and multivariate analysis must be used. This involves more complex equations giving the risk factors a weighting to represent their relative importance. If these are wrong, or the risk factors interact in unexpected ways, then the analysis falls down.

The most common technique is to calculate 'odds ratios' (ORs) or 'relative risks' (RRs) for the risk of causing disease that may be attributed to the various known risk factors. These terms are often almost interchangeable and reasonably self-explanatory. For example, if we find an OR of 2 for asbestos exposure being associated with cancer of the larynx, then this means that, other things being equal, an asbestos worker is twice as likely as some other employee to develop laryngeal neoplasia, but the OR itself is an estimate and should be quoted with 95% confidence limits. 'Confidence intervals' are an important concept. Our study has inevitably picked only a sample of all people exposed, for example, to asbestos, giving a mean risk for developing laryngeal neoplasia. The true mean of everyone in a genetically and environmentally similar population will, we hope, be fairly close but is unlikely to coincide exactly. We would like to have some measure of how far the true figure may vary from that described and to that end 95% confidence limits can be calculated for the mean of the population. This means we can be 95% confident that the true mean risk, for everyone exposed whether in our study or not, lies between certain limits; this gives us a measure of the precision of our measurements and we would like the confidence interval to be fairly narrow. This issue is important for applying our findings more widely than the confines of our own work. If the 95% confidence limits for the OR for asbestos exposure cover the range 0–4, then we can be 95% confident that the true risk lies within this range – which is not very useful as there may be no risk at all!

Cross-sectional studies give a snapshot picture of a disease, being undertaken at one stage in time. This is therefore valid for that period, but patterns of disease will change with time. For countries with virtually no cases of cancer of the larynx registered in a given year, such as Mongolia,[93] the value of such data is very limited. Pooled over a number of countries, or in countries with a higher incidence of this disease, it is more useful.

Errors

Errors in findings may be of three types: random error, measurement error and systematic error. Random error is always with us and is unavoidable. Measurement error reflects mistakes by observers, e.g. missing a lesion on a chest radiograph. This can only be addressed by everyone being vigilant. Systematic error lies in our designing our study incorrectly, or using tools that regularly make untrue readings, or in poor statistical analysis. Probability and errors are two very important issues. We are accustomed to 'P values', typically 'P <0.05'. This refers to 'false-positive' findings of differences which do not truly exist. These are also referred to as type 1 or alpha errors. 'P <0.05' tells us that we are 95% certain that the difference we have found has not arisen due to chance. There is still the other 0.05, or 5%; if we conducted the experiment 20 times we 'ought to' get it wrong once – and how do we know our present experiment is not that 1 in 20? The second issue is the 'false-negative', where we fail to detect a difference which truly exists. This is also referred to as a type 2 or beta error, and reflects the fact that the study was not 'powerful enough' to detect the difference. In biological and medical sciences this has often been regarded as a lesser failing, but if we conduct otherwise meticulous studies which do not detect real differences we are not going to achieve true answers to our questions. The concept of 'power' depends on the magnitude of the 'risk' caused by the risk factor. If everyone who smoked developed cancer of the larynx within a matter of years, the answer would be obvious. If this is a rare event not occurring for many years we need large numbers.

Unsuitable studies

We require information from which we can make inferences applicable to other populations. A description of a single case or of a series of cases validly reports what happened to those individuals but is only otherwise useful in suggesting avenues of future more rigorous study. Small snapshot series, such as trauma as a cause of cancer of the larynx,[21] may be confusing if not taken in context; almost all the traumatized larynges were those of smokers. One frequently quoted retrospective study found asbestos to be apparently a very powerful risk factor,[82] which was not consistently borne out by many of the subsequent studies (see below).

Summary

In summary, on reading the epidemiological literature we need to be aware of how the survey was conducted, and on how great a scale, to give that study a weighting in our overall analysis. We can use prospective controlled cohort studies or retrospective case-controlled studies to derive information, but the analysis is complex and depends on our identifying the various confounding variables and including them in our (usually multivariate) analysis. Correctly used, this is a powerful tool, but elegant mathematical algorithms are only as good as the information given to them.

Demographic factors

To describe epidemiology accurately, we need accurate data. Almost all countries of the world now provide cancer registries to the World Health Organization (WHO).[8] The validity of these figures depends on the accuracy of the national registry. For many countries this will be of good quality, but not for all. Laryngeal cancer is relatively uncommon, making it particularly important to have accurate data. These figures describe only whole countries; within most countries there will be regions of relatively high incidence and others of low incidence.

Nonetheless, there are certain countries consistently with very high rates, such as Brazil, Spain, Italy, France, India and black populations in the USA, Hungary and Poland.[15,91] Countries with particularly low incidences include Japan, Sweden, Norway, China and Ireland.[15,91] Regional data are available for many, though not all, countries. In general, the incidence is higher amongst inhabitants of heavily industrialized cities and laryngeal cancer is usually more common in urban than in rural populations.[80] Migrating from country to town was found to lead to a later increase in a prospective study in Finland,[85] particularly in unmarried men. However, Chiang Mai province in Thailand, hardly an industrial area, at one time had the highest incidence in the world[58,74] and still has a high incidence in both sexes,[89] which is linked to smoking; and laryngeal carcinoma is found in Aboriginal populations,[5] demonstrating that no part of the human race is exempt from this condition.

Patterns of disease change with time and certainly changes in incidence and mortality due to laryngeal cancer have been described.[45] Such findings need to be interpreted in the light of the age distribution of the population. A country with few older people and a predominantly young population is likely to have an apparently low incidence of most solid tumors, and therefore figures take the age distribution into account. A clear area for concern is when neoplasms become more frequent amongst younger people such as laryngeal cancer in the Turin region in Italy.[4]

The larynx is anatomically divided into three main regions: supraglottis, glottis and subglottis. The relative incidences of tumors in these three sites also varies between populations. In North America, Australia and Sweden most laryngeal cancers are glottic whereas supraglottic tumors are more common in Finland, Italy, France and Spain. In the USA, the percentage of cancer occurrence amongst glottis, supraglottis and subglottis is reported as follows: glottic, 59%; supraglottic, 40%; subglottis, 1%.[6]

Clearly defined subgroups within a larger population may have a different incidence due to their behavior. The Mormons of Utah[28,77] and the Parsi in Bombay[42,43] have a far lower incidence due to their religious regulations forbidding smoking and drinking. Many diseases follow a gradient, increasing as one passes down the social classes in society. In New York, Jews of high social class have a far lower mortality than poor Roman Catholics and blacks. This may be expected because tobacco and alcohol consumption is lower among Jews than among non-Jews. Californian Adventists also have a truly low risk of cancer of the larynx due to proscription from use of all types of tobacco and alcoholic beverages.[80]

Age and sex

Cancer of the larynx has long been described as being most common in adult male smokers with a peak incidence in the sixth and seventh decades.[6] Standard texts long described this tumor as being far, far more common in men than women. Generally, the male to female ratio is 10:1 but it may be very different in some locations. For example, in Bombay it has been estimated to be 4.5:1, in Norway 7:1, in Finland 21:1.[16] These observations may well change in the coming years as the effect of the relative increase in women's smoking and drinking in early adult life onwards becomes apparent. More than 20% of laryngeal cancers now occur in women[12,46] and although the incidence rates are still considerably lower among women, the increase in incidence among women has been proportionally greater than that among men.[22] Laryngeal cancer has been described to occur during pregnancy; nonetheless, the age and sex of the pregnant woman makes her an unlikely candidate for laryngeal malignancies.[32]

Supraglottic cancer has been described as being proportionately more common in women,[73,83] a retrospective study documenting a male-to-female ratio of 3–5:1 both in whites and blacks for the supraglottis as against 9.2:1 among whites and 11.8:1 among blacks for glottic lesions.[96] Laryngeal cancer is rare in childhood and adolescence but not unknown.[31,57,75] It is interesting that factors such as tobacco and alcohol are less significant in the over 70s and that there is a far higher proportion of women affected in this age group.[50]

Patients without a history of tobacco and alcohol use who developed laryngeal cancer showed different characteristics compared with smokers or drinkers. They were an average of 10 years older, they showed no male predominance and their lesions were located in the glottis, which permitted early diagnosis and higher survival rate.[1]

Hormonal factors

Some *in vitro* studies have suggested that sex hormones may have a growth regulatory role in cancer of the larynx, explaining the difference in incidence between men and women.[36,55] Whilst it is clear that male sex hormones account for the change in the voice at puberty and the difference between the voices of men and women, evidence to implicate androgens as carcinogens is much more sketchy. The laryngopharyngeal mucosa normally possesses steroid hormone receptors;[55,69] hence, it is not surprising that occasionally cancers have been found with such receptors. A large retrospective Swedish study[72] found female alcoholics to have a sevenfold increased risk of laryngeal cancer compared with other women; this rather implies that women exposed to the same degree of the same risk factors may well get the same rate of disease. Overall there is no convincing evidence that laryngeal cancer is in any way a hormone-dependent neoplasm.

Genetic factors

Any disease will be a reflection of exogenous, and endogenous, genetic factors. Hence whilst smoking is the most clearly defined risk factor for cancer of the larynx, many heavy smokers will never develop this disease and some non-smokers will. Passive smoking is a concept hotly debated in the media, but relatively difficult to delineate as a risk factor. Evidently individuals have a widely varying susceptibility which will reflect their genetic makeup. This observation is strongly underlined by the existence of 'cancer-prone families'.[51] Laryngeal cancer has been described as a part of multiple cancer in Lynch syndromes-II.[52] Tracing relatives of patients with variety of carcinomas has been used as a means to attempt to identify cancer-prone families. A large case-controlled study in Brazil found the relative risk (RR) of developing a head and neck cancer to be doubled if a first-degree relative had had such a tumor.[34] Such information can lead to the identification of genes associated with an increased risk of carcinoma, potentially a very fruitful line of inquiry. As cancer of the larynx is much rarer than, for example, cancer of the colon, relatively less work has been undertaken but there are a number of interesting findings. Epidermal growth factor receptor (EGFR) has been found to be overexpressed in laryngeal cancers;[2] as in many other malignancies, alterations to the protein coded by the p53 tumor suppressor gene have been described.[49] With time, differing mutations are likely to be found for differing populations, for example in one series of oral cancers in India, more than 95% of samples showed oncogene involvement,[66] whereas this is rare in Western cancers.[33] Increased susceptibility to mutagen-induced chromosomal damage and decreased DNA repair capability in lymphocytes from patients with untreated upper aerodigestive tract cancer have been reported.[68,79] Substantial effect-measure modification was observed for smokers who demonstrated mutagen sensitivity whilst little evidence for such interaction was found between alcohol drinking and mutagen sensitivity. However, it is not clear if increased mutagen sensitivity might be due to the neoplastic disease process.

Increased susceptibility could be to all cancers, or merely to cancer of the larynx. Given that it is not uncommon to have two synchronous primary tumors in the upper aerodigestive tract, genetic factors could render the whole of that epithelial lining susceptible. Genetic factors and the influence of environmental factors other than tobacco and alcohol are difficult to separate.[18,86]

Racial differences are well documented in the USA where American blacks have a higher incidence of most cancers.[35] This contributes to their greater mortality rate, although such other factors as availability and usage of medical services are significant.

Extrinsic and environmental risk factors

Tobacco

Study upon study from around the world in widely differing populations demonstrate that there is no longer any question about the exposure to tobacco smoke as the major cause of laryngeal cancer, as well as many other diseases. Laryngeal cancer would be a very rare disease if people did not smoke; it is thus in most cases a preventable disease. Typically, it has previously affected men far more than women, but this may merely be because men have always smoked more.

Exposure to cigarette smoke may be active, i.e. by smoking, or passive. Passive smoking is a concept hotly debated in the media, but relatively difficult to delineate as a risk factor. In Denmark passive smoking has been estimated as accounting for 0.6% of cases of carcinoma of the bronchus[26] but similar estimates are not yet available for the less common laryngeal cancers.

For smokers, the quantity of tobacco consumption and the period for which exposure has been occurring are directly proportional to the incidence of laryngeal cancer.[14,95] In a study based on the mortality rates among US veterans there was evidence of 0.6 deaths per 100 000 person-years among non-smokers, up to 15 deaths per 100 000 among those who had smoked 40 or more cigarettes daily.[63]

There are popular myths that pipe and cigar smokers are less at risk, also that the smokers who do not inhale have a lower risk of developing lung and laryngeal cancer. Rothman *et al.*[63] reported a mortality rate of 5.0 among pipe and cigar smokers. Non-inhalers of smoke also had a decreased risk for laryngeal cancer relative to inhalers (RR = 0.66).[88] 'The less harmful cigarette' is supposedly one with a filter and low tar tobacco (light tobacco).[37,94] A study compared the risk of laryngeal squamous cell carcinoma between light and dark tobacco smokers in Uruguay, stating that the relative risk for the dark tobacco users was 2.5 times higher than that for light tobacco users.[23]

The causative agents are polycyclic aromatic hydrocarbons, which are found in tar from tobacco. The best known are benzopyrene, benzanthracene and methylcholanthrene. These are broken down to produce carcinogenic epoxides, which bind to DNA and RNA. Since the whole respiratory tract is exposed to this, it follows that the whole epithelium may undergo 'field change' towards malignancy. All parts of the upper respiratory tract have been exposed to the same carcinogenic agents, and are handling them in a manner genetically predetermined for that individual; hence it is not surprising if two distant sites both succumb to the effects of carcinogens and both produce a malignancy. Other factors that are likely to come into play are the type of the tobacco, temperature, the nutritional state of the individual exposed, and the individual's genetic makeup. While smoking is clearly the major risk factor and the epithelium is exposed to well documented carcinogens, the variation between individuals and populations in their response to repeated exposure over time is enormous. Within the continent of Europe the tremendous variation in incidence of laryngeal cancer between the north of Europe and the south of Europe[10] simply cannot be explained by tobacco alone. Smoking is increasing in some southern European countries such as Italy,[48] particularly amongst women. Strangely, for two smoking-related malignancies, the incidence (and mortality) for lung and laryngeal cancers do not necessarily correlate well across geographic regions of Europe. In some regions where lung cancer has declined, laryngeal cancer has maintained or even increased in incidence.[59] Cadiz in Spain has a particularly high incidence[29] for reasons which are unclear.

Following stopping smoking, the risks decline from year to year, but ex-smokers do not decline to nearly the same risk as those who have never smoked until some 15 years after ceasing to smoke.[78] The risk is not altogether abolished. This fits with the molecular biology understanding of carcinogenesis as a multistage process, and would suggest that, up to a point, changes will reverse but beyond that point become irreversible.

Alcohol

Alcohol is generally regarded as the second major risk factor for laryngeal cancer. Yet pure ethyl alcohol is not thought to be carcinogenic.[95] Since smoking and drinking go together, it is more difficult to separate out the effects due to alcohol alone. Alcohol is regarded as a promoting factor or cocarcinogen.[7]

The current suspected causes in alcoholics are a deficiency of riboflavin, changes in immunoglobulin and other immune molecule levels, poor nutrition, cirrhosis and vitamin deficiency.

Mortality studies find that cancer of the larynx is more common in alcoholics than non-drinkers.[7] For smokers who are also heavy drinkers, the incidence of laryngeal cancer is increased 25–50 times.[7] Scandinavian data[25] from population registries estimate that eliminating alcohol consumption would reduce the incidence of laryngeal cancer by 29%. Alcohol abuse is associated with decreased survival after diagnosis, after controlling for other factors.[19]

There is some evidence that cigarette smoking tends to cause vocal cord or other endolaryngeal cancers, whilst drinking and possibly cigars and pipes may affect the supraglottis, or the epilarynx, more.[16]

Irradiation

An individual may be exposed to radiation either therapeutically in hospital, or through their environment, whether this is their place of employment or the place in which they live. Exposure to radiation from a place of work is now much better controlled than in the past. A classic study from 1939 demonstrated pitchblende workers having increased mortality from lung and laryngeal cancer.[61]

The main contemporary concern is therefore the use of therapeutic irradiation. This may be divided into irradiation in clinical situations where it is no longer used and, secondly, irradiation as used at present for tumors of the larynx and pharynx.

A feature of the history of this subject has been the long lag time between exposure to irradiation and the latest development of an irradiation malignancy. Hence, external beam irradiation was at one time practiced for thyrotoxicosis, skin malignancies, mycoses, tuberculous lymph nodes (scrofula), and was later reported as the cause of induced laryngeal cancer. It has also been described following radioactive iodine used in therapeutic doses, for example in Graves' disease.[7] Similarly, juvenile laryngeal papilloma was at one time treated with irradiation and led to later malignant degeneration.[7]

The question of radiation-induced cancer of the larynx following previous treatment for laryngeal or hypopharyngeal cancer is more difficult. Most clinicians would probably feel that recurrences of the primary tumor, or manifestations of residual primary tumor, present in the first few years following irradiation.

By definition, therefore, radiation-induced cancer ought to recur after at least 5 symptom-free years following the previous radiotherapy treatment. The interval between irradiation and subsequent malignancy may be quite long, and tumors developing in irradiated fields have been reported to have latencies of up to 40 years.[64] The quality and modality of the irradiation is likely to influence the likelihood of such a tumor forming. Current hyperfractionation regimens and modern, more accurate linear accelerators might be expected to target the treatment more accurately and, with less of the irradiation being wasted on adjacent healthy tissue, one would anticipate a lower incidence of radiation-induced cancers.

Nonetheless, only a small minority of previously irradiated patients will demonstrate such a cancer. Again there must be an interplay of other factors: smoking, genetic makeup and perhaps other factors.

Diet and nutritional factors

There are two aspects to this issue: first, poor general nutrition as a risk factor and, secondly, certain foodstuffs as potential preventative agents.

Many patients presenting with cancer of the larynx are middle-aged smokers who have a heavy alcohol intake. As previously suggested, this will often be associated with relatively poor nutritional state. In a recent study, poor nutrition was identified as a strong independent risk factor.[97] Separating out dietary deficiency on its own is a difficult matter. Cancer of the larynx is not enormously common in many countries in which malnutrition is common, although many of these countries are also likely to have the greatest potential problems with the accuracy of their databases.

There is now quite strong epidemiological evidence for a protective effect of a high dietary intake of vegetables and fruit against malignancies in a variety of sites.[81] Although most of the studies assessed in a recent review were case controlled,[81] there are some cohort studies. The reduction in risk of cancer seems to be most marked for epithelial cancers, particularly the alimentary and respiratory tracts. Raw forms of fruit and vegetables may be more beneficial than cooked.[9,13,81] Relatively high dietary fat has been implicated in breast and colon cancer,[27] but has not been noted as a factor in cancer of the larynx. The proposed mechanisms of prevention are through antioxidants in foodstuffs.[9,13,27]

The presence of vitamins, such as A and C, may explain the protective effect of dietary fruits and vegetables.[47] Vitamin A, in particular, has been shown to have an inhibitory effect on the development of epithelial tumors by controlling cell differentiation.[70] In fact, its deficiency leads to epithelial metaplasia. Vitamin A derivatives have been used for the treatment of epithelial leukoplakia,[11] and a number of studies have found vitamin A associated with a reduced risk of human cancers,[56] thought to be through its precursor β-carotene, again because it is an antioxidant. In a case-control study, people in the intermediate third of β-carotene intake had an OR of 1.4 and people in the lowest third had an OR of 1.8 as compared to the highest third.[84] Retinoids, analogs of retinol, a precursor of vitamin A, have been shown to suppress *in vitro* expression of malignant phenotypes,[20] yet Mayne *et al.*[56] consider retinol, another vitamin A compound, to enhance carcinogenesis.

In a recent Chinese population-based control-study a dose–response relationship between the salt-preserved meat and fish consumption and the increased risk of laryngeal cancer has been observed.[98]

Occupational factors

There are many substances thought to be carcinogens, cocarcinogens or other promotive factors. It is very difficult to prove that an individual patient has developed laryngeal cancer because of these, and it is difficult to separate out their effects from smoking. However, cancer of the larynx is more common in industrial areas and a number of agents have been suspected of being involved.

The most likely to be associated with the development of laryngeal cancer are asbestos, wood dust, cement dust and tar products.[47]

The debate over whether or not asbestos is truly a risk factor illustrates some of the problems of methodology. Two early studies[71,82] found an apparently very strong link, using a sample (possibly very skewed) and looking retrospectively. Many of the later studies, some much larger and conducted prospectively, have not borne this out at all.[39,87] One recent study which did show an increased risk was a population-based case-control study finding an OR of 2.0 related to asbestos exposure, although no dose–response relationship with frequency or duration of exposure.[98] There is some evidence of histological change due to asbestos[44] but this does not necessarily imply progression to malignancy. Overall it seems best to apply the Scottish verdict of 'not proven', rather than 'guilty' or 'innocent'.

With regard to galvanizers, paint-sprayers and enamel workers, one study[92] did not find an increased incidence, whilst a more recent study[54] did implicate these substances. A review of 25 studies examining carcinogenicity of sulphuric acid vapor was inconclusive.[67]

Dry cleaning, with exposure to perchloroethylene[2,85,89] was found to give an OR of 2.7 for developing cancer of the larynx; this large study[90] is one of the all too few quoting confidence intervals.

Various other environmental factors have been implicated in laryngeal cancer, such as steam and heat inhalation, thermal burns, organic chemical compounds (polycyclic aromatic hydrocarbons, nitrosamines) which are produced in coal, iron and rubber industries, insecticides (benzopyrenes), alkylating substances produced in mustard gas factories, chemical fumes (vinyl chloride, formaldehyde), fibers in textile manufacturing and the leather industry, nickel and chromate mining.[7]

Interestingly, air pollution indoors and in the place of work due to emissions of fossil fuel from stove heating with oil, coal, gas and wood has been found to be associated with an OR of 2.0 (after adjustment for tobacco and alcohol) for laryngeal cancer after an exposure of more than 40 years.[24]

Multiple primary cancers

In general, second primary cancers have been described in 10–35% of patients with head and neck cancers.[60] Cancer of the larynx is associated with substantial excess risk of a second cancer in the upper alimentary tract and lung. The more frequent association of cancers of the larynx and lung suggests that these lesions might share biologic properties and susceptibility to some environmental factors, such as cigarette smoking and certain occupational factors as well as genetic factors.[62] Because of the high mortality of lung cancer, it is uncommon to discover a second primary laryngeal cancer before the lung cancer becomes fatal. A recent study reported an increased risk of second aerodigestive cancers (including cancer of the larynx) from 2% per patient per year to more than 14% after more than 10 years, in patients free of disease (small cell lung cancer) for more than 2 years.[40]

The risk of developing a second primary laryngeal cancer following other cancers has also been investigated. In particular, an increased risk for laryngeal cancer has been observed in patients with bladder cancer.[65]

The future

Laryngeal cancer in theory could be subjected to a screening program of examining patients' larynges. Being a relatively rare tumor, this is unlikely ever to be appropriate at a population level. The pragmatic approach would appear to be the widely practiced pattern of recommending referral of adults hoarse for 3 weeks or more. This has several weaknesses:

- firstly, awareness of primary care physicians of the need to make such referrals; and
- secondly, patients' willingness or otherwise to present to their primary care physician.

In particular, the at-risk group of heavy smokers and drinkers who neglect their health are often poorly compliant with screening or preventive strategies. Screening might be appropriate to groups of workers defined as being at risk and is to some extent undertaken in industrial environments. Identifying and screening cancer-prone families might become a fruitful area as clinical genetics advances.

Survival rates for European countries vary somewhat between countries. There appears little improvement in survival rates since the 1970s, although it can be argued that survival of head and neck cancer patients is in general improving.[41]

There are a number of areas requiring future research. The importance of diet and/or alcohol in their own right, separate from tobacco, is hard to determine. Passive smoking will be extremely hard to define as a risk factor for cancer of the lung, let alone cancer of the larynx. The fate of patients with chronic laryngitis and dysplasia would seem to be an area needing further prospective attention. Whilst these do not appear to constitute the largest group of patients presenting with malignancy, their long-term progress might provide useful information on the pathogenesis of this disease.

References

1. Agudelo D, Quel M, León X, Diez S, Burgués J. Laryngeal carcinoma in patients without a history of tobacco and alcohol use. *Head Neck* 1997; **19**: 200–4.
2. Almadori G, Cadoni G, Maurizi M *et al.* Oncogenes and cancer of the larynx. EGFR, p21 ras and HPV-DNA infections. *Acta Otorhinolaryngol Ital* 1995; **15(Suppl 46)**: 1–22.
3. Altman DG. Better reporting of randomised controlled trials: the CONSORT statement. *Br Med J* 1998; **313**: 570–1.
4. Amasio E, Aversa S, Bisi O *et al.* Epidemiologia descrittiva del cancro laringeo, ipofaringeo nella città di Torino. *Acta Otorhinolaryngol Ital* 1983; **3**: 417–25.

5. Atkinson L. Some features of the epidemiology of cancer of the larynx in Australia and Papua New Guinea. *Laryngoscope* 1975; **85:** 1173–84.
6. Austen DF. Larynx. In: Schottenfeld D, Fraumani JF, eds. *Cancer Epidemiology and Prevention.* Philadelphia: Saunders, 1982.
7. Ballenger JJ. *Diseases of the Nose, Throat, Ear, Head, and Neck,* 14th edn. Philadelphia: Lea & Febiger, 1991: 682–746.
8. Barclay THC, Rao NN. The incidence and mortality rates for laryngeal cancer from total cancer registries. *Laryngoscope* 1975; **85:** 254–8.
9. Berrino F, Crosignani F. Epidemiology of malignant tumours of the larynx and lung. *Ann Ist Sup Sanita* 1992; **28:** 107–20.
10. Berrino F, Sant M, Verdecchia A, Capocaccia R, Hakulinen T, Esteve J. *Survival of Cancer Patients in Europe: the EUROCARE Study.* Lyon: IARC Scientific Publications, 1995.
11. Bollag W. Retinoids and cancer. *Cancer Chemother Pharmacol* 1979; **3:** 207–15.
12. Boring CC, Squires TS, Heath CW. Cancer statistics for African-Americans. *CA Cancer J Clin* 1992; **42:** 7–17.
13. Boyle P, Macfarlane GJ, Zheng T, Maisonneuve P, Evstifeeva T, Scully C. Recent advances in epidemiology of head and neck cancer. *Curr Opin Oncol* 1992; **4:** 471–7.
14. Cann CI, Fried MP. Determinants and prognosis of laryngeal cancer. *Otolaryngol Clin North Am* 1984; **17:** 139–50.
15. Cann CI, Rothman KJ, Fried MP. The epidemiology of laryngeal cancer. In: Fried MP, ed. *The Larynx. A Multidisciplinary Approach,* 2nd edn. St Louis: Mosby, 1996: 425–36.
16. Cantrell RW. The current status of laryngeal cancer. In: Inouye T, Fukuda H, Sato T, Hinohara T, eds. *Recent Advances in Bronchoesophagology. Proceedings of the 6th World Congress on Bronchoesophagology, Tokyo.* Amsterdam: Excerpta Medica, 1990: 3–12.
17. Cattaruzza MS, Maisonneuve P, Boyle P. Epidemiology of laryngeal cancer. *Oral Oncol Eur J Cancer* 1996; **32B:** 293–305.
18. Copper MP, Jovanovic A, Nauta JJP *et al.* Role of genetic factors in the etiology of squamous cell carcinoma of the head and neck. *Arch Otolaryngol Head Neck Surg* 1995; **121:** 157–60.
19. Deleyiannias FW, Thomas DB, Vaughan TL, Davis S. Alcoholism: independent predictor of survival in patients with head and neck cancer. *J Natl Cancer Inst* 1996; **88:** 542–9.
20. De Luca L, Maestri N, Bonanni F, Nelson D. Maintenance of epithelial cell differentiation. The mode of action of vitamin A. *Cancer* 1972; **30:** 1326–31.
21. Denecke HJ, Jahnke V. Carcinom nach pharyngotrachealem Trauma und Hautlappenplastik. *HNO* 1974; **22:** 236–7.
22. DeRienzo DP, Greenberg SD, Fraire AE. Carcinoma of the larynx. Changing incidence in women. *Arch Otolaryngol Head Neck Surg* 1991; **117:** 681–4.
23. De Stefani E, Correa P, Oreggia F *et al.* Risk factors for laryngeal cancer. *Cancer* 1987; **60:** 3087–91.
24. Dietz A, Senneweld E, Maier H. Indoor air pollution by emissions of fossil fuel single stoves: possibly a hitherto underrated risk factor in the development of carcinomas in the head and neck. *Otolaryngol Head Neck Surg* 1995; **112:** 308–15.
25. Dreyer L, Winther JF, Andersen A, Pukkala E. Avoidable cancers in the Nordic countries. Alcohol consumption. *APMIS* 1997; **76(Suppl):** 48–67.
26. Dreyer L, Winther JF, Pukkala E, Andersen A. Avoidable cancers in the Nordic countries. Tobacco smoking. *APMIS* 1997; **76(Suppl):** 9–47.
27. El-Bayoumy K, Chung FL, Richie J Jr *et al.* Dietary control of cancer. *Proc Soc Exp Biol Med* 1997; **216:** 211–23.
28. Enstrom JE. Cancer and total mortality among active Mormons. *Cancer* 1978; **42:** 1943–51.
29. Errezola M, Lopez-Abente G, Escolar A. Geographical patterns of cancer mortality in Spain. *Recent Results Cancer Res* 1989; **114:** 154–62.
30. Ferlito A, Friedmann I. Squamous cell carcinoma. In: Ferlito A, ed. *Neoplasms of the Larynx.* Edinburgh: Churchill Livingstone, 1993: 113–33.
31. Ferlito A, Rinaldo A, Marioni G. Laryngeal malignant neoplasms in children and adolescents. *Int J Pediatr Otorhinolaryngol* 1999; **49:** 1–14.
32. Ferlito A, Devaney SL, Carbone A *et al.* Pregnancy and malignant neoplasms of the head and neck. *Ann Otol Rhinol Laryngol* 1998; **107:** 991–8.
33. Field JK, Malliri A, Jones AJ, Spandidos DA. Mutations in the p53 gene at codon 249 are rare in squamous cell carcinoma of the head and neck. *Int J Oncol* 1992; **1:** 253–6.
34. Foulkes WD, Brunet JS, Kowalski LP, Narod SA, Franco EL. Family history of cancer is a risk factor for squamous cell carcinoma of the head and neck in Brazil: a case-control study. *Int J Cancer* 1995; **63:** 769–73.
35. Garfinkel L. The epidemiology of cancer in black Americans. *Stat Bull Metrop Insur Co* 1991; **72:** 11–17.
36. Grenman R, Virolainen E, Shapiro A, Carey T. In vitro effects of tamoxifen on UM-SCC head and neck cancer cell lines: correlation with the estrogen and progesterone receptor content. *Int J Cancer* 1987; **39:** 77–81.
37. Hoffmann D, Tso TC, Gori GB. The less harmful cigarette. *Prev Med* 1980; **9:** 287–96.
38. Hoffman HT, Karnell LH, Funk GF, Robinson RA, Menck HR. The National Cancer Data Base report on cancer of the head and neck. *Arch Otolaryngol Head Neck Surg* 1998; **124:** 951–62.
39. Imbernon E, Goldberg M, Bonenfant S *et al.* Occupational respiratory cancer and exposure to asbestos: a case-control study in a cohort of workers in the electricity and gas industry. *Am J Ind Med* 1995; **28:** 339–52.
40. Johnson BE, Linnoila RI, Williams JP *et al.* Risk of second aerodigestive cancers increases in patients who survive free of small-cell lung cancer for more than 2 years. *J Clin Oncol* 1995; **13:** 101–11.
41. Jones AS, Houghton DJ, Beasley NJP, Husband DJ. Improved survival in patients with head and neck cancer in the 1990s. *Clin Otolaryngol* 1998; **23:** 319–25.
42. Jussawalla DJ, Deshpande VA, Haenszel W, Natekar MV. Differences between the Parsi community and the total population of greater Bombay: a critical appraisal. *Br J Cancer* 1970; **24:** 56–66.

43. Jussawalla DJ, Yeole BB, Natekar MV, Rajagopalan TR. Differences in site patterns of cancer in Sindhi and Parsi sub-groups and the general population of greater Bombay. *Indian J Cancer* 1980; **17**: 78–88.
44. Kambic V, Radsel Z, Gale N. Alterations in the laryngeal mucosa after exposure to asbestos. *Br J Ind Med* 1989; **46**: 717–23.
45. Kleinsasser O. *Tumors of the Larynx and Hypopharynx*. Stuttgart: Thieme, 1988: 2–24.
46. Kokoska MS, Piccirillo JF, Haughey BH. Gender differences in cancer of the larynx. *Ann Otol Rhinol Laryngol* 1995; **104**: 419–24.
47. Koufman JA, Burke AJ. The etiology and pathogenesis of laryngeal carcinoma. *Otolaryngol Clin North Am* 1997; **30**: 1–19.
48. La Vecchia C, Harris RE, Wynder EL. Comparative epidemiology of cancer between the United States and Italy. *Cancer Res* 1988; **48**: 7285–93.
49. Lavieille JP, Brambilla E, Riva-Lavieille C, Reyt E, Charachon R, Brambilla C. Immunohistochemical detection of p53 protein in preneoplastic lesions and squamous cell carcinoma of the head and neck. *Acta Otolaryngol (Stockh)* 1995; **115**: 334–9.
50. León X, Quer M, Agudelo D *et al*. Influence of age on laryngeal carcinoma. *Ann Otol Rhinol Laryngol* 1998; **107**: 164–9.
51. Lynch HT, Mulcahy GM, Harris RE, Guirgis HA, Lynch JF. Genetic and pathologic findings in a kindred with hereditary sarcoma, breast cancer, brain tumours, leukaemia, lung, laryngeal and adrenal cortical carcinoma. *Cancer* 1978; **41**: 2055–64.
52. Lynch HT, Kriegler M, Christiansen TA, Smyrk T, Lynch JF, Watson P. Laryngeal carcinoma in a Lynch syndrome II kindred. *Cancer* 1988; **62**: 1007–13.
53. Maier H, Tisch M. Epidemiology of laryngeal cancer: results of the Heidelberg case-control study. *Acta Otolaryngol Suppl (Stockh)* 1997; **527**: 160–4.
54. Maier H, Tisch M, Enderle G, Dietz A, Weidauer H. Occupational exposure to paint, lacquer and solvents, and cancer risk in the area of the upper aero-digestive tract. *HNO* 1997; **45**: 905–8.
55. Matsuoka H, Sugimachi K, Ueo H, Kuwano H, Nakano S, Nakayama M. Sex hormone response of a newly established squamous cell line derived from clinical esophageal carcinoma. *Cancer Res* 1987; **47**: 4134–40.
56. Mayne ST, Graham S, Zheng TZ. Dietary retinol: prevention or promotion of carcinogenesis in humans? *Cancer Causes Control* 1991; **2**: 443–50.
57. McGuirt WF, Little JP. Laryngeal cancer in children and adolescents. *Otolaryngol Clin North Am* 1997; **30**: 207–14.
58. Menakanit W, Muir CS, Jain DK. Cancer in Chiang Mai, North Thailand. A relative frequency study. *Br J Cancer* 1971; **25**: 225–36.
59. Moulin JJ, Mur JM, Cavelier C. Comparative epidemiology, in Europe, of cancers related to tobacco (lung, larynx, pharynx, oral cavity). *Bull Cancer* 1985; **72**: 155–8.
60. Olofsson J. Routines for follow-up and the risk of multiple primaries. In: Ferlito A, ed. *Neoplasms of the Larynx*. Edinburgh: Churchill Livingstone, 1993: 591–8.
61. Peller S. Lung cancer among mine workers in Joachimsthal. *Hum Biol* 1939; **11**: 130–43.
62. Rinaldo A, Marchiori C, Faggionato L, Saffiotti U, Ferlito A. The association of cancers of the larynx with cancers of the lung. *Eur Arch Otorhinolaryngol* 1996; **253**: 256–9.
63. Rothman KJ, Cann CI, Flanders D, Fried MP. Epidemiology of laryngeal cancer. *Epidemiol Rev* 1980; **2**: 195–209.
64. Sakamoto A, Sakamoto G, Sugano H. History of cervical radiation and incidence of carcinoma of the pharynx, larynx, and thyroid. *Cancer* 1979; **44**: 718–23.
65. Salminen E, Pukkala E, Teppo L, Pyrhonen S. Subsequent primary cancers following bladder cancer. *Eur J Cancer* 1994; **30A**: 303–7.
66. Saranath D, Bhoite LT, Deo MG. Molecular lesions in human oral cancer: the Indian scene. *Eur J Cancer* 1993; **29**: 107–12.
67. Sathiakumar N, Delzell E, Amoateng Adjepong Y, Larson R, Cole P. Epidemiological evidence on the relationship between mists containing sulphuric acid and respiratory tract cancer. *Crit Rev Toxicol* 1997; **27**: 233–51.
68. Schantz SP, Hsu TC, Ainslie N, Moser RP. Young adults with head and neck cancer express increased susceptibility to mutagen-induced chromosome damage. *JAMA* 1989; **262**: 3313–15.
69. Sesti G, Marini MA, Briata P *et al*. Androgens increase insulin receptors mRNA levels, insulin binding, and insulin responsiveness in HEP-2 larynx carcinoma cells. *Mol Cell Endocrinol* 1992; **86**: 111–18.
70. Shekelle B, Lepper M, Liu S *et al*. Dietary vitamin A and risk of cancer in the Western Electric Study. *Lancet* 1981; **2**: 1185–90.
71. Shettigara PT, Morgan RW. Asbestos, smoking and laryngeal cancer. *Arch Environ Health* 1975; **30**: 517–19.
72. Sigvardsson S, Hardell L, Przybeck TR, Cloninger R. Increased cancer risk among Swedish female alcoholics. *Epidemiology* 1996; **7**: 140–3.
73. Silvestri F, Bussani R, Stanta G, Cosatti C, Ferlito A. Supraglottic versus glottic laryngeal cancer: epidemiological and pathological aspects. *ORL J Otorhinolaryngol Relat Spec* 1992; **54**: 43–8.
74. Simarak S, de Jong UW, Breslow N *et al*. Cancer of the oral cavity, pharynx/larynx, and lung in North Thailand: case control study and analysis of cigar smoke. *Br J Cancer* 1977; **36**: 130–40.
75. Simon M, Kahn T, Schneider A, Pirsig W. Laryngeal carcinoma in a 12 year-old child. Association with human papillomavirus 18 and 33. *Arch Otolaryngol Head Neck Surg* 1994; **120**: 277–82.
76. Sinard RJ, Netterville JL, Garrett CG, Ossoff RH. Cancer of the larynx. In: Myers EN, Suen JY, eds. *Cancer of the Head and Neck*. Philadelphia: Saunders, 1996: 381–421.
77. Smart CR, Lyon JL, Skolnick M, Wilson ML, Edwards CB, Cowan LR. Cancer of the head and neck in Utah. *Am J Surg* 1974; **128**: 463–5.
78. Spitz MR, Fueger JJ, Goepfert H, Hong WK, Newell GR. Squamous cell carcinoma of the upper aerodigestive tract. A case comparison analysis. *Cancer* 1988; **61**: 203–8.
79. Spitz MR, Fueger JJ, Halabi S, Schantz SP, Sample D, Hsu TC. Mutagen sensitivity in upper aerodigestive tract

cancer: a case-control analysis. *Cancer Epidemiol Biomarkers Prev* 1993; **2**: 329–33.

80. Staszewski J. Epidemiology of cancer of the larynx. In: Ferlito A, ed. *Cancer of the Larynx*, Vol. I. Boca Raton: CRC Press, 1985: 1–34.
81. Steinmetz KA, Potter JD. Vegetables, fruit and cancer. I. Epidemiology. *Cancer Causes Control* 1991; **2**: 325–57.
82. Stell PM, McGill T. Exposure to asbestos and laryngeal cancer. *J Laryngol Otol* 1975; **89**: 513–17.
83. Stephenson WT, Barnes DE, Holmes FF, Norris CW. Gender influences subsite of origin of laryngeal carcinoma. *Arch Otolaryngol Head Neck Surg* 1991; **117**: 774–8.
84. Tavani A, Negri E, Franceschi S, Barbone F, La Vecchia C. Attributable risk for laryngeal cancer in northern Italy. *Cancer Epidemiol Biomarkers Prev* 1994; **3**: 121–5.
85. Tenkanen L, Teppo L. Migration, marital status and smoking as risk determinants of cancer. *Scand J Soc Med* 1987; **15**: 67–72.
86. Trizna Z, Schantz S. Hereditary and environmental factors associated with risk and progression of head and neck cancer. *Otolaryngol Clin North Am* 1992; **25**: 1089–101.
87. Tsai SP, Waddell LC, Gilstrap EL, Ransdell JD, Ross CE. Mortality amongst maintenance employees potentially exposed to asbestos in a refinery and petrochemical plant. *Am J Ind Med* 1996; **29**: 89–98.
88. Tuyns AJ, Estève J, Raymond L *et al.* Cancer of the larynx/hypopharynx, tobacco and alcohol: IARC international case-control study in Turin and Varese (Italy), Zaragoza and Navarra (Spain), Geneva (Switzerland) and Calvados (France). *Int J Cancer* 1988; **41**: 483–91.
89. Vatanasapt V, Martin N, Sriplung H *et al.* Cancer incidence in Thailand, 1988–1991. *Cancer Epidemiol Biomarkers Prev* 1995; **4**: 475–83.
90. Vaughan TL, Stewart PA, Davis S, Thomas DB. Work in dry cleaning and the incidence of cancer of the oral cavity, larynx and oesophagus. *Occup Environ Med* 1997; **54**: 692–5.
91. Waterhouse JAH. Epidemiology. In: Ferlito A, ed. *Neoplasms of the Larynx*. Edinburgh: Churchill Livingstone, 1993: 49–64.
92. Wilke L. Laryngological screening of industrial workers (galvanizers, spray painters, enamellers). In: Wigand ME, Steiner W, Stell PM, eds. *Functional Partial Laryngectomy: Conservation Surgery for Carcinoma of the Larynx*. New York: Springer, 1984: 42–3.
93. World Health Organization. *1996 World Health Statistics Annual/Annuaire de Statistiques Sanitaires Mondiales*. Geneva: WHO, 1998.
94. Wynder EL, Stellman SD. Impact of long-term filter cigarette usage on lung and larynx cancer risk: a case control study. *J Natl Cancer Inst* 1979; **62**: 471–7.
95. Wynder EL, Covey LS, Mabuchi K, Mushinski M. Environmental factors in cancer of the larynx: a second look. *Cancer* 1976; **38**: 1591–601.
96. Yang PC, Thomas DB, Daling JR, Davis S. Differences in the sex ratio of laryngeal cancer incidence rates by anatomic subsite. *J Clin Epidemiol* 1989; **42**: 755–8.
97. Zatonski W, Becher H, Lissowska J, Wahrendorf J. Tobacco, alcohol and diet in the etiology of laryngeal cancer: a population-based case-control study. *Cancer Causes Control* 1991; **2**: 3–10.
98. Zheng W, Blot WJ, Shu XO *et al.* Diet and other risk factors for laryngeal cancer in Shanghai, China. *Am J Epidemiol* 1992; **136**: 178–91.

Experimental laryngeal carcinogenesis

Umberto Saffiotti

Experimental animal models for laryngeal carcinogenesis

The study of the induction of malignant transformation and tumor development in the laryngeal epithelium has gained substantial knowledge from clinical, pathological and epidemiological observations in human subjects. The experimental induction of tumors in specific target tissues of different organs of experimental animals, under controlled conditions, has provided a basis for understanding the histogenesis of induced tumors, the stages of carcinogenesis, the activity of specific carcinogenic agents and cofactors, and their underlying molecular mechanisms. A link between whole animal models and the molecular mechanisms of carcinogenesis is represented by the development of cell culture models for the target cells – the cells of origin of the induced tumors – that can be used to induce neoplastic transformation in culture, without interference by other cell types, in relatively short time periods, and under conditions that make it possible to investigate and dissect molecular events and the roles of controlling genes.

Studies on carcinogenesis in the laryngeal epithelium – at the animal, cellular and molecular level – have been relatively scarce in comparison with similar studies on tracheobronchial epithelia, but the latter can be useful indicators for the development of mechanism studies in animals and in cultured epithelial cells related to the target cells of the larynx. The literature on laryngeal carcinogenesis was reviewed in 1975, 1985, 1993,[90,92,121] and presently. In the 1990s no new reports on larynx carcinogenesis in long-term animal experiments were found. However, in the past decade, new directions of research have been addressed to the development of cell culture models and to the study of molecular mechanisms.

Laryngeal carcinogenesis in experimental animals was obtained by topical exposure to polycyclic aromatic hydrocarbons and to tobacco smoke products, by systemic or topical administration of *N*-nitrosamines and *N*-nitrosamides, and by combined treatments with different carcinogens and cofactors, including tissue injury and the consequent regeneration and inflammation. The experimental carcinogens active in the larynx are representative of classes of compounds present in cigarette smoke, the major causative factor for laryngeal cancer in humans as shown by epidemiologic studies. Human studies have also suggested a role for excessive alcohol intake, and possibly for occupational asbestos exposure. More recently, several studies indicated a role for the human papilloma virus in laryngeal carcinogenesis.

Of the molecular mechanisms that have been investigated so far for laryngeal carcinogenesis, particular attention has been given to the role of tumor suppressor genes. Other molecular studies concern epidermal growth factor receptor, retinoic acid receptors, p21 *ras* protein expression, and gene products controlling the pathways of metabolic activation of carcinogens.

In carcinogenesis research, it is important to distinguish etiologic factors from pathogenetic factors and mechanisms. For example, if altered genetic control mechanisms are identified in the process of cell transformation from normal to neoplastic phenotypes, they may be due to somatic mutations induced by exogenous factors in oncogenes or in tumor suppressor genes, or they may involve accumulation of mutations through damaged DNA repair mechanisms, in turn dependent on altered genetic controls, as in the case of a 'mutator phenotype'.[63]

Animal models for laryngeal carcinogenesis were first developed in the course of experimental studies addressed to establishing methods for carcinogenesis in the whole respiratory tract. Anatomic and cellular characteristics distinguish the epithelia of the different segments of the respiratory tract – larynx, trachea, bronchi, bronchioles and alveoli – and require special methods for the study of each segment at the cellular level, whilst at the same time providing certain unified criteria, justified by the common embryologic origin of the laryngobronchial tract.[111] Experimental methods for the induction of respiratory epithelial tumors were developed by long-term investigations, especially since the 1960s, when the incidence of respiratory tract cancers was seen to increase dramatically in the population of many countries.

The Syrian golden hamster, extensively investigated since the 1950s as an animal model for carcinogenesis in various organs and tissues,[108] was found to be particularly suitable for respiratory tract carcinogenesis studies because of its lack of spontaneous respiratory tumors, its resistance to pulmonary infections,[21,93] and its susceptibility to respiratory carcinogenesis by different agents. The histopathology and histogenesis of hamster respiratory tumors, induced by polycyclic aromatic hydrocarbons, closely resemble the corresponding human pathology.[93,121] It was in the hamster that the laryngeal carcinogenic effects of polycyclic aromatic hydrocarbons, *N*-nitroso compounds, tobacco smoke and combined multifactorial treatments were demonstrated.

As for other species, no laryngeal tumors in rats were reported in a large series of carcinogenesis tests on many *N*-nitroso compounds.[61] Over 400 compounds of widely different chemical structure were thoroughly tested for carcinogenicity in 2-year studies in rats and mice of both sexes by the National Toxicology Program in the USA, and none of them revealed any carcinogenic effect on the larynx; only a few laryngeal tumors were found, unrelated to experimental treatment (quoted in reference 90).

The current evidence points to the Syrian golden hamster as the species of choice for laryngeal carcinogenesis studies. The genetic basis for its susceptibility remains to be investigated. The susceptibility of humans for laryngeal cancer is well known. It would be interesting to investigate the possible cellular and molecular basis of the susceptibility of the laryngeal epithelium in hamsters and the apparent resistance in some other species, such as the rat, in comparison with human subjects with or without laryngeal cancer. Genetic differences may involve the role of specific genes and gene products, expressed in the larynx, including those which control some critical steps in the activation of carcinogens or cofactors. Molecular epidemiology studies may reveal a subset of the human population at high risk for laryngeal cancer. In the future, specific cell lines of laryngeal epithelium could be established from these animal species with different susceptibility, and they could be studied for molecular mechanisms in comparison with cultures of human laryngeal epithelium. Methods for the latter will be discussed below.

Polycyclic aromatic hydrocarbons

Initial studies showed that a small number of invasive laryngeal squamous cell carcinomas could be induced in hamsters treated with many (17–45) weekly intratracheal instillations of the polycyclic aromatic hydrocarbon, 7,12-dimethylbenz[*a*]anthracene (DMBA), in a colloidal gelatin suspension, which also produced marked inflammatory lung reactions.[21] Benzo[*a*]pyrene, a less toxic polycyclic hydrocarbon which is commonly present in air pollution, combustion products and cigarette smoke, was shown to induce some laryngeal tumors in hamsters that received intratracheal instillations of this carcinogen suspended in a solution of the nonionic surfactant Tween 60.[40]

Substantial human respiratory exposure to polycyclic hydrocarbons occurs by inhalation of air containing fine dispersed particles of combustion products, as in the case of cigarette smoke and of certain occupational exposures (e.g. roofing tars). The carcinogens are attached or adsorbed to solid particles, such as carbon and other inorganic materials, and penetrate with them into the distal airways, where the particles are deposited and internalized and the soluble carcinogen then eluted out near target cells. In order to provide an experimental model for such exposures, Saffiotti and coworkers developed a method for attaching carcinogens to fine carrier particles for intratracheal instillation in the hamster.[88,89,93,95] This most effective method for respiratory tract carcinogenesis by polycyclic hydrocarbons is based on adsorbing the carcinogen (usually benzo[*a*]pyrene) on fine particles (mostly <1 μm) of a carrier mineral dust, usually hematite (ferric oxide) and suspending the particles in a buffered saline suspension for intratracheal instillation in hamsters.[93] The mixed dust was prepared by grinding together crystalline benzo[*a*]pyrene and hematite to a fine particle size. An even finer dispersion of the carcinogen on the carrier particles was obtained by a nucleation procedure, slowly adding a solution of benzo[*a*]pyrene in acetone to a large volume of water containing the hematite particles in suspension at low temperature. Under these conditions, the benzpyrene crystallizes on the surface of the carrier particles, which are then filtered, dried and resuspended.[88,89] The purpose of this method is to provide for the distribution and uptake of the carcinogen into the distal airways, with minimal inflammatory reaction, as extensively studied in the Syrian golden hamster. The liposoluble carcinogen, eluted out of the particles in the alveolar and interstitial macrophages and in the airway epithelium, diffuses towards the hilum and the proximal airways and induces preneoplastic lesions (epithelial hyperplasia and squamous metaplasia) and tumors (carcinomas in situ and invasive carcinomas, mostly epidermoid) in the epithelia of the bronchi, trachea and larynx.[37,38,52,53,88,89,93–95,97]

A series of experiments with this hamster model showed that the carcinogenic response in the larynx is dependent on the dose of benzo[*a*]pyrene, but independent of the dose of the carrier dust, hematite.[96,104] Even a single intratracheal instillation proved sufficient to induce tracheal and bronchial tumors (but not laryngeal tumors); repeated instillations were much more effective, even for lower total doses, and the response was proportional to the number of doses,[98] as well as to the dose level per instillation.[96] An analysis of a series of experiments in a total of 887 hamsters of both sexes, treated by intratracheal instillations of benzo[*a*]pyrene/hematite, showed that out of a total of 359 respiratory tract tumors, 14 (4%) occurred in the larynx (11 squamous cell carcinomas, one adenocarcinoma, and two benign polyps).[70,89]

Of course, the larynx represents the shortest segment of the respiratory airways, and the area of its epithelium is a small fraction of that of the tracheobronchial tree. The ratio of malignant to benign tumors was high in the larynx and bronchi, and much lower in the trachea and the bronchiolar–alveolar region; the ratio of squamous to secretory cell tumors (polyps, adenomas and adenocarcinomas) was highest in the larynx and trachea, intermediate in the bronchi and low in the bronchiolar–alveolar region.[70] A later experiment in which three groups of hamsters received 10 intratracheal instillations, every 2 weeks, each of 3 mg benzo[*a*]pyrene carried respectively by 3, 6 or 9 mg of hematite, resulted in a higher yield of laryngeal tumors (6 polyps, 6 squamous cell papillomas and 16 squamous cell carcinomas, in a total of 197 hamsters) representing 19% of the total respiratory tumors; the different amounts of hematite did not affect the tumor yield.[104]

Another polycyclic aromatic hydrocarbon present in cigarette tar, 7*H*-dibenzo[*c,g*]carbazole (DBC), was also studied in hamsters. Ground with equal weights of hematite and suspended in saline, it was given either by 15 intratracheal instillations of 3 mg DBC each, or by 30 instillations of 0.5 mg DBC each. The instillations were given once weekly in both groups. The group with the lower total dose, fractionated in twice as many instillations, developed a higher yield of squamous cell carcinomas in the larynx, trachea and bronchi than the first group. In the larynx there were seven carcinomas in 45 effective hamsters in the lower total dose group and three carcinomas in 35 hamsters in the higher total dose group.[103] This apparent discrepancy may be explained by the combined reaction to mechanical injury due to the higher number of instillations, as discussed below. It is interesting that, when tested without the hematite carrier dust, DBC still induced some laryngeal carcinomas (as well as tracheal and bronchial carcinomas), whereas benzo[*a*]pyrene did not.[105]

When different mineral particles of graded particle size classes (from 0.5–1 μm to 15–30 μm) were tested as carriers of benzo[*a*]pyrene in Syrian golden hamsters by 25 weekly intratracheal instillations, laryngeal tumors were effectively induced with hematite at all sizes, with carbon only at the finest size, and not at all with aluminum oxide.[27] In other experiments, hematite was again very effective, as were magnesium oxide, titanium dioxide (crystalline form not specified) and talc, whereas aluminum oxide and carbon were poorly effective.[117,118] Niemeier *et al.*[75] tested a series of mineral particles, including crystalline silica (quartz) and various silicates, suspended in saline together with benzo[*a*]pyrene and instilled intratracheally in hamsters; the yield of laryngeal tumors was comparable or higher than the yield obtained with hematite.[97]

Experiments in rats, treated with intratracheal instillations of benzo[*a*]pyrene or DMBA dispersed in colloidal casein suspensions with India ink particles, resulted in significant induction of bronchogenic carcinomas, but no indication was given of the induction of laryngeal tumors.[106] Also in rats, 15 intratracheal instillations of benzo[*a*]pyrene with hematite resulted in high yields of bronchogenic carcinomas, which were mostly epidermoid carcinomas, but also included adenocarcinomas and small cell undifferentiated carcinomas; no laryngeal tumors were reported.[11]

N-Nitroso compounds

Carcinogens characterized by the presence of the *N*-nitroso group (=N–NO) include two categories of compounds, nitrosamides and nitrosamines, known for their capacity to alkylate DNA bases and to induce tumors in experimental animals in a wide range of organs and tissues by topical or systemic administration. *N*-Nitrosamides are direct-acting alkylating agents, whereas *N*-nitrosamines require metabolic activation in target tissues.[61] Strong carcinogenic activity for the larynx was demonstrated in several experiments with diethylnitrosamine (DEN), following subcutaneous injection in Syrian golden hamsters of both sexes. Of 290 respiratory tract tumors induced by DEN in adult hamsters, 67 (23%) were laryngeal tumors; their incidence varied from 72% in a high-dose group to 17% in a low-dose group. When newborn hamsters were similarly treated with DEN, the same proportion of tumors developed in the larynx: 27 (23%) laryngeal tumors out of 115 respiratory tumors. All the DEN-induced tumors were histologically benign, papillary in structure and lined with either squamous or columnar mucous epithelium or sometimes with mixed areas of differentiation.[68–70,92]

N-Nitrosoheptamethyleneimine[62] and ethylnitrosovinylamine,[33] given systemically, induced high incidences of laryngeal tumors in Syrian golden hamsters. *N*-Nitrosodi-n-propylnitrosamine,[81] *N*-nitrosomethyl-n-propylnitrosamine[82] and 2,2'-dimethyldipropylnitrosamine[2] also produced relatively high incidences of tumors of the larynx.

The tobacco-specific nitrosamines, *N*'-nitrosonornicotine (NNN) and 4-(methylnitrosamino)-1-(3-pyridyl)-1-butanone (NNK), injected subcutaneously in hamsters, induced nasal, tracheal and lung tumors, but no laryngeal tumors were reported in these tests.[41]

The *N*-nitrosamide, *N*-methyl-*N*-nitrosourea (MNU), administered by weekly intratracheal instillations, induced laryngeal carcinomas in several studies.[39,41,46,120] MNU was used as a topical carcinogen by delivery to a circumscribed region of the trachea for histogenesis studies.[46,101,122,133] Even a single instillation of MNU directly to the larynx (0.2 ml of 1% MNU in 0.015 N sodium citrate) in 5-week-old hamsters, with or without cannulation injury to the epithelium, induced a few laryngeal tumors;[53] this protocol was used for studies on multifactorial carcinogenesis, described below.

Nitrosamines are present in many foodstuffs as well as in tobacco smoke and in certain occupational exposures.[61] In recent years, human epidemiologic studies provided evidence that dietary intake of nitrosamines results in significantly increased risks for cancer of the lung (with a slight prevalence of adenocarcinoma), larynx and oropharynx (see references in reference 20).

Cigarette smoke

The induction of laryngeal cancer by cigarette smoke, well documented by human epidemiology, was reproduced experimentally in several animal studies, in which the Syrian golden hamster proved to be the species of choice, as was the case with carcinogenesis by polycyclic aromatic hydrocarbons carried by mineral particles. This analogy is not surprising, since the latter is an experimental model for the exposure to carcinogens present in tobacco smoke.

Experimental evidence of laryngeal carcinogenesis by cigarette smoke was first reported by Dontenwill and colleagues,[23,24] who provided extensive histologic documentation of preneoplastic lesions (leukoplakia, papillomatous leukoplakia, pseudoepitheliomatous leukoplakia) and carcinomas induced in hamsters that had been exposed to cigarette smoke inhalation twice daily (the incidence of laryngeal carcinomas reached up to 16% in males). In the inbred Syrian golden hamster strain BIO15.16, selected as susceptible to respiratory carcinogenesis, microinvasive laryngeal carcinomas were induced in 19% of the animals following inhalation of cigarette smoke for up to 100 weeks, whereas the more resistant strain BIO87.20 developed an incidence of only 4% under similar conditions of exposure.[9] Inhalation exposure to smoke from American and British reference cigarettes induced laryngeal cancer in 40–50% of the hamsters of the susceptible BIO15.16 strain.[10,43,44] The histopathology of the induced preneoplastic lesions and of the early and invasive carcinomas of the larynx in the hamsters was shown to be closely similar to the corresponding human pathology.[23,24,44,127] By contrast, rats proved to be highly resistant to laryngeal carcinogenesis by tobacco smoke inhalation.[19,130] These animal models have now been available for some two decades, but they have not yet been used to investigate the underlying molecular lesions, nor the genetic basis of the marked host differences in susceptibility in laryngeal carcinogenesis.

Hamsters exposed to the inhalation of a mixture of four major vapor phase components of cigarette smoke (isoprene, methyl chloride, methyl nitrite and acetaldehyde) for up to 23 months developed significant incidences of laryngeal tumors (one papilloma and six carcinomas out of 31 males and six carcinomas out of 32 females).[29] The authors attribute the effect mostly to acetaldehyde, which was found to be highly carcinogenic for the nasal mucosa in separate rat experiments.

Methods for detection of carcinogen–DNA adducts have been used to measure such adducts in larynges exposed to cigarette smoke inhalation. In rats exposed for 32 weeks, the levels of total DNA adducts in the larynx increased by 10- to 20-fold in comparison with controls.[32] In human subjects, carcinogen–DNA adducts were identified in the larynges of cigarette smokers, but not in nonsmokers, and appeared to derive predominantly from polycyclic aromatic hydrocarbons; their levels depended on the expression in the target tissue of the specific metabolizing enzyme P450(CYP)2C9/10.[4] The adducts were found to decline only slowly after cessation of smoking.[83] A strong correlation was found in human laryngeal specimens between total DNA adducts and the combined levels of CYP2C and CYP1A1.[119]

Glutathione *S*-transferases (GSTs) are enzymes involved in the metabolism of xenobiotics, including many carcinogens as well as chemotherapeutic agents. Several polymorphic genes, including those encoding for GSTs, have been reported to be involved in modifying the risk for respiratory cancers.[72,125] GSTs occur as isoenzymes of different classes, designated α, μ, π, σ and θ. The *GSTM1* gene encodes for class μ GST involved in the detoxification of polycyclic aromatic hydrocarbons.[125] Lack of class μ GST has been suggested to confer an increased risk for lung cancer in smokers.[102] The frequency of this phenotype was measured in 78 laryngeal cancers and matched controls, and found to be significantly lower than the frequency in controls (33% vs 55.1%, $P < 0.01$).[55] The anticarcinogenic activity of the chemopreventive agent oltipraz has been suggested to be due to its ability to induce GSTs of the classes α, μ and π.[18]

Recent studies on other enzyme control mechanisms related to metabolic activation of carcinogens are discussed below.

Combined exposures

Combined or synergistic effects of different carcinogens and/or cofactors in respiratory carcinogenesis were investigated in a number of studies, but only some of them reported detailed results on tumors in the larynx.

Inhalation exposure to cigarette smoke was studied in hamsters that had previously received an 'initiating' treatment with a carcinogen. Two intralaryngeal instillations of DMBA followed by 45 weeks of cigarette smoke inhalation resulted in incidences of 45% papillomas and 7.5% carcinomas of the larynx, whereas DMBA alone induced only 12.5% papillomas and smoke alone no tumors.[42] In a similar experiment, a low dose of benzo[*a*]pyrene and hematite (ferric oxide) followed by smoke inhalation resulted in 5% papillomas, whereas the single treatments induced no tumors.[42]

A study of DEN given systemically in hamsters (12 subcutaneous injections) followed by lifetime inhalation of cigarette smoke showed increased incidences of papillomas and of early lesions in the larynx in comparison to single factors,[129] but another analogous study did not show significant effects.[24]

Experiments were conducted to study the interaction of *N*-nitroso compounds, benzo[*a*]pyrene and topical tissue injury. DEN (6 mg, given as 12 subcutaneous injections, each of 0.5 mg) was followed 5 weeks later by a course of intratracheal instillations with benzo[*a*]pyrene/hematite (2 mg each in 0.2 ml saline for up to 15 instillations).[70] Whereas the treatments with only DEN or only benzo[*a*]-pyrene/ hematite at these doses resulted in relatively low incidences of laryngeal tumors (respectively in 17% and 11% of the animals) with long latent periods, the combined treatment induced laryngeal tumors in 61% of the animals with shortened latent periods. In hamsters treated with a higher dose of DEN (total of 12 mg), a higher incidence of laryngeal tumors was induced (50%), but the addition of the secondary treatment with benzo[*a*]pyrene/hematite produced no further significant increase of tumors of the larynx (52%). By contrast, this secondary treatment greatly enhanced the induction of peripheral lung tumors, even with repeated intratracheal injections of hematite without benzo[*a*]pyrene (calculated from original records).[70]

These experiments pointed to the importance of complex interactions in respiratory carcinogenesis and suggested a role for less specific factors, including noncarcinogenic particulates (such as hematite) and repeated mucosal injury and repair due to multiple cannulations, with consequent inflammation and stimulated epithelial cell proliferation. It was pointed out that these complex tissue reactions require that the results of the combined-treatment experiments be interpreted with caution.[90,97,121]

In order to clarify the role of tissue injury in the hamster model, studies were made to determine the roles, as separate variables, of instillations of benzo[*a*]pyrene (BP), hematite particles or saline and of the mechanical effects of cannulation (with a blunt 19-gauge stainless steel cannula fitted with a plastic stop) inserted respectively either at the level of the larynx or down to the tracheal carina. These treatments were given as such or after pretreatment with a single intralaryngeal instillation (0.2 ml of a 0.1% solution in sodium citrate) of the *N*-nitrosamide, *N*-methyl-*N*-nitrosourea (MNU). The resulting morphological and cytokinetic effects and tumor induction were analyzed.[52,53] Cannulation by itself induced areas of abrasion of the surface epithelium and underlying submucosa which were evident in the larynx alone after intralaryngeal cannulation and in both the larynx and the trachea after intratracheal cannulation. The tissue reactions to these mucosal wounds were described in detail.[48–53,65] The wound surface was rapidly covered by migration of surrounding epithelial secretory cells (small granule mucous cells), followed by marked epithelial cell proliferation (hyperplasia) and accompanied by a moderate underlying inflammatory reaction. The resulting effects of the interactions of the carcinogens and cofactors were discussed in the original report[53] and in a subsequent review[90] and are briefly summarized here.

In these studies, laryngeal tumors (papillomas, carcinomas in situ or invasive carcinomas) were induced only in animals treated with one of the two carcinogens (MNU or BP) or both, whereas no tumors occurred in any of the 101 larynges from animals that received no carcinogens, even if they had received the course of 15 intratracheal cannulations. When wounding extended to the trachea was compared with wounding limited to the larynx, increased induction of all tumor types in the larynx was found for the groups given both MNU and BP, and in the groups given only one carcinogen, indicating that the inflammatory and hyperplastic/metaplastic lesions in the larynx, which were much more marked following intratracheal than intralaryngeal cannulations, contributed to the carcinogenic response in the larynx. Instillations of saline or of hematite in saline did not result in consistent significant effects in the larynx. The strongest effect on laryngeal carcinogenesis in this multifactorial protocol was shown by the instillation of BP. In the presence of MNU pretreatment, laryngeal and/or tracheal wounding and instillation of hematite in saline, the addition of BP to the instillations shortened the latent period and increased the incidence of laryngeal papillomas and, more strikingly, induced a tenfold increase in the incidence of carcinomas. In the absence of MNU, BP/hematite intratracheal instillations induced 12 carcinomas in 34 larynges examined, whereas none was induced without BP. The dose of MNU was selected as pretreatment by single intralaryngeal instillation, because it gave a low response in the respiratory tract, resulting in one papilloma and one carcinoma in situ in 34 larynges examined, and no tumors in the trachea and lung; it had, however, remarkable effects at distant sites, inducing by itself benign and malignant tumors in the oral and pharyngeal mucosa, esophagus, forestomach, pancreas, biliary tract and large intestine. The MNU pretreatment, when combined with repeated instillations of BP/hematite, had a strong effect on carcinogenesis in the lung and trachea, but not in the larynx. However, repeated intratracheal instillations of saline after MNU pretreatment induced one papilloma and three carcinomas in situ as well as considerable inflammatory and hyperplastic/metaplastic lesions in the 32 larynges examined, compared with no tumors in the 31 larynges of the corresponding group without MNU.

The experimental evidence that multiple factors, including polycyclic aromatic hydrocarbon and *N*-nitroso carcinogens, mineral particles and epithelial injury interact in the mechanisms of laryngeal carcinogenesis suggests a close relevance to human carcinogenesis by cigarette smoke, which involves a complex combination of such factors. The marked species differences in susceptibility to respiratory carcinogenesis in experimental animals point to the critical role of genetic factors, which may well correspond to genetic controls of susceptibility to cigarette smoke and other environmental carcinogens in the human population.

The role of the human papilloma virus (HPV)

The role of HPV in laryngeal carcinogenesis was indicated by several studies in which DNA from one or more types of HPV was detected in laryngeal tumors. This subject was recently extensively reviewed and critically discussed.[115] Studies on benign recurrent laryngeal papillomas (which may include localization in the trachea and bronchi) showed that almost all contain HPV DNA. The virus types HPV-6 and HPV-11 are causally associated with over 90% of the benign papillomas. The accepted mode of transmission of this viral infection is from mother to child at the time of birth from active condylomatous lesions. Latent infection with HPV can be found in asymptomatic patients, and activation of viral expression, caused by various factors, results in increased transcription of early genes and development of a papilloma. The permissive tissue for papilloma viruses is the squamous epithelium, but areas of squamous metaplasia in the columnar epithelium of the airways are frequent.[8] Carcinomas can also develop in laryngeal papilloma patients, and a high risk for such malignant conversion was demonstrated following radiation therapy for papillomas. It was suggested that heavy smoking also increases the risk of malignant conversion in papilloma patients. In this respect, HPV can act as a cocarcinogen with radiation and chemical carcinogens. Some precancerous lesions of the larynx were also found to be positive for HPV and 54.4% of them were positive for p53 expression. Three out of 57 cases were positive for both.[31]

The question whether HPV also plays a causal role in the induction of laryngeal carcinomas was reviewed by Steinberg and DiLorenzo,[115] who reported several positive studies, but discussed methodological problems and concluded that the role of HPV in laryngeal carcinogenesis is possible, but not yet fully clarified. HPV-6, 11, 16 and 18 were the most frequent types detected in laryngeal carcinomas.[99,128] In a study of 100 formalin-fixed and paraffin-embedded laryngeal carcinomas, 63.4% of the glottic and 10.2% of the supraglottic carcinomas were found positive.[3] In another series of 36 laryngeal carcinomas, HPV DNA was detected in 22.2% of the cases (with the high-risk types HPV-16 and 18 only detected in 5.5% of the cases); the frequency of detection was higher (50%) in women than in men (8%).[99] Very strong evidence that HPVs can cause human carcinomas is provided by extensive studies on cervical carcinoma, but even in this case HPV infection alone is insufficient to bring about complete malignant transformation, suggesting a multistep model for the development of HPV-associated cancer.[115]

Cellular models for laryngeal carcinogenesis

Carcinogenesis research in recent years has been aimed at elucidating cellular and molecular mechanisms underlying the process of transformation from normal to neoplastic cells in various tissues and cell types. When considering the appropriate choice of cellular and molecular models to investigate the carcinogenic process in the larynx, one needs to consider what types of cells are representative of the laryngeal epithelium as a target for carcinogenesis. The normal epithelium of the larynx, of course, includes both the stratified squamous epithelium on the anterior surface of the epiglottis and on the vocal cords and a wider area of pseudostratified ciliated columnar epithelium with secretory cells on the remainder of the laryngeal surface. The former is similar to the epithelium of the oropharyngeal mucosa and the latter is similar to the epithelium of the tracheobronchial mucosa with which it shares embryological origin and development. Islets of metaplastic squamous epithelium are found throughout the larynx in 50% of normal human larynges.[8] The vast majority of human benign laryngeal tumors are squamous cell papillomas, associated with HPV types 6 and 11, and they often occur at sites where the squamous and the secretory epithelium are juxtaposed.[45] As for malignant laryngeal tumors, most of them are squamous cell carcinomas, which derive either from areas of stratified squamous epithelium or from metaplastic areas in the columnar epithelium, or directly from the latter. Experimental studies on the tracheal epithelium have shown that the secretory cells of the columnar epithelium (small granule mucous cells) are functional stem cells, capable of replicating and differentiating into ciliated cells as well as squamous cells.[12,47–51,64,66] The ability of secretory cells to extend and restore epithelial integrity after cell injury and to divide and differentiate into different cell types was demonstrated in the early stages of experimental laryngeal and tracheal carcinogenesis.[52,53]

Cellular and molecular mechanisms of differentiation may distinguish the pathways to transformation in laryngeal cells of squamous epithelial origin from those in cells derived from the columnar secretory epithelium. The response of the larynx to polycyclic aromatic hydrocarbon carcinogens is similar to that of the trachea. Moreover, following systemic administration, the carcinogen diethylnitrosamine induces the same type of response in the larynx and in the trachea, no carcinogenic response in the oropharynx, and a marked response in the nasal epithelium.[70,89] In these respects, the epithelium of the larynx clearly behaves as an integral part of the respiratory tract.

Extensive experience has been gathered on methods for the culture and transformation of squamous epithelia (including oral keratinocytes) and of respiratory secretory epithelia (including tracheal and bronchial epithelia). More recently, many studies were devoted to cultures of human laryngeal keratinocytes and of human laryngeal papilloma cells,[22,67,85,86,116] and to cultures of oral/laryngeal keratinocytes and their premalignant and malignant derivatives, including the establishment of human head and neck squamous cell carcinoma (HNSCC) cell lines. These studies were thoroughly reviewed in 1996 by Sacks,[87] who discussed various specialized culture techniques, such as raft cultures, explant-organ cultures, and three-dimensional cultures of multicellular tumor spheroids, and the opportunities they offer for molecular analysis. Out of 98 reported HNSCC cell lines, 12 were of laryngeal origin.[87]

A comparative study of different types of cells of origin in the laryngeal epithelium, especially squamous and secretory, and of their susceptibility to transformation is clearly feasible, using either human cells or cells from appropriate experimental animal models, but it has not been done yet, to this writer's knowledge. It could provide important insights into the mechanisms of laryngeal carcinogenesis.

Cellular mechanisms in the growth and neoplastic transformation of respiratory tract epithelia have been widely investigated for tracheobronchial cells. Initial studies, starting in the 1950s and especially developed in the 1970s, showed that tracheobronchial epithelial cells from several mammalian species could be maintained in organ cultures (reviewed in reference 56). Effective methods were established for the culture and transformation of tracheobronchial epithelia from Syrian golden hamsters[17,47,71,91,110,112] and from rats.[76,113,114] Neoplastic transformation was induced by *N*-methyl-*N*'-nitro-*N*-nitrosoguanidine (MNNG) treatment in rat tracheal epithelial cells, either cultured with a fibroblast feeder layer[124] or without feeder layer in a specially developed serum-free medium.[123]

Methods were developed for the explant culture of human bronchial epithelial cells.[5,35,36] These methods made it possible to investigate structural and functional characteristics of the target respiratory epithelia in normal human cells and their ability to metabolize carcinogens. Subsequently, clonal growth of epithelial cells from normal human bronchus was obtained using appropriately designed culture media[60] and later a serum-free defined medium.[59] Immortalization of human bronchial cell cultures into established cell lines was obtained by transfection with plasmids containing the SV40 early region genes, or by infection with SV40 virus or with adenovirus-12-SV40 hybrid virus.[84] These immortalized cell lines were not tumorigenic in nude mice and retained features of human bronchial epithelial cells. Neoplastic transformation of the immortalized human bronchial cells was induced by transfection with a plasmid containing c-*raf*-1 and c-*myc* protooncogenes, and the transformed cell lines gave rise to multidifferentiated carcinomas in nude mice.[78,79]

An experimental model for laryngeal carcinogenesis was described by Tsutsumi *et al.*,[126] who studied combined effects of HPV and a chemical carcinogen in primary cultures of human laryngeal epithelial cells (HLEC), presumably of keratinocyte origin (although the segment of the larynx and the type of epithelium from which the cells were obtained were not specified, the cells were isolated in a serum-free keratinocyte growth medium). These cells were transfected with cloned full-length HPV-16 DNA, and from these cells, two cell lines (called HLEC-16 cell lines) were subsequently isolated, which were immortalized but not tumorigenic in nude mice and did not proliferate in a selective medium (DMEM with 1.6 mM Ca^{2+} and 10% fetal bovine serum). When the transfected cultures, at 70% confluence, were exposed to the carcinogenic nitrosamide *N*-methyl-*N*'-nitro-*N*-nitrosoguanidine (MNNG) at 1.0 µg/ml for 3 hours, and then grown in the selective medium, proliferating colonies were isolated which were calcium- and serum-resistant. One of these transformed cell lines was found to be tumorigenic in nude mice, giving rise to poorly differentiated squamous cell carcinomas. Neither p53 mutations nor p53 protein were detected in the tumor cells.[126]

Studies on molecular mechanisms

Molecular mechanisms of neoplastic transformation in various tissues and cell types have increasingly become the focus of carcinogenesis research. The early concepts of initiation and promotion, derived from mouse skin carcinogenesis[7] and liver carcinogenesis models,[26,80] and the concept of independent progression of individual tumors through stages up to the acquisition of the ability to invade and metastasize,[30] have now been developed, modified and extended to studies of many other organs and cells and to the identification of some of the underlying genetic lesions. Major differences among cell types invite caution in extrapolating molecular models from one organ to another, but more cohesive patterns are likely to emerge from further comparisons and from the elucidation of pathways of gene expression and activation in specific tissues and cells.

In recent years, considerable attention has been given to the occurrence of DNA lesions involving the repetitive nucleotide sequences called microsatellites, which are very frequent in human DNA. Variations in the number of repetitive unit sequences in each microsatellite, indicating microsatellite instability, have been found in various types of cancers but not in adjacent normal tissues, and have come to represent a sensitive indicator for genetic instability in human tumors.[63] Genetic stability, required for the accurate transfer of genetic information during cell division, appears to depend on several 'stability genes' involved in DNA replication, DNA repair and chromosomal segregation. Mutations in the stability genes may generate secondary mutations and this cascade of mutations may accumulate during tumor progression, as in the model of mutator phenotype proposed by Loeb.[63]

A multistage molecular progression model for carcinogenesis of head and neck squamous cell carcinoma (HNSCC) has recently been proposed.[15,87] Derived by analogy from a well documented model for colon carcinogenesis,[28] it stimulated a study of the progression of genetic lesions by microsatellite analysis at ten major chromosomal loci showing frequent loss of heterozygosity and loss in a putative tumor suppressor locus.[15] Alteration of microsatellite markers can be detected by polymerase chain reaction for the presence of new alleles (shifts) or loss of heterozygosity (LOH). The results of this analysis – on specimens of benign squamous hyperplasia, dysplasia, carcinoma in situ and invasive carcinoma – suggested progressive accumulation of genetic events, some of which were already present in about 30% of the benign hyperplastic lesions. Progression was thought to involve clonal outgrowth of a subpopulation of cells with yet additional genetic alterations.[15] In a parallel study,[6] using microsatellite analysis of allelic loss on chromosomes 9p and 3p (identified as early events in the progression of HNSCC), specimens were examined from eight female patients with multiple head and neck tumors (only one with a laryngeal cancer), which were either distinct synchronous or metachronous tumors. The results showed that in at least three of the eight cases the multiple primary tumors had identical clonal markers, suggesting that they arose from the same clone.

A further step in these studies was made with the unexpected observation that microsatellite DNA alterations can be detected not only in the tumor tissue, but also in DNA from paired serum samples, when compared with normal DNA from peripheral blood lymphocytes.[74] This phenomenon is due to the fact that a tumor-specific microsatellite shift can still be seen when tumor DNA is highly diluted with normal DNA. In six of 21 patients with HNSCC, serum DNA showed one or more microsatellite alterations precisely matching those in the primary tumors. This novel approach may provide a way to monitor the development of genetic lesions in the progression of carcinogenesis directly in patients.

Much further research is needed in order to elucidate the individual genes, mutations, gene products and their functions, that are specifically involved in carcinogenesis of the laryngeal epithelium. Sacks[87] pointed out the value of cellular models for such studies, while cautioning that, even for normal cells, 'cells derived from various sites within the oral cavity may possess different biochemical and biological properties based on their tissue of origin'.

Tumor suppressor genes, oncogenes and other molecular markers

Analysis of the spectrum of mutations in the p53 tumor suppressor gene has provided clues to the etiology and molecular pathogenesis of many types of human cancer.[34] A comprehensive analysis of p53 mutations in 2567 tumors and cell lines of various organ sites, confirmed by DNA sequencing, included 42 squamous carcinomas of the pharynx/larynx.[34] In pharynx/larynx carcinomas, the p53 mutation prevalence was relatively low (34%), but the spectrum of mutations was considerably different from the spectrum in oral and nasopharynx carcinomas and was quite similar to the spectrum of lung cancers in smokers (as opposed to non-smokers), with the highest frequencies of base substitutions being represented by G:C to T:A transversions (29%), G:C to A:T transitions (23%) and A:T to G:C transitions (17%). This pattern of mutations is suggestive of tobacco combustion products as the active carcinogens.[34]

The mutant p53 protein, which is detectable by immunohistochemical analysis, was observed in squamous cell carcinomas, carcinomas in situ, dysplastic, hyperplastic and (in some cases) normal-appearing mucosa of the head and neck of human subjects exposed to tobacco and alcohol. Localization of p53 was most frequent in the pharynx and larynx, and in dysplasias, carcinomas in situ and invasive carcinomas.[57,58]

Analysis of precancerous lesions and squamous cell carcinomas of the larynx by either p53 immunohistochemical staining or by DNA image cytometry for altered ploidy showed that nearly all carcinomas and 77% of the precancerous lesions were positive by either method; when the results of both methods were combined, only one precancerous lesion was negative, suggesting that p53 mutation and altered ploidy are early events in laryngeal carcinogenesis.[73] Immunohistochemical analysis with a monoclonal antibody specific for p53 protein was applied to formalin-fixed, paraffin-embedded sections of 69 head and neck carcinoma samples, 18 of which were laryngeal primaries, in patients who had been treated with definitive local therapy (surgery and/or radiotherapy). Nuclear localization of p53 protein was positive (defined as ≥10% of tumor cells showing nuclear reactivity) in 52% of the total 69 tumors and in 39% of the laryngeal primaries. The survival and the times to tumor recurrence or to second primaries were lower in the p53-positive group and the rate of second primaries was higher in the p53-positive group as compared with the p53-negative group.[107]

The inactivation of tumor suppressor genes is often manifested by allelic loss (loss of heterozygosity at nearby genetic mapping sites, detected by polymerase chain reaction). A study of 37 supraglottic laryngeal squamous cell carcinomas showed allelic losses in the p53 gene (56% of the tumors), the retinoblastoma gene (59%) and the p13–14 region of chromosome 3 (64%), suggesting that these suppressor genes play a major role in the mechanisms of laryngeal carcinogenesis.[100] In a study of 60 samples of head and neck squamous cell carcinomas (including six laryngeal carcinomas, and also including lymph node metastases), p53 overexpression detected immunohistochemically and p53 mutations detected by single-strand conformational polymorphism did not correspond in several cases, which were positive by one type of reaction and negative by the other, suggesting that both alterations may have a distinct role in the genesis of the tumors.[131]

Using polymerase chain reaction assays that can detect one mutant cancer cell among 10 000 normal cells, p53 mutations were searched for in histologic sections from the surgical margins and lymph nodes from 25 cases of head and neck squamous cell carcinomas (including seven laryngeal carcinomas).[14] In 13 of the 25 cases, sections of surgical margins, which were histologically negative for carcinoma, revealed the presence of p53 mutations in at least one margin; in five of these 13 patients, the carcinoma recurred locally. Analysis of the histologically negative lymph nodes showed that 21% were positive for p53 mutations specific for the primary tumor.[14]

The pattern of p53 mutations was examined by sequence analysis in 129 patients with primary head and neck squamous cell carcinoma (35% of which were laryngeal). Again, the most common mutations were GC→TA, GC→AT and AT→GC. The percentage of patients with p53 mutations was lowest for patients with no history of tobacco and alcohol use, intermediate for patients with tobacco but no alcohol use, and highest for patients with a history of both tobacco and alcohol use.[13]

The present 'state of the art' in the study of carcinogenesis mechanisms related to the role of tumor suppressor genes was clearly described in a recent review[77] which discusses the mechanisms of p53 and also of p21, an inhibitor of cyclin-dependent kinases, both of which induce cell cycle arrest in G_1 and prevent apoptosis in response to genotoxic damage. The role of another putative tumor suppressor gene, p16, related to cell-cycle regulation and the pRb suppressor, remains hypothetical.[77]

Studies on other molecular markers for head and neck cancers were also recently reviewed,[77] including epidermal growth factor receptor (EGFR), cyclin D1, proliferating cell nuclear antigen (PCNA), markers of squamous cell differentiation (cytokeratins, involucrin and transglutaminase I) and genetic susceptibility markers.

Specific studies on laryngeal carcinomas investigated EGFR expression, which was found at significantly higher levels in 103 primary laryngeal squamous cell carcinomas in comparison with 42 normal laryngeal tissue specimens ($P < 0.001$), and at higher levels in patients who had a recurrence than in recurrence-free patients ($P < 0.05$).[1] In the same study, p21 *ras* expression was analyzed in 43 laryngeal cancers and seven normal mucosa specimens, and found to be higher in the neoplastic tissue than in normal mucosa. No correlation was found between EGFR and p21 *ras* expression.[1] Genetic controls for enzymatic pathways for carcinogen activation offer further biologic markers of susceptibility. In addition to glutathione *S*-transferases, *N*-acetyltransferase polymorphism, through monogenic inheritance of the *NAT2* locus, determines a phenotype ('slow acetylator') that has been related to individual susceptibility to head and neck carcinogenesis, since it was found more frequently in patients with carcinoma of the larynx than in controls.[25,54]

The correlation of markers for molecular mechanisms of carcinogenesis with the epidemiologic patterns of cancer susceptibility (molecular epidemiology) has received progressively more focused attention in recent years for various types of cancer, including head and neck and specifically laryngeal cancers.[54]

The early observation that vitamin A (retinyl palmitate by oral administration) not only controlled cell differentiation in the respiratory epithelium, but also markedly inhibited respiratory carcinogenesis induced by benzo[*a*]pyrene in the hamster model,[95] led to extensive studies on retinoids biology and on cancer chemoprevention. Such studies contributed to the molecular understanding of laryngeal carcinogenesis, especially through the role of the nuclear retinoic acid receptors (RAR). The expression of RAR-β, which was found to be most frequently lacking in carcinomas, seems to play a major role in aerodigestive tract carcinogenesis.[77] Future research in this area may identify the genes involved in this process and thus clarify the pathway(s) by which the receptor may suppress carcinogenesis.[132] The field of laryngeal cancer chemoprevention is discussed in detail in Chapter 58.

Conclusions

Our understanding of the process of carcinogenesis in the larynx has expanded considerably in the last decade with the development of methods for epithelial cell culture and for the investigation of molecular mechanisms. Specific studies on the larynx have often been shared with studies on the two adjacent types of epithelium, the oropharyngeal squamous epithelium and the tracheobronchial columnar secretory epithelium.

Both experimental and human clinical evidence show that the larynx is susceptible to the independent multifocal development of preneoplastic lesions and multiple primary tumors, a phenomenon that has been termed field cancerization when first described for oral carcinogenesis.[109] This analogy has been recently reexamined in studies aimed at identifying molecular markers as common or distinct in primary tumors of the head and neck and in second primaries occurring in the same individual.[6,15,16,54,77] Significant proportions of cases of second primaries were found to either share some identical clonal markers (supporting a single clonal origin for at least some of the multiple tumors) or to show discordant markers (indicating multiple independent primaries). In view of the multistep nature of the carcinogenic process with accumulation of mutations in subsequent stages, the molecular characterization of progressive stages of laryngeal carcinogenesis and of second primaries deserves further study.

In conclusion, we can presently think of laryngeal carcinogenesis as a process that is:

- induced by different exogenous carcinogens acting singly or synergistically, among which those present in cigarette smoke have a prominent role;
- conditioned by other factors, including excessive alcohol intake and dietary factors, among which retinoids have a preventive role;
- dependent on mutations in specific oncogenes and tumor suppressor genes and on the role of specific growth factors and receptors; and
- affecting multiple sites in the laryngeal mucosa which may develop into separate foci of preneoplastic and neoplastic lesions.
- related to the role of human papilloma virus in benign recurrent papillomas, and possibly in malignancies.

The fundamental process of turning a normal laryngeal epithelial cell into a neoplastic cell is reproducible under cell culture conditions. A detailed analysis of the molecular events controlling and determining laryngeal cell transformation in the target cells, in culture and in the more complex milieu of living tissues, has become a feasible goal with current methods of cellular and molecular biology. The specific differentiation programs of cells located in different parts of the larynx relate it to the cell biology and carcinogenesis, respectively, of the oropharynx and of the tracheobronchial tract. More specific studies on the larynx will elucidate its potential differences from adjacent tissues in relation to carcinogenesis and provide effective models for its possible prevention.

References

1. Almadori G, Cadoni G, Maurizi M *et al.* Oncogeni e cancro della laringe. EGFR, p21 ras ed infezioni da HPV-DNA. *Acta Otorhinolaryngol Ital* 1995; **15(Suppl 46)**: 1–22.
2. Althoff J, Eagen M, Grandjean C. Carcinogenic effect of 2,2'-dimethyldipropylnitrosamine in Syrian hamsters. *J Natl Cancer Inst* 1975; **55**: 1209–11.
3. Arndt O, Brock J, Kundt G, Müllender A. Der Nachweis humaner Papillomvirus (HPV) DNA in formalinfixierten Plattenepithelkarzinomen des Larynx mit der Polymerase Chain Reaction (PCR). *Laryngorhinootologie* 1994; **73**: 527–32.
4. Badawi AW, Stern SJ, Lang NP, Kadlubar FF. Cytochrome P-450 and acetyltransferase expression as biomarkers of carcinogen-DNA adduct levels and human cancer susceptibility. *Prog Clin Biol Res* 1996; **395**: 109–40.
5. Barrett LA, McDowell EM, Frank AL, Harris CC, Trump BF. Long-term organ culture of human bronchial epithelium. *Cancer Res* 1976; **36**: 1003–10.
6. Bedi GC, Westra W, Gabrielson E, Koch W, Sidransky D. Multiple head and neck tumors: evidence for a common clonal origin. *Cancer Res* 1996; **56**: 2484–7.
7. Berenblum I, Shubik P. A new, quantitative approach to the study of the stages of chemical carcinogenesis in the mouse's skin. *Br J Cancer* 1947; **1**: 383–91.
8. Berkowitz BKB, Hickey SA, Moxham BJ. Embryology and anatomy. In: Ferlito A, ed. *Neoplasms of the Larynx.* Edinburgh: Churchill Livingstone, 1993: 27–48.
9. Bernfeld P, Homburger F, Russfield AB. Strain differences in the response of inbred Syrian hamsters to cigarette smoke inhalation. *J Natl Cancer Inst* 1974; **53**: 1141–57.
10. Bernfeld P, Homburger F, Soto E, Pai KJ. Cigarette smoke inhalation studies on inbred Syrian golden hamsters. *J Natl Cancer Inst* 1979; **63**: 675–89.
11. Blair WH. Chemical induction of lung carcinomas in rats. In: Karbe E, Park JF, eds. *Experimental Lung Cancer. Carcinogenesis and Bioassays.* New York: Springer-Verlag, 1974: 199–206.
12. Boren HG, Paradise LJ. Cytokinetics of the lung. In: Harris CC, ed. *Pathogenesis and Therapy of Lung Cancer.* New York: Marcel Dekker, 1978: 369–418.
13. Brennan JA, Boyle JO, Koch WM *et al.* Association between cigarette smoking and mutation of the p53 gene in squamous-cell carcinoma of the head and neck. *N Engl J Med* 1995; **332**: 712–17.
14. Brennan JA, Mao L, Hruban RH *et al.* Molecular assessment of histopathological staging in squamous-cell carcinoma of the head and neck. *N Engl J Med* 1995; **332**: 429–35.
15. Califano J, van der Riet P, Westra W *et al.* Genetic progression model for head and neck cancer: implications for field cancerization. *Cancer Res* 1996; **56**: 2488–92.
16. Chung KY, Mukhopadyay T, Kim J *et al.* Discordant p53 gene mutations in primary head and neck cancers and corresponding second primary cancers of the upper aerodigestive tract. *Cancer Res* 1993; **53**: 1676–83.
17. Clamon GH, Sporn MB, Smith JM, Saffiotti U. α- and β-retinyl acetate reverse metaplasias of vitamin A deficiency in hamster trachea in organ culture. *Nature* 1974; **250**: 64–6.
18. Clapper ML, Everly LC, Strobel LA, Townsend AJ, Engstrom PF. Coordinate induction of glutathione *S*-transferase α, μ and π expression in murine liver after a single administration of oltipraz. *Mol Pharmacol* 1994; **45**: 469–74.
19. Dalbey WE, Nettesheim P, Griesemer R, Caton JE, Guerin MR. Chronic inhalation of cigarette smoke by F344 rats. *J Natl Cancer Inst* 1980; **64**: 383–90.
20. De Stefani E, Deneo-Pellegrini H, Carzoglio JC, Ronco A, Mendilaharsu M. Dietary nitrosodimethylamine and the risk of lung cancer: a case control study from Uruguay. *Cancer Epidemiol Biomarkers Prev* 1996; **5**: 679–82.
21. Della Porta G, Kolb L, Shubik P. Induction of tracheobronchial carcinomas in the Syrian golden hamster. *Cancer Res* 1958; **18**: 592–7.
22. DiLorenzo TP, Steinberg BM. Laryngeal keratinocytes show variable inhibition of replication by TGF-beta. *J Cell Sci* 1990; **96**: 115–19.
23. Dontenwill W. Tumorigenic effect of chronic cigarette smoke inhalation on Syrian golden hamsters. In: Karbe E, Park JF, eds. *Experimental Lung Cancer. Carcinogenesis and Bioassays.* New York: Springer-Verlag, 1974: 331–59.
24. Dontenwill W, Chevalier HJ, Harke HP, Lafrenz U, Reckzeh G, Schneider B. Investigations on the effects of chronic cigarette-smoke inhalation in Syrian golden hamsters. *J Natl Cancer Inst* 1973; **51**: 1781–832.
25. Drosdz M, Gierek T, Jendryczko A, Pilch J, Piekarslea J. *N*-Acetyltransferase phenotype of patients with cancer of the larynx. *Neoplasma* 1987; **34**: 481–4.
26. Farber E. The sequential analysis of liver cancer induction. *Biochim Biophys Acta* 1980; **605**: 149–66.
27. Farrell RL, Davis GW. Effect of particulate benzo[*a*]pyrene carrier on carcinogenesis in the respiratory tract of hamsters. In: Karbe E, Park JF, eds. *Experimental Lung Cancer. Carcinogenesis and Bioassays.* New York: Springer-Verlag, 1974: 186–98.
28. Fearon ER. Vogelstein B. A genetic model for colorectal tumorigenesis. *Cell* 1990; **61**: 759–67.
29. Feron VJ, Kuper CF, Spit BJ, Reuzel PGJ, Woutersen RA. Glass fibers and vapor phase components of cigarette smoke as cofactors in experimental respiratory tract carcinogenesis. In: Mass MJ, Kaufman DG, Siegfried JM, Steele VE, Nesnow S, eds. *Cancer of the Respiratory Tract. Predisposing Factors. (Carcinogenesis: A Comprehensive Survey).* Vol. 8. New York: Raven Press, 1985: 93–118.
30. Foulds L. *Neoplastic Development,* Vol. 1. New York: Academic Press, 1969.

31. Fouret P, Dabit D, Sibony M *et al.* Expression of p53 protein related to the presence of human papillomavirus infection in precancer lesions of the larynx. *Am J Pathol* 1995; **146:** 599–604.
32. Gairola CG, Gupta RC. Cigarette smoke-induced DNA adducts in the respiratory and nonrespiratory tissues of rats. *Environ Mol Mutagen* 1991; **17:** 253–7.
33. Green U, Althoff J. Carcinogenicity of vinylethylnitrosamine in Syrian golden hamsters. *J Cancer Res Clin Oncol* 1982; **102:** 227–33.
34. Greenblatt MS, Bennett WP, Hollstein M, Harris CC. Mutations in the p53 tumor suppressor gene: clues to cancer etiology and molecular pathogenesis. *Cancer Res* 1994; **54:** 4855–78.
35. Harris CC. Chemical carcinogenesis and experimental models using human tissues. *Beitr Pathol* 1976; **158:** 389–404.
36. Harris CC, Autrup H, Stoner GD, Trump BF. Carcinogenesis studies in human respiratory epithelium. An experimental model system. In: Harris CC, ed. *Pathogenesis and Therapy of Lung Cancer.* New York: Marcel Dekker, 1978: 559–607.
37. Harris CC, Sporn MB, Kaufman DG, Smith JM, Jackson FE, Saffiotti U. Histogenesis of squamous metaplasia in the hamster tracheal epithelium caused by vitamin A deficiency or benzo[*a*]pyrene-ferric oxide. *J Natl Cancer Inst* 1972; **48:** 743–61.
38. Harris CC, Kaufman DG, Sporn MB *et al.* Localization of benzo[*a*]pyrene-3*H* and alterations in nuclear chromatin caused by benzo[*a*]pyrene-ferric oxide in the hamster respiratory epithelium. *Cancer Res* 1973; **33:** 2842–8.
39. Herrold KM. Upper respiratory tract tumors induced in Syrian hamsters by *N*-methyl-*N*-nitrosourea. *Int J Cancer* 1970; **6:** 217–22.
40. Herrold KM, Dunham LJ. Induction of carcinoma and papilloma of the tracheobronchial mucosa in the Syrian golden hamster by intratracheal instillations of benzo[*a*]pyrene. *J Natl Cancer Inst* 1962; **28:** 467–91.
41. Hoffmann D, Castonguay A, Rivenson A, Hecht SS. Comparative carcinogenicity and metabolism of 4-(methylnitrosamino)-1-(3-pyridyl)-1-butanone and *N*'-nitrosonornicotine in Syrian golden hamsters. *Cancer Res* 1981; **41:** 2386–93.
42. Hoffmann D, Rivenson A, Hecht SS, Hilfrich J, Kobayashi N, Wynder EL. Model studies in tobacco carcinogenesis with the Syrian golden hamster. *Prog Exp Tumor Res* 1979; **24:** 370–90.
43. Homburger F. 'Smokers' larynx' and carcinoma of the larynx in Syrian hamsters exposed to cigarette smoke. *Laryngoscope* 1975; **85:** 1874–81.
44. Homburger F, Soto E. Animal model of human disease: carcinoma of the larynx in hamsters exposed to cigarette smoke. *Am J Pathol* 1979; **95:** 845–8.
45. Kashima HK, Leventhal BG. Recurrent respiratory papillomatosis. In: Ferlito A, ed. *Neoplasms of the Larynx.* Edinburgh: Churchill Livingstone, 1993: 89–95.
46. Kaufman DG, Madison RM. Synergistic effects of benzo(a)pyrene and *N*-methyl-*N*-nitrosourea on respiratory carcinogenesis in Syrian golden hamsters. In: Karbe E, Park JF, eds. *Experimental Lung Cancer. Carcinogenesis and Bioassays.* New York: Springer-Verlag, 1974: 207–18.
47. Kaufman DG, Baker MS, Harris CC *et al.* Coordinated biochemical and morphologic examination of hamster tracheal epithelium. *J Natl Cancer Inst* 1972; **49:** 783–92.
48. Keenan KP, Combs JW, McDowell EM. Regeneration of hamster tracheal epithelium after mechanical injury. I. Focal lesions: quantitative morphologic study of cell proliferation. *Virchows Arch B* 1982; **41:** 193–214.
49. Keenan KP, Combs JW, McDowell EM. Regeneration of hamster tracheal epithelium after mechanical injury. II. Multifocal lesions: stathmokinetic and autoradiographic studies of cell proliferation. *Virchows Arch B* 1982; **41:** 215–29.
50. Keenan KP, Combs JW, McDowell EM. Regeneration of hamster tracheal epithelium after mechanical injury. III. Large and small lesions: comparative stathmokinetic and single pulse and continuous thymidine labeling autoradiographic studies. *Virchows Arch B* 1982; **41:** 231–52.
51. Keenan KP, Wilson TS, McDowell EM. Regeneration of hamster tracheal epithelium after mechanical injury. IV. Histochemical, immunological, and ultrastructural studies. *Virchows Arch B* 1983; **43:** 213–40.
52. Keenan KP, Saffiotti U, Stinson SF, Riggs CW, McDowell EM. Morphological and cytokinetic responses of hamster airways to intralaryngeal or intratracheal cannulation with instillation of saline or ferric oxide particles in saline. *Cancer Res* 1989; **49:** 1521–7.
53. Keenan KP, Saffiotti U, Stinson SF, Riggs CW, McDowell EM. Multifactorial hamster respiratory carcinogenesis with interdependent effects of cannula-induced mucosal wounding, saline, ferric oxide, benzo[*a*]pyrene and *N*-methyl-*N*-nitrosourea. *Cancer Res* 1989; **49:** 1528–40.
54. Khuri FR, Lippman SM, Spitz MR, Lotan R, Hong WK. Molecular epidemiology and retinoid chemoprevention of head and neck cancer. *J Natl Cancer Inst* 1997; **89:** 199–211.
55. Lafuente A, Pujol F, Carretero P, Villa JP, Cuchi A. Human glutathione *S*-transferase μ (GSTμ) deficiency as a marker for the susceptibility to bladder and larynx cancer among smokers. *Cancer Lett* 1993; **15:** 49–54.
56. Lane BP. In vitro studies. In: Harris CC, ed. *Pathogenesis and Therapy of Lung Cancer.* New York: Marcel Dekker, 1978: 419–41.
57. Lavieille JP, Brambilla E, Riva-Lavieille C, Charachon R, Brambilla C. Immunohistochemical detection of p53 protein in preneoplastic lesions and squamous cell carcinoma of the head and neck. *Acta Otolaryngol (Stockh)* 1995; **115:** 334–9.
58. Lavieille JP, Lubin R, Soussi T, Reyt E, Brambilla C, Riva C. Analysis of p53 antibody response in patients with squamous cell carcinoma of the head and neck. *Anticancer Res* 1996; **16:** 2385–8.
59. Lechner JF, Haugen A, McClendon IA, Pettis EW. Clonal growth of normal adult human bronchial epithelial cells in a serum-free medium. *In Vitro* 1982; **18:** 633–42.
60. Lechner JF, Haugen A, Autrup H, McClendon IA, Trump BF, Harris CC. Clonal growth of epithelial cells from normal adult human bronchus. *Cancer Res* 1981; **41:** 2294–304.

61. Lijinsky W. *Chemistry and Biology of* N *-nitroso Compounds.* Cambridge: Cambridge University Press, 1992.
62. Lijinsky W, Ferrero A, Montesano R, Wenyon CEM. Tumorigenicity of cyclic nitrosamines in Syrian golden hamsters. *Cancer Res Clin Oncol* 1970; **74:** 185–9.
63. Loeb LA. Microsatellite instability: marker of a mutator phenotype in cancer. *Cancer Res* 1994; **54:** 5059–63.
64. McDowell EM, Trump BF. Histogenesis of preneoplastic and neoplastic lesions in tracheobronchial epithelium. *Surv Synth Path Res* 1983; **2:** 235–79.
65. McDowell EM, Keenan KP, Huang M. Effects of vitamin A-deprivation on hamster tracheal epithelium. A quantitative morphologic study. *Virchows Arch B* 1984; **45:** 197–219.
66. McDowell EM, Becci PJ, Schürch W, Trump BF. The respiratory epithelium. VII. Epidermoid metaplasia of hamster tracheal epithelium during regeneration following mechanical injury. *J Natl Cancer Inst* 1979; **62:** 995–1008.
67. Mendelsohn MG, DiLorenzo TP, Abramson AL, Steinberg BM. Retinoic acid regulates, in vitro, the two normal pathways of differentiation of human laryngeal keratinocytes. *In Vitro Cell Dev Biol* 1991; **27A:** 137–41.
68. Montesano R, Saffiotti U. Carcinogenic response of the respiratory tract of Syrian golden hamsters to different doses of diethylnitrosamine. *Cancer Res* 1968; **28:** 2197–210.
69. Montesano R, Saffiotti U. Carcinogenic response of the hamster respiratory tract to single subcutaneous administrations of diethylnitrosamine at birth. *J Natl Cancer Inst* 1970; **44:** 413–17.
70. Montesano R, Saffiotti U, Shubik P. The role of topical and systemic factors in experimental respiratory carcinogenesis. In: Hanna MG, Nettesheim P, Gilbert JR, eds. *Inhalation Carcinogenesis. Atomic Energy Commission Symposium Series, No. 18.* Oak Ridge: Atomic Energy Commission, 1970: 353–68.
71. Mossman BT, Craighead JE. Long-term maintenance of differentiated respiratory epithelium in organ culture. I. Medium composition. *Proc Soc Exp Biol Med* 1975; **149:** 227–33.
72. Mulder TPJ, Manni JJ, Roelofs HMJ, Peters WHM, Wiersma A. Glutathione *S*-transferases and glutathione in human head and neck cancer. *Carcinogenesis* 1995; **16:** 619–24.
73. Munck-Wickland E, Kuylenstierna R, Lindholm J, Auer G. p53 immunostaining and image cytometry DNA analysis in precancerous and cancerous squamous epithelial lesions of the larynx. *Head Neck* 1977; **19:** 107–15.
74. Nawroz H, Koch W, Anker P, Stroun M, Sidransky D. Microsatellite alterations in serum DNA of head and neck cancer patients. *Nat Med* 1996; **2:** 1035–7.
75. Niemeier RW, Mulligan LT, Rowland J. Cocarcinogenicity of foundry silica sand in hamsters. In: Goldsmith DF, Winn DM, Shy CM, eds. *Silica, Silicosis, and Cancer.* New York: Praeger, 1986: 215–27.
76. Pai SB, Steele VE, Nettesheim P. Neoplastic transformation of primary tracheal epithelial cell cultures. *Carcinogenesis* 1983; **4:** 369–74.
77. Papadimitrakopoulou VA, Shin DM, Hong WK. Molecular and cellular biomarkers for field cancerization and multistep process in head and neck tumorigenesis. *Cancer Metastasis Rev* 1996; **15:** 53–76.
78. Pfeifer AMA, Mark GE III, Malan Shibley L, Graziano SL, Amstad P, Harris CC. Cooperation of c-*raf*-1 and c-*myc* protooncogenes in the neoplastic transformation of simian virus 40 large tumor antigen-immortalized human bronchial epithelial cells. *Proc Natl Acad Sci USA* 1989; **86:** 10075–9.
79. Pfeifer AMA, Jones RT, Bowden PE *et al.* Human bronchial epithelial cells transformed by the c-*raf*-1 and c-*myc* protooncogenes induce multidifferentiated carcinomas in nude mice: a model for lung carcinogenesis. *Cancer Res* 1991; **51:** 3793–801.
80. Pitot HC, Sirica AE. The stages of initiation and promotion in hepatocarcinogenesis. *Biochim Biophys Acta* 1980; **605:** 191–215.
81. Pour P, Krüger FW, Cardesa A, Althoff J, Mohr U. Carcinogenic effect of di-*N*-propylnitrosamine in Syrian golden hamsters. *J Natl Cancer Inst* 1973; **51:** 1019–27.
82. Pour P, Krüger FW, Cardesa A, Althoff J, Mohr U. Tumorigenicity of methyl-*N*-propylnitrosamine in Syrian golden hamsters. *J Natl Cancer Inst* 1974; **52:** 457–62.
83. Randerath E, Miller RH, Mittal D, Avitts TA, Dunsford HA, Randerath K. Covalent DNA damage in tissues of cigarette smokers as determined by ^{32}P-postlabeling assay. *J Natl Cancer Inst* 1989; **81:** 341–7.
84. Reddel RR, Ke Y, Gerwin BI *et al.* Transformation of human bronchial epithelial cells by infection with SV40 or adenovirus-12 SV40 hybrid virus, or transfection via strontium phosphate coprecipitation with a plasmid containing SV40 early region genes. *Cancer Res* 1988; **48:** 1904–9.
85. Reppucci AD, DiLorenzo TP, Abramson AL, Steinberg BM. *In vitro* modulation of human laryngeal papilloma cell differentiation by retinoic acid. *Otolaryngol Head Neck Surg* 1991; **105:** 528–32.
86. Romani VG, Abramson AL, Steinberg BM. Laryngeal papilloma cells in culture have an altered cytoskeleton. *Acta Otolaryngol (Stockh)* 1987; **103:** 345–52.
87. Sacks PG. Cell, tissue and organ culture as *in vitro* models to study the biology of squamous cell carcinomas of the head and neck. *Cancer Metastasis Rev* 1996; **15:** 27–51.
88. Saffiotti U. Experimental respiratory tract carcinogenesis. *Prog Exp Tumor Res* 1969; **11:** 302–33.
89. Saffiotti U. Experimental respiratory tract carcinogenesis and its relation to inhalation exposure. In: Hanna MG, Nettesheim P, Gilbert JR, eds. *Inhalation Carcinogenesis. Atomic Energy Commission Symposium Series, No. 18.* Oak Ridge: Atomic Energy Commission, 1970: 27–54.
90. Saffiotti U. Experimental carcinogenesis. In: Ferlito A, ed. *Neoplasms of the Larynx.* Edinburgh: Churchill Livingstone, 1993: 69–77. [In Table 5.1 of this reference, a typographical error should be corrected: for Group 12, no MNU pretreatment was given.]
91. Saffiotti U, Harris CC. Carcinogenesis studies on organ cultures of animal and human respiratory tissues. In: Griffin AC, Shaw CR, eds. *Carcinogens: Identification and Mechanisms of Action.* New York: Raven Press, 1979: 65–82.
92. Saffiotti U, Kaufman DG. Carcinogenesis of laryngeal carcinoma. *Laryngoscope* 1975; **85:** 454–67.

93. Saffiotti U, Cefis F, Kolb LH. A method for the experimental induction of bronchogenic carcinoma. *Cancer Res* 1968; **28:** 104–24.
94. Saffiotti U, Cefis F, Kolb LH, Shubik P. Experimental studies on the conditions of exposure to carcinogens for lung cancer induction. *J Air Pollution Control Assoc* 1965; **15:** 23–5.
95. Saffiotti U, Montesano R, Sellakumar AR, Borg SA. Studies of experimental lung cancer: inhibition by vitamin A of the induction of tracheobronchial squamous metaplasia and squamous cell tumors. *Cancer* 1967; **20:** 857–64.
96. Saffiotti U, Montesano R, Sellakumar AR, Kaufman DG. Respiratory carcinogenesis induced in hamsters by different dose levels of benzo[*a*]pyrene and ferric oxide. *J Natl Cancer Inst* 1972; **49:** 1199–204.
97. Saffiotti U, Stinson SF, Keenan KP, McDowell EM. Tumor enhancement factors and mechanisms in the hamster respiratory tract carcinogenesis model. In: Mass MJ, Kaufman DG, Siegfried JM, Steele VE, Nesnow S, eds. *Cancer of the Respiratory Tract. Predisposing factors. (Carcinogenesis: A Comprehensive Survey,* Vol. 8). New York: Raven Press, 1985: 63–92.
98. Saffiotti U, Montesano R, Sellakumar AR, Cefis F, Kaufman DG. Respiratory tract carcinogenesis in hamsters induced by different numbers of administrations of benzo[*a*]pyrene and ferric oxide. *Cancer Res* 1972; **32:** 1073–81.
99. Salam MA, Rockett J, Morris A. General primer-mediated polymerase chain reaction for simultaneous detection and typing of human papillomavirus DNA in laryngeal squamous cell carcinomas. *Clin Otolaryngol* 1995; **20:** 84–8.
100. Scholnick SB, Sun PC, Shaw ME, Haughey BH, el-Mofty SK. Frequent loss of heterozygosity for Rb, TP53, and chromosome arm 3p, but not NME1 in squamous cell carcinomas of the supraglottic larynx. *Cancer* 1994; **73:** 2472–80.
101. Schreiber H, Schreiber K, Martin DH. Experimental tumor induction in a circumscribed region of the hamster trachea: correlation of histology and exfoliative cytology. *J Natl Cancer Inst* 1975; **54:** 187–97.
102. Seidegard J, Pero RW, Miller DG, Beattie EJ. A glutathione transferase in human leukocytes as a marker for the susceptibility to lung cancer. *Carcinogenesis* 1986; **7:** 751–3.
103. Sellakumar A, Shubik P. Carcinogenicity of 7*H*-dibenzo[*c,g*]carbazole in the respiratory tract of hamsters. *J Natl Cancer Inst* 1972; **48:** 1641–6.
104. Sellakumar A, Montesano R, Saffiotti U, Kaufman DG. Hamster respiratory carcinogenesis induced by benzo[*a*]pyrene and different dose levels of ferric oxide. *J Natl Cancer Inst* 1973; **50:** 507–10.
105. Sellakumar A, Stenback F, Rowland J, Shubik P. Tumor induction by 7*H*-dibenzo[*c,g*]carbazole in the respiratory tract of Syrian hamsters. *J Toxicol Environ Health* 1977; **3:** 935–9.
106. Shabad LM. Experimental cancer of the lung. *J Natl Cancer Inst* 1962; **28:** 1305–32.
107. Shin DM, Lee JS, Lippman SC *et al.* p53 expression: predicting recurrence and second primary tumors in head and neck squamous cell carcinoma. *J Natl Cancer Inst* 1996; **88:** 519–29.
108. Shubik P, Della Porta G, Pietra G *et al.* Factors determining the neoplastic response induced by carcinogens. In: Brennan MG, Simpson WL, eds. *Biological Interactions in Normal and Neoplastic Growth.* Boston: Little, Brown, 1962: 285–97.
109. Slaughter DP, Southwick HW, Smejkal W. Field cancerization in oral stratified squamous epithelium: clinical implications of multicentric origin. *Cancer* 1953; **6:** 963–8.
110. Smith JM, Sporn MB, Berkowitz DM, Kakefuda T, Callan E, Saffiotti U. Isolation of enzymatically active nuclei from epithelial cells of the trachea. *Cancer Res* 1971; **31:** 199–202.
111. Sorokin SP. The cells of the lung. In: Nettesheim P, Hanna MG, Deatherage JW Jr, eds. *Morphology of Experimental Respiratory Carcinogenesis. Atomic Energy Commission Symposium Series No. 21.* Oak Ridge: Atomic Energy Commission, 1970: 3–43.
112. Sporn MB, Clamon GH, Dunlop NM, Newton DL, Smith JM, Saffiotti U. Activity of vitamin A analogues in cell cultures of mouse epidermis and organ cultures of hamster trachea. *Nature* 1975; **253:** 47–50.
113. Steele VE, Marchok AC, Nettesheim P. Transformation of tracheal epithelium exposed *in vitro* to *N*-methyl-*N'*-nitro-*N*-nitrosoguanidine (MNNG). *Int J Cancer* 1977; **20:** 234–8.
114. Steele VE, Marchok AC, Nettesheim P. Oncogenic transformation in epithelial cell lines derived from tracheal explants exposed *in vitro* to *N*-methyl-*N'*-nitro-*N*-nitrosoguanidine. *Cancer Res* 1979; **39:** 3805–11.
115. Steinberg BM, DiLorenzo TP. A possible role for human papillomaviruses in head and neck cancer. *Cancer Metastasis Rev* 1996; **15:** 91–112.
116. Steinberg BM, Abramson AL, Meade RD. Culture of human laryngeal papilloma cells in vitro. *Otolaryngol Head Neck Surg* 1982; **90:** 728–35.
117. Stenbäck F, Rowland J, Sellakumar A. Carcinogenicity of benzo[*a*]pyrene and dusts in the hamster lung (instilled intratracheally with titanium oxide, aluminum oxide, carbon and ferric oxide). *Oncology* 1976; **33:** 29–34.
118. Stenbäck F, Sellakumar A, Shubik P. Magnesium oxide as a carrier dust in benzo[*a*]pyrene-induced lung carcinogenesis in Syrian hamsters. *J Natl Cancer Inst* 1975; **54:** 861–7.
119. Stern SJ, Degawa M, Martin MV *et al.* Metabolic activation, DNA adducts, and H-*ras* mutations in human neoplastic and non-neoplastic laryngeal tissue. *J Cell Biochem Suppl* 1993; **17F:** 129–37.
120. Stinson SF, Lilga JC. Morphogenesis of neoplasms induced in the hamster trachea with *N*-methyl-*N*-nitrosourea. *Cancer Res* 1980; **40:** 609–13.
121. Stinson SF, Saffiotti U. Experimental laryngeal carcinogenesis. In: Ferlito A, ed. *Cancer of the Larynx.* Boca Raton: CRC Press, 1985: 5–54.
122. Stinson SF, Reznik-Schüller HM, Reznik G, Donahoe R. Spindle cell carcinoma of the hamster trachea induced by *N*-methyl-*N*-nitrosourea. *Am J Pathol* 1983; **111:** 21–6.

123. Thomassen DG, Saffiotti U, Kaighn ME. Clonal proliferation of rat tracheal epithelial cells in serum-free medium and their responses to hormones, growth factors and carcinogens. *Carcinogenesis* 1986; **7:** 2033–9.
124. Thomassen DG, Gray TE, Mass MJ, Barrett JC. High frequency of carcinogen-induced early, preneoplastic changes in rat tracheal epithelial cells in culture. *Cancer Res* 1983; **43:** 5956–63.
125. To Figueras J, Gené M, Gomez-Catalán J *et al.* Glutathione S-transferase M1 (GSTM1) and T1 (GSTT1) polymorphisms and lung cancer risk among Northwestern Mediterraneans. *Carcinogenesis* 1997; **18:** 1529–33.
126. Tsutsumi K, Iwatake H, Suzuki T. An experimental model of multistep laryngeal carcinogenesis: combined effect of human papillomavirus type 16 genome and *N*-methyl-*N'*-nitro-*N*-nitrosoguanidine. *Acta Otolaryngol Suppl (Stockh)* 1996; **522:** 89–93.
127. Vaughan CW, Homburger F, Shapshay SM, Soto E, Bernfeld P. Carcinogenesis in the upper aerodigestive tract. *Otolaryngol Clin North Am* 1980; **13:** 403–12.
128. Watts SL, Brewer EE, Fry TL. Human papillomavirus DNA types in squamous carcinomas of the head and neck. *Oral Surg Oral Med Oral Pathol* 1991; **71:** 701–7.
129. Wehner AP, Busch RH, Olson RJ. Effects of diethylnitrosamine and cigarette smoke on hamsters. *J Natl Cancer Inst* 1976; **56:** 749–56.
130. Wehner AP, Dagle GE, Milliman EM *et al.* Inhalation bioassays of cigarette smoke in rats. *Toxicol Appl Pharmacol* 1981; **61:** 1–17.
131. Xu L, Chen YT, Huvos AG *et al.* Overexpression of p53 protein in squamous cell carcinomas of head and neck without apparent gene mutations. *Diagn Mol Pathol* 1994; **3:** 83–92.
132. Xu X-C, Sozzi G, Lee JS *et al.* Suppression of retinoic acid receptor β in non-small-cell lung cancer in vivo: implications for lung cancer development. *J Natl Cancer Inst* 1997; **89:** 624–9.
133. Yarita T, Nettesheim P. Effects of carcinogen dose on the characteristics of the tracheal tumor response induced by *N*-nitroso-*N*-methylurea in hamsters. *Int J Cancer* 1978; **22:** 298–303.

Immunologic disorders of laryngeal cancer

G Christoph Mahnke and
Thomas P U Wustrow

Current management of squamous cell carcinoma (SCC) of the larynx consists mainly of surgery and radiotherapy. Despite these interventions, patients often suffer from locoregional recurrence and/or distant metastasis. Only to some extent is the clinical course predictable by the primary tumor size at first diagnosis and the degree of lymph node involvement. Often the disease takes a completely unexpected course for the better or worse. Therefore, several other factors seem to influence the interaction between tumor and tumor host. In this interaction immunological factors are often the key events. Analysis of the pathophysiology of the immune system may thus facilitate the identification of factors that influence the clinical course of the disease, allowing for a more precise prognosis in the individual patient and for an adjustment of the aggressiveness of the therapy.

The immune system of patients with laryngeal cancer is exposed to a great variety of damaging factors (Table 37.1). Of predominant importance is the long-term influence of alcohol and tobacco. Malnutrition and local viral infections cause further immunological disarray. Given that patients with laryngeal cancer are mostly in their fifth to seventh decades of life, age must also be considered as a factor taking its toll on the immune defense. Once the diagnosis of laryngeal cancer is established, the patient undergoes therapy. Although usually intended to fight the tumor, therapy can often have harmful effects on the immune system, which therapists need to be aware of.

These factors frequently act as cofactors. It is thus often difficult to determine if they impose a cumulative damage to the immune system and how they may promote carcinogenesis in laryngeal cancer. The resulting immunologic disorders are of a great variety. Some are causative whilst others may be a sequel of the malignancy. A third group may be completely unrelated to the tumor.

Table 37.1 Factors with damaging effects on the immune system

External factors
Alcohol
Tobacco
Malnutrition
Viral infections
Age
Therapy-related factors
Surgery
Anesthesia
Radiotherapy
Chemotherapy
Tumor factors

In this chapter, the present knowledge of how these factors influence the immune system and how, in turn, the imposed damage facilitates the development of laryngeal cancer are discussed.

Alcohol

The role of alcohol and nicotine in the development of laryngeal cancer has been documented extensively in epidemiologic studies.[69,75,97,137,181,211,232,248,281,283] Although the role of alcohol is even greater in carcinomas of the oro- and hypopharynx, it is obvious that alcohol is also of significant importance for the development of laryngeal cancer due to its systemic effects.[248] Early investigations probably underestimated the etiologic importance of alcohol and attributed the principal cause to tobacco.[116,254,282,283] However, recent studies point to a greater role of alcohol, particularly when ingested in high quantities.[32,63,151,152,248] The amount of alcohol consumption varies highly according to regional customs. About 10% of the Western population has a high alcohol intake (80 g/day or more in males). In these cases alcohol provides up to 43% of the caloric intake.[101,155,160] The amount of alcohol consumed also determines the extent of malnourishment. Chronic alcohol consumption significantly increases the risk of other malignant diseases (partially by concomitant immunosuppression),[29,283] infections[2] and liver damage.[206] It is also viewed as a strong cofactor for carcinogens contained in tobacco smoke and as a promoter of tumorigenesis.[171]

Local effects

Alcohol may exert its carcinogenic potential and its immunosuppressive effects at the larynx through different mechanisms:

- Acetaldehyde, an early metabolite of alcohol inhibits different functions of the immune system[133] and can cause DNA alterations in human cells.[141] Alcoholic beverages also contain a variety of other carcinogenic substances.[249]
- In chronic alcohol users the secretion of saliva is reduced, which in turn causes histologic alterations of the salivary glands and of the mucosa of the upper aerodigestive tract.[124,143,144] Lacking the protective effect of the saliva, the mucosa is exposed to carcinogens such as polycyclic aromatic hydrocarbons, which may then penetrate and cause a malignant transformation.[259]
- The lack of saliva also results in a mucosal inflammation with an increased infiltration of granulocytes and macrophages. These cells can produce superoxide and hydroxyl radicals and H_2O_2, substances which can cause malignant degeneration in epithelial cells already containing procarcinogens.
- Alcohol directly facilitates the conversion of procarcinogens into carcinogens and mitogens by an enhanced induction of microsomal enzymes.[36,135]
- Repair of the alcohol-induced mucosal damage may be delayed by the release of inhibitory substances due to a direct effect of alcohol similar to mechanisms reported for the carcinogenesis at the liver.[237]

Direct systemic effects of alcohol consumption

Alcohol consumption also has a damaging systemic effect on the immune system. This effect can be a direct effect or can be a result of the injury of other organ systems. Chronic consumption of high amounts of alcohol directly causes a great variety of defects in the regulation of the immune system.[20,224] Almost all components of the immune defense mechanism may be affected. This includes the mononuclear macrophages,[166,266] the IgG-Fc-receptor,[166,167] the antigen-stimulated antibody response[4] and the antigen-specific antibody response.[275–278] High alcohol intake can cause a polyclonal activation of B-cells with subsequent hypergammaglobulinemia.[12,60]

The formation of polymorphonuclear leukocytes in the bone marrow is decreased as a result of chronic alcohol consumption. This in turn explains the granulocytopenia found in 8% of all alcoholics.[136] Long-term feeding with alcohol in animal studies caused atrophy of the thymus and the spleen[107,241] and subsequent reduction of the total number of T-cells.[171] The chronic intake of alcohol in high doses may also have an effect on the dynamics of the formation, differentiation and half-life of T-cells since their number is reduced in alcoholics.[86,89,139,224] Alcohol has an inhibiting effect on the Fc-receptor, thereby causing a decrease in the activity of natural killer (NK) cells and in the antibody-dependent cell-mediated cytotoxicity (ADCC).[229,258] The alcohol-related inhibition of the IL-2 effect in cells with IL-2 receptors results in a suppression of the T-lymphocyte proliferation. More precisely, alcohol inhibits the interaction between IL-2 and IL-2R[114] and the T-lymphocyte proliferation in a late phase.[154] Alcohol further decreases the formation of colonies of bone marrow cells[200,245] and the glycosylation of immunoglobulins.

Indirect systemic effects

Indirect effects of alcohol on the immune system are caused by the alteration of other organ systems such as metabolism, endocrine function, gastrointestinal and liver function. Furthermore, chronic alcohol consumption also exerts an effect on the neocortex of the central nervous system which, through neuroimmunological mechanisms, can alter the number and activity of T-lymphocytes.[200]

Short-term ingestion of high amounts of alcohol causes a decrease in the number of T-lymphocytes, mostly of the suppressor type, and of the IgM-positive B-lymphocytes,[266] probably secondary to an elevation of endogenous steroid levels.[108] The impact of high alcohol consumption on the immune system is increased if the alcohol intake is combined with age- or work-related stress. It also depends on body weight and physical activity. In addition to the age-related decrease of the function of the immune system as shown, for example, by a decreased mitogen induced or IL-2-dependent T-cell proliferation, alcohol can cause further significant immunosuppression.[43]

Interestingly, alcohol-induced immunosuppression is more pronounced in young and old mice as compared to middle-aged animals, most likely due to higher levels of the alcohol dehydrogenase.[59] Development of cancer is thus significantly facilitated by the combined immunosuppressive effect of alcohol and aging.

The indirect effects of alcohol on the immune system as exerted through alterations of the gastrointestinal system vary depending on quantity and duration of the alcohol consumption and the condition of the gastrointestinal system.[11] These indirect effects are to a large degree a function of alcohol-induced malnourishment, the consequences of which are discussed below. Regular alcohol consumption causes an increased intestinal bacterial colonization and permeability which in turn results in an increased uptake of antigens. Coexisting alcoholic liver damage renders the reticuloendothelial system dysfunctional so that these antigens are not eliminated adequately. Hyperimmunoglobulinemia may be the result.[148] Chronic consumption of high amounts of alcohol delays the gastric emptying and decreases the secretion of gastric acid with successive bacterial colonization of the jejunum.[250] Due to an increased intestinal permeability, the uptake of bacterial endotoxins is increased. As a result, the serum levels of IL-1, IL-6 and TNF are elevated.

Tobacco

Epidemiologic data show that the relative risk for laryngeal cancer correlates with the amount of tobacco consumption. Although most epidemiologic studies of head and neck cancer do not differentiate between different sites, it seems clear that in the development of cancer of the larynx tobacco plays a larger role than alcohol as opposed to cancer of the oro- and hypopharynx where alcohol consumption is the main culprit.[250]

The immune response is altered by cigarette smoke,[22,182] which may be one of the pathways facilitating carcinogenesis. As a result of the influence of tobacco smoke, the levels of IgG, IgM and IgE are decreased.[83] In smokers, the number of leukocytes and lymphocytes, in particular, is increased in the peripheral blood and the CD4/CD8 ratio is significantly decreased.[157,158] Chronic influence of tobacco smoke causes a decrease in the mitogen-induced proliferation of lymphocytes.[187] These observations may result from a decreased number of T-lymphocytes which occurs in strong smokers or by an increased erythropoiesis and stimulation of the bone marrow secondary to a decreased oxygen saturation in the blood.

NK cells show a reduced activity in smokers[188] as well as in patients with head and neck cancer.[279] Immune surveillance and antitumor immunity are to a large extent a function of these immune system components and their activity may be used as a prognostic parameter to predict lymph node involvement.[90] The decreased NK cell activity may either precede, and thereby cause, the occurrence of a carcinoma, or it may be an important factor in the malignant transformation and in the development of metastases.

The antigen-specific antibody production in both undivided and Sephadex-divided lymphocyte cultures is significantly decreased in patients with laryngeal cancer who have a high tobacco consumption when compared to age- and sex-matched controls.[275,277–279]

The accumulation of Langerhans cells in the mucosa reflects part of the immunologic reaction to tobacco smoke.[38] However, Langerhans cells may have different harmful effects on the epithelium. Their release of collagenase can destroy important structures of the mucosa.[205] Release of IL-1 may stimulate the proliferation of fibroblasts, the emission of arachidonic acid derivatives from fibroblasts and the acute phase protein response.[7] The Langerhans cells may also release prostaglandin E, which can modify a multitude of different functions of inflammatory cells and subepithelial cells,[7] explaining the immunologic alterations of the mucosal reactivity caused by exposure to tobacco smoke.

Tobacco smoke contains a variety of substances which are potential antigens for Langerhans cells in particular and the immune system in general.[123] Tobacco-glycoprotein (TGP), which has been isolated from tobacco leaves and condensate of tobacco smoke, may play an important role in this pathway.[16] Biochemically it is a polyphenol containing a glycoprotein resembling rutin. Immunologically it acts as an antigen, inducing an IgE response which has been proven in smokers.[16] It also promotes the proliferation of human T-lymphocytes and the differentiation of B-lymphocytes.[80] Consequently B-lymphocytes increasingly differentiate into plasma cells and produce IgM, IgG and IgA independently of mitogens and T-lymphocytes, although the exact mechanism is as yet unclear. It appears that the TGP-induced T-lymphocyte proliferation is IL-2 independent;[80] nevertheless, an increased expression of the high-affinity receptor for IL-2 through the low-affinity receptor might be possible. Alternatively, the regulation could proceed with IL-4. T-lymphocytes can directly be activated by an antigenic effect of TGP, given its presence in a variety of fruits and vegetables such as green peppers, tomatoes, cocoa, coffee and aubergines.[16,17] The immune response to TGP could therefore also be discussed as a secondary response.

Experimental studies have shown a mitogenic effect of TGP on B-lymphocytes[44] and an inhibitory effect on the classical pathway of complement activation by binding to C2.[73] The proliferation of vascular smooth muscle cells and, by means of the factor XII-dependent metabolism, the activation of clotting and fibrinolysis are facilitated by TGP.[15] As a result, active serum proteases, kallikrein, thrombin and bradykinin are activated. By these mechanisms the well-documented cardiovascular and pulmonary damage caused by high tobacco consumption can be explained.

The production of tumor necrosis factor (TNF) in monocytes and alveolar macrophages is decreased by tobacco smoke,[179] although this may reflect a generally decreased immune response rather than a specific effect of tobacco smoke.

Malnutrition

Malnourishment or undernourishment is a frequent problem in patients with laryngeal cancer. Several factors contribute to this situation. In large laryngeal tumors odynophagia and dysphagia or tumor-related pain can be a reason for a reduction in the oral intake. Cancer may also cause anorexia or cachexia and thereby aggravate malnutrition.

Of greater importance is the effect of the regularly coexisting chronic intake of alcohol. Ingestion of high amounts of alcohol has an effect on the nutritional intake, reducing absorption, consumption, storage and excretion of nutritional contents, thus often resulting in nutritional deficiency. Alcoholics require increased quantities of protein.[155] Bioavailability, storage capacity and increased secretion of nutritional contents all act as causes of malnutrition in alcoholics,[179,243] which in turn can lead to immunosuppression.[267,268] Omission of meals or intake of meals of inferior quality or quantity leads to vitamin and mineral deficiency, especially of vitamin A,[96,101,160,202] vitamin C,[33,96,101] thiamin,[96,101,160,202] folic acid[160] and niacin.[101] Alcoholics have a high renal excretion of zinc,[160] calcium, magnesium and phosphate.[33] Decreased intake of these minerals or increased excretion causes significant alterations of the concentrations of antioxidant substances such as α-tocopherol, retinol, β-carotene, selenium and zinc,[24,87] resulting in significant inhibiting effects on the immune system. Most of the described alcohol-induced alterations of the immune system are due to malnutrition.[165]

The importance of nutrition is reflected by the observation that malnourished patients have an increased rate of infections of 22.4% (as compared to 7.3% in well-nourished patients). Recovery from tumor therapy is achieved more rapidly in patients who receive hyperalimentation. The process of tumor development, tumor growth and metastasis is influenced by the immune system which can be altered by the imbalance of certain nutrients.[265]

The nutritional state influences cell growth, cell function, metabolism, inflammatory reactions, cell–cell interactions and pharmacologic reactivity. Malnutrition, either partial or complete, can result in a disturbed immune function and in decreased antibacterial defense mechanisms.[41,42,54,55] The skin reactivity is decreased in malnourished patients.[54,61] In the long run, a diet selectively deficient in proteins causes atrophy of the thymus and other lymphatic organs[225,273] and immunosuppression[39,153] independent of calorie intake. Even after only 2–3 days a protein-deficient diet results in lower serum levels for transferrin and the complement factor C3. The number of lymphocytes as measured by E- and EAC-rosettes and their function (as measured by mitogen-induced proliferation) decreases[195] after 5–8 days. At this point the delayed cutaneous hypersensitivity and the alloreactive cytotoxic T-cell function are also decreased.[39] The number of CD4 T-cells is reduced, causing a fall in the IL-2 secretion.[40] The function of macrophages is disturbed, particularly with regard to chemotaxis, phagocytosis[198] and intracellular bactericidal mechanisms such as the production of superoxide anions (O_2^-).[197,198] This is probably a result of an insufficient IFN-γ production which is required for activation of these cells.[173] The mechanism of phagocytosis is diminished, most likely secondary to alterations of the cell membrane and thereby of the receptor expression for IgG (Fc), complement and mannose groups of oligosaccharides.[197,198]

The translocation of bacteria and endotoxins is amplified by the immunosuppression itself,[21] by systemic chemotherapy, by intravenous hyperalimentation,[5,284] by viral infections and by antibiotic therapy. The result of this increased translocation in malnutrition is infections, delayed wound-healing and an increased morbidity and mortality.[57,142] Under the influence of endotoxins, the metabolic rate is increased thus aggravating the nutritional deficiency, and the immune system is activated, particularly the B-lymphocytes. Both serum protein levels and immunologic function[6] can be restored by increasing the dietary protein content, especially when applied intragastrically. The content of arginine in the diet appears to be of particular importance for an increase in the number of T-helper cells,[55] for the correction of immune suppression caused by malnutrition[13,208] and for a decreased tumor growth.[201] Oral intake of φ-3-fatty acids,[247] vitamin A, C and E, iron, zinc and other minerals also improves

Table 37.2 Immunologic alterations caused by malnutrition

Nutritional deficit	*Immunologic function/effect*	*Reference*
Protein/calories	Thymus atrophy	273
	↓ Skin testing	225
	↓ Mitogenic lymphocyte response	130
	↓ CD4 cells	39
	↓ IL-2 production	42
	↓ B-cell number	35
	↓ IFN-γ production	173
Fatty acids	↓ Mitogenic lymphocyte response	245
w-6-Fatty acids	↓ Skin testing	273
	↓ T-cell function	18
	↑ Tumor growth	70
w-3-Fatty acids	↓ T-cell function	64
	↓ B-cell function	64
	↓ IL-1 production by macrophages	64
Vitamin A	↓ Lymphatic organs	122
	↓ Mitogenic lymphocyte response	176
	↓ IFN-α/β production	26
	↓ B-cell function	184
Vitamin E	↑ Tumor growth	120
	↑ Chromosomal breaks	37
Selenium	↑ Tumor growth	251
Zinc	Thymus atrophy	264
	↓ Skin testing	225
Copper	Thymus atrophy	194
	↓ B-cell function	193
	↓ T-helper cells	138
	↓ IL-1 and IL-2 production	76
	↓ Neutrophil function	
Nucleotides	↓ IL-2 production	
	↓ Macrophage function	

the immune response. The main immunologic alterations caused by malnutrition are summarized in Table 37.2.[18,26,35,37,39,42,64,70,76,120,122,130,138,173,176,184,193,194,225,245,251,264,273]

Arginine, fish oil and nucleotides yield a general increase of immunity. Further studies are required to show whether controlled nutrition can have a positive effect on the immune system inasmuch as malnutrition has a detrimental effect. This applies particularly to the function of endogenous growth factors, hormones, cytokines and cells of the immune system. Through the concept of dietetic prevention of carcinogenesis, new promising therapeutic approaches may become available, including:

- the inhibition of tumor neogenesis by alteration of cell metabolism;
- the removal of active carcinogenic substances;
- the inhibition of tumor progression by alterations of cell differentiation;
- the prevention of gene activation and cell proliferation by tumor-promoting substances; and
- the prevention of tumor development and tumor growth by correction of dietetically related immunosuppression.

If disease-specific nutritional contents are eventually defined, the dietetically-induced immunosuppression may be better controlled, thus preventing the development of laryngeal cancer, strengthening the immune system, slowing tumor growth and lowering recurrence rates.

Viral infections

Viral infections can not only result in immunosuppression and, according to Thomas and Burnet, thereby facilitate the development of cancer by a decreasing immunosurveillance, but they can also directly or indirectly act as cofactors in the development of malignant tumors. Oncogenes can be activated and suppressor oncogenes can be inhibited by viral infections, although the precise mechanism of viral carcinogenesis in laryngeal cancer has yet to be described.

The measles virus was the first to be shown to induce immunosuppression[255] of both the cellular and the humoral immune system. Since the immunosuppression lasts for up to 6 weeks it can be the cause of bacterial infections such as otitis media or of a reactivation of latent processes such as tuberculosis. There are multiple other viruses that may cause a decreased immunity such as cytomegalovirus, hepatitis B virus, adenovirus and influenza virus. Although some of these viruses have a cytotoxic lymphotropic effect, causing some damage of immunocompetent cells, this may not be a sufficient explanation for the immunosuppressive effect. Other mechanisms have been implicated. These include:

- the disruption of the immune system by inhibition of macrophages and activation of T-suppressor cells;
- the destruction of the microenvironment in the affected mucosa;
- an immunosuppression by host factors such as prostaglandins or viral proteins; and
- immunological derangement due to structural homologies between immunoregulatory molecules and viral sequences.

Human immunodeficiency virus (HIV)

Patients suffering from immunosuppression are at a significantly higher risk for SCC of the oral cavity.[185] In general, the rate of epithelial carcinomas is increased in HIV-positive patients.[23,163,216] Present epidemiologic data are limited by the low life expectancy of AIDS patients. However, advances in retroviral therapy and an increased survival in such patients may increase the incidence of squamous cell carcinomas of the larynx.[1,50]

Human papilloma virus (HPV)

HPV has long been implicated as a factor in the carcinogenesis of laryngeal cancer. HPV DNA, particularly of types 4, 6, 11, 16, 30, and 33, has been identified in verrucous carcinomas of the larynx,[1,28] in several laryngeal SCC,[58,98,113,164,186] and in precancerous lesions.[145] The prevalence of HPV in normal tissue of the upper aerodigestive tract varies between 0 and 64%.[81,213,226] It is unlikely that HPV infection alone can cause cancer[287] in the absence of other cofactors such as alcohol, tobacco, irradiation or other immunosuppressive factors.

Asymptomatic and persisting virus infections have not yet received attention even though they may have a significant impact on the immune system. HPV studies in children have detected antibodies against certain proteins.[104,125] Animal studies in mice have shown that in congenital infections the virus spreads to almost all tissues, including the thymus,[228] thereby possibly affecting the cell-mediated immune response. A generalized immunosuppression may be caused by lymphotropic viruses through their effect on antigen-representing cells.[244] The experimental therapeutic approach of adoptive immune therapy suppresses the virus-specific cytotoxic T-cell response so that persisting infection is overcome by lifelong immunity.[103,180]

Herpes simplex virus (HSV)

HSV is also discussed as a factor in the carcinogenesis of laryngeal cancer since increased antibody titers against HSV,[99,126,219] particularly IgA and IgM,[218] have been found in these patients. However, increased HSV titers have also been found in smokers without laryngeal cancer.[218] Infection with HSV is correlated with several defects of the cellular immunity including a decreased NK cell activity necessary for the control of HSV.[71] It is, however, unclear whether the immune defect precedes the viral infection or if it is caused by it. HSV may still contribute to the development of carcinomas by decreasing immunity and by direct mutagenic mechanisms.[82,220]

Age

The function of the immune system declines with age. This decline, particularly of the cellular immunity, commences during puberty with the involution of the thymus gland. The delayed skin reaction is clearly decreased after the age of 50.[25,119] With increasing age the mitogenic reactivity decreases in both animals[100,177] and humans.[172,260] Factors contributing to the process of aging include a decrease in number and function of cooperating T- and B-cells and macrophages[280] and a reduced production of different lymphokines such as IL-1, IL-2 and IL-3.[102,114,158] The macrophage function is reduced in old age,[79] thus causing interferences with cellular and humoral immunity and in turn increasing the risk of malignant diseases.[280]

The age-related decline of the immune defense may be one explanation for the higher incidence of viral and fungal infections and malignancies in older patients. However, the alterations of the local and systemic immune system and its effects on tumorigenesis and tumor growth are not well understood. Here the role of several factors needs to be defined, including the decreased production of mucous, the reduced activity of cilias and the increased activity of proteases with successively increased inactivation of fibronectin, immunoglobulin A and other local factors. The influence of age on the immune system underlines the need for control groups matched for age. Decisions relating to the treatment of laryngeal cancer are at present frequently based on subjective clinical experience. Objective parameters for the evaluation of the immune system would allow one to adjust the treatment of laryngeal cancer in older patients more precisely.

The impact of cancer therapy on the immune system

The immune system in patients with laryngeal cancer is not only affected by preexisting external factors but also by the different therapeutic modalities themselves. Oncologic therapy may therefore not just treat the malignant tumor but may also promote tumor growth and spread due to its immunosuppressive adverse effects. Often, too little attention is paid to this dilemma.

Surgery

Surgical traumatization

The precise surgical resection of laryngeal cancer with maximal functional organ preservation is the most effective and desirable form of treatment. An unwanted side effect of the surgical trauma, as of any trauma, is a decrease in immunity through several mechanisms,[95,161,183,222] which involves different immunologic pathways. Postoperative anergy is closely correlated to an increased morbidity.[45,150,190] Following surgery, skin reaction,[149,222] mitogenic reaction to phytohemagglutinin (PHA) and the activity of the macrophage-inhibiting factor (MIF) are reduced.[112,183,222] This is most likely due to an increased activity of suppressor cells, an altered function of monocytes and neutrophils and suppressor factors in the serum.[149] B-cell functions are also inhibited.[178] Other reasons for the postoperative immunosuppression are a decrease in the number of lymphocytes,[222] especially T-cells,[95] mononuclear cells and a reduced production of IL-1, IL-2,[3,68] and IL-3,[74] probably secondary to increased postoperative steroid levels.[53,74,117,121,257] Following surgical trauma a variety of other substances with immunosuppressive effects are found in increased concentrations, including histamine, thromboxane A2, prostaglandin I_2 and TNF-α. The postoperative production of IL-6 is increased, perhaps due to TNF-α, IL-1 or endotoxins. One effect of IL-6 is the enhanced activation or secretion of TGF-β by monocytes,[159] which in turn induces immunosuppression reversible by anti-IL-6 antibodies.[10] As a result of surgery of the larynx, the NK cell activity is significantly reduced. This may increase the risk for distant metastasis[94,210] as an effect induced by the tumor cells itself and by postoperatively increased suppressor cells with adherent characteristics. An increased rate of postoperative metastasis has been reported in clinical and experimental studies, warranting research into mechanisms to modify the suppressor cells.[62,189,192,235] A potential stimulator of the immune response is Tuftsin, which increases the postoperatively reduced activity of NK cells, enhances the macrophage-dependent cytotoxicity and perhaps induces suppressor macrophages.[189,210] It may therefore be a useful substance in a perioperative immunoadjuvant therapy. Another immune-potentiating substance is Ge-132 which has an IFN-γ effect shown to alleviate immunosuppression postoperatively in experimental studies.[174]

Blood loss and blood transfusion

Intraoperative blood loss does cause a suppression of the immune system, in particular if it is greater than 500 ml.[27] Effects include a decrease in the IL-2 release and the mitogenic lymphocyte response[8,230] as well as a significant increase in the serum levels of TGF-β.[8] TGF-β and its isoforms β_{1-3} have both a suppressive and a stimulating effect on the immune system. They stimulate some macrophage-mediated reactions[9] and the release of monokines[256] and suppress the IL-2 secretion and the mitogenic T-cell response.[147] Another effect of intraoperative blood loss is an increase in TNF and IL-6,[66] which promote the release and activation of TGF-β.[286] The release of PGE_2 is increased by TGF-β which induces further immunosuppression.[239] A partial reversal of the immunosuppression induced by blood loss is possible with anti-TGF-β antibodies[8] and with inhibitors of the cyclooxygenase.[65,216] This points to an important role of TGF-β in prolonged postoperative immunosuppression.

As a result of extensive blood loss, allogenic blood transfusion may be indicated. However, this can cause further immunosuppression and an increased rate of perioperative infections. The selective removal of leukocytes and thrombocytes by filters helps to reduce this effect.[106] In patients with organ transplants, blood transfusions have been shown to advantageously suppress immunity. The activity of T-suppressor cells is increased[223] whereas the total number of T-cells, the number of IL-2 receptor-positive T-helper cells[140] and the activity of NK cells are reduced.[78,115] Other effects of blood transfusions are an increased production of PGE_2,[270] an altered macrophage function[115] and a significant increase in serum steroid levels, which in turn lowers the total number of leukocytes.[271] For the immunosuppressive effect, the interval between allogenous blood transfusions and time of operative trauma may be important as may be the bacterial colonization of the wound. Not only blood transfusion but also frequent donation of blood[128] or donation of two units within 3–4 days[146] as needed for autologous blood transfusion causes a decreased activity of NK cells.

Anesthesia

Ever since the early days of anesthesia in 1916 a possible effect of anesthetics on the development, growth and metastasis of tumors has been discussed. It later became clear that the more important cause of immunosuppression after general anesthesia is the surgical trauma rather than the anesthetics. Nevertheless, anesthetics do alter several functions of the immune system.[169,261,262] Under the influence of volatile anesthetics the permeative activity of neutrophils is decreased.[170] Different anesthetics and analgesics reduce the activity of phagocytes[168] and the mitogen-induced proliferation of lymphocytes.[31] The cytotoxicity of leukocytes against tumor cells is decreased *in vitro* by local anesthetics,[118] barbiturates[131] and halothane.[52]

General anesthesia with halothane or nitric oxide suppresses the immune response,[118,209] as shown by a reduction in the mitogenic lymphocyte reaction[175] and for 7–10 days in the number of B-cells.[27] Ether and cyclopropamide have been shown to lower mitogenic lymphocyte response and the number of T- and B-cells up to 10 days postoperatively. *In vitro*, the decreased immune response starts in the early phase of anesthesia and lasts until 5 days postoperatively.[222] *In vivo* studies such as skin testing display a decreased response over 5 days after general anesthesia and normalization in the second to third week. Uncontrolled stress due to either surgery itself or anesthesia can cause a significant immunosuppression as shown by a decreased mitogenic lymphocyte response,[129] decreased NK cell activity,[215] decreased tumor rejection[253] and increased tumor growth.[221] The stress-related steroid release also affects tumor growth and distant metastasis.[47,246]

In addition to the described direct pharmaceutical effects of the medications used during anesthesia, there may be other indirect effects on the immune system. The behaviour of tumor cells and tumor infiltrating lymphocytes may be influenced by the redistribution of the blood flow with changes in blood pressure, temperature, and oxygenation during anesthesia.[111] In experimental studies, a reactivation of tumor cells and an increased rate of distant metastasis following general anesthesia has been shown.[214,252] However, halothane does not accelerate tumor growth even in repeated operations.[51] It actually seems to inhibit tumor growth by destroying cytoplasmic actin-like microfilaments,[240] by a calmodulin-inhibitor-like effect[207] or by modification of proteinase inhibitors.[269]

Radiotherapy

Radiation therapy exerts its immunosuppressive effect by several mechanisms. It has a myeloablative effect, depending on single doses, dose rate, fractionation, type of radiation and the field of radiation. The effects of this local and locoregional immunosuppression are not yet well defined. The simultaneous application of chemotherapy further increases the myelotoxic effects and the immunosuppression, especially if 5-fluorouracil and carboplatin are given.

Radiotherapy locally reduces the saliva production, increases its viscosity and decreases the pH. As a result, the local defense mechanism of the upper aerodigestive tract is rendered less efficient. The adverse effects of radiotherapy such as odynophagia, nausea or mucositis may indirectly decrease immunity by causing malnutrition. In addition, bacterial, fungal or latent viral infections can further weaken the immune defense.[34]

Even though the fields exposed to radiotherapy are comparatively small in laryngeal cancer, a damaging effect on the highly radiosensitive lymphocytes has been documented by a reduced mitogenic reactivity after PHA stimulation,[231,242] probably due to the rapid blood flow in the neck region. Whilst skin testing remains unaffected,[48,85,91] the total number of T-cells is reduced for several years. This may be an explanation for the development of secondary carcinomas or distant metastasis despite local tumor control.[72,217] Locoregional control is significantly better after a combination therapy of surgery and postoperative radiotherapy. However, the addition of radiation therapy was in some studies correlated with an increased risk for distant metastasis.[109,234] Other studies do not find an increased rate of distant metastasis after postoperative radiotherapy.[49,156] At present, studies on the development of secondary carcinomas are not available.

The total number of T-cells is decreased after radiotherapy[105,182] for a long time.[274] The number of CD8+ cells and NK cells (Leu 7^+) increases during radiotherapy.[274] Different cells seem to be more susceptible to the effects of radiotherapy than others. This has been shown in patients with Hodgkin's disease and breast cancer treated by radiotherapy where a relative radioresistance of CD8+

cells with a capacity for an early recovery, as compared to CD4+ cells, has been found.[110,191] T-cells circulating in the peripheral blood after extensive operations with significant blood loss are mostly in an early stage of maturation. In this stage they are more sensitive to irradiation and recovery takes even longer.[274] A pre-therapeutically decreased number of T-cells is correlated with a significantly shorter disease-free survival. Also, the rate of recurrence is higher in patients whose T-cells do not normalize rapidly. This has led to the conclusion that the post-radiotherapeutic immune reactivity seems to have a significant effect on the prognosis. A post-radiotherapeutic increase of CD8+ cells is correlated with an increased disease-free survival, since cytotoxic cells can then become effective for the destruction of tumor cells.[274]

Radiotherapy seems to decrease the adherence of tumor cells among themselves. This may increase motility. Since radiotherapy also increases the permeability of connective tissue and basal membranes, tumor cells may thus be transferred as microthrombi and cause distant metastasis. Radiotherapy also has a long-term disabling effect on the immune function of the nontumorous cervical lymph nodes, which is due to radiation-induced lymphopenia and lasts for a long time. These barriers will subsequently fail to provide local tumor control. Also, because of the immunologic effects, the indication for primary or postoperative radiotherapy has to be assessed thoroughly, particularly in cases with a low probability for regional metastasis such as completely resected small primary tumors or N1 stage metastases.

Chemotherapy

Chemotherapy is applied in advanced laryngeal carcinomas and experimentally as inductive anterior chemotherapy. It does have a significant immunosuppressive effect. Depending on the substances used, numerous different malignancies have been described after chemotherapy.[84] Following the application of methotrexate and adriamycin, lymphocyte reactivity is reduced for 24–48 hours, whereas skin testing with 2,4-dinitrochlorobenzene (DNCB) remains unaffected.[203] Due to the long-term application the effect is also long-lasting.

Tumor-related immunosuppression

The primary tumor itself and possible second carcinomas induce several alterations in the immune system. The activity of peripheral lymphocytes is reduced by exposure to tumor cells,[92,93] cell-free extracts of solid tumors,[162] serum of cancer patients[88] and supernatant fluid of tumor cell cultures.[77,204,236] Immunological dysfunctions include an inhibition of the mitogen and antigen proliferation,[199,272] the NK cell function[238] and the lymphokine activated killer (LAK) cell function.[92,93] The tumor cell-induced immunosuppression is due to different mechanisms such as direct activation of T-suppressor cells,[14,19] mediators like TGF-β,[127,196] prostaglandins,[132,227] glycoproteins,[204] plasma fibronectin,[212] p53 products,[134] peptides resembling p15 and showing homologies to the envelope proteins of retroviruses[46] and other suppressor molecules derived from tumor cells.[30,56] The observation that SCC of the larynx continues to grow in the presence of high numbers of activated lymphocytes indicates functional defects of these cells. However, there are also factors, released by the tumor itself, which suppress inherent defense mechanisms for tumor regression. For example, laryngeal cancer cells produce a soluble factor (SCIF – squamous carcinoma inhibitory factor) which inhibits the LAK activity.[233] These soluble suppressor factors are produced in increasing amounts with increasing proximity of the primary tumor to the lymph node.[263] The immune reactivity of lymph nodes is thus not only influenced by the primary tumor but also by other lymph nodes in a hierarchical manner since these also produce inhibiting factors. The suppressing factors of tumor cells may also interfere with the DNA synthesis, especially in T-cells if IL-2 is required. An IL-2 induced T-suppressor activity has been described in SCC of the larynx.[67]

The insufficient immune response in tumor-infiltrated and tumor-draining cervical lymph nodes is due to a variety of factors including tumor-induced suppressor cells and immuno-inhibitory factors, lack of precursors of immunocompetent cells or the inability of these cells to differentiate or induce mechanisms of activation in the altered tumor area. It has been shown that in SCC of the larynx the suppression of blood group-related antigens is suppressed and that immature carbohydrate chains are accumulated.[285] Of further importance could be the removal of antigen-reactive T-cells, the inactivation of antigen-reactive T-cells, a suppression of antigen-reactive T-cells by regulatory cells or an inability to produce cytokines. On the other hand, lymphocytes derived from tumor-infiltrated cervical lymph nodes of patients with SCC of the larynx are unable to produce IL-1β or TNF-α and only very little IFN-γ, which is not caused by suppressor cells.[132] Tumor cells seem to produce immunosuppressive factors which support tumor growth and distant metastasis. An inactivation of these tumor-derived suppressor factors may offer new therapeutic perspectives.

Therapeutic perspectives

Different immune therapeutic approaches have been described for the treatment of laryngeal cancer. These include immunoprophylaxis, passive, nonspecific or adoptive specific immunotherapy, immune reconstructive therapy, immune modulation, immune depletion and immunologic gene therapy.

The therapeutic approach of immune prophylaxis utilizes the patient's own immunity by immunizing against viral or tumoral antigens associated with carcinomas. In passive immune therapy, cytotoxic, blocking or antibody-toxin conjugates are applied. Unspecific immune therapy exerts its effect through an improved allocation of cytotoxic antibodies, inhibition of blocking antibodies, for example with cyclophosphamide or by plasmapheresis, and increasing activity of macrophages with BCG, *Cryptosporidium parvum* or zymosan. Unspecific immune therapy can also be an improvement of cell-mediated immunity by *Bordetella pertussis*, lipopolysaccharide (LPS) or Lectines, immune stimulation by various pharmaceuticals or bacterial vaccines and immune potentiation with levamisole, thymosin, thymopoietin or OK-432. In adoptive specific immune therapy, immunologic competence is transferred by cells, cell products or antibodies. Potential cell products in this respect are transfer factor, interferon, cytokines, especially IL-2 and TNF, combinations of different cytokines and combinations of cytokines with chemotherapeutics. Cells reinfused for adoptive specific immune therapy could be tumor-infiltrating lymphocytes, cytotoxic T-cells, NK cells, LAK cells or monocytes that are purified and expanded *in vitro*. Antibodies available for this mode of therapy can bind growth factors, receptors of receptor antagonists, for example the EGF, transferrin or IL-2 receptors. Immunity can be restored by improved nutrition, blood transfusion or with GM-CSF or IL-3. A modulation of the immune system is possible with IL-4, IL-4 and IL-6, IL-12 and interferon. Currently great interest is paid to advances in immunologic gene therapy through genetic modifications of tumor-infiltrating lymphocytes or alloantigens caused by antisense genes and suppressor genes. The discussion of all information available on this topic would require a separate review.

Conclusions

The immune system of patients with squamous cell carcinoma of the larynx is challenged by a great variety of factors causing numerous dysfunctions with prognostic relevance. The individual role of these factors deserves future investigations, in particular with regard to potential therapeutic approaches. At present, different therapies that modify the immune system are at least conceptually available. However, long-term studies need to clarify if and how patients with laryngeal cancer can benefit from these forms of treatment and how dysfunctions of the immune system can be corrected without causing excessive reactions. The surgeon treating laryngeal cancer should consider whether immune-stimulating or reconstructive measures are indicated in patients with decreased immunity and whether less traumatic procedures with less blood loss have a beneficial effect on the tumor immunologic situation and therefore on the overall survival. This gives minimal-invasive or functional surgery a new meaning by making it biologically adjusted surgery, biologically preservative reconstructive surgery or biologically functional surgery. In laryngeal cancer it is not only the radical removal of the primary tumor that is of concern but also the regional lymph nodes and their importance for other lymph nodes and the primary tumor as well as the immunity of the patient as a whole. Holistic therapeutic concepts need to take these factors into consideration and preserve and – by biological immunotherapy – restore the tumor-specific immunity. Survival rates and quality of life may then improve even in problematic cases.

References

1. Abramson AL, Brandsma J, Steinberg B, Winkler B. Verrucous carcinoma of the larynx. Possible human papilloma virus etiology. *Arch Otolaryngol* 1985; **111**: 709–15.
2. Adams HG, Jordan C. Infection in the alcoholic. *Med Clin North Am* 1984; **68**: 179–200.
3. Akiyoshi T, Koba F, Arinaga S, Miyazaki S, Wada T, Tsuji H. Impaired production of interleukin-2 after surgery. *Clin Exp Immunol* 1985; **59**: 45–9.
4. Aldo-Benson M. Mechanisms of alcohol-induced suppression of B-cell response. *Alcohol Clin Exp Res* 1989; **13**: 469–75.
5. Alexander JW, Gonce SJ, Miskell PW, Peck MD, Sax H. A new model for studying nutrition in peritonitis. The adverse effect of overfeeding. *Ann Surg* 1989; **209**: 334–40.
6. Alexander JW, MacMillan BG, Stinnett JD *et al.* Beneficial effects of aggressive protein feeding in severely burned children. *Ann Surg* 1980; **192**: 505–17.
7. Arenzana-Seisdedos F, Barbey S, Virelizier JL, Kornprobst M, Nezelof C. Histiocytosis X purified (T6+) cells from bone marrow granuloma produced interleukin 1 and prostaglandin E2 in culture. *J Clin Invest* 1986; **77**: 326–9.
8. Ayala A, Meldrum DR, Perrin MM, Chaudry IH. The release of transforming growth factor-β following haemorrhage: its role as a mediator of host immunosuppression. *Immunology* 1993; **79**: 479–84.
9. Ayala A, Perrin MM, Wagner MA, Chaudry IH. Enhanced susceptibility to sepsis after simple hemorrhage: depression of Fc and C3b receptor mediated phagocytosis. *Arch Surg* 1990; **125**: 70–5.
10. Ayala A, Knotts JB, Ertel W, Perrin MM, Morrison MH, Chaudry IH. Role of interleukin 6 and transforming growth factor-β in the induction of depressed splenocyte responses following sepsis. *Arch Surg* 1993; **128**: 89–95.
11. Bagasra O, Howeedy A, Dorio R, Kajdacsy-Balla A. Functional analysis of T-cell subsets in chronic experimental alcoholism. *Immunology* 1987; **61**: 63–9.
12. Bailey RJ, Krasner N, Eddleston ALWF *et al.* Histocompatibility antigens, autoantibodies, and immunoglobulins in alcoholic liver disease. *Br Med J* 1976; **2**: 727–9.
13. Barbul A, Wasserkrug HL, Seifter E, Rettura G, Levenson SM, Efron G. Immunostimulatory effects of arginine in normal and injured rats. *J Surg Res* 1980; **29**: 228–35.
14. Bear HD. Tumor-specific suppressor T-cells which inhibit the in vitro generation of cytolytic T-cells from immune and early tumor-bearing host spleens. *Cancer Res* 1986; **46**: 1805–12.
15. Becker CG, Dubin T. Activation of factor XII by tobacco glycoprotein. *J Exp Med* 1977; **146**: 457–67.
16. Becker CG, Dubin T, Wiedemann HP. Hypersensitivity to tobacco antigen. *Proc Natl Acad Sci USA* 1976; **73**: 1712–16.

17. Becker CG, Van Hamont N, Wagner M. Tobacco, cocoa, coffee and ragweed: cross-reacting allergens that activate factor-XII-dependent pathways. *Blood* 1981; **58:** 861–4.
18. Bennett M, Uauy R, Grundy SM. Dietary fatty acid effects on T-cell-mediated immunity in mice infected with *Mycoplasma pulmonis* or given carcinogens by injection. *Am J Pathol* 1987; **126:** 103–13.
19. Berd D, Mastrangelo MJ. Effect of low dose cyclophosphamide on the immune system of cancer patients: reduction of T-suppressor function without depletion of the CD8+ subset. *Cancer Res* 1987; **47:** 3317–21.
20. Berenyi MR, Straus B, Cruz D. In vitro and in vivo studies of cellular immunity in alcoholic cirrhosis. *Dig Dis Sci* 1974; **19:** 199–205.
21. Berg RD, Wommack E, Deitch EA. Immunosuppression and intestinal bacterial overgrowth synergistically promote bacterial translocation. *Arch Surg* 1988; **123:** 1359–64.
22. Berger LR. Cigarette smoking and the acquired immunodeficiency syndrome. *Ann Intern Med* 1988; **108:** 638. [Letter]
23. Biggar RJ, Burnett W, Mikl J, Nasca P. Cancer among New York men at risk of acquired immunodeficiency syndrome. *Int J Cancer* 1989; **43:** 979–85.
24. Bjorneboe GEA, Johnsen J, Bjorneboe A *et al.* Some aspects of antioxidant status in blood from alcoholics. *Alcohol Clin Exp Res* 1988; **12:** 806–10.
25. Bleumink E, Nater JP, Schraffordt Koops H, The TH. A standard method for DNCB sensitization testing in patients with neoplasms. *Cancer* 1974; **33:** 911–15.
26. Bowman A, Fergusson RJ, Allan SG *et al.* Potentiation of cisplatin by alpha-interferon in advanced non-small cell lung cancer (NSCLC): a phase II study. *Ann Oncol* 1990; **1:** 351–3.
27. Boynet R, Arthur JR. Effects of selenium and copper deficiency on neutrophil function in cattle. *J Comp Pathol* 1981; **91:** 271–6.
28. Brandsma JL, Steinberg BM, Abramson AL, Winkler B. Presence of human papillomavirus type 16 related sequences in verrucous carcinoma of the larynx. *Cancer Res* 1986; **46:** 2185–8.
29. Breeden JH. Alcohol, alcoholism and cancer. *Med Clin North Am* 1984; **68:** 163–77.
30. Brotherick I, Shenton BK, Kirby JA *et al.* Production of immunosuppressive factors by a cultured tumour cell line and their effect on lymphocyte proliferation and cell cycle response. *Surg Oncol* 1993; **2:** 241–8.
31. Bruce DL. Halothane action on lymphocytes does not involve cyclic AMP. *Anesthesiology* 1976; **44:** 151–4.
32. Brugere J, Guenel P, Leclerc A, Rodriguez J. Differential effects of tobacco and alcohol in cancer of the larynx, pharynx and mouth. *Cancer* 1986; **57:** 391–5.
33. Bunout D, Gattás V, Iturriaga H, Pérez C, Pereda T, Ugarte G. Nutritional status of alcoholic patients: its possible relationship to alcoholic liver damage. *Am J Clin Nutr* 1983; **38:** 469–73.
34. Bustamante CI, Wade JC. Herpes simplex virus infection in the immunocompromised cancer patient. *J Clin Oncol* 1991; **9:** 1903–15.
35. Cannon PR. The importance of proteins in resistance to infection. *JAMA* 1945; **128:** 360–2.
36. Capel ID, Jenner M, Pinnock MH, Williams DC. The effect of chronic alcohol intake upon the hepatic microsomal carcinogen-activation system. *Oncology* 1978; **35:** 168–70.
37. Carney JM, Starke-Reed PE, Oliver CN *et al.* Reversal of age-related increase in brain protein oxidation, decrease in enzyme activity and loss in temporal and spatial memory by chronic administration of the spin-trapping compound *N*-tert-butyl-alpha-phenylnitrone. *Proc Natl Acad Sci USA* 1991; **88:** 3633–6.
38. Casolaro MA, Bernaudin JF, Saltini C, Ferrans VJ, Crystal RG. Accumulation of Langerhans cells on the epithelial surface of the lower respiratory tract in normal subjects in association with cigarette smoking. *Am Rev Respir Dis* 1988; **137:** 406–11.
39. Chandra RK. Immunocompetence in undernutrition. *J Pediatr* 1972; **81:** 1194–200.
40. Chandra RK. Numerical and functional deficiency in T-helper cells in protein energy malnutrition. *Clin Exp Immunol* 1983; **51:** 126–35.
41. Chandra RK. Nutrition, immunity, and infection: present knowledge and future directions. *Lancet* 1983; **1:** 688–91.
42. Chandra RK. Trace elements and immune responses. *Immunol Today* 1983; **4:** 322–5.
43. Chang MP, Norman DC. Immunotoxicity of alcohol in young and old mice. II. Impaired T cell proliferation and T cell-dependent antibody responses of young and old mice fed ethanol-containing liquid diet. *Mech Ageing Dev* 1991; **57:** 175–86.
44. Choy JW, Becker CG, Siskind GW, Francus T. Effects of tobacco glycoprotein (TGP) on the immune system. I. TGP is a T-independent B cell mitogen for murine lymphoid cells. *J Immunol* 1985; **134:** 3193–8.
45. Christou NV, Meakins JG. Neutrophil function in anergic surgical patients: neutrophil adherence and chemotaxis. *Ann Surg* 1979; **190:** 557–64.
46. Cianciolo GJ, Copeland TD, Oroszlan S, Snyderman R. Inhibition of lymphocyte proliferation by synthetic peptide homologous to retroviral envelope protein. *Science* 1985; **230:** 453–5.
47. Clarke RSJ, Johnston H, Sheridan B. The influence of anaesthesia and surgery on plasma cortisol, insulin and free fatty acids. *Br J Anaesth* 1970; **42:** 295–9.
48. Clement JA, Kramer S. Immunocompetence in patients with solid tumors undergoing cobalt 60 irradiation. *Cancer* 1974; **34:** 193–6.
49. Constable WC, Marks RD, Robbins JP, Fitz-Hugh GS. High dose pre-operative radiotherapy and surgery for cancer of the larynx. *Laryngoscope* 1972; **82:** 1861–8.
50. Cremer KJ, Spring SB, Gruber J. Role of human immunodeficiency virus type 1 and other viruses in malignancies associated with acquired immunodeficiency disease syndrome. *J Natl Cancer Inst* 1990; **82:** 1016–24.
51. Cullen BF, Sundsmo JS. Failure of halothane anaesthesia to alter growth of sarcoma in mice. *Anesthesiology* 1974; **41:** 580–4.
52. Cullen BF, Duncan PG, Ray-Keil L. Inhibition of cell-mediated cytotoxicity by halothane and nitrous oxide. *Anesthesiology* 1976; **44:** 386–90.

53. Culpepper JA, Lee F. Regulation of IL-3 expression by glucocorticoids in cloned murine T-lymphocytes. *J Immunol* 1985; **135:** 3191–7.
54. Daly JM, Reynolds J, Sigal RK, Shou J, Liberman MD. Effect of dietary protein and amino acids on immune function. *Crit Care Med* 1990; **18:** 86–93.
55. Daly JM, Reynolds J, Thom A *et al.* Immune and metabolic effects of arginine in the surgical patient. *Ann Surg* 1988; **208:** 512–23.
56. Deal H, Steele JK, Stammers AT, Singhai R, Levi JG. Preadministration of a T-suppressor factor enhances tumour immunity in DBA/2 mice. *Cancer Immunol Immunother* 1989; **28:** 193–8.
57. Deitch EA, Winterton J, Li M, Berg R. The gut as a portal of entry for bacteremia. Role of protein malnutrition. *Ann Surg* 1987; **205:** 681–92.
58. Dekmezian RH, Batsakis JG, Goepfert H. In situ hybridization of papillomavirus DNA in head and neck squamous cell carcinomas. *Arch Otolaryngol Head Neck Surg* 1987; **113:** 819–21.
59. Domiati-Saad R, Jerrells TR. The influence of age on blood alcohol levels and ethanol-associated immunosuppression in a murine model of ethanol consumption. *Alcohol Clin Exp Res* 1993; **17:** 382–8.
60. Drew PA, Clifton PM, LaBrooy JT, Shearman DJC. Polyclonal B cell activation in alcoholic patients with no evidence of liver dysfunction. *Clin Exp Immunol* 1984; **57:** 479–86.
61. Edelman R, Suskind R, Olson RE, Sirisinha S. Mechanisms of defective delayed cutaneous hypersensitivity in children with protein-calorie malnutrition. *Lancet* 1973; **1:** 506–8.
62. El Rifi K, Bacon B, Mehigan J, Hoppe E, Cole WH. Increased incidence of pulmonary metastases after celiotomy. Counteraction by heparin. *Arch Surg* 1965; **91:** 625–34.
63. Elwood JM, Pearson JCG, Skippen DH, Jackson SM. Alcohol, smoking, social and occupation factors in the aetiology of cancer of the oral cavity, pharynx and larynx. *Int J Cancer* 1984; **34:** 603–12.
64. Endres S, Ghorbani R, Kelley VE *et al.* The effect of dietary supplementation with n-3 polyunsaturated fatty acids on the synthesis of interleukin-1 and tumor necrosis factor by mononuclear cells. *N Engl J Med* 1989; **320:** 265–71.
65. Ertel W, Morrison MH, Ayala A, Perrin MM, Chaudry IH. Blockade of prostaglandin production increases cachectin synthesis and prevents depression of macrophages functions following hemorrhagic shock. *Ann Surg* 1991; **213:** 265–71.
66. Ertel W, Morrison MH, Ayala A, Perrin MM, Chaudry IH. Anti-TNF monoclonal antibodies prevent haemorrhage-induced suppression of Kupffer cell antigen presentation and MHC class II antigen expression. *Immunology* 1991; **74:** 290–7.
67. Eura M, Maehara T, Ikawa T, Ishikawa T. Suppressor cells in the effector phase of autologous cytotoxic reactions in cancer patients. *Cancer Immunol Immunother* 1988; **27:** 147–53.
68. Faist E, Mewes A, Strasser T *et al.* Alteration of monocyte function following major injury. *Arch Surg* 1988; **123:** 287–92.
69. Feldman JG, Hazan M. A case-control investigation of alcohol, tobacco, and diet in head and neck cancer. *Prev Med* 1975; **4:** 444–63.
70. Fernandes G, Venkatraman J. Micronutrient and lipid interactions in cancer. *Ann N Y Acad Sci* 1990; **587:** 78–91.
71. Ferson M, Edwards A, Lind A, Milton GW, Hersey P. Low natural-killer cell activity and immunoglobulin levels associated with smoking in human subjects. *Int J Cancer* 1979; **23:** 603–9.
72. Fidler IJ, Zeidman I. Enhancement of experimental metastasis by x-ray: a possible mechanism. *J Med* 1972; **3:** 172–7.
73. Firpo A, Polley MJ, Becker CG. The effect of tobacco derived products on the human complement system. *Immunobiology* 1983; **164:** 318.
74. Fishman P, Nedivi R, Djaldetti M, Sredni B, Kayzer S, Chaimoff C. Kinetics of cortisol, interleukin-2 and interleukin-3-like activity levels following surgical intervention. *Nat Immun* 1993; **12:** 35–40.
75. Flanders WD, Rothman KJ. Interaction of alcohol and tobacco in laryngeal cancer. *Am J Epidemiol* 1982; **115:** 371–9.
76. Flynn A, Loftus MA, Finke JH. Production of interleukin-1 and interleukin-2 in allogeneic mixed lymphocyte cultures under copper, magnesium and zinc deficient conditions. *Nutr Res* 1984; **4:** 673–9.
77. Fontana A, Hengartner H, De Tribolet N, Weber E. Glioblastoma cells release interleukin 1 and factors inhibiting interleukin 2-mediated effects. *J Immunol* 1984; **132:** 1837–44.
78. Ford CD, Warnick CT, Sheets S, Quist R, Stevens L. Blood transfusion lowers natural killer cell activity. *Transplant Proc* 1987; **19:** 1456–7.
79. Fox RA. Immunology of aging. In: Brockelhurst JC, ed. *Textbook of Geriatric Medicine and Gerontology.* New York: Churchill Livingstone, 1985: 82–104.
80. Francus T, Klein RF, Staiano-Coico L, Becker CG, Siskind GW. Effects of tobacco glycoprotein (TGP) on the immune system. *J Immunol* 1988; **140:** 1823–9.
81. Fukushima K, Ogura H, Watanabe S, Yabe Y, Masuda Y. Human papillomavirus type 16 DNA detected by the polymerase chain reaction in non-cancer tissues of the head and neck. *Eur Arch Otorhinolaryngol* 1994; **251:** 109–12.
82. Galloway DA, McDougall JK. The oncogenic potential for herpes simplex viruses: evidence for a 'hit and run' mechanism. *Nature* 1983; **302:** 21–4.
83. Gerrard JW, Ko CG, Myers A, Heiner DC, Mink J, Dosman JA. Immunoglobulin levels in smokers and nonsmokers. *Ann Allergy* 1980; **44:** 261–2.
84. Gertz MA, Noöl P, Kyle RA. Second malignancies after chemotherapy and transplantation. *Crit Rev Oncol Hematol* 1993; **14:** 107–25.
85. Ghossein NA, Bosworth JL, Bases RE. The effect of radical radiotherapy on delayed hypersensitivity and the inflammatory response. *Cancer* 1975; **35:** 1616–20.
86. Gilhus NE, Matre R. In vitro effect of ethanol on subpopulations of human blood mononuclear cells. *Int Arch Allergy Appl Immunol* 1982; **68:** 382–6.

87. Girre C, Hispard E, Therond P, Guedj S, Bourdon R, Dally S. Effect of abstinence from alcohol on the depression of glutathione peroxidase activity and selenium and vitamin E levels in chronic alcoholic patients. *Alcohol Clin Exp Res* 1990; **14:** 909–12.
88. Glasgow AH, Nimberg RB, Menzoian JO *et al.* Association of anergy with an immunosuppressive peptide fraction in the serum of patients with cancer. *N Engl J Med* 1974; **291:** 1263–7.
89. Gluckman SJ, Dvorak VC, Mac Gregor RR. Host defenses during prolonged alcohol consumption in a controlled environment. *Arch Intern Med* 1977; **137:** 1539–43.
90. Gonzalez FM, Vargas JA, Gea-Banacloche JC *et al.* Study of spontaneous cytotoxic activity in laryngeal carcinoma: prognostic value. *Acta Otorrinolaringol Esp* 1995; **46:** 431–6.
91. Gross L, Manfredi OL, Protos AA. Effect of cobalt-60 irradiation upon cell-mediated immunity. *Radiology* 1973; **106:** 653–6.
92. Guillou PJ, Sedman PC, Ramsden CW. Inhibition of lymphokine-activated killer cell generation by cultured tumour cell lines in vitro. *Cancer Immunol Immunother* 1989; **28:** 43–53.
93. Guillou PJ, Ramsden CW, Somers SS, Sedman PC. Suppression of the generation of lymphokine-activated killer (LAK) cells by serum-free supernatants of in vitro maintained tumour cell lines. *Br J Cancer* 1989; **59:** 515–21.
94. Hanna N, Fidler IJ. Role of natural killer cells in the destruction of circulating tumor emboli. *J Natl Cancer Inst* 1980; **65:** 801–9.
95. Hansbrough JF, Bender EM, Zapata-Sirvent R, Anderson J. Altered helper and suppressor lymphocyte populations in surgical patients. A measure of postoperative immunosuppression. *Am J Surg* 1984; **148:** 303–7.
96. Hillers VN, Massey LH. Interrelationships of moderate and high alcohol consumption with diet and health status. *Am J Clin Nutr* 1985; **41:** 356–62.
97. Hinds MW, Thomas DB, O'Reilly HP. Asbestos, dental X-rays, tobacco, and alcohol in the epidemiology of laryngeal cancer. *Cancer* 1979; **44:** 1114–20.
98. Hoffmann M, Kahn T, Mahnke CG, Goeroegh T, Lippert BM, Werner JA. Prevalence of human papillomavirus in squamous cell carcinoma of the head and neck determined by polymerase chain reaction and southern blot hybridization: proposal for optimized diagnostic requirements. *Acta Otolaryngol (Stockh)* 1998; **118:** 138–44.
99. Hollinshead AC, Lee O, Chretien PB, Tarpley JL, Rawls WE, Adam E. Antibodies in herpesvirus non-virion antigens in squamous carcinomas. *Science* 1973; **182:** 713–15.
100. Hori Y, Perkins EH, Halsall MK. Decline in phytohemagglutinin responsiveness of spleen cells from aging mice. *Proc Soc Exp Biol Med* 1973; **144:** 48–53.
101. Hurt RD, Higgins JA, Nelson RA, Morse RM, Dickson RE. Nutritional status of a group of alcoholics before and after admission to an alcoholism treatment unit. *Am J Clin Nutr* 1981; **34:** 386–92.
102. Inamizu T, Chang MP, Makinodan T. Influence of age on the production and regulation of interleukin-1 in mice. *Immunology* 1985; **55:** 447–55.
103. Jamieson BD, Ahmed R. T-cell tolerance: exposure to virus in utero does not cause a permanent deletion of specific T cells. *Proc Natl Acad Sci USA* 1988; **85:** 2265–8.
104. Jenison SA, Firzlaff JM, Langenberg A, Galloway DA. Identification of immunoreactive antigens of human papillomavirus type 6b by using *Escherichia coli*-expressed fusion proteins. *J Virol* 1988; **62:** 2115–23.
105. Jenkins VK, Ray P, Ellis H, Griffiths CM, Perry RR, Olson MH. Lymphocyte response in patients with head and neck cancer. Effect of clinical stage and radiotherapy. *Arch Otolaryngol* 1976; **102:** 596–600.
106. Jensen LS, Andersen AJ, Christiansen PM *et al.* Postoperative infection and natural killer cell function following blood transfusion in patients undergoing elective colorectal surgery. *Br J Surg* 1992; **79:** 513–16.
107. Jerrells TR, Smith W, Eckardt MJ. Murine model of ethanol-induced immunosuppression. *Alcoholism* 1990; **14:** 546–50.
108. Jerrells TR, Peritt D, Marietta C, Eckardt MJ. Mechanisms of suppression of cellular immunity induced by ethanol. *Alcohol Clin Exp Res* 1989; **13:** 490–3.
109. Jesse RH, Lindberg RD. The efficacy of combining radiation therapy with a surgical procedure in patients with cervical metastasis from squamous cancer of the oropharynx and hypopharynx. *Cancer* 1975; **35:** 1163–6.
110. Job G, Pfreundschuh M, Bauer M, Zum-Winkel K, Hunstein W. The influence of radiation therapy on T-lymphocyte subpopulations defined by monoclonal antibodies. *Int J Radiat Oncol Biol Phys* 1984; **10:** 2077–81.
111. Johnson R, Fowler JF, Zanelli GD. Changes in mouse blood pressure, tumor blood flow, and core and tumor temperatures following Nembutal or urethane anesthesia. *Radiology* 1976; **118:** 697–703.
112. Jubert AV, Lee ET, Hersh EM, McBride CM. Effects of surgery, anesthesia and intraoperative blood loss on immunocompetence. *J Surg Res* 1973; **15:** 399–403.
113. Kahn T, Schwarz E, zur Hausen H. Molecular cloning and characterization of the DNA of a new human papillomavirus (HPV 30) from a laryngeal carcinoma. *Int J Cancer* 1986; **37:** 61–5.
114. Kaplan DR. A novel mechanism of immunosuppression mediated by ethanol. *Cell Immunol* 1986; **102:** 1–9.
115. Kaplan J, Sarnaik S, Gitlin J, Lusher J. Diminished helper/suppressor lymphocyte ratios and natural killer cell activity in recipients of repeated blood transfusions. *Blood* 1984; **64:** 308–10.
116. Keane WM, Atkins JP Jr, Wetmore R, Vidas M. Epidemiology of head and neck cancer. *Laryngoscope* 1981; **91:** 2037–45.
117. Kelso A, Munck A. Glucocorticoid inhibition of lymphokine secretion by alloreactive T lymphocyte clones. *J Immunol* 1984; **133:** 784–91.
118. Kemp AS, Berke G. Inhibition of lymphocyte-mediated cytolysis by local anesthetics benzyl and salicyl alcohol. *Eur J Immunol* 1973; **3:** 674–7.

119. Kenefick TC. Delayed hypersensitivity skin test in head and neck cancer. *J Laryngol Otol* 1976; **90:** 935–43.
120. Kline K, Sanders BG. Modulation of immune suppression and enhanced tumorigenesis in retrovirus tumor challenged chicken treated with vitamin E. *In Vivo* 1989; **3:** 161–6.
121. Knudsen PJ, Dinarello CA, Strom TB. Glucocorticoids inhibit transcriptional and post-transcriptional expression of interleukin-1 in U937 cells. *J Immunol* 1987; **139:** 4129–34.
122. Krishnan S, Bhuyan UN, Talwar GP, Ramalingaswami V. Effect of vitamin A and protein-calorie undernutrition on immune responses. *Immunology* 1974; **27:** 383–92.
123. Kudielka IJ, Schneider A, Braun R *et al.* Antibodies against the human papillomavirus type 16 early proteins in human sera: correlation of anti-E7 reactivity with cervical cancer. *J Natl Cancer Inst* 1989; **81:** 1698–704.
124. Kulkarni AD, Fanslow WC, Drath DB, Rudolph FB, van Buren CT. Influence of dietary nucleotide restriction on bacterial sepsis and phagocytic function in mice. *Arch Surg* 1986; **121:** 169–72.
125. Kulkarni SS, Bhateley DC, Zander AR *et al.* Functional impairment of T-lymphocytes in mouse radiation chimeras by a nucleotide-free diet. *Exp Hematol* 1984; **12:** 694–9.
126. Kumari TV, Shanmugam J, Prabha B, Vasudevan DM. Prevalence of antibodies against herpes simplex and adenovirus in oral and cervical cancer patients. *Indian J Med Res* 1982; **75:** 590–2.
127. Kuppner MC, Hamou MF, Sawamura Y, Bodmer S, De Tribolet N. Inhibition of lymphocyte function by glioblastoma-derived transforming growth factor β2. *J Neurosurg* 1989; **71:** 211–17.
128. Lasek W, Plodziszewska M, Jakobisiak M. The effect of blood donation on natural killer activity in man. *J Clin Lab Immunol* 1987; **22:** 165–8.
129. Laudenslager ML, Ryan S, Drugan RC, Hyson RL, Maier SF. Coping and immunosuppression: inescapable but not escapable shock suppresses lymphocyte proliferation. *Science* 1983; **221:** 568–70.
130. Law DK, Dudrick SJ, Abdou NI. The effects of protein calorie malnutrition on immune competence of the surgical patient. *Surg Gynecol Obstet* 1974; **139:** 257–66.
131. Lee KW, Singh J, Taylor RB. Subclasses of T-cells with different sensitivities to cytotoxic antibody in the presence of anesthetics. *Eur J Immunol* 1976; **5:** 259–62.
132. Letessier EM, Sacchi M, Johnson JT, Herberman RB, Whiteside TL. The absence of lymphoid suppressor cells in tumor-involved lymph nodes of patients with head and neck cancer. *Cell Immunol* 1990; **130:** 446–58.
133. Levallois C, Mani JC, Balmes JL. Sensitivity of human lymphocytes to acetaldehyde: comparison between alcoholic and control subjects. *Drug Alcohol Depend* 1987; **20:** 135–42.
134. Levine AJ, Momand J, Finlay CA. The p53 tumour suppressor gene. *Nature* 1991; **351:** 453–6.
135. Lindahl-Magnusson P, Leary P, Gresser I. Interferon inhibits DNA synthesis induced in mouse lymphocyte suspensions by phytohaemagglutinin or by allogeneic cells. *Nature* 1972; **237:** 120–1.
136. Liu YK. Effects of alcohol on granulocytes and lymphocytes. *Semin Hematol* 1980; **17:** 130–6.
137. Luce D, Guenel P, Leclerc A, Brugere J, Point D, Rodriguez J. Alcohol and tobacco consumption in cancer of the mouth, pharynx, and larynx: a study of 316 female patients. *Laryngoscope* 1988; **98:** 313–16.
138. Lukasewycz OA, Prohaska JR, Meyer SG, Schmidtke JR, Hatfield SM, Marder P. Alterations in lymphocyte subpopulations in copper-deficient mice. *Infect Immun* 1985; **48:** 644–7.
139. Lundy J, Wanebo H, Pinsky C, Strong E, Oettgen H. Delayed hypersensitivity reactions in patients with squamous cell cancer of the head and neck. *Am J Surg* 1974; **128:** 530–3.
140. MacRae JD, Lampe H, Banerjee D. Blood transfusions and phenotypic immune profile in head and neck cancer patients undergoing surgical resection. *J Otolaryngol* 1991; **20:** 310–14.
141. MacSween RNM. Alcohol and cancer. *Br Med Bull* 1982; **38:** 31–3.
142. Maddaus MA, Wells CL, Platt JL, Condie RM, Simmons RL. Effect of T cell modulation on the translocation of bacteria from the gut and mesenteric lymph node. *Ann Surg* 1988; **207:** 387–98.
143. Maier H, Born IA, Mall G. Effect of chronic ethanol and nicotine consumption on the function and morphology of the salivary glands. *Klin Wochenschr* 1988; **66(Suppl 11):** 140–50.
144 Maier H, Born IA, Veith S, Adler D, Seitz HK. The effect of chronic ethanol consumption on salivary gland morphology and function in the rat. *Alcohol Clin Exp Res* 1986; **10:** 425–7.
145. Maitland NJ, Cox MF, Lynas C, Prime SS, Meanwell CA, Scully C. Detection of human papillomavirus DNA in biopsies of human oral tissue. *Br J Cancer* 1987; **56:** 245–50.
146. Marquet RL, Hoynck van Papenbrecht MA, Busch OR, Jeekel J. Blood donation leads to a decrease in natural killer cell activity: a study in normal blood donors and cancer patients. *Transfusion* 1993; **33:** 368–73.
147. Massague J. The transforming growth factor-beta family. *Annu Rev Cell Biol* 1990; **6:** 597–641.
148. McGregor RR. Alcohol and immune defense. *JAMA* 1986; **256:** 1474–9.
149. McLaughlin GA, Wu AV, Saporoschetz AB, Nimberg RB, Mannick JA. Correlation between anergy and a circulating immunosuppressive factor following major surgical trauma. *Ann Surg* 1979; **190:** 297–304.
150. McLean LD, Meakins JG, Tagucki K, Duignan JP, Dhillon KS, Gordon J. Host resistance in sepsis and trauma. *Ann Surg* 1975; **182:** 207–17.
151. McMichael AJ. Increases in laryngeal cancer in Britain and Australia in relation to alcohol and tobacco consumption trends. *Lancet* 1978; **1:** 1244–7.
152. McMichael AJ. Laryngeal cancer and alcohol consumption in Australia. *Med J Aust* 1979; **1:** 131–4.
153. McMurray DN, Yetley EA, Burch T. Effect of malnutrition

and BCG vaccination on macrophage activation in guinea pigs. *Nutr Res* 1981; **1:** 373–84.
154. Meagher RC, Sieber R, Spivak JL. Suppression of hematopoietic-progenitor-cell proliferation by ethanol and acetaldehyde. *N Engl J Med* 1982; **307:** 845–9.
155. Mendenhall CL, Anderson S, Weesner RE, Goldberg SJ, Crolic KA. Protein-calorie-malnutrition associated with alcoholic hepatitis. *Am J Med* 1984; **67:** 211–22.
156. Merino OR, Lindberg RD, Fletcher GH. An analysis of distant metastases from squamous cell carcinoma of the upper respiratory and digestive tracts. *Cancer* 1977; **40:** 145–51.
157. Miller LG, Goldstein G, Murphy M, Ginns LC. Reversible alterations in immunoregulatory T cells in smoking. Analysis by monoclonal antibodies and flow cytometry. *Chest* 1982; **82:** 526–9.
158. Miller RA, Stutman O. Decline, in aging mice, of the anti-2,4,6-trinitrophenyl (TNP) cytotoxic T cell response attributable to loss of Lyt 2, interleukin 2-producing helper cell function. *Eur J Immunol* 1981; **11:** 751–6.
159. Miller-Graziano CL, Szabo G, Griffey K, Mehta B, Kodys K, Catalano D. Role of elevated monocyte transforming growth factor beta (TGF-beta) production in posttrauma immunosuppression. *J Clin Immunol* 1991; **11:** 95–102.
160. Mills PR, Shenkin A, Anthony RS *et al.* Assessment of nutritional status and in vivo immune responses in alcoholic liver disease. *Am J Clin Nutr* 1983; **38:** 849–59.
161. Miyazaki S, Akiyouishi T, Arinaga S. Depression of the generation of cell-mediated cytotoxicity by suppressor cells after surgery. *Clin Exp Immunol* 1983; **54:** 573–97.
162. Mohagheghpour N, Parhami B, Dowlatshahi K, Kadjehnouri D, Elder JH, Chisari FV. Immunoregulatory properties of human esophageal tumor extract. *J Immunol* 1979; **122:** 1350–8.
163. Monfardini S, Vaccher E, Pizzocaro G *et al.* Unusual malignant tumours in 49 patients with HIV infection. *AIDS* 1989; **3:** 449–52.
164. Morgan DW, Abdullah V, Quiney R, Myint S. Human papillomavirus and carcinoma of the laryngopharynx. *J Laryngol Otol* 1991; **105:** 288–90.
165. Morgan MY, Levine JA. Alcohol and nutrition. *Proc Nutr Soc* 1988; **47:** 85–98.
166. Mørland B, Mørland J. Reduced Fc-receptor function in human monocytes exposed to ethanol in vitro. *Alcohol Alcohol* 1984; **19:** 211–17.
167. Mørland B, Mørland J. Effects of ethanol on human monocyte IgG Fc receptors. *Scand J Immunol* 1987; **26:** 187–92.
168. Moudgil GC. Effect of premedicants, intravenous anaesthetic agents and local anaesthetics on phagocytosis in vitro. *Can Anaesth Soc J* 1981; **28:** 597–602.
169. Moudgil GC. Update on anaesthesia and the immune response. *Can Anaesth Soc J* 1986; **33:** 54–60.
170. Moudgil GC, Gordon J, Forrest JB. Comparative effects of volatile anaesthetic agents and nitrous oxide on human leucocyte chemotoxins in vitro. *Can Anaesth Soc J* 1984; **31:** 631–7.
171. Mufti SI, Prabhala R, Moriguchi S, Sipes IG, Watson RR. Functional and numerical alterations induced by ethanol in the cellular immune system. *Immunopharmacology* 1988; **15:** 85–94.
172. Murasko DM, Weiner P, Nelson B, Silver R, Matour J, Kaye D. Decline in mitogen induced proliferation of lymphocytes with increasing age. *Clin Exp Immunol* 1987; **70:** 440–5.
173. Murray HW. Interferon-gamma, the activated macrophage, and the host defense against microbial challenge. *Ann Intern Med* 1988; **108:** 595–608.
174. Nakada Y, Kosaka T, Kuwabara M, Tanaka S, Sato KI, Koide F. Effects of 2-carboxythylgerumanium sesquioxide (Ge-132) as an immunological modifier of post-surgical immunosuppression in dogs. *J Vet Med Sci* 1993; **55:** 795–9.
175. Nakama S, Tanaka M, Tanaka T. Effect of halothane or pentobarbital anesthesia on blastogenesis of peripheral blood lymphocytes in dogs. *Jpn J Vet Anesth Surg* 1990; **21:** 71–7.
176. Nauss KM, Mark DA, Suskind RM. The effect of vitamin A deficiency on the in vitro cellular immune response of rats. *J Nutr* 1979; **109:** 1815–23.
177. Nielsen HE. The effect of age on the response of rat lymphocytes in mixed leukocyte culture, to PHA, and in the graft-vs.-host reaction. *J Immunol* 1974; **112:** 1194–200.
178. Nohr CW, Christou NV, Rode H, Gordon J, Meakins JL. In vivo and in vitro humero-immunity in surgical patients. *Ann Surg* 1984; **200:** 373–80.
179. Odeleye OE, Eskelson CD, Mufti SI, Watson RR. Vitamin E protection against nitrosamine-induced esophageal tumor incidence in mice immunocompromised by retroviral infection. *Carcinogenesis* 1992; **13:** 1811–16.
180. Oldstone MBA, Blount P, Southern PJ, Lampert PW. Cytoimmunotherapy for persistent virus infection reveals a unique clearance pattern from the central nervous system. *Nature* 1986; **321:** 239–43.
181. Olsen J, Sabroe S, Fasting U. Interaction of alcohol and tobacco as risk factors in cancer of the laryngeal region. *J Epidemiol Community Health* 1985; **39:** 165–8.
182. Order SE. The effects of therapeutic irradiation on lymphocytes and immunity. *Cancer* 1977; **39:** 737–43.
183. Park SK, Brody JI, Wallace HA, Blakemore WS. Immunosuppressive effect of surgery. *Lancet* 1971; **1:** 53–5.
184. Pasatiempo AMG, Taylor CE, Ross AC. Vitamin A status and the immune response to pneumococcal polysaccharide: effects of age and early stages of retinol deficiency in rats. *J Nutr* 1991; **121:** 556–62.
185. Penn I. Cancer is a complication of severe immunosuppression. *Surg Gynecol Obstet* 1986; **162:** 603–10.
186. Pérez-Ayala M, Ruiz-Cabello F, Esteban F *et al.* Presence of HPV 16 sequences in laryngeal carcinomas. *Int J Cancer* 1990; **46:** 8–11.
187. Petersen BH, Steimel LF, Callaghan JT. Suppression of mitogen-induced lymphocyte transformation in cigarette smokers. *Clin Immunol Immunopathol* 1983; **27:**135–40.
188. Phillips B, Marshall ME, Brown S, Thompson JS. Effect of smoking on human natural killer cell activity. *Cancer* 1985; **56:** 2789–92.

189. Phillips JH, Nishioka K, Babacock GF. Tuftsin-induced enhancement of murine and human natural cell-mediated cytotoxicity. *Ann NY Acad Sci* 1983; **419:** 192–204.
190. Pietsch JB, Meakins JL, MacLean LD. The delayed hypersensitivity response: application in clinical surgery. *Surgery* 1977; **82:** 349–55.
191. Posner MR, Reinherz E, Lane H, Mauch P, Hellman S, Schlossman SF. Circulating lymphocyte populations in Hodgkin's disease after mantle and paraaortic irradiation. *Blood* 1983; **61:** 705–8.
192. Proberts JC, Thompson RW, Bagshan MA. Patterns of spread of distant metastases in head and neck carcinoma. *Cancer* 1974; **33:** 127–34.
193. Prohaska JR, Lukasewycz OA. Copper deficiency suppresses the immune response of mice. *Science* 1981; **213:** 559–61.
194. Prohaska JR, Downing SW, Lukasewycz OA. Chronic dietary copper deficiency alters biochemical and morphological properties of mouse lymphoid tissues. *J Nutr* 1983; **113:** 1583–90.
195. Qazzaz ST, Mamattah JHK, Ashcroft T, McFarlane H. The development and nature of immune deficit in primates in response to malnutrition. *Br J Exp Pathol* 1981; **62:** 452–60.
196. Ranges GE, Figari IS, Espevik T, Palladino MA Jr. Inhibition of cytotoxic T cell development by transforming growth factor β and reversal by recombinant tumor necrosis factor α. *J Exp Med* 1987; **166:** 991–8.
197. Redmond HP, Shou J, Kelly CJ *et al.* Immunosuppressive mechanisms in protein-calorie malnutrition. *Surgery* 1991; **110:** 311–17.
198. Redmond HP, Leon P, Lieberman MD *et al.* Impaired macrophage function in severe protein-energy malnutrition. *Arch Surg* 1991; **126:** 192–6.
199. Remacle-Bonnet MM, Pommier GJ, Kaplanski S, Rance RJ, Depieds RC. Inhibition of normal allogenic lymphocyte mitogenesis by a soluble inhibitor extracted from human clonic carcinoma. *J Immunol* 1996; **117:** 1145–51.
200. Renoux G, Biziere K, Renoux M, Guillaumin JM. The production of T-cell-inducing factors in mice controlled by the brain neocortex. *Scand J Immunol* 1983; **17:** 45–50.
201. Rettura G, Padawer J, Barbul A, Levenson SM, Seifter E. Supplemental arginine increases thymic cellularity in normal and murine sarcoma virus-inoculated mice and increases the resistance to murine sarcoma virus tumor. *JPEN J Parenter Enteral Nutr* 1979; **3:** 409–16.
202. Rissanen A, Sarlio Lähteenkorva S, Alfthan G, Gref CG, Keso L, Salaspuro M. Employed problem drinkers: a nutritional risk group? *Am J Clin Nutr* 1987; **45:** 456–61.
203. Roth JA, Eilber FR, Morton DL. Effect of adriamycin and high-dose methotrexate chemotherapy on in vivo and in vitro cell-mediated immunity in cancer patients. *Cancer* 1978; **41:** 814–19.
204. Roth JA, Grimm EA, Gupta RK, Ames RS. Immunoregulatory factors derived from human tumors. I. Immunologic and biochemical characterization of factors that suppress lymphocyte proliferative and cytotoxic responses in vitro. *J Immunol* 1982; **128:** 1955–62.
205. Rousseau-Merck MF, Barbey S, Mouly H, Bazin S, Nezelof C. Collagenolytic activity of eosinophilic granuloma in vitro. *Experientia* 1979; **35:** 1226–8.
206. Rubin E, Lieber CS. Alcoholism, alcohol, and drugs. *Science* 1971; **172:** 1097–102.
207. Rudnick S, Stevenson GW, Hall SC, Espinoza-Delgado I, Stevenson HC, Longo D. Halothane potentiates the anti-tumor activity of gamma-interferon and mimics calmodulin blocking agents. *Anesthesiology* 1991; **74:** 115–19.
208. Saito H, Trocki O, Wang SL, Gonce SJ, Joffe SN, Alexander JW. Metabolic and immune effects of dietary arginine supplementation after burn. *Arch Surg* 1987; **122:** 784–9.
209. Salo M. Effect of anesthesia and surgery on the number of and mitogen-induced transformation of T- and B-lymphocytes. *Ann Clin Res* 1978; **10:** 1–13.
210. Schantz SP, Romsdahl MM, Babcock GF, Nishioka K, Goepfert H. The effect of surgery on natural killer cell activity in head and neck cancer patients: in vitro reversal of a postoperatively suppressed immunosurveillance system. *Laryngoscope* 1985; **95:** 588–94.
211. Schottenfeld D, Gantt RC, Wyner EL. The role of alcohol and tobacco in multiple primary cancer of the upper digestive system larynx, and lung: a prospective study. *Prev Med* 1974; **3:** 277–93.
212. Schultz JC, Shahidi NT. Inhibition of human lymphocyte reactivity by plasma fibronectin in vitro. *Transfusion* 1990; **30:** 791–8.
213. Scully C, Maitland NJ, Cox MF, Prime SS. Human papillomavirus DNA and oral mucosa. *Lancet* 1987; **1:** 336. [Letter]
214. Shapiro J, Jersky J, Katzav S, Feloman M, Segal S. Anesthetic drugs accelerate the progression of postoperative metastases of mouse tumours. *J Clin Invest* 1981; **68:** 678–87.
215. Shavit Y, Lewis J, Terman G, Gale R, Leibeskind J. Opioid peptides mediate the suppressive effect of stress on natural killer cell cytotoxicity. *Science* 1984; **224:** 188–90.
216. Shelby J, Marushack MM, Nelson EW. Prostaglandin production and suppressor cell induction in transfusion-induced immune suppression. *Transplantation* 1987; **43:** 113–16.
217. Sheldon PW, Begg AC, Fowler JF, Lansley IF. The incidence of lung metastases in C3H mice after treatment of implanted solid tumours with x-rays or surgery. *Br J Cancer* 1974; **30:** 342–8.
218. Shillitoe EJ, Greenspan D, Greenspan JS, Hansen LS, Silverman S. Neutralizing antibody to herpes simplex virus type 1 in patients with oral cancer. *Cancer* 1982; **49:** 2315–20.
219. Silverman NA, Alexander JC, Hollinshead AC, Chretien PB. Correlation of tumor burden with in vitro lymphocyte reactivity and antibodies to herpesvirus tumor-associated antigens in head and neck squamous carcinoma. *Cancer* 1976; **37:** 135–40.
220. Skinner GR. Transformation of primary hamster

embryo fibroblasts by type 2 herpes-simplex virus: evidence for a 'hit and run' mechanism. *Br J Exp Pathol* 1976; **57**: 361–76.

221. Sklar LS, Anisman H. Stress and coping factors influence tumor growth. *Science* 1979; **205**: 513–15.
222. Slade MS, Simmons RL, Yunis E, Greenberg LJ. Immunodepression after major surgery in normal patients. *Surgery* 1975; **78**: 363–72.
223. Smith MD, Williams JD, Coles GA, Salaman JR. The effects of blood transfusion on T suppressor cells in renal dialysis patients. *Transplant Proc* 1981; **13**: 181–3.
224. Smith WI Jr, Van Thiel DH, Whiteside T *et al.* Altered immunity in male patients with alcoholic liver disease: evidence for defective immune regulation. *Alcohol Clin Exp Res* 1980; **4**: 199–206.
225. Smythe PM, Brereton Stiles GG, Grace HJ *et al.* Thymolymphatic deficiency and depression of cell-mediated immunity in protein-calorie malnutrition. *Lancet* 1971; **2**: 939–46.
226. Snijders PJF, van den Brule AJC, Meijer CJLM, Walboomers JMM. Papillomaviruses and cancer of the upper digestive and respiratory tracts. *Curr Top Microbiol Immunol* 1994; **186**: 177–98.
227. Snyderman CH, Klapan I, Milanovich M *et al.* Comparison in vivo and in vitro prostaglandin E2 production by squamous cell carcinoma of the head and neck. *Otolaryngol Head Neck Surg* 1991; **111**: 189–96.
228. Southern PJ, Blount P, Oldstone MBA. Analysis of persistent virus infections by in situ hybridization to whole-mouse sections. *Nature* 1984; **312**: 555–8.
229. Stacey NH. Inhibition of antibody-dependent cell-mediated cytotoxicity by ethanol. *Immunopharmacology* 1984; **8**: 155–61.
230. Stephan RN, Kupper TS, Geha AS, Baue AS, Chaudry IH. Hemorrhage without tissue trauma produces immunosuppression and enhances susceptibility to sepsis. *Arch Surg* 1987; **122**: 62–8.
231. Stjernswärd J, Yondel M, Vanky F, Wigzell H, Sealy R. Lymphopenia and change in distribution of human B and T lymphocytes in peripheral blood induced by irradiation for mammary carcinoma. *Lancet* 1972; **1**: 1352–6.
232. Stockwell HG, Lyman GH. Impact of smoking and smokeless tobacco on the risk of cancer of the head and neck. *Head Neck Surg* 1986; **9**: 104–10.
233. Strasnick B, Lagos N, Lichtenstein A, Mickel RA. Suppression of lymphokine-activated killer cell cytotoxicity by a soluble factor produced by squamous tumors of the head and neck. *Otolaryngol Head Neck Surg* 1990; **103**: 537–49.
234. Strong MS, Vaughan CW, Kayne HL *et al.* A randomized trial of preoperative radiotherapy in cancer of the oropharynx and hypopharynx. *Am J Surg* 1978; **136**: 494–500.
235. Sugarbaker EV, Ketcham AS. Mechanisms and prevention of cancer dissemination. An overview. *Semin Oncol* 1977; **4**: 19–32.
236. Sugimura K, Ueda Y, Takeda K *et al.* A cytokine, lymphocyte blastogenesis inhibitory factor (LBIF), arrests mitogen stimulated T lymphocytes at early G1 phase with no influence on interleukin 2 production and interleukin 2 receptor light chain expression. *Eur J Immunol* 1989; **19**: 1357–64.
237. Takada A, Nei J, Takase S, Matsuda Y. Effects of ethanol on experimental hepatocarcinogenesis. *Hepatology* 1986; **6**: 65–72.
238. Tartter PI, Steinberg B, Baron DM, Martinelli G. Transfusion history, T cell subsets and natural killer cytotoxicity in patients with colorectal cancer. *Vox Sang* 1989; **56**: 80–4.
239. Tashjian AH Jr, Voelkel EF, Lazzaro M *et al.* Alpha and beta human transforming growth factors stimulate prostaglandin production and bone resorption in cultured mouse calvaria. *Proc Natl Acad Sci USA* 1985; **82**: 4535–8.
240. Telser A, Hinkley RE. Cultured neuroblastoma cells and halothane. *Anesthesiology* 1977; **46**:102–10.
241. Tennenbaum JI, Ruppert RD, Pierre RL, Greenberger NJ. The effect of chronic alcohol on the immune responsiveness of rats. *J Allergy* 1969; **44**: 272–81.
242. Thomas JW, Coy P, Lewis HS, Yuen A. Effect of therapeutic irradiation on lymphocyte transformation in lung cancer. *Cancer* 1971; **27**: 1046–50.
243. Thomson AD, Pratt OE. Interaction of nutrients and alcohol: absorption, transport, utilization and metabolism. In: Watson RR, Watzl B, eds. *Nutrition and Alcohol.* Boca Raton: CRC Press, 1992: 75–99.
244. Tishon A, Borrow P, Evans C, Oldstone MBA. Virus-induced immunosuppression. I. Age at infection relates to a selective or generalized defect. *Virology* 1993; **195**: 397–405.
245. Tisman G, Herbert VJ. In vitro myelosuppression and immunosuppression by ethanol. *J Clin Invest* 1973; **52**: 1410–14.
246. Toolan HW. Growth of human tumors in cortisone-treated laboratory animals: the possibility of obtaining permanently transplantable human tumors. *Cancer Res* 1953; **13**: 389–94.
247. Trocki O, Heyd TJ, Waymack JP, Alexander JW. Effects of fish oil on postburn metabolism and immunity. *JPEN J Parenter Enteral Nutr* 1987; **11**: 521–8.
248. Tuyns AJ. Epidemiology of alcohol and cancer. *Cancer Res* 1979; **39**: 2840–3.
249. Tuyns AJ. Alcohol. In: Schottenfeld D, Fraumeni JF, eds. *Cancer Epidemiology and Prevention.* Philadelphia: Saunders, 1982: 519–35.
250. Tuyns AJ, Esteve J, Raymond L *et al.* Cancer of the larynx/hypopharynx, tobacco and alcohol. *Int J Cancer* 1988; **41**: 483–91.
251. Van Vleet JF, Watson RR. Effects of selenium and vitamin E on resistance to infectious disease. In: Watson RR, ed. *Nutrition, Disease Resistance, and Immune Function.* New York: Dekker, 1984: 299–312.
252. Varani J, Lovett EJ III, Lundy J. A model of tumour cell dormancy: effects of anaesthesia and surgery. *J Surg Oncol* 1981; **17**: 9–14.
253. Vistainer MA, Volpicelli JR, Seligman MEP. Tumor rejection in rats after inescapable or escapable shock. *Science* 1982; **216**: 437–9.

254. Vogler WR, Lloyd JW, Milmore BK. A retrospective study of etiological factors in cancer of the mouth, pharynx and larynx. *Cancer* 1962; **15:** 246–58.
255. Von Pirquet C. Verhalten der kutanen Tuberkulinreaktion während der Masern. *Dtsch Med Wochenschr* 1908; **30:** 1297–300.
256. Wahl JS, Hunt DA, Wakefield LM *et al.* Transforming growth factor type β induces monocyte chemotaxis and growth factor production. *Proc Natl Acad Sci USA* 1987; **84:** 5788–92.
257. Wahl SM, Altman LC, Rosentreich DL. Inhibition of in vitro lymphokine synthesis by glucocorticoids. *J Immunol* 1975; **115:** 476–82.
258. Walia AS, Pruitt KM, Rodgers JD, Lamon EW. In vitro effect of ethanol on ce655. *Immunopharmacology* 1987; **13:** 11–24.
259. Wallenius K. Experimental oral cancer in the rat. With special reference to the influence of saliva. *Acta Pathol Microbiol Scand* 1966; **180(Suppl):** 1–91.
260. Walters CS, Claman HN. Age-related changes in cell-mediated immunity in BALB/c mice. *J Immunol* 1975; **115:** 1438–43.
261. Walton B. Anaesthesia, surgery and immunology. *Anaesthesia* 1978; **33:** 322–48.
262. Walton B. Effects of anaesthesia and surgery on immune status. *Br J Anaesth* 1979; **51:** 37–43.
263. Wang MB, Lichtenstein A, Mickel RA. Hierarchical immunosuppression of regional lymph nodes in patients with head and neck squamous cell carcinoma. *Otolaryngol Head Neck Surg* 1991; **105:** 517–27.
264. Watson RR. Nutrition, disease resistance, and age. *Food Nutr News* 1979; **51:** 1–4.
265. Watson RR. *Nutrition, Disease Resistance and Immune Function.* New York: Dekker, 1984.
266. Watson RR, Prabhala RH, Abril E, Smith TL. Changes in lymphocyte subsets and macrophage functions from high, short-term dietary ethanol in C57/BL6 mice. *Life Sci* 1988; **43:** 865–70.
267. Watzl B, Watson RR. Role of alcohol abuse in nutritional immunosuppression. *J Nutr* 1992; **122:** 733–7.
268. Watzl B, Watson RR. Role of nutrients in alcohol-induced immunomodulation. *Alcohol Alcohol* 1993; **28:** 89–95.
269. Waxler B, Zhang X, Wezeman FH. Anesthetic agents modify tissue proteinase inhibitor content and tumor behavior. *J Lab Clin Med* 1993; **123:** 53–8.
270. Waymack JP, Gallon L, Barcell U, Trocki O, Alexander JW. Effect of blood transfusions on immune function. III. Alterations in macrophage arachidonic acid metabolism. *Arch Surg* 1987; **122:** 56–60.
271. Waymack JP, Fernandes G, Cappelli PJ *et al.* Alterations in host defense associated with anesthesia and blood transfusions. II. Effect on response to endotoxin. *Arch Surg* 1991; **126:** 59–62.
272. Whitehead JS, Kim YS. An inhibitor of lymphocyte proliferation produced by a human colonic adenocarcinoma cell line in culture. *Cancer Res* 1980; **40:** 29–35.
273. Winick M, Noble A. Cellular response in rats during malnutrition at various ages. *J Nutr* 1966; **89:** 300–6.
274. Wolf GT, Amendola B, Diaz RE *et al.* Definite vs. adjuvant radiotherapy. Comparative effects on lymphocyte subpopulations in patients with head and neck squamous carcinoma. *Arch Otolaryngol* 1985; **111:** 716–26.
275. Wustrow TPU. *Zellbiologische und immunologische Untersuchungen des Plattenepithel-karzinoms im Kopf-Halsbereich.* Habilitationsschrift Ludwig-Maximilians-Universität München.
276. Wustrow TPU. Antigenspezifische Antikörperbildung zur Bestimmung der Immunreaktion von Patienten mit Kopf-Halskarzinomen. *Laryngorhinootologie* 1989; **68:** 169–80.
277. Wustrow TPU. Antigen-specific plaque formation of cultured mononuclear cells in head and neck cancer. *Acta Otolaryngol (Stockh)* 1991; **111:** 420–7.
278. Wustrow TPU. Verminderte antigenspezifische B-Zell-Antwort bei Rauchern und Trinkern. *Otorhinolaryngol Nova* 1991; **1:** 173–81.
279. Wustrow TPU, Zenner HP. Natural killer (NK) cell activity in patients with carcinoma of the larynx and hypopharynx. *Laryngoscope* 1985; **95:** 1391–400.
280. Wustrow TPU, Denny T, Fernandes G, Good RA. Changes in macrophages and their functions with aging in C57Bl/6J, AKR/J and SJL/J mice. *Cell Immunol* 1982; **69:** 227–34.
281. Wynder EL, Bross IJ, Day E. A study of environmental factors in cancer of the larynx. *Cancer* 1956; **9:** 86–110.
282. Wynder EL, Bross IJ, Feldmann RM. A study of the etiological factors in cancer of the mouth. *Cancer* 1957; **10:** 1300–23.
283. Wynder EL, Covey LS, Mabuchi K, Mushinski M. Environmental factors in cancer of the larynx. *Cancer* 1976; **38:** 1591–601.
284. Yamazaki K, Maiz A, Moldawer LL, Bistrian BR, Blackburn GL. Complications associated with the overfeeding of infected animals. *J Surg Res* 1986; **40:** 152–8.
285. Yokota M, Ito N, Hatake K, Yane K, Miyahara H, Matsunaga T. Aberrant glycosylation based on the neo-expression of poly-*N*-acetyllactosamine structures in squamous cell carcinomas of the head and neck. *Histochem J* 1997; **29:** 555–62.
286. Zhou DH, Munster A, Winchurch RA. Pathologic concentrations of interleukin 6 inhibit T cell responses via induction of activation of TGF-beta. *FASEB J* 1991; **5:** 2582–5.
287. Zur Hausen H. Papillomaviruses in anogenital cancer as a model to understand the role of viruses in human cancers. *Cancer Res* 1989; **49:** 4677–81.

Specific immunologic aspects of laryngeal cancer

William J Richtsmeier

There are two major questions to be addressed in this chapter in addition to what we collectively know about squamous cell carcinoma of the upper aerodigestive tract. The first question is whether there is a comprehensive understanding of the immunology of laryngeal cancer. The second question is whether laryngeal cancer is different than other cancers of the upper aerodigestive tract.

The answer to the first question is that we do not have comprehensive understanding of cancer immunology at the time of this writing. There is a great deal we do know about cancer in general, but there is still much to be learned about head and neck cancer. What is presented here is a collective 'work in progress'.

All cancers, especially squamous cell carcinoma of the head and neck, are extremely complex both in their physiologic characteristics, which distinguish the malignant phenotype from other normal epithelial activities, and in their molecular biology. The discussion of laryngeal cancer in this chapter will review what we know about the body's response to cancer of the larynx. Woven into the dialogue is what we know about the biology of head and neck cancer in general and it will also discuss aspects of other human cancers and experimental cancers which help explain our current understanding, attempting to put laryngeal cancer in a proper perspective. Aspects of natural immunity[30] and immunology reflected by immunostaining of lymphocyte populations and pathologic analysis are reviewed elsewhere.[7,25]

Laryngeal cancer is different from other cancers of the head and neck in survival rates stage for stage. However, I feel that this is largely explained by the early recognition of laryngeal cancers due to the symptoms they cause on speech and swallowing. The staging system for laryngeal cancer for the most part involves function, which is different from all the other anatomic sites in the upper aerodigestive tract where staging is fundamentally a size criterion. In this discussion I specifically refer to upper aerodigestive tract cancers which are smoking related. Therefore, nasopharyngeal carcinoma, carcinoma of the paranasal sinuses, skin cancers and nonsquamous cancers of the pharyngoesophagus may very well have a different biology. Although there are many significant parallels, cancer of the larynx, I believe, is not fundamentally different in biology from cancer of the oral cavity, oropharynx, or hypopharynx. Nasopharyngeal cancer is an exception to the lower pharynx and larynx. Cancer of the larynx also begins in an organ that is particularly well defined both in its ability to help diagnose it at an early stage and for the limited lymphoid tissue that accompanies it. A carcinoma of the tonsil or a carcinoma of the tongue base may be thought of as being N1 when it first becomes an invasive cancer since the malignant squamous tissue is engulfed by a sea of lymphoid tissue immediately adjacent to it. It is therefore a primary failure of the immune system to respond to it, whereas, laryngeal cancer truly becomes N1 when the metastases occur in the neck. Another explanation for the relative high survival rates of laryngeal cancer compared to other upper aerodigestive tract cancers has to do with ease with which oncologic procedures are understood by all surgeons. A laryngectomy is a straightforward operation understood relatively easily by everyone, whereas one person's composite resection or tongue base resection may well be quite different from that of another surgeon.

Squamous cell carcinoma of the head and neck is a tumor where immunosuppression has been observed for many years. Is there evidence that the immune system can control cancers? There are several indirect types of

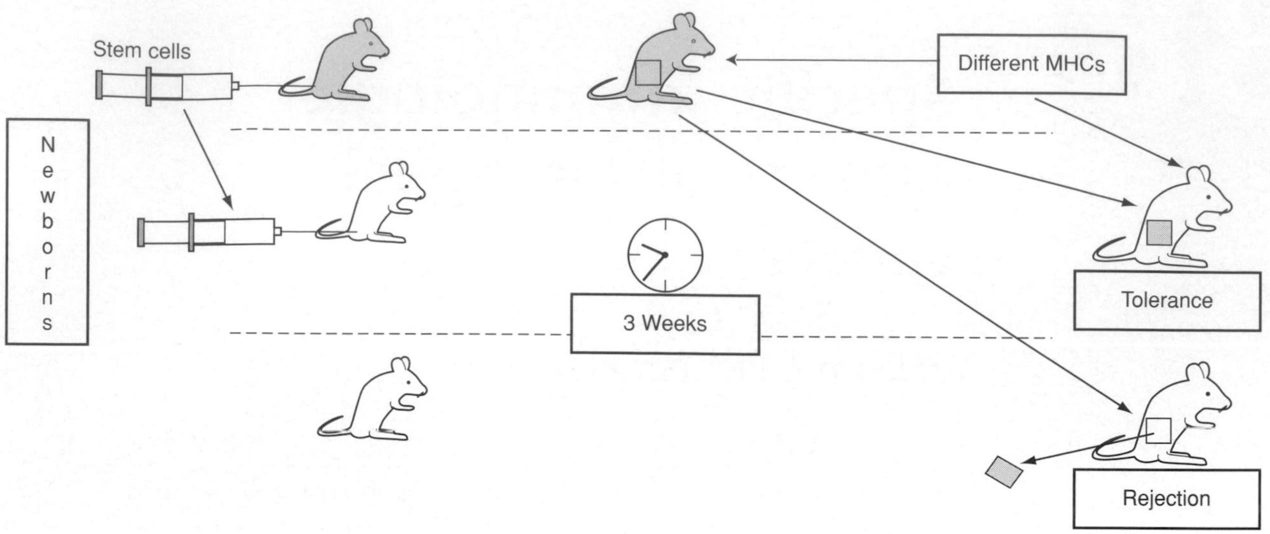

Figure 38.1 *Metawar's original experiments. In this diagram the stem cells from the dark mouse are injected into mice that are immunologically distinct as diagrammed by being a different shade. Three weeks later, mice who received stem cells can receive skin grafts from the dark mice without a rejection phenomenon. Litter mates from the same white mice will reject the darker skin grafts.*

observations that suggest that it does. First, we commonly see patients who have had a presumptive regression of a primary cancer because they present with a regional lymph node with no detectable primary. Second, there are rare cases of spontaneous tumor regression usually in the face of infection. Unfortunately, this author has seen only one documented case of spontaneous regression of head and neck squamous cell carcinoma (which occurred in the setting of a local infection). Third, there are observations of other cancers that seem to regress in the face of immune reactions. Malignant melanoma is one such cancer. Another cancer closer to squamous cell carcinoma is keratoacanthoma. Patel *et al.*[23] feel that keratoacanthoma is a squamous cell carcinoma in regression as demonstrated by increased IL-2 receptors, increased infiltrating CD4+ T-lymphocytes and increased adhesion molecules. Whether this perspective is true or not, the immune activity observed in keratoacanthoma is what one would expect to exist in the immune control of cancer.

There are reports of small series of patients who have responded to cytokine therapy, indicating that restoration of the immune system may be beneficial in the therapy of larynx cancer.[11,12,27] As yet there is no controlled series showing significant benefit.

Laryngeal-associated immunosuppression

In the 1960s, systemic immunosuppression in the form of failure to respond to delayed hypersensitivity skin testing was identified in a head and neck cancer patient by a number of authors. This fundamental cell-mediated immunity depression appeared to persist as the cancers were unsuccessfully treated, and remain as the single most powerful biologic predictors of successful therapeutic outcome. How can larynx cancer contribute to systemic immunosuppression? To understand this we need to look at the basics of the immune response.

Our original observations on the immune response go back to the pretransplant era where immunologically different animals (dizygotic twins) who shared a common placenta could tolerate grafts of entire organs well after the neonatal period. It is presumed that these animals shared blood cells *in utero* via a common placenta circulation. Therefore, tolerance was thought to be induced during this period of *in utero* exposure.

To investigate this neonatal tolerance further, experiments were performed in immunologically distinct mice (mice with different major histocompatibility antigens) to test this theory. Stem cells removed from one distinct group of mice were injected into newborn mice of a separate species. Litter mates of the recipient mice would reject a skin graft from the first group of mice after maturing for 3 weeks (Fig 38.1). By contrast, mice that received stem cell injections in the newborn period would become tolerant to and accept skin grafts from the donor mice. It was presumed that maturation of the immune system occurred during the 3-week period. Subsequent experiments indicated that T-lymphocytes matured in the thymus as a critical event in the acquisition of immune competence. These concepts dominated our thinking for 40 years.

Investigations into neonatal tolerance and immune maturation were revisited by Matzinger and colleagues[8,19,20] in an experiment where they could utilize the unique antigen which occurs only on the outside of male cells of mice in an inbred strain. Other than this male, Hy antigen, all the mice were immunologically

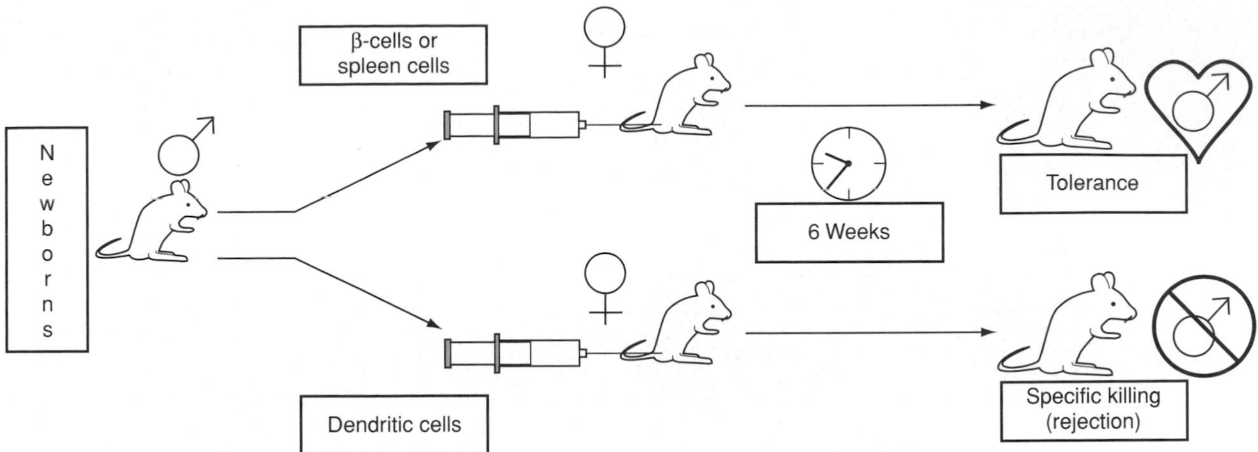

Figure 38.2 *Experiments by Matzinger reveal that dendritic cells are the key cells conferring immune rejection and B-cells confer tolerance. In his experiments a specific male antigen (Hy), not present on female mice, is the only difference between the animals even though female mice for diagrammatic purposes are shown to be darker in color than the white male mice. They are otherwise immunologically exactly the same. Dendritic cells from the male mice are injected into the female mice. After 6 weeks, specific killing of male antigen cells is measured. The dendritic cells confer specific male killing, whereas B-cells or spleen cells, containing large numbers of B-cells, confer tolerance.*

identical. This antigen allowed extremely specific control of experiments in cell-mediated immunity and cellular killing. In their experiments, purified cells from donor mice expressing the male antigen were injected into recipient female mice in control animals who received no injection as newborns. Mean specific male cell killing rates were induced in the 40–60% range in control, 'mature' animals. These measures are made by removing cells from female mice older than 6 weeks and testing their ability to kill cells from the male mice. Even though we would see experimentally that injection of spleen cells could induce tolerance, injection of purified professional antigen-processing cells such as dendritic cells on day 1 induced specific male killing rates of 40% – the same as those induced in adults. By contrast, when mice were induced with B-cells, they developed no specific male killing even when they were again primed as adults. In mice that received dendritic cells in day 1 and then B-cells on day 7, they developed essentially the same amount of specific killing seen with dendritic cells alone. A diagram of this experiment is presented in Fig 38.2, underscoring the fundamental difference between the B-cells and dendritic cells. From this experiment and a series of others, it appears that dendritic cells are the fundamental antigen-presenting cells in the newborn period.[28]

Dendritic cells

Dendritic cells have been shown to be the critical antigen-processing cells in mature individuals. They are of bone marrow macrophage/monocyte origin and their biology is reviewed.[18,19,21] Dendritic cells lack the monocyte differentiation marker CD14 but express many adhesion molecules which can be intensified by culture with GM-CSF. They express class II MHC molecules constitutively as well as class I. Dendritic cells are found in every tissue but they have been given different names in various tissues such as Langerhans cells in skin or veiled cells in lymph, where the dendritic cells may differentiate slightly. They are active in head and neck tissues.[26] How certain subsets of dendritic cells get to and differentiate in tissues is still an area of investigation. The interaction of dendritic cells and T-cells is discussed later.

The roll of dendritic cells in the response to tumors has been investigated by some authors.[9] Isolated tumor antigens can be selectively exposed to dendritic cells. In such experiments, tumor-peptide pulsed dendritic cells from control animals stimulated T-cells effectively but dendritic cells from tumor-bearing animals that were tumor-peptide pulsed could not. Although the exact mechanism of dendritic cell failure in these tumors is not known, the dendritic cell dysfunction in mice infected with the retrovirus, Rauscher leukemia virus, is due to downregulation of class II MHC.[10] The similarities between retroviral infections and squamous cell carcinoma is discussed below in the context of the retroviral substance p15E.

With the interest in dendritic cells as playing a central role in the immune response to tumors, ways of using them in adoptive immunotherapy has become of great interest. The induction of tumor immunity using dendritic cells derived from peripheral blood has been described by several laboratories[1,13,24] but there are no reports as yet investigating laryngeal cancer. Part of the reason for this is that head and neck squamous cell carcinoma has the disadvantage of not having a unique surface antigen available to stimulate dendritic cells.

Other immunologic observations would extend the concept that dendritic cells are the professional

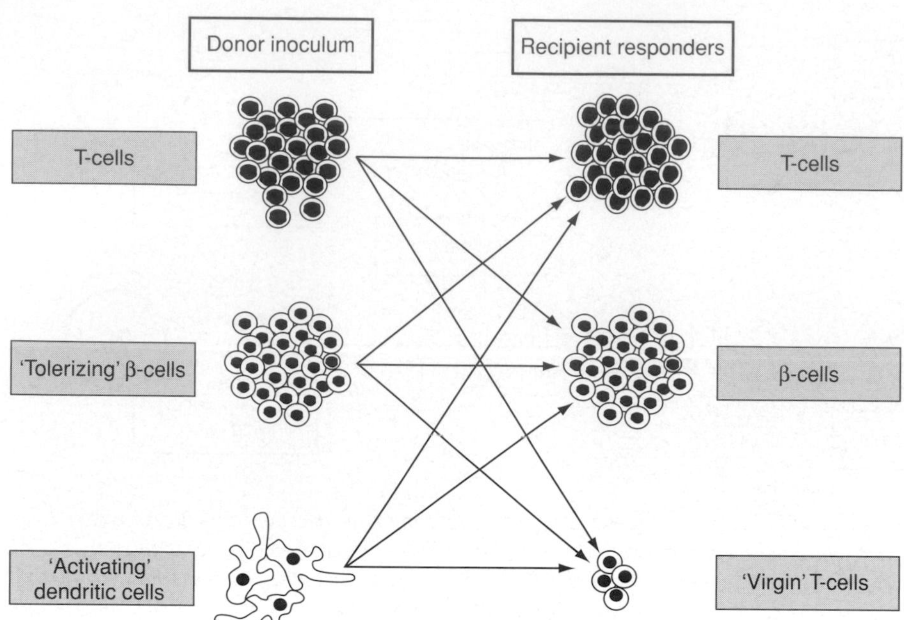

Figure 38.3 *The possible immunologic interactions between donor inoculum cells in recipient responder cells. The experiment reveals that it is much more likely that T-cells or tolerizing B-cells from the donor will interact with the T- and B-cells of the recipient mice, more than the few donor 'activating' dendritic cells. Only the virgin T-cells, which are also relatively low in number, can respond to the dendritic cells. The high incidence of tolerizing B-cells is much more likely to come in contact with the virgin T-cells. Under circumstances where dendritic cells are not concentrated, the newborn inoculum of white blood cells is more likely to be tolerizing than to be immunologically activating.*

antigen-presenting cell regardless of age. B-cells, on the other hand, can induce tolerance at virtually any age, identifying a fundamental difference in the immune system as to which cell processes the antigen. The type of encounter that occurs can be seen in Fig 38.3 where the donor inoculum cells seen on the left have a smaller or larger chance of coming in contact with the virgin T-cell, which is the only cell that can respond to a new antigen and create a new immunologic reaction. T-cells that come in contact with the antigen must have previously counted this antigen to produce any significant response and, therefore, do not participate in most of the response. B-cells, which are in relative abundance, particularly in the newborn period, when they come in contact with a virgin T-cell will cause that T-cell to become tolerant. The relatively uncommon dendritic cells in the normal inoculum of spleen cells are much more likely to encounter a T-cell or B-cell rather than a virgin T-cell to induce the response which would be measured in the above experiment. This would explain the experiments where stem cells that were injected most likely included large amounts of the tolerizing B-cells and few, if any, dendritic cells.

Danger signals

In these immunologic experiments it is important to understand that the dendritic cell itself does not have any innate ability to select the antigen which it is presenting. In these experiments with inbred mice, the antigen being presented is a self-antigen made in its own ribosomes and expressed partially by chance in combination with the class II major histocompatibility antigen. Figure 38.4 demonstrates the mechanisms involved in the interaction between the dendritic cell and the T-cell. On the right side of the dendritic cell, the antigen can be seen being either pinocytosed at the cell membrane as shown in number 1, manufactured inside the cell as an internal antigen as shown in number 2, or synthesized to be expressed on the surface of the cells shown in number 3. Male Hy antigen is the type shown in 3 and is the antigen used in the experiments by Matzinger.[19] To be involved in the immune response, the antigen must be expressed in conjunction with the major histocompatibility antigen as the first signal to the T-cell. To activate the T-cell, a second signal must occur. In mice this occurs between the CD28-B7.1 (or the CD28-B7.2) complex. This second signal is apparently inducible and requires the dendritic cell to sense some problem or potential danger. The activation of the second signal by the third 'danger' signal gives us the perspective that if the first signal (i.e. the antigen MH2 complex) is presented in the absence of signal 2, the T-cell will either die or go back to an inactive state and no reaction to that antigen will occur. Therefore, normal antigens that are expressed on the surface of cells in the absence of a danger signal simply never have the immune system activated. This mechanism would dictate that normal internal antigens and normal cell surface antigens are never identified as immunogenic.

Matzinger's perspective is that the danger signal is primarily conveyed by reactions to infection, primarily those expressed in the heat shock proteins. Heat shock proteins can then activate message 2 and antigens that are caught on the surface in conjunction with MHC complex will initiate some T-cell reaction. The relative abundance of reaction to that antigen will be a statistical problem but the type of reactivity is primarily run by the inducibility of signal 2. It is Matzinger's contention (and those who have gone before her) that the primary activating force of the immune system is infection. Since the common result of infection is fever, most circumstances of the immune system would appear to work quite well; at least with

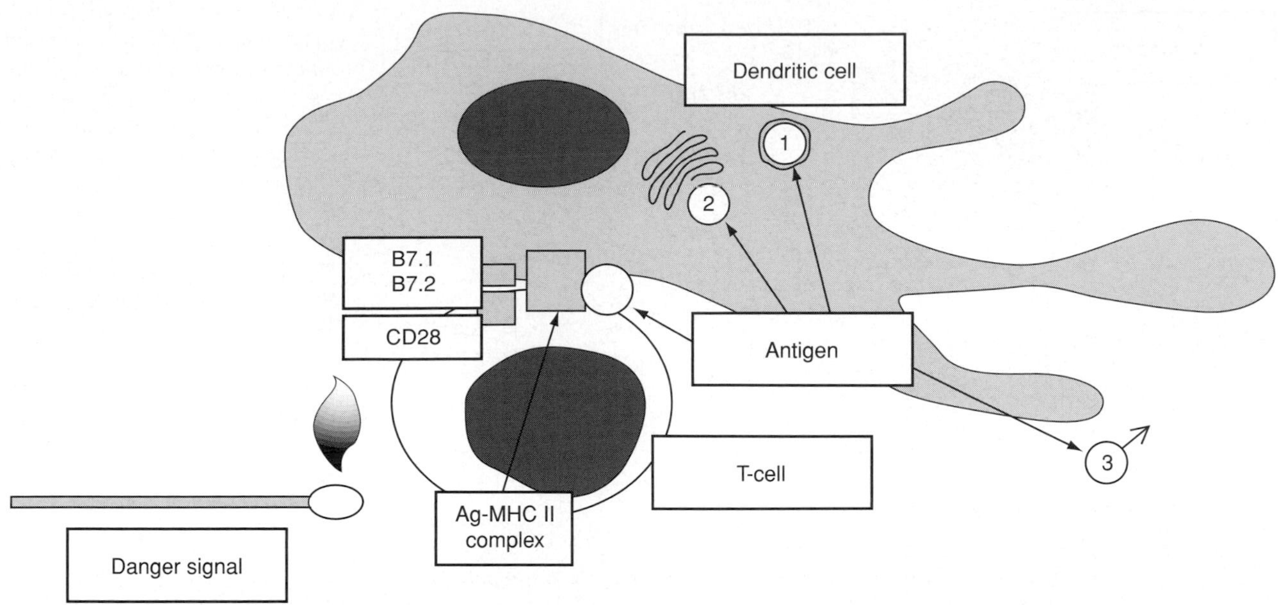

Figure 38.4 *The mechanisms of activation of the dendritic cells are shown as it interacts with a T-cell. In this circumstance the antigen, which can be acquired from a variety of mechanisms, is eventually expressed with the MHC complex. To form a response, the B7.1 or B7.2 CD28 complex must combine for the T-cells to see it as an important response. Activation of this complex requires some type of 'danger signal' seen by the dendritic cells. Danger signals include primarily heat shock protein, but also TNFα or exposure to one of the superantigens such as staphylococcal enterotoxin.*

regard to cell-mediated immunity. Under normal circumstances the immune system is as much at risk of overreacting to itself as it is to not identifying a true danger. Unfortunately, cancer rarely induces a danger signal in its early stages and when a long enough period of antigen exposure without a danger signal is endured, then tolerance is induced.

B-cells which can commonly encounter an antigen cannot express signal 2 and therefore can never induce a new response in a virgin T-cell. They can, however, reactivate memory T-cells that have already been induced by a dendritic cell and their ability to concentrate antigens through expression of antibodies on their surface makes them extremely efficient in this manner.

Cellular interactions causing immunosuppression

Another question regarding immunity in the newborn system was addressed by Sarzotti *et al.*[29] In this series of experiments they looked at the cytotoxic T-lymphocyte (CTL) response to a retrovirus. They vaccinated mice in the newborn period in various doses and found that high dose inocula of 10 virus doses per mouse or above induced virtually no cytotoxicity, whereas virus doses which are small, such as one virus per mouse or less, induce substantial amounts of cytotoxicity. During these responses, they also measured IL-4 and interferon-γ. In responding, mice with low inoculum had high interferon-γ sera titers similar to those seen in immune responses in the adult. Conversely, newborns induced with high inoculum had low interferon-γ titer and high IL-4 titers. The observation is that wherever IL-4 was high, interferon-γ was low and vice versa. This experiment leaves confirmation of two types of responses for the immune system. Type 1 occurs with relatively low antigen exposure in the newborn. It produces effective CTL and induces interferon-γ, IL-2, and TNF-α. Type II, which occurs at high antigen exposure in the newborn, induces tolerance or serologic type response, and produces IL-4, IL-5 and IL-10. IL-10 has been shown to have an effect on dendritic cells.

One question is, how can tumors escape detection by the immune system or in fact induce tolerance? Figure 38.5 shows mechanisms by which this can occur. At the top of the diagram, it is shown in different human cell cultures that tumor cells can produce IL-10, causing dendritic cells to become less responsive to express antigens or virgin T-cells.[14] Similarly, a retroviral antigen p15E has been shown to be expressed by squamous cell carcinoma of the head and neck.[2–6] This protein has been shown to adversely affect dendritic cells similar to the effect of IL-10.[15]

Tumor products causing immunosuppression

The activation of the second signal was studied in an experimental system in mice: the experiments of molecule CTLA-4, which is a normal expressed molecule that has a higher affinity for B7.1 or B7.2 than does the normal CD28 complementary molecule on the T-cell. Free CTLA-4 then combines and covers up the second message. Leach *et al.*[12a] utilized antibody to CTLA-4 to induce significant

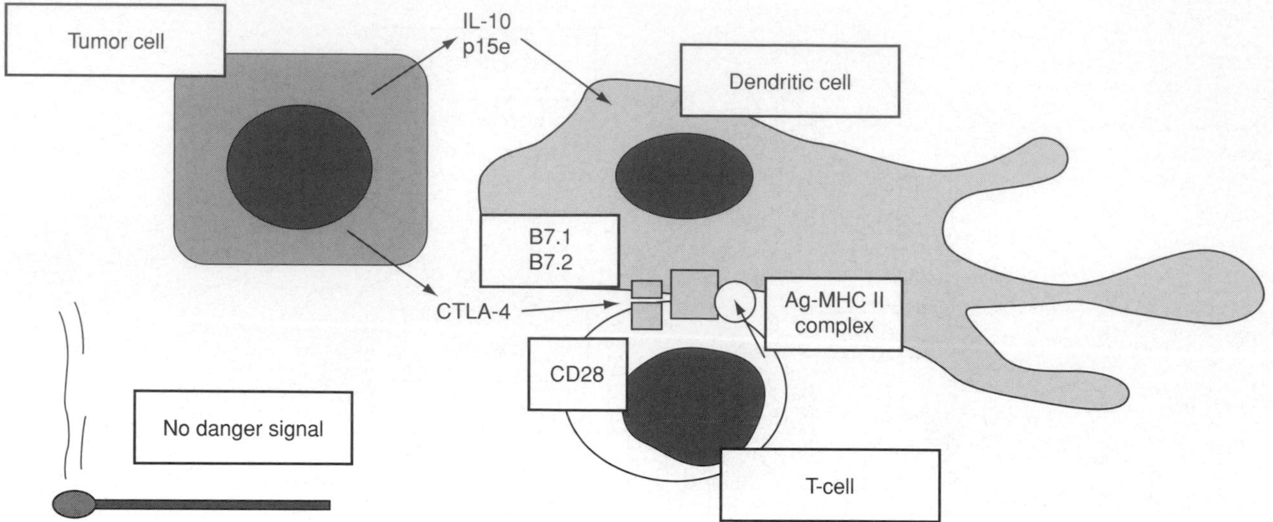

Figure 38.5 *The dendritic cell–T-cell response is inactivated by tumor cells through several methods. First, the tumor cell may make substances such as IL-10 or p15E, both of which inhibit dendritic cell function. Tumor cells may make a molecule that binds to the CD28 complex more tightly than B7.1 or B7.2. Lastly, tumor cells for the most part fail to initiate the immune response by not releasing heat shock protein, in contrast to that usually released by infection.*

depression of tumor growth in both mouse carcinomas and sarcomas known to produce CTLA-4. Other mechanisms for turning off the second signal or editing the activation of it by inhibiting the danger signal may also be a strategy used by larynx cancer but is yet to be investigated.

Another mechanism of tumor-induced immunosuppression observed in head and neck squamous cell carcinoma is the production of a substance similar to p15E, a retroviral membrane protein.[4] This substance described by Nelson *et al.*[22] has been shown to have significant areas of homology with proteins produced by tumors.[30,31] P15E causes a number of immunosuppressive activities, including the inhibition of macrophage migration, dendritic cell function and lymphocyte proliferation. P15E also has homology with important immune mediators such as IFN-α and TGF-β. This agent has been identified in head and neck squamous cell carcinoma using immunohistochemical techniques.[32] The cross-reaction of the antibodies made against p15E with tumor-produced products is an interesting observation. In the retrovirus infection situation, treatment with antibodies to p15E inhibits virus-transformed tumor growth in mice using the Rauscher virus transformed myeloid cell line RMB-1.[16,17] In this system, the tumor cells express the antigen on the surface of the cells and antibodies can interact with intact cells and free immunosuppressive material. The most active tumor growth suppressing antibodies are those demonstrating cell surface identification of p15E-like material. Research in our laboratories indicates that cell lines derived from human squamous cell carcinoma do not express the antigen homologous to p15E on the cell surface even though they do make it as detected by FACS analysis and it can be detected in the region of naturally occurring squamous cell carcinomas.

Wustrow and Mahnke[33] review external causes of immunosuppression such as alcohol, tobacco, malnutrition, viruses and age. They also review research of other authors who have demonstrated that other molecules produced by squamous cell carcinoma can be immunosuppressive, such as prostaglandin. These molecules are listed in Table 38.1.

Table 38.1 Potential agents of squamous cell carcinoma associated immunosuppression

Agent	*Mechanism*
Histamine	H2-receptor-mediated activation of T-suppression cells
Prostaglandin	Inhibition of LAK cell generation
p15E (and similar proteins)	Inhibition of dendritic cell and macrophage function and leukocyte proliferation
IL-10	Dendritic cell and macrophage inhibition
TNF-α	Cachexia
IFN-α, IL-1	Tachyphylaxis
Circulating Ag–Ab complexes	Arthus reaction
IgA antitumor antibodies	No Fc inflammation initiation
Dendritic cell tolerance	Dendritic cell ratios
EBV-B cell clones	Constitutive cytokine production, B-cell suppression
Anti CD40-Abs	TNF receptor family activation of dendritic cells

Conclusions

In summary, laryngeal cancer is perceived by this author as being similar to other head and neck squamous cell carcinomas in many ways. The primary immune response to such cancers requires a series of events involving dendritic cells, which can be interrupted by the host or the tumor. It is critical that the host sees tumor antigens in the context of a setting similar to an infection. It is possible to present antigens to dendritic cells to augment the response to tumors. Currently there is no proven immune therapy that can replace standard therapy.

References

1. Celluzzi CM, Mayordomo JI, Storkus WJ, Lotze MT, Falo LD Jr. Peptide-pulsed dendritic cells induce antigen-specific, CTL-mediated protective tumor immunity. *J Exp Med* 1996; **183:** 283–7.
2. Cianciolo GJ. Antiinflammatory proteins associated with human and murine neoplasms. *Biochim Biophys Acta* 1986; **865:** 69–82.
3. Cianciolo GJ, Phipps D, Snyderman R. Human malignant and mitogen-transformed cells contain retroviral p15E-related antigen. *J Exp Med* 1984; **159:** 964–9.
4. Cianciolo GJ, Copeland TD, Oroszlan S, Snyderman R. Inhibition of lymphocyte proliferation by a synthetic peptide homologous to retroviral envelope proteins. *Science* 1985; **230:** 453–5.
5. Cianciolo GJ, Lostrom ME, Tam M, Snyderman R. Murine malignant cells synthesize a 19,000-dalton protein that is physicochemically and antigenically related to the immunosuppressive retroviral protein, p15E. *J Exp Med* 1983; **158:** 885–900.
6. Cianciolo GJ, Hunter J, Silva J, Haskill JS, Snyderman R. Inhibitors of monocyte responses to chemotaxins are present in human cancerous effusions and react with monoclonal antibodies to the p15E structural protein of retroviruses. *J Clin Invest* 1981; **68:** 831–44.
7. Cortesina G, Sacchi M, Galeazzi E, De Stefani A. Immunology of head and neck cancer: perspectives. *Head Neck* 1993; **15:** 74–7.
8. Fuchs EJ, Matzinger P. Is cancer dangerous to the immune system? *Immunology* 1996; **8:** 271–80.
9. Gabrilovich DI, Ciernik IF, Carbone DP. Dendritic cells in antitumor immune responses. *Cell Immunol* 1996; **170:** 101–10.
10. Gabrilovich DI, Patterson S, Timofeev AV, Harvey JJ, Knight SC. Mechanism of dendritic cell dysfunction in retroviral infection of mice. *Clin Immunol Immunopathol* 1996; **80:** 139–46.
11. Hadden JW. Immunology of squamous cell carcinoma of the aerodigestive tract and the prospects for immunotherapy. *Int J Immunother* 1995; **11:** 1–14.
12. Hadden JW, Endicott J, Baekey P, Skipper P, Hadden EM. Interleukins and contrasuppression induce immune regression of head and neck cancer. *Arch Otolaryngol Head Neck Surg* 1994; **120:** 395–403.

12a. Hurwitz AA, Yu TF, Leach DR, Allison JP. CTLA-4 blockade synergises with tumor-derived granulocyte-macrophage colony-stimulating factor for treatment of an experimental mammary carcinoma. *Proc Natl Acad Sci USA* 1998; **95:** 10067–71.

13. Inaba K, Inaba M, Romani N *et al.* Generation of large numbers of dendritic cells from mouse bone marrow cultures supplemented with granulocyte/macrophage colony-stimulating factor. *J Exp Med* 1992; **176:** 1693–702.
14. Kim J, Modlin RL, Moy RL *et al.* IL-10 production in cutaneous basal and squamous cell carcinomas. *J Immunol* 1995; **155:** 2240–7.
15. Kleinerman ES, Lachman LB, Knowles RD, Snyderman R, Cianciolo GJ. A synthetic peptide homologous to the envelope proteins of retroviruses inhibits monocyte-mediated killing by inactivating interleukin 1. *J Immunol* 1987; **139:** 2329–37.
16. Lang MS, Hovvenkamp E, Savelkoul HFJ, Knegt P, van Ewijk W. Immunotherapy with monoclonal antibodies directed against the immunosuppressive domain of p15E inhibits tumor growth. *Clin Exp Immunol* 1995; **102:** 468–75.
17. Lang MS, Oostendorp RAJ, Simons PJ, Boersma W, Knegt P, van Ewijk W. New monoclonal antibodies against the putative immunosuppressive site of retroviral p15E. *Cancer Res* 1994; **54:** 1831–6.
18. Massard G, Tongio MM, Wihlm JM, Morand G. The dendritic cell lineage: a ubiquitous antigen-presenting organization. *Ann Thorac Surg* 1996; **61:** 252–8.
19. Matzinger P. Tolerance, danger, and the extended family. *Annu Rev Immunol* 1994; **12:** 991–1045.
20. Matzinger P. Immunology. Memories are made of this? *Nature* 1994; **269:** 605–6.
21. McWilliam AS, Nelson DJ, Holt PG. The biology of airway dendritic cells. *Immunol Cell Biol* 1995; **73:** 405–13.
22. Nelson M, Nelson DS, Cianciolo GJ, Snyderman R. Effects of CKS-17, a synthetic retroviral envelope peptide, on cell-mediated immunity in vivo: immunosuppression, immunogenicity, and relation to immunosuppressive tumor products. *Cancer Immunol Immunother* 1989; **30:** 113–18.
23. Patel A, Halliday GM, Cooke BE, Barnetson RSC. Evidence that regression in keratoacanthoma is immunologically mediated: a comparison with squamous cell carcinoma. *Br J Dermatol* 1994; **131:** 789–98.
24. Porgador A, Snyder D, Gilboa E. Induction of antitumor immunity using bone marrow-generated dendritic cells. *J Immunol* 1996; **156:** 2918–26.
25. Richtsmeier WJ. Immunology of head and neck cancer. *Bull Am Coll Surg* 1997; **82:** 32–7.
26. Richtsmeier WJ, Bowers WE, Ellsworth CA, Sorge K, Berkovitz M. Dendritic cell identification in head and neck lymphoid tissue. Newly recognized cells control T-lymphocyte functions. *Arch Otolaryngol* 1984; **110:** 701–6.
27. Richtsmeier WJ, Koch WM, McGuire WP, Poole ME, Chang EH. Phase I–II study of advanced head and neck squamous cell carcinoma patients treated with recombinant human interferon gamma. *Arch Otolaryngol Head Neck Surg* 1990; **116:** 1271–7.
28. Ridge JP, Fuchs EJ, Matzinger P. Neonatal tolerance revisited: turning on newborn T cells with dendritic cells. *Science* 1996; **271:** 1723–6.

29. Sarzotti M, Robbins DS, Hoffman PM. Induction of protective CTL responses in newborn mice by a murine retrovirus. *Science* 1996; **271**: 1726–8.
30. Schantz SP, Brown BW, Lira E, Taylor DL, Beddingfield N. Evidence for the role of natural immunity in the control of metastatic spread of head and neck cancer. *Cancer Immunol Immunother* 1987; **25**: 141–5.
31. Scheeren RA, Oostendorp RAJ, van der Baan S, Keehnen RMJ, Scheper RJ, Meijer CJLM. Distribution of retroviral p15E-related proteins in neoplastic and non-neoplastic human tissues, and their role in the regulation of the immune response. *Clin Exp Immunol* 1992; **89**: 94–9.
32. Simons PJ, Oostendorp RAJ, Tas MPR, Drexhage HA. Comparison of retroviral p15E-related factors and interferon-α in head and neck cancer. *Cancer Immunol Immunother* 1994; **38**: 178–84.
33. Wustrow TPU, Mahnke CG. Causes of immunosuppression in squamous cell carcinoma of the head and neck. *Anticancer Res* 1996; **16**: 2433–68.

Molecular biology of laryngeal cancer

Thomas E Carey and Carol R Bradford

Laryngeal cancer can be treated successfully in a decreasing proportion of cases, depending on the location and extent of the tumor at the time of diagnosis. For stage I carcinomas, most series report 5-year survival figures of 90%, regardless of whether surgery or radiation treats the tumor. The proportion of cases cured by standard treatment modalities, either alone or in combination, drops off to roughly 70% of stage II, 50% of stage III and 30–40% of stage IV carcinomas. Another way of looking at these same figures is that at each stage there is a fraction of tumors that are refractory to standard therapy. These might be tumors that have spread beyond the margin of resection in the case of surgery or that are resistant to radiation. If we could identify at the time of diagnosis those tumors that are radiation resistant, these might be more successfully treated by surgical resection or might be candidates for combined chemotherapy and radiation or even genetic therapy to increase their susceptibility to radiation. Similarly, if we could predict from genetic changes those tumors most likely to have spread from the primary site, then we would know that cure is unlikely by surgery alone and adjunctive therapy must be added. We envision in the near future that all tumors will be screened for genetic markers as part of the diagnostic workup and that the genetic profile that determines the biologic behavior of each tumor will be used to select the most effective treatment. Treatments will specifically target those genetic changes or make use of the most effective existing treatment based on the probability of susceptibility or resistance.

There are approximately 11 000 new cases of laryngeal cancer per year in the USA, representing just over 1% of all new cancer diagnoses. National Cancer Institute statistics indicate that cancer of the larynx causes 0.82% of all cancer deaths in the USA. Thus, the incidence of death is almost as high as the incidence rate in spite of the deceptive 5-year survival rates for early-stage disease. The incidence of laryngeal carcinoma in men and women in the USA increased significantly from 1947 to 1984. In men, the incidence has increased from 5.6 to 9.0 per 100 000 population and in women, from 0.5 to 1.5 per 100 000 population. Rates of larynx cancer are even higher in other parts of the world. Furthermore, the conventional treatments that combine laryngectomy and radiation therapy are associated with profound functional morbidity affecting communication, taste, smell, swallowing, cosmesis, intimacy and overall quality of life. Many laryngectomees suffer isolation and withdraw from society. The poor cure rates and morbidity of treatment demonstrate the need for a better understanding of the molecular biology that determines individual tumor behavior and frustrates the best efforts of the physician.

The optimal treatment of cancer should preserve the best possible function of the tissues. It should not cripple or disfigure the patient or destroy his or her quality of life. It should also be balanced so that sufficient therapy is given to cure the disease without causing unnecessary morbidity. However, the desire to avoid morbidity must not result in undertreatment, nor should it ignore the probability of systemic disease that must also be controlled. In the case of advanced laryngeal cancer, total laryngectomy in combination with radiation therapy is still the most effective therapy for advanced disease. However, this radical surgical approach is now being rivaled by organ-sparing procedures consisting of combined chemotherapy and radiation that can be used even on tumors thought too large to be adequately treated by radiation alone. However, even this advance has yet to prove itself superior to conventional therapy except in the area of quality of life. Thus it is clear that we need to understand the molecular basis for tumor behavior and to make use of the knowledge to selectively destroy tumor cells by the most effective means.

Identifying molecular markers of disease progression

The molecular basis for malignant behavior of laryngeal cancers is still being defined. Nevertheless, we do have substantial knowledge of genetic molecular changes that specifically arise in this tumor type and we are beginning to make progress toward using this information to more effectively treat tumors. In this chapter we will not attempt to be exhaustive, but rather to touch on a few important discoveries that may have therapeutic relevance in the near future.

There are several common methods of identifying molecular genetic markers in human tumors. These are the following:

- Cytogenetic characterization is used to identify large consistent chromosome changes that are in some cases associated with changes in gene expression, either overexpression of a gene or loss of expression through mutation and chromosome loss. Conventional cytogenetic analysis is now being supplemented by fluorescence *in situ* hybridization (FISH) analysis wherein a fluorescently labeled DNA probe is hybridized either to a chromosome spread or even the nucleus of a tumor cell to detect changes in gene copy number or chromosome number. Comparative genomic hybridization is also used to investigate regions of genetic gain and loss. The latter is accomplished by isolating DNA from the tumor cells, labeling it with a fluorescent dye and then mixing it with normal DNA labeled with a different colored dye and hybridizing the mixture to normal chromosomes. If the tumor DNA is red and the normal is green, then areas of gain in the tumor will stain red on the target chromosomes and areas of loss in the tumor will stain green on the target chromosomes.
- Loss of heterozygosity studies can detect small regions of chromosome loss by use of highly polymorphic markers that differ on individual chromosomes. Thus, if the markers at any particular locus differ in the normal tissue from an individual (for many markers the probability of heterozygosity is 60–80%), then absence of one of the markers in that patient's tumor can be readily determined by polymerase chain reaction (PCR) amplification of normal and tumor DNA. Loss of heterozygosity is generally considered to mark areas where an inactivated tumor suppressor gene might be found.
- Immunohistology studies are used to search for overexpression or absence of gene products that are known to be involved in cell proliferation or loss of cell cycle control.

Often these methods are used in combination to good success. We will illustrate examples in the next sections of this chapter.

Chromosome alterations identify genes altered in tumor cells

In the leukemias and lymphomas, cytogenetic changes tend to be relatively simple, consistent for each leukemic subtype, and directly associated with the behavior of the tumor. Most leukemias have balanced rearrangements and at the breakpoint two genes are often brought into proximity, resulting in the expression of a fusion protein or up-regulation of a protein that regulates cell growth. A few examples follow. The first identified product of a chromosome translocation is the up-regulated expression of the c-*myc* protein in Burkitt lymphomas that is the result of translocation between one of the active immunoglobulin genes on chromosome 14, 22 or 2 and c-*myc* on chromosome 8. In this case the active promoter region of the immunoglobulin genes drives c-*myc* expression and this increases cell proliferation. A second example is the fusion protein that is the product of the Philadelphia chromosome (Ph′) tumor-specific chromosome translocation. This is found in chronic myelogenous leukemias. The Ph′ rearrangement is a t(9;22) translocation that results in a fusion protein encoded by sequences from both chromosomes. The fusion protein is an activated *bcr-abl* kinase. This deregulates the activity of the c-*abl* encoded kinase, leading to inappropriate phosphorylation of substrates and activation of growth control pathways. In follicular lymphomas a t(14;18) translocation activates the *bcl-2* gene on chromosome 18. Bcl-2 is an anti-apoptotic protein that prevents cells from undergoing programmed cell death. These cytogenetic changes are so specific that they are used to classify the leukemias and to determine the most appropriate treatment. Sometimes the treatment is directly related to the genetic change. Such an example is the t(15;17) translocation in promyelomonocytic leukemia that results in aberrant behavior of the retinoic acid receptor. This leukemia responds to treatment with retinoic acid. Similarly, in tumors with amplified expression of *bcl-2*, transfection with *bcl-*x_S, a gene that encodes a pro-apoptotic protein in the *bcl-2* family, results in increased sensitivity to chemotherapeutic agents or radiation.[45] Thus, although the genetic changes in the solid tumors are more complicated, it is very likely that characterization of the genetic changes in these tumors will identify target genes that will determine response to therapy in larynx cancer.

From chromosome aberration to altered gene to improved therapy

Working in head and neck tumors, including larynx cancers, we and others have identified a panel of consistent chromosome changes that are related to specific molecular changes in gene expression. For example, loss of the short arm of chromosome 9 is one of the most common consistent chromosome changes in head and neck cancers occurring in approximately 70% of all tumors of this type.[47,48,50] It is also an early event found in tumors with only minimal rearrangements and in high frequency in preinvasive head and neck tumors.[47] Continuing analysis has demonstrated that this genetic change results in loss of one copy of a gene cluster at 9p21 that involves the p16 gene, the p15 gene[34,38,47] and p19ARF, an alternatively spliced gene from the same region. The p16 gene (so-called because it encodes a protein of 16 kDa) had already been identified as a gene called MTS1 for multiple tumor suppressor gene-1 because it was inactivated in a large proportion of tumor types. p16 protein was soon identified as one of the cyclin-dependent kinase inhibitors. It was first called INK4 (inhibitor of kinase 4), later CDKN2 (cyclin-dependent kinase inhibitor 2), and more recently CKI2 (cyclin kinase inhibitor 2). This protein forms a complex with cyclin D1 (or cyclin E) and the appropriate cyclin-dependent kinase (CDK4 or CDK6), thereby blocking activation of the kinase. The CDKs become activated by binding to cyclins and then can phosphorylate other proteins allowing cells to progress through the cell cycle. For example, activation of CDK4 by cyclin D1 results in phosphorylation of the retinoblastoma protein, Rb, which then releases the transcription factor E2F. E2F binds to promoter elements in DNA and activates expression of proteins such as DNA polymerase delta (also known as PCNA – proliferating cell nuclear antigen) that are required for entry into the cell cycle. Thus the loss of p16 CKI2 in head and neck tumors results in increased likelihood of entry into and passage through the cell cycle.

Another example of a consistent chromosome change that is associated with loss of cell cycle control is amplification of the long arm of chromosome 11.[22,42,48] In an elegant series of experiments beginning with chromosome analysis, Akervall *et al.*[2,4,5] showed that rearrangement of chromosome 11q was associated with poor survival in head and neck cancers and then went on to demonstrate the predictive value of this for therapy. Typically, such tumors in their hospital are treated by radiotherapy with salvage surgery for failure or a combination of surgery and radiation that is planned in advance. Previously, cyclin D1 (CCND1) had been mapped to 11q13 and it seemed likely that this was a candidate gene possibly responsible for the aggressive nature of tumors with rearrangements of this region. Using antibodies specific for cyclin D1 Akervall and coworkers showed amplified expression of the protein in tumors with 11q rearrangements.[5] Then to confirm the association of CCND1 amplification they used FISH and showed that in some tumors with amplified expression there were multiple copies of the gene.[3] What is perhaps the most interesting aspect of this study is the translational portion. They examined the status of 11q in a small series of patients who were treated with chemotherapy. In spite of the poor survival associated with 11q abnormalities in patients given standard therapy, in the group treated with chemotherapy, those with 11q defects had the best response to therapy, suggesting that genetic markers might be useful in selecting patients for one or another treatment.[2] Clearly this is an area for active research. Other investigators have used immunohistochemistry to detect overexpression of cyclin D and have confirmed the poor prognosis associated with this molecular event. However, based on the very preliminary findings of the Akervall group with chemotherapy, and with what is known about the function of cyclin D1 in allowing cells to progress through the cell cycle, overexpression of cyclin D1 may result in higher growth fraction and greater susceptibility to chemotherapy. By contrast, tumors with this molecular change may be more likely to escape from local therapies of radiation and surgery. Thus, using molecular genetics, it may be possible to identify prognostic indicators that portend poor outcome when treated with one therapy, but the same marker may be a predictive factor for response to a different therapy.

In the molecular genetic studies in our own laboratory we observed that loss of chromosome 18q is a common genetic change in head and neck tumors, including larynx cancers.[18,24,48] Furthermore, we noted that this was more common in our series which was biased toward more advanced tumors, but was uncommon in reports from laboratories studying very early tumors.[1,32] This suggested that 18q loss might be a change associated with tumor progression and therefore may be a marker of biologically advanced disease if found in an early-stage tumor. In fact, we noted that of all patients whose tumors were examined for 18q loss, those with loss had decreased survival relative to those whose tumors showed no loss.[24] To pursue this question further, Pearlstein *et al.*[35] examined a series of stage III patients for loss of heterozygosity on distal 18q. In multivariant analysis it was shown that 18q loss was statistically significantly associated with reduced survival and that this was independent of stage, site and nodal status. Frank *et al.*[18] then examined a series of tumor cell lines derived from primary tumors and recurrent or metastatic tumors in the same patients and found that 18q loss developed with progression in many cases. We hypothesize that 18q harbors a tumor suppressor gene that when both copies are inactivated allows more aggressive tumor growth, invasion or spread. Our current studies are focused on determining the minimal region of loss to find the locus of this gene and to determine how it affects tumor behavior. In the meantime we are attempting to determine if loss of 18q, like overexpression of cyclin D1, can be used to identify patients at risk of more aggressive disease than their tumor stage would suggest. If so, can this information be used to improve outcome by selecting such patients for aggressive systemic therapy?

p53 regulates cell cycle and apoptosis

The p53 gene is one of the most commonly mutated genes in cancers induced by carcinogens. This gene product was first discovered as a protein that could be coprecipitated by antibodies against the SV-40 viral-transforming T-antigen. Subsequently, p53 was shown to be overexpressed in many cancer cells and it was thought to be an oncogene product or growth factor that drove tumor cell growth. However, when the gene was cloned and sequenced it was determined that the p53 sequence in most tumor cells was different from that in normal cells, indicating that the tumors contained mutant p53. Similarly, loss of heterozygosity studies showed that one chromosome copy containing the locus of p53 was often lost in tumor cells. This suggested that p53 was a tumor suppressor gene, like the retinoblastoma gene which had a similar pattern of loss of one copy of the gene and an inactivating mutation in the other copy. Eventually it was deduced that p53 was a negative regulator of the cell cycle and that transfection and overexpression of wild-type p53 could cause cells with mutant p53 to die or become sensitive to chemotherapy or radiation. It was also found that the mutant forms of p53 protein lack the proper conformation for recognition by proteins that regulate the rapid degradation of p53 in normal cells. Thus most cases of overexpressed p53 in tumors are cases in which p53 is mutated. Further study of p53 demonstrated that it has multiple important functions in regulating the cell cycle such as signaling cells to arrest at the G1 and G2 checkpoints in the cell cycle, as well as to signal cells to undergo programmed cell death. It contains a DNA binding domain and can act as a transcription factor, regulating the expression of several other proteins including the cyclin-dependent kinase inhibitors. In fact, up-regulation of the cyclin-dependent kinase inhibitor p21 is regulated by p53 and is necessary for cell cycle arrest at the G1/S border of the cell cycle. This checkpoint is critical since it prevents cells from replicating DNA until the DNA has been checked for correct base pairing and sequence. This checkpoint is also critical for DNA repair to occur. p53 also controls programmed cell death or apoptosis by up-regulating expression of pro-apoptotic proteins, thus it can signal the cell to die if extensive DNA damage is present. In fact, p53 expression is up-regulated by DNA damaging agents such as radiation and chemical carcinogens. Because of these important roles in regulating the cell cycle and regulating cell death and DNA repair after damage it is a critical protein in maintaining the integrity of the genome in each cell.

Gene therapy with p53 in head and neck cancer

As introduced in the preceding section, p53 plays an important role in the maintenance of genomic integrity through the induction of either cell growth arrest or apoptosis following exposure to DNA-damaging agents. The p53-dependent G1/S checkpoint allows the cell to repair damaged DNA before DNA synthesis. In addition to inducing increased DNA repair time, recent findings suggest that p53 also participates in DNA repair processes. If DNA repair fails, p53 may induce programmed cell death or apoptosis by effects on the Bcl-2 family of proteins.[19,28,31] However, wild-type p53 function is abrogated by mutations in a wide variety of human malignancies, including laryngeal squamous cell carcinoma (HNSCC).[8,52] In fact, p53 mutations are associated with rapid tumor cell proliferation, highly malignant behavior and poor prognosis.[6,8,25,33]

However, recent findings suggest that this poor prognostic factor can be turned to a therapeutic advantage. The growth of HNSCC can be suppressed by the introduction of a wild-type p53 gene via a recombinant adenovirus *in vitro* and in nude mice.[26] This effect is in part the result of induction of apoptosis in cells expressing the wild-type p53 gene.[27] Clayman *et al.*[13] have applied this strategy to preclinical models by using adenovirus-mediated transfer of the p53 gene into SCC cell lines and tumors in nude mice and have shown dramatic tumor regression. In fact there are several clinical protocols that are based on the concept that p53 can be a therapeutic agent. One currently in progress uses infection of HNSCC tumors with an adenovirus vector that causes expression of wild-type p53. Another relies on the inability of cells with mutant p53 to resist infection with adenovirus such that only mutant tumor cells will be killed by the viral infection. These are significant and exciting examples of the application of therapy based on molecular genetics for treating SCC tumors.

p53 is an important component of apoptosis pathways induced by anticancer agents.[30,46] It may well be that the best use of expressing p53 in tumors will be in combination with other therapeutic agents. Exciting recent studies[11,36,37,51] have demonstrated that p53 can be delivered specifically to tumor cells after systemic administration using targeting liposomes coated with transferrin which binds to the transferrin receptor that is overexpressed on many tumor cells.[51] This vector induces high-level expression of p53 and sensitizes the tumor cells to the cytotoxic effects of either chemotherapy or radiation.[11,37] Of greatest interest is the demonstration that this strategy can be used to target lung metastases and presumably also micrometastases in other tissues.[36]

Alterations in the apoptotic pathway and response to therapy

The treatment and response of locally advanced laryngeal cancer with chemotherapy or radiation is limited by the emergence of resistant cancer cells. The molecular mechanisms responsible for this resistance are partly understood although many aspects remain largely unknown. Alterations in the pathways of apoptosis involving the p53 and *bcl-2* family of genes are becoming better understood.[19,31] Apoptosis, or programmed cell death, is a normal physiologic process by which cellular life span is controlled and certain cells are programmed for elimination. It is a major mechanism for preserving homeostatic balance between cell birth and death in a given cell population. Many anticancer drugs kill cancer cells primarily by inducing apoptosis.[16,17,21,39,43] Resistance to chemotherapy has been associated with decreased susceptibility to apoptosis.[14] Like p53, the *bcl-2* gene products have an important role in the programmed cell death pathway.[17] The *bcl-2* gene, located on chromosome 18q21, encodes an integral membrane protein of 25 kDa. *bcl-2* has been shown to inhibit cell death after chemotherapy and radiation,[12] and overexpression of Bcl-2 can confer resistance to various chemotherapeutic agents.[15,20,23,29,40] The p53 protein can regulate apoptosis by down-regulating Bcl-2 expression and stimulating expression of *bax*, a gene which encodes a dominant-inhibitor of the Bcl-2 protein. In fact it is becoming clear that induction of apoptosis or inhibition of apoptosis is regulated by the ratio of pro-apoptotic proteins such as Bax, Bad and others to the anti-apoptotic proteins Bcl-2, and Bcl-x_L.[41] Interestingly, alternative splicing of the *bcl-x* gene results in two *bcl-x*-derived mRNA species, which encode either an anti-apoptotic protein called Bcl-x_L[41] or a pro-apoptotic protein called Bcl-x_S.[7,45] The Bcl-x_L protein protects cancer cells from p53-mediated apoptosis. Bcl-x_S functions as a dominant negative inhibitor of both Bcl-x_L and Bcl-2 and as a promoter of apoptosis.[45,53]

Bcl-x_L and Bcl-2 may provide differential protection from apoptosis induced by the DNA-damaging agents, γ-irradiation and cisplatin according to studies performed by Simonian *et al.*[43] Ionizing radiation and cisplatin, two agents used in the treatment of head and neck cancer, induce apoptosis in all phases of the cell cycle by causing nonspecific DNA damage. Dose response and time course experiments revealed that Bcl-x_L and Bcl-2 provided similar protection at each dose of γ-irradiation. Bcl-x_L, however, conferred increased survival compared to Bcl-2 when the cells were treated with cisplatin. A recent study of 121 head and neck tumors from patients undergoing curative therapy revealed that tumors with mutated p53 were twice as likely to recur locally after radiation.[25] Thus, both p53 and the Bcl-2 family may have important effects in determining the response to therapy in head and neck cancer.

Predicting response to therapy from molecular markers in larynx cancer

Bradford *et al.*[9] have studied the expression of p53, PCNA and other markers including the Bcl-2 family of proteins in tissue specimens obtained from the largest prospectively randomized controlled multi-institutional trial of larynx cancer comparing surgery and radiation to chemotherapy and radiation, the so-called VA larynx cancer trial.[49] This trial was designed to determine if chemotherapy and radiation could be used to preserve the larynx in patients with advanced laryngeal cancer. In fact the survival was equivalent in both arms. Thus, the combination of chemotherapy and radiation resulted in saving of the larynx in a significant proportion of cases.[44,49] However, it was clear from this trial that not all tumors respond to chemotherapy or radiation and those individuals ended up with laryngectomy. Similarly, some patients treated with surgery and radiation failed to be rendered disease free.[49] An important question we asked was whether there are molecular markers that could be used to predict which form of therapy would be most effective for an individual patient's tumor.

Surprisingly the first finding from the studies by Bradford *et al.*[9] were counter-intuitive. The patients whose tumors overexpressed p53, and presumably contained mutant p53, were more likely to preserve their larynx on the chemotherapy arm. This is in contrast to the observation that tumors with p53 mutation are less susceptible to radiation.[25] This provoked us to perform further investigation and we found that laryngeal tumor cell lines with mutant p53 are more sensitive to cisplatin than are cell lines with wild-type p53 (S Zhu *et al.*, unpublished data). Similarly, experiments on cell lines, selected for resistance to multiple rounds of exposure to cisplatin, demonstrated that the mutant p53 populations were killed by cisplatin and only wild-type p53-containing cells survived (D Trask *et al.*, unpublished data). These observations are now being confirmed by sequencing of the p53 gene in the laryngeal tumors previously tested for p53 expression. As the immunohistology experiments suggested, those tumors with wild-type p53 are far less likely to respond to cisplatin and those patients are also less likely to preserve their larynges after combined therapy (S Zhu *et al.*, unpublished data). We have observed that *bcl-x_L* is more likely than *bcl-2* to be overexpressed in head and neck tumors. Furthermore, it appears that this gene product is also associated with reduced organ preservation. Our preliminary data in laryngeal tumors show that of those with overexpression of *bcl-x_L*, the majority (13/16) failed to respond to combined chemoradiation, whereas 10/11 with low *bcl-x_L* did respond with larynx preservation (C R Bradford *et al.*, unpublished data).

In summary, our results indicate that examination of gene expression and mutational status of appropriate genes may predict the response of individual tumors to therapy. These results also strongly suggest that the tumor cells that are sensitive to radiation and to chemotherapy are different. The majority of published work indicates that tumors with mutant p53 are more likely to be resistant to radiation and many thought that because cisplatin is considered to be radiomimetic, tumors with mutant p53 would also be resistant to cisplatin. Our data suggest instead that these tumor cells are the most sensitive to cisplatin and that this finding predicts a synergy between chemotherapy with cisplatin-based regimens and radiation since each will kill a different tumor cell population. Reports in the literature support this position. Transfection of a mutant p53 gene into a cisplatin-resistant ovarian cell line conferred significantly increased sensitivity to cisplatin.[10] The challenge before us now is to translate the growing body of knowledge on the *in vivo* and *in vitro* biology of chemotherapy and radiation sensitivity into clinically meaningful strategies for organ preservation and cure.

References

1. Ah-See KW, Cooke TG, Pickford IR, Soutar D, Balmain A. An allelotype of squamous carcinoma of the head and neck using microsatellite markers. *Cancer Res* 1994; **54:** 1617–21.
2. Akervall JA, Brun E, Michalides R, Dictor MR, Balm A, Wennerberg JP. Overexpression of cyclin D1 correlates with response to neoadjuvant treatment with cisplatin and 5-fluorouracil in squamous cell carcinoma of the head and neck. In: Akervall J. *Prognostic Factors in Squamous Cell Carcinoma of the Head and Neck with Emphasis on 11q13 Rearrangements and Cyclin D1 Overexpression.* Thesis, University of Lund, 1998: 83–91.
3. Akervall JA, Borg A, Dictor MR *et al.* Multiple genetic mechanisms are involved in overexpression of cyclin D1 in squamous cell carcinoma of the head and neck. In: Akervall J. *Prognostic Factors in Squamous Cell Carcinoma of the Head and Neck with Emphasis on 11q13 Rearrangements and Cyclin D1 Overexpression.* Thesis, University of Lund, 1998: 93–103.
4. Akervall JA, Jin Y, Wennerberg JP *et al.* Chromosomal abnormalities involving 11q13 are associated with poor prognosis in patients with squamous cell carcinoma of the head and neck. *Cancer* 1995; **76:** 853–9.
5. Akervall JA, Michalides RJ, Mineta H *et al.* Amplification of cyclin D1 in squamous cell carcinoma of the head and neck and the prognostic value of chromosomal abnormalities and cyclin D1 overexpression. *Cancer* 1997; **79:** 380–9.
6. Atula S, Kurvinen K, Grénman R, Syrjänen S. SSCP pattern indicative for p53 mutation is related to advanced stage and high-grade of tongue cancer. *Eur J Cancer B Oral Oncol* 1996; **32B:** 222–9.
7. Boise LH, Gonzáles-García M, Postema CE *et al. bcl-x*, a *bcl-2*-related gene that functions as a dominant regulator of apoptotic cell death. *Cell* 1993; **74:** 597–608.
8. Bradford CR, Zhu S, Poore J *et al.* p53 mutation as a prognostic marker in advanced laryngeal carcinoma. Department of Veterans Affairs Laryngeal Cancer Cooperative Study Group. *Arch Otolaryngol Head Neck Surg* 1997; **123:** 605–9.
9. Bradford CR, Zhu S, Wolf GT *et al.* Overexpression of p53 predicts organ preservation using induction chemotherapy and radiation in patients with advanced laryngeal cancer. Department of Veterans Affairs Laryngeal Cancer Study Group. *Otolaryngol Head Neck Surg* 1995; **113:** 408–12.
10. Brown R, Clugston C, Burns P *et al.* Increased accumulation of p53 protein in cisplatin-resistant ovarian cell lines. *Int J Cancer* 1993; **55:** 678–84.
11. Chang EH, Jang Y-J, Hao Z *et al.* Restoration of the G1 checkpoint and the apoptotic pathway mediated by wild-type p53 sensitizes squamous cell carcinoma of the head and neck to radiotherapy. *Arch Otolaryngol Head Neck Surg* 1997; **123:** 507–12.
12. Chiou SK, Rao L, White E. Bcl-2 blocks p53-dependent apoptosis. *Mol Cell Biol* 1994; **14:** 2556–63.
13. Clayman GL, El-Naggar AK, Roth JA *et al.* In vivo molecular therapy with p53 adenovirus for microscopic residual head and neck squamous carcinoma. *Cancer Res* 1995; **55:** 1–6.
14. Dive C, Hickman JA. Drug-target interactions: only the first step in the commitment to programmed cell death. *Br J Cancer* 1991; **64:** 192–6.
15. Dole M, Nuñez G, Merchant AK *et al.* Bcl-2 inhibits chemotherapy-induced apoptosis in neuroblastoma. *Cancer Res* 1994; **54:** 3253–9.
16. Eastman A. Activation of programmed cell death by anticancer agents: cisplatin as a model system. *Cancer Cells* 1990; **2:** 275–80.
17. Fisher DE. Apoptosis in cancer therapy: crossing the threshold. *Cell* 1994; **78:** 539–42.
18. Frank CJ, McClatchey KD, Devaney KO, Carey TE. Evidence that loss of chromosome 18q is associated with tumor progression. *Cancer Res* 1997; **57:** 824–7.
19. Haldar S, Negrini M, Monne M, Sabbioni S, Croce CM. Down-regulation of *bcl-2* by p53 in breast cancer cells. *Cancer Res* 1994; **54:** 2095–7.
20. Herod JJO, Eliopoulos AG, Warwick J, Niedobitek G, Young LS, Kerr DJ. The prognostic significance of *bcl-2* and p53 expression in ovarian carcinoma. *Cancer Res* 1996; **56:** 2178–84.
21. Hickman JA. Apoptosis induced by anticancer drugs. *Cancer Metastasis Rev* 1992; **11:** 121–39.
22. Jin Y, Mertens F, Mandahl N *et al.* Chromosome abnormalities in eighty-three head and neck squamous cell carcinomas: influence of culture conditions on karyotypic pattern. *Cancer Res* 1993; **53:** 2140–6.
23. Kamesaki S, Kamesaki H, Jorgensen T, Tanizawa A, Pommier Y, Cossman J. Bcl-2 protein inhibits etoposide-induced apoptosis through its effects on events subsequent to topoisomerase II-induced DNA strand breaks and their repair. *Cancer Res* 1993; **53:** 4251–6.
24. Kelker W, Van Dyke DL, Worsham MJ *et al.* Loss of 18q and homozygosity for the DCC locus: possible markers for clinically aggressive squamous cell carcinoma. *Anticancer Res* 1996; **16:** 2365–72.
25. Koch WM, Brennan JA, Zahurak M *et al.* p53 mutation and locoregional treatment failure in head and neck squamous cell carcinoma. *J Natl Cancer Inst* 1996; **88:** 1580–6.
26. Liu TJ, Zhang WW, Taylor DL, Roth JA, Goepfert H, Clayman GL. Growth suppression of human head and neck cancer cells by the introduction of a wild-type p53 gene via a recombinant adenovirus. *Cancer Res* 1994; **54:** 3662–7.
27. Liu TJ, El-Naggar AK, McDonnell TJ *et al.* Apoptosis induction mediated by wild-type p53 adenoviral gene

transfer in squamous cell carcinoma of the head and neck. *Cancer Res* 1995; **55:** 3117–22.

28. Lotem J, Sachs L. Hematopoietic cells from mice deficient in wild-type p53 are more resistant to induction of apoptosis by some agents. *Blood* 1993; **82:** 1092–6.
29. Lotem J, Sachs L. Regulation of *bcl-2*, c-*myc*, and *p53* of susceptibility to induction of apoptosis by heat shock and cancer chemotherapy compounds in differentiation-competent and -defective myeloid leukemia cells. *Cell Growth Differ* 1993; **4:** 41–7.
30. Lowe SW, Ruley H, Jacks T, Housman DE. p53-dependent apoptosis modulates the cytotoxicity of anticancer agents. *Cell* 1993; **74:** 957–67.
31. Miyashita T, Krajewski S, Krajewska M *et al.* Tumor suppressor p53 is a regulator of *bcl-2* and *bax* gene expression *in vitro* and *in vivo*. *Oncogene* 1994; **9:** 1799–805.
32. Nawroz H, van der Riet P, Hruban RH, Koch W, Ruppert JM, Sidransky D. Allelotype of head and neck squamous cell carcinoma. *Cancer Res* 1994; **54:** 1152–5.
33. Nylander K, Nilsson P, Mehle C, Roos G. *p53* mutations, protein expression and cell proliferation in squamous cell carcinomas of the head and neck. *Br J Cancer* 1995; **71:** 826–30.
34. Papadimitrakopoulou V, Izzo J, Lippman SM *et al.* Frequent inactivation of *p16INK4a* in oral premalignant lesions. *Oncogene* 1997; **14:** 1799–803.
35. Pearlstein RP, Benninger MS, Carey TE *et al.* Loss of 18q predicts poor survival of patients with squamous cell carcinoma of the head and neck. *Genes Chromosomes Cancer* 1998; **21:** 333–9.
36. Pirollo KF, Xu L, Tang WH, Chang EH. Systemically delivered, tumor-targeted wt*p53* gene therapy in combination with radiation results in tumor regression. *Proc Am Assoc Cancer Res* 1999; **40:** A1318, 203.
37. Pirollo KF, Hao ZM, Rait A *et al.* *p53* mediated sensitization of squamous cell carcinoma of the head and neck to radiotherapy. *Oncogene* 1997; **14:** 1735–46.
38. Reed AL, Califano J, Cairns P *et al.* High frequency of *p16 (CDKN2/MTS-1/INK4A)* inactivation in head and neck squamous cell carcinoma. *Cancer Res* 1996; **56:** 3630–3.
39. Reed JC. Bcl-2 and the regulation of programmed cell death. *J Cell Biol* 1994; **124:** 1–6.
40. Reed JC. Regulation of chemoresistance by the bcl-2 oncoprotein in non-Hodgkin's lymphoma and lymphocytic leukemia cells. *Ann Oncol* 1994; **5(Suppl 1):** 61–5.
41. Schott AF, Apel IJ, Nuñez G, Clarke MF. Bcl-xl protects cancer cells from p53-mediated apoptosis. *Oncogene* 1995; **11:** 1389–94.
42. Schuuring E, Verhoeven E, Mooi WJ, Michalides RJAM. Identification and cloning of two overexpressed genes, *U21B31/PRAD1* and *EMS1*, within the amplified chromosome 11q13 region in human carcinomas. *Oncogene* 1992; **7:** 355–61.
43. Simonian PL, Grillot DAM, Nuñez G. Bcl-2 and Bcl-x_L can differentially block chemotherapy induced cell death. *Blood* 1997; **90:** 1208–16.
44. Spaulding MB, Fisher SG, Wolf GT. Tumor response, toxicity, and survival after neoadjuvant organ-preserving chemotherapy for advanced laryngeal carcinoma. The Department of Veterans Affairs Cooperative Laryngeal Cancer Study Group. *J Clin Oncol* 1994; **12:** 1592–9.
45. Sumantran VN, Ealovega MW, Nuñez G, Clarke MF, Wicha MS. Overexpression of Bcl-x_S sensitizes MCF-7 cells to chemotherapy-induced apoptosis. *Cancer Res* 1995; **55:** 2507–10.
46. Symonds H, Krall L, Remington L *et al.* p53-dependent apoptosis suppresses tumor growth and progression *in vivo*. *Cell* 1994; **78:** 703–11.
47. van der Riet P, Nawroz H, Hruban RH *et al.* Frequent loss of chromosome 9p21–22 early in head and neck cancer progression. *Cancer Res* 1994; **54:** 1156–8.
48. Van Dyke DL, Worsham MJ, Benninger MS *et al.* Recurrent cytogenetic abnormalities in squamous cell carcinomas of the head and neck region. *Genes Chromosomes Cancer* 1994; **9:** 192–206.
49. Wolf GT, Hong WK, Fisher SG *et al.* Induction chemotherapy plus radiation compared with surgery plus radiation in patients with advanced laryngeal cancer. The Department of Veterans Affairs Laryngeal Cancer Study Group. *N Engl J Med* 1991; **324:** 1685–90.
50. Worsham MJ, Benninger MJ, Zarbo RJ, Carey TE, Van Dyke DL. Deletion 9p22-pter and loss of Y as primary chromosome abnormalities in a squamous cell carcinoma of the vocal cord. *Genes Chromosomes Cancer* 1993; **6:** 58–60.
51. Xu L, Pirollo KF, Chang EH. Transferrin-liposome-mediated p53 sensitization of squamous cell carcinoma to radiation *in vitro*. *Hum Gene Ther* 1997; **8:** 467–75.
52. Zhang LF, Hemminki K, Szyfter K, Szyfter W, Söderkvist P. p53 mutations in larynx cancer. *Carcinogenesis* 1994; **15:** 2949–51.
53. Zhu S, Trask DD, Wolf GT, Carey TE, Wicha MS, Bradford CR. Bcl-x_S transfer increases the chemosensitivity of laryngeal carcinoma cells *in vitro*. *Head Neck* 1998; **20:** 485.

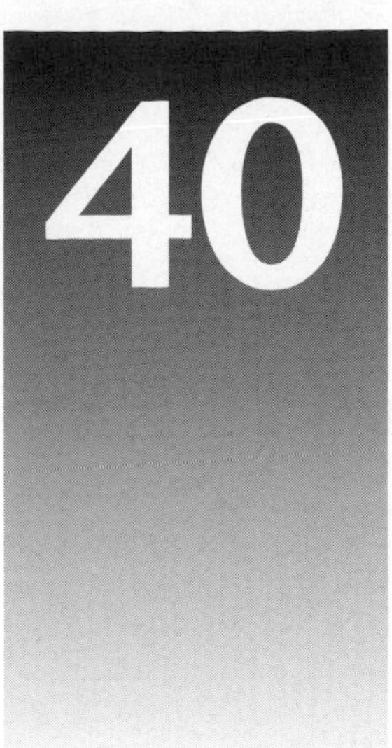

Pathology of malignant laryngeal tumors

Kenneth O Devaney

As the preceding chapter has demonstrated, the molecular biology of malignancies of the larynx is an area of great excitement and intense interest amongst researchers. Does this mean that the relatively more humble gross and light microscopic appearances of laryngeal tumors – that is, the pathology of these tumors – has been supplanted by these newer modalities to such an extent as to be rendered useless? Actually, for the foreseeable future, the answer would seem to be a clear no. Whilst we certainly attach great significance to the clinical stage of a given laryngeal tumor, there remain data to be attained both from pathologic staging of the patient's disease and from a study of the precise histologic features of the tumor itself.

Despite the advances made in diagnostic imaging, it has become apparent that not all patients are accurately staged by radiology alone; accordingly, some percentage of individuals with laryngeal cancer prove to have more advanced disease than that predicted by preoperative evaluation.[4,55,67]

The usual sort of laryngeal malignancy – a keratinizing squamous carcinoma – would seem to be a relatively homogeneous entity; whilst varying degrees of keratinization may be found in different tumors, little is added to the prognosis by making such a grading of the degree of keratinization. However, this is not why histologic study of laryngeal malignancies continues to be of central consequence; instead, it is of paramount importance to distinguish these commonly encountered keratinizing squamous lesions from the less commonly encountered malignancies, such as unusual variants of carcinoma, sarcomas and hematopoietic lesions, for the simple reason that these other (less frequently encountered) lesions may be treated in radically different ways than are the conventional squamous tumors. It should be apparent by now that these other tumor types are defined not by their clinical appearance, but by their microscopic appearances, making the role of the pathologist a well nigh essential one in the evaluation of this patient population.

In this section, the pathologic attributes of laryngeal malignancies will be explored so as to provide a backdrop against which subsequent discussions of diagnosis and treatment of these lesions will be cast.

Gross pathology

In general, the sorts of gross specimens handled by pathologists fall into two categories: those small diagnostic specimens obtained to confirm an initial clinical suspicion of malignancy and to histologically subtype that malignancy, and those larger specimens (laryngectomy or partial laryngectomy) that are removed at the time of definitive therapy for laryngeal cancer.

The pathologist often receives small diagnostic biopsy specimens that are not fixed in formalin. Whilst this is perfectly appropriate for a deep biopsy specimen of an 'obvious' malignancy (placed in quotes, of course, because not all such suspicious lesions ultimately prove to be malignant), very superficial mucosal based lesions may be difficult to analyze microscopically if they are poorly oriented. That is to say, it can be challenging to distinguish a superficially invasive lesion from a noninvasive one when the histologic sections are not taken in a plane perpendicular to the mucosal surface. In this setting – when obtaining a superficial mucosal biopsy – perhaps a page might be taken from the gastroenterologists, who often orient their endoscopic biopsies on a piece of paper before fixing them, and so preserve a sense of where the superficial-most portion of the tissue is, which in turn will permit the pathologist to select the most appropriate plane for sectioning.

The large (therapeutic) specimens, by contrast, require a much greater attention to anatomic detail. Much of our understanding of the patterns of spread of laryngeal carcinoma is derived directly from pathologic examination of large specimens, from laryngectomy.[6,28,44,61,63,69,84] The product of a total laryngectomy specimen will, in modern practice, be processed by the surgical pathologist in such a way as to provide the sorts of details as regards the size of the tumor, the extent of disease, the adequacy of the surgical margins, and the presence or absence of metastatic deposits.

A word about surgical margins is required here – in the typical (large, relative to a tiny biopsy) laryngectomy specimen, the sheer surface area of area of margin for potential microscopic examination would fill dozens to hundreds of individual tissue cassettes (which each have, incidentally, a size of only 3 cm by 2 cm, with a few millimeters in depth). As a practical matter, such a total embedding of the entire surgical margin is impracticable; as a consequence, the surgical pathologist will of necessity sample only selected portions of the margin for microscopic study. Knowing this, the prudent surgeon particularly concerned about the close approximation of tumor to a particular margin will clearly identify that margin to the pathologist by means of a suture, personal visit to the pathology suite at the time of the dissection of the specimen, or some other suitable means so as to insure that the area of interest is sampled. After all, pathologists are not mind-readers and so cannot always know without some prompting where the clinically significant areas for sampling in a particular case may lie.

In both small and large specimens, an initial impression will be formed with regard to the gross extent of disease. As it is believed that most malignancies encountered in the larynx begin as in situ carcinomas of the overlying mucosa, then breach the enveloping basement membrane to become 'early' (superficially invasive carcinomas), and finally invade deeply into the adjacent soft tissues and so yield a mass which may be appreciated on naked eye examination, it is obviously going to be much easier to make such an assessment microscopically when a well oriented gross specimen has been properly processed for microscopic study.[19,41]

Routine light microscopy

It is at the light microscopic level that it first becomes possible to carry out two critical tasks: first, to distinguish benign (pseudomalignant) processes from true malignancies;[98,99] then, once a deceptive benign lesion has been excluded, to distinguish amongst the various subtypes of malignant laryngeal tumors.[35,39]

Whether at the time of frozen section (intraoperative consultation), or with the study of permanent (formalin-fixed) sections, the analysis carried out by the microscopist is the same. A series of questions are asked:

- Is the cellularity low or high?
- Are the cells of interest (the 'abnormal' cells, by light microscopy) cytologically benign, or are they cytologically atypical?
- Do these cells all seem to be the same size, or is their size wildly variable?
- What is the shape of the cells of interest: are they round, polygonal, or spindle-shaped?
- Are the cells individual units, or do they appear to form coherent masses?
- Are there areas of necrosis, or readily apparent mitotic figures?
- Finally, what of the background in which the cells are disposed: is it fibrous, cartilaginous, or inapparent?

This is something of an oversimplification perhaps, but it gives one the flavor of the multifaceted analysis going on behind the surgical pathologist's silent study of a difficult slide.

Once an impression of a malignant tumor has been formed, the pathologist next turns to a determination of the specific tissue type of malignancy. As alluded to above, most laryngeal malignancies will ultimately prove to be keratinizing squamous carcinomas; a significant minority of tumors, however, will prove to be other tumor types, and it is with regard to these other tumors that the remainder of this section will be devoted. To begin with

Table 40.1 Laryngeal cancer – general categories of tumor types

Epithelial
Carcinomas, carcinosarcomas – primary as well as metastatic
Mesenchymal
Sarcoma
Hematopoietic
Lymphomas
Leukemias
Multiple myeloma

Table 40.2 Epithelial malignancies of the larynx

Squamous carcinoma – keratinizing and non-keratinizing, as well as basaloid squamous, lymphoepithelial and verrucous
Neuroendocrine carcinoma – including carcinoid, small cell carcinoma, large cell neuroendocrine carcinoma and malignant paraganglioma
Salivary-gland-type carcinoma – including adenoid cystic carcinoma, mucoepidermoid carcinoma and acinic cell carcinoma
Adenocarcinoma – type not further subclassified
Adenosquamous carcinoma
Carcinosarcoma – also known as sarcomatoid carcinoma, spindle cell carcinoma and pseudosarcoma

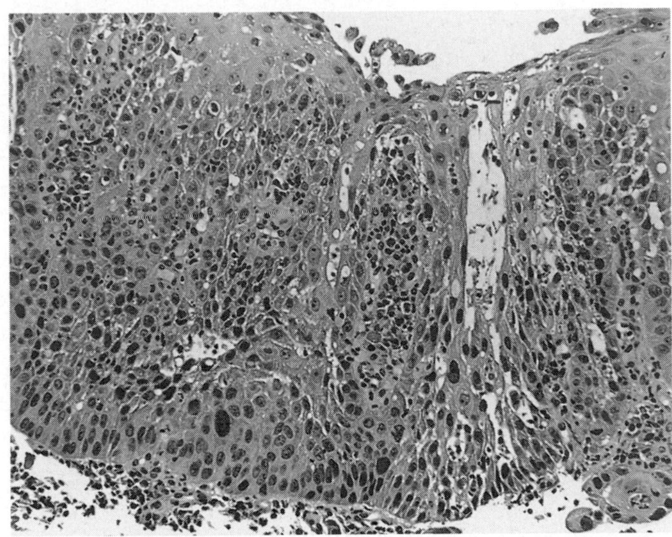

Figure 40.1 *This laryngeal lesion is an in situ squamous carcinoma, marked by a disorganized proliferation of cytologically atypical squamous cells which are still confined by a basement membrane (hematoxylin and eosin, original magnification ×220).*

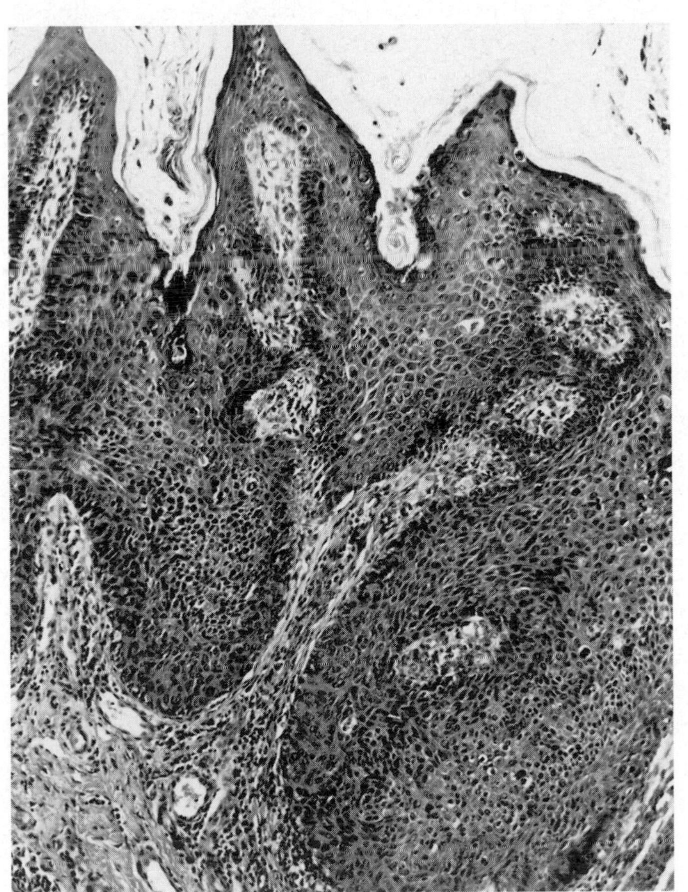

Figure 40.2 *In this superficially invasive squamous carcinoma, bulbous masses grow down into the submucosa, but retain their connection with the overlying epithelium (hematoxylin and eosin, original magnification ×110).*

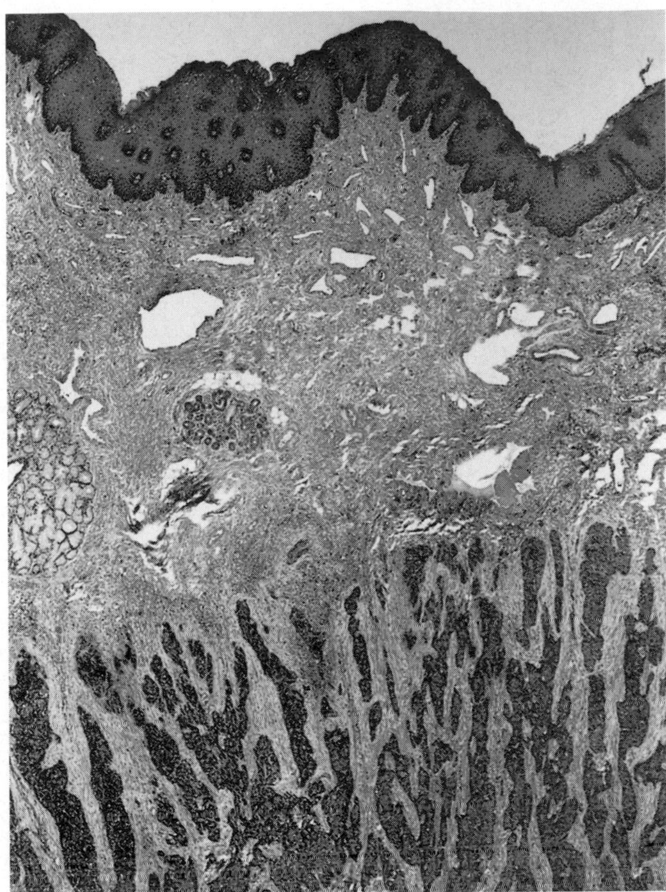

Figure 40.3 *Some biopsies of invasive squamous carcinoma show a distinct invasive component (bottom) with an uninvolved overlying epithelium (top) (hematoxylin and eosin, original magnification ×40).*

a broad generalization, tumors can usually be relegated, by a synthesis of the light microscopic features discussed in the paragraph above, to one of three categories: epithelial, mesenchymal, or hematopoietic (see Table 40.1).

To begin with the epithelial tumors (see Table 40.2), keratinizing squamous carcinomas are clearly the most common form of laryngeal malignancy, accounting for 12 000–14 000 new diagnoses of laryngeal cancer in the USA each year (Figs 40.1–40.5).[6,19,35,38,39,41] Less common patterns of squamous malignancies include the basaloid squamous carcinomas (Fig 40.6), the lymphoepithelial carcinomas (Fig 40.7) and the verrucous carcinomas (Fig 40.8).[37,42,97] It is with regard to these variants that the power of light microscopy to recognize prognostically significant subtypes of tumors becomes apparent, for, it turns out, the verrucous carcinomas appear to be indolent lesions that are much less aggressive than conventional squamous carcinomas, whereas, by contrast, the basaloid squamous and lymphoepithelial carcinomas are more aggressive than conventional carcinomas.

Another subtype of epithelial malignancies is the family of neuroendocrine carcinomas, a group of tumors ranging

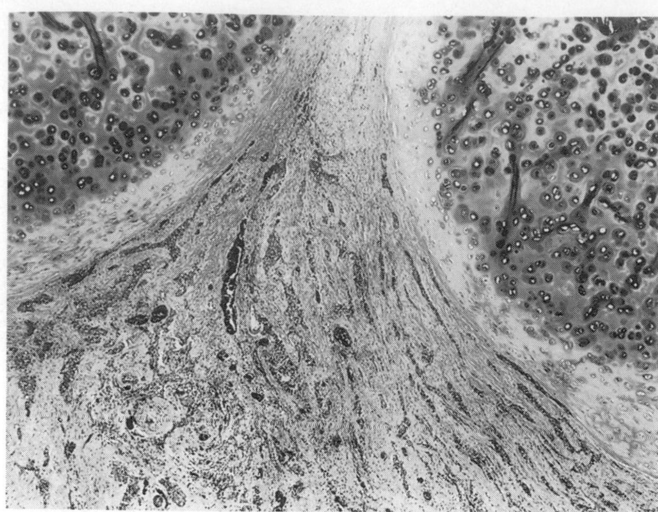

Figure 40.4 *The invasive pattern of a conventional laryngeal squamous carcinoma is highly variable; as shown here, cartilage often forms a relative barrier to spread of tumor, with the cords of invasive tumor surrounding and engulfing the islands of chondroid material (hematoxylin and eosin, original magnification ×40).*

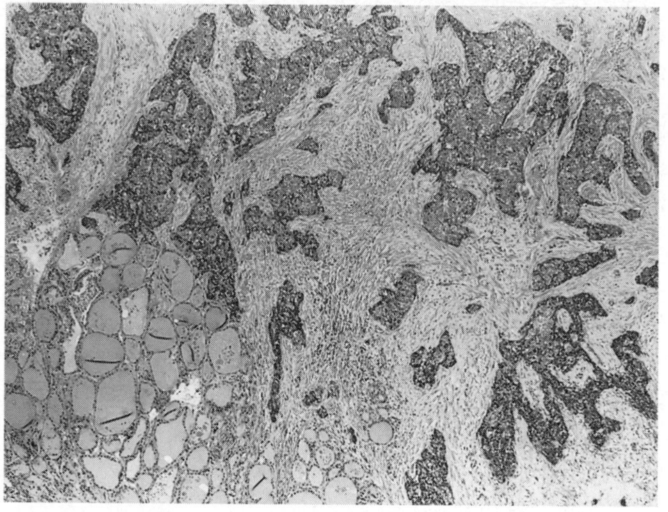

Figure 40.5 *One microscopic measure of the extralaryngeal spread of a squamous carcinoma is its identification, shown here, invading an adjacent structure such as the thyroid gland (left of figure) (hematoxylin and eosin, original magnification ×110).*

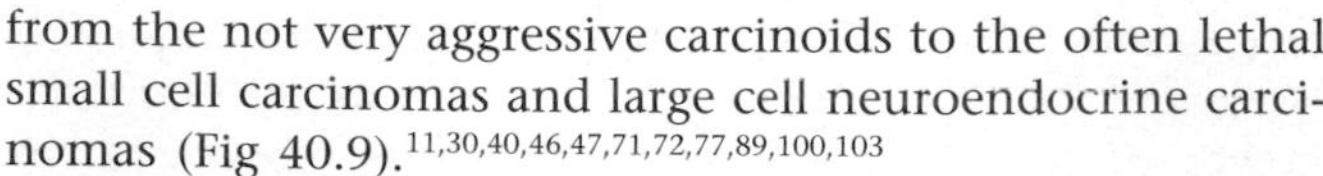

from the not very aggressive carcinoids to the often lethal small cell carcinomas and large cell neuroendocrine carcinomas (Fig 40.9).[11,30,40,46,47,71,72,77,89,100,103]

Finally, the least common variants of carcinoma include:

- the salivary-gland-type carcinomas, whose patterns include adenoid cystic carcinoma (Fig 40.10), mucoepidermoid carcinoma and acinic cell carcinoma;
- adenocarcinomas, which cannot be further subclassified;

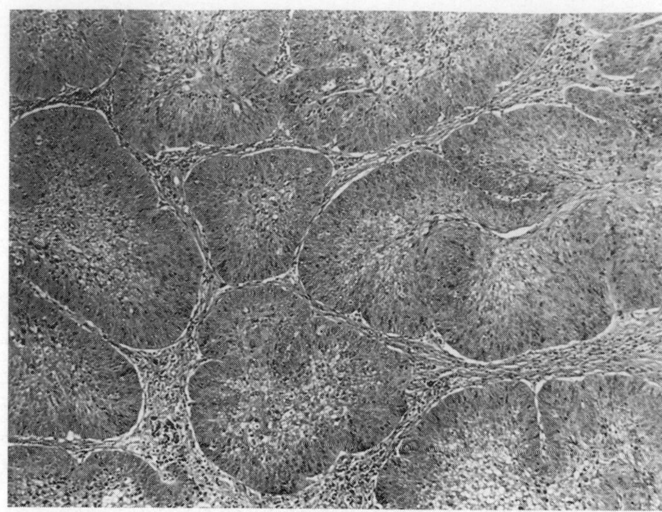

Figure 40.6 *The basaloid pattern of squamous carcinoma is distinguished by its architecture; islands of tumor cells show, at their peripheries, a pronounced pattern of palisading of tumor cells, an appearance reminiscent of that of a cutaneous basal cell carcinoma (hematoxylin and eosin, original magnification ×110).*

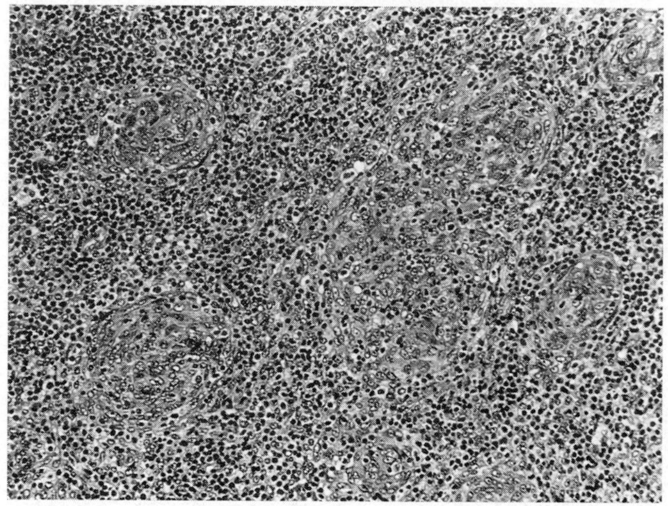

Figure 40.7 *The tumor cells of a lymphoepithelial carcinoma may be partially obscured, as here, by the dense accompanying (benign) lymphoid infiltrate (hematoxylin and eosin, original magnification ×110).*

- adenosquamous carcinomas, which combine features of a cytologically malignant squamous lesion with those of a cytologically malignant gland-forming lesion.

The behavior of these tumors is variable, with the salivary-gland-type tumors following a more indolent course whereas the adenocarcinomas (not further subclassified) seem to behave in a more aggressive fashion.[18,58,78,87,88,94,95,102] One rare epithelial malignancy, the carcinosarcoma, combines histologic features of a

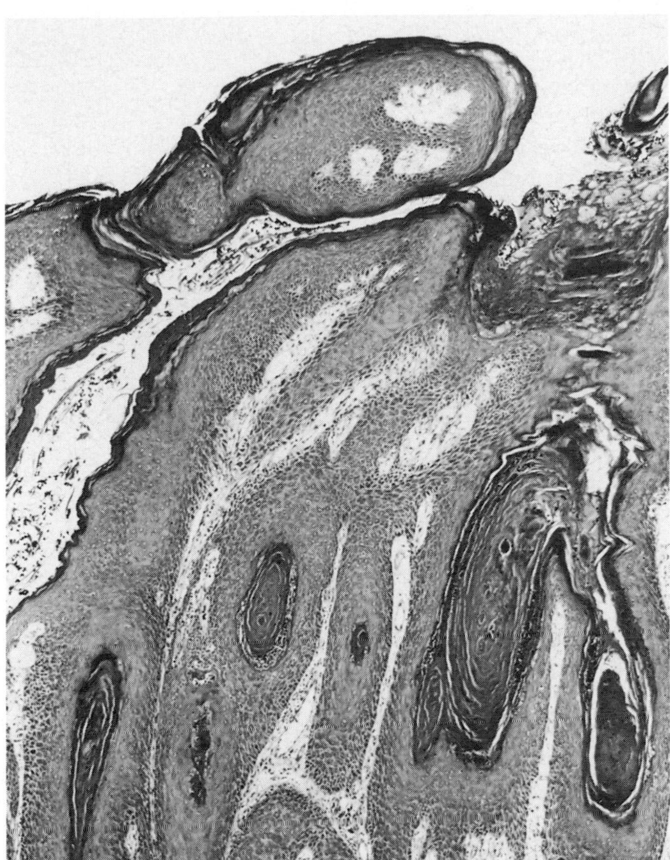

Figure 40.8 *The very well differentiated verrucous carcinoma is marked by an exophytic (papillary) external component and an accompanying invasive component marked by broad pegs of invasive tumor composed of keratinizing cells which lack a pronounced degree of cytologic atypia (hematoxylin and eosin, original magnification ×40).*

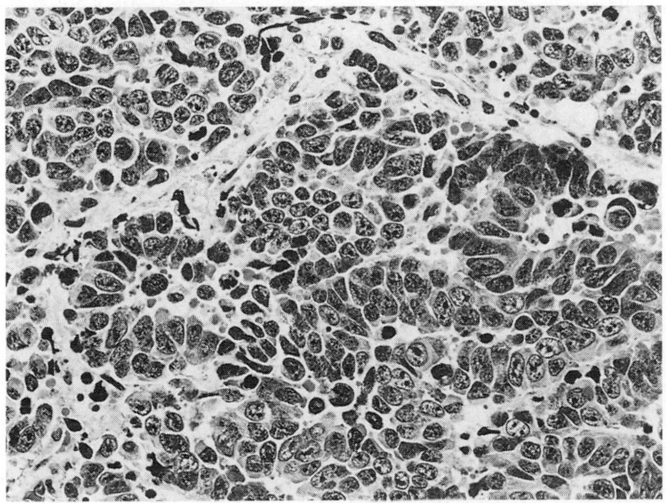

Figure 40.9 *Large cell neuroendocrine carcinoma cells are closely packed, arranged in islands and cords (an arrangement reminiscent of a carcinoid tumor) and – individually – have limited quantities of cytoplasm, hyperchromatic cytologically malignant nuclei and prominent nucleoli (hematoxylin and eosin, original magnification ×320).*

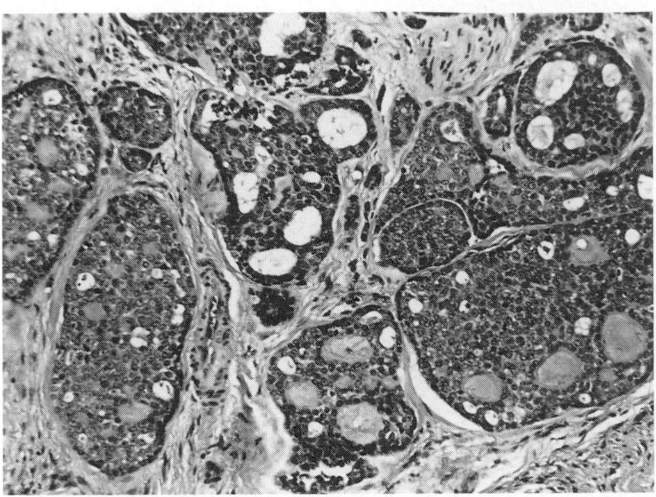

Figure 40.10 *Adenoid cystic carcinoma of the larynx, like its major salivary gland counterpart, is composed of relatively monomorphous small round cells arranged in islands perforated by spaces - a 'cribriform' growth pattern (hematoxylin and eosin, original magnification ×110).*

carcinoma with those of a sarcoma. When such tumors form polypoid exophytic masses projecting into the airway, they actually have a surprisingly good prognosis following excision; the more invasive tumors, however, are much more aggressive lesions.[3,33,104]

Whilst substantially less common than epithelial tumors, the mesenchymal malignancies (sarcomas) provide a bewildering array of different histologic patterns (see Table 40.3).[48] By a wide margin, chondrosarcomas are the most frequently encountered laryngeal sarcomas (Fig 40.11); less common patterns include osteosarcoma, malignant fibrous histiocytoma (MFH), fibrosarcoma, liposarcoma, angiosarcoma, synovial sarcoma and rhabdomyosarcoma.[2,7,13,20,23–26,29,36,70,80–82,101] Also traditionally included among the sarcomas is Kaposi's sarcoma (although, at present, there is some question as to whether or not this lesion might not actually be related to an infectious process and so is not a true sarcoma after all; for the present, the traditional classification of this

Table 40.3 Mesenchymal malignancies of the larynx
Chondrosarcoma
Osteosarcoma
Malignant fibrous histiocytoma
Fibrosarcoma
Liposarcoma
Angiosarcoma
Synovial sarcoma
Rhabdomyosarcoma
Kaposi's sarcoma

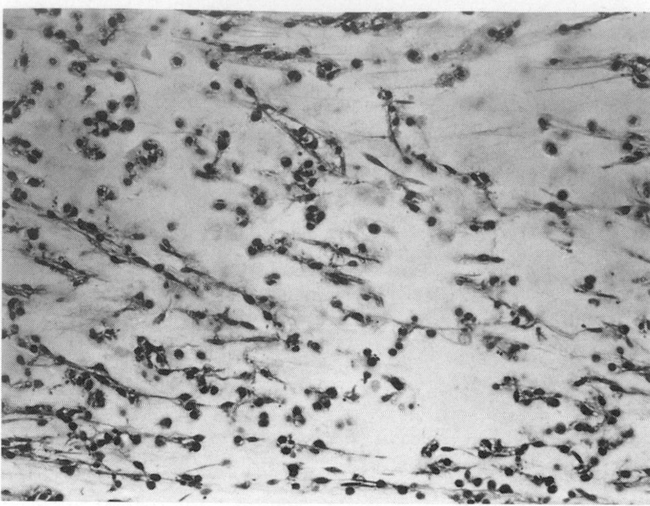

Figure 40.11 *This low-grade chondrosarcoma of the larynx exhibits a somewhat cellular proliferation set in a chondroid matrix; this tumor lacks both the pronounced cellularity and marked cytologic atypia of a high-grade chondrosarcoma (hematoxylin and eosin, original magnification ×220).*

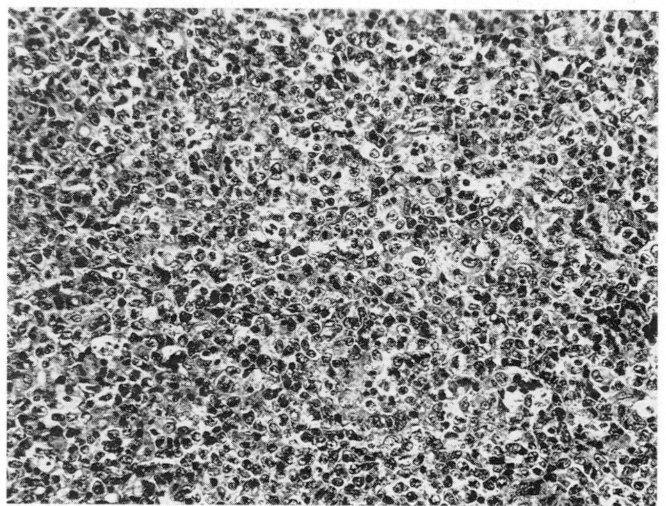

Figure 40.12 *Here, a densely cellular diffuse malignant lymphoma is shown, replacing and obscuring the underlying architecture of the laryngeal soft tissues (hematoxylin and eosin, original magnification ×220).*

tumor as a sarcoma will be retained).[65,86] In general, the chondrosarcomas are more often low-grade tumors than high-grade aggressive malignancies; the remaining sarcoma types usually are high-grade tumors, with a well established capacity both for local recurrence and metastasis.

Even less frequent than sarcomas are hematopoietic malignancies presenting as clinically significant lesions of the larynx; most of these lesions prove to be non-Hodgkin's lymphomas (Fig 40.12), although occasional cases of leukemia and multiple myeloma have been

Table 40.4 Hematopoietic malignancies of the larynx

Lymphocytic leukemia – acute and chronic
Myelogenous leukemia – acute and chronic
Non-Hodgkin's lymphoma – includes follicular, diffuse, small lymphocytic, large cell anaplastic, lymphoblastic, and peripheral T-cell types
Multiple myeloma
? Hodgkin's disease

reported in this region (see Table 40.4).[14,17,32,56,75,90,93,96] Whilst Hodgkin's disease has not been described in the larynx proper, there is no reason to think that such an occurrence may not be reported in the future.

In reality, not all lesions can be placed into neatly designated categories; there will be the occasional patient in whom no more satisfying diagnosis than 'carcinoma (or sarcoma), type not further subclassified' or even 'malignant tumor, not further subclassified' will be rendered. Fortunately, the number of such cases will be small.

The pathologic staging of disease – distinguishing superficially invasive or in situ carcinoma from extensively invasive tumor (see Figs 40.1, 40.2 and 40.5), assessing the adequacy of surgical excision, and studying any associated lymph nodes for the presence or absence of metastatic deposits – is the next step in the process.

Once a lesion has been assigned to a histologic category and a pathologic staging has been carried out, some attempt at light microscopic grading will usually be made by the pathologist. This, however, is not always a simple matter; whilst grading systems have been developed for all three types of malignancies – epithelial, mesenchymal, and hematopoietic – these grading systems often appear to compete with one another and so it often occurs that

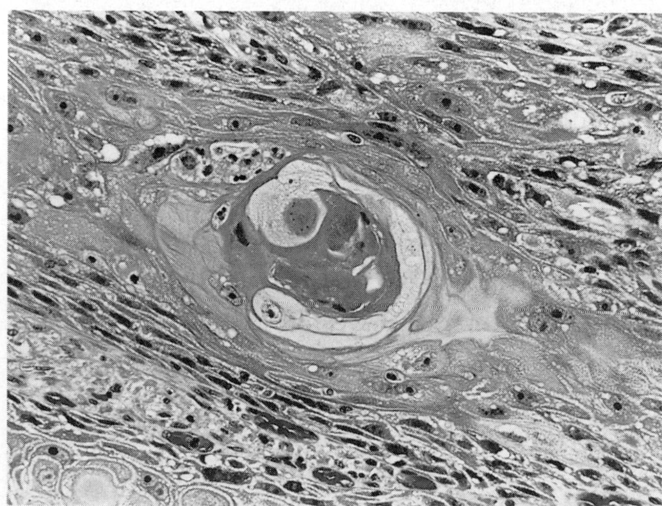

Figure 40.13 *Well differentiated squamous carcinoma (hematoxylin and eosin, original magnification ×320).*

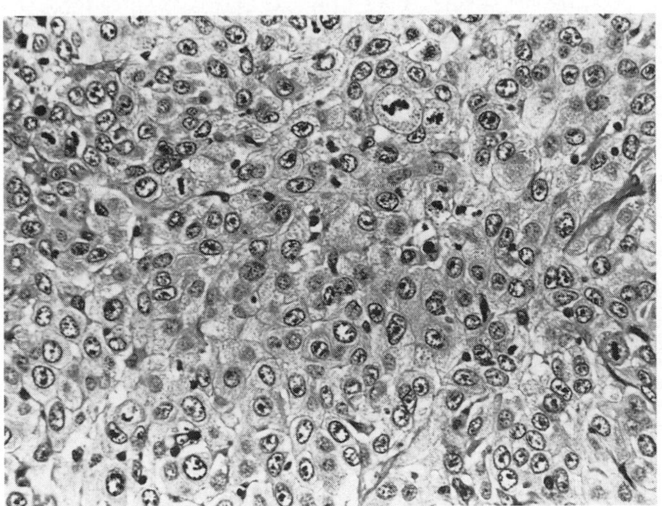

Figure 40.14 *Poorly differentiated squamous carcinoma (hematoxylin and eosin, original magnification ×320).*

one center favors one grading system over another.[12,15,16,54,85,92] Take, as an example, the conventional keratinizing squamous carcinoma of the larynx; in Fig 40.13 is seen a well differentiated (highly keratinized) tumor, whereas Fig 40.14 shows a poorly differentiated (poorly keratinized) variant of squamous carcinoma. Such distinctions actually do not add a great deal to the prognosis of the lesion – the clinical/pathologic stage has proven to be a more powerful prognostic factor. Nonetheless, malignancies continue to be closely studied by pathologists for any subtle microscopic findings – the degree of mitotic activity, for example, or the pattern of the advancing edge of the invasive tumor – which might shed further light on the behavior of these tumors. No striking factors have yet been uncovered for the carcinomas, although it should be noted that histologic grading is a more important feature of the sarcomas.

Although not a common occurrence, the pathologist dealing with laryngeal malignancies will on occasion encounter metastatic deposits which mimic – both clinically and histologically – primary laryngeal tumors.[1,8] Often, the best protection against such an occurrence is a thorough clinical evaluation prior to biopsy, so as to afford the pathologist the maximum information possible at the time of tissue examination.

In brief, this is the message to be derived from this section on light microscopy: tumor classification systems change with time; moreover, the prognosis attached to a particular histologic tumor type may also be expected to change as therapy changes (Hodgkin's disease, for example, has changed from being a uniformly fatal tumor at the beginning of this century to its present status as one of the potentially curable cancers). Those involved in the care of patients with laryngeal malignancies will probably be best served by first determining the microscopic tissue type or tumor type, then correlating this tumor type with the prognostic attributes of the tumor known at that time, and then finally act upon this information so as to design the best therapy possible for that particular tumor type.

Immunohistochemistry

The epithelial nature of a typical keratinizing squamous carcinoma is rarely in doubt, and so in the majority of such lesions it is not necessary to resort to the use of ancillary diagnostic techniques such as immunohistochemistry for confirmation of a diagnosis. There are instances, however – as, for example, the poorly differentiated nonkeratinizing carcinoma – where the knowledge of a tumor's immunoprofile is of tremendous aid in the elucidation of a correct diagnosis. Today, immunohistochemical studies are sufficiently widely available, either in individual laboratories or as a service provided by a reference laboratory, as to be all but universally employed in the diagnostic process.[22,53,68,76,83,91]

In an ideal situation, a tumor's immunoprofile will allow the pathologist to divine the derivation of that tumor, that is, immunohistochemistry at its best will permit the separation of lymphomas from carcinomas from sarcomas. In practice, unfortunately, this is not always the case; it should be confessed at this time that immunohistochemical studies do not always yield a clear, unequivocal statement as to the identity of a poorly differentiated tumor. It has been established by dint of a great deal of practical experience with these immunostains over the past decade and a half that two confounding factors may arise:

- first, technical problems may interfere with the accuracy of the results obtained; and

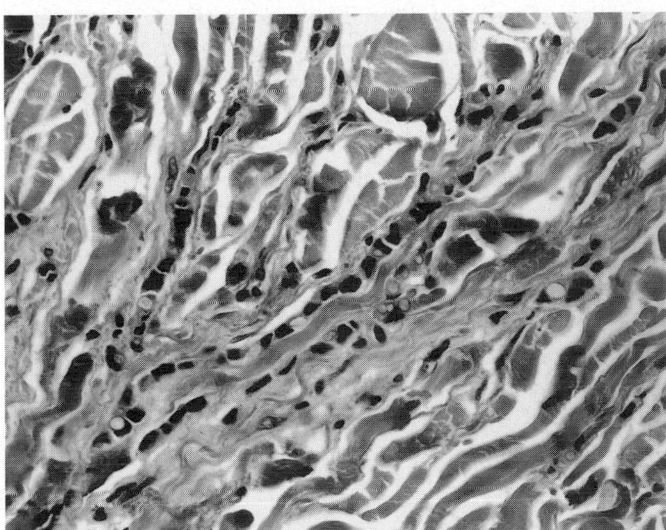

Figure 40.15 *This is an invasive poorly differentiated carcinoma; its malignant (epithelial) nature is in some danger of being overlooked on routine light microscopy, and so might be highlighted by immunohistochemistry (hematoxylin and eosin, original magnification ×320).*

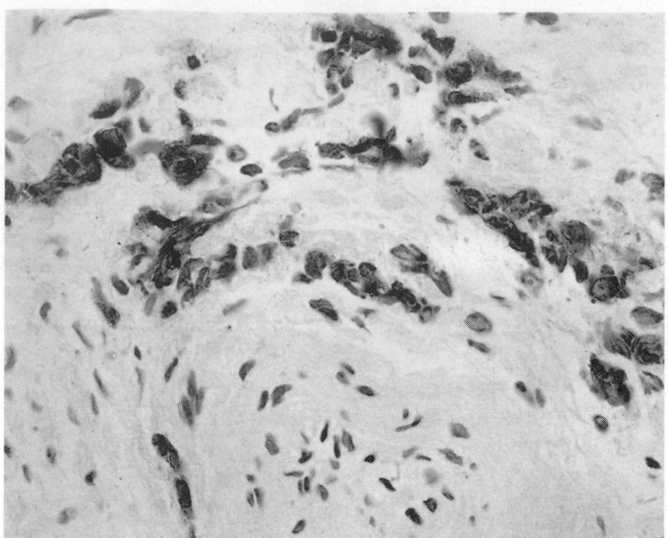

Figure 40.16 *The invasive carcinoma seen in the preceding figure (Fig 40.15) is clearly delineated here by immunoperoxidase staining of the tumor cells with antibody to cytokeratin (antibody to cytokeratin, original magnification ×320).*

- second, it is always essential that the pathologist correlates the results of immunostaining with the light microscopic findings, as the immunostaining results taken in isolation may lead one astray.

With the foregoing caveats in mind, here are some generalizations with regard to the application of immunohistochemical stains to the diagnosis of tumors of uncertain lineage. Cytokeratin is a reasonably reliable marker for epithelial tumors (Figs 40.15 and 40.16), while leukocyte common antigen (CD45/CD45RB) is both a sensitive and specific marker for lymphoid lesions. Epithelial members of the neuroendocrine carcinoma family of lesions may be delineated by their positivity with antibodies such as chromogranin, neuron-specific enolase, or synaptophysin. Among the sarcomas, desmin and actin are found in muscle tumors, whilst CD31 and CD34 appear in vascular tumors; vimentin is a nonspecific marker that may be found in a variety of sarcomas (and a minority of carcinomas). Finally, in view of the fact that thyroid tumors sometimes invade the larynx and so mimic primary tumors, antibody to thyroglobulin may be employed to identify such deceptive tumors (see Table 40.5).[9,10,21,49,50,57,62,64,66,73]

A final caution would seem to be in order. Most immunostains, at the time of their initial marketing as diagnostic probes, have been touted as 'magic bullets' that lend an unerring accuracy to the diagnostic process. Almost without exception, these tumor-specific claims have been diluted for each new antibody within a few years of its initial marketing by virtue of the discovery of 'exceptions to the rule'.[5,27,31,52] Of all of the antibodies discussed above, only leukocyte common antigen (LCA) has shown a consistent high specificity for lymphoid lesions. Even here, however, problems may arise; a minority of malignant lymphomas may be LCA negative, requiring the use of additional antibodies (directed against T-cell- and B-cell-specific epitopes) for the elucidation of such a tumor's lymphoid nature. The message is clear: immunostaining of problem tumors has become an essential modality in most surgical pathologists' practices, but the results of these stains must be interpreted judiciously, with the light microscopic appearances of the lesion ever present in the pathologist's mind's eye, for correlation with these immunostaining results.

Table 40.5 Diagnostic immunohistochemistry – some commonly used antibodies

Cytokeratin – epithelial lesions
Leukocyte common antigen (LCA) – lymphoid lesions
Muscle-specific actin – skeletal muscle lesions
Smooth muscle actin – smooth muscle lesions
Desmin – smooth and skeletal muscle lesions
Vimentin – mesenchymal lesions
CD31 or CD34 – vascular lesions
Chromogranin, neuron-specific enolase, or synaptophysin – neuroendocrine lesions
Thyroglobulin – lesions of the thyroid gland

The definitive pathology report

Custom will, of course, vary from one hospital to another, but in general terms the well prepared pathology report of a laryngeal description will touch on these areas:

- a description of the *type* of specimen examined (biopsy, partial laryngectomy, total laryngectomy, or other procedure);
- a gross report of the anatomic *site(s)* and *side(s)* of involvement – glottis, supraglottic, transglottic, or pyriform sinus;
- the *extent* of disease (drawn from a correlation of both gross and microscopic observations) – including a note as to the presence or absence of tumor extension *beyond the confines* of the larynx proper (or, alternatively, destroying thyroid cartilage), as well as the *gross dimensions* of the tumor in three planes);
- the status of the *surgical margins* of excision, that is, whether they are involved or free of tumor (often either a gross or, if quite close, microscopic assessment of the closest approach of tumor to a surgical margin);
- if present, an evaluation of the regional lymph *nodes* with notice of the number of positive nodes as well as the maximum *diameter* of the largest positive node (many centers note as well in the positive nodes the presence or absence of tumor spread *beyond* the confines of the node *capsule*).

It should be apparent that this analysis will be limited only by the pathologist's skills as an anatomist and so liberal consultation should be sought with the attending surgeon for orientation of such a specimen prior to dissection should any uncertainty exist as to the pertinent anatomic landmarks.

Future directions in the pathology of malignant laryngeal tumors

The preceding chapter has elucidated many of the elegant mechanisms by which molecular biologic techniques are being enlisted in the battle for a greater understanding of the development and progression of laryngeal cancer, and so it is not our goal here to reduplicate that effort. One observation seems pertinent and that relates to the availability of the sophisticated molecular techniques. General pathology laboratories do not, at present, always offer a full range of such studies to the clinician caring for patients with laryngeal malignancies. It may be predicted that one of two things will occur: either the methods of the molecular investigators will become sufficiently reproducible among less highly trained personnel (probably through increased automation), or, alternatively, markers which today are identifiable only in advanced laboratories may be translated to a more readily accessible medium, as for example immunohistochemistry.[34,43,45,51,59,60,74] One observation seems unassailable, however, and that is that the partnership between surgeon and pathologist, while not always the most amicable of marriages,[79] seems destined to continue for the foreseeable future.

References

1. Abemayor E, Cochran AJ, Calcaterra TC. Metastatic carcinoma to the larynx. *Cancer* 1983; **52:** 1944–8.
2. Allsbrook WC, Harmon JD. Liposarcoma of the larynx. *Arch Pathol Lab Med* 1985; **109:** 294–6.
3. Appelman HD, Oberman HA. Squamous cell carcinoma of the larynx with sarcoma-like stroma. A clinicopathologic assessment of spindle cell carcinoma and 'pseudosarcoma'. *Am J Clin Pathol* 1965; **44:** 135–45.
4. Archer CR, Yeager VL, Herbold DR. Improved diagnostic accuracy in laryngeal cancer using a new classification based on computed tomography. *Cancer* 1984; **53:** 44–57.
5. Azumi N, Battifora H. The distribution of vimentin and keratin in epithelial and nonepithelial neoplasms. A comprehensive immunohistochemical study on formalin- and alcohol-fixed tumors. *Am J Clin Pathol* 1987; **88:** 286–96.
6. Barnes L, Johnson JT. Pathologic and clinical considerations in the evaluation of major head and neck specimens resected for cancer. *Pathol Annu* 1986; **21(part 1):** 173–250.
7. Batsakis JG, Fox JE. Rhabdomyosarcoma of the larynx. *Arch Otolaryngol* 1970; **91:** 136–40.
8. Batsakis JG, Luna MA, Byers RM. Metastases to the larynx. *Head Neck Surg* 1984; **7:** 458–60.
9. Battifora H. Recent progress in the immunohistochemistry of solid tumors. *Semin Diagn Pathol* 1984; **1:** 251–71.
10. Battifora H. Clinical applications of the immunohistochemistry of filamentous proteins. *Am J Surg Pathol* 1988; **12(Suppl 1):** 24–42.
11. Benisch BM, Tawfik B, Breitenbach EE. Primary oat cell carcinoma of the larynx: an ultrastructural study. *Cancer* 1975; **36:** 145–8.
12. Broders AC. Squamous cell epithelioma of the lip. *JAMA* 1920; **74:** 656–64.
13. Canalis RF, Green M, Konard HR, Hirose FM, Cooper S. Malignant fibrous xanthoma (xanthofibrosarcoma) of the larynx. *Arch Otolaryngol* 1975; **101:** 135–7.
14. Chen KTC. Localized laryngeal lymphoma. *J Surg Oncol* 1984; **26:** 208–9.
15. Chung CK, Stryker JA, Abt AB, Cunningham DE, Strauss M, Connor GH. Histologic grading in the clinical evaluation of laryngeal carcinoma. *Arch Otolaryngol* 1980; **106:** 623–34.
16. Costa J, Wesley RA, Glatstein E, Rosenberg SA. The grading of soft tissue sarcomas. Results of a clinicohistopathologic correlation in a series of 163 cases. *Cancer* 1984; **53:** 530–41.
17. Costen JB. Plasmacytoma. A case with original lesion of the epiglottis and metastasis to the tibia. *Laryngoscope* 1951; **61:** 266–70.
18. Crissman J, Rosenblatt A. Acinous cell carcinoma of the larynx. *Arch Pathol Lab Med* 1978; **102:** 233–6.
19. Crissman JD, Gnepp DR, Goodman ML, Hellquist H, Johns ME. Preinvasive lesions of the upper aerodigestive tract: histologic definitions and clinical implications. *Pathol Annu* 1987; **22(part 1):** 311–52.
20. Dahm LJ, Schaefer SD, Carder HM, Vellios F. Osteosarcoma of the soft tissue of the larynx: report of a case with light and electron microscopic studies. *Cancer* 1978; **42:** 2343–51.
21. DeLellis RA, Dayal Y. The role of immunohistochemistry in the diagnosis of poorly differentiated malignant neoplasms. *Semin Oncol* 1987; **14:** 173–92.
22. DeLellis RA, Kwan P. Technical considerations in the immunohistochemical demonstration of intermediate filaments. *Am J Surg Pathol* 1988; **12(Suppl 1):** 17–23.
23. Devaney K. Fibrous and histiocytic neoplasms. In: Ferlito A, ed. *Surgical Pathology of Laryngeal Neoplasms*. London: Chapman and Hall, 1996: 295–320.
24. Devaney K. Vascular neoplasms. In: Ferlito A, ed. *Surgical Pathology of Laryngeal Neoplasms*. London: Chapman and Hall, 1996: 341–74.
25. Devaney K, Ferlito A. Cartilaginous and osteogenic neoplasms. In: Ferlito A, ed. *Surgical Pathology of Laryngeal Neoplasms*. London: Chapman and Hall, 1996: 393–424.
26. Devaney K, Ferlito A, Silver C. Cartilaginous tumors of the larynx. *Ann Otol Rhinol Laryngol* 1995; **104:** 251–5.
27. Devaney K, Abbondanzo SL, Shekitka KM, Wolov RB, Sweet DE. MIC2 detection by antibody to HBA71 in tumors of bone and adjacent soft tissues. *Clin Orthop Relat Res* 1995; **310:** 176–87.
28. Djalilian M, Weiland LH, Devine KD, Beahrs OH. Significance of jugular vein invasion by metastatic carcinoma in radical neck dissection. *Am J Surg* 1973; **126:** 566–9.
29. Dodd-o JM, Wieneke KF, Rosman PM. Laryngeal

rhabdomyosarcoma. Case report and literature review. *Cancer* 1987; **59**: 1012–18.

30. Doglioni C, Ferlito A, Chiamenti C, Viale G, Rosai J. Laryngeal carcinoma showing multidirectional epithelial neuroendocrine and sarcomatous differentiation. *ORL J Otorhinolaryngol Relat Spec* 1990; **52**: 316–26.
31. Dranoff G, Bigner DD. A word of caution in the use of neuron-specific enolase expression in tumor diagnosis. *Arch Pathol Lab Med* 1984; **108**: 535.
32. East D. Laryngeal involvement in multiple myeloma. *J Laryngol Otol* 1978; **92**: 61–5.
33. Ellis GL, Langloss JM, Heffner DK, Hyams VJ. Spindle-cell carcinoma of the aerodigestive tract. An immunohistochemical analysis of 21 cases. *Am J Surg Pathol* 1987; **11**: 335–42.
34. Ensley JF. Molecular medicine: the forest, trees, and leaves. *Arch Otolaryngol Head Neck Surg* 1993; **119**: 1173–7.
35. Ferlito A. Histological classification of larynx and hypopharynx cancers and their clinical implications. Pathologic aspects of 2052 malignant neoplasms diagnosed at the ORL Department of Padua University from 1966 to 1976. *Acta Otolaryngol Suppl (Stockh)* 1976; **342**: 1–88.
36. Ferlito A. Histiocytic tumors of the larynx. A clinicopathologic study with review of the literature. *Cancer* 1978; **42**: 611–22.
37. Ferlito A, Recher G. Ackerman's tumor (verrucous carcinoma) of the larynx: a clinicopathologic study of 77 cases. *Cancer* 1988; **46**: 1617–30.
38. Ferlito A, Devaney K, Rinaldo A. The squamous neoplastic component in unconventional squamous carcinomas of the larynx. *Ann Otol Rhinol Laryngol* 1996; **105**: 926–32.
39. Ferlito A, Rinaldo A, Devaney KO. Malignant laryngeal tumors: phenotypic evaluation and clinical implications. *Ann Otol Rhinol Laryngol* 1995; **104**: 587–98.
40. Ferlito A, Milroy CM, Wenig BM, Barnes L, Silver CE. Laryngeal paraganglioma versus atypical carcinoid tumor. *Ann Otol Rhinol Laryngol* 1995; **104**: 78–83.
41. Ferlito A, Carbone A, De Santo LW *et al.* 'Early' cancer of the larynx: the concept as defined by clinicians, pathologists, and biologists. *Ann Otol Rhinol Laryngol* 1995; **103**: 245–50.
42. Ferlito A, Weiss LM, Rinaldo A *et al.* Lymphoepithelial carcinoma of the larynx, hypopharynx, and trachea. *Ann Otol Rhinol Laryngol* 1997; **106**: 437–44.
43. Frank CJ, McClatchey KD, Devaney KO, Carey TE. Evidence that loss of chromosome 18q is associated with tumor progression. *Cancer Res* 1997; **57**: 1–4.
44. Glanz HK. Carcinoma of the larynx. *Adv Otorhinolaryngol* 1984; **32**: 1–123.
45. Glassman AB. Cytogenetics. An evolving role in the diagnosis and treatment of cancer. *Clin Lab Med* 1997; **17**: 21–37.
46. Gnepp DR, Ferlito A, Hyams V. Primary anaplastic small cell (oat cell) carcinoma of the larynx. *Cancer* 1983; **51**: 1731–45.
47. Goldman NC, Hood CI, Singleton GT. Carcinoid of the larynx. *Arch Otolaryngol* 1969; **90**: 64–7.
48. Gorenstein A, Neel HB III, Weiland LH, Devine KD. Sarcomas of the larynx. *Arch Otolaryngol* 1980; **106**: 8–12.
49. Gould VE. Synaptophysin. A new and promising pan-neuroendocrine marker. *Arch Pathol Lab Med* 1987; **111**: 791–4.
50. Hagn C, Schmid KW, Fischer-Colbrie R, Winkler H. Chromogranin A, B, and C in human adrenal medulla and endocrine tissues. *Lab Invest* 1986; **55**: 405–11.
51. Hall EJ. The gene as theme in the paradigm of cancer. *Br J Radiol* 1993; **66**: 1–11.
52. Herrera GA, Turbat-Herrera EA, Lott RL. S-100 protein expression by primary and metastatic adenocarcinomas. *Am J Clin Pathol* 1988; **89**: 168–76.
53. Hsu SM, Raine L, Fanger H. Use of avidin-biotin-peroxidase complex (ABC) in immunoperoxidase techniques: a comparison between ABC and unlabeled antibody (PAP) procedures. *J Histochem Cytochem* 1981; **29**: 557–80.
54. Jakobsson PA, Eneroth CM, Killander D. Histologic classification and grading of carcinoma of the larynx. *Acta Radiol Ther* 1973; **12**: 1–8.
55. Johns ME, Farrior E, Boyd JC, Cantrell RW. Staging of supraglottic cancer. *Arch Otolaryngol* 1982; **108**: 700–2.
56. Jones RV. Laryngeal involvement in acute leukemia. *J Laryngol Otol* 1968; **82**: 123–8.
57. Kahn HJ, Marks A, Thom H, Baumal R. Role of antibody to S100 protein in diagnostic pathology. *Am J Clin Pathol* 1983; **79**: 341–7.
58. Kaznelson DJ, Schindel J. Mucoepidermoid carcinoma of the air passages: report of three cases. *Laryngoscope* 1979; **89**: 115–21.
59. Kiechle FL. Diagnostic molecular pathology in the twenty-first century. *Clin Lab Med* 1996; **16**: 213–22.
60. Killeen AA. Quantification of nucleic acids. *Clin Lab Med* 1997; **17**: 1–19.
61. Kirchner JA, Carter D. Intralaryngeal barriers to the spread of cancer. *Acta Otolaryngol (Stockh)* 1987; **103**: 503–13.
62. Kurtin PJ, Pinkus GS. Leukocyte common antigen – a diagnostic discriminant between hematopoietic and nonhematopoietic neoplasms in paraffin sections using monoclonal antibodies: correlation with immunologic studies and ultrastructural localization. *Hum Pathol* 1985; **16**: 353–65.
63. Lam KH. Extralaryngeal spread of cancer of the larynx. A study with whole-organ section. *Head Neck Surg* 1983; **5**: 410–24.
64. Leader M, Collins M, Patel J, Henry K. Vimentin: an evaluation of its role as a tumour marker. *Histopathology* 1987; **11**: 63–72.
65. Levy FE, Tansek KM. AIDS-associated Kaposi's sarcoma of the larynx. *Ear Nose Throat J* 1990; **69**: 177–84.
66. Listron MB, Dalton LW. Comparison of keratin monoclonal antibodies MAK-6, AE1:AE3, and CAM-5.2. *Am J Clin Pathol* 1987; **88**: 297–301.
67. Merritt RM, Williams MF, James TH, Porubsky ES. Detection of cervical metastasis. A meta-analysis comparing computed tomography with physical examination. *Arch Otolaryngol Head Neck Surg* 1997; **123**: 149–52.
68. Mesa-Tejada R, Pascal RR, Fenoglio CM. Immunoperoxidase: a sensitive immunohistochemical

technique as a 'special stain' in the diagnostic pathology laboratory. *Hum Pathol* 1977; **8:** 313–20.

69. Micheau C, Luboinski B, Sancho H, Cachin Y. Modes of invasion of cancer of the larynx. A statistical, histological, and radioclinical analysis of 120 cases. *Cancer* 1976; **38:** 346–60.
70. Miller LH, Santaella-Latimer L, Miller T. Synovial sarcoma of the larynx. *Trans Am Acad Ophthalmol Otolaryngol* 1975; **80:** 448–51.
71. Mills SE, Johns ME. Atypical carcinoid tumor of the larynx. A light microscopic and ultrastructural study. *Arch Otolaryngol* 1984; **110:** 58–62.
72. Mills SE, Cooper PH, Garland TA, Johns ME. Small cell undifferentiated carcinoma of the larynx. Report of two cases and review of 13 additional cases. *Cancer* 1983; **51:** 116–20.
73. Milroy CM, Ferlito A. Immunohistochemical markers in the diagnosis of neuroendocrine neoplasms of the head and neck. *Ann Otol Rhinol Laryngol* 1996; **104:** 413–18.
74. Milroy CM, Ferlito A, Devaney KO, Rinaldo A. The role of DNA measurements of head and neck tumors. *Ann Otol Rhinol Laryngol* 1997; **106:** 801–4.
75. Morgan K, MacLennan K, Narula A, Bradley PJ, Morgan DAL. Non-Hodgkin's lymphoma of the larynx (stage 1E). *Cancer* 1989; **64:** 1123–7.
76. Niemi M, Korhonen LK. Histochemical methods in diagnostic pathology. *Int Pathol* 1972; **13:** 11–28.
77. Ohsawa M, Kurita Y, Horie A, Kurita K. Malignant chemodectoma (paraganglioma) of the larynx. A case report with electron microscopy and biochemical assay. *Acta Pathol Jpn* 1983; **33:** 1279–88.
78. Olofsson J, van Nostrand AWP. Adenoid cystic carcinoma of the larynx: a report of four cases and a review of the literature. *Cancer* 1977; **40:** 1307–13.
79. Pack GT. Functions and dysfunctions of the surgical pathologist. *Surgery* 1962; **52:** 752–5.
80. Prasad JN. Fibrosarcoma of the larynx. *J Laryngol Otol* 1972; **86:** 267–74.
81. Pratt LW, Goodof II. Hemangioendotheliosarcoma of the larynx. *Arch Otolaryngol* 1968; **87:** 484–9.
82. Quinn HJ. Synovial sarcoma of the larynx treated by partial laryngectomy. *Laryngoscope* 1984; **94:** 1158–61.
83. Regezi JA, Batsakis JC. Diagnostic electron microscopy of head and neck tumors. *Arch Pathol Lab Med* 1978; **102:** 8–14.
84. Robbins KT, Michaels L. Feasibility of subtotal laryngectomy based on whole-organ examination. *Arch Otolaryngol* 1985; **111:** 356–60.
85. Russell WO, Cohen J, Enzinger F *et al.* A clinical and pathologic staging system for soft tissue sarcomas. *Cancer* 1977; **40:** 1562–70.
86. Schiff NF, Annino DJ, Woo P, Shapshay SM. Kaposi's sarcoma of the larynx. *Ann Otol Rhinol Laryngol* 1997; **106:** 563–7.
87. Spiro RH, Hajdu SI, Lewis JS, Strong EW. Mucus gland tumors of the larynx and laryngopharynx. *Ann Otol* 1976; **85:** 498–503.
88. Squires JE, Mills SE, Cooper PH, Innes DJ, McLean WC. Acinic cell carcinoma: its occurrence in the laryngotracheal junction after thyroid radiation. *Arch Pathol Lab Med* 1981; **105:** 266–8.
89. Stanley RJ, DeSanto LW, Weiland LH. Oncocytic and oncocytoid carcinoid tumors (well differentiated neuroendocrine carcinomas) of the larynx. *Arch Otolaryngol Head Neck Surg* 1986; **112:** 529–35.
90. Swerdlow JB, Merl SA, Davey FR, Gacek RR, Gottlieb AJ. Non-Hodgkin's lymphoma limited to the larynx. *Cancer* 1984; **53:** 2546–9.
91. Taylor CR. Immunoperoxidase techniques. *Arch Pathol Lab Med* 1978; **102:** 113–21.
92. The Non-Hodgkin's Lymphoma Pathologic Classification Project. National Cancer Institute sponsored study of classifications on non-Hodgkin's lymphomas. Summary and description of a Working Formulation for clinical usage. *Cancer* 1982; **49:** 2112–35.
93. Ti M, Villafuente R, Chase PH, Dosik H. Acute leukemia presenting as a laryngeal obstruction. *Cancer* 1972; **34:** 427–30.
94. Tomita T, Lotuaco L, Talbott L, Watanabe I. Mucoepidermoid carcinoma of the subglottis. An ultrastructural study. *Arch Pathol Lab Med* 1977; **101:** 145–8.
95. Toomey JM. Adenocarcinoma of the larynx. *Laryngoscope* 1967; **77:** 931–61.
96. Vassallo J, Altemani AM, Cardinalli IA *et al.* Granulocytic sarcoma of the larynx preceding chronic myeloid leukemia. *Pathol Res Pract* 1993; **189:** 1084–9.
97. Wain SL, Kier R, Vollmer RT, Bossen EH. Basaloid-squamous carcinoma of the tongue, hypopharynx, and larynx: report of 10 cases. *Hum Pathol* 1986; **17:** 1158–66.
98. Wenig BM, Devaney K, Bisceglia M. Inflammatory myofibroblastic tumor of the larynx: a clinicopathologic study of eight cases simulating a malignant spindle cell neoplasm. *Cancer* 1995; **76:** 2217–29.
99. Wenig BM, Devaney K, Wenig BL. Nonneoplastic lesions of the oropharynx and larynx which may simulate malignancy. *Pathol Annu* 1995; **30(part 1):** 143–87.
100. Wenig BM, Hyams VJ, Heffner DK. Moderately differentiated neuroendocrine carcinoma of the larynx. A clinicopathologic study of 54 cases. *Cancer* 1988; **62:** 2658–76.
101. Wenig BM, Weiss SW, Gnepp DR. Laryngeal and hypopharyngeal liposarcoma. A clinicopathologic study of 10 cases with a comparison of soft-tissue counterparts. *Am J Surg Pathol* 1990; **14:** 134–41.
102. Whicker JH, Neel HB III, Weiland LH, Devine KD. Adenocarcinoma of the larynx. *Ann Otol* 1974; **83:** 487–90.
103. Woodruff JM, Huvos AG, Erlandson RA, Shah JP, Gerald FP. Neuroendocrine carcinomas of the larynx. *Am J Surg Pathol* 1985; **9:** 771–90.
104. Zarbo RJ, Crissman JD, Venkat H, Weiss MA. Spindle-cell carcinoma of the upper aerodigestive tract mucosa. An immunohistologic and ultrastructural study of 18 biphasic tumors and comparison with seven monophasic spindle-cell tumors. *Am J Surg Pathol* 1986; **10:** 741–53.

Classification and staging of laryngeal cancer

Jay F Piccirillo and Peter D Lacy

A comprehensive multidisciplinary approach to the evaluation of patients with laryngeal cancer is essential for accurate classification, staging and prediction of outcomes. Those who should be involved include the surgical, radiation and medical oncologist; speech pathologist; nutritionist; social worker; and clinical nurse specialist. Together these professionals provide each patient with a thorough and organized diagnostic evaluation and treatment plan. Improvement in management is hampered by less than ideal methods for the evaluation, classification and staging of patients with laryngeal cancer. This chapter will address the general principles of evaluation, classification and staging of patients with laryngeal cancer. It will also highlight deficiencies with the present systems and suggest what improvements can be made.

Evaluation

An accurate history and physical examination on initial presentation, together with subsequent laboratory and radiographic tests, provide the basis for tumor classification, staging, prediction of outcomes and treatment planning. Psychosocial, nutritional, specific medical and anesthetic assessments with specific intervention when indicated are vital to achieving optimal outcomes. No treatment, irrespective of whether it is with curative or palliative intent, should be started until the patient and attending physician both have a clear understanding of the goals of treatment and have discussed openly the treatment options available with recognition of individual patient preferences.

History

Many patients are referred to the head and neck oncologic specialist with an established diagnosis of laryngeal cancer. However, a careful history provides the basis for a complete differential diagnosis, which ensures that all possibilities are considered prior to establishing a definitive diagnosis and planning treatment. Symptoms indicate where particular emphasis should be placed in physical examination and subsequent laboratory or radiographic investigation. By determining the duration, type and rate of progression of symptoms and signs, the degree of functional impairment experienced by the patient and some aspects of a tumor's biological behavior (see below) can be assessed. This, in turn, will provide estimates of prognosis and aid in the selection of treatment. For example, the symptom of bone pain or the sign of jaundice suggests the presence of bone metastasis or impaired liver function and necessitates a complete metastatic evaluation.

Etiology

Risk factors for the development of laryngeal cancer include the use of tobacco products, alcohol, environmental exposure to carcinogenic agents, dietary deficiencies and previous radiotherapy to the neck. Whilst exposure to these agents may point towards a malignant diagnosis, their presence has little tumor-specific prognostic importance. Rather, these factors may have greater significance with respect to comorbidity and other host-specific factors.

Physical examination

The clinician uses the physical examination to assess the structural integrity of the larynx, and the presence of nodal and distant metastases. The examiner must correlate pathologic findings on examination with the patient's clinical presentation. Careful inspection and palpation of the surfaces and cavities of the head and neck localizes and characterizes the pathology causing the patient's symptoms. For example, the gloved finger may detect a firm mass in the base of the tongue, representing extension of tumor beyond the larynx responsible for a patient's ankyloglossia. The examiner should give special attention to abnormalities in the texture and color of the mucosal linings of the upper aerodigestive tract. Areas of ulceration or leukoplakia are suspicious for malignancy. Likewise, a mass that is abnormally firm in consistency or fixed to adjacent structures is characteristic of a malignant process. Clinical assessment of nodal disease in the neck is based on determination of the size, number and consistency of palpable nodes. The examination of the head and neck confirms the exact size and location of the laryngeal tumor and, together with radiographic evaluation, forms the basis for the tumor, nodes, metastases (TNM) staging system.[1] The examination also identifies any other pathology, including synchronous tumors.

The introduction of fiberoptic technology has greatly enhanced the clinician's access to the many recesses of the upper aerodigestive tract in the office setting. The use of the flexible nasopharyngolaryngoscope can greatly increase diagnostic reliability even in the hands of the novice.[85] Videolaryngoscopy can further refine the technique by providing permanent documentation of the examination which allows subsequent review without subjecting the patient to further discomfort. Videostroboscopy provides detailed information regarding laryngeal function and as with laryngoscopy, can be recorded for later review. Both provide the added benefit of patient education.[58,98]

Patients undergoing a total or near-total laryngectomy will require voice rehabilitation postoperatively. Adequate manual dexterity and vision for care of a tracheoesophageal fistula and valve are essential for success using valved speech and for written communication in the postoperative period before speech rehabilitation. Literacy is also important and all these functions should be assessed preoperatively to predict any communication difficulties that may arise. Availability of and accessibility to the speech pathologist is also of great importance for success using all forms of voice rehabilitation. Patients should meet with other laryngectomees to prepare them for the alteration in physical appearance of the head and neck after surgery. This visit also allows the patient to see what communication options may be possible postoperatively and help both physician and patient in setting realistic goals of treatment. The patient can discuss his/her concerns and fears at this time with someone who has been in the same situation. This is invaluable and often greatly boosts patient morale. A willing group of volunteers is available through various laryngectomy societies and support groups for this purpose.

Comorbidity

Associated diseases, which are present but not related to the cancer, are called comorbidities. These conditions will often affect diagnosis, prognosis and treatment planning. A review of the past medical history and current medications will identify specific comorbidities. The severity of the comorbidity can be assessed through the subjective complaints of the patient and objective findings from physical examination and diagnostic testing. Communication with the primary care physician helps in understanding a patient's general medical condition and the clinician is well advised to utilize medical consultation for patients who have newly diagnosed or possibly suboptimally treated complex medical problems.

Alcohol and tobacco abuse are common in many laryngeal cancer patients and should not be overlooked. Alcohol abuse can create many medical and psychologic problems during treatment. Patients actively abusing alcohol should undergo detoxification to avoid withdrawal reaction during therapy. Nicotine withdrawal can lead to problems with anxiety, sleep disturbances and headache. Withdrawal can be avoided with the judicious use of transdermal or oral nicotine supplements.

Performance status

Assessment of performance status is important in the medical evaluation of the laryngeal cancer patient. Performance status is a global assessment of a patient's ability for self-care and ambulation. Performance status has been shown to be an important prognostic factor in a wide variety of cancers.[97] Poor performance status, as established by the Specific Activities Scale, has proven to be one of the strongest predictors of postoperative medical complications.[100] Changes in performance status enable the clinician to evaluate the impact of interventions on the patient's health status. In addition to health status, measurements of health-related quality of life should also be assessed as an integral part of the pre- and post-treatment assessment.

Research is currently underway in an effort to develop valid tools for the measurement of performance status,[67] although a number of tools have already been developed to provide reliable performance status data. These include the Karnofsky Performance Status (KPS) Scale,[82] the Eastern Cooperative Oncology Group (ECOG) Scale,[143] the Spitzer Quality of Life Index[126] and the Host (AJCC) Scale.[1] The prognostic impact of KPS for patients with laryngeal cancer is discussed in greater detail later in this chapter. In its third edition,[2] the AJCC stated 'the host performance status or the condition of the patient does not enter into determination of stage of the tumor but may be a factor in deciding type and time of treatment'. They go on to describe and suggest the use of three scales: AJCC, KPS and ECOG. Surprisingly, the recommendation to include performance status measures when evaluating patients with cancer was removed from the fourth edition.[3]

Metastatic workup

Laryngeal cancer is generally considered a regional disease due to the tendency of nodal spread. However, the possibility of systemic metastasis should not be overlooked, particularly in patients with a large primary tumor, bulky neck disease, or locoregional recurrence.[10] The lungs are the most common sites of metastasis (45%), followed by the skeletal system (25%) and liver (6%).[20,121] Although chest radiography is adequate routine screening for pulmonary metastasis in asymptomatic patients, the additional sensitivity of computed tomography (CT) can be invaluable in patients with pulmonary symptoms or questionable lesions on the chest radiograph. In patients with abnormal liver function studies, CT scan of the abdomen is useful in ruling out metastatic liver disease. The usefulness of bone scanning in the asymptomatic patient has been questioned by several authors.[105] Lack of specificity has made the validity of the test suspect.[117] Although the presence of metastatic disease has a profound impact on outcome and choice of treatment, restricting the use of adjunctive testing to patients with suspicious symptoms or abnormal laboratory results seems appropriate.

Nutritional assessment

Patients with laryngeal neoplasms may present with nutritional deficiencies secondary to the disruption of the normal anatomic pathways for dietary intake or to the systemic effects of cancer. Frequently, these patients are known abusers of alcohol and tobacco products, which results in further nutritional compromise. Malnutrition can compromise immunologic function, inhibit wound healing, and increase susceptibility to infection. Regardless of the chosen course of treatment, most patients with nutritional deficiencies will benefit from nutritional support.

Choosing the appropriate form of support requires a thorough baseline nutritional assessment. Although a registered dietitian is indispensable in generating accurate baseline measures, the physician can quickly identify the high-risk patient based on readily available data. A patient who experiences a 10% or greater decrease in their usual weight and is found to have a serum albumin less than 3.2 mg/dl or a total lymphocyte count less than 1500 cells/ml is considered malnourished and may benefit from supplementation.[35] Additional data may be obtained to more clearly define a patient's specific nutritional needs. In order to administer the safest, most cost-effective form of support for the individual patient, the type of initial antineoplastic therapy and duration of nutritional support must be considered.

The prognostic nutritional index (PNI) has been studied as an indicator of postoperative complications in patients with head and neck cancer.[71] The PNI combines data from anthropomorphic measurements, laboratory evaluation, and measures of immune function to establish an accurate assessment of a patient's nutritional status. The triceps skin fold thickness, serum albumin and transferrin levels, and the number of positive responses to delayed-hypersensitivity skin testing are combined using the formula

$$\text{PNI} = 158\% - 0.78(\text{TSF}) - 16.6(\text{ALB}) - 0.2(\text{TFN}) - 5.8(\text{DH})$$

where TSF is triceps skin fold, ALB is serum albumin, TFN is serum transferrin and DH is delayed hypersensitivity. Patients with advanced-stage head and neck cancer and a PNI greater than 20% were shown to be at increased risk for one or more complications after surgery.[71]

The goals of nutritional support must be established prior to implementing supplementation. A reversal of the catabolic state seen in many cancer patients is a primary goal of nutritional support. Increases in serum transferrin and prealbumin provide the earliest evidence of anabolic metabolism.[53] Increase in lean body mass has been suggested as a goal for pretreatment supplementation. However, due to the metabolic demands of the tumor, attempts to meet this goal have been less than satisfactory. There is an obvious need to balance the optimization of nutritional status with prompt therapy of the malignancy. A low threshold for initiating nutritional supplementation should be maintained due to the high complication rate associated with malnutrition.[54]

Once the need for nutritional supplementation has been established, the route of supplementation is selected. Whenever possible, the natural alimentary tract is used for nutritional support. The implementation of tube feedings has been shown to be more effective than *ad libitum* oral supplementation.[93] Anorexia, lethargy and tumor bulk may compromise the preoperative effectiveness of oral supplementation, whilst postoperatively, structural alterations affecting deglutition and ability to protect the airway may continue to impair oral intake. Traditionally, the nasogastric tube has been used for supplementation in these two situations. However, technical improvement in the fluoroscopic and endoscopic placement of gastrostomy tubes has provided an alternative for patients requiring long-term tube feedings. In our experience, patient satisfaction is greater with the gastrostomy than nasogastric tube. One study has shown a decrease in postoperative complications and length of stay with the use of gastrostomy when compared with the use of a nasogastric tube.[59] The use of total parenteral nutrition (TPN) in head and neck cancer may be necessary when the bowel is temporarily unavailable for supplementation, such as in the jejunal free-tissue transfer patients, and in such cases, TPN should be implemented in a timely fashion to achieve optimal results.

Psychosocial assessment

Psychological investment in the head and neck region is greater than any other site of the body.[17] Patients with laryngeal cancer suffer the same life-threatening illness of any cancer patient, yet unlike many other cancer patients, they are unable to conceal their affliction from public view. Treatments resulting in dysfunction or disfigurement of the structure of the head and neck and difficulties in communication will have great psychological impact on the patient and may lead to social isolation. Preoperative psychosocial evaluation can identify patients at risk for developing psychiatric problems throughout the course of the disease.[87] Preoperative assessment should focus on coping skills, family support, identification of personality disorders, psychiatric illness and substance abuse.

Patients undergoing treatment for laryngeal cancer frequently have problems with self-esteem due to a change in self-image.[57] These effects are greatest after major disfiguring surgery. Emotional maturity and ability to cope with changes in body image will directly affect patients' psychological health in the postoperative period. Reactive anxiety and depression are the most common psychiatric problems seen in cancer patients.[32] Patients with preexisting anxiety or depressive disorders are at risk for developing major psychiatric problems as a result of oncologic therapy and it should always be remembered that suicidal ideation is not uncommon.

Radiologic evaluation

The advent of computed tomography (CT) and magnetic resonance imaging (MRI) has largely supplanted plain films, tomography, fluoroscopy and laryngography for assessing tumors of the larynx.[23] Both CT and MRI are useful for assessing the deep tissue extension of laryngeal tumors. Imaging studies are most often used in patients with T2 tumors or greater.[34] Although CT will not show minor mucosal abnormalities, it is capable of showing the submucosal extent of the tumor in the subglottis and inferior surfaces of the true and false vocal cords. CT is excellent for showing bony changes and gross cartilage destruction as is seen in small T4 laryngeal tumors invading the thyroid or cricoid cartilages. However, CT is very poor at detecting microinvasion of cartilage or small lesions adjacent to cartilage.[7,23,72,83,84,99] MRI has multiplanar imaging capabilities and better soft tissue contrast than CT, allowing it to better distinguish inflammatory changes from fibrosis or recurrent tumor,[106] and it is more sensitive than CT in detecting neoplastic invasion of cartilage.[13] Positron emission tomography (PET) is a relatively new radiologic imaging technique that is based on the uptake and metabolism of a glucose analog in different tissues. Its applications in head and neck oncology have not yet been clearly defined, but it appears to have capabilities superior to CT or MRI for the diagnosis of tumor recurrence.[6,8]

Accurate assessment of the physical extent of tumor involvement and regional spread is critical in treatment planning for laryngeal cancers. Radiologic criteria for malignant nodal involvement were correlated with pathologic specimens in several studies.[84,130,136] Nodal size >1 cm and presence of central necrosis were shown to be the most reliable criteria.[136] CT has been shown to alter the clinical description of neck disease in 20–30% of cases, most patients being upstaged from the clinical examination.[130] The impact of technology on cancer staging and statistics is referred to as stage migration and is discussed later in the chapter. The presence of extensive local or regional metastatic disease on CT will affect treatment planning.

A standard PA chest radiograph, with or without a lateral view, must form part of a patient's initial assessment. Should multiple metastatic nodes be evident, subsequent, more complex and costly radiologic studies are unlikely to alter treatment planning and patient outcome. If a chest radiograph is suspicious but not diagnostic of pulmonary metastases, then CT or MRI may be of benefit to confirm the diagnosis.

Future development in radiographic techniques may prove beneficial to the evaluation of the laryngeal cancer patient. MR angiography has shown promise in assessing flow in the carotid artery and in determining the presence of invasive tumor within the lumen.[64,86] It may also prove useful in evaluating both donor and recipient vascular bed suitability when planning free-tissue transfer in reconstructive procedures. B-mode ultrasound has been successfully used to demonstrate carotid artery adventitia invasion when CT had failed to do so.[56] Recent studies have supported the utility of ultrasound-guided needle aspiration in increasing the yield of aspiration cytology in cervical lymph nodes.[135]

Cytology

In patients with a known primary tumor and clinically positive neck disease, fine needle aspiration (FNA) cytology adds little to the diagnostic evaluation. However, in the patient with a neck mass of unknown etiology, aspiration cytology can save the time, expense and possible complications of an extensive workup for malignant disease and open biopsy. Several studies have shown the excellent diagnostic accuracy of aspiration cytology.[81,116] To achieve this high degree of diagnostic accuracy, the cytopathologist must be well trained in the interpretation of head and neck aspiration cytology. As in other areas of medicine, if the findings of FNA do not correlate with the clinical picture, the clinician should pursue further diagnostic evaluation until he or she is confident in the findings.

Endoscopy

Traditionally, the preoperative evaluation of the laryngeal cancer patient has included panendoscopy (laryngoscopy, bronchoscopy and esophagoscopy) to detect the presence of synchronous lesions. This is typically performed in the operating room when the patient is undergoing biopsy of the primary lesion. In the interests of reducing costs, clinicians have attempted to reduce the use of operating room time. Many biopsies are performed in the office setting and fiberoptic technology has helped improve the effectiveness of this practice.[12] Thus, many clinicians have supplanted esophagoscopy and bronchoscopy with barium swallow and chest radiography. In one study, where patients were selected for endoscopy on the basis of having one or more risk factors for a second primary, panendoscopy revealed a synchronous lesion in <2% of cases.[73] The cost-effectiveness of routine panendoscopy was prospectively evaluated in 100 patients.[14] Results of the study showed a one-third savings in total cost and reduction in unnecessary procedures if bronchoscopy and endoscopy were reserved for symptomatic patients. It should be noted that Japanese investigators have been able to increase the yield of esophagoscopy with the addition of Lugol's solution to endoscopic evaluation.[74,96]

In an effort to address the current environment of cost-effective therapy, a preoperative chest radiograph may be used as an alternative to bronchoscopy. A chest CT scan is then obtained only when suspicious lesions are found on chest radiography. The barium swallow may be reserved for patients with swallowing complaints and those with risk factor for esophageal pathology. Esophagoscopy would then be necessary for biopsy of suspicious areas on the barium swallow or for inadequate examinations. We feel this type of preoperative workup could reduce costs without compromising patient care.

Future directions

The incorporation of the findings of molecular biology into the clinical practice of head and neck oncology has yet to become a reality. Several tumor markers are being investigated at present. For example, a new tumor antigen, A9/alpha 6 beta 4 integrin has recently been shown to have prognostic value in patients with squamous cell carcinoma.[140,141] In this study, the loss of blood group antigen expression and high A9/alpha 6 beta 4 integrin expression was related to early tumor recurrence. The authors suggested that this finding identified patients with worse prognosis who might benefit from aggressive primary therapy. Assays for mutations in the p53 gene have also shown promise in screening for head and neck cancer.[118] As molecular biologic techniques become more refined and their results more clinically applicable, the incorporation of such techniques into clinical practice will become a reality.

Post-treatment follow-up

Follow-up of individuals treated for laryngeal cancer currently focuses on surveillance for new or recurrent disease. A review of nationwide practices in patients with head and neck cancer shows that the majority of clinicians see patients monthly in the first postoperative year.[88] Sixty per cent of respondents recommend an annual chest radiograph, whereas other testing is reserved for symptomatic patients. The majority of second malignant tumors present in the lung, lending support to the annual chest radiograph.[90] In a meta-analysis of 40 287 head and neck cancer patients, Haughey *et al.* found a 14.2% prevalence of second malignant tumors with the majority presenting as metachronous lesions.[68] Based on these results, the authors emphasized aggressive follow-up to ensure detection of these lesions. A prospective study of 428 head and neck cancer patients showed improved survival when recurrence was detected with routine follow-up rather than self-referral (58 vs 32 months, $P<0.05$).[33] The necessity for surveillance of recurrent disease in the postoperative period is essential. In addition to tumor surveillance, recent literature has increasingly emphasized the importance of assessing quality of life in the postoperative period.

Laryngeal cancer and its treatment have tremendous impact on a patient's quality of life. Clinicians have long recognized the importance of survival, pain control and minimizing impairment in bodily functions, such as speech and swallowing. However, studies have recently shown the importance of body image, social acceptance and sexual function on patient satisfaction.[70,79] Disease-specific quality of life questionnaires provide much information on the outcomes of various treatment regimens. These data will help treatment planning in the future, but can also benefit the individual patient. Many of the current questionnaires will identify specific areas of dysfunction in the individual patient. The clinician can then direct treatment and counseling efforts in these specific areas.

Tumor classification

A series of rules for classifying tumors have evolved in order to describe the morphologic extent of tumor. The standardization of cancer classification has allowed for the uniform collection and reporting of cancer-related information in cancer registries. The objectives of cancer classification have been stated by the UICC and AJCC and include:

- aiding the clinician in planning treatment;
- giving some indication of prognosis;
- assisting in the evaluation of end results;
- facilitating the exchange of information between treatment centers; and
- assisting in the continuing investigation of cancer.

To investigate the reasons for and value of cancer classification one of the authors (JFP) surveyed, by mailed questionnaire, 101 physicians specializing in the care of patients with head and neck cancer.[102] Of the five stated purposes of cancer staging, assisting in the evaluation of end results was rated most important overall. However, a considerable degree of variation existed among the respondents in the rank order of importance of the five purposes.

History of classification and staging

The tumor, nodes, metastases (TNM) system for classification of malignant tumors was developed by Pierre Denoix in France between 1943 and 1952.[31a] In 1953, the International Union against Cancer (UICC) and the International Congress of Radiology, in a joint meeting, agreed upon a general technique for classification of tumors by anatomic extent of disease using the TNM system. A special TNM committee was set up and in 1958, published its first recommendations for the clinical classification of laryngeal cancers. Between 1960 and 1967, this Committee published nine brochures for classification of tumors in 23 different anatomic sites and in 1968 these were combined in a booklet *Le Livre Poche* (pocket book),[133] which has undergone a number of revisions since then in consultation with the American Joint Committee on Cancer (AJCC).

The TNM system was adopted in the USA in 1959, when the American Colleges of Surgeons and Radiology, the College of American Pathologists, the American Cancer Society and the National Cancer Institute sponsored the formation of the American Joint Committee on Cancer (AJCC) Staging and End Results Reporting. The stated purpose of the AJCC was 'to develop systems for the clinical classification of cancer which would be of value to practicing American physicians'. It published its first *Manual for Staging of Cancer* in 1977 and further editions appeared in 1983, 1988, and 1992. In 1988, the AJCC reached agreement with the UICC for a common TNM and stage classification system, thereby resolving many minor differences that prevented the creation of a single system. The AJCC *Manual for Staging of Cancer* (5th edition)[4] is now identical to the UICC TNM staging system.[77]

Present TNM system

Anatomy

The anterior limit of the larynx consists of the lingual surface of the suprahyoid epiglottis, the thyrohyoid membrane, the anterior commissure and the anterior wall of the subglottic region, which includes the thyroid cartilage, the cricothyroid membrane and the anterior arch of the cricoid cartilage. The posterior and lateral limits include the laryngeal aspect of the arytenoepiglottic folds, the arytenoid and interarytenoid regions and the posterior surface of the subglottic space, represented by the mucous membrane covering the cricoid cartilage. The superolateral limits comprise the tip and lateral borders of the epiglottis. The larynx is bounded inferiorly by a line passing through the inferior edge of the cricoid cartilage.

Table 41.1 Anatomic sites and subsites of the larynx

Site	*Subsite*
Supraglottis	Ventricular bands (false cords) Arytenoids Syprahyoid epiglottis (both lingual and laryngeal aspects) Infrahyoid epiglottis Arytenoepiglottic folds (laryngeal aspect)
Glottis	True vocal cords including anterior and posterior commissures
Sublottis	Subglottis

These definitions exclude tumors arising from the lateral or posterior pharyngeal wall, the pyriform sinus, the postcricoid area, the vallecula, and the base of tongue.

For the purposes of classification, the larynx is divided into three distinct anatomic regions: the supraglottis, the glottis and the subglottis. Until the latest editions of the AJCC and UICC manuals there still were differences in anatomic descriptions of laryngeal subsites. However, these systems are now identical in all aspects of TNM staging. The supraglottis comprises the epiglottis (both lingual and laryngeal aspects), the laryngeal aspect of the arytenoepiglottic folds, the arytenoids and false cords. A horizontal plane passing through the apex of the ventricle separates the supraglottis from the glottis. From here, the glottis extends 1 cm inferiorly to encompass the true vocal cords, including the anterior and posterior commissures. The subglottis extends from the lower boundary of the glottis to the lower margin of the cricoid cartilage. The anatomic sites and subsites of the larynx are summarized in Table 41.1.

Rules for morphologic classification

The logic of cancer classification is to develop standard criteria for morphologic extent of neoplasms across different anatomic sites. Despite the variability in clinical presentation, tumors from all sites can be classified in general terms according to the morphologic extent of tumor (T), regional nodal involvement (N) and presence of distant metastatic disease (M). Classification must be distinguished from staging, which is the grouping of tumors, with similar crude survival rates to aid in statistical analysis and reporting.

The TNM system classifies a cancer's gross morphology or macroscopic spread from primary to distant sites according to three dimensions: tumor, node and metastasis.

Tumor (T) is the extent of primary tumor, described in five categories: Tis, T1, T2, T3 and T4 (with Tis representing carcinoma in situ).

Node (N) is the extent of regional lymph node spread, described in four N categories: N0, N1, N2 and N3.

Table 41.2 Primary tumor categories (T)

TX	Primary tumor cannot be assessed
T0	No evidence of primary tumor
Tis	Carcinoma in situ
	Supraglottis
T1	Tumor limited to one site of the supraglottis with normal vocal cord mobility
T2	Tumor invades mucosa of more than one adjacent subsite of the supraglottis or glottis or region outside the supraglottis (e.g. mucosa of base of tongue, vallecula, medial wall of pyriform sinus) without fixation of the larynx
T3	Tumor limited to larynx with vocal cord fixation and/or invades any of the following: postcricoid area, pre-epiglottic tissues, deep base of tongue
T4	Tumor invades through thyroid cartilage and/or extends into soft tissues of the neck, thyroid, and/or esophagus
	Glottis
T1	Tumor limited to the vocal cord(s), which may involve the anterior or posterior commissures, with normal vocal cord mobility T1a: Tumor limited to one vocal cord T1b: Tumor involves both vocal cords
T2	Tumor extends to the supraglottis and/or subglottis and/or with impaired vocal cord mobility
T3	Tumor limited to the larynx with vocal cord fixation
T4	Tumor invades through the thyroid cartilage and/or extends to other tissues beyond the larynx
	Subglottis
T1	Tumor limited to the subglottis
T2	Tumor extends to the vocal cord(s) with normal vocal cord mobility
T3	Tumor limited to the larynx with vocal cord fixation
T4	Tumor invades through the thyroid cartilage and/or extends to other tissues beyond the larynx

Metastasis (M) is the presence of distant metastases, dichotomized as M0 (not present) or M1 (present).

Tumor categories

The definitions for the T categories for the larynx subsites, as described in the AJCC *Manual for Staging of Cancer*,[4] are shown in Table 41.2.

The general criteria for categorizing tumors of the larynx are surface spread, size of the tumor, vocal cord function and cartilage invasion. Unlike cancers of the oral cavity,[21,125] microscopic depth of invasion is not used for tumor classification of the larynx. Size of the tumor is related to the number of cancer cells, which may be related to the age of the tumor and its rate of growth.

Table 41.3 Regional lymph node categories

NX	Regional lymph nodes cannot be assessed
N0	No regional lymph node metastasis
N1	Metastasis in a single ipsilateral lymph node 3 cm or less in greatest dimension
N2	Metastasis in a single ipsilateral lymph node, more than 3 cm but less than 6 cm in greatest dimension; or in multiple ipsilateral lymph nodes, none more than 6 cm in greatest dimension; or in bilateral or contralateral lymph nodes none more than 6 cm in greatest dimension N2a: Metastasis in a single ipsilateral lymph node, more than 3 cm but less than 6 cm in greatest dimension N2b: Metastasis in multiple ipsilateral lymph nodes, none more than 6 cm in greatest dimension N2c: Metastasis in bilateral or contralateral lymph nodes none more than 6 cm in greatest dimension
N3	Metastasis in a lymph node more than 6 cm in greatest dimension

Unfortunately, the terms 'early' and 'late' are often interchanged with localized and advanced (or widespread) implying some regular progression with time. This implication erroneously leads to the idea that, left untreated, stage I progresses directly to stage II, then to stage III, etc.

Assumptions about age of tumor (i.e. 'early' or 'late') based on its size is fraught with hazard since rate of growth, cell removal or loss, and host resistance factors all impact on size of tumor.[109] The use of the term 'early cancer' should, therefore, be avoided. Instead, localized or advanced should be used since these terms accurately describe the observation of morphologic extent.

Node categories

The general criteria for the classification of regional lymph node spread is based on size, number, distribution and level of involvement (Table 41.3). Size is one of the most important criteria in node classification. It is believed that a superficial node that is >0.5 cm in diameter becomes palpable whereas a deeper node must reach 1 cm in diameter before it becomes palpable.[112]

Level of lymph node involvement is generally discussed in terms of station or echelon.[108] Station refers to a regular stopping place in a stage of progression. The first station is the cluster of lymph nodes receiving direct drainage of a specific site or organ. The second stage refers to those nodes that commonly receive lymph drainage from other lymph nodes rather than directly from the site or organ. Level of lymph node involvement has been shown to be of prognostic importance.[124,129] but is not included in the N classification.

Table 41.4 Distant metastasis categories (M)

MX	Presence of distant metastasis cannot be assessed
M0	No distant metastasis
M1	Distant metastasis

Table 41.5 Histopathologic grade (G)

GX	Grade cannot be assessed
G1	Well differentiated
G2	Moderately differentiated
G3	Poorly differentiated
G4	Undifferentiated

Metastasis categories

Metastasis is classified as present or absent, i.e. M0 or M1. When a metastatic workup has not been completed and the probability of metastasis is low, the designation MX should be used (Table 41.4).

Histopathologic grade

Although it does not form part of the staging system, it is recommended that histopathologic grade (G), using the Broders classification (Table 41.5),[18] be recorded. Other tumors of the head and neck may originate from tissues of glandular epithelium, odontogenic, lymphoid, various soft tissue, or bone and cartilage origin. Only laryngeal tumors of squamous cell origin are included in the AJCC TNM cancer staging system. Because tumors of squamous cell origin always display histopathologic differentiation, grades of G1, G2 or G3 are always used. Tumors containing areas of undifferentiation adjacent to areas of squamous differentiation are classified as poorly differentiated.

Optional descriptors

Table 41.6 shows optional descriptors but no specific recommendation for their recording is made by the AJCC or UICC.

TNM system for unified stage grouping

For each cancer, the individual T, N and M category ratings are combined in tandem to form expressions, such as T2N1M0 or T3N2M1. Because five categories of T, four categories of N, and two categories of M create 40 possible combinations for the TNM expressions, stage groupings (I, II, III and IV) are created to ease statistical analyses (Table 41.7).[1,19] The various combinations were selected based on the observation that patients with localized tumors had higher survival rates than patients with widespread tumors.

When there is no nodal involvement, the stage is determined by the extent of primary tumor. Thus, T1 = stage I; T2 = stage II; T3 = stage III; and T4 = stage IV. With nodal spread, stage is essentially determined by extent of nodal involvement. Thus N1 is classified as stage III for T1–3 and stage IV when T = 4. When N is greater than N1, then stage is stage IV.

Table 41.6 Optional descriptors

Lymphatic invasion (L)	
LX	Lymphatic invasion cannot be assessed
L0	No lymphatic invasion
L1	Lymphatic invasion
Venous invasion (V)	
VX	Venous invasion cannot be assessed
V0	No venous invasion
V1	Microscopic venous invasion
V2*	Macroscopic venous invasion
Residual tumor (R) classification†	
RX	Presence of residual tumor cannot be assessed
R0	No residual tumor
R2	Microscopic residual tumor
R3	Macroscopic residual tumor

*Macroscopic involvement of the wall of veins (with no tumor within the veins) is classified as V2.
†The absence or presence of residual tumor after treatment is described by the symbol R.

Table 41.7 Stage grouping for larynx cancer according to UICC and AJCC

Stage 0	Tis	N0	M0
Stage I	T1	N0	M0
Stage II	T2	N0	M0
Stage III	T3	N0	M0
	T1	N1	M0
	T2	N1	M0
	T3	N1	M0
Stage IVA	T4	N0	M0
	T4	N1	M0
	Any T	N2	M0
Stage IVB	Any T	N3	M0
Stage IVC	Any T	Any N	M1

Cancer statistics

Definition of starting time

A definition of the starting time or 'zero' time[40,45] forms the basis for the calculation or measurement of survival and other outcome measures. Various starting times are commonly used:

- date of diagnosis;
- date of first visit to physician or clinic;

- date of hospital admission; and
- date of treatment initiation.

If the time to recurrence of a tumor after apparent complete remission is being studied, the starting time is the date of apparent complete remission.

The most convenient starting time for studies which are evaluating treatment effectiveness is the date of first antineoplastic treatment. For untreated patients, the most comparable date is the time at which it was decided that no tumor-directed treatment would be given. For both treated and untreated laryngeal cancer patients, the above times from which survival rates are calculated will usually coincide with the date of the initial staging of cancer.

Classifications of treatment

The classification of treatment for laryngeal cancer is based on the type, timing and sequence of treatment. The extraction of this data from the medical record has been carefully and completely described elsewhere.[43,45–47] Treatment modalities include surgery, radiotherapy and chemotherapy. Within each treatment type, subtypes can be easily defined (i.e. supraglottic laryngectomy is a specific type of surgical treatment, brachytherapy is a specific form of radiotherapy, and methotrexate therapy is a type of chemotherapy). Treatment timing can be defined as initial or subsequent and treatments can be used singly or in combination. Initial treatment refers to the first course of antineoplastic therapy. Initial therapy can be either single or combination. Subsequent treatment is any treatment used after initial treatment and initiated as a result of persistence, recurrence, or some other clinical aspect in the tumor. Using this classification, therapy which included surgery and postoperative radiotherapy could be classified either as initial combination therapy or initial surgery and subsequent radiotherapy depending on the clinical scenario. In the first scenario, surgery and postoperative radiotherapy are classified as initial combination therapy when the decision to use radiotherapy was made prior to surgery. In the second scenario, postoperative radiotherapy is classified as subsequent therapy when the decision to use radiotherapy was made after surgery and as a result of findings at surgery (i.e. tumor too extensive for complete removal or extracapsular lymph node spread of tumor).

Classification of staging times

The following rules for classification are recommended by the AJCC and UICC. Five classification times, clinical, pathologic, retreatment, autopsy and surgical, are described for each site.

Clinical classification (cTNM or just TNM)

This classification is based on evidence acquired before treatment. Such evidence arises from physical examination, imaging, endoscopy, biopsy and other relevant findings. In other words, all information available prior to the first definitive treatment is used.

Pathologic classification (pTNM)

Pathologic classification is based on the evidence acquired before treatment, supplemented or modified by the additional evidence acquired from pathologic examination of a resected specimen.

Retreatment classification (rTNM)

Retreatment classification is used after a disease-free interval and when further definitive treatment is planned. All information available at the time of retreatment should be used in determining the stage of the recurrent tumor or new primary.

Autopsy classification (aTNM)

If classification of a cancer is done after the death of a patient and a postmortem examination has been done, all pathologic information should be used.

Surgical classification (sTNM)

A fifth classification, based on examination of the tumor during surgical exploration or surgical treatment is sometimes used.[52]

Description of outcome

Vital status

The post-zero-time vital status for each patient can be classified as alive, dead, or unknown (i.e. lost to follow-up). Survival time is the time from the starting point to the terminal event, to the end of the study, or to the date of last observation. Vital status at survival time can be further described as:

- alive – tumor-free; no recurrence;
- alive – tumor-free; after recurrence;
- alive with persistent, recurrent, or metastatic disease;
- alive with primary tumor;
- dead – tumor-free;
- dead – with cancer (primary, recurrent, or metastatic disease);
- dead – postoperative; and
- unknown – lost to follow-up.

Completeness of follow-up is crucial in any study of survival time.

Calculation of survival rates

The survival rate is the primary outcome measure in cancer statistics. There are several ways to measure survival rates.[37]

Direct method

The simplest procedure for summarizing patient survival is to calculate the percentage of patients alive at the end of a specified interval, such as 5 years.

Actuarial or life-table method

This method provides a means for using all follow-up information accumulated up to the closing date of the study. This method also provides information on the pattern of survival or the manner in which deaths reduce the patient group size during the total period of observation.

Observed survival rate

The observed survival rate accounts for all deaths, regardless of cause, and is a true reflection of total mortality.

Adjusted survival rate

The adjusted survival rate is the proportion of the initial patient group that escaped death due to cancer if all other causes of death were not operating. The use of adjusted survival rate is particularly important in comparing patient groups that may differ with respect to factors such as sex, age, race and socioeconomic status.

Relative survival rate

The relative survival rate is the ratio of the observed survival rate to the expected rate for a group of people in the general population similar with respect to sex, age, race and the calendar period of observation.

Quality of life

Although survival rate is the standard outcome measure in oncology, it does not capture the essence of clinical practice and human illness.[91,92] Important information collected in daily practice includes patient-based measures of symptoms, functional capacity, social and emotional consequences of disease and its treatment, and satisfaction with care.[41] A hierarchical definition of patient outcome has been described by Fries and Spitz.[55] In this arrangement, mortality and morbidity form the first two levels of description of patient outcome. The next level of patient outcome is described by the health status of the patient.

Health status can be described by the physical, functional and emotional limitations experienced by an individual.[69,75] Health-related quality of life (HRQOL) represents the fourth level of patient outcome. A definition of HRQOL on which all patients, physicians and researchers can agree may be impossible to obtain. However, during the past decade sufficient research has been conducted over a wide range of conditions and by a large number of investigators that a common core description of HRQOL may now be possible.[5,65] Health-related quality of life includes a suitable description of the health status of the patient and the value, importance, or utility, placed on that condition by the patient.[31] Patient satisfaction with medical care is viewed as the final level or feature of patient outcome.

Cost

Patient outcomes may also be described in terms of the resources utilized or monies spent to obtain a certain health outcome state.[132] There are three different dimensions in which to consider economic analysis of medical care:

- type of analysis;
- point of view; and
- types of costs and benefits.[36]

The three types of analyses are cost-identification, cost-effectiveness and cost-benefit. There are four points of view associated with economic analysis: provider, payer, patient and society. The four types of costs and benefits are direct medical, direct nonmedical, indirect morbidity and mortality, and intangible.

Problems with the present classification system for cancer

Many problems and weaknesses of the current cancer staging system have been identified.[9,42,78,102,110,119] These problems can be classified as to whether they describe problems with the current TNM system or problems relevant to cancer staging overall. Proposals for improvements for each of these problems are suggested below.

Problems with the current TNM system

Definition criteria

The most important problems with the current TNM system arise from ambiguity and variability of the actual definitions for the various T, N and M categories. More explicit definitions and criteria need to be created to reduce ambiguity that prevents the standardized collection of tumor information. Specifically, improved definitions are needed for the T definitions for supraglottic and glottic tumors and vocal cord function.[102] For example, cord fixation mandates a T3 classification, regardless of whether the primary site is supraglottis, glottis, or subglottis. Obviously, a supraglottic or subglottic tumor that causes cord fixation is more advanced than a glottic tumor. Thus T3 tumors across subsites are not of equal anatomic extent.

New definitions with explicit criteria should be created for other morphologic characteristics, such as exophytic and endophytic, depth of invasion, and microscopic

Table 41.8 Certainty (C) factor definitions

C1	Evidence from standard diagnostic means – e.g. inspection, palpation and standard radiography, intraluminal endoscopy for tumors of certain organs
C2	Evidence obtained by special diagnostic means – e.g. radiographic imaging in special projections, tomography (CT), ultrasonography, lymphography, angiography; scintigraphy; magnetic resonance imaging (MRI); endoscopy, biopsy, and cytology
C3	Evidence from surgical exploration, including biopsy and cytology
C4	Evidence of the extent of disease following definitive surgery and pathologic examination of the resected specimen
C5	Evidence from autopsy

Example: degrees of C may be applied to the T, N and M categories. A case might be described as T3C2, N2C1, M0C2.

characteristics of the tumor border for excised tumors. For patients with clinically positive regional neck disease, criteria for the classification of clinical nodal disease should include size of largest node, quality of nodal disease (e.g. soft, mobile, firm, immobile, matted, etc.), and neck level of furthest node from primary tumor. The five level nodal classification system described by Suen and Goepfert[131] and used at the Memorial Sloan-Kettering Cancer Center[115] could be used for this purpose. Microscopic pathologic examination of nodal disease should also report status of node capsule (e.g. intact or capsule breached).

Staging methods

As discussed above, multiple procedures are available for the classification of laryngeal tumors. Whilst it is well recognized that the validity of any classification system depends on the diagnostic methods used,[120] no specific recommendations on what these methods should be to ensure consistent and accurate classification have been given by the AJCC. The UICC, however, does address this issue with the C-factor, or certainty factor.[76] This reflects the validity of classification according to the diagnostic methods employed. The C-factor definitions, which are optional descriptors, are shown in Table 41.8. As can be seen, C1, C2 and C3 refer to the cTNM and specify further how classification was performed, whereas C4 is equivalent to pTNM.

Stage groupings

The original and current stage groupings were created based on presumed prognosis.[1] No prospective, multivariate analysis was performed to create the four stage groupings from the various combinations of T, N and M. The grouping together of the various T, N and M combinations into stages was thought by many of the respondents in the previously described survey[102] to be inconsistent and biologically inaccurate. For example, one major shortcoming of the stage groupings is the combination of patients with no regional disease (e.g. T3N0), with those who have nodal disease (e.g. T1N1, T2N1, or T3N1). New stage groupings, based on multivariate studies of the relative impact of the T, N and M categories should be undertaken.

One system, referred to as the Tumor and Node Integer System (TANIS), calculates the stage grouping by adding the T, N and M values. This system was shown to have a statistically significant association with survival for patients with squamous cell tumors of the oral cavity.[122]

Observer variability

Observer variability and measurement error can create significant problems with the use of a staging system. For instance, in a retrospective medical record review of outcomes for 193 patients with laryngeal carcinoma, one of the authors (JFP) identified 44 examples of two or more physicians staging the same patients differently.[104] Through education and establishment of 'Validated TNM Physician' programs, observer variability may be reduced. These educational training sessions could utilize videotapes demonstrating cancers in various head and neck sites and demonstration neck mannequins to aid in the examination and estimation of size and character of various regional nodal presentations.

Inclusion of CT/MRI scans

The proper role and criteria for sophisticated roentgenographic and other imaging techniques in the anatomic staging of patients is not clear and this ambiguity creates further problems with the current system. More clinical studies need to be conducted to examine the relative prognostic impact of these studies on classification and therapeutic decisions.

Stage migration

The change in stage grouping of a patient because of inclusion of additional diagnostic information is referred to as stage migration. Stage migration can occur whenever the diagnostic data used to assign disease stages are different for compared patient groups.[50] The situation most commonly arises when advances in diagnostic technology can be applied only to relatively recent groups of patients. Because the sensitive new methods can identify 'silent' or 'subclinical' tumor spread that would have been previously undetected, the new technological data allow patients in the more recent cohort with silent spread to 'migrate' or 'shift' from localized stages with generally good prognoses (i.e. TNM stages I and II) into advanced stages with generally worse prognoses (i.e. TNM stages III and IV).[101]

Table 41.9 Effects of stage migration on 6-month survival rates in lung cancer

Old-data TNM stage (1953–64)*	*Stage migration*	*New-data TNM stage* (1977)*
I: 32/42 (76)	I: 22/24 (92)	I: 22/24 (92)
	II: 1/1 (100)	
	III: 9/17 (53)	
II: 17/25 (68)	II: 12/17 (71)	II: 13/18 (72)
	III: 5/8 (63)	
III: 23/64 (36)	III: 23/64 (36)	III: 37/89 (42)
Total 72/131 (55)	Total 72/131 (55)	Total 72/131 (55)

*TNM denotes tumor, nodes, metastases. Values are numbers of patients, with percentages in parentheses.
Reproduced with permission from Feinstein AR, Sosin DM, Wells CK. The Will Rogers phenomenon. Stage migration and new diagnostic techniques as a source of misleading statistics for survival in cancer. *N Engl J Med* 1985; **312:** 1604–8. [50]

To better illustrate this phenomenon, consider the 131 patients with lung cancer studied by Feinstein *et al.*[50] Patients in this study were classified by TNM in two different ways. The first used only clinical examination and results of simple laboratory tests. In the second method, results from recently developed radiological investigations, such as CT, liver–spleen scanning and abdominal ultrasound were also used. With the improved diagnostic capability of the more recently developed tests, more advanced disease was diagnosed. Patients therefore migrated from a lower TNM stage to a higher stage with the addition of new diagnostic methods. The effects of this migration are shown in Table 41.9.

The table gives the 6-month survival rates for the same cohort of patients using the different classification criteria. The middle column identifies those patients who migrated because of the greater ability of the newer classification techniques to detect covert disease. As can be seen, patients migrate to higher TNM stages as the result of the advanced technology, causing a rise in the survival rate for each individual TNM stage, but the overall survival rate remains the same.

Another example of stage migration can be seen with the addition of CT scanning to the diagnostic workup of patients with glottic tumors. Consider a patient with a small glottic tumor involving the anterior commissure, as determined on endoscopy, and no nodal disease. This tumor will be classified as a T1 tumor and stage I disease. However, there may be cartilage invasion detectable only by CT scanning. By showing thyroid cartilage invasion, CT scanning changes the classification of this tumor from T1 to T4 and changes the stage classification from I to IV. Similarly stage II and III patients may also be upstaged or migrate after more advanced disease is demonstrated by CT. The net result of this migration is that the survival rates rise within each stage, because the patients 'migrating' represent a more morphologically advanced subset of the group they are leaving yet a less advanced subset of the group they are joining. The survival rate for the overall cohort remains the same since there is only movement of individual patients between stages. Thus, comparison of survival rates between two temporally distinct cohorts (i.e. before and after the advent of CT scanning) may lead to false conclusions about treatment effectiveness.

This stage migration is also known as the Will Rogers phenomenon.[50] This is in reference to a comment made by the American humorist, who, when reflecting on the geographic migration in the USA during the economic depression of the 1930s, said: 'When the Okies left Oklahoma and moved to California, they raised the average intelligence level in both states.'

Problems relevant to cancer staging overall

The current system fails to address other areas important to cancer description, prognosis and treatment evaluation. These areas include host- or patient-based prognostic variables and the lack of a formal mechanism to collect data on biological markers.

Exclusion of host factors

Despite an excellent description of a tumor's size and extent of anatomic spread, the TNM system does not account for the clinical biology of the cancer,[11,42] which is manifested by both the structural form of the tumor and its physiologic function in the patient. Human tumors do not necessarily or always spread in an orderly fashion.[109] Thus, the clinical biology of the tumor can not be fully described by the extent or size of the tumor alone.

The tumor's morphologic structure can be reported for gross anatomy (TNM categories) and microscopic forms (cell type, degree of differentiation, etc.), and also for biomolecular attributes (tumor markers, ploidy, etc.). The functional effects of the tumor can be described by clinical entities that create severity of illness in the patient. These functional effects are manifested by the type, duration and severity of cancer symptoms (e.g. weight loss, fatigue)[38,39,95] and the performance or functional

Table 41.10 Host performance scale

H	The physical state (performance scale) of the patient, considering all cofactors determined at the time of stage classification and subsequent follow-up examinations
H0	Normal activity
H1	Symptomatic and ambulatory; cares for self
H2	Ambulatory more than 50% of time; occasionally needs assistance
H3	Ambulatory 50% or less of the time; nursing care needed
H4	Bedridden; may need hospitalization

status of the host.[127,142] Another important aspect of clinical biology is the comorbidity of the patient who is the 'setting' in which the cancer occurs. Although unrelated to the cancer itself, the patient's concomitant disease can affect the clinical course of the cancer, as well as choice of treatment and prognosis.[27,63,113,114,139] Each aspect of the clinical features of cancer will be discussed below.

Performance status

At the time of diagnosis, a patient may have symptoms and other functional effects of the cancer that are manifested in overall performance status or physical capacity. As discussed earlier, the Karnofsky Performance Status (KPS) Scale,[82] Spitzer Quality of Life Index,[126] the Eastern Cooperative Oncology Group Scale,[143] and the Host (AJCC) scale[1] (Table 41.10) are examples of rating scales that have been used in oncology to assess a patient's functional capacity for work and for daily activities of self-care.

Prognosis for cancer patients is much better if they have ample functional capacity and can perform activities of self-care than if function and activities are impaired. The patient's performance status can affect not only prognosis, but also the choice of treatments. Patients with decreased functional capacity may be deemed 'too sick' for one treatment (e.g. surgery) and receive an alternative (e.g. irradiation). The widely cited[94] prognostic impact of the KPS can be illustrated with the observed survival results shown in Fig 41.1 for 763 patients with previously untreated larynx cancer.[127]

In Fig 41.2, the survival results are presented according to high, medium, or low KPS ratings. The results led Stell to comment:[127]

> *Performance status is a very important prognostic factor...more significant in fact than T status. Furthermore, assessment of performance status requires no technology.*

Symptoms as an index of biologic behavior

Cancer symptoms (and certain physical signs) provide important prognostic information[38,95] because they reflect some of the tumor's biologic behavior. Although a patient's symptoms are regularly noted in medical-student histories, presented at tumor boards, and used in the 'clinical judgment' of experienced clinicians, the patient's presenting symptoms are generally not cited, categorized, or analyzed in the evaluation of prognosis and therapy.

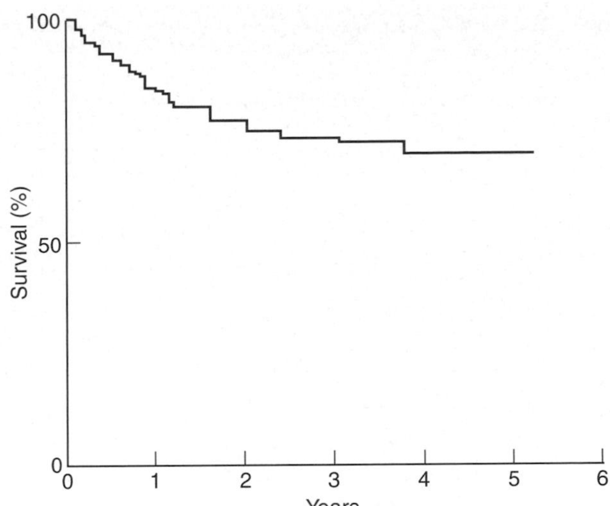

Figure 41.1 *Survival rates for 763 patients with previously untreated larynx cancer. (Reproduced with permission from Myers EN, Suen JY, eds.* Cancer of the Head and Neck, *3rd edn. Philadelphia: Saunders, 1996; adapted from Stell PM. Prognostic factors in laryngeal carcinoma.* Clin Otolaryngol *1988;* ***13:*** *399-409.[127])*

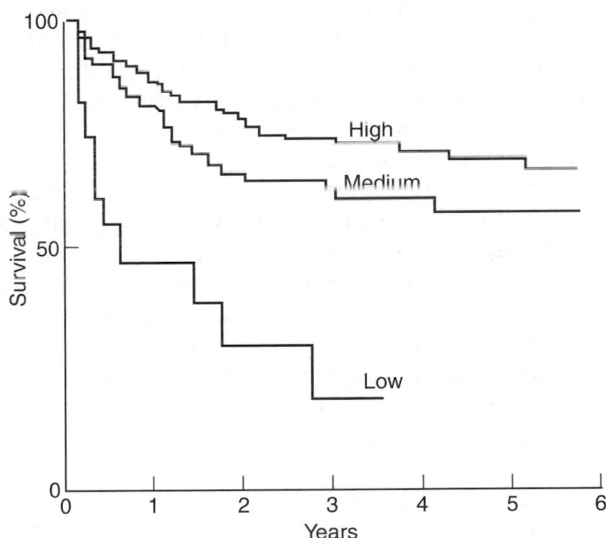

Figure 41.2 *Survival results according to performance status. (Reproduced with permission from Myers EN, Suen JY, eds.* Cancer of the Head and Neck, *3rd edn. Philadelphia: Saunders, 1996; adapted from Stell PM. Prognostic factors in laryngeal carcinoma.* Clin Otolaryngol *1988;* ***13:*** *399-409.[127])*

Table 41.11 Five-year survival rates in larynx cancer according to symptom stage

	Feinstein et al.[51] *(1977)*		*Piccirillo et al.*[104] *(1994)*		*J F Piccirillo (unpublished observations, October 1998)*	
Symptom stage	*Total patients*	*Survival rate (%)*	*Total patients*	*Survival rate (%)*	*Total patients*	*Survival rate (%)*
Primary	37/48	77	91/115	79	154/225	68
Systemic	38/68	56	30/62	48	74/144	51
Distant	21/76	28	6/16	38	16/4	734
Total	96/192	50	127/193	66	244/416	59

One main reason for the neglect of symptoms has been their variability.[41] Because tumors with similar morphologic properties can be accompanied by different symptoms, physicians have often concluded that symptoms are too subjective to merit scientific consideration. A second reason for the scientific exclusion of symptoms has been the assumed absence of a suitable taxonomy for classifying the symptoms into appropriate subgroups. This assumption is incorrect, however, because several taxonomies have been created to classify symptoms, as illustrated in the following example of the prognostic importance of symptoms.

One taxonomic system, proposed more than 25 years ago,[38] is based on the type, duration and severity of symptoms and physical signs. Symptoms and physical signs are classified as primary, systemic and distant, based on their presumed mechanism. This taxonomy has been used to show the prognostic importance of symptoms in a variety of cancers.[25,44,49] Primary symptoms are related to a tumor at its primary site. For example, symptoms such as hoarseness and voice change are classified as primary symptoms. Systemic symptoms are due to effects of the tumor away from the primary site. Weight loss and fatigue are examples of systemic symptoms. Distant symptoms, when accompanied by appropriate laboratory documentation of distant spread, imply the cancer has extended beyond its primary locus. Distant symptoms of cancer of the larynx include a tender neck mass or visual changes from invasion of the base of skull.

In a hierarchical arrangement that resembles the TNM system, patients with distant symptoms are classified as distant, regardless of the presence of primary or systemic symptoms. Patients with systemic symptoms, but no distant symptoms, are classified as systemic, regardless of the presence or absence of primary symptoms. Patients with primary symptoms alone are classified as primary. Primary symptoms can be further classified as local if they can be attributed to the tumor at the primary site (examples include hoarseness and voice change) or perilocal, which can be attributed to inflammation surrounding the tumor at its primary site (examples include throat irritation, fullness, hemoptysis and otalgia). Patients without any pertinent symptoms are classified as asymptomatic.

Table 41.11 shows the results of three studies that demonstrate the prognostic importance of symptoms in cancer of the larynx. In one study of 192 patients with cancer of the larynx,[51] the total 5-year survival was 50% (96/192), but the rates ranged from 77% (37/48) in the primary symptom stage, to 56% (38/68) in the systemic symptom stage, and 28% (21/76) in the distant symptom stage. In a later study of cancer of the larynx,[104] the total 5-year survival rate was 66% (127/193), with rates of 79% (91/115), 48% (30/62), and 38% (6/16) in the primary, systemic, and distant stages, respectively. Within the primary stage, the survival rate varied between 80% (65/81) and 76% (26/34) in the local and perilocal groups, respectively. The third set of results is from current research at Washington University. In this project, 416 patients with laryngeal cancer who received initial treatment between 1980 and 1992 were studied. The overall 5-year survival rate was 59% (244/416) with rates ranging from 68% (154/225) in the primary symptom group, to 51% (74/144) in the systemic group, to 34% (16/47) in the distant symptom group (J F Piccirillo, unpublished data, October 1998). Within the primary group, the survival rate varied between 70% (125/178) and 62% (29/47) in the local and perilocal groups, respectively. In each of these studies, the prognostic gradients described by symptoms were statistically significant, even when controlling for other known prognostic variables, including TNM stage.

To demonstrate that symptoms offer discrete prognostic information, the conjoined effects of symptom and TNM stage on 5-year survival rates are shown in Table 41.12. To maximize the sample size in each of the 16 conjoined cells, the 1994 and 1977 cohorts (Table 41.11) were combined. The marginal row and column totals give the 5-year survival rates as a function of TNM stage and symptom stage. There are clear prognostic gradients for both variables. The 5-year survival rate varies between 74% (165/222) for those with TNM stage I disease to 33% (31/95) for those with TNM stage IV disease and from 73% (190/259) for those with only local symptoms (stage 1) to 35% (22/63) for those with distant symptoms (stage 4). However, the important information of Table 41.12 is in the individual cells. Within each TNM stage, the symptom stages produce a distinctive prognostic gradient (except in those cells with small numbers of patients). For example,

Table 41.12 Five-year survival rates in conjunction with symptom and anatomic stages*

	TNM anatomic stage				
Symptom stage†	*I*	*II*	*III*	*IV*	*Total*
1	123/159 (77%)	44/62 (71%)	21/35 (60%)	2/3 (67%)	190/259 (73%)
2	16/23 (70%)	22/30 (73%)	14/22 (64%)	3/6 (50%)	55/81 (68%)
3	23/37 (62%)	29/53 (55%)	35/70 (50%)	17/46 (37%)	104/206 (50%)
4	3/3 (100%)	4/4 (100%)	6/16 (38%)	9/40 (23%)	22/63 (35%)
Total	165/222 (74%)	99/149 (66%)	76/143 (53%)	31/95 (33%)	371/609 (61%)

*Multivariate logistic regression analysis confirmed the independent significance of TNM anatomic stage ($\chi^2 = 18.1$; $P < 0.0001$) and symptom stage ($\chi^2 = 10.3$; $P = 0.0013$).
†Symptom stage: 1, local; 2, perilocal; 3, systemic; 4, distant.

Table 41.13 Charlson Weighted Index of Comorbidity

Assigned weights for each disease	*Disease*
1	Myocardial infarct Congestive heart failure Peripheral vascular disease Cerebrovascular disease Dementia Chronic pulmonary disease Connective tissue disease Ulcer disease Mild liver disease Diabetes
2	Hemiplegia Moderate or severe renal disease Diabetes with end organ damage Any tumor Leukemia
3	Lymphoma
6	Metastatic solid tumor Acquired immunodeficiency syndrome (AIDS)

The cumulative total equals the score. Example: chronic pulmonary (1) and lymphoma (2) = total score (3).
Reprinted with permission from *J Chronic Dis*, **40**, Charlson ME, Pompei P, Ales KL, MacKenzie CR, A new method of classifying prognostic comorbidity in longitudinal studies: development and validation, 373–83, 1987. Elsevier Science Inc.[24]

Table 41.14 Five-year survival rates according to Charlson Weighted Index of Comorbidity

Charlson Comorbidity Score	*5-Year survival rate (%)*
0	84/114 (74%)
1	28/43 (65%)
2	10/15 (67%)
3	2/12 (17%)
4	2/4 (50%)
5	1/1 (100%)
6	0/2 (0%)
7	0/1 (0%)
8	0/1 (0%)
Total	127/193 (66%)

χ^2 linear trend = 24.7, $P = 0.002$.

within TNM stage I, the gradient goes from 77% to 62% from symptom stage 1 to symptom stage 3, and correspondingly, in TNM stage II, from 71% to 55%. If symptoms merely reflected anatomic extent of disease, the small, localized tumors of stage I would produce only mild symptoms, while the large, extensive tumors of stage IV would produce severe symptoms. On the contrary, many patients with small tumors had severe symptoms, and those with large tumors often had only mild symptoms. Furthermore, symptoms help demarcate unique prognostic groups within TNM groups which are supposedly homogenous. Symptom severity, a reflection of the clinical biology of the tumor, may help explain why some patients in stage I do poorly and some in TNM stage IV do well.

Comorbidity

Although not a feature of the cancer itself, comorbidity is an important attribute of the patient. The concomitant disease(s) other than the cancer can strongly affect the patient's survival and also treatment options. The cancers

Table 41.15 Modified Kaplan–Feinstein comorbidity index

Cogent comorbid ailment	*Grade 3 (severe decompensation)*	*Grade 2 (moderate decompensation)*	*Grade 1 (mild decompensation)*
Hypertension	Severe or malignant; papilledema; encephalopathy; or diastolic pressure 130 mmHg or higher	Diastolic pressure 115–129 mmHg; or at any level below 130 mmHg, with sedentary cardiovascular or symptomatic effects such as headaches, vertigo, epistaxis	Diastolic pressure 90–114 mmHg, without secondary effects or symptoms
Cardiac	Within past 6 months: congestive heart failure, myocardial infarction, significant arrhythmias, or hospitalization required for angina pectoris or angina-like chest pain	Congestive heart failure more than 6 months ago; or angina pectoris not requiring hospitalization	Myocardial infarction more than 6 months ago; ECG evidence of coronary disease; or atrial fibrillation
Cerebral or psychic	Recent stroke, comatose state, or suicidal state	Old stroke, with residua; recent transient ischemic attacks; or recent episode of status epilepticus	Old stroke without residua; past transient ischemic attacks; or frequent epileptic seizures
Respiratory	Marked pulmonary insufficiency (i.e. cyanosis, CO_2 narcosis); or recurrent status asthmaticus	Moderate pulmonary insufficiency (i.e. dyspnea on slight exertion); recurrent pneumonia; or recurrent asthmatic attacks with chronic obstructive pulmonary disease	Mild pulmonary insufficiency; recent active tuberculosis; chronic lung disease manifested only on x-ray or function tests; or recurrent asthmatic attacks without underlying lung disease
Renal	Uremia; renal decompensation with secondary anemia, edema, hypertension	Azotemia, manifested by elevated BUN (>25 mg%) and/or creatinine (>3.0 mg%) without secondary effects; nephrotic syndrome; recurrent renal infections; hydronephrosis	Proteinuria (tests of 3+ or 4+ on two or more urinalyses, or excretion of >1 g on 24-hour urine collection); recurrent lower urinary infections or renal stones
Hepatic	Hepatic failure (ascites, icterus, encephalopathy); or esophageal varices	Compensated hepatic failure (cutaneous spiders, palmar erythema, hepatomegaly or other clinical evidence of chronic liver disease)	Chronic liver disease manifested on biopsy or by persistently elevated BSP (>25% retention) or bilirubin (>3 mg%)
Gastrointestinal	Recent major bleeding controlled by 6 or more units of blood transfusion	Moderate bleeding, requiring transfusion but less than 6 units of blood; recent acute pancreatitis; or chronic malabsorption syndrome	Slight bleeding, not requiring transfusion; episodes of symptomatic cholelithiasis; chronic pancreatitis; or peptic ulcer
Peripheral vascular	—	Recent amputation or gangrene of extremity	Old amputation; intermittent claudication
Malignancy	Uncontrolled	Controlled (i.e. successful previous resection or other therapy); Kaposi sarcoma	—
Locomotor impairment (regardless of cause)	Bed-to-chair existence	Moderately impaired (confined to home, nursing home, or convalescent setting)	Slightly impaired (some limitation of activity)
Alcoholism	Severely decompensated (i.e. more than one episode of delirium tremens or alcoholic seizures)	Moderately decompensated (i.e. single episode of delirium tremens or seizures); recurrent hospitalization for alcohol-associated ailments such as gastritis or pancreatitis; nutritionally caused cachexia or anemia; or significant behavior problems	Mildly decompensated (i.e. 'drinking problem'); may have bad hospitalizations for acute intoxication but no documented alcohol-associated ailments
Miscellaneous	Uncontrolled systemic 'collagen disease' (e.g. lupus erythematosus)	Controlled systemic 'collagen disease'	Recurrent epistaxis requiring transfusion; chronic active infection not specified elsewhere

Reprinted with permission from *J Chronic Dis*, **27**, Kaplan MH, Feinstein AR. The importance of classifying initial co-morbidity in evaluating the outcome of diabetes mellitus, 387–404, 1974. Elsevier Science Inc.[80]

Table 41.16 Impact of prognostic comorbidity on 5-year survival rates*

Prognostic comorbidity	*Rectum cancer*[49]	*Larynx cancer*[51]	*Endometrial cancer*[139]	*Prostate cancer*[25]	*Larynx cancer*[104]	*Larynx cancer (J F Piccirillo, unpublished data, October 1998)*
Absent	85/264 (32%)	93/172 (54%)	102/131 (78%)	137/229 (60%)	123/166 (74%)	230/376 (61%)
Present	6/54 (11%)	3/20 (15%)	3/11 (27%)	6/38 (16%)	4/27 (15%)	16/47 (34%)
Total	91/318 (29%)	96/192 (50%)	105/142 (74%)	143/267 (54%)	127/193 (66%)	246/423 (58%)
χ^2	9.76	10.94	3.54	25.41	36.27	12.6
P value	0.0018	0.0009	0.0599	<0.0001	<0.0001	<0.0001

*Denominators, number of patients in each category; numerators, corresponding number of 5-year survivors. Numbers in parentheses indicate 5-year survival rates.

for which comorbidity is particularly important are those cancers that are not rapidly fatal and that affect middle-aged or older people. The cancers where comorbidity has been shown to be important or could be expected to be important based on the above statement include: oral cavity, pharynx, larynx,[51,104] breast,[113,114] prostate,[25,27] bladder, ovary, uterus[139] and non-Hodgkin's lymphoma. Based on recent cancer incidence rates,[15] these cancers represent almost two-thirds of all adult cancers. Several comorbidity instruments have been validated and are available for use.

The Charlson Comorbidity Index[21] (Table 41.13) was created from studies of 1-year mortality for patients admitted to a medical unit of a teaching hospital. It is a weighted index that takes into account the number and seriousness of comorbid diseases. The scoring system for this instrument assigns weights of 1, 2, 3 and 6 for each of the existing comorbid diseases present at initial assessment and derives from that a total score that determines the patient's overall prognostic status. The prognostic impact of comorbidity, according to the Charlson Index, for patients with laryngeal cancer, is shown in Table 41.14. A progressive reduction in survival is seen with increasing comorbidity. This effect remains significant even after controlling for TNM stage.

Another comorbidity instrument, the Kaplan–Feinstein Comorbidity Index (KFI),[80] categorizes patients into one of four comorbidity groups. The KFI was developed from a study of the impact of comorbidity on outcomes for patients with diabetes mellitus. Specific diseases and conditions were classified according to their severity of organ decompensation:

- mild (grade 1);
- moderate (grade 2); and
- severe (grade 3) or none if no comorbidity was present.

The overall Comorbidity Severity Score (0–3) is defined by the grade of the highest ranked single ailment. One exception to this rule is in the case where two or more grade 2 ailments occur in different organ systems, in which case the patient's Comorbidity Severity Score is designated grade 3. The original KFI was modified to include diabetes and other endocrine disorders, dementia, Parkinson's disease, HIV/AIDS, peripheral vascular disease and obesity. The modified KFI form is shown in Table 41.15.

Severe comorbidity is also referred to as prognostic comorbidity. Examples of prognostic comorbidity, are significant cardiac disease, severe hypertension, far advanced tuberculosis, severe liver disease and recent severe stroke. The impact of prognostic comorbidity for four different cancers, regardless of the TNM stage of the tumor, is shown in Table 41.16. In each of the six case series, the 5-year survival rates were significantly reduced for the patients with prognostic comorbidity and significantly elevated when prognostic comorbidity was absent. For each series, the impact of prognostic comorbidity remained significant, even when other prognostic factors were considered. For instance, in cancer of the larynx,[85,104] survival rates were significantly different within TNM stages based on the presence or absence of prognostic comorbidity.

The American Society of Anesthesiologists (ASA)[111] devised a system for the collection and tabulation of statistical data to classify preoperative condition. Total operative risk depends not only on the proposed surgery and skill of the surgeon but also on the physical status of the patient. The ASA classification index was strictly limited to a definition of preoperative physical status.[107] Vacanti *et al.*[134] found that operative mortality (deaths within the first 48 postoperative hours) was significantly associated with ASA physical status category and Marx *et al.*[89] found that operative mortality (deaths within the first 7 postoperative days) was significantly related to ASA score (Table 41.17).

Consequently, the presence of comorbidity, rather than the TNM stage, may determine the selection of treatment and the patient's eventual outcome. In fact, in the previ-

Table 41.17 Mortality rates according to American Society of Anesthesiologists (ASA)

	Vacanti et al.[134]		*Marx et al.*[89]	
Physical status class	*Deaths/anesthetic procedures*	*Mortality rate (%)*	*Deaths/anesthetic procedures*	*Mortality rate (%)*
I	43/50 703	0.08	11/18 320	0.06
II	34/12 601	0.27	50/10 609	0.47
III	66/3626	1.82	168/3820	4.40
IV	66/850	7.76	252/1073	23.48
V	57/608	9.38	164/323	50.77
Total	266/68 388	0.39	645/34 145	1.89

ously cited study of larynx cancer,[104] comorbidity was prognostically more important than TNM stage. Nevertheless, comorbidity data are not currently collected or included in cancer statistics. As demonstrated in Tables 41.16 and 41.17 and in the reports previously cited, the omission continues to produce major imprecision in classification of patients, and in the subsequent interpretation of both 5-year survival rates and therapeutic effectiveness.

Reasons for the exclusion of host factors

Despite the numerous examples of the importance of patient factors to prognosis and evaluation of treatment effectiveness, these variables continue to be excluded from the standard system for cancer classification. There are multiple reasons for the exclusion of these important patient-based variables:

- belief in the exclusive importance of morphology;
- desire to avoid soft data;
- previous lack of a taxonomy for patient-based variables;
- desire to avoid multiple variables and components to a staging system; and
- desire to keep the system simple for clinical practice.[102]

Incorporation of additional prognostic variables into cancer staging system

The incorporation of additional, prognostically important variables into a cancer staging system has been regarded as a cumbersome and time-consuming activity that could impair the physician's documentation of the patient's pretherapeutic condition. Many tumor registry technicians would probably agree with the reply received from an otolaryngology professor who was asked if he thought performance status should be included in a cancer staging system: 'It is difficult enough just to get TNM reported on all patients by all physicians.'[128] The unwillingness to obtain and include important clinical information, which often requires no new technology or investigation and is readily available, is peculiarly inexplicable in an era when clinicians have been willing to order a plethora of additional laboratory and imaging tests, many of which have not been validated as useful in the care of patients.

In addition to presenting problems in data collection, the inclusion of additional prognostic variables also presents problems in data analysis. Because the TNM system is based on a 'bin' model,[19] the number of bins increases rapidly as additional prognostic variables are added. For example, if the presence or absence of prognostic comorbidity were directly added to the TNM staging system for larynx cancer, the number of bins would increase from 40 to 80 [i.e. (5T × 4N × 2M) × 2]. The inclusion of new factors in the TNM system was therefore deemed not practical. Furthermore, before the advent of computers and appropriate statistical programs, the analysis of multiple variables and the identification of independent prognostic variables were difficult. Limiting the staging system to one component – anatomic extent of tumor – was therefore a practical necessity.

Multivariable regression analyses, such as Cox's proportional-hazard method,[28] however, can now be done easily with microcomputers and independent prognostic variables can be readily identified. Independent prognostic variables are those that significantly contribute to predictions of prognosis even after controlling for other known prognostic variables. In addition to identifying the important prognostic variables, the 'output' from these analyses quantifies the relative impact (or 'weight') for each of the prognostic variables.[66] Interactions between variables can also be examined. These outputs can be used to construct clinical prediction models to estimate prognosis.[26,123] The operational rules for the clinical prediction models can then be stored in microcomputers and the myriad of important individual data can be entered to produce a prognostic estimate.[48] This multivariable regression process has obvious analytic appeal, but may not seem appealing to clinicians because of the reliance on microcomputers and 'black-box' mathematics.[103]

A different form of multivariable analysis, referred to as conjunctive consolidation[44] or targeted-cluster analysis, can be used to incorporate additional prognostic factors without relying on cryptic mathematical equations or increasing the number of bins.[44,138] In this form of analysis, a staging system is created through the combination of multiple prognostic variables, based on biologic sensibility and statistical criteria. It is the process of cross-table analysis of the conjoined effect of two clinical predictive variables on the outcome of interest. Individual conjoined cells represent a group of patients with the same attributes for the two clinical variables creating the cell. Adjacent cells are then consolidated according to both statistical and biological rules.[44] A full description of this procedure is given elsewhere.[16,62,137]

One of the most important characteristics of this type of analysis is that it allows a staging system to include multiple prognostic variables (e.g. symptom severity, prognostic comorbidity and TNM system), yet maintains a discrete number of stages (usually three or four). A second important characteristic of conjunctive consolidation is that it is an uncomplicated analytical technique that seems more relevant and meaningful to clinicians than the results of regression equations or neural networks. The use of conjunctive consolidation to create the clinical severity (CS) staging system for cancer of the larynx has been described by one of the authors (JFP) previously.[104] Data from that study is combined with data from current research at Washington University (F J Piccirillo, unpublished data, October 1998) to demonstrate how the TNM system could be expanded with the inclusion of symptom severity and prognostic comorbidity. These three variables are combined, using conjunctive consolidation, to create the Clinical Severity Staging (CS) System.

The goal of the CS staging system project was twofold:

- to demonstrate the prognostic importance of symptom severity and comorbidity; and
- to demonstrate that a composite CS staging, created by the addition of symptom severity and comorbidity to the TNM system, could substantially improve the prognostic precision of laryngeal cancer staging.

The first step in the creation of the CS system was the creation of a functional severity (FS) system. The term functional severity is used for the conjunction of symptom severity and comorbidity since this represents the functional aspects of the cancer. As seen in Table 41.18, the conjoined impact of symptom severity and comorbidity is shown. Within each category of symptom stage, the survival rates were substantially lowered when prognostic comorbidity was present. For example, patients with local (stage 1) symptoms had a 76% (181/237) 5-year survival rate without prognostic comorbidity, but this was reduced to 41% (9/22) when prognostic comorbidity was present. Because both symptom severity and prognostic comorbidity were independently important, categories of each variable were combined using the conjunctive consolidation techniques described above. Thus the eight groups generated by the conjunction between symptom stage and prognostic comorbidity, were consolidated into three composite, FS stages, labeled as alpha, beta and gamma.

Table 41.18 Five-year survival rates in conjunction with symptom severity and prognostic comorbidity stages

*Symptom stage**		*Prognostic comorbidity stage* *Absent*		*Present*	*Total*
1	Alpha	181/237 (76%)	Gamma	9/22 (41%)	190/259 (73%)
2		53/73 (73%)		2/8 (25%)	55/81 (68%)
3	Beta	96/173 (55%)		8/33 (24%)	104/206 (50%)
4		21/53 (40%)		1/10 (10%)	22/63 (35%)
Total		351/536 (65%)		20/76 (27%)	371/609 (61%)

*1, local; 2, perilocal; 3, systemic; 4, distant.
Alpha, Beta, and Gamma refer to the names of the three categories of the new composite Functional Severity Staging System.

Next, the prognostic impact of FS was examined within each TNM stage. As shown in Table 41.19, within each vertical column of TNM anatomic stage, the FS staging system defined important and consistent prognostic gradients. The 5-year survival rates ranged from 81% to 40% in stage I, from 77% to 12% in stage II, from 59% to 38% in stage III, and from 56% to 8% in stage IV.

These results demonstrate the profound prognostic heterogeneity that can exist among patients who are in the same TNM stage. The 12 categories created by the conjunction of FS and TNM stage (Table 41.19) were then consolidated to form four groups which represent the stages of the CS system as shown in Table 41.20.

Table 41.19 Five-year survival rates in conjunction with functional severity and TNM anatomic stages

Functional severity stage	*TNM anatomic stage* *I*	*II*	*III*	*IV*	*Total*
Alpha	134/166 (81%)	65/84 (77%)	30/51 (59%)	5/9 (56%)	234/310 (75%)
Beta	23/36 (64%)	32/48 (67%)	37/68 (54%)	25/74 (34%)	117/226 (52%)
Gamma	8/20 (40%)	2/17 (12%)	9/24 (38%)	1/12 (8%)	20/73 (27%)
Total	165/222 (74%)	99/149 (66%)	76/143 (53%)	31/95 (33%)	371/609 (61%)

Alpha, Beta and Gamma refer to the names of the three categories of the new composite Functional Severity Staging System as defined in Table 41.18.

Table 41.20 Five-year survival rates in conjunction with functional severity and TNM anatomic stages

Functional severity stage	*TNM anatomic stage*			
	I	*II*	*III*	*IV*
Alpha	134/166 (81%)	65/84 (77%)	30/51 (59%)	5/9 (56%)
Beta	23/36 (64%)	32/48 (67%)	37/68 (54%)	25/74 (34%)
Gamma	8/20 (40%)	2/17 (12%)	9/24 (38%)	1/12 (8%)

Stages of composite Clinical Severity Staging System (CS):

stage A; stage B; stage C; stage D.

The 5-year survival rates as a function of CS are shown in Table 41.21. As can be seen, the survival gradient was significant ($\chi^2 = 27.7$; $P < 0.001$), with an overall difference in rates between stages A and D of 49%.

The CS staging system contains the same number of stages as the TNM system (four) but incorporates two more prognostic variables. As a result, the CS produces a larger range in overall survival (49% vs. 41%) and a larger χ^2 linear trend value (91.6 vs. 54.6). The main value of conjunctive consolidation is that it allows the incorporation of additional prognostic variables (i.e. symptom severity and prognostic comorbidity) into the existing TNM staging system without increasing the number of bins exponentially. As stated by Burke and Henson,[19] '...to increase our prognostic accuracy, the current system must be enhanced by the creation of a system that contains the TNM variables as well as the new predictive variables'.

Lack of a formal mechanism to collect data on biologic markers of behavior

Tumor cell differentiation and other biologic markers of tumor behavior have been shown in a variety of studies to have prognostic importance in cancers of the head and neck.[22,29,30,60,61] Nevertheless, no agreement has been reached for the uniform collection of biologic markers of tumor behavior and reporting of survival results. Until such time, the true prognostic importance of each of these different markers will remain unknown and will prevent their inclusion into a formal staging system.

Table 41.21 Five-year survival rates in composite Clinical Severity Staging System (CS)

Stage	*Five-year survival rate*
A	134/166 (81%)
B	65/84 (77%)
C	122/203 (60%)
D	50/156 (32%)
Total	371/609 (61%)

$\chi^2 = 91.6$; $P < 0.001$.

Persistence and recurrence

The problems and suggestions for improvement of classification and staging at initial presentation also apply to patients with tumor persistence and recurrence.

Persistence of residual tumor

The residual tumor (R) classification, as described above (see Table 41.6) is an additional descriptor in tumor classification but does not affect the cTNM. It is a strong predictor of prognosis,[3] but only gives information regarding tumor status and the effects of therapy after treatment. It should only be regarded as an indicator of success of first antineoplastic therapy.

Recurrence

Patients presenting with laryngeal tumor recurrence (i.e. tumor after a clinically tumor-free period) represent a distinct group of patients who have varied outcomes depending on a number of host, tumor and treatment factors. The AJCC allows for the classification of recurrent tumors using the rTNM system. The authors attempted to use this system to classify patients with recurrent laryngeal tumors in current research at Washington University (J F Piccirillo, unpublished data, October 1998). However, in a number of situations, the rTNM system proved unusable as it failed to accurately document key information, relevant to the specific situation of recurrence. For example, normal laryngeal anatomy is essential when assessing vocal cord mobility and cannot be properly defined in a patient with a previous unilateral cordectomy. Also, local tumor recurrence causing contralateral cord fixation represents a more extensive tumor than a tumor causing ipsilateral vocal cord fixation, although both would be classified as T3, assuming no cartilage invasion. These difficulties present problems, particularly when surgery has been used as initial therapy. Previous radiotherapy will also make clinical and radiological evaluation difficult.

In current research at Washington University (J F Piccirillo, unpublished data, October 1998), the authors studied the prognostic importance of a variety of patient, tumor and treatment factors in a series of 124 patients presenting with recurrence from a treated population of 424 patients with squamous cell tumors of the larynx. The overall 2-year survival rate was 40% (49/124). Three factors were statistically significant independent predictors of survival for patients with recurrence:

Table 41.22 Two-year survival rates after recurrence as a function of significant variables

Variable	*Category*	*Patients (no.)*	*Survivors (no.)*	*Percentage*	*χ^2 linear trend*
Total		124	49	40	
TNM stage	I	35	23	66	
	II	27	12	44	$\chi^2 = 19.8$
	III	32	10	31	$P < 0.001$
	IV	30	4	13	
Extent of recurrence	Local	59	33	56	
	Regional	35	13	37	$\chi^2 = 17.7$
	Distant	30	3	10	$P < 0.001$
Initial treatment*	Surgery	25	15	60	
	Radiation	49	27	55	$\chi^2 = 22.4$
	Combined	46	7	15	$P < 0.001$

*Four patients had other treatments and are omitted.

Table 41.23 Two-year survival rates in conjunction with TNM anatomic stage and extent of recurrence

TNM stage	*Extent of recurrence*		
	Local	*Regional*	*Distant*
I	18/27 (67%)	4/6 (67%)	1/2 (50%)
II	10/18 (56%)	3/7 (43%)	0/3 (0%)
III	5/9 (56%)	4/11 (36%)	1/11 (9%)
IV	1/6 (17%)	2/11 (18%)	1/13 (8%)
Total	34/60 (57%)	13/35 (37%)	3/29 (10%)

Stages of Composite Recurrence Staging System:
stage A; stage B; stage C; stage D.

- TNM stage of the initial laryngeal tumor;
- morphological extent of recurrence (i.e. whether it was a local, regional – including loco-regional – or distant recurrence); and
- type of initial antineoplastic treatment (Table 41.22).

Both TNM stage and extent of recurrence provide independent prognostic information which is readily available for all patients with recurrence and requires no extra investigation or technology. TNM stage gives important information regarding the initial tumor, and extent of recurrence divides the morphologic presentation into three separate groups, independent of the initial tumor. To use both variables in a staging system, the two variables were combined using conjunctive consolidation as shown in Table 41.23.

The shaded areas define cells with similar survival rates for different combinations of TNM stage and extent of recurrence, forming four separate groups of a new composite staging system with distinct and statistically significantly different survival rates. In cells with small numbers, clinical judgment was also used to help allocate different combinations to new stage groups. For example, the survival rate for patients with TNM stage I and distant recurrence is 50%, which might suggest inclusion in a better survival group than group D. However, there are only two patients in this group and, because the presence of distant recurrence signifies a universally poor prognosis, it is reasonable to assign this combination of TNM stage and extent of recurrence to group D. Table 41.24 shows 2-year survival rates as a function of this new Composite Recurrence Larynx Staging System (CRLSS).

Thus, two independent variables are used to create a staging system for recurrent larynx tumors, which, because of the use of conjunctive consolidation, has only four groups instead of 12. The staging system has a range of survival of 54% (range 67–13%) and each prognostic group is more homogenous with respect to survival rate than would be the case using only one prognostic variable.

Table 41.24 Two-year survival rates by CRLSS stages

CRLSS stage	*2-Year survival rate*
A	22/33 (67%)
B	15/27 (56%)
C	7/18 (39%)
D	6/46 (13%)
Total	50/124 (40%)

$\chi^2 = 40.1$; $P < 0.001$.

Further work may lead to refinements in this staging system. Obviously, validation is an important issue and testing in another setting is necessary before the CRLSS is deemed accurate and clinically useful to practicing Otolaryngologists. Research is presently underway at Washington University to prospectively validate the CRLSS. With no workable staging system presently available for patients presenting with laryngeal recurrence, the CRLSS may be a valuable tool to aid both patient and physician when planning treatment. As a simple, accurate and effective method to describe patients presenting with recurrence, it allows consistent exchange of information on similar patient groups between different treatment centers.

The future

With advances in technology and increased ease in both collection of and accessibility to information from many different sources (e.g. medical records, radiology, pathology, etc.), classification and staging procedures will become more sophisticated. The new systems must describe not only the morphologic extent of tumor (as with the present TNM system), but also include other variables with independent prognostic significance. The new systems may take the form of an AJCC-type manual with specific directions for each tumor site. A more likely system, in the authors' opinion, would be a series of computer software staging packages that cannot only give estimates of prognosis, but can also give an indication of the accuracy of those estimates based on the amount of information used to generate them.

Conclusions

Patients with laryngeal cancers present a significant challenge to health care professionals. Because of the anatomic complexity of the head and neck, the various treatment options available, and the functional limitations resulting from treatment, the initial evaluation, treatment and follow-up of the patient with laryngeal cancer requires a multidisciplinary team approach. When excellence in delivery of treatment is coupled with complete and valid assessments of extent of disease, severity of illness, psychosocial situation and patient preference, successful outcomes can usually be achieved.

The AJCC/UICC TNM system is an excellent method for the classification of extent of tumor. Nevertheless, other features of the patient with laryngeal cancer are important for prognosis, treatment selection and evaluation of therapeutic effectiveness. Improvements in the management of patients with head and neck cancer will result from improvements in their evaluation, classification and treatment. Many improvements in the evaluation and classification are possible by the incorporation of currently available information without the need for any additional investigation or new technology. What is needed is the recognition of the importance of this information and its formal acceptance and incorporation into the present methods of classification and staging of laryngeal tumors.

References

1. American Joint Committee on Cancer. *Manual for Staging of Cancer*, 2nd edn. Philadelphia: JB Lippincott, 1983.
2. American Joint Committee on Cancer. Beahrs OH, Henson DE, Hutter RVP, Myers MH, eds. *Manual for Staging of Cancer*, 3rd edn. Philadelphia: JB Lippincott, 1988.
3. American Joint Committee on Cancer. Beahrs OH, Henson DE, Hutter RVP, Kennedy BJ, eds. *Manual for Staging of Cancer*, 4th edn. Philadelphia: JB Lippincott, 1992.
4. American Joint Committee on Cancer. Fleming ID, Cooper JS, Henson DE *et al.*, eds. *Manual for Staging of Cancer*, 5th edn. Philadelphia: Lippincott-Raven, 1997.
5. Anonymous. The Portugal Conference. Measuring quality of life and functional status in clinical and epidemiological research. Proceedings. *J Chronic Dis* 1987; **40:** 459–650.
6. Anzai Y, Carroll WR, Quint DJ *et al.* Recurrence of head and neck cancer after surgery or irradiation: prospective comparison of 2-deoxy-2-[F-18]fluoro-D-glucose PET and MR imaging diagnoses. *Radiology* 1996; **200:** 135–41.
7. Archer CR, Sagel SS, Yeager VL, Martin S, Friedman WH. Staging of carcinoma of the larynx: comparative accuracy of CT and laryngography. *Am J Roentgenol* 1981; **136:** 571–5.
8. Bailet JW, Abemayor E, Jabour BA, Hawkins RA, Ho C, Ward PH. Positron emission tomography: a new, precise imaging modality for detection of primary head and neck tumors and assessment of cervical adenopathy. *Laryngoscope* 1992; **102:** 281–8.
9. Bailey BJ. Beyond the 'new' TNM classification. *Arch Otolaryngol Head Neck Surg* 1991; **117:** 369–70.
10. Barnes L. Pathology of the head and neck: general considerations. In: Myers EN, Suen JY, eds. *Cancer of the Head and Neck*, 3rd edn. Philadelphia: Saunders, 1996: 17–32.
11. Barr LC, Baum M. Time to abandon TNM staging of breast cancer? *Lancet* 1992; **339:** 915–17.
12. Bastian RW, Collins SL, Kaniff T, Matz GJ. Indirect videolaryngoscopy versus direct endoscopy for larynx and pharynx cancer staging. Toward elimination of preliminary direct laryngoscopy. *Ann Otol Rhinol Laryngol* 1989; **98:** 693–8.
13. Becker M, Zbaren P, Laeng H, Stoupis C, Porcellini B, Vock P. Neoplastic invasion of the laryngeal cartilage: comparison of MR imaging and CT with histopathologic correlation. *Radiology* 1995; **194:** 661–9.
14. Benninger MS, Enrique RR, Nichols RD. Symptom-directed selective endoscopy and cost containment for evaluation of head and neck cancer. *Head Neck* 1993; **15:** 532–6.
15. Boring CC, Squires TS, Tong T, Montgomery S. Cancer statistics, 1994. *CA Cancer J Clin* 1994; **44:** 7–26.
16. Breiman L, Freidman JH, Olshen RA, Stone CJ. *Classification and Regression Trees*. Blemont: Wadsworth International Group, 1984.
17. Breitbart W, Holland J. Psychosocial aspects of head and neck cancer. *Semin Oncol* 1988; **15:** 61–9.
18. Broders AC. The grading of carcinoma. *Minn Med* 1925; **8:** 726–30.
19. Burke HB, Henson DE. The American Joint Committee on Cancer. Criteria for prognostic factors and for an enhanced prognostic system. *Cancer* 1993; **72:** 3131–5.
20. Calhoun KH, Fulmer P, Weiss R, Hokanson JA. Distant metastases from head and neck squamous cell carcinomas. *Laryngoscope* 1994; **104:** 1199–205.
21. Cancer Registries Amendment Act of 1992. 42 USC. 201. 1992.
22. Carey TE, Kimmel KA, Schwartz DR, Richter DE, Baker SR, Krause CJ. Antibodies to human squamous cell carcinoma. *Otolaryngol Head Neck Surg* 1983; **91:** 482–91.

23. Castelijns JA, van den Brekel MWM, Niekoop VA, Snow GB. Imaging of the larynx. *Neuroimaging Clin North Am* 1996; **6:** 401–15.
24. Charlson ME, Pompei P, Ales KL, MacKenzie CR. A new method of classifying prognostic comorbidity in longitudinal studies: development and validation. *J Chronic Dis* 1987; **40:** 373–83.
25. Clemens JD, Feinstein AR, Holabird N, Cartwright S. A new clinical-anatomic staging system for evaluating prognosis and treatment of prostatic cancer. *J Chronic Dis* 1986; **39:** 913–28.
26. Concato J, Feinstein AR, Holford TR. The risk of determining risk with multivariable models. *Ann Intern Med* 1993; **118:** 201–10.
27. Concato J, Horwitz RI, Feinstein AR, Elmore JG, Schiff SF. Problems of comorbidity in mortality after prostatectomy. *JAMA* 1992; **267:** 1077–82.
28. Cox DR. Regression methods and life tables (with discussion). *J R Stat Soc B* 1972; **34:** 187–220.
29. Crissman JD. Tumor–host interactions as prognostic factors in the histologic assessment of carcinomas. *Pathol Annu* 1986; **21:** 29–52.
30. Crissman JD, Liu WY, Gluckman JL, Cummings G. Prognostic value of histopathologic parameters in squamous cell carcinoma of the oropharynx. *Cancer* 1984; **54:** 2995–3001.
31. De Haes JCJM, van Knippenberg FCE. Quality of life of cancer patients: review of the literature. In: Aaronson NK, Beckmann J, eds. *The Quality of Life of Cancer Patients.* New York: Raven Press, 1987: 167–82.
31a. Denoix PF, Schwartz D. Regeles generales de classification des cancers et de presentation des resultats therapeutics. *Acad Chir (Paris)* 1959; **85:** 115–21.
32. Derogatis LR, Morrow GR, Fetting J *et al.* The prevalence of psychiatric disorders among cancer patients. *JAMA* 1983; **249:** 751–7.
33. De Visscher AV, Manni JJ. Routine long-term follow-up in patients treated with curative intent for squamous cell carcinoma of the larynx, pharynx, and oral cavity. Does it make sense? *Arch Otolaryngol Head Neck Surg* 1994; **120:** 934–9.
34. Dillon WP, Harnsberger HR. The impact of radiologic imaging on staging of cancer of the head and neck. *Semin Oncol* 1991; **18:** 64–79.
35. Dudrick SJ, O'Donnell JJ, Weinmann-Winkler S. Nutritional management of head and neck tumor patients. In: Thawley SE, Panje WR, eds. *Comprehensive Management of Head and Neck Tumors.* Philadelphia: Saunders, 1987: 14–24.
36. Eisenberg JM. Clinical economics. A guide to the economic analysis of clinical practices. *JAMA* 1989; **262:** 2879–86.
37. Entrom JE, Austin DF. Interpreting cancer survival rates. *Science* 1977; **195:** 847–51.
38. Feinstein AR. Symptoms as an index of biological behaviour and prognosis in human cancer. *Nature* 1966; **209:** 241–5.
39. Feinstein AR. A new staging system for cancer and a reappraisal of 'early' treatment and 'cure' by radical surgery. *N Engl J Med* 1968; **279:** 747–53.
40. Feinstein AR. *Clinical Judgment.* Melbourne: Krieger, 1974.
41. Feinstein AR. Clinical biostatistics. XLI. Hard science, soft data, and the challenges of choosing clinical variables in research. *Clin Pharmacol Ther* 1977; **22:** 485–98.
42. Feinstein AR. On classifying cancers while treating patients. *Arch Intern Med* 1985; **145:** 1789–91.
43. Feinstein AR, Spitz H. The epidemiology of cancer therapy. I. Clinical problems of statistical surveys. *Arch Intern Med* 1969; **123:** 171–86.
44. Feinstein AR, Wells CK. A clinical-severity staging system for patients with lung cancer. *Medicine* 1990; **69:** 1–33.
45. Feinstein AR, Pritchett JA, Schimpff CR. The epidemiology of cancer therapy. II. The clinical course: data, decisions, and temporal demarcations. *Arch Intern Med* 1969; **123:** 323–44.
46. Feinstein AR, Pritchett JA, Schimpff CR. The epidemiology of cancer therapy. III. The management of imperfect data. *Arch Intern Med* 1969; **123:** 448–61.
47. Feinstein AR, Pritchett JA, Schimpff CR. The epidemiology of cancer therapy. IV. The extraction of data from medical records. *Arch Intern Med* 1969; **123:** 571–90.
48. Feinstein AR, Rubinstein JF, Ramshaw WA. Estimating prognosis with the aid of a conversational-mode computer program. *Ann Intern Med* 1972; **76:** 911–21.
49. Feinstein AR, Schimpff CR, Hull EW. A reappraisal of staging and therapy for patients with cancer of the rectum. II. Patterns of presentation and outcome of treatment. *Arch Intern Med* 1975; **135:** 1454–62.
50. Feinstein AR, Sosin DM, Wells CK. The Will Rogers phenomenon. Stage migration and new diagnostic techniques as a source of misleading statistics for survival in cancer. *N Engl J Med* 1985; **312:** 1604–8.
51. Feinstein AR, Schimpff CR, Andrews JFJ, Wells CK. Cancer of the larynx: a new staging system and a re-appraisal of prognosis and treatment. *J Chronic Dis* 1977; **30:** 277–305.
52. Ferlito A, Harrison DFN, Bailey BJ, DeSanto LW. Are clinical classifications for laryngeal cancer satisfactory? *Ann Otol Rhinol Laryngol* 1995; **104:** 741–7.
53. Fletcher JP, Little JM, Guest PK. A comparison of serum transferrin and serum prealbumin as nutritional parameters. *JPEN J Parenter Enteral Nutr* 1987; **11:** 144–7.
54. Flynn MB, Leightty FF. Preoperative outpatient nutritional support of patients with squamous cancer of the upper aerodigestive tract. *Am J Surg* 1987; **154:** 359–62.
55. Fries JF, Spitz PW. The hierarchy of patient outcome. In: Spilker B, ed. *Quality of Life Assessments in Clinical Trials.* New York: Raven Press, 1990: 25–35.
56. Gaffney RJ, Viani L, McShane DP. B-mode ultrasound demonstration of non-luminal carotid artery invasion by tumour. *J Laryngol Otol* 1992; **106:** 73–4.
57. Gamba A, Romano M, Grosso IM *et al.* Psychosocial adjustment of patients surgically treated for head and neck cancer. *Head Neck* 1992; **14:** 218–23.
58. Gates GA, Painter C. Objective assessment of laryngeal function. In: Cummings CW, Fredrickson JM, Krause CJ, Harker LA, Schuller DE, eds. *Otolaryngology – Head and Neck Surgery.* Update II. Vol. 1. St Louis: Mosby Year Book, 1990: 3–9.
59. Gibson S, Wenig BL. Percutaneous endoscopic gastrostomy in the management of head and neck carcinoma. *Laryngoscope* 1992; **102:** 977–80.

60. Goldsmith MM, Cresson DH, Askin FB. The prognostic significance of stromal eosinophilia in head and neck cancer. *Otolaryngol Head Neck Surg* 1987; **96:** 319–24.
61. Goldsmith MM, Cresson DH, Arnold LA, Postma DS, Askin FB, Pillsbury HC. DNA flow cytometry as a prognostic indicator in head and neck cancer. *Otolaryngol Head Neck Surg* 1987; **96:** 307–18.
62. Gordon T. Editorial: hazards in the use of the logistic function with special reference to data from prospective cardiovascular studies. *J Chronic Dis* 1974; **27:** 97–102.
63. Greenfield S, Aronow HU, Elashoff RM, Watanbe D. Flaws in mortality data. The hazards of ignoring comorbid disease. *JAMA* 1988; **260:** 2253–5.
64. Grevers G, Balzer JO, Vogl TJ. Magnetic resonance angiography: a new procedure for vascular imaging in the area of the head-neck. *Laryngorhinootologie* 1993; **72:** 116–24.
65. Guyatt G, Feeny D, Patrick D. Issues in quality of life measurement in clinical trials. *Controlled Clin Trials* 1991; **12:** S81–90.
66. Harrell FE Jr, Lee KL, Matchar DB, Reichert TA. Regression models for prognostic prediction: advantages, problems, and suggested solutions. *Cancer Treat Res* 1985; **69:** 1071–7.
67. Hassan SJ, Weymuller EA Jr. Assessment of quality of life in head and neck cancer patients. *Head Neck* 1993; **15:** 485–96.
68. Haughey BH, Gates GA, Arfken CL, Harvey J. Meta-analysis of second malignant tumors in head and neck cancer: the case for an endoscopic screening protocol. *Ann Otol Rhinol Laryngol* 1992; **101:** 105–12.
69. *Healthy People 2000.* U.S. Department of Health and Human Services Publication DHHS 91–50212. Washington, DC: Public Health Service, 1991.
70. Hess M, Kugler J, Kalveram KT, Vosteen KH. The effect of functional impairments and autonomic symptoms on the quality of life after the therapy of tumors in the ENT area. *Laryngorhinootologie* 1990; **69:** 647–52.
71. Hooley R, Levine H, Flores TC, Wheeler T, Steiger E. Predicting postoperative head and neck complications using nutritional assessment. The prognostic nutritional index. *Arch Otolaryngol* 1983; **109:** 83–5.
72. Hoover LA, Calcaterra TC, Walter GA, Larrson SG. Preoperative CT scan evaluation for laryngeal carcinoma: correlation with pathological findings. *Laryngoscope* 1984; **94:** 310–15.
73. Hordijk GJ, Bruggink T, Ravasz LA. Panendoscopy: a valuable procedure? *Otolaryngol Head Neck Surg* 1989; **101:** 426–8.
74. Ina H, Shibuya H, Ohashi I, Kitagawa M. The frequency of a concomitant early esophageal cancer in male patients with oral and oropharyngeal cancer. Screening results using Lugol dye endoscopy. *Cancer* 1994; **73:** 2038–41.
75. Institute of Medicine. *Disability in America. Toward a National Agenda for Prevention.* Washington, DC: National Academy Press, 1991.
76. International Union Against Cancer. Hermanek P, Sobin LH, eds. *TNM Classification of Malignant Tumours*, 4th edn. Berlin: Springer-Verlag, 1992.
77. International Union Against Cancer. Sobin LH, Wittekind C, eds. *TNM Classification of Malignant Tumours*, 5th edn. New York: Wiley, 1997.
78. Jacobs CD. Biophysiology of antineoplastic chemotherapy for head and neck cancer. In: Cummings CW, Fredrickson JM, Harker LA, Krause CJ, Schuller DE, eds. *Otolaryngology – Head and Neck Surgery*, Vol. 4. St Louis: Mosby, 1986: 51–72.
79. Jones E, Lund VJ, Howard DJ, Greenberg MP, McCarthy M. Quality of life of patients treated surgically for head and neck cancer. *J Laryngol Otol* 1992; **106:** 238–42.
80. Kaplan MH, Feinstein AR. The importance of classifying initial co-morbidity in evaluating the outcome of diabetes mellitus. *J Chronic Dis* 1974; **27:** 387–404.
81. Karayianis SL, Francisco GJ, Schumann GB. Clinical utility of head and neck aspiration cytology. *Diagn Cytopathol* 1988; **4:** 187–92.
82. Karnofsky DA, Abelmann WH, Craver LF, Burchenal JH. The use of the nitrogen mustards in the palliative treatment of carcinoma. *Cancer* 1948; **1:** 634–56.
83. Katsantonis GP, Archer CR, Rosenblum BN, Yeager VL, Friedman WH. The degree to which accuracy of preoperative staging of laryngeal carcinoma has been enhanced by computed tomography. *Otolaryngol Head Neck Surg* 1986; **95:** 52–62.
84. Kazkayasi M, Onder T, Ozkaptan Y, Can C, Pabuscu Y. Comparison of preoperative computed tomographic findings with postoperative histopathological findings in laryngeal cancers. *Eur Arch Otorhinolaryngol* 1995; **252:** 325–31.
85. Lancer JM, Moir AA. The flexible fibreoptic rhinolaryngoscope. *J Laryngol Otol* 1985; **99:** 767–70.
86. Langman AW, Kaplan MJ, Dillon WP, Gooding GA. Radiologic assessment of tumor and the carotid artery: correlation of magnetic resonance imaging, ultrasound, and computed tomography with surgical findings. *Head Neck* 1989; **11:** 443–9.
87. Lucente FE, Strain JJ, Wyatt DA. Psychological problems of the patient with head and neck cancer. In: Thawley SE, Panje WR, eds. *Comprehensive Management of Head and Neck Tumors.* Philadelphia: Saunders, 1987: 69–78.
88. Marchant FE, Lowry LD, Moffitt JJ, Sabbagh R. Current national trends in the posttreatment follow-up of patients with squamous cell carcinoma of the head and neck. *Am J Otolaryngol* 1993; **14:** 88–93.
89. Marx GF, Mateo CV, Orkin LR. Computer analysis of postanesthetic deaths. *Anesthesiology* 1973; **39:** 54–8.
90. McDonald S, Haie C, Rubin P, Nelson D, Divers LD. Second malignant tumors in patients with laryngeal carcinoma: diagnosis, treatment, and prevention. *Int J Radiat Oncol Biol Phys* 1989; **17:** 457–65.
91. McNeil BJ, Weichselbaum R, Pauker SG. Fallacy of the five-year survival in lung cancer. *N Engl J Med* 1978; **299:** 1397–401.
92. McNeil BJ, Weichselbaum R, Pauker SG. Speech and survival: tradeoffs between quality and quantity of life in laryngeal cancer. *N Engl J Med* 1981; **305:** 982–7.
93. Meguid MM, Campos AC, Hammond WG. Nutritional support in surgical practice. Part 1. *Am J Surg* 1990; **159:** 345–58.
94. Mendelsohn J. Principles of neoplasia. In: Wilson JD,

Braunwald E, Isselbacher KJ *et al.* eds. *Harrison's Principles of Internal Medicine*, 12th edn. New York: McGraw-Hill, 1991: 1021–2.

95. Neel HB, Taylor WF, Pearson GR. Prognostic determinants and a new view of staging for patients with nasopharyngeal carcinoma. *Ann Otol Rhinol Laryngol* 1985; **94:** 529–37.
96. Okumura T, Aruga H, Inohara H *et al.* Endoscopic examination of the upper gastrointestinal tract for the presence of second primary cancers in head and neck cancer patients. *Acta Otolaryngol Suppl (Stockh)* 1993; **501:** 103–6.
97. Orr ST, Aisner J. Performance status assessment among oncology patients: a review. *Cancer Treat Res* 1986; **70:** 1423–9.
98. Painter C. Semi-automated voice evaluation. *Am J Otolaryngol* 1991; **12:** 329–42.
99. Parsons CA, Chapman P, Counter RT, Grundy A. The role of computed tomography in tumours of the larynx. *Clin Radiol* 1980; **31:** 529–33.
100. Pelczar BT, Weed HG, Schuller DE, Young DC, Reilley TE. Identifying high-risk patients before head and neck oncologic surgery. *Arch Otolaryngol Head Neck Surg* 1993; **119:** 861–4.
101. Pfister DG, Wells CK, Chan CK, Feinstein AR. Classifying clinical severity to help solve problems of stage migration in nonconcurrent comparisons of lung cancer therapy. *Cancer Res* 1990; **50:** 4664–9.
102. Piccirillo JF. Purposes, problems, and proposals for progress in cancer staging. *Arch Otolaryngol Head Neck Surg* 1995; **121:** 145–9.
103. Piccirillo JF, Feinstein AR. Black-box mathematics and medical practice. *Arch Otolaryngol Head Neck Surg* 1993; **119:** 147–55.
104. Piccirillo JF, Wells CK, Sasaki CT, Feinstein AR. New clinical severity staging system for cancer of the larynx. Five-year survival rates. *Ann Otol Rhinol Laryngol* 1994; **103:** 83–92.
105. Piepenburg R, Bockisch A, Hach A *et al.* Importance of whole body skeletal scintigraphy within the scope of staging of neoplasms in the ENT area. *Laryngorhinootologie* 1992; **71:** 605–10.
106. Piollet H, Lufkin RB, Hanafee W. Magnetic resonance imaging of tumors of the upper aerodigestive tract. *Oncology (Huntingt)* 1989; **3:** 80–8, discussion 93–4.
107. Ross AF, Tinker JH. Anesthesia risk. In: Miller RD, ed. *Anesthesia*, 3rd edn. New York: Churchill Livingstone, 1995: 723–4.
108. Rouviere H. *Anatomy of the Human Lymphatic System.* Transl. Tobias MJ, ed. Ann Arbor: Edwards Bros, 1938.
109. Rubin P. A unified classification of cancers: an oncotaxonomy with symbols. *Cancer* 1973; **31:** 963–82.
110. Rucci L, Gammarota L, Gallo O. Carcinoma of the anterior commissure of the larynx: II. Proposal of a new staging system. *Ann Otol Rhinol Laryngol* 1996; **105:** 391–6.
111. Saklad M. Grading of patients for surgical procedures. *Anesthesiology* 1941; **2:** 281–4.
112. Sako K, Pradier RM, Marchetta FC, Pickren JW. Fallibility of palpation in the diagnosis of metastases to cervical nodes. *Surg Gynecol Obstet* 1964; **118:** 989.
113. Satariano WA. Comorbidity and functional status in older women with breast cancer: implications for screening, treatment, and prognosis. *J Gerontol* 1992; **47:** 24–31.
114. Satariano WA, Ragland DR. The effect of comorbidity on 3-year survival of women with primary breast cancer. *Ann Intern Med* 1994; **120:** 104–10.
115. Shah JP, Strong E, Spiro RH, Vikram B. Surgical grand rounds. Neck dissection: current status and future possibilities. *Clin Bull* 1981; **11:** 25–33.
116. Shaha A, Webber C, Marti J. Fine-needle aspiration in the diagnosis of cervical lymphadenopathy. *Am J Surg* 1986; **152:** 420–3.
117. Sham JS, Tong CM, Choy D, Yeung DW. Role of bone scanning in detection of subclinical bone metastasis in nasopharyngeal carcinoma. *Clin Nucl Med* 1991; **16:** 27–9.
118. Sidransky D, Boyle J, Koch W. Molecular screening. Prospects for a new approach. *Arch Otolaryngol Head Neck Surg* 1993; **119:** 1187–90.
119. Smith C. The questionable practice of clinical staging. *Perspect Biol Med* 1976; **19:** 273–7.
120. Snow GB, Gerritsen GJ. TNM classification according to the UICC and AJCC. In: Ferlito A, ed. *Neoplasms of the Larynx.* Edinburgh: Churchill Livingstone, 1993: 425–34.
121. Snow GB, Balm AJ, Arendse JW *et al.* Prognostic factors in neck node metastasis. In: Larson DL, Ballantyne AJ, Guillamondegui OM, eds. *Cancer in the Neck: Evaluation and Treatment.* New York: Macmillan, 1986: 53.
122. Snyderman CH, Wagner RL. Superiority of the T and N integer score (TANIS) staging system for squamous cell carcinoma of the oral cavity. *Otolaryngol Head Neck Surg* 1995; **112:** 691–4.
123. Sox HC Jr, Blatt M, Higgins MC, Marton KI. *Medical Decision Making.* London: Butterworths, 1965.
124. Spiro RH, Alfonso AE, Farr HW, Strong EW. Cervical node metastasis from epidermoid carcinoma of the oral cavity and oropharynx. A critical assessment of current staging. *Am J Surg* 1974; **128:** 562–7.
125. Spiro RH, Huvos AG, Wong GY, Spiro JD, Gnecco CA, Strong EW. Predictive value of tumor thickness in squamous carcinoma confined to the tongue and floor of the mouth. *Am J Surg* 1986; **152:** 345–50.
126. Spitzer WO, Dobson AJ, Hall J *et al.* Measuring the quality of life of cancer patients: a concise QL-index for use by physicians. *J Chronic Dis* 1981; **34:** 585–97.
127. Stell PM. Prognostic factors in laryngeal carcinoma. *Clin Otolaryngol* 1988; **13:** 399–409.
128. Stell PM. Letter to author, (JFP) March, 1992.
129. Stell PM, Morton RP, Singh SD. Cervical lymph node metastases: the significance of the level of the lymph node. *Clin Oncol* 1983; **9:** 101–7.
130. Stevens MH, Harnsberger HR, Mancuso AA, Davis RK, Johnson LP, Parkin JL. Computed tomography of cervical lymph nodes. Staging and management of head and neck cancer. *Arch Otolaryngol* 1985; **111:** 735–9.
131. Suen JY, Goepfert H. Standardization of neck dissection nomenclature. *Head Neck Surg* 1987; **10:** 75–7.
132. Torrance GW. Measurement of health state utilities for

economic appraisal. A review. *J Health Econ* 1986; **5:** 1–30.

133. Union Internationale Contre le Cancer. *TNM Classification of Malignant Tumours.* Geneva: UICC, 1968.
134. Vacanti CJ, VanHouten RJ, Hill RC. A statistical analysis of the relationship of physical status to postoperative mortality in 68,388 cases. *Anesth Analg* 1970; **49:** 564–6.
135. van den Brekel MWM, Stel HV, Castelijns JA, Croll GJ, Snow GB. Lymph node staging in patients with clinically negative neck examinations by ultrasound and ultrasound-guided aspiration cytology. *Am J Surg* 1991; **162**: 362–6.
136. van den Brekel MWM, Stel HV, Castelijns JA *et al.* Cervical lymph node metastasis: assessment of radiologic criteria. *Radiology* 1990; **177:** 379–84.
137. Vandenbroucke JP. Should we abandon statistical modeling altogether? *Am J Epidemiol* 1987; **126:** 10–13.
138. Walter SD, Feinstein AR, Wells CK. A comparison of multivariable mathematical methods for predicting survival – II. Statistical selection of prognostic variables. *J Clin Epidemiol* 1990; **43:** 349–59.
139. Wells CK, Stoller JK, Feinstein AR, Horwitz RI. Comorbid and clinical determinants of prognosis in endometrial cancer. *Arch Intern Med* 1984; **144:** 2004–9.
140. Wolf GT, Carey TE. Tumor antigen phenotype, biologic staging, and prognosis in head and neck squamous carcinoma. *Monogr Natl Cancer Inst* 1992; **13:** 67–74.
141. Wolf GT, Carey TE, Schmaltz SP *et al.* Altered antigen expression predicts outcome in squamous cell carcinoma of the head and neck. *J Natl Cancer Inst* 1990; **82:** 1566–72.
142. Zelen M. Keynote address on biostatistics and data retrieval. *Cancer Chemother Rep* 1973; **4:** 31–42.
143. Zubrod CG, Schneiderman M, Frei E. Appraisal of methods for the study of chemotherapy of cancer in man: comparative therapeutic trial of nitrogen mustards and triethylene thiophosphoramide. *J Chronic Dis* 1960; **11:** 7–30.

Laryngeal epithelial changes: diagnosis and therapy

Alfio Ferlito, Imrich Friedmann and Alessandra Rinaldo

Several laryngeal epithelial changes, indicated in the literature as precancerosis, precancerous lesions, precursors of invasive cancer, preneoplastic lesions, premalignant lesions, latent cancer, etc., express our inability to relate morphologic changes to biologic potential.[35]

Laryngeal epithelial changes present a major challenge to clinician and pathologist and therefore the evaluation of these lesions in a biopsy specimen demands their closest cooperation[18] coupled with a knowledge of a well defined and agreed terminology.

Normal histology

The anterior (or lingual) epiglottic surface, the upper half of the posterior (or laryngeal) epiglottic surface, the superior margin of the aryepiglottic folds and the vocal cords (or vocal folds) are covered by stratified squamous epithelium. There is no keratin layer on the surface of the epithelium. The ventricular folds (or false cords), ventricle, saccule (the appendix of the laryngeal ventricle) and subglottic region are lined with pseudostratified ciliated columnar ('respiratory') epithelium, with interspersed goblet cells. Seromucous glands are present in the lamina propria and are particularly numerous on the posterior epiglottic surface, false cords, ventricle, saccule and subglottis.

Epithelial changes

The two normal epithelia of the larynx are subject to a spectrum of abnormal epithelial proliferation. The following terminology has evolved.

Leukoplakia

The term means 'white plaque' and is a clinical term describing any white lesion on a mucous membrane. The term cannot be considered a pathologic diagnosis. It is not indicative of underlying malignant neoplasm.[64]

Erythroplakia

This is a clinical term describing any reddish patch of raised epithelium. It may be indicative of an underlying malignant tumor.[64]

Erythroleukoplakia

This clinical term describes mixed forms of white and red mucosal changes. It is not applicable as a histological diagnosis.

Pachydermia

This is another descriptive clinical term used in the past to indicate large areas involved by leukoplakia, not applicable as a histological diagnosis.

Squamous metaplasia

This is a term describing the replacement of respiratory epithelium by stratified squamous epithelium, a change common even in the subglottic region of the nonsmoking, non-bronchitic urban adult[60] and in the human fetal larynx.[57] The process usually involves only the superficial epithelium, but may occur in the epithelium of the seromucous laryngeal glands. Squamous metaplasia is usually the result of persistent trauma or chronic irritation. There is no evidence that it is a potentially dangerous lesion. No treatment is necessary.

Squamous cell hyperplasia

This is a benign change in which the epithelium becomes thicker without cellular atypia. Such thickening is due to an increase in the prickle cell and/or basal cell layers. Squamous cellular differentiation is well preserved and this type of epithelial change is reversible. Squamous cell hyperplasia usually represents a response to injury and is not a precancerous lesion. Excisional biopsy is the treatment of choice.

Pseudoepitheliomatous hyperplasia

This term describes an exuberant reactive or reparative overgrowth of squamous epithelium with epithelial extension into the stroma. The hyperplastic epithelium may simulate well differentiated squamous cell carcinoma, especially when it appears detached from the surface. The absence of any atypical epithelial cells and the presence of an inflammatory infiltrate are useful features for correct diagnosis. The pseudoepitheliomatous reaction may be associated with a granular cell tumor, various specific chronic inflammatory conditions (tuberculosis in particular), mycotic diseases and occasionally primary eosinophilic granuloma of the larynx.[27] There is no evidence that pseudoepitheliomatous hyperplasia is a potentially malignant lesion and treatment depends on the nature of the subepithelial disease.

Keratosis

This is a pathological feature resulting from the production of keratin on the surface of the epithelium. Squamous differentiation is well preserved and a granular layer is often apparent. Keratinization may be without nuclei (orthokeratosis) or with nuclei (parakeratosis). Hyperplasia of the stratum spinosum or prickle cell layer (acanthosis) occurs in combination with keratinization, and the proportions of acanthosis and keratinization can vary considerably. The basal membrane remains intact. There may be inflammatory cells in the lamina propria. Since the laryngeal mucosa is not normally keratinized, the term hyperkeratosis is redundant and should be avoided.[2,64] Excisional biopsy using scissors, scalpel and laser, or surgical stripping are generally satisfactory forms of treatment. Although keratosis is reported to have a potential for malignant change into cancer, it must not be regarded as a precancerous lesion from the histologic and photometric standpoints.[32] Keratosis may be associated with dysplasia (keratinizing dysplasia) or occur on the surface of squamous cell carcinoma (keratinizing squamous cell carcinoma). Papillary keratosis may be confused with verrucous carcinoma.[3] In conclusion, simple keratosis is a lesion with no inherent risk of progression.

Dyskeratosis

This represents a faulty or premature and abnormal keratinization of individual squamous cells scattered throughout the thickness of the squamous epithelium. It is most frequently associated with subsequent invasive carcinoma. Blackwell *et al.*[5] believe that dyskeratosis does imply an increased malignant potential.

Laryngeal intraepithelial neoplasia (LIN) or dysplasia or atypia

These terms describe the presence of atypical cytological features in the laryngeal squamous epithelium. Dysplasia is a process of qualitative alteration in a malignant direction in the appearance of cells.[37,64] The time-honored designation 'dysplasia' has been largely replaced by the term 'intraepithelial neoplasia' because the epithelial changes are considered to be morphologic manifestation of a neoplastic process.[15,28] Three grades of dysplasia are recognized, based on the degree of cellular atypia and structural alterations, i.e. mild, moderate and severe.

Friedmann and Ferlito[28] have used the term laryngeal intraepithelial neoplasia (LIN) to include both dysplasia and carcinoma in situ. In their scheme, LIN I is the equivalent of mild dysplasia, LIN II of moderate dysplasia and LIN III of severe dysplasia and carcinoma in situ. Concerning the esophagus and stomach, other authors have used the terms high-grade dysplasia and carcinoma in situ as interchangeable terms.[10] The Working Group on epithelial hyperplastic laryngeal lesions of the European Society of Pathology suggests a different system of classification of epithelial abnormalities.[34] Its adoption by expert pathologists should not be undertaken lightly and uncritically.[31]

LIN I (mild or minimal dysplasia)

The general tendency of the squamous epithelium to show stratification is preserved and the superficial layers show cytoplasmic differentiation (maturation) with easily visible intracellular bridges and keratinization. The orientation of the cells in the lower layers is not maintained and 'nuclear crowding' is conspicuous, with some pleomorphism and an increased nuclear–cytoplasmic ratio. Nucleoli are prominent and mitoses are occasionally found.[28] Mild dysplasia should be differentiated from immature squamous metaplasia, where nuclear pleomorphism is absent and there are no abnormal mitotic figures.

Overdiagnosis of LIN I may occur and depends largely on the experience or lack of it of the pathologist. The patient should be observed for several months and the biopsy repeated if clinically indicated. This may also apply to LIN II cases and rather rarely to LIN III.

It is a fact that there exists considerable interobserver variability of the histopathologic diagnosis of precancer, leading to anxiety and unnecessary, often costly, investigations.

Terms such as borderline lesions or atypical squamous cells of undetermined significance abound, especially in cervical smear reports. Exfoliative cytology, although rewarding, has found little or no place in the diagnosis of laryngeal malignancy.[24]

LIN II (moderate dysplasia)

Histologic changes are similar to those of mild dysplasia, but the undifferentiated (immature) cells extend to two-thirds of the thickness of the epithelium; differentiation and stratification are still seen in the superficial third of the epithelium. Mitotic figures are more numerous.[28]

LIN III (severe dysplasia and carcinoma in situ)

The non-stratified, undifferentiated cells occupy from over two-thirds of the epithelium up to its full thickness; this is usually accompanied by a more obvious degree of nuclear pleomorphism including the presence of bizarre large nuclei. Mitotic figures are seen with increasing frequency in all layers and they are often of abnormal appearance. There is no keratinization in the majority of cases, but a thin layer of keratin is occasionally seen on the surface, with a complete lack of orientation of the cells underneath.

The initial microscopic change is believed to be in the basal layer of the epithelium and the neoplastic change gradually extends until it reaches the surface; as it extends towards the surface it also spreads laterally in all directions within the epithelial layers. The lesion is always contained at its deep aspect by the basal lamina[28] and the ducts are also frequently involved. In carcinoma in situ, all layers of the epithelium are replaced by malignant cells. Stratification is lacking and cellular polarity may be vertical.[33]

The first descriptions of this lesion were published early in this century[39] and the term carcinoma in situ (also called intraepithelial, or superficial, or preinvasive carcinoma, or stage 0) was introduced by Broders in 1932.[6] The annual incidence of laryngeal carcinoma in situ is only 0.4 cases per 100 000 in the general population.[15] Published reports of cases of carcinoma in situ indicate that there are considerable discrepancies regarding its incidence. The rates range from nil to 15% of the total number of carcinomas of the larynx collected from the literature.[20] The incidence of this neoplasm is often overestimated.[20] Two possible factors explain the discrepancies:

- carcinoma in situ may accompany an undiagnosed invasive lesion; and
- carcinoma in situ may be incorrectly diagnosed by pathologists.[26]

Besides, the diagnosis of carcinoma in situ is very subjective.

The lesion may be multicentric in origin and may be found in all laryngeal regions, though it is most frequent in the vocal cords and particularly in the anterior half of the true vocal cords.

The diagnosis of carcinoma in situ on the basis of a small biopsy specimen can only be accepted with reserve.[17] Multiple sections should be processed in order to rule out invasion. Carcinoma in situ may rarely occur as an isolated lesion, but it is more commonly associated with invasive cancer. Areas suggesting carcinoma in situ have been found in spindle cell carcinoma and in basaloid squamous cell carcinoma. LIN III lesions have an abnormal aneuploid DNA content indicating neoplastic change.[13] Severe dysplasia and squamous cell carcinoma in situ are defined by Crissman *et al.*[15] as squamous intraepithelial neoplasia grade 3 (SIN). Ferlito *et al.*[20] agreed with the notion that carcinoma in situ is a form of intraepithelial neoplasm and the term 'laryngeal intraepithelial neoplasia' (LIN) would encompass both carcinoma in situ and all grades of dysplasia. Like cervical intraepithelial neoplasia, its laryngeal counterpart may be defined as 'a spectrum of intraepithelial change which begins as a generally well differentiated neoplasm, traditionally classified as mild dysplasia, and ends with invasive carcinoma'.[7] Blackwell *et al.*[4,5] found that biopsies demonstrating severe dysplasia did not differ significantly from biopsies demonstrating carcinoma in situ, implying that severe dysplasia and carcinoma in situ both represent intraepithelial neoplastic change.

Such an approach has significant implications: the changes occurring in laryngeal intraepithelial neoplasia are considered as a morphologic manifestation of a neoplastic process, not as a precancerous lesion.[14,21,25]

For classification purposes, three stages of carcinoma in situ, similar to those described for the more common squamous cell carcinoma, have been distinguished:

- well differentiated (grade I);
- moderately well differentiated (grade II); and
- poorly differentiated (grade III).

Among these variants, the first is the least common and the second is the most common.

The World Health Organization[54] accepts the term papillary carcinoma in situ (non-invasive papillary carcinoma) to indicate exophytic papillary tumors composed of cores of fibrovascular stroma covered by squamous epithelium with cytological features similar to those of the conventional carcinoma in situ.

Carcinoma in situ is regarded more as a histopathologic than as a clinical entity[42] and under the International Union Against Cancer (UICC)[38] and American Joint Committee on Cancer (AJCC)[1] it is represented by 'Tis'.

Many invasive cancers of the larynx do not pass through the stage of carcinoma in situ and are invasive from the start, unlike cervical intraepithelial neoplasia.[64]

The accurate diagnosis of carcinoma in situ requires a full excisional biopsy.[56] Usually the inclusion of cases of cancer with microinvasion distorts findings on the outcome and prognosis of this lesion.

It is equally difficult to accurately forecast the development of laryngeal malignancy in its different stages. The role of p53 expression has been widely studied with somewhat contradictory results. Nylander *et al.*[46] found no indication of a clinical or prognostic significance of p53 expression in squamous cell carcinoma of the head and neck, in contrast to the conclusion of Field *et al.*[23] who concluded that overexpression of this gene correlated 'with a very poor prognosis' but in patients classified with 'end-stage disease'. It is of no real help to patient or surgeon. Kushner *et al.*[41] in a recent report expressed a view that there is a significant correlation between staging for p53 and Ki-67 proteins and dysplasia of the squamous epithelium from the floor of the mouth leading to dysregulation of cell proliferation at this site.

Histologic understaging of carcinoma in situ ('false carcinoma in situ') is a frequent finding in laryngeal pathology. Carcinoma in situ and microinvasive carcinoma can coexist in the same specimen.[15] The true extent of the tumor can only be established on examination of the whole surgical specimen, and the diagnosis is only correct and final if the surgical specimen reveals 'true' carcinoma in situ.

A wide variability in the choice of primary treatment for laryngeal carcinoma in situ, including postbiopsy observation alone, vocal cord stripping, laryngofissure–cordectomy, radiation therapy, laser laryngoscopy, partial or complete laryngectomy and diathermocoagulation has been found.[20]

Excisional biopsy with the carbon dioxide laser (i.e. removal of the entire lesion together with a rim of healthy tissue) is ideal for both diagnosis and treatment of this lesion; if the margins are not free, re-excision or radiotherapy remain alternative options.[29] No benefit was achieved by stopping smoking after LIN III lesions had developed, indicating that the genetic changes induced by smoke had already taken place, and that these were irreversible.[61] Radiotherapy has a definite, though secondary role in the treatment of all LIN cases. Patients treated with stripping often have a recurrence and this procedure is not sufficient for a conclusive diagnosis and treatment. Laser surgery and laryngofissure with cordectomy have been advocated by several authors who considered that the pretreatment diagnosis of carcinoma in situ may not be confirmed on the surgical specimen and has to be changed to microinvasive carcinoma.

A fundamental distinction must be made between laryngeal epithelial abnormalities according to whether or not they show a significant risk of progressing to become an invasive neoplasm. Severe dysplasia and carcinoma in situ (LIN III) do carry this risk, whereas such laryngeal aberrations as squamous metaplasia, squamous cell hyperplasia, pseudoepitheliomatous hyperplasia and keratosis without atypia do not. These abnormalities in the surface epithelium have been erroneously considered as premalignant, but their prognosis is excellent. Metaplastic, hyperplastic and dysplastic conditions are commonly found in the larynx in combination with in situ and invasive carcinoma. Cancer of the larynx may develop simultaneously at different sites after prolonged exposure to a carcinogen ('field cancerization' theory). The entire laryngeal epithelial surface, or 'field', is exposed to repeated, carcinogenic insults and independent synchronous tumors can occur. Multiple intralaryngeal primary cancers are not uncommon and are explained by the concept of field cancerization. The occurrence of a second cancer in the larynx should therefore not necessarily be considered as a failure to treat the first laryngeal primary, since the second cancer may represent a new primary malignancy (e.g. involving the vocal cord contralateral to a previously diseased cord, or a supraglottic cancer occurring after vocal cord disease).[51]

Very close follow-up, especially in the first year, is essential.[44,52] The appearance of a new malignancy may be a recurrence or a new expression of carcinogenesis.

Early cancer

The development of human laryngeal squamous cell carcinoma is a multistage progressive process and is often accompanied by cancer of the head and neck, and of the lung.[51] The hypothesis of a genetic or environmental etiology is feasible for this multiple condition.

The natural history of neoplastic development in some experimental models, and presumably in humans too, may be separated into three distinct stages: initiation, promotion and progression.[50] Initiation is the first stage of carcinogenesis and involves a direct attack on the cell's DNA by the initiating agent. It is not a reversible process. Carcinogens that act in this first phase are called initiators. The second carcinogenic stage is promotion and it may begin after some time, even several years; this is a reversible process that may be modulated by various environmental factors. The factors taking effect in this second phase are called promoters. Together, these two phases of carcinogenesis are also called the induction phase. Animal studies seem to have demonstrated that if a promoter is administered prior to the administration of an initiator, the carcinogenic process fails to take place. Many known active carcinogens have the capacity both to initiate and to promote the malignant process.[50] Tobacco smoke, for example, is a complete carcinogen; it contains both initiators (hydrocarbons) and promoters (phenols), and it is essentially a weak carcinogen; lengthy exposure is required to obtain an effective dose[63] and the relative risk diminishes after giving up smoking.[8] The effects of complete carcinogens are irreversible. Other carcinogenic agents are called incomplete carcinogens because they are only capable of initiation.

The natural history of laryngeal cancer also includes the third stage called progression, which is divided into two different substages: the first includes epithelial abnormalities, such as dysplasia and carcinoma in situ, potentially capable of progression into an invasive neoplasm; the second is characterized by the presence of an invasive cancer. Most of the natural history of neoplastic development occurs subclinically, during the so-called latency period, and it probably takes many years for the cancer to reach a clinically apparent phase. The initially visible tumor usually coincides with the stage of the disease called progression, which may appear clinically limited.

Usually, Tis, T1, T2 and favorable T3 lesions are erroneously included under the umbrella term of 'early' tumors, as opposed to extensive T3 and T4 tumors which are classified as 'advanced'.[19] It appears evident that various non-early cancers are included under the term 'early' in many textbooks and papers. It has, indeed, become a clinical convention to describe Tis and T2 as early cancers, whereas early cancer includes only T1 lesions and so excludes Tis and T2.

The term 'early' cancer is often erroneously and ambiguously used to describe a variety of lesions ranging from severe dysplasia to genuine neoplastic disease invading the muscle or cartilage structures. Such careless terminology is regrettable because it not only causes confusion in the nomenclature, making it difficult to compare findings in the medical literature. It can also prompt erroneous prognostic conclusions and therapeutic decisions.

The term 'early invasive cancer' should be restricted to a minimally invasive neoplastic lesion that does not extend into the adjacent muscle or cartilaginous structures, but still is capable of metastasis. When the infiltration has reached muscle or cartilage, the lesion is no longer an early invasive cancer, confined to the lamina propria.[19] It often includes a prominent in situ component with only focal invasion of the lamina propria, in which case it is called 'microinvasive' carcinoma. There is some controversy over the definition of the depth of invasion, in millimeters, for a cancer to be considered as microinvasive.[28] Some authors state that the term microinvasive carcinoma should be used when carcinoma in situ has infiltrated the stroma by 1–2 mm.[15,48] More recently, Crissman defined microinvasive carcinoma as a focus of 2–3 mm of stromal invasion.[12] However, it may be extensive, giving rise to the so-called 'carpet' or 'superficial extending' carcinoma.[9,62] In any case, the lesion tends to spread superficially rather than in a deeply infiltrating direction.[19] In other words, 'early' cancer is a superficially invasive lesion involving the lamina propria, thus representing more than a carcinoma in situ, but less than a deeply infiltrating carcinoma.[22] The tumor called 'superficial extending carcinoma' also qualifies as an early cancer. Early laryngeal cancers are lesions confined to the mucosa, regardless of any presence or absence of lymph node metastases.

It is important to make a clear distinction between preinvasive lesions (dysplasia and carcinoma in situ) and early invasive carcinoma because, whilst the former are characterized by atypical or malignant cytologic features restricted to the laryngeal squamous epithelium without metastatic potential, the latter may metastasize. In the natural history of laryngeal cancer, however, dysplasia and carcinoma in situ of the laryngeal mucosa may subsequently evolve into an invasive neoplasm. It is also a fact that laryngeal cancers may develop directly as invasive neoplasms, without going through the dysplasia–carcinoma in situ evolutionary stages.[64] Early cancers of the larynx may occur in the glottis.

In biologic terms, early cancer – unlike carcinoma in situ – is capable of metastasizing, via either lymphatic or vascular channels. For the purposes of biologic staging, carcinoma in situ belongs to stage I, whereas early cancer comes under stage II.[53]

In conclusion, 'early' laryngeal cancers are 'invasive' carcinomas ('microinvasive' or 'superficial extending' carcinomas) confined to the lamina propria, but potentially capable of forming lymph node metastases.

Invasion of the pre-epiglottic space has been observed histologically in 24 specimens of the 25 (96%) cancers (squamous cell carcinoma) originally classified as 'early' cancer, originating below the hyoepiglottic ligament. They were clinically understaged. Cervical metastasis occurred in 12 of the 24 patients (50%) with pre-epiglottic space invasion.[65] Pre-epiglottic space invasion should be considered as equivalent to the spread of cancer outside the larynx and should therefore be graded as T4,[30] although both the UICC[38] and the AJCC[1] imply a T3 stage for tumor invading this space.

Early vocal cord cancer has a high cure rate by various treatments; there is no treatment of choice, but a choice of treatments. Excellent control is possible with stripping, endoscopic laser surgery, radiotherapy, laryngofissure–cordectomy, or with the association of two treatments (stripping and radiotherapy; laser surgery and radiotherapy).[16,36,40,45,47,49,55,58] Radiotherapy provides a better postoperative voice than laryngofissure–cordectomy. Endoscopic laser resection of early laryngeal cancer results in a vocal function that is acceptable to patients and is rated by them as normal or almost normal;[43] it is not significantly different from the post-radiotherapy voice.[11]

The treatment of early cancer, involving the supraglottic region, may be different from that of carcinoma in situ, because lymph node metastases may be present.[19] Supraglottic laryngectomy is a valid procedure for T1 supraglottic cancer with lymph node metastasis. Stell and Dalby[59] pointed out that radiotherapy and surgery produce similar survival rates for patients with no clinically detectable nodal metastasis. Both forms of treatment give equally good results and the choice of treatment depends on the patient's fitness and on locally available expertise.[59] Selective lateral neck dissection of levels II, III and IV is indicated for early supraglottic cancer staged clinically as N0 or N1. Steiner and Ambrosch[58] and Zeitels *et al.*[66] believe that the CO_2 laser is an excellent alternative treatment for early supraglottic cancer, but several clinically 'early' supraglottic cancers are actually T3 cancers.

References

1. American Joint Committee on Cancer (AJCC). *Manual for Staging of Cancer*, 5th edn. Philadelphia: Lippincott, 1997.
2. Barnes L, Gnepp DR. Diseases of the larynx, hypopharynx and esophagus. In: Barnes L, ed. *Surgical Pathology of the Head and Neck*. Vol I. New York: Dekker, 1985: 156–9.
3. Barnes L, Peel RL. *Head and Neck Pathology. A Text/Atlas of Differential Diagnosis*. New York: Igaku-Shoin, 1990.
4. Blackwell KE, Calcaterra TC, Fu Y-S. Laryngeal dysplasia: epidemiology and treatment outcome. *Ann Otol Rhinol Laryngol* 1995; **104:** 596–602.
5. Blackwell KE, Fu Y-S, Calcaterra TC. Laryngeal dysplasia. A clinicopathologic study. *Cancer* 1995; **75:** 457–63.

6. Broders AC. Carcinoma in situ contrasted with benign penetrating epithelium. *JAMA* 1932; **99**: 1670–4.
7. Buckley CH, Butler EG, Fox H. Cervical intraepithelial neoplasia. *J Clin Pathol* 1982; **35**: 1–13.
8. Cann CI, Fried MP, Rothman KJ. Epidemiology of squamous cell cancer of the head and neck. *Otolaryngol Clin North Am* 1985; **18**: 367–88.
9. Carbone A, Volpe R, Barzan L. Superficial extending carcinoma (SEC) of the larynx and hypopharynx. *Pathol Res Pract* 1992; **188**: 729–35.
10. Chejfec G. Atypias, dysplasias, and neoplasias of the esophagus and stomach. *Semin Diagn Pathol* 1985; **2**: 31–41.
11. Cragle SP, Brandenburg JH. Laser cordectomy or radiotherapy: cure rates, communication, and cost. *Otolaryngol Head Neck Surg* 1993; **108**: 648–54.
12. Crissman JD. Upper aerodigestive tract. In: Henson DE, Albores-Saavedra J, eds. *Pathology of Incipient Neoplasia.* Philadelphia: Saunders, 1993: 44–63.
13. Crissman JD, Fu YS. Intraepithelial neoplasia of the larynx: a clinicopathological study of six cases with DNA analysis. *Arch Otolaryngol Head Neck Surg* 1986; **112**: 522–8.
14. Crissman JD, Zarbo RJ. Quantitation of DNA ploidy in squamous intraepithelial neoplasia of the laryngeal glottis. *Arch Otolaryngol Head Neck Surg* 1991; **117**: 182–8.
15. Crissman JD, Zarbo RJ, Drozdowicz S, Jacobs J, Ahmad K, Weaver A. Carcinoma in situ and micro-invasive squamous carcinoma of the laryngeal glottis. *Arch Otolaryngol Head Neck Surg* 1988; **114**: 299–307.
16. Eckel HE, Thumfart WF. Laser surgery for the treatment of larynx carcinomas: indications, techniques, and preliminary results. *Ann Otol Rhinol Laryngol* 1992; **101**: 113–18.
17. Ferlito A. Carcinoma in situ. [Letter to editor] *Clin Otolaryngol* 1977; **2**: 292.
18. Ferlito A. Precancerous lesions of the larynx: diagnostic and therapeutic problems. In: Sacristán T, Alvarez-Vincent JJ, Bartual J, Antolí-Candela F, Rubio L, eds. *Proceedings of the XIV World Congress of Otorhinolaryngology Head and Neck Surgery, Madrid.* Amsterdam: Kugler & Ghedini, 1991: 2315–18.
19. Ferlito A. The natural history of early vocal cord cancer. *Acta Otolaryngol (Stockh)* 1995; **115**: 345–7.
20. Ferlito A, Polidoro F, Rossi M. Pathological basis and clinical aspects of treatment policy in carcinoma-in-situ of the larynx. *J Laryngol Otol* 1981; **95**: 141–54.
21. Ferlito A, Doglioni C, Rinaldo A, Devaney KO. What is the earliest non-invasive malignant lesion of the larynx? *ORL J Otorhinolaryngol Relat Spec* 2000; **62**: 57–9.
22. Ferlito A, Carbone A, DeSanto LW *et al.* 'Early' cancer of the larynx: the concept as defined by clinicians, pathologists, and biologists. *Ann Otol Rhinol Laryngol* 1996; **105**: 245–50.
23. Field JK, Pavelic ZP, Spandidos DA, Stambrook PJ, Jones AS, Gluckman JL. The role of the p53 tumor suppressor gene in squamous cell carcinoma of the head and neck. *Arch Otolaryngol Head Neck Surg* 1993; **119**: 1118–22.
24. Friedmann I. Exfoliative cytology as an aid in the diagnosis of tumours of the throat, nose and ear. *J Laryngol Otol* 1951; **65**: 1–9.
25. Friedmann I. Nose, throat and ears. In: Symmers WStC, ed. *Systemic Pathology.* Vol 1. Edinburgh: Churchill Livingstone, 1986: 210–49.
26. Friedmann I. Precursors of squamous cell carcinoma. In: Ferlito A, ed. *Surgical Pathology of Laryngeal Neoplasms.* London: Chapman & Hall, 1996: 107–21.
27. Friedmann I, Ferlito A. Primary eosinophilic granuloma of the larynx. *J Laryngol Otol* 1981; **95**: 1249–54.
28. Friedmann I, Ferlito A. *Granulomas and Neoplasms of the Larynx.* Edinburgh: Churchill Livingstone, 1988: 111–22.
29. Gillis TM, Incze J, Strong MS, Vaughan CW, Simpson GT. Natural history and management of keratosis, atypia, carcinoma in situ, and micro-invasive cancer of the larynx. *Am J Surg* 1983; **146**: 512–16.
30. Gregor RT. The preepiglottic space revisited: is it significant? *Am J Otolaryngol* 1990; **11**: 161–4.
31. Helliwell TR. Commentary. 'Risky' epithelium in the larynx – a practical diagnosis? *Histopathology* 1999; **34**: 262–5.
32. Hellquist H, Olofsson J. Photometric evaluation of laryngeal epithelium exhibiting hyperplasia, keratosis and moderate dysplasia. *Acta Otolaryngol (Stockh)* 1981; **92**: 157–65.
33. Hellquist H, Lundgren J, Olofsson J. Hyperplasia, keratosis, dysplasia and carcinoma in situ of the vocal cords – a follow-up study. *Clin Otolaryngol* 1982; **7**: 11–27.
34. Hellquist H, Cardesa A, Gale N, Kambic V, Michaels L. Criteria for grading in the Ljubljana classification of epithelial hyperplastic laryngeal lesions. A study by members of the Working Group on Epithelial Hyperplastic Lesions of the European Society of Pathology. *Histopathology* 1999; **34**: 226–33.
35. Henson DE, Albores-Saavedra J. Introduction. In: Henson DE, Albores-Saavedra J, eds. *Pathology of Incipient Neoplasia*, 2nd edn. Philadelphia: Saunders, 1993: 1–7.
36. Hirano M, Mori K. Transoral laser resection in team practice for early cancer of larynx. In: Shah JP, Johnson JT, eds. *Proceedings of the Fourth International Conference on Head and Neck Cancer, Toronto.* Madison: Omnipress, 1996: 277–83.
37. Hyams VJ, Batsakis JG, Michaels L. *Tumors of the Upper Respiratory Tract and Ear. Atlas of Tumor Pathology.* 2nd series, fascicle 25. Washington, DC: Armed Forces Institute of Pathology, 1988: 52–5.
38. International Union Against Cancer. Sobin LH, Wittekind Ch, eds, *TNM Classification of Malignant Tumours*, 5th edn. New York: Wiley-Liss, 1997.
39. Jackson C. Cancer of the larynx: is it preceded by a recognizable precancerous condition? *Ann Surg* 1923; **77**: 1–14.
40. Kanonier G, Rainer T, Fritsch E, Thumfart WF. Radiotherapy in early glottic carcinoma. *Ann Otol Rhinol Laryngol* 1996; **105**: 759–63.
41. Kushner J, Bradley G, Jordan RK. Patterns of p53 and Ki-67 protein expression in epithelial dysplasia from the floor of the mouth. *J Pathol* 1997; **183**: 419–23.
42. Maran AGD, Mackenzie IJ, Stanley RE. Carcinoma in situ of the larynx. *Head Neck Surg* 1984; **7**: 28–31.
43. McGuirt WF, Blalock D, Koufman JA, Feehs RS. Voice analysis of patients with endoscopically treated early

laryngeal carcinoma. *Ann Otol Rhinol Laryngol* 1992; **101:** 142–6.

44. Murty GE, Diver JP, Bradley PJ. Carcinoma in situ of the glottis: radiotherapy or excisional biopsy? *Ann Otol Rhinol Laryngol* 1993; **102:** 592–5.
45. Nguyen C, Naghibzadeh B, Black MJ, Rochon L, Shenouda G. Glottic micro-invasive carcinoma: is it different from carcinoma in situ? *J Otolaryngol* 1996; **25:** 223–6.
46. Nylander K, Stenling R, Gustafsson H, Zackrisson B, Roos G. p53 expression and cell proliferation in squamous cell carcinomas of the head and neck. *Cancer* 1995; **75:** 87–93.
47. Olsen KD, Thomas JV, DeSanto LW, Suman VJ. Indications and results of cordectomy for early glottic carcinoma. *Otolaryngol Head Neck Surg* 1993; **108:** 277–82.
48. Padovan IF. Premalignant laryngeal lesions – a laryngologist's viewpoint. *Can J Otolaryngol* 1974; **3:** 543–5.
49. Peretti G, Cappiello J, Nicolai P, Smussi C, Antonelli A. Endoscopic laser excisional biopsy for selected glottic carcinomas. *Laryngoscope* 1994; **104:** 1276–9.
50. Pitot HC. The natural history of neoplastic development: the relation of experimental models to human cancer. *Cancer* 1982; **49:** 1206–11.
51. Rinaldo A, Marchiori C, Faggionato L, Saffiotti U, Ferlito A. The association of cancers of the larynx with cancers of the lung. *Eur Arch Otorhinolaryngol* 1996; **253:** 256–9.
52. Rothfield RE, Myers EN, Johnson JT. Carcinoma in situ and micro-invasive squamous cell carcinoma of the vocal cords. *Ann Otol Rhinol Laryngol* 1991; **100:** 793–6.
53. Schantz SP. Biological staging of head and neck cancer. *Curr Opin Otolaryngol Head Neck Surg* 1993; **1:** 107–13.
54. Shanmugaratnam K. *Histological Typing of Tumours of the Upper Respiratory Tract and Ear. World Health Organization. International Classification of Tumours*, 2nd edn. Berlin: Springer-Verlag, 1991.
55. Shapshay SM, Hybels RL, Bohigian RK. Laser excision of early vocal cord carcinoma: indications, limitations, and precautions. *Ann Otol Rhinol Laryngol* 1990; **99:** 46–50.
56. Small W Jr, Mittal BB, Brand WN *et al.* Role of radiation therapy in the management of carcinoma in situ of the larynx. *Laryngoscope* 1993; **103:** 663–7.
57. Stafford ND, Davies SJ. Epithelial distribution in the human fetal larynx. *Ann Otol Rhinol Laryngol* 1988; **97:** 302–7.
58. Steiner W, Ambrosch P. Transoral laser microsurgery for early laryngeal cancer. In: Shah JP, Johnson JT, eds. *Proceedings of the Fourth International Conference on Head and Neck Cancer, Toronto.* Madison: Omnipress, 1996: 284–8.
59. Stell PM, Dalby JE. The treatment of early (T1) glottic and supra-glottic carcinoma: does partial laryngectomy have a place? *Eur J Surg Oncol* 1985; **11:** 263–6.
60. Stell PM, Gregory I, Watt J. Morphology of the human larynx. II. The subglottis. *Clin Otolaryngol* 1980; **5:** 389–95.
61. Stenersen TC. *Prognostic Factors in Laryngeal Preneoplastic Lesions.* Thesis. University of Oslo, 1994.
62. Sulfaro S, Volpe R, Barzan L *et al.* Superficial extending carcinoma of the larynx. *Laryngoscope* 1988; **98:** 1127–32.
63. Vaughan CW, Homburger F, Shapshay SM, Soto E, Bernfeld P. Carcinogenesis in the upper aerodigestive tract. *Otolaryngol Clin North Am* 1980; **13:** 403–12.
64. Wenig BM. *Atlas of Head and Neck Pathology.* Philadelphia: Saunders, 1993.
65. Zeitels SM, Vaughan CW. Preepiglottic space invasion in 'early' epiglottic cancer. *Ann Otol Rhinol Laryngol* 1991; **100:** 789–92.
66. Zeitels SM, Koufman JA, Davis RK, Vaughan CW. Endoscopic treatment of supraglottic and hypopharynx cancer. *Laryngoscope* 1994; **104:** 71–8.

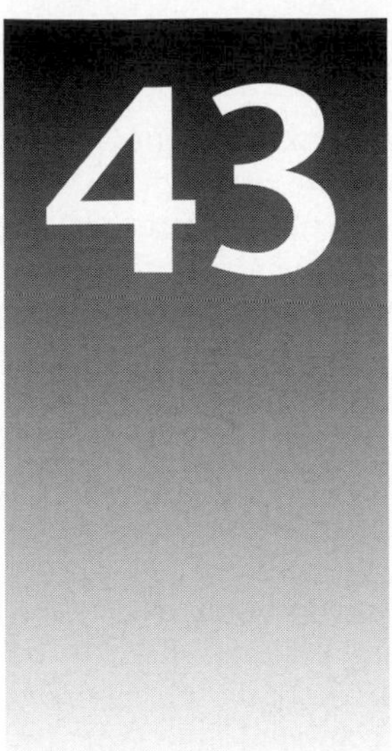

Cancer of the supraglottis

Carl E Silver and Alfio Ferlito

Anatomy

The supraglottic region of the larynx extends from the aryepiglottic folds to the most inferior portions of the ventricles. The surface consists mostly of mucosa covering both lingual and laryngeal surfaces of the epiglottis, with the remainder covering the ventricles, ventricular bands (false vocal cords), aryepiglottic folds, arytenoids and the area between the ventricular bands and aryepiglottic folds. The cartilages of the supraglottic region include the entire epiglottis, the cuneiform and corniculate cartilages and most of the arytenoid cartilages except for the vocal processes and basal portions, which are within the glottis. The body of the hyoid bone and the anterior two-thirds of the upper halves of the thyroid alae are within the supraglottis. The fibroelastic quadrangular membrane extends from the lateral borders of the epiglottis to the medial surfaces of the arytenoid cartilages. The superior border of this membrane is thickened, to form the aryepiglottic ligaments. Inferiorly, the membrane is thickened into the ventricular ligament, which, together with the overlying mucosa, forms the ventricular band. Inferior to the ventricular ligament, the membrane is deficient, permitting the mucosa of the ventricle to invaginate between the true and false vocal cords. The inferior portion of the epiglottis, or petiole, is attached to the inner surface of the midline of thyroid cartilage, where it blends with the fibres of Broyles' tendon.

The supraglottic space is a potential space between the mucosa and the quadrangular membrane. The paraglottic space is formed between the quadrangular membrane and the internal perichondrium of thyroid cartilage. The ventricle penetrates into the paraglottic space from beneath the ventricular ligament. The supraglottic portion of the paraglottic space is divided by the ventricle into medial and lateral portions. The supraglottic paraglottic space is continuous with the glottic and subglottic portions of the paraglottic space only through the narrow portion lateral to the ventricle. This factor may play a role in containing the spread of cancer from supraglottic to glottic portions of the larynx. The paraglottic space is also narrowly continuous anteriorly with the pre-epiglottic space, although it is also rare for cancer to spread from pre-epiglottic to paraglottic spaces. The pre-epiglottic space lies anterior to the epiglottis. It is bounded superiorly by the hyoepiglottic ligament, anteriorly by the thyrohyoid membrane and thyroid cartilage, and posteriorly by the epiglottic cartilage and thyroepiglottic ligament. The space is filled with fat and areolar tissue anterior and lateral to the epiglottis, and it contains the saccule. The epiglottic cartilage contains deep lacunae that are filled with mucous glands. These lacunae permit ready spread of cancer from the laryngeal surface of the epiglottis into the paraglottic space. A less frequent route is laterally around the edge of the epiglottis. Anatomically, the entire pre-epiglottic space is confined to the supraglottic portion of the larynx, above the true vocal cords.

Pathology

Approximately 90% of supraglottic cancers are squamous cell carcinomas and can be graded as well, moderately or poorly differentiated. Other less common cancers include verrucous squamous cell carcinoma, spindle cell carcinoma, basaloid squamous cell carcinoma, neuroendocrine carcinomas, those of minor salivary gland origin, and sarcomas. This discussion is confined to the natural history, treatment and prognosis of squamous cell carcinoma of the supraglottis, except in instances where the same principles may be applied to other tumors involving the same areas. Most supraglottic carcinomas, in distinction to other laryngeal cancers, tend to grow with pushing margins, and despite frequent invasion of the pre-epiglottic space, tend to remain confined to the supraglottic portions of the larynx. The behavior of supraglottic tumors has been related to several factors, regional, gross and cytologic, as well as to anatomy of the supraglottis. Exophytic tumors tend to have 'pushing' margins and to remain confined to the supraglottis. These lesions are most often relatively well differentiated.[40,52,53] Ulcerative tumors tend to be less well differentiated, and have greater tendency to spread transglottically. Supraglottic tumors either predominantly involve the epiglottis or they involve the more posterior and lateral aspects of the supraglottic region (false cords, arytenoids and aryepiglottic folds). Supraglottic cancers have thus been divided into suprahyoid supraglottic cancers (suprahyoid epiglottis, aryepiglottic fold and arytenoid) and infrahyoid supraglottic cancers (infrahyoid epiglottis, ventricular fold and ventricle). Infrahyoid cancers are more common and display a clear tendency to spread into the fatty-areolar tissue of the pre-epiglottic space.[12,26,66] The tendency for invasion of the pre-epiglottic space has also been observed histologically in specimens of epiglottic cancer originally and clinically understaged as T1 and T2.[24] While the pre-epiglottic space is frequently invaded by supraglottic cancer, the hyoid bone remains tumor free except in far advanced lesions. In 112 supraglottic lesions reported by Kirchner,[38] the hyoid bone was only removed in two cases. Timon *et al.*[81] reported hyoid bone involvement by squamous cell carcinoma in 11 cases of 755 whole-organ laryngeal specimens examined. The lesion was localized in the supraglottic area in 172 cases and hyoid involvement occurred in four cases.

Suprahyoid epiglottic cancers tend to invade the tongue base and pyriform sinus rather than the pre-epiglottic space. Lesions occurring more laterally and posteriorly in the supraglottic region also lack the tendency to spread to the pre-epiglottic space. They tend to be less invasive than similar growths in other parts of the larynx.[37] Occasionally lateral supraglottic tumors penetrate the quadrangular membrane where they can travel laterally to the ventricle through the paraglottic space, thus extending transglottically.[83] Lesions may travel laterally along the medial surface of the aryepiglottic fold as far the arytenoid, usually without involving the arytenoid cartilage itself. Cartilaginous involvement occurs only when there is extensive involvement of the mucosa over the arytenoid.[41] Massive invasion of the upper aspect of the arytenoid cartilage causes fixation of the vocal cord in supraglottic cancers.

Kirchner[38] demonstrated the rarity of involvement of the thyroid cartilage in supraglottic cancer, although it occurs in a small number of cases. Han and Yamashita[31] found its infiltration in 9 of 100 cases of supraglottic cancer studied.

Spread of supraglottic cancer to the glottis

It is common knowledge that the supraglottic larynx arises embryologically from the buccopharyngeal anlage (branchial arches III and IV), while the glottis and subglottis derive from the tracheobronchial anlage (arches V and VI), but this does not justify the false assumption that supraglottic cancers do not extend to the glottic region. Certainly, supraglottic cancers have a marked tendency to remain confined above the glottis, particularly in their earlier stages, and in their less invasive forms. Nevertheless, a cancer may invade any neighboring tissue, regardless of its embryological origin. Supraglottic cancers may infiltrate the glottic plane as well as the subglottic region. Some authors have repeatedly postulated an anatomical barrier between the supraglottic and glottic regions[8,10,59,60] but numerous pathological studies, including whole-organ sections, have shown that there is no such barrier.[38,39,55] Kirchner[38] believes that 'whole-organ sections have failed to demonstrate an anatomic structure within the fundus of the ventricle that could qualify as a barrier to downward spread of cancer from the ventricular band'.

In a recent analysis of the literature, Ferlito *et al.*[20] evaluated the various reports and theories regarding a fixed anatomic or embryologic barrier to spread of supraglottic cancer to the glottis. The authors noted that:

> *... although the concept of a barrier between supraglottic and glottic regions of the larynx has been frequently repeated in the literature ... there is no evidence of an anatomical structure that could qualify as a barrier to the downward extension of supraglottic cancer on whole organ sections and in numerous other adequate histological studies .... Supraglottic cancers may cross the ventricle and extend down in the vocal cord ... sometimes without being visible endoscopically.*

The authors concluded that there is no anatomic structure qualifying as a barrier between the supraglottis and the glottis and that, although the supraglottis and the glottis have different embryological derivations, the exact location of the demarcation line has not been established. The more advanced supraglottic cancers have quite a high tendency to invade the glottic region, and basing supraglottic laryngectomy on embryological characteristics would be questionable. Nevertheless, Ferlito *et al.*[20] felt that supraglottic laryngectomy 'represents a safe and effective method for treating cancer confined to the supraglottis, regardless of any unjustified embryological considerations'.

Supraglottic cancer often remains confined to the supraglottic area (Figs 43.1–43.4). But if a supraglottic cancer invades the paraglottic space instead of the pre-epiglottic space, inferior invasion to the glottis can easily occur,[45] and has often been reported.[19,40,52,65,66,80] This is because the paraglottic space extends into the glottis along the medial surface of the thyroid cartilage (see above). In the Olofsson and van Nostrand series,[66] six of 25 (24%) of the supraglottic cancers invaded the glottic region. More recently, Han and Yamashita[31] investigated the manner of spread of supraglottic cancer by the whole-organ serial section study of surgical specimens from 100 supraglottic cancers and found the glottis involved in 48 cases and the

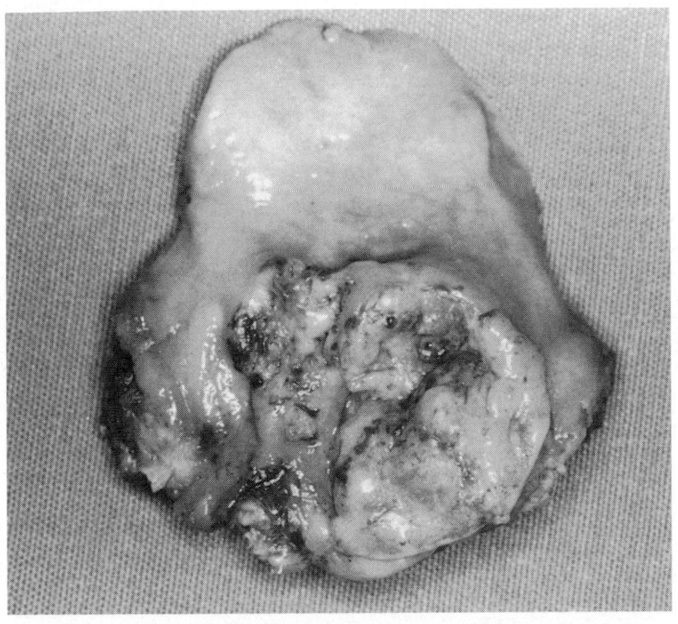

Figure 43.1 *Supraglottic laryngectomy specimen showing basaloid squamous carcinoma.*

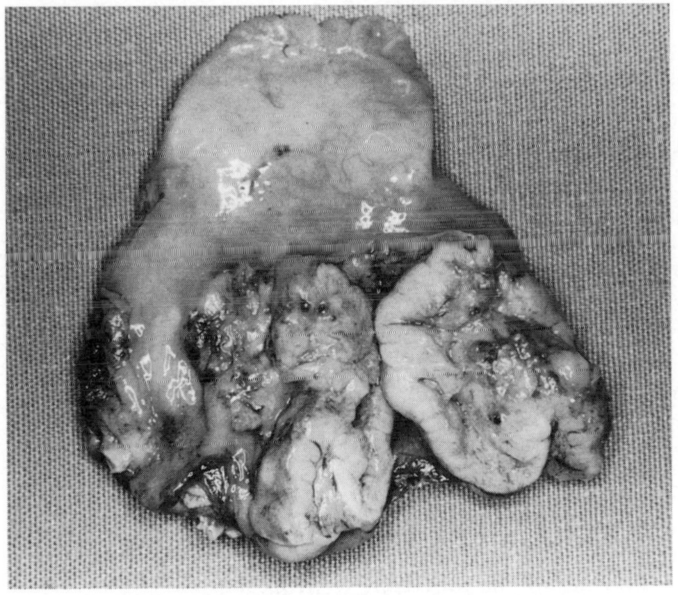

Figure 43.2 *Supraglottic carcinoma of exophytic type.*

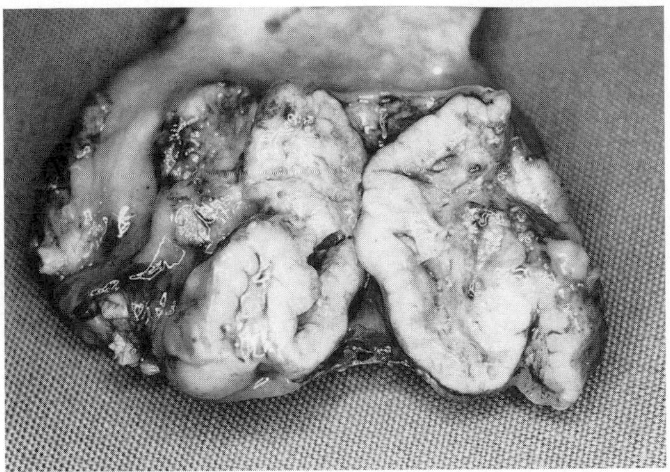

Figure 43.3 *A particular of the previous figure.*

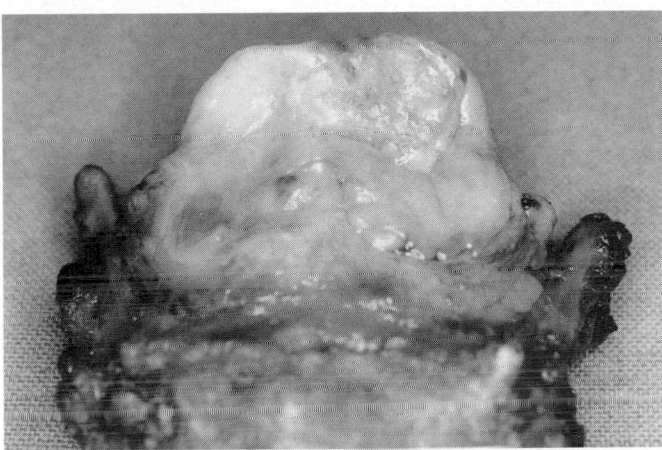

Figure 43.4 *Neoplastic lesion involving the lingual surface of the epiglottis.*

anterior commissure in 12. Weinstein *et al.*[87] evaluated the spread of supraglottic cancer to the glottic level by whole-organ sections of total laryngectomy specimens from 37 patients with previously untreated supraglottic cancers. Twenty (54%) specimens were noted to have extension of the cancer to the glottic level.

Staging of supraglottic cancer

Staging systems are methods of correlating various tumor characteristics with prognosis. At present the most commonly applied versions of the TNM system are those of the International Union Against Cancer (UICC),[33] and the American Joint Committee on Cancer (AJCC) published in 1997,[4] and virtually unified in 1987 (see Table 43.1).

Treatment of supraglottic cancer

Curable squamous cell supraglottic cancer is treated either by surgery or irradiation, alone or in combination. Either modality may be used in combination with chemotherapy. Because of the tendency for many supraglottic carcinomas to remain confined above the vocal cords, partial laryngectomy (conservation surgery) of various sorts has been a mainstay of treatment for these lesions.[9,11,32,51,56,78] Radiation therapy is an alternative to partial laryngectomy. More advanced tumors may require total or near total laryngectomy, often in combination with radiation therapy. The larynx preservation protocol developed by the Department of Veterans Affairs Laryngeal Study Group

Table 43.1 Classification of the primary tumor (T) for supraglottis

UICC	
Tx	Primary tumour cannot be assessed
TO	No evidence of primary tumour
Tis	Carcinoma in situ
T1	Tumour limited to one subsite of supraglottis, with normal vocal cord mobility
T2	Tumour invades mucosa of more than one adjacent subsite of supraglottis or glottis or region outside the supraglottis (e.g. mucosa of base of tongue, vallecula, medial wall of piriform sinus) without fixation of the larynx
T3	Tumour limited to larynx with vocal cord fixation and/or invades any of the following: postcricoid area, pre-epiglottic tissues, deep base of tongue
T4	Tumour invades through thyroid cartilage, and/or extends into soft tissues of the neck, thyroid, and/or esophagus

is an alternative to laryngectomy and postoperative irradiation for advanced lesions.[17] The incidence of cervical metastasis, often bilateral, is high in supraglottic carcinoma, and must be considered in any treatment plan.

Radiation therapy

Radiotherapy as an alternative to surgery

Radiation alone may be employed in the treatment of supraglottic cancer amenable to conservation surgery. For more advanced lesions, irradiation is less effective as primary treatment, but is an important adjuvant to surgical therapy, particularly in cases with lymph node metastasis.

The superiority of surgery over primary irradiation for supraglottic lesions, particularly those that were bulky and in more advanced stages, was emphasized in the older literature. Vermund,[85] in 1970, reviewed 544 supraglottic tumors staged T2, T3 and T4N0, reported in the contemporaneous literature. The combined series yielded 5-year survival of 32% for lesions treated with primary irradiation as opposed to 64% for primary surgery. Other reports indicated surgical cure rates about double those of radiotherapy.[15,36,64]

Goepfert *et al.*,[27] in 1975, reported results with radiotherapy equivalent to surgery for supraglottic lesions that would have been amenable to partial laryngectomy. They achieved initial control of primary tumor with normal voice ranging from 88.5% of T1 lesions to 60% of T4 lesions. This group, at the M. D. Anderson Cancer Center, felt that most T2 and many T3 lesions could be treated effectively with primary irradiation. The main contraindications to treatment with irradiation were bulky or infiltrative tumors with cord fixation, marked edema, or extensive pre-epiglottic space invasion. Since 1984, the M.D. Anderson group has employed hyperfractionated therapy of 110 or 120 cGy twice daily for all patients with T2 and T3 supraglottic tumors selected for primary radiation treatment. In 1990, the group reported that actuarial 2-year local control rate was 90%, with 84% local-regional control. Five of the six failures were successfully salvaged with surgery, yielding total 2-year local-regional control in 96% of patients.[46] In the same year, Mendenhall *et al.*,[54] at the University of Florida, reported local control in 100% of T1, 81% of T2, 61% of T3, and 50% of T4 supraglottic tumors.

The advent of the sophisticated imaging techniques of CT (computed tomography) and MRI (magnetic resonance imaging) have provided a means of better distinguishing which supraglottic tumors could be satisfactorily managed by radiation therapy. Successful radiation treatment of primary supraglottic carcinoma is generally correlated with the volume of tumor, with best results obtained with superficial and low-volume tumor.[25,49] Studies at the University of Florida have indicated overall local control of 83% for lesions less than 6 cc in volume, and 46% for lesions 6 cc or larger.[34,49]

A major disadvantage of primary radiotherapy treatment for supraglottic carcinoma is that subsequent conservation surgery for salvage becomes most difficult in cases of radiation failure. Som[75] reported five cases of supraglottic laryngectomy after high-dose primary radiotherapy. One developed flap necrosis with rupture of the carotid artery and three others developed perichondritis with elevation of skin flaps and prolonged postoperative courses. One of these had persistent laryngeal stenosis. DeSanto *et al.*[18] studied a large number of radiation failures treated at the Mayo Clinic. They noted that tumor recurrence is often recognized too late to utilize conservation surgery and concluded that the concept of 'radiate and watch', which was designed to save larynges, had resulted in more total laryngectomies than would have been necessary if the patients had been treated by conservation surgery in the first place.

Radiotherapy as adjuvant treatment

Irradiation may be used as an adjunct to surgery in an effort to increase cure rates, either as preoperative low-dose irradiation or as postoperative radiation therapy. There is little evidence that adjuvant radiotherapy is helpful following supraglottic laryngectomy, for suitable primary lesions, without palpable cervical metastatic disease. In past studies, Biller *et al.*[7] and Ogura and Biller[61] found no significant difference between patients with supraglottic carcinoma treated surgically with and without preoperative radiotherapy of 1500–3000 cGy over a period of 2–3 weeks. Som[75] found little justification for assuming the additional hazards of radiation for lesions that, treated by surgery alone, had 70% curability with preservation of laryngeal function. Ogura *et al.*,[64] however, reported better results in patients with clinically positive lymph nodes treated with preoperative radiotherapy than by surgery alone.

The current trend is to employ postoperative rather than preoperative irradiation, most often in cases with extralaryngeal spread of tumor, extensive pre- and paraglottic space involvement and in patients with positive lymph nodes. Nevertheless, postoperative irradiation presents a significant risk after supraglottic subtotal laryngectomy. Bocca *et al.*[10] reported chondronecrosis, laryngeal edema and severe respiratory stenosis in patients treated with radiotherapy after this procedure. A modified irradiation protocol, with 5500 cGy in 30 fractions delivered over 6 weeks, with an increased dose of electron beam therapy to the neck, when indicated, has been employed at the M. D. Anderson Cancer Center to minimize these problems.[28] Nevertheless, the possibility of postirradiation complications may influence the choice of procedure for management of the primary tumor in patients with lesions suitable for conservation surgery, but with extensive cervical node disease.

Surgical treatment of supraglottic cancer

Conservation surgery

As discussed above, a majority of supraglottic squamous cell carcinomas are at least moderately differentiated, with pushing margins. The tumors have little tendency to extend inferiorly to the glottis or laterally to the thyroid cartilage, but they have a marked propensity for invasion of the pre-epiglottic space. These lesions are often suitable for 'conservation' surgery, by which the tumor containing portions of larynx are removed with oncologically adequate margins, while preserving the essential functions of the larynx. A partial laryngectomy can be considered a 'conservation' procedure if, following the procedure, the patient is able to speak without artificial devices, swallow without aspiration, and breathe through an intact airway without tracheotomy.

Supraglottic tumors must be distinguished from tumors primarily originating in the ventricle, which penetrate readily into the paraglottic space from where extensive submucosal spread, cartilage invasion, and extralaryngeal spread occur. The latter lesions are transglottic, a term which has some ambiguity as it may be applied to supraglottic carcinomas that cross anterior or posterior to the ventricle to involve the glottic level, as well as to the true transventricular tumors just described. Conservation surgery has been employed for supraglottic tumors with glottic involvement as well as for transventricular (transglottic) carcinomas that extend into the paraglottic space, but results of treatment are considerably better for the supraglottic than for the transglottic lesions. Conservation surgery for supraglottic carcinoma usually consists of resection of a horizontal half of the larynx above the vocal cords (supraglottic laryngectomy), but may be extended to include glottic and infraglottic regions (subtotal or three-quarter laryngectomy and supracricoid laryngectomy). Extended supraglottic laryngectomy may be used in patients with tongue base carcinoma involving the vallecula and the lingual face of epiglottis.[79]

Standard supraglottic laryngectomy (SSL)

Excision of cancer of the epiglottis by lateral pharyngotomy was first performed by Trotter in the early twentieth century.[82] Development of this procedure was continued by Colledge[16] and Orton,[67] but the procedure remained obscure until the publications in 1947 and 1952 of the work of Alonso.[2,3] Alonso's procedure required a temporary pharyngostoma because of difficulty in approximating the base of the tongue to the cut surface of the larynx after resection. This feature as well as other limitations of the time hampered popular acceptance.

In 1958, Ogura[60] published his technique for SSL and radical neck dissection, with primary closure using a muscle flap and skin graft. The results of treatment of 15 patients with epiglottic carcinoma, with no local recurrence and preservation of the larynx in all cases, were reported. This paper was instrumental in stimulating interest in the procedure. In 1959, Som[74] described a similar procedure with primary closure obtained by direct approximation of local tissues, without a skin graft. Sixteen patients were treated, with only one local recurrence.

Acceptance of the procedure by the surgical community was still hampered by concern for the narrow inferior resection margins obtained by SSL. In 1968, Bocca *et al.*[10] reported results of 124 supraglottic laryngectomies with 72.7% survival in the 33 cases followed for 5 years or longer. Because of favorable results reported in an increasingly large number of patients, by the 1970s, supraglottic laryngectomy had become widely accepted in the USA.

The standard supraglottic laryngectomy consists of resection of the epiglottis, hyoid bone, thyrohyoid membrane, upper half of thyroid cartilage and supraglottic mucosa, with lines of transection going through both aryepiglottic folds, the valleculae, and the ventricles. Thus, lesions confined to the laryngeal surface of the epiglottis or false vocal cords without extension onto the lingual surface of the epiglottis, aryepiglottic folds, or arytenoid region are amenable to this resection.

A major consideration has been the inferior extent of the tumor. As stated above, surgeons were initially reluctant to employ this procedure for tumors extending below the petiole. As better understanding of the marked barrier to spread of supraglottic tumor to the vocal cords increased, surgeons became willing to accept narrower inferior resection margins. It has become apparent that lesions arising low in the vestibule are actually more suitable for supraglottic laryngectomy than lesions involving the suprahyoid portion of the epiglottis, as the latter are more likely to extend superiorly and laterally beyond the confines of conventional supraglottic laryngectomy, leading to recurrence. Inferiorly, however, a margin of only 2–3 mm of normal mucosa is adequate to prevent recurrence at the glottic level.

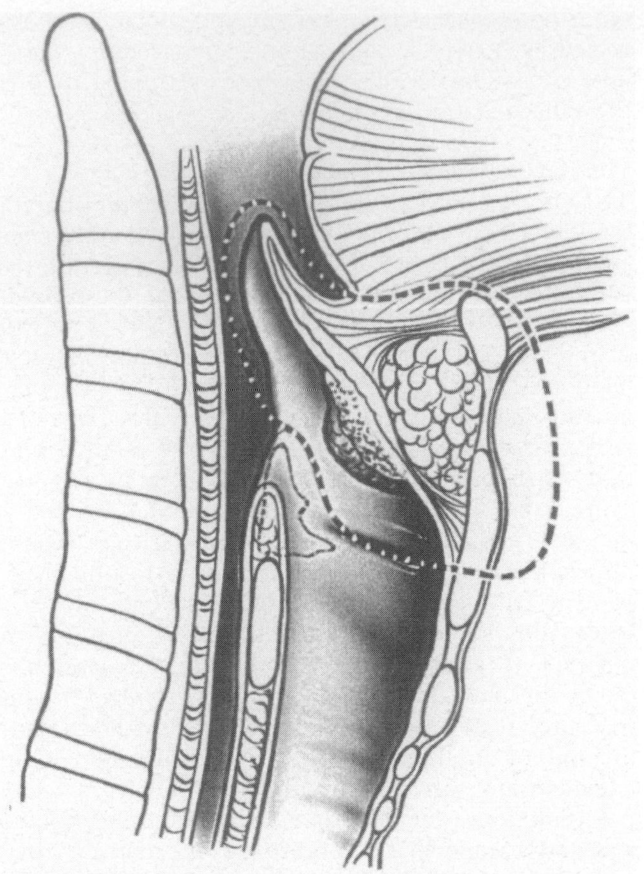

Figure 43.5 *Lines of resection for standard supraglottic laryngectomy. (Reproduced with permission from Silver CE, Ferlito A.* Surgery for Cancer of the Larynx and Related Structures, *2nd edn. Philadelphia: Saunders, 1996.)*

Evaluation of a supraglottic tumor for partial laryngectomy may be hampered by the bulk of the tumor, which may obscure the inferior margin of the tumor as viewed from above by indirect or direct laryngoscopy. Fiberoptic laryngoscopy or endoscopic examination with a small right-angle telescope, as well as thin axial CT sections may be helpful in determining the lower limit, as well as in ruling out the presence of cartilage involvement or extralaryngeal spread. The greatest difficulty in evaluating inferior extension of tumor occurs with lesions that extend to the anterior commissure. Once the anterior commissure is involved, thyroid cartilage involvement (in the midline) and extralaryngeal spread occur readily. While this may be demonstrated by CT, occasionally cartilaginous involvement may be inapparent until the perichondrium is elevated at surgery, revealing the underlying thyroid cartilage to be invaded by tumor. This finding makes total laryngectomy mandatory.

Vocal cord fixation due to invasion of the cricoarytenoid joint or to extension of tumor into the paraglottic space is a contraindication to SSL. Fixation of the cord may simply be due to the bulk of the tumor. Such cases are amenable to SSL. As the mechanism of fixation may not be apparent preoperatively, exploratory lateral pharyngotomy with the option of converting to total laryngectomy is worthwhile in questionable cases. As it is often impossible to establish preoperatively, with certainty, the suitability of a given lesion for conservation surgery, consent for possible total laryngectomy should be obtained in all cases.

The technique of SSL is demonstrated in Fig 43.5. Neck dissection, often bilateral, is usually performed in conjunction with supraglottic laryngectomy (see below).

The conventional supraglottic resection may be extended posteriorly to include resection of the arytenoid. The line of resection traverses the cricoarytenoid joint and vocal process of the arytenoid. This procedure is used for lesions that grow posteriorly along the vestibular fold or aryepiglottic fold to involve the mucosa over the arytenoid or, occasionally, the upper portion of the cartilage itself. Lesions with extensive arytenoid cartilage or cricoarytenoid joint involvement require total laryngectomy, as do lesions that extend across the posterior commissure to the opposite arytenoid.

The results of several published series are summarized in Table 43.2.[1,9,13,30,32,46–48,51,63,71,75,76,78] Cure rates consistently ranging approximately from 70 to 90% are obtained in the treatment of primary supraglottic carcinoma, with the added benefit of preservation of laryngeal function. It is difficult to compare results from different series treated by different methods (supraglottic laryngectomy, extended supraglottic laryngectomy, combined treatment – surgery and radiotherapy, radiotherapy and surgery).

The success of salvage procedures after failure of SSL is questionable. Local recurrences almost always involve the base of the tongue and pharyngeal structures and rarely involve the vocal cords.[10,75] They are often difficult to manage by any combination of modalities. The experience at our departments has indicated that failure due to lymph node metastasis is more common than from local recurrence. Extracapsular spread is the most important factor affecting the prognosis of patients with supraglottic cancer.[58]

Subtotal laryngectomy (subtotal glottic–supraglottic laryngectomy, three-quarter laryngectomy)

Subtotal, or three-quarter, laryngectomy theoretically consists of resection of both a vertical and horizontal half of the larynx. Beyond this basic definition, however, the procedure and its indications have varied as used by various authors, and at different times. In 1965 Ogura and Dedo[62] described a procedure for resection of T2 supraglottic cancers involving the arytenoids and glottis with minimal subglottic extent. The resection continued downward to include the true vocal cord, with the arytenoid if necessary. The cord was reconstructed with a triangular wedge of thyroid cartilage, which was then covered with a flap of hypopharyngeal mucosa. A more extensive 'subtotal laryngectomy' was described by Iwai,[35] in Japan, for T3 transglottic lesions of the larynx. The

Table 43.2 Results of supraglottic laryngectomy

Series	*Year*	*Follow-up (years)*	*No. of patients*	*Percentage survival*	*Remarks*
Som[75]	1970	5	75	68	
Ogura *et al.*[63]	1980	3	119	67	The series includes also patients treated with partial laryngopharyngectomy (11 cases) and extended subtotal supraglottic laryngectomy (8 cases). 74% of the patients received low-dose (3000 rad) preoperative irradiation
Burnstein and Calcaterra[13]	1985	2	41	90	Follow-up was available on 40 patients. 17 patients received postoperative radiation therapy and 1 patient received preoperative irradiation. The series includes conventional and extended supraglottic laryngectomies
Maceri *et al.*[48]	1985	2	25	80	
Strijbos *et al.*[76]	1987	5	57	80	The 10-year actuarial survival rate was 59%
Robbins *et al.*[71]	1988	5	34	89	The series includes cases of intermediate stage (T2 and T3). 32 patients underwent conventional supraglottic laryngectomy, whilst 2 patients had an extended supraglottic laryngectomy. 23 patients received postoperative radiotherapy and 2 patients received preoperative irradiation
Lee *et al.*[46]	1990	5	60	91	50 patients (83%) received adjunctive postoperative radiation therapy
Lutz *et al.*[47]	1990	2	102	77	Surgery alone
Bocca[9]	1991	5	487	78	
Suárez *et al.*[78]	1995	3	193	74.3	94 patients (48.7%) received postoperative irradiation
Gregor *et al.*[30]	1996	5	26	81	Postoperative irradiation was given in some cases
Herranz-González *et al.*[32]	1996	5	110	72.6	Postoperative radiotherapy was used in 42 patients (38%)
Maurice *et al.*[51]	1996	5	87	68.5	56 patients received postoperative radiation therapy
Adamopoulos *et al.*[1]	1997	3	92	83.6	Postoperative radiotherapy only in T3 T4, N+ patients (40%)

vertical component of the resection included not only the vocal cord, but also the ipsilateral thyroid ala and possibly part of the cricoid. The glottis was reconstructed by rotating the superior cornu of thyroid cartilage to replace the resected portion of laryngeal framework, with resurfacing by a flap of hypopharyngeal mucosa. Sekula[72] reported on a variety of subtotal laryngectomies performed at his clinic in Cracow, Poland, for the resection of tumors with supraglottic and glottic involvement. The procedures were often performed within 'narrow limits of safety' as far as tumor margins were concerned. The author pointed to favorable early results and to the advantages of offering these procedures to patients who would otherwise have refused total laryngectomy. Some severe problems with postoperative deglutition were encountered.

Friedman *et al.*[23] developed a subtotal laryngectomy, which consisted of horizontal partial laryngectomy with vertical extension for supraglottic carcinomas extending onto the arytenoid and/or the vocal cord, as well as for transglottic cancers with minimal subglottic extension and minimal cephalic extension onto the ventricle and false cord. The procedure was employed in selected patients with vocal cord fixation as well as previous radiation therapy, the key factor in selection of patients being unequivocal preoperative demonstration by computed tomography of the absence of cartilage invasion.

The best known procedure is that described by Biller and Lawson,[5] in 1984. This resection combines the supraglottic laryngectomy with hemilaryngectomy (three-quarter laryngectomy). Reconstruction is accomplished with a large flap of thyroid cartilage pedicled on the inferior constrictor muscle. The procedure is suitable for glottic tumors with superior extension, supraglottic tumors with inferior extension, or tumors that originated within the ventricle with bidirectional spread. It is limited to lesions 2 cm or less in diameter without vocal cord fixation, subglottic extension, anterior commissure or cartilage involvement or prior radiation therapy. The technique is demonstrated in Fig 43.6.

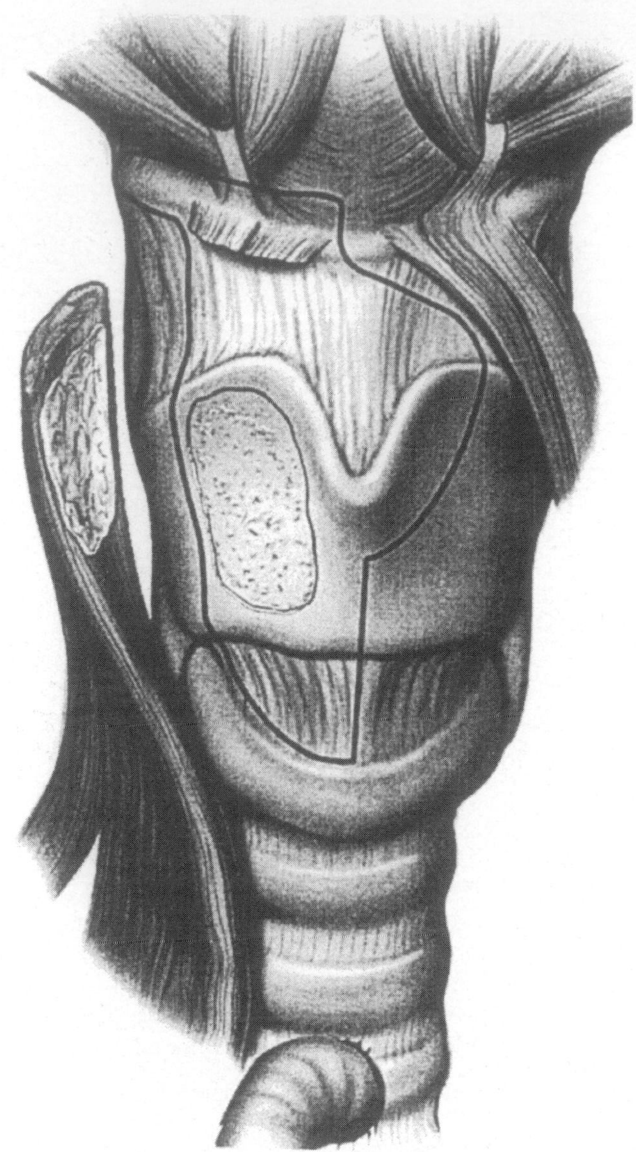

Figure 43.6 *Lines of resection for subtotal laryngectomy. (Reproduced with permission from Silver CE, Ferlito A.* Surgery for Cancer of the Larynx and Related Structures, *2nd edn. Philadelphia: Saunders, 1996.)*

Results of subtotal laryngectomy are difficult to evaluate because of small numbers of cases reported and variations in indications. Sekula[72] and Iwai,[35] who used this procedure for resection of transglottic tumors in their relatively small series of cases, achieved cure rates between 60 and 70%. Ogura and Dedo[62] reported no recurrences and good laryngeal function in four patients followed 9–21 months after the procedure described above. Friedman and Katsantonis[22] reported 3-year survival of 70% in a series of 24 patients with similar tumors, some with fixed vocal cords.

Five patients operated on by Biller and Lawson[5] were free of tumor for periods longer than 1.5 years, at the time of their report. The authors noted the procedure to be more efficacious in treatment of either glottic or supraglottic tumors that did not invade the paraglottic space deeply, than for true ventricular tumors with significant paraglottic space involvement.

Supracricoid laryngectomy with cricohyoidopexy

Segmental resection of the larynx from the cricoid cartilage to the hyoid bone has been popular in Europe, but not in the USA, for the past 15 years. The concept of a partial laryngeal resection in which reconstruction was accomplished by suturing the hyoid bone to the cricoid cartilage was first described by Majer and Rieder in 1959.[50] The procedure was refined and reported by Piquet *et al.*[69] in 1974, and has been used extensively in Europe.[42,44,70] It has been employed for supraglottic carcinomas with pre-epiglottic space, paraglottic space and thyroid cartilage involvement that were not amenable to conventional or extended supraglottic subtotal laryngectomy.

Laccourreye *et al.*[42] listed the indications for supracricoid laryngectomy with cricohyoidopexy as follows:

- T1 and T2 supraglottic lesions extending to the ventricle, the infrahyoid epiglottis and the posterior third of the false vocal cord;
- T1 and T2 supraglottic lesions extending to the glottis and the anterior commissure with or without impaired mobility of the true vocal cord;
- T3 transglottic cancers with marked limitation of the true vocal cord; and
- selected cases of T4 transglottic carcinomas invading the thyroid cartilage.

These authors consider the following as contraindications to the procedure:

- subglottic extent greater than 10 mm anteriorly and 5 mm posteriorly, as these tumors involve the cricoid cartilage;
- preoperative clinical examination that reveals arytenoid cartilage fixation, as these lesions invade either the posterior intrinsic laryngeal muscles, the cricoarytenoid joint, or the arytenoid cartilage;
- massive invasion of the pre-epiglottic space observed preoperatively, either during the clinical examination or with CT (limited invasion of the pre-epiglottic space is not considered a contraindication, as this compartment is totally resected during the procedure);
- supraglottic and transglottic lesions that involve the pharyngeal wall, vallecula, base of the tongue, postcricoid and arytenoid region; and
- cricoid cartilage invasion.

The technique of supracricoid laryngectomy with cricohyoidopexy is demonstrated in Fig 43.7.

Laccourreye *et al.*[42] reported results of treatment of 68 patients operated at the Laennec Hospital in Paris between 1974 and 1986. The minimum follow-up was 18 months, and 39 patients were followed for at least 3 years. There were no local recurrences. Four (5.88%) of 68 patients developed neck recurrence. All had preoperatively palpa-

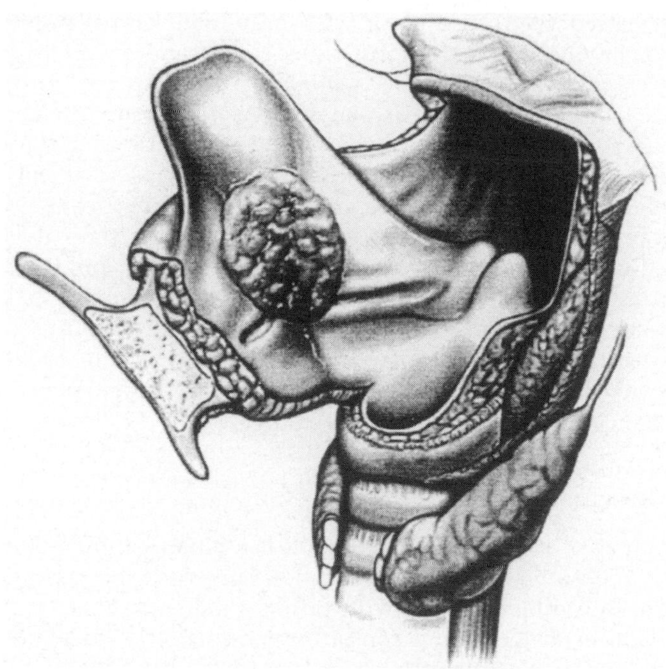

Figure 43.7 *Demonstration of extent of resection in supracricoid laryngectomy. (Reproduced with permission from Silver CE, Ferlito A.* Surgery for Cancer of the Larynx and Related Structures, *2nd edn. Philadelphia: Saunders, 1996.)*

ble cervical lymph nodes, and all had been treated, at the time of primary resection, with radical neck dissection and postoperative radiation therapy. Eight (11.76%) patients developed distant metastases. The 3-year actuarial survival rate was 71.4%. Ten patients died of second primaries, two of distant metastases, and two of intercurrent disease.

Laccourreye *et al.*[44] reported results in 19 patients with infrahyoid epiglottic squamous cell carcinoma with gross pre-epiglottic space invasion, not amenable to SSL for various reasons, including massive invasion of the petiole, invasion of the anterior commissure, invasion of the true vocal cord, involvement of the floor of the ventricle or marked limitation of true vocal cord mobility. In most of the patients one arytenoid was either totally or partially removed. The 5-year actuarial survival was 84.2%. There was only one instance of local recurrence and one of nodal recurrence. The 5-year actuarial rate of distant metastasis was 5.6% and of second primary tumors, 30%. A second primary tumor was the cause of death in five of six patients who succumbed.

In the series of 68 patients, all patients were decannulated within 8 weeks with the exception of one patient who died of a ruptured aortic aneurism on the third postoperative day. The average time of decannulation was 7 days. Normal postoperative deglutition was achieved by 50 (75%) of 67 patients within the first postoperative month. Physiologic phonation without tracheostomy was achieved in all patients within the same time period. Fifteen patients required temporary gastrostomy, and in two, permanent gastrostomy was required – one because of resection of the base of the tongue for a second primary tumor. Laccourreye *et al.*[44] found that swallowing problems occurred with significantly greater frequency in patients who underwent partial or complete resection of an arytenoid.

In this study, various complications were found related to postoperative radiation therapy. These included persistent laryngeal edema in four of 19 patients, reduced mobility of the remaining arytenoid in three and chondroradionecrosis in two. There was one instance each of glottic stenosis and of cervical fibrosis with phrenic nerve paralysis.

In 1997, Naudo *et al.*[57] reported their experience presenting a retrospective analysis over a 20-year period of 124 patients who consecutively underwent supracricoid partial laryngectomy with cricohyoidopexy. Their functional results with regard to respiration and deglutition were comparable with the results achieved with horizontal supraglottic laryngectomy.

In 1998, Laccourreye *et al.*[43] reviewed their experience with neoadjuvant chemotherapy and supracricoid partial laryngectomy with crycohyoidopexy in a series of 60 patients with an isolated, untreated, advanced supraglottic/transglottic invasive squamous cell carcinoma classified as T3–T4 lesion. The Kaplan–Meier 5-year actuarial survival, local failure, nodal failure and distant metastasis estimates were 72.7%, 8.3%, 9.2% and 9.8%, respectively.

Complications and sequelae of conservation surgery

Aspiration is actually the most significant early postoperative complication, being present at least to some degree in approximately 20–80% of patients.[8,21,32,71,73,75–77] Chronic aspiration frequently leads to pneumonia and atelectasis and if aspiration continues to be a problem conversion to a total laryngectomy is required. Aspiration of food and, in particular, of liquids, is the most common problem after supraglottic laryngectomy. Aspiration is frequent in patients who underwent extensive supraglottic laryngectomy, in particular in those cases when the arytenoid cartilage has been removed.

Airway obstruction occurs infrequently. It may arise from differing causes. The most common type occurs in the early postoperative period and is due to lymphedema of unresected supraglottic mucosa. This problem is prevented by removing the entire false vocal cord at the time of initial resection, even if inclusion of this structure is not necessary to ensure an adequate resection margin. Loss of the supraglottic structures not only removes the anatomic protection of the laryngeal introitus, but also interrupts the sequential sensory input of the swallowing mechanism. This sensory derangement is the most important factor in loss of adequate deglutition after supraglottic resections.[84] Deficiency in sensory reception can be compensated for by the residual structures, provided damage to the external branch of the superior laryngeal nerve as well as the recurrent laryngeal nerve is avoided.[86] In extensive resections for larger tumors, which may include arytenoid resection and tongue base excision, injury to these nerves as well as erratic healing, edema and scarring may combine to further reduce sphincteric function.

The true extent of the aspiration problem may not be appreciated by many surgeons. Flores *et al.*[21] determined that relatively normal swallowing could be expected in only 85–90% of patients after supraglottic laryngectomy. Approximately half the remaining patients can swallow and cough well enough to prevent pneumonia, but are unable to ingest sufficient food to maintain adequate nutrition and require either gastrostomy or completion laryngectomy. The remaining 5–7% develop persistent pulmonary infection and require completion laryngectomy.

Corrective surgical measures may be taken to prevent or treat the incompetent glottic insufficiency that may follow supraglottic laryngectomy, particularly in elderly patients or in those with more extensive resections. These include thyroid cartilage implants,[6] laryngeal suspension[14,29] and cricopharyngeal myotomy.[21]

Pharyngocutaneous fistula is an uncommon complication in supraglottic laryngectomy for supraglottic carcinoma (2–12% of the cases).[13,32,46,76] Postoperative complications also include hemorrhage, wound abscess, seroma and delayed wound healing.[32]

Treatment of advanced lesions – total and near total laryngectomy

Because of the tendency to remain confined above the glottis, advanced supraglottic lesions may still be technically amenable to conservation surgery, the advanced stage being mainly due to extensive lymph node disease. Nevertheless, some primary tumors are so extensive as to require total, or near total laryngectomy. Transglottic spread of tumor, extensive extralaryngeal invasion, thyroid cartilage invasion and tongue base involvement requiring more than 3 cm of tongue base resection are all contraindications to supraglottic laryngectomy and its variations. As stated above, at times the presence of extensive lymph node disease, which will mandate postoperative irradiation, as well as unsuitability of the patient for conservation surgery, will determine the indication for total laryngectomy. Not all surgeons agree that the need for postoperative irradiation is a contraindication to conservation surgery. Nevertheless, the difficulties with this combination of modalities have been discussed above, and the need for postoperative irradiation is a factor to consider in determining treatment of the primary tumor.

Thus a discussion of results of total laryngectomy for management of supraglottic carcinoma would be rather meaningless, as factors related to the primary tumor are not the major cause of treatment failure. The majority of total laryngectomies are indicated because of the patient's predicted inability to tolerate partial laryngectomy, rather than because of tumor factors.

Results of treatment of supraglottic cancer by near total laryngectomy are of some interest. In 1998, Pearson *et al.*[68] reviewed their experience with near total laryngectomy for laryngeal and pyriform sinus cancer and found that local control of cancer was similar to that expected with total laryngectomy or laryngopharyngectomy. Conversational voice was achieved in 85% of patients surviving beyond 1 year. Local recurrence rate was 7%. It may be concluded from this report that local recurrence is no more prevalent after near total laryngectomy than it is after total laryngectomy. The procedure, which produces better functional results than total laryngectomy, has value for patients who are not sufficiently healthy to withstand supraglottic laryngectomy, or in whom extensive cervical metastatic disease may discourage performance of supraglottic laryngectomy.

Conclusions

Supraglottic cancer of the larynx is a curable tumor that is often amenable to conservation surgery. Most tumors are well differentiated, with pushing margins. There is a high incidence of invasion of the pre-epiglottic space, but the entire pre-epiglottic space is removed by supraglottic laryngectomy. Total laryngectomy may be indicated for lesions with transglottic spread, thyroid cartilage invasion or extralaryngeal spread. Lack of patient suitability for supraglottic laryngectomy may also be an indication for total or near total laryngectomy. Several conservation procedures are available for treatment of the primary tumor. These include standard supraglottic laryngectomy, supraglottic laryngectomy extended to include an ipsilateral arytenoid, the vallecula with or without a portion of the base of the tongue, the medial wall of the pyriform sinus, 'subtotal' laryngectomy and supracricoid laryngectomy. Satisfactory local control rates are obtained with all these procedures for appropriate lesions.

References

1. Adamopoulos G, Yotakis I, Apostolopoulos K, Manolopoulos L, Kandiloros D, Ferekidis E. Supraglottic laryngectomy – series report and analysis of results. *J Laryngol Otol* 1997; **111:** 730–4.
2. Alonso JM. Conservative surgery of cancer of the larynx. *Trans Am Acad Ophthalmol Otolaryngol* 1947; **51:** 633–42.
3. Alonso JM, Jackson CL. Conservation of function in surgery of cancer of the larynx: bases, techniques and results. *Trans Am Acad Ophthalmol Otolaryngol* 1952; **56:** 722–5.
4. American Joint Committee on Cancer (AJCC). *Manual for Staging of Cancer*, 5th edn. Philadelphia: Lippincott, 1997.
5. Biller HF, Lawson W. Partial laryngectomy for transglottic cancers. *Ann Otol Rhinol Laryngol* 1984; **93:** 297–300.
6. Biller HF, Lawson W, Sacks S. Correction of posterior glottic incompetence following partial laryngectomy. *Ann Otol Rhinol Laryngol* 1982; **91:** 448–9.
7. Biller HF, Ogura JH, Davis WH, Powers WE. Planned preoperative irradiation for carcinoma of the larynx and laryngopharynx treated by total and partial laryngectomy. *Laryngoscope* 1969; **79:** 1387–95.

8. Bocca E. Supraglottic cancer. *Laryngoscope* 1975; **85:** 1318–26.
9. Bocca E. Surgical management of supraglottic cancer and its lymph node metastases in a conservative perspective. *Ann Otol Rhinol Laryngol* 1991; **100:** 261–7.
10. Bocca E, Pignataro O, Mosciaro O. Supraglottic surgery of the larynx. *Ann Otol* 1968; **67:** 1005–26.
11. Bocca E, Pignataro O, Oldini C. Supraglottic laryngectomy: 30 years of experience. *Ann Otol Rhinol Laryngol* 1983; **92:** 14–18.
12. Bryce DP. The management of laryngeal cancer. *J Otolaryngol* 1979; **8:** 105–26.
13. Burnstein FD, Calcaterra TC. Supraglottic laryngectomy: series report and analysis of results. *Laryngoscope* 1985; **95:** 833–6.
14. Calcaterra T. Laryngeal suspension after supraglottic laryngectomy. *Arch Otolaryngol* 1971; **94:** 306–9.
15. Coates HL, DeSanto LW, Devine KD, Elveback LR. Carcinoma of the supraglottic larynx. A review of 221 cases. *Arch Otolaryngol* 1976; **102:** 686–9.
16. Colledge L. Repair of pharyngeal defects after operation for removal of malignant tumors. *Proc R Soc Med* 1931; **24:** 14.
17. Department of Veterans Affairs Layngeal Cancer Study Group. Induction chemotherapy plus radiation compared with surgery plus radiation in patients with advanced laryngeal cancer. *N Engl J Med* 1991; **324:** 1685–90.
18. DeSanto LW, Lillie JC, Devine KD. Surgical salvage after radiation for laryngeal cancer. *Laryngoscope* 1976; **86:** 649–57.
19. Ferlito A. Histological classification of larynx and hypopharynx cancers and their clinical implications. Pathologic aspects of 2052 malignant neoplasms diagnosed at the ORL Department of Padua University from 1966 to 1976. *Acta Otolaryngol Suppl (Stockh)* 1976; **342:** 1–88.
20. Ferlito A, Oloffson J, Rinaldo A. The barrier between the supraglottis and the glottis: myth or reality? *Ann Otol Rhinol Laryngol* 1997; **106:** 716–19.
21. Flores TC, Wood BG, Levine HL, Koegel L Jr, Tucker HM. Factors in successful deglutition following supraglottic laryngeal surgery. *Ann Otol Rhinol Laryngol* 1982; **91:** 579–83.
22. Friedman WH, Katsantonis GP. Subtotal laryngectomy with contralateral laryngoplasty. In: Silver CE, ed. *Laryngeal Cancer.* New York: Thieme, 1991: 183–92.
23. Friedman WH, Katsantonis GP, Siddoway JR, Cooper MH. Contralateral laryngoplasty after supraglottic laryngectomy with vertical extension. *Arch Otolaryngol* 1989; **107:** 742–5.
24. Friedmann I, Ferlito A. Precursors of squamous cell carcinoma. In: Ferlito A, ed. *Neoplasms of the Larynx.* Edinburgh: Churchill Livingstone, 1993: 97–111.
25. Gilbert RW, Birt D, Shulman H *et al.* Correlation of tumor volume with local control in laryngeal carcinoma treated by radiotherapy. *Ann Otol Rhinol Laryngol* 1987; **96:** 514–18.
26. Glanz H. Carcinoma of the larynx. *Adv Otorhinolaryngol* 1984; **32:** 1–123.
27. Goepfert H, Jesse RH, Fletcher GH, Hamberger A. Optimal treatment for the technically resectable squamous cell carcinoma of the supraglottic larynx. *Laryngoscope* 1975; **85:** 14–32.
28. Goepfert H, Lee N, Wendt C, Peters L. Treatment of cancer of the supraglottic larynx. In: Silver CE, ed. *Laryngeal Cancer.* New York: Thieme, 1991: 176–82.
29. Goode R. Laryngeal suspension in head and neck surgery. *Laryngoscope* 1976; **86:** 349–54.
30. Gregor RT, Oei SS, Baris G, Keus RB, Balm AJM, Hilgers FJM. Supraglottic laryngectomy with postoperative radiation versus primary radiation in the management of supraglottic laryngeal cancer. *Am J Otolaryngol* 1996; **17:** 316–21.
31. Han DM, Yamashita K. The manner of spread of supraglottic carcinoma. *Larynx Jpn* 1991; **2:** 175–86.
32. Herranz-González J, Gavilán J, Martínez-Vidal J, Gavilán C. Supraglottic laryngectomy: functional and oncologic results. *Ann Otol Rhinol Laryngol* 1996; **105:** 18–22.
33. International Union Against Cancer. Sobin LH, Wittekind Ch, eds. *TNM Classification of Malignant Tumours*, 5th edn. New York: Wiley-Liss, 1997.
34. Isaacs JH Jr, Mancuso AA, Mendenhall WM, Parsons JT. Deep spread patterns in CT staging of T2–4 squamous cell laryngeal carcinoma. *Otolaryngol Head Neck Surg* 1988; **99:** 455–64.
35. Iwai H. Limitations of conservation surgery in carcinoma involving the arytenoid. In: Alberti PW, Bryce DP, eds. *Workshops from the Centennial Conference on Laryngeal Cancer.* New York: Appleton-Century-Crofts, 1976: 426–31.
36. Jankovic I, Merkas Z. Radiotherapy as the primary approach in the treatment of laryngeal cancer. In: Alberti PW, Bryce DP, eds. *Workshops from the Centennial Conference on Laryngeal Cancer.* New York: Appleton-Century-Crofts, 1976: 881–8.
37. Kirchner JA. One hundred laryngeal cancers studied by serial sections. *Ann Otol* 1969; **78:** 689–709.
38. Kirchner JA. Spread and barriers to spread of cancer within the larynx. In: Silver CE, ed. *Laryngeal Cancer.* New York: Thieme, 1991: 6–13.
39. Kirchner JA. Glottic-supraglottic barrier: fact or fantasy? *Ann Otol Rhinol Laryngol* 1997; **106:** 700–4.
40. Kirchner JA, Som ML. Clinical and histological observations on supraglottic cancer. *Ann Otol* 1971; **80:** 638–45.
41. Kirchner JA, Som ML. The anterior commissure technique of partial laryngectomy: clinical and laboratory observations. *Laryngoscope* 1975; **85:** 1308–17.
42. Laccourreye H, Laccourreye O, Weinstein G, Menard M, Brasnu D. Supracricoid laryngectomy with cricohyoidopexy: a partial laryngeal procedure for selected supraglottic and transglottic carcinomas. *Laryngoscope* 1990; **100:** 735–41.
43. Laccourreye O, Brasnu D, Blacabe B, Hans S, Seckin S, Weinstein G. Neo-adjuvant chemotherapy and supracricoid partial laryngectomy with cricohyoidopexy for advanced endolaryngeal carcinoma classified as T3–T4: 5-year oncologic results. *Head Neck* 1998; **20:** 595–9.
44. Laccourreye O, Brasnu D, Merite-Drancy A *et al.* Cricohyoidopexy in selected infrahyoid epiglottic carcinomas presenting with pathological preepiglottic space

invasion. *Arch Otolaryngol Head Neck Surg* 1993; **119:** 881–6.

45. Lam KH, Wong J. The preepiglottic and paraglottic spaces in relation to spread of carcinoma of the larynx. *Am J Otolaryngol* 1983; **4:** 81–91.
46. Lee NK, Goepfert H, Wendt CD. Supraglottic laryngectomy for intermediate-stage cancer: U.T. M.D. Anderson Cancer Center experience with combined therapy. *Laryngoscope* 1990; **100:** 831–6.
47. Lutz CK, Johnson JT, Wagner RL, Myers EN. Supraglottic carcinoma: patterns of recurrence. *Ann Otol Rhinol Laryngol* 1990; **99:** 12–17.
48. Maceri DR, Lampe HB, Makielski KH, Passamani PP, Krause CJ. Conservation laryngeal surgery. A critical analysis. *Arch Otolaryngol* 1985; **111:** 361–5.
49. Mancuso AA. Evaluation and staging of laryngeal and hypopharyngeal cancer by computed tomography and magnetic resonance imaging. In: Silver CE, ed. *Laryngeal Cancer.* New York: Thieme, 1991: 46–94.
50. Majer H, Rieder W. Technique de laryngectomie permettant de conserver la perméabilité respiratoire la crico-hyoido-pexie. *Ann Otolaryngol Chir Cervicofac* 1959; **76:** 677–83.
51. Maurice N, Delol J, Makeieff M, Arnoux A, Crampette L, Guerrier B. La laryngectomie horizontale supraglottique. Technique, indications, résultats carcinologiques et suites fonctionnelles précoces. A propos de 87 cas. *Ann Otolaryngol Chir Cervicofac* 1996; **113:** 203–11.
52. McDonald TJ, DeSanto LW, Weiland LH. Supraglottic larynx and its pathology as studied by whole laryngeal sections. *Laryngoscope* 1976; **86:** 635–48.
53. McGavran M, Mauer W, Ogura J. The incidence of cervical lymph node metastases from epidermoid carcinoma of the larynx and their relationship to certain characteristics of the primary tumor; a study based on the clinical and pathological findings in 96 patients treated by primary en bloc laryngectomy and radical neck dissection. *Cancer* 1961; **14:** 55–66.
54. Mendenhall WM, Parsons JT, Stringer SP, Cassisi NJ, Million RR. Carcinoma of the supraglottic larynx: a basis for comparing the results of radiotherapy and surgery. *Head Neck* 1990; **12:** 204–9.
55. Million RR, Cassisi NJ, Mancuso AA. Larynx. In: Million RR, Cassisi NJ, eds. *Management of Head and Neck Cancer. A Multidisciplinary Approach,* 2nd edn. Philadelphia: Lippincott, 1994: 431–97.
56. Myers EN, Alvi A. Management of carcinoma of the supraglottic larynx: evolution, current concepts, and future trends. *Laryngoscope* 1996; **106:** 559–67.
57. Naudo P, Laccourreye O, Weinstein G, Hans S, Laccourreye H, Brasnu D. Functional outcome and prognosis factors after supracricoid partial laryngectomy with cricohyoidopexy. *Ann Otol Rhinol Laryngol* 1997; **106:** 291–6.
58. Nicolai P, Redaelli de Zinis LO, Tomenzoli D *et al.* Prognostic determinants in supraglottic carcinoma: univariate and Cox regression analysis. *Head Neck* 1997; **19:** 323–34.
59. Ogura JH. Surgical pathology of cancer of the larynx. *Laryngoscope* 1955; **65:** 867–926.
60. Ogura JH. Supraglottic subtotal laryngectomy and radical neck dissection for carcinoma of the epiglottis. *Laryngoscope* 1958; **68:** 983–1003.
61. Ogura JH, Biller H. Pre-operative irradiation for laryngeal and laryngopharyngeal cancers. *Laryngoscope* 1970; **80:** 802–10.
62. Ogura JH, Dedo HH. Glottic reconstruction following subtotal glottic–supraglottic laryngectomy. *Laryngoscope* 1965; **75:** 865–78.
63. Ogura JH, Marks JE, Freeman RB. Results of conservation surgery for cancers of the supraglottis and pyriform sinus. *Laryngoscope* 1980; **90:** 591–600.
64. Ogura JH, Sessions DG, Spector GJ. Conservation surgery for epidermoid carcinoma of the supraglottic larynx. *Laryngoscope* 1975; **85:** 1808–15.
65. Olofsson J. Aspects on laryngeal cancer based on whole organ sections. *Auris Nasus Larynx* 1985; **12(Suppl II):** 166–71.
66. Olofsson J, van Nostrand AWP. Growth and spread of laryngeal and hypopharyngeal carcinoma with reflections on the effect of preoperative irradiation. 139 cases studied by whole organ serial sectioning. *Acta Otolaryngol Suppl (Stockh)* 1973; **308:** 1–84.
67. Orton HB. Lateral transthyroid pharyngotomy. *Arch Otolaryngol* 1930; **12:** 320–38.
68. Pearson BW, Olsen KD, DeSanto LW, Salassa JR. Results of near total laryngectomy. *Ann Otol Rhinol Laryngol* 1998; **107:** 820–5.
69. Piquet JJ, Desaulty A, Decroix G. Crico-hyoido-pexie. Technique opératoir et résults fonctionels. *Ann Otolaryngol Chir Cervicofac* 1974; **91:** 681–9.
70. Piquet JJ, Darras JA, Berrier A, Roux X, Garcette L. Les larygectomies sub-totales fonctionnelles avec crico-hyoïdo-pexie. Technique, indication, résultats. *Ann Otolaryngol Chir Cervicofac* 1986; **103:** 411–15.
71. Robbins KT, Davidson W, Peters LJ, Goepfert H. Conservation surgery for T2 and T3 carcinomas of the supraglottic larynx. *Arch Otolaryngol* 1988; **114:** 421–6.
72. Sekula J. The subtotal operation in the treatment of cancer of the larynx. *Laryngoscope* 1967; **77:** 1996–2006.
73. Sessions DG, Ogura JH, Ciralsky RH. Late glottic insufficiency. *Laryngoscope* 1975; **85:** 950–9.
74. Som ML. Surgical treatment of carcinoma of the epiglottis by lateral pharyngotomy. *Trans Am Acad Ophthalmol Otolaryngol* 1959; **63:** 28–47.
75. Som ML. Conservation surgery for carcinoma of the supraglottis. *J Laryngol Otol* 1970; **84:** 655–78.
76. Strijbos M, van den Broek P, Manni JJ, Huygen PLM. Supraglottic laryngectomy: short- and long-term functional results. *Clin Otolaryngol* 1987; **12:** 265–70.
77. Suárez C, Rodrigo JP, Herranz J, Diaz C, Fernandez JA. Complications of supraglottic laryngectomy for carcinomas of the supraglottis and the base of the tongue. *Clin Otolaryngol* 1996; **21:** 87–90.
78. Suárez C, Rodrigo JP, Herranz J, Llorente JL, Martínez JA. Supraglottic laryngectomy with or without postoperative radiotherapy in supraglottic carcinomas. *Ann Otol Rhinol Laryngol* 1995; **104:** 358–63.
79. Suárez C, Rodrigo JP, Herranz J, Rosal C, Alvarez JC. Extended supraglottic laryngectomy for primary base of

tongue carcinomas. *Clin Otolaryngol* 1996; **21:** 37–41.
80. Szlezak L. Histological serial block examination of 57 cases of laryngeal cancer. *Oncologia* 1966; **20:** 178–94.
81. Timon CI, Gullane PJ, Brown D, Van Nostrand AWP. Hyoid bone involvement by squamous cell carcinoma: clinical and pathological features. *Laryngoscope* 1992; **102:** 515–20.
82. Trotter W. A method of lateral pharyngotomy for the exposure of large growths in the epilaryngeal region. *J Laryngol Otol* 1920; **35:** 289–95.
83. Tucker GF Jr. The anatomy of laryngeal cancer. *J Otolaryngol* 1974; **3:** 417–31.
84. Tucker H. Deglutition following partial laryngectomy. In: Silver CE, ed. *Laryngeal Cancer.* New York: Thieme, 1991: 197–200.
85. Vermund H. Role of radiotherapy in cancer of the larynx as related to the TNM system of staging. *Cancer* 1970; **24:** 485–504.
86. Ward PH. Complications of laryngeal surgery: etiology and prevention. *Laryngoscope* 1988; **98:** 54–7.
87. Weinstein GS, Laccourreye O, Brasnu D, Tucker J, Montone K. Reconsidering a paradigm: the spread of supraglottic carcinoma to the glottis. *Laryngoscope* 1995; **105:** 1129–33.

Cancer of the glottis

Javier Gavilán

Clinical characteristics of glottic cancer

The glottis includes the vocal cords and the slit – *rima glottidis* – between them; it also contains the anterior and posterior commissures (Fig 44.1). Unfortunately, there is no agreement on the location of the anatomic boundaries of the glottis. For clinical purposes, the glottis is limited superiorly by a horizontal plane passing across the floor of the ventricle. Histologically, the junction of the squamous epithelium of the vocal cord with the respiratory epithelium of the ventricle is the border. The lower limit is more difficult to define because there is no clear anatomic landmark at the glottic–subglottic junction. The histologic barrier between the glottis and subglottis is the conus elasticus. At the 1974 centennial laryngeal meeting, the glottic to subglottic boundary was set at the inferior phonatory surface of the vocal cord where the squamous epithelium changes to columnar-type epithelium. At the midcord level this line is approximately 5 mm below the superior surface of the cord. However, this boundary has proven impractical for clinical purposes and the UICC has standardized the inferior level of the glottis as 1 cm inferior to the superior surface of the vocal cord.[6]

Local spread

The patterns of local and regional spread of laryngeal tumors are influenced by the site of origin of the primary tumor. Glottic tumors usually arise on the free margin of the membranous cord and extend horizontally toward the anterior and posterior commissures. Tumors primarily arising at the anterior commissure are uncommon and require a different approach because of the special anatomic characteristics of this area. Posterior glottic tumors are rare, although this may be due to the less symptomatic nature of the posterior third of the glottis making early diagnosis less common.

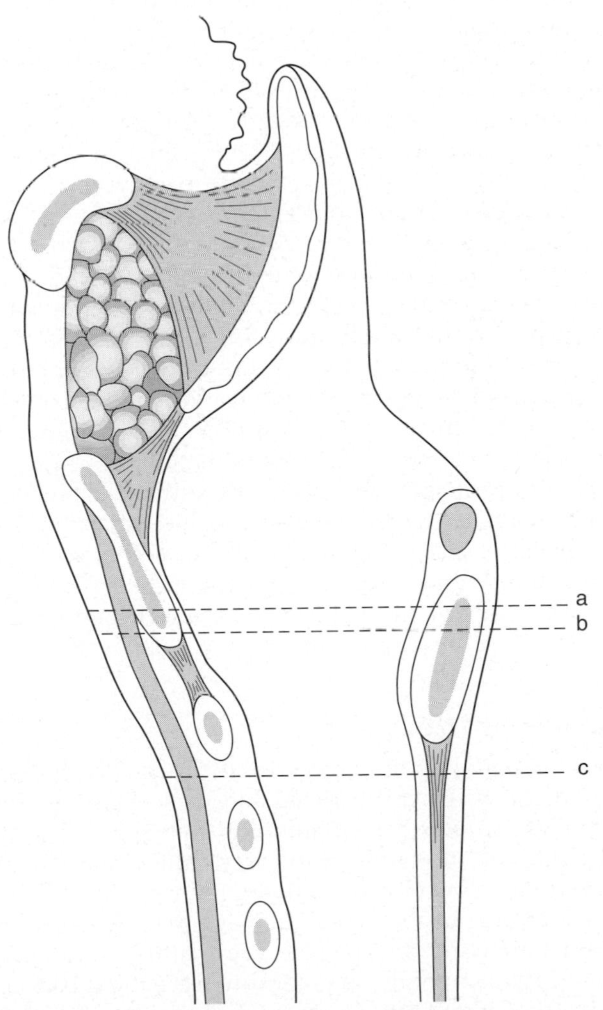

Figure 44.1 *Schematic representation of the larynx with its major subdivisions: (a) supraglottis; (b) glottis; (c) subglottis.*

Glottic tumors may invade the opposite vocal cord through the anterior commissure. They may also extend to the posterior commissure, infiltrating the vocal process or the anterior face of the arytenoid cartilage. Vertical growth is initially delayed by embryologic and anatomic barriers. The different origin of the supraglottis with respect to the glottis and subglottis provides a natural barrier to cephalad spread of primary glottic cancer, whilst the conus elasticus acts as an important barrier to inferior tumor spread. After a period of time confined to Reinke's space, the tumor may infiltrate the vocal ligament and vocalis muscle, reaching the paraglottic space. This space is bounded by the thyroid ala anterolaterally, quadrangular membrane medially, pyriform mucosa posteriorly, and conus elasticus inferiorly[70] and constitutes a veritable avenue for tumor dissemination to the supraglottis or to the subglottic area.

Invasion of the anterior commissure also constitutes an open door to intra- and extralaryngeal dissemination. The anterior junction of the vocal ligaments and overlying mucosa attaches to the posterior plate of the thyroid cartilage – Broyles' tendon – in an area devoid of inner perichondrium.[9] The close proximity between cartilage and mucosa at this point results in lower protection against tumor invasion of the cartilage.[71] Tumors invading this region may easily extend superiorly to the supraglottis. They can also invade the anterior subglottic wedge, which is a triangular-shaped zone with the apex terminating just below the anterior commissure tendon and is delineated inferiorly by the anterior arch of the cricoid cartilage.[8] From here, the cricothyroid membrane can be penetrated, allowing the tumor to extend extralaryngeally. Exteriorization can also occur after cartilage invasion at the thyroid and epiglottic cartilages anteriorly or by cricoid invasion posteriorly. When the laryngeal cartilages are involved, the ossified portion shows the least resistance to tumor dissemination.[39,51] Also, the epiglottic cartilage has numerous natural dehiscences which facilitate the dissemination of the tumor into the pre-epiglottic space. The mucous glands and blood vessels of the larynx may also influence the local spread of the tumor by creating lines of least resistance which facilitate extralaryngeal dissemination.[7,56]

Regional spread

The lymphatics of the larynx form two highly compartmentalized systems: superficial and deep. The superficial system constitutes an intramucosal network connecting both sides of the larynx with very little clinical importance from an oncologic standpoint. By contrast, the deep system creates a submucosal drainage web, which is critical for tumor spread. The true vocal cords are devoid of submucosal lymphatics and constitute a natural barrier in the vertical lymphatic drainage of the larynx. Therefore, glottic tumors rarely present with regional lymphatic metastasis at the time of diagnosis and tend to metastasize only when deeper invasion involves the paraglottic space with subsequent access to lymphatic channels. The incidence of regional metastasis then increases proportionately. The probability of metastasis from glottic carcinoma is less than 5% for T1 cancer, 7% for T2, about 14% for T3, and 33% for T4 tumors.[12] A positive midline deep lymph node – delphian node – occurs in 1–5% of glottic lesions with cordal fixation and subglottic extension.[54] The appropriate selection of treatment in every situation requires the careful consideration of all these facts. Whilst operations for early glottic cancer do not require neck dissection, with cordal fixation the treatment plan should include the neck. In patients with extensive subglottic extension, the paratracheal nodes and the thyroid gland should also be resected with the primary tumor.

Diagnosis

Symptoms

Hoarseness is the cardinal symptom of glottic cancer and appears early because of interference with the normal phonatory function of the larynx. The smooth normal mucosa is essential for the production of a normal voice. With early invasion the vocal cords fail to perform properly due to irregularities and altered mobility. The patient notices changes in the quality of the voice. The symptom is persistent and necessitates a careful examination of the larynx in any patient who is hoarse longer than 2 weeks. Laryngeal irritation and voice deterioration may force the patient to clear the throat frequently. As the tumor grows, hoarseness becomes more evident and vocal cord mobility decreases. When the vocal cord is fixed, the voice becomes a harsh whisper.

Cough is frequently associated with glottic tumors but has no diagnostic significance. With advanced glottic lesions, dyspnea and stridor may appear. Bulky ulcerated tumors may also produce hemoptysis. Halitosis is frequently present in patients with large fungating tumors with areas of necrosis.

Pain is another late symptom of glottic tumors. It may reveal invasion of the cartilaginous framework of the larynx with extralaryngeal spread. Referred pain, usually to the ipsilateral ear, is mediated by the tenth nerve and is characteristic of advanced tumors with extralaryngeal involvement or neck metastasis. Odynophagia also denotes advanced lesions and appears when there is supraglottic involvement or extralaryngeal spread to the pharynx, pyriform sinus, esophageal inlet, or tongue base. Dysphagia is a very late symptom and also suggests hypopharyngeal or tongue base invasion.

Neck nodes seldom develop in early stages with glottic cancer. When present, they denote deep invasion. Jugular nodes and delphian nodes are the first to appear. Differential diagnosis of a midline neck mass should include laryngeal framework invasion from glottic cancer with spread to extralaryngeal tissue. Finally, weight loss is an ominous late symptom, which indicates extralaryngeal tumor extension or distant metastasis.

Office examination

In most instances, the diagnosis of glottic cancer is made by a thorough clinical examination which includes indirect mirror inspection of the larynx, rigid telescopic examination, fiberoptic nasolaryngoscopy, and palpation of the neck. In addition to this, direct laryngoscopy and imaging studies may be required for the accurate assessment of tumor extension. Precise evaluation of the larynx and neck in this manner is fundamental for treatment planning, particularly when partial laryngectomy is considered.

Mirror examination of the larynx provides a comprehensive view of the larynx and pharynx. However, this method has been widely replaced by rigid telescopic examination, which provides an excellent overview of the larynx and pharynx and offers the advantage of close-up views and documentation. Laryngeal indirect examination should include specific information on symmetry, motion and surface characteristics of the following structures: tongue base, vallecula, epiglottis, aryepiglottic folds, arytenoids, false vocal cords, true vocal cords, subglottis, upper tracheal rings, lateral and posterior hypopharyngeal walls and pyriform sinuses (Fig 44.2). When a patient with glottic cancer is examined it is advisable to document the lesion with videolaryngoscopy or a photograph. If documentation is not available, the tumor should be depicted on a drawing indicating the site of origin of the primary tumor as well as its local extension. Invasion of adjacent laryngeal subsites and extralaryngeal involvement should be precisely described. The clinical status of the neck should also be indicated. Cervical palpation must be methodical, including not only the lateral aspects of the neck but also the larynx and other midline structures. If lymph nodes are present, they must be described according to their number, size, location, mobility, consistency and tenderness.

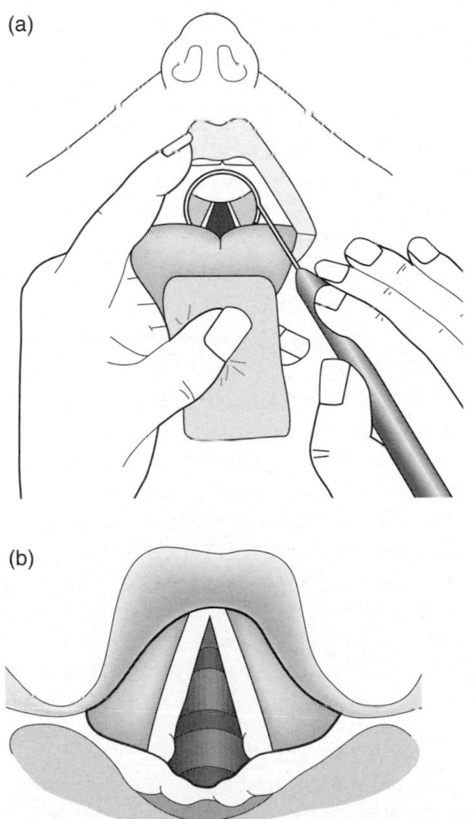

Figure 44.2 *Office examination with mirror or telescopes provides a comprehensive view of the larynx and pharynx. (a) Clinical examination. (b) Endolaryngeal image.*

Office examination may also include flexible fiberoptic endoscopy, which can be helpful to obtain additional information on hard-to-see sites, such as the anterior commissure, the infrahyoid epiglottis, the ventricles and the subglottis. The office examination can be completed with laryngostroboscopy to assess specific details of vocal cord motion, particularly in superficial lesions suspicious of deep invasion.

Cordal mobility is a keystone of laryngeal examination in patients with cancer of the larynx. Information on the dynamic function of the larynx may only be obtained while the patient is awake by asking him or her to phonate. The mobility of the vocal cords must be accurately recorded since it holds the clue to tumor classification and treatment. Not only gross movements but all details relating to cordal mobility must be studied: arytenoid function, false cord mobility, and mucosal wave pattern must be documented. The importance of a precise study of vocal cord mobility cannot be overemphasized. Cordal mobility creates the separation between early tumors and advanced lesions, and is the keystone of partial laryngeal surgery. All this information must be obtained before direct laryngoscopy is performed and treatment is decided.

'Impaired motion' is a controversial concept in glottic cancer. In some instances there will be disagreement, even within a group of experts, on whether there is normal mobility or impaired motion. The same may happen between impaired motion and fixation. In these cases additional information may be obtained with video documentation, laryngostroboscopy, direct laryngoscopy and imaging techniques. However, when there is doubt about mobility, the only reliable determinant that a lesion is biologically a T1 cancer or a higher stage is histologic data about muscle invasion.[13] The problem is that discussions about 'impaired mobility' may lead to selection of a wrong treatment option.

Direct laryngoscopy

Direct laryngoscopy is not needed in all patients with glottic cancer. However, the accurate assessment of the extent of the primary lesion frequently requires examination under general anesthesia with an operating microscope. As a general rule, diagnostic direct laryngoscopy should not be performed to resolve what cannot be clarified in the office but as a means to refine information on tumor extent. It is best to obtain as much information as possible from office examination before a direct laryngoscopy is performed. Patients who are difficult to explore in the office are usually also difficult to examine under general anesthesia.

When direct laryngoscopy is performed for glottic cancer, supraglottic and subglottic extension, as well as involvement of the anterior commissure and arytenoid cartilages, must be carefully evaluated. The precise identification of tumor extension at these sites is fundamental in patients in whom partial laryngectomy is contemplated. A systematic routine examination is also performed including evaluation of all areas in the larynx, pharynx and esophageal inlet. Special telescopes may be used to look around corners or reach into portions of the larynx obscured by the bulk of the tumor. A biopsy is usually taken at the time of direct laryngoscopy. This should be made by the physician responsible for the treatment and must be performed with extreme care to preserve the chances for partial laryngeal surgery. Patients selected for transoral removal should be treated at the time of diagnostic direct laryngoscopy.

Imaging studies

Sometimes, the three-dimensional extent of glottic cancer cannot be adequately perceived by clinical examination alone. In these cases imaging studies may be helpful in assessing the local extension of the lesion. However, in most patients with glottic cancer the clinical and endoscopic examinations provide all the critical information required for staging and treatment planning. Office examination is usually more informative than any imaging study, which should be reserved for special situations requiring more detailed information than that obtained with clinical exploration alone. In our practice, imaging studies are not a standard part of the diagnostic workup for glottic cancer.

Current diagnostic imaging studies include CT and MRI scans. Other studies such as plain films, xerograms and laryngograms are seldom used nowadays. CT scans have been used for evaluation of pre-epiglottic space involvement and thyroid cartilage invasion. However, its sensitivity is too low to be used as a standard tool for treatment planning, particularly when partial laryngectomy is contemplated. A normal CT scan does not preclude focal thyroid invasion through ossified cartilage without changes in the radiologic pattern of calcification. The precise plane of transition from false to true cords on a CT scan is obscure. Motion cannot be evaluated either. MRI scanning provides three-dimensional images in axial, coronal and sagittal planes. They may be helpful in assessing subglottic extension of a primary glottic lesion and seem to be superior to CT scanning in detecting cartilage invasion. However, the usefulness of MRI is limited in radiated patients and is restricted by claustrophobia, movement artifacts, and occasional local field distortions due to nearby paramagnetic materials such as dental implants.[57] Both CT and MRI scans have been used to provide information on the status of cervical lymph nodes in N0 patients without significant success from a clinical standpoint.[17,33] Modern imaging techniques can give some information on the situation of the lymph nodes in the neck, but clinically negative necks include both nonpalpable and microscopic disease. There are CT and MRI clues – node size, central necrosis, nodal confluence, pericapsular extension – that may help with the identification of some nonpalpable nodes, but true microscopic disease cannot be detected with conventional imaging studies. Some reports suggest that ultrasound alone[1] or in combination with fine-needle aspiration cytology,[73] is superior to palpation and can be more helpful than CT and MRI. However, further evidence is required before these methods can be routinely applied to the clinical practice. In conclusion, we do not believe that imaging techniques currently play a significant role in treatment planning for glottic cancer.

Treatment planning

The primary goal in cancer treatment is control of the tumor. However, when feasible, issues other than death become relevant and should be included as secondary objectives. With glottic cancer these are voice preservation, quality of the voice, success with first treatment, avoidance of tracheostomy, quality of life, and cost. In order to successfully achieve all these goals it is vitally important to follow some basic principles which constitute the foundations of laryngeal cancer treatment and establish the basic philosophy of laryngeal oncology (Table 44.1). The commandments of this 'oncologic decalog' summarize the knowledge of my mentors and teachers and condense my personal experience in the treatment of patients with laryngeal cancer.[14,21]

Table 44.1 The oncologic decalog for laryngeal cancer treatment

1. Life is more important than voice.
2. There is no treatment of choice but choices of treatment.
3. Cancer of the larynx is not a single disease, but a spectrum of lesions.
4. Cancer of the larynx is highly curable.
5. The first treatment is the most likely to succeed.
6. There must be a physician responsible for the treatment from the beginning to the end.
7. More is not always better. The use of combined therapy must be justified and protocols must be reserved for advanced disease.
8. Classifications are made for end-stage reporting, not for treatment planning.
9. Postoperative radiotherapy is not a substitute for free surgical margins.
10. Survival statistics are inappropriate to measure success in early glottic cancer.

Selection of the treatment modality

The basic principle of laryngeal oncology states that there is no *treatment of choice* for patients with glottic cancer, but *choices of treatment*. Every cancer, every patient and every situation require a personal solution based on particular factors relating to the tumor, the patient and the treatment team. The main reason for this is that cancer of the larynx is not a single disease but a spectrum of lesions. This assertion holds true even for the limited field of early glottic cancer, where multiple options exist for the treatment of T1 lesions. The group of T1 glottic cancers includes such a broad range of lesions that there cannot be one treatment that is optimal for every tumor. A T1 glottic cancer may range from a small superficial tumor located on the free edge of a mobile cord to a bulky tumor involving both vocal cords and the anterior commissure. By no means all these lesions could be managed with a single approach. Furthermore, two patients with exactly the same laryngeal tumor may have different personal situations, general health and preferences. Finally, even with the same lesion and the same patient conditions, there are still some factors relating to the treatment team which may determine the therapeutic option selected. Consequently, the management of glottic cancer requires a thorough evaluation of the tumor, analysis of the options, awareness of the consequences, communication between patient and physician, estimates of probable outcomes, and precise execution of treatment.[13]

The importance of first treatment and personal responsibility

Since glottic cancer is highly curable, all attempts should be made to cure the patient with the first treatment because this is the one most likely to succeed. As a general rule, the initial treatment offers the best opportunity for cure and sometimes the only opportunity for cure. To improve the results of treatment there must be a rule of personal responsibility. This has been frequently underestimated due to the importance acquired by tumor boards and committees in most institutions. The individualized approach that we recommend assumes that the patient has a physician who is responsible for the treatment from the beginning. Consultation to tumor boards and other specialists is essential during the treatment process, but the physician who starts the treatment should be responsible to the end. This responsibility begins with the diagnosis, since direct laryngoscopy and biopsy constitute an essential part of the treatment in many instances. Some patients can be cured by endoscopic removal at the time of the biopsy, others may benefit from partial laryngeal surgery, and in selected cases a total laryngectomy can be avoided by using a voice preserving operation. In all cases precise evaluation of the larynx is essential to assess the local extent of the lesion and to identify the structures not involved by the tumor.

Combined therapy

Combined surgery and postoperative radiotherapy is considered a standard approach for advanced glottic cancer in many institutions although its impact on survival has not yet been demonstrated. Postoperative radiotherapy is also frequently used for N-positive necks after neck dissection. However, there is lack of scientific evidence supporting its usefulness in terms of improved survival.[15] Therefore, our group only uses combined therapy for selected patients in whom this approach might offer some predictable benefit to the patient (e.g. extranodal involvement) and not as a standard treatment.

Every effort should be made to avoid positive margins in the surgical specimen. Although positive margins are less likely with glottic cancers than with other head and neck tumors,[37] survival of patients with positive surgical margins decreases by approximately 50%.[37,47,66] The surgeon should not rely on postoperative radiotherapy for positive margins and the tumor must be completely excised during the operation. In our experience radiation therapy is not a substitute for free margins. A skilled pathologist is essential in laryngeal surgery, particularly when conservation surgery is contemplated. Frozen section is an important guiding tool in partial laryngeal surgery. If the pathologist finds positive margins in a well-oriented and labeled surgical specimen, the surgeon must go on until safe margins are found.

Report of results

Cancer of the larynx is a highly curable disease. This is particularly true for glottic cancer, something that must be borne in mind for treatment planning and end results reporting. Since few people die from early glottic cancer, survival statistics are inappropriate to measure success and other criteria are needed for the accurate evaluation of the outcome of different treatment modalities. Success with the first treatment and voice quality should be routinely evaluated as a measure of treatment amelioration. The usual mixing of results from first treatment and salvage is inappropriate to compare the outcome of different treatment options. Quality of life issues should also be included in the treatment evaluation since they reflect the patient's personal opinion about the disease and the impact of treatment. In this respect, avoidance of a permanent stoma should be regarded as an important advantage between two treatments with equal oncologic effectiveness.[16] Finally, cost is another important issue in treatment planning. Most glottic cancers can be successfully treated with a single-modality treatment and therefore multimodality options should be restricted to specific situations that may justify the use of combined therapy. Likewise, innovative protocols should only be used in a controlled environment under strict surveillance and should not be considered a standard approach until their results have been sufficiently proved. This applies particularly to the so-called organ-preservation protocols.[36,62,68]

Life is more important than voice

A final consideration concerning treatment planning refers to the importance of voice in patients with cancer of the larynx. It has been previously mentioned that voice preservation must be a secondary goal of treatment for patients with glottic cancer. The term secondary assumes the fact that every effort has been made to cure the patient from the primary tumor. No attempt should be made to treat a patient with glottic cancer using a conservative method, either surgery, radiotherapy, chemotherapy, or a combination of them, that has fewer chances of cure than a radical method – e.g. total laryngectomy – because voice can be preserved. The golden rule of glottic cancer treatment should always be 'life first, voice second'. In summary, voice is very important, but life is even more important.

Classification and staging

Clinical classification for laryngeal cancer is a controversial issue.[18] In spite of its multiple categories, the TNM staging system is incomplete and unreliable. In addition, the TNM classification system was designed for end-stage reporting and should not be used for treatment planning. In other words, the TNM stage of a tumor does not dictate its treatment plan.

However, in practice the TNM system is frequently used as a prospective method for treatment selection without considering many other variables which are relevant to the final decision. For treatment selection the binomial patient–physician, not the classification, is the ultimate responsible for the final decision. Factors other than those related to the tumor itself should be taken into consideration. To emphasize this concept, we use a complementary classification to the TNM system, which is lightly referred to in our own practice as the 'OLE' system (Table 44.2). This classification includes most variables relating to the patient and to the treatment team, highlighting the fact that we are not just treating cancers: we treat patients.

Table 44.2 'OLE' classification including clinical factors useful in the selection of treatment for patients with laryngeal cancer

O	Occupation Organization Operating room Other factors not included in the TNM classification: patient's preference, previous treatment, distance from treatment facility, follow-up reliability, pathologist availability, concomitant diseases, etc.
L	Lung disease Laboratory facilities Life quality
E	Expectations Expense Emotional situation Experience

Treatment options

Two distinct groups can be defined concerning treatment for glottic cancer: early tumors and advanced lesions. In both groups surgery and radiotherapy are standard options for initial management. This chapter deals with the surgical options for the treatment of glottic cancer and presumes a surgical bias from the author. I assume this bias which is based on the principles previously stated and decades of experience accumulated with many patients. I believe that a surgical bias in the initial treatment results in more cures and more voices preserved if partial laryngectomy is precisely utilized. By contrast, a radiotherapeutic bias will produce some better voices in early disease and some avoidance of stomas in advanced tumors, with a significant long-term cost in lives, retreatment, voices and expense.[57] However, this surgical bias does not prevent us from using radiotherapy for the treatment of some early glottic cancers or to help in controlling the high-risk neck in patients with advanced lesions that have metastasized. In summary, the selection of the treatment method will depend on the particular characteristics of the tumor, the personal preferences of the patient, and the thorough review of the options.

Early glottic cancer

According to Ferlito and associates, early glottic cancer is a minimally invasive neoplastic lesion that does not invade the muscle or cartilage and is confined to one or both vocal cords.[19] The clinical manifestation of early glottic cancer is cordal mobility. The pathologic characteristic of these tumors is infiltration of the lamina propria without extension into the adjacent muscle or cartilage. Early glottic tumors should therefore be distinguished, both clinically and pathologically, from carcinoma in situ, which does not involve the lamina propria. However, from a therapeutic standpoint carcinoma in situ of the vocal cords is usually included in the group of early tumors since its management involves the same options as for the remaining tumors in the group.

According to the previous definition, carcinoma in situ is a preinvasive lesion that has not yet acquired the capacity for metastasis, whereas early laryngeal cancers are potentially capable of invading the lymphatic channels and metastasizing to the neck. This is true for early supraglottic cancers, with approximately 30% of T1 tumors presenting with lymph node metastasis at the time of diagnosis.[32] By contrast, the sparse lymphatic drainage of the true cords limits metastatic spread, making early glottic cancer synonymous with localized cancer and avoiding the necessity of including the neck in the treatment plan of early tumors of the vocal cords.

Treatment options for early glottic cancer include radiation therapy, transoral removal and conservation surgery. Each method has its place and no option exists to the exclusion of another. Radiotherapy for laryngeal cancer is addressed in a different chapter and no further comments on this topic will be made here.

Transoral removal of selected early glottic cancers was proposed in the nineteenth century and was first described in 1920 by Lynch.[48] The concept has been accepted as a current standard treatment option for T1 glottic lesions. The oncologic safety of transoral removal for early glottic carcinoma has been sufficiently proved[53,55,69,76] and, although it is currently performed with lasers, endoscopic surgery can be accomplished using microscissors or electrocautery, since the laser is just the latest available tool. To be safe, endoscopic surgery must provide a complete exposure of the lesion through the laryngoscope and allow the *en bloc* removal of the tumor. The lesion should not reach the anterior commissure since there is a significant rate of failure associated with transoral removal of glottic lesions in this area.[42,69] Free margins must be documented in the patient's tissue by means of frozen sections and the well-oriented specimen must be submitted to the pathologist for microscopic study. When the margins are insecure or the exposure inadequate, endoscopic removal should not be considered a viable option and partial laryngectomy or radiotherapy must be selected, according to tumor conditions and patient preferences.

Partial laryngectomy is a good option for lesions that do not fulfill the criteria for transoral removal. Cordectomy is the basic operation from which the remaining partial vertical laryngectomies derive. Although most cordectomies are currently being performed with laser through a transoral approach, some patients still can benefit from an open approach. Frontolateral laryngectomy, anterior frontal laryngectomy and hemilaryngectomy are variations of the basic procedure. They are designed to securely remove specific lesions not amenable to cordectomy while preserving laryngeal functions. All of them are performed through a thyrotomy or laryngofissure. The structures resected in each procedure are shown in Fig 44.3.

The cordectomy removes the entire vocal cord from the anterior commissure to the vocal process of the arytenoid and from the subglottis to the false vocal cord (Fig 44.3a). The frontolateral laryngectomy is a cordectomy in which the angle of the thyroid cartilage is included in the resection to encompass the anterior commissure and the tendon within the specimen (Fig 44.3b). The anterior frontal laryngectomy is used to remove the anterior portion of both vocal cords together with the anterior commissure (Fig 44.3c). Finally, the hemilaryngectomy, as presently performed, consists of the vertical resection of the supracricoid and infrahyoid hemilarynx (Fig 44.3d). The amount of thyroid ala resected and the inclusion of the arytenoid in the specimen depend on the type of procedure performed.

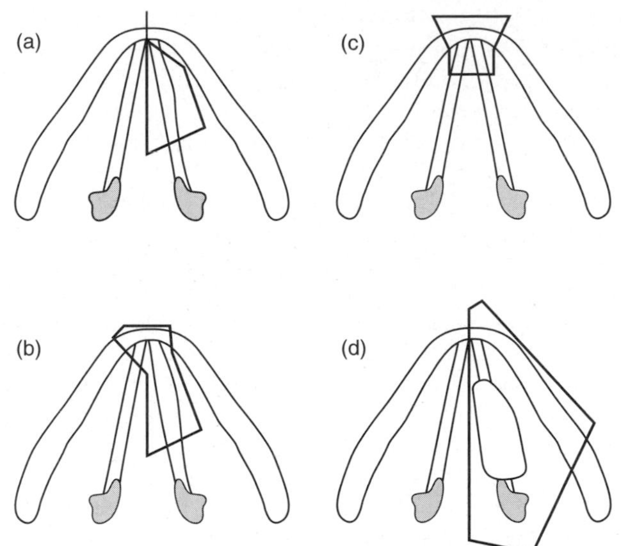

Figure 44.3 *Diagram of conventional partial vertical procedures. (a) Cordectomy; (b) Frontolateral laryngectomy; (c) Anterior frontal laryngectomy; (d) Hemilaryngectomy.*

Advanced glottic cancer

Advanced tumors of the vocal cords – T3 and T4 – constitute a completely different scenario for two reasons:

- local extension usually prevents the classic partial operations, except for some selected early T3 lesions in which hemilaryngectomy can be performed; and
- access of the tumor to the lymphatic channels of the neck results in high probability of lymph node metastasis.

Four treatment options are available for advanced glottic cancers: open surgery, endoscopic removal, radiotherapy and combined treatments.

Open surgery

Surgical treatment for advanced glottic cancer has been classically associated with total laryngectomy and its subsequent mutilation. However, some alternatives to total laryngectomy are currently available. One is hemilaryngectomy, that can be used for selected early T3 lesions, since vocal cord fixation by itself is not a contraindication to this operation as has been shown by anatomic and clinical studies.[41,45] Another option is the supracricoid subtotal laryngectomy with cricohyoidopexy – CHP – described by Majer and Rieder in 1959,[49] and modified by Piquet *et al.* in 1974.[61] The latter has been called cricohyoidoepiglottopexy – CHEP – and includes the preservation of the upper two-thirds of the epiglottis to facilitate swallowing after the operation. Although frequently used for early tumors, CHP and CHEP can be used for selected T3 glottic lesions and true T4 anterior commissure tumors clinically staged as T1. The last voice-preserving option for advanced glottic tumors is the near-total laryngectomy described by Pearson *et al.* in 1980.[59] This operation fills the gap between the classic functional procedures and the conventional total laryngectomy. It is an oncologically radical operation that allows a lung-powered voice by creating an internal physiologic, non-prosthetic, tracheopharyngeal shunt. Since the cricoid is always sacrificed on the tumor side, a permanent stoma is always required.

Quality of life issues are frequently used against total laryngectomy, although few studies have documented the actual impact of voice and stoma upon the quality of life in patients undergoing surgical treatment for cancer of the larynx. A classic study by McNeil *et al.*[50] documented the fear of laryngectomy by the public in a theoretical situation by asking healthy firemen whether they would be willing to compromise their chance of survival by 20% in order to have a chance to keep a lung-powered glottic voice. About one-fifth of them said they would take that chance. However, in a recent study on quality of life performed by our group on 67 patients surgically treated for cancer of the larynx, this impression could not be confirmed.[4] The study includes patients treated with cordectomy, supraglottic laryngectomy, near-total laryngectomy and total laryngectomy. No difference was found in role adjustment between total laryngectomy, supraglottic (all of them decannulated and with good voice) and near-total laryngectomy (good voice but a permanent stoma) groups. Only patients who had a cordectomy adjusted more favorably than the others. The fact that the patients in the total laryngectomy, near-total laryngectomy and supraglottic groups had nearly the same perception about quality of life suggests that neither voice nor stoma is a primary determinant of quality of life in patients with laryngeal cancer. In fact, patients in the cordectomy group adjusted better, regardless of a worse voice quality, than patients in the supraglottic group. It is difficult to understand why the supraglottic group had such a poor adjustment and did not fall in the in-between position between cordectomy patients and the total laryngectomy group, as was initially predicted. An explanation can be found in the fact that a large percentage of supraglottic patients received radiotherapy as part of their treatment whereas cordectomy patients were not irradiated. It must be emphasized that this study showed a significant impact of postoperative radiotherapy on quality of life. Patients receiving postoperative radiotherapy adjusted less favorably than nonirradiated patients. A recent study by DeSanto *et al.*[16] showed a similar impact of voice, although the stoma was a primary determinant of quality of life in their patients.

Transoral removal

Laser endoscopic removal has gained popularity among head and neck surgeons and its indications have been extended, including the removal of large laryngeal and hypopharyngeal tumors.[67] Transoral removal of advanced glottic tumors requires a piecemeal resection of the lesion which is excised in several fragments. This policy violates many of the well-established classic oncologic principles and its safety has not been sufficiently proved by scientific studies. Laser is simply a surgical tool that allows a bloodless field but lacks any miraculous properties in terms of local control of cancer. Therefore, piecemeal removal of tumors should not be recommended as a standard method for advanced glottic cancer treatment until further studies are conducted. In addition, the neck must be treated after laser resection has been completed, thus increasing the treatment time and the number of procedures performed in the same patient. In summary, what can be good for early lesions may not be useful for advanced tumors.

Radiotherapy

Radical radiation with surgery for salvage is the preferred option for the management of advanced glottic lesions in many institutions. The rationale for this option is that some advanced tumors will be cured by radiotherapy alone, thus allowing a normal voice. It is assumed that under a careful follow-up the failures can be detected early and salvage surgery applied successfully. The concept is alluring, although its validity has not fulfilled the initial expectations. When compared to surgery, radiation for advanced glottic tumors leads to a higher failure rate and a greater percentage of retreatments.[29]

We agree with those who think that this is a very attractive concept for those patients in whom it succeeds[11] and also with those who state that radiation in large lesions is a risky gamble against cure, to retain a voice and avoid a stoma.[57] We have already mentioned that voice and stoma are secondary goals of treatment and that no effort should be made to save voices by risking lives. On the other hand, the complications and long-term complaints of radiotherapy are higher than those of surgery alone. Finally, whilst good radiation therapy requires a well trained team of therapists, physicists, and technicians along with a technically sophisticated and reliable equipment at their disposal, surgery relies only on one person. Therefore, to be comparable and reproducible the results of radiotherapy must consider all these variables.

In summary, radiation therapy is another option for the treatment of glottic cancer, with its advantages and disadvantages. Once again, a personal decision after a thorough evaluation of the options is fundamental to select radiotherapy as the initial treatment.

Combined treatment

Combined surgery and radiotherapy may be useful for advanced lesions. In our practice the indications for radiotherapy are usually related to the findings in the neck. Only large nodes with extranodal involvement are treated

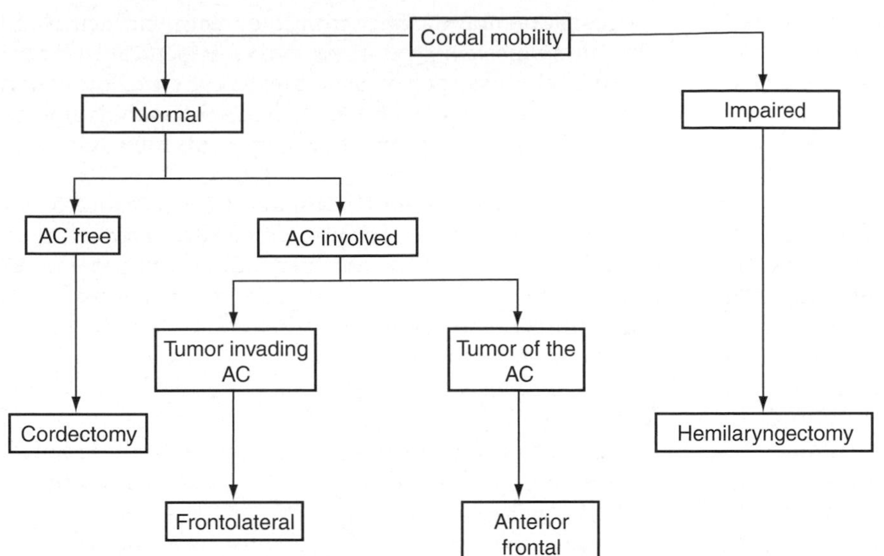

Figure 44.4 *Decision matrix for the selection of conventional partial vertical laryngectomy. (AC = anterior commissure.)*

with postoperative radiation. Small nodes in patients undergoing functional neck dissection are not routinely treated with postoperative radiotherapy, regardless of the number of nodes. Combined therapy is seldom used for the primary tumor after initial surgery. Only large tumors with massive infiltration of extralaryngeal soft tissues are treated postoperatively with radiotherapy.

Several protocols including radiotherapy, chemotherapy and salvage surgery have been designed for the so-called 'organ preservation' in patients with advanced laryngeal cancer.[36,62,68] These have not showed a significant improvement in survival or voice preservation when compared to standard approaches using surgery and radiotherapy, alone or in combination, and therefore should only be used in well designed research projects until their usefulness is sufficiently demonstrated. When feasible, surgery is the best 'organ-preservation' approach and for advanced lesions cure remains the main concern.

Finally, it is important to emphasize that surgical treatment after radiation and chemotherapy must be performed following the initial margins of the lesion. We do not believe that inoperable cancer can be made operable either with radiation or chemotherapy. 'Down-staging' the tumor for surgery by means of chemoradiation protocols is not safe because human tumors are not reduced from the periphery, as could be supposed from the radiobiologic theory.

Conservation surgery

The clues for the adequate selection of partial laryngectomy are cordal mobility and the anterior commissure (Fig 44.4). Cordal mobility creates the dividing line between hemilaryngectomy and the remaining partial vertical procedures. If the affected cord moves, then hemilaryngectomy is not needed and should be avoided because it offers no oncologic benefit and has worse functional results. When there is normal mobility cordectomy is indicated for tumors not extending to the anterior commissure (Fig 44.3a). Tumors involving the anterior commissure and up to one-third of the opposite vocal cord are best treated by means of a frontolateral laryngectomy (Fig 44.3b). The anterior frontal operation – also called the anterior commissure variation – is indicated for those rare tumors that start and stay at the anterior commissure (Fig 44.3c). Hemilaryngectomy is used in selected patients with cordal cancer extending either onto the arytenoid or into the floor of the ventricle (Fig 44.3d). Finally, supracricoid reconstructive laryngectomy may also be used for early lesions.

The surgeon must be extremely careful when contemplating conservation surgery for radiation failures because, even when the recurrence is detected early, it is usually difficult to evaluate the actual extension of the disease and how it was at the beginning. When partial vertical laryngectomy is used as a salvage procedure for radiation failures, one must be sure that the tumor was initially suitable for conservation surgery. If there is any doubt, functional surgery should not be tried. In addition, complications are more frequent in patients who have been previously irradiated.

Cordectomy

Laryngofissure and cordectomy consists of resection of the vocal cord through an open cervical approach.[23] The conventional laryngofissure and cordectomy removes the entire vocal cord from the anterior commissure to the vocal process of the arytenoid, and from the subglottis to the false cord. Some surgeons also include part of the ventricular band in the resection. This 'cordobandectomy' gives an extra margin where it is less needed: superiorly. For embryologic reasons the glottis can be divided from the supraglottis, cutting through the ventricle without violating sound principles of cancer surgery. Likewise, hemilaryngectomy offers no benefit in the treatment of early glottic tumors on mobile cords. The lateral extra margin obtained with hemilaryngectomy is not needed in early glottic cancer because cancer cannot spread very far laterally and still leaves a mobile cord.

These 'extra safe' operations are probably due to the discomfort produced in the surgeon by the small resection margins obtained with conservation surgery of the larynx. However, the oncologic safety of conservation surgery has stood the test of time and histologic free margins of more than 2 mm produce results generally comparable to widely clear margins.[3]

The tracheostomy is another 'extra-safe' maneuver usually linked to laryngofissure and cordectomy. Most surgeons consider the tracheostomy to be a required part of the surgical technique. Our experience does not support this idea. No tracheostomy was initially performed in the last 70 patients treated with laryngofissure and cordectomy at La Paz Hospital, and none of them required a tracheostomy during the postoperative period. A needed tracheostomy can save the patient's life. An unnecessary tracheostomy is only a source of infection and discomfort for the patient. It can extend the recovery period without providing a benefit other than the surgeon's reassurance. Therefore, for laryngofissure and cordectomy, it is more the surgeon than the patient who 'needs' the tracheostomy.

Indications

The major indication for laryngofissure and cordectomy is an early glottic tumor confined to the membranous portion of the vocal cord. There must be no limitation to cordal mobility. The procedure has been also used for larger tumors involving the anterior commissure or the vocal process of the arytenoid. However, these tumors are best treated using more extensive procedures, such as the anterior frontal laryngectomy or the hemilaryngectomy.

Laryngofissure and cordectomy is also used for the treatment of radiation failures. In these cases multiple frozen sections of the surgical margins are required to be sure that the tumor has been completely removed. The complication rate in such instances is higher than in nonirradiated patients.

Chronological age alone is not a contraindication to laryngofissure and cordectomy. The patient's general health and pulmonary function are more important variables than age alone. Some older patients might have radiotherapy recommended for two reasons:

- they would not be at risk for a second tumor for as long a period as younger patients; and
- older patients are less capable of adapting to the partial loss of the sphincteric function of the larynx.

On the other hand, some elderly patients may do better with laryngofissure and cordectomy rather than undergo a full course of radiotherapy.

Occupation and distance from the treatment facility are also important considerations for treatment selection.[12] Patients who use their voice a great deal are good candidates for radiotherapy. Patients living far away from the treatment center may prefer surgery to shorten the treatment time.

Today the majority of the tumors that are suitable for laryngofissure and cordectomy are usually removed by a transoral approach. However, depending on anatomic or tumor conditions, a number of patients still can benefit from an open cordectomy.

Surgical technique

The procedure is performed under general endotracheal anesthesia with transoral or transnasal intubation. To facilitate sectioning the cord from the vocal process of the arytenoid, the anesthesiologist must use the thinnest possible tube.

A collar incision at the level of the cricothyroid membrane is preferred. A vertical incision provides good exposure of the surgical field, but the aesthetic results are much better with a horizontal skin incision. Skin flaps are elevated on the plane superficial to the fascia overlying the strap muscles. The superior flap is raised up to the level of the hyoid bone. The dissection of the inferior skin flap is carried down to the level of the first tracheal ring, completely exposing the thyroid isthmus.

A midline vertical incision is made between the sternohyoid muscles, and the strap muscles are retracted laterally, exposing the thyroid cartilage and the isthmus of the thyroid gland. The thyroid isthmus is divided between clamps, ligated and lateralized by permanent sutures to the sternocleidomastoid muscles on each side, leaving the anterior surface of the cervical trachea just below the skin (Fig 44.5).The external perichondrium of

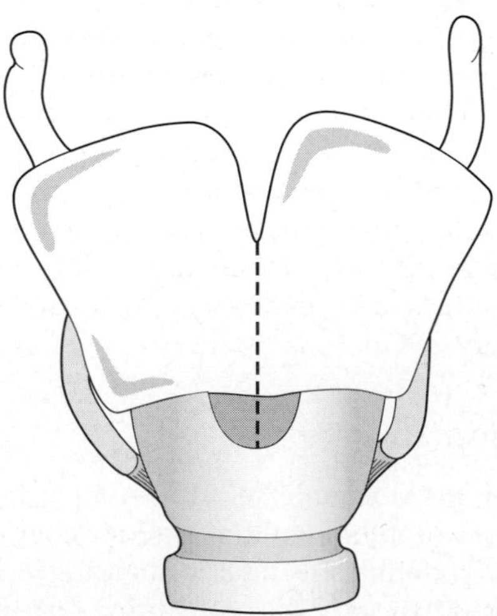

Figure 44.5 *The larynx is widely exposed showing the cricoid cartilage and the first tracheal ring. The dotted line indicates the incision over the thyroid cartilage and cricothyroid membrane.*

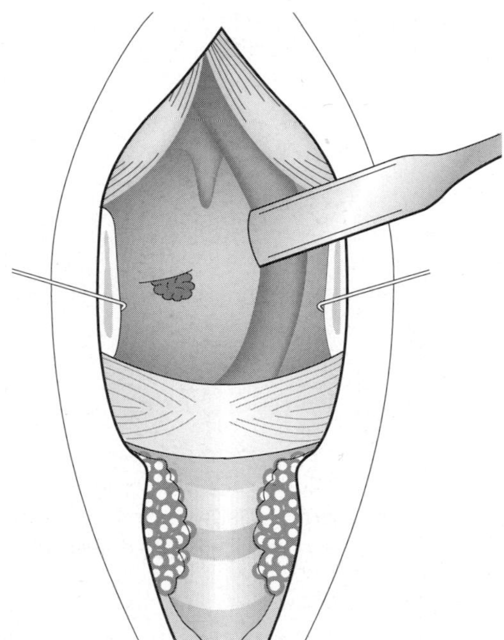

Figure 44.6 *The thyrotomy has been completed and both thyroid alae are retracted laterally. The endolarynx is inspected and the extent of the tumor is assessed under direct vision.*

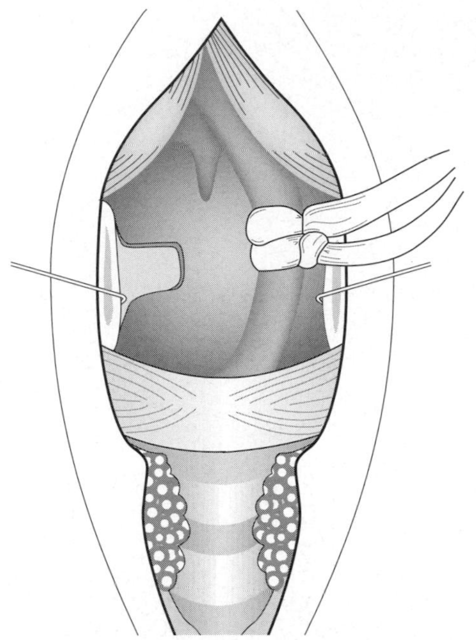

Figure 44.7 *The vocal cord has been removed from the ventricle superiorly to the subglottis inferiorly. The lateral boundary of the resection is the internal perichondrium of the thyroid ala.*

the thyroid cartilage is incised vertically in the midline and dissected laterally for a few millimeters. The thyroid cartilage is then divided strictly in the midline.

The delphian node is removed for histologic examination and the cricothyroid membrane is opened with a midline vertical incision. The thyroid laminae are slightly retracted laterally with skin hooks and the cricothyroid incision is continued superiorly. Under direct vision the vocal cords are separated exactly in the midline and the incision is extended superiorly until satisfactory view of the endolarynx is obtained (Fig 44.6). A self-retaining retractor placed in the superior angle of the thyroid cartilage widely separates the thyroid laminae, exposing the entire endolarynx.

The endotracheal tube is retracted towards the normal side with a Langenbeck retractor and the limits of the resection are marked. The lower cut is made first so that blood, running in a downward direction, will not obstruct the vision of the upper incision. This cut is made in the subglottis below the inferior limit of the vocal cord, leaving a free margin from the tumor of at least 5 mm. The upper incision is made through the ventricle. Both cuts should be carried deep to the internal perichondrium of the thyroid ala. Using a sharp dissector, a cleavage plane is opened between the thyroid ala and the vocal cord. The anterior commissure is then separated from the thyroid cartilage. Finally, an incision is made through the vocal process of the arytenoid. The cordectomy is thus completed (Fig 44.7) and the specimen can be oriented and submitted to the pathologist.

Resurfacing of the surgical defect is usually not necessary. If the uninvolved cord was released from its anterior insertion, it should be refixed to the anterior edge of the thyroid ala with a suture passing through the perichondrium or through the cartilage. The cricothyroid membrane is repaired and the two halves of the thyroid cartilage are carefully approximated in the midline, using sutures through the perichondrium. The strap muscles are sutured in the midline, the platysma muscle is approximated, and skin clips are used for the skin.

Anterior frontal laryngectomy

The anterior commissure is a potential route of spread for invasive glottic cancer into the thyroid cartilage. Tumors arising at this area are rare and may remain limited to their site of origin or extend along the surface of one or both vocal cords, the so-called horseshoe lesions. The surgical treatment of tumors located in the anterior commissure requires the inclusion of a wedge of thyroid cartilage *en bloc* with the primary tumor. All tumors located within 3 mm of the anterior limit of the vocal cord should be treated with surgical techniques that avoid midline laryngofissure for laryngeal exposure.[2]

Indications

The anterior frontal laryngectomy is indicated for glottic carcinomas arising at the anterior commissure. The tumor can extend along the surface of one or both vocal cords, but normal mobility of both vocal cords is mandatory. The operation is not strictly limited by subglottic or supraglottic extension. However, the following should be

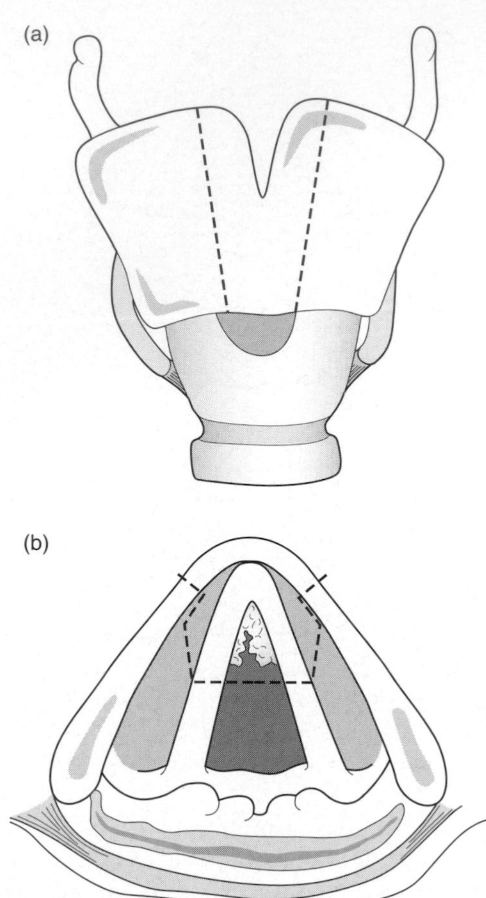

Figure 44.8 *(a) The larynx has been widely exposed and the thyroid cartilage is divided vertically 5–6 mm from the midline (dotted line). (b) The vocal cords are incised vertically beyond the posterior limit of the tumor (dotted line).*

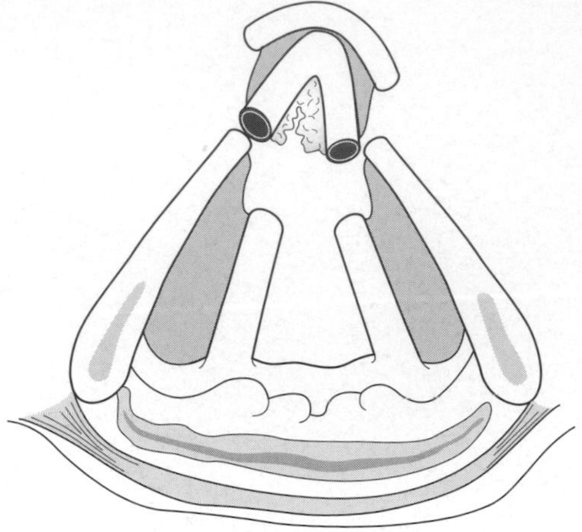

Figure 44.9 *The thyroid cartilage is retracted laterally and the larynx is opened. The resection is completed under direct vision of the tumor margins.*

considered contraindications to anterior frontal laryngectomy: vocal cord mobility impairment, extensive subglottic spread, and proven cartilage invasion. If the surgical pathologist reports cartilage invasion at the time of surgery, the technique should be modified according to tumor extension.

As with other partial laryngectomies, the anterior frontal technique should be used with extreme care as a salvage procedure after radiation failures. Even when the recurrence is detected early, it is difficult to evaluate the actual extension of the disease and a wide resection is oncologically safer. On the other hand, complications are more likely to occur in previously irradiated patients.

Surgical technique

A tracheostomy is previously performed using an independent horizontal incision. The operation is continued under general anesthesia and endotracheal intubation through the tracheostomy. A horizontal incision is made at the level of the cricothyroid membrane. The skin flaps are raised and the strap muscles are retracted laterally, exposing the thyroid cartilage. The external perichondrium of the thyroid cartilage is incised vertically in the midline and dissected laterally 10–15 mm from the midline. The cricothyroid membrane is divided with a scalpel.

Using an oscillating saw, each thyroid ala is divided vertically 5–6 mm from the midline, or more if tumor extension in one side demands a more posterior cartilage cut (Fig 44.8). These cuts involve only the cartilage, preserving the internal perichondrium. Using small hooks, the posterior portion of the thyroid alae is reflected laterally and the inner perichondrium is elevated until the level of insertion of the cords in the arytenoid cartilages. Using a headlight and working from below, a vertical incision is made in the inner perichondrium and vocal cord beyond the posterior limit of the tumor (Fig 44.9). This first cut should be made in the side of less glottic tumor involvement. After the cut is completed, both sides of the thyroid alae are retracted laterally and the larynx is entered. Tumor extension is now carefully assessed under direct vision and the resection is completed on the side of greater involvement. Frozen sections of the surgical margins are analyzed and the well-oriented and fully labeled specimen is submitted to the pathologist.

Reconstruction of the anterior commissure area is very important. The remaining portions of the vocal cords are reattached without tension to the perichondrial flaps. A suspension stitch is used to fix the epiglottis to the pre-epiglottic area. A silicon keel is placed between both thyroid plates to avoid web formation (Fig 44.10). No stitches are placed through the keel, to facilitate its removal 5 or 6 weeks after the operation. The thyroid alae are closed by one or two perforating stitches placed above and below the silicon keel. The strap muscles are approximated in the midline, the platysma muscle is sutured and skin clips are used for the skin. Suction drain and feeding tube are usually not necessary.

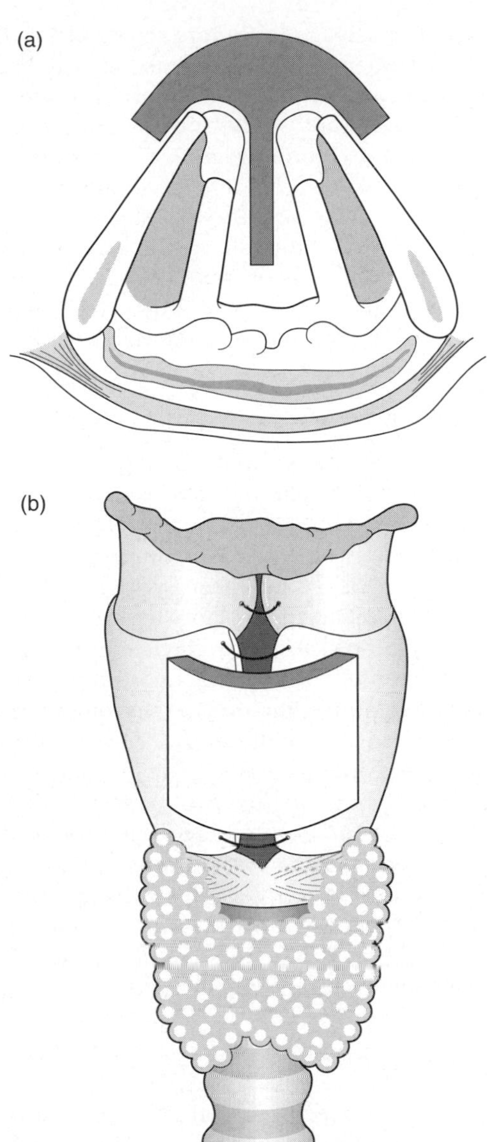

Figure 44.10 *(a) A silicon keel is placed to avoid web formation at the anterior commissure area. (b) The thyroid alae are approached using two stitches placed above and below the silicon keel. An additional stitch is used to reattach the epiglottis to the pre-epiglottic space.*

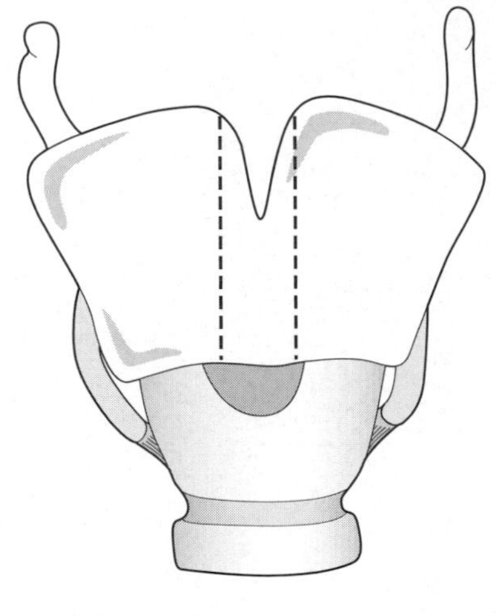

Figure 44.11 *The larynx is approached as for a basic cordectomy but the thyrotomy is lateralized to include a strip of thyroid cartilage with the anterior commissure in the resection. The dotted lines show the thyroid cartilage incisions.*

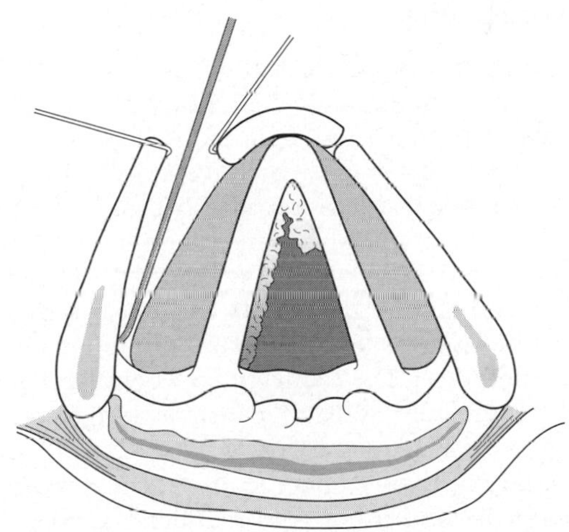

Figure 44.12 *The internal perichondrium is elevated from the thyroid ala as far posteriorly as necessary before the vocal cord is divided.*

Frontolateral laryngectomy

The frontolateral laryngectomy is simply a cordectomy in which a vertical strip of thyroid cartilage and the most anterior portion of the opposite vocal cord are removed. Although some surgeons also include the entire arytenoid in the resection, we seldom remove more than the vocal process because hemilaryngectomy is preferred for tumors extending back onto the arytenoid.

Indications for frontolateral laryngectomy include unilateral vocal cord tumors involving the anterior commissure and up to one-third of the opposite vocal cord. Vocal cord mobility must be preserved and the tumor should not involve the subglottis.

Technically, the operation is similar to laryngofissure and cordectomy except for the inclusion of a vertical strip of thyroid cartilage in the resection (Figs 44.11 and 44.12). Reconstruction of the anterior commissure is very important in order to achieve the best functional results. The remaining vocal cord and the ventricular band should be sutured anteriorly to the edge of the thyroid cartilage (Fig 44.13). This prevents retraction of the remaining vocal cord and promotes healing at the anterior commissure area. A tracheostomy is usually performed.

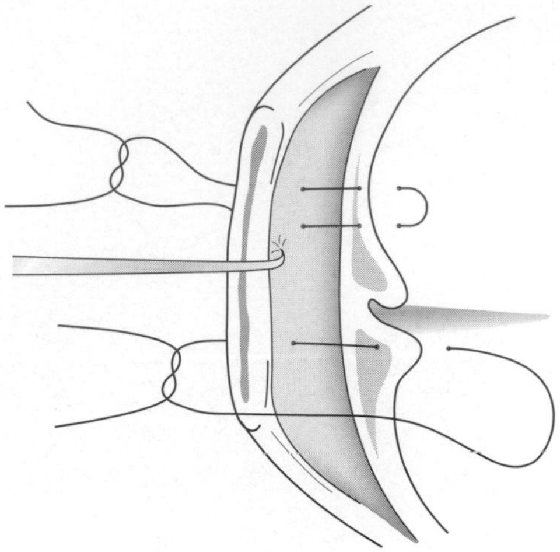

Figure 44.13 *The remaining vocal cord and ventricular band are fixed anteriorly to the edge of the thyroid cartilage to prevent retraction. This maneuver also prevents web formation at the anterior commissure area causing functional impairment.*

Hemilaryngectomy

Hemilaryngectomy was originally described as the resection of a true anatomic half of the larynx, including the thyroid ala, arytenoid and half of the cricoid cartilage. This procedure, developed by Gluck, fell into disuse during the early twentieth century because of its devastating effect on laryngeal function and high recurrence rate. Later modifications were developed to improve the functional and oncologic results of hemilaryngectomy. These operations introduced new and more flexible reconstructive methods. The concept of hemilaryngectomy evolved to include vertical partial laryngectomies in which less than half of the larynx is resected. Today the term hemilaryngectomy refers to the vertical resection of the supracricoid and infrahyoid hemilarynx.

Indications

Hemilaryngectomy is indicated for glottic carcinomas not amenable to less extensive vertical partial procedures. The major indication for hemilaryngectomy in our practice is glottic cancer either with posterior or limited superior extension. Posteriorly, the vocal process and anterior surface of the arytenoid may be involved, but invasion of the cricoarytenoid joint, posterior surface of the arytenoid, or interarytenoid area is a contraindication. Tumors that extend superiorly involving the ventricle are still amenable to hemilaryngectomy. However, extension to the false cord across the ventricle is a contraindication to this operation. Subglottic extension should be no more than 5 mm posterolaterally and 10 mm anteriorly. Hemilaryngectomy should not be attempted when more than one-third of the contralateral vocal cord is involved across the anterior commissure. Hemilaryngectomy is also possible in some selected T3 glottic tumors.

When used as a salvage procedure for radiation failure, the surgical specimen must encompass all the tissue in which the tumor was initially present. If there is any doubt, hemilaryngectomy should not be attempted.

Chronological age alone is not a contraindication. However, patients older than 70 years should be carefully evaluated because their capacity to adapt to the partial loss of the sphincteric function of the larynx is diminished, increasing the risk of aspiration. For the same reason, hemilaryngectomy is contraindicated in patients with severe chronic obstructive pulmonary disease.

Surgical technique

In our practice hemilaryngectomy includes the resection of the ipsilateral thyroid ala, the involved vocal cord, the ventricle, the false cord and the arytenoid (Fig 44.3d). Only the cricoid cartilage is preserved on the involved side.[24]

After the skin incision has been made, the flaps are elevated in the subplatysmal plane to the level of the hyoid bone superiorly and the clavicle inferiorly. The larynx is fully exposed and the tracheostomy performed. The external perichondrium of the thyroid cartilage is incised vertically in the midline and elevated from the thyroid ala on the involved side. The perichondrium is also raised 1 or 2 mm on the contralateral side. If the tumor does not invade the anterior commissure, a midline thyrotomy is performed. For tumors involving the anterior commissure the cartilage cut is lateralized 5 mm to 1 cm from the midline on the contralateral side. The endolarynx is inspected and the extent of the tumor is assessed under direct vision (Fig 44.14).

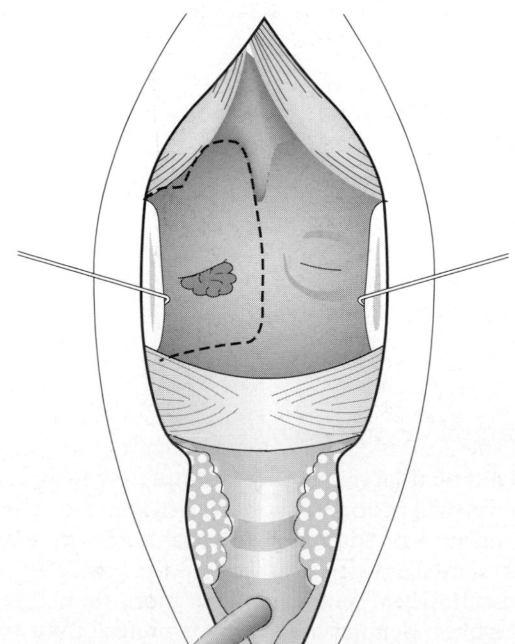

Figure 44.14 *The larynx has been opened in the midline and the tumor margins are assessed under direct vision. The dotted line shows the resection limits of the hemilarynx.*

The larynx is then rotated, exposing the thyroid cartilage on the involved side, and a vertical cartilage cut is made at the junction of the posterior and middle thirds of the thyroid ala. The cartilage cut is made down to but not through the soft tissues within the larynx. At this stage, the external surface of the pyriform sinus is seen through the lateral cartilage cut. The remaining posterior third of the thyroid ala, along with the superior and inferior cornua, remain attached to the inferior constrictor muscle and will be used during reconstruction to anchor the epiglottis.

The cricothyroid membrane is exposed and the delphian node is resected for histologic examination. Then, the limits of the resection are marked (Fig 44.14). The inferior incision is started at the cricothyroid membrane and continued horizontally along the upper border of the cricoid cartilage back to the cricoarytenoid joint. Superiorly, a horizontal cut is made across the aryepiglottic fold along the upper border of the thyroid ala and above the false cord. The incision is continued through the thyrohyoid membrane. These two incisions are connected with a posterior cut which includes the entire arytenoid on the surgical specimen. This cut runs in the midline through the interarytenoid mucosa and muscle, taking care not to injure the mucosa of the anterior surface of the hypopharynx and pyriform sinus. The specimen is now completely free and can be removed.

Reconstruction begins by suturing the uninvolved vocal cord anteriorly to the thyroid cartilage. Then, the epiglottis is dissected and mobilized inferiorly until it covers the surgical defect without tension. To prevent partial devascularization of the epiglottic flap, the lingual epiglottic mucosa should not be injured during the dissection. The epiglottis is then rotated laterally and sutured to the cut edges of the thyroid cartilage, cricothyroid membrane and upper edge of the cricoid cartilage (Fig 44.15). Finally, the perichondrium is approximated and the strap muscles are sutured in the midline. The tracheostomy tube is secured in place and a light pressure dressing is applied. A nasogastric feeding tube is placed and no drains are usually inserted.

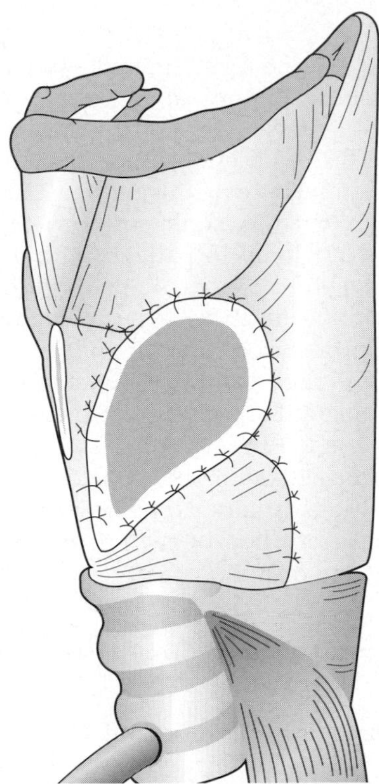

Figure 44.15 *The hemilarynx is reconstructed by suturing the lateral border of the epiglottis to the cut edge of the thyroid cartilage, cricothyroid membrane and upper edge of the cricoid cartilage. The cricothyroid muscle is used to reinforce the suture.*

Supracricoid laryngectomy with cricohyoidopexy or cricohyoidoepiglottopexy

The supracricoid subtotal laryngectomy with cricohyoidopexy – CHP – entails *en bloc* excision of all tissues between the superior border of the cricoid cartilage and the inferior surface of the hyoid bone. The specimen includes the entire thyroid cartilage, both true and false cords together with the epiglottis and the pre-epiglottic space, and both paraglottic compartments. Only the arytenoid on the less involved side is preserved. Reconstruction is achieved by approaching the cricoid cartilage to the hyoid bone. For glottic tumors without supraglottic involvement, the upper two-thirds of the epiglottis can be preserved. This modification is known as cricohyoidoepiglottopexy – CHEP (Fig 44.16).

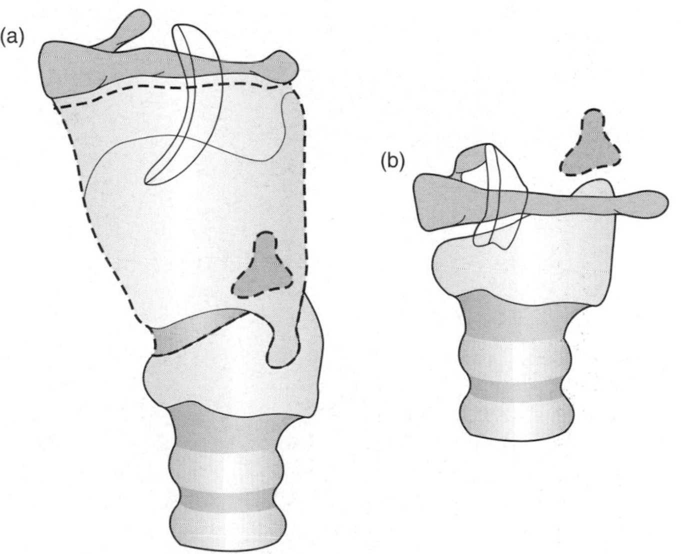

Figure 44.16 *(a) CHEP removes all laryngeal tissues between the superior border of the cricoid cartilage and the inferior surface of the hyoid bone. Only the upper two-thirds of the epiglottis and the arytenoid on the less involved side are preserved. (b) Reconstruction is achieved by suturing the cricoid cartilage underneath the hyoid bone.*

Indications

Indications for CHP and CHEP include glottic, transglottic, and supraglottic tumors, along with some selected hypopharyngeal lesions. For glottic cancer, CHEP has been mainly used for T2 lesions and bilateral T1 tumors with anterior commissure involvement.[43] However, the operation is considered by some surgeons as an alternative to total laryngectomy in patients with a fixed vocal cord.[8] The pre-epiglottic space, the posterior commissure, and one arytenoid must be free of tumor invasion. Limited supraglottic involvement is not a contraindication to CHEP, although extensive invasion of the supraglottis and pre-epiglottic space require the removal of the epiglottis using the CHP.

Arytenoid cartilage fixation and subglottic involvement are contraindications to any supracricoid subtotal laryngectomy, since preservation of the cricoid cartilage is an essential part of the operation.

Surgical technique for supracricoid laryngectomy with CHEP

An apron incision is performed and the skin flaps are elevated deep to the platysma muscle until adequate exposure of the hyoid bone and strap muscles is obtained. Neck dissection is performed according to the clinical scenario. A tracheostomy is placed at the level of the third or fourth tracheal ring.

The strap muscles are divided inferior to the hyoid bone and at the level of the thyroid gland. A horizontal cut is made in the external perichondrium of the cricoid, 2 mm below the upper border of the cartilage. The cut is continued laterally until the inferior thyroid cornu, dividing the lateral cricothyroid muscle. The internal perichondrium of the cricoid cartilage is elevated anterolaterally (Fig 44.17).

The larynx is then skeletonized as for a total laryngectomy, dividing the insertion of the inferior pharyngeal constrictor muscle on both sides of the thyroid cartilage. The superior laryngeal neurovascular bundle is identified and the vessels are ligated and divided on both sides. The pyriform sinus is elevated from the thyroid cartilage.

The larynx is now entered, cutting with a scalpel just above the upper border of the thyroid cartiliage. This cut includes the epiglottis, 1 cm above the petiole. The cut is continued above the false cords to the level of the arytenoids. On the less involved side an incision is then made immediately anterior to the arytenoid, across the false and true cords. Preservation of the arytenoid on the tumor side will depend on tumor extension (Fig 44.18). To include the arytenoid in the resection, a posterior cut is made in the midline through the interarytenoid mucosa and muscle, preserving the pyriform sinus. Then, the cricoarytenoid joint is separated and the resection is completed inferiorly along the upper border of the cricoid cartilage.

The reconstruction is performed by placing a series of sutures through the cricoid cartilage, epiglottis and hyoid bone (Fig 44.19). The cricoid must be 'telescoped' underneath the hyoid bone to achieve good results (Fig 44.16). Suprahyoid- or infracricoid-releasing maneuvers are seldom necessary, but should be performed when needed to avoid excessive tension at the suture line.

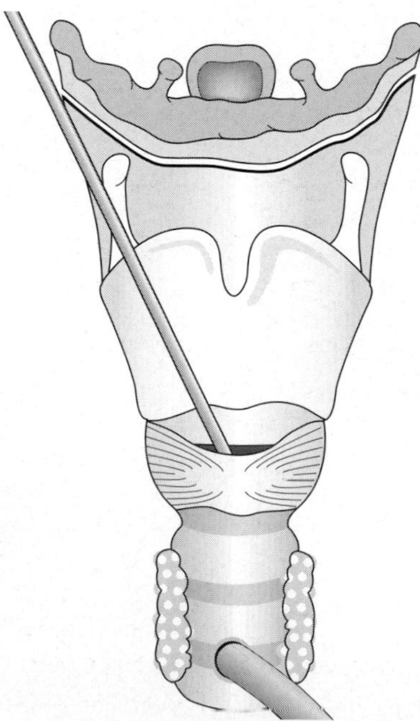

Figure 44.17 *The strap muscles are sectioned below the hyoid bone. The internal perichondrium of the cricoid cartilage is elevated anterolaterally.*

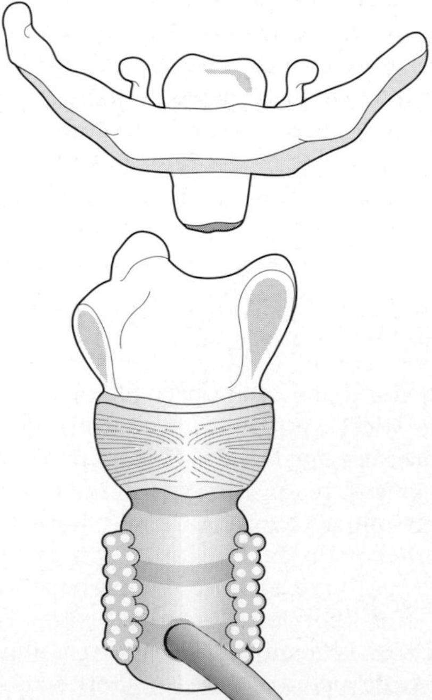

Figure 44.18 *The specimen has been removed preserving the right arytenoid cartilage and the upper two-thirds of the epiglottis.*

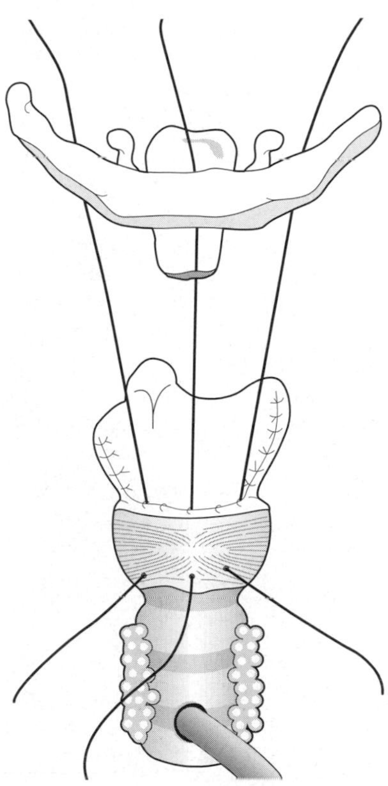

Figure 44.19 *The mucosa is sutured to the cut edges of the cartilage and the cricoid is approached to the hyoid and epiglottis by means of three sutures.*

Other procedures

Other partial laryngeal resections have been described for the surgical treatment of early glottic tumors. All of them constitute technical variations of the basic cordectomy and resemble some of the aforementioned procedures.

Bilateral cordectomy with cartilage resection and epiglottic reconstruction has been called 'near-total' laryngectomy by Tucker.[72] This procedure should be distinguished from the near-total operation described by Pearson *et al.*[59] Tucker's 'near-total' technique is a modified anterior frontal laryngectomy with epiglottic reconstruction, whereas the near-total laryngectomy described by Pearson is a radical procedure including the removal of the entire larynx except for an arytenoid and part of the vocal cord. The former is indicated for early glottic cancers whereas the latter can be used for selected advanced glottic lesions, as well as for some hypopharyngeal and supraglottic tumors.

Radical surgery

Advanced lesions require a more aggressive approach. However, total laryngectomy is not the only operation for large glottic tumors. Some subtotal procedures – such as near-total laryngectomy – may be performed in selected patients.

Near-total laryngectomy

Near-total laryngectomy provides a functional alternative to total laryngectomy in selected cases of lateralized cord-fixing laryngeal and pharyngeal cancers not amenable to conventional conservation operations. From a surgical point of view, the operation resembles more a total than a partial laryngectomy since the entire larynx is resected except for a narrow posterolateral strip connecting the trachea to the pharynx. This tracheopharyngeal bridge includes the arytenoid and a small portion of the vocal cord from the uninvolved side. The recurrent laryngeal nerve is also preserved and a dynamic shunt is created. The glottic portion of the shunt is partially sphincteric and prevents aspiration.

Indications

Indications for near-total laryngectomy are either oncologic or physiologic. Oncologic indications include unilateral cord-fixing tumors unsuitable for conventional conservation procedures. The patient must have an uninvolved laryngeal ventricle on the less involved side and a free ipsilateral arytenoid. Also, the interarytenoid space must be free of tumor invasion.

Physiologic indications include patients whose tumors are candidates for conservation surgery but will not tolerate it for reasons of age or health. In our practice, the most frequent physiologic indication is poor cardiopulmonary function in elderly patients unsuitable for standard partial laryngectomy.[26]

Surgical technique

The need to include the neck in the treatment plan will determine the neck incision. The skin flaps are elevated in the subplatysmal plane until adequate exposure of the hyoid bone and strap muscles is obtained. The tracheostomy is placed through a separate incision at the level of the third or fourth tracheal ring.

For an easier understanding of the surgical technique of near-total laryngectomy we prefer to describe the operation as the combination of two different procedures in the same patient. On the side of the tumor the larynx is approached as for a total laryngectomy, whereas on the less involved side the operation resembles a supraglottic laryngectomy.[25,52]

On the tumor side the neurovascular bundles are divided and the larynx is freed from its muscular attachments as if a total laryngectomy was being performed. Removal of the strap muscles, hyoid bone and thyroid lobe will be dictated by the size and location of the tumor.

On the less involved side, the larynx is approached through the vallecula – as for supraglottic laryngectomy – in all patients in which this area is not invaded by the tumor. First of all, a midline thyrotomy is performed and the thyroid ala is removed. If the tumor involves the anterior commissure, the cartilage cut is lateralized

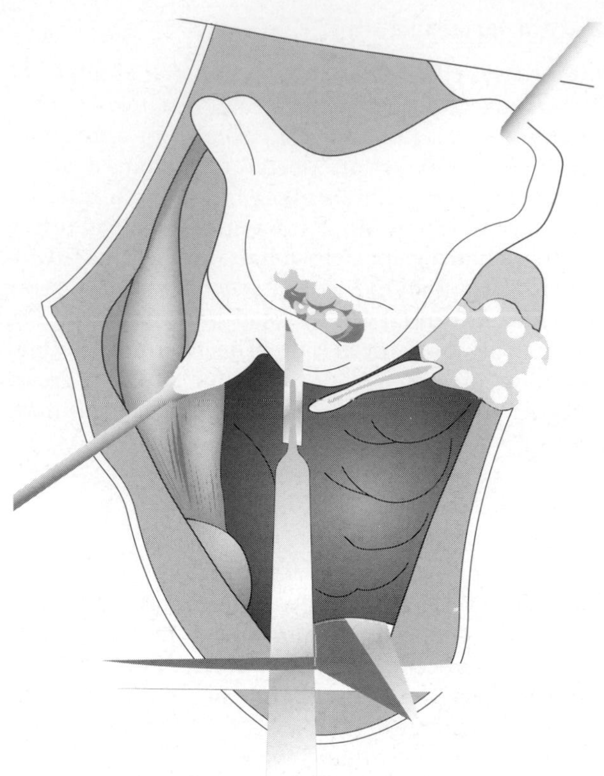

Figure 44.20 *Under direct vision, the true vocal cord is divided posterior to the tumor, allowing safe resection margins.*

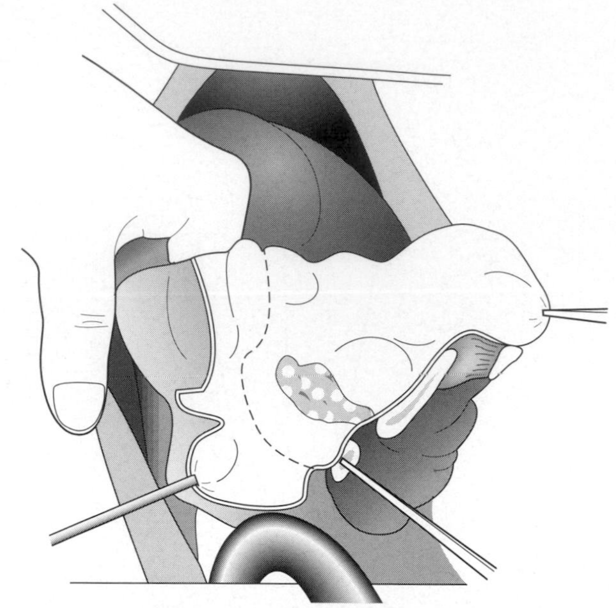

Figure 44.21 *Posteriorly, the incision runs on the front surface of the cricoid plate (dotted line). A finger inserted in the hypopharynx helps fracturing the cricoid cartilage. The interarytenoid muscle and the posterior cricoarytenoid muscle are transected until the mucosa of the pyriform sinus is visible.*

towards the normal side. The cartilage cut is made down to but not through the soft tissue within the larynx. The pharynx is opened from the lateral wall of the pyriform sinus, extending the pharyngotomy to the vallecula. By reflecting the hyoid bone upwards and the mucosa of the pyriform sinus laterally, a good view of the endolarynx is obtained. Under direct vision, the aryepiglottic fold is transected. The cut runs close to the superior and anterior surface of the arytenoid cartilage, towards the posterior end of the ventricle. This cut is continued anteriorly along the bottom of the ventricle to the point were the vocal cord will be divided (Fig 44.20). Until here, the operation on the less involved side has been developed as for a standard supraglottic laryngectomy.[31] Now both approaches must be connected with the single step which is characteristic of the near-total operation.

The amount of vocal cord that can be preserved must be decided at this moment. If necessary, the transection can be sited as far posteriorly as the vocal process of the arytenoid. Even in these cases the shunt can be easily created. Once the vocal cord has been divided, the incision is carried inferiorly and medially, transecting the cricoid arch near the midline. The cut is continued laterally below the cricoid cartilage on the side of the tumor. The incision is then curved upwards on the front surface of the posterior cricoid plate and, pushing with a finger from behind, the cricoid is easily fractured (Fig 44.21). The interarytenoid muscle is sectioned and the specimen is fully rotated towards the side of the tumor, exposing the posterior cricoarytenoid muscle. The muscle is transected until the mucosa of the pyriform sinus is visible. The specimen is finally released by cutting the last attachments between the pyriform sinus and the larynx.

Reconstruction begins after confirmation that the resection margins are clear of tumor. Before creating the shunt, some residual cricoid cartilage has to be resected in order to allow tubing. Care must be taken to preserve the mucosa and to avoid injury to the recurrent laryngeal nerve. Therefore, the portion of the cricoid located near the cricothyroid joint should be left undisturbed. If the remaining tissue at the level of the shunt is not wide enough to be tubed around a 12-gauge catheter, then a triangular augmentation mucosal flap from the pyriform sinus can be designed (Fig 44.22). The flap is rotated and sewn to the laryngeal remnant, increasing the diameter of the shunt. The pyriform sinus is then reconstructed with interrupted absorbable sutures.

A 12-gauge catheter is placed along the shunt and the mucosa is sutured in a tubular fashion (Fig 44.23). The only role of this catheter is to serve as a calibrating device to obtain the adequate shunt diameter, especially at the glottic level. Moving the calibrating catheter up and down while creating the shunt will give the surgeon an idea of the diameter of the shunt. Making the shunt too wide will cause aspiration problems; if it is too tight it will delay or even prevent phonation. Once the shunt has been created, the catheter should be removed to avoid mucosal

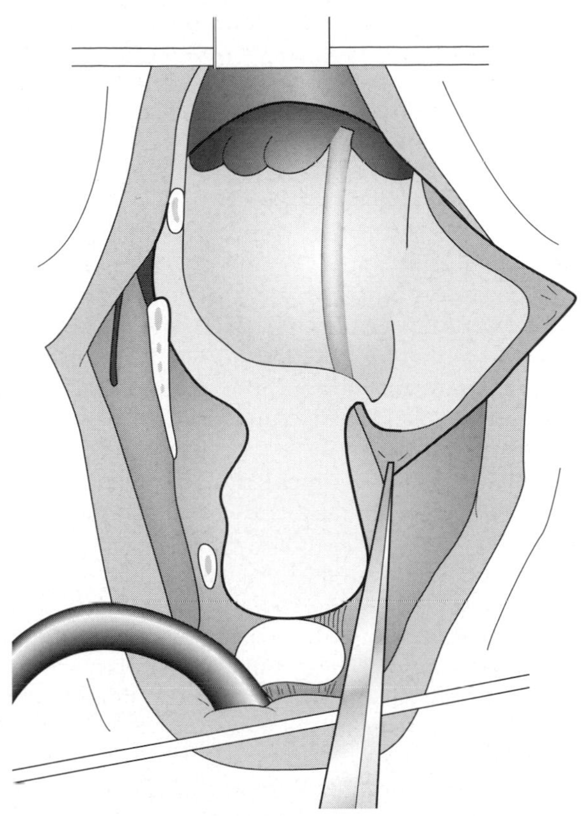

Figure 44.22 *The operation has been completed and the laryngeal remnant and pyriform sinus are visible. A triangular mucosal flap can be obtained from the hypopharynx to enlarge the shunt when necessary.*

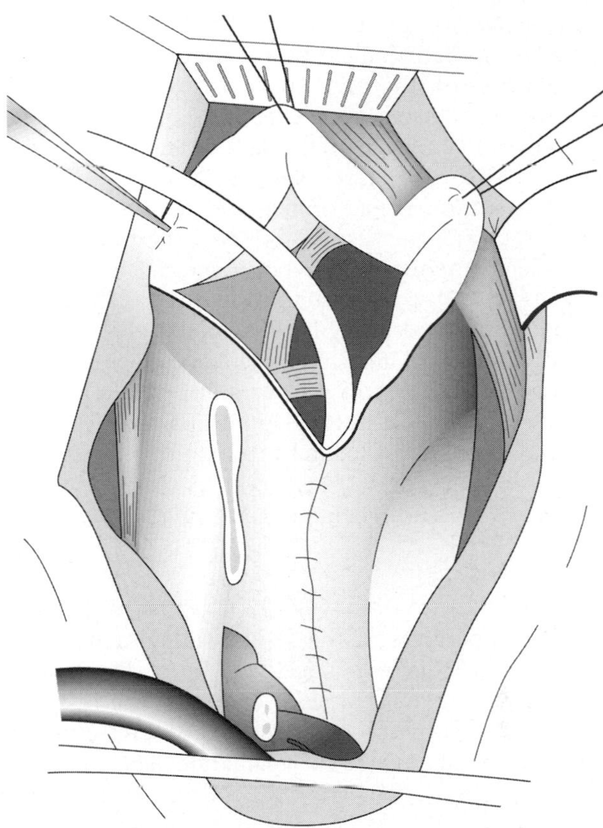

Figure 44.23 *The shunt is tubed around a 12-gauge catheter. The catheter is removed upon completion of the shunt to avoid mucosal damage. The anterior wall of the hypopharynx is then closed in the usual fashion.*

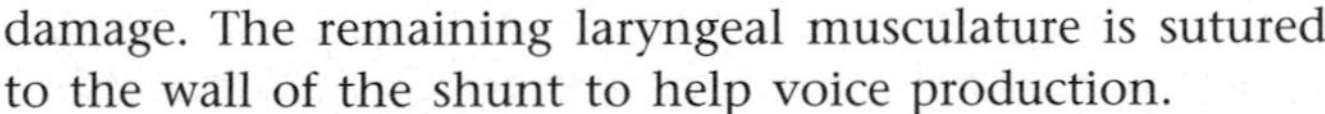

damage. The remaining laryngeal musculature is sutured to the wall of the shunt to help voice production.

A T-shaped closure of the pharynx is performed with interrupted absorbable sutures, similar to closure in a total laryngectomy. If possible, the closure is reinforced with a second muscular layer. The stoma is constructed by suturing the skin to the tracheal walls and a cuffed tracheostomy tube is placed.

Total laryngectomy

In spite of all the previously described partial techniques, some tumors can only be safely treated with total laryngectomy. This operation produces a total loss of normal phonatory elements and results in a complete separation of breathing from swallowing. Speech restoration after total laryngectomy may be accomplished either by physiologic, surgical, or prosthetic methods which are discussed elsewhere in this book.

Total laryngectomy is indicated for advanced glottic tumors with vocal cord fixation not amenable to near-total laryngectomy. In practice total laryngectomy is also frequently used as a salvage operation after radiation failure although partial procedures are theoretically possible in some selected cases. In most patients requiring total laryngectomy, the neck should also be included in the treatment plan since deep invasion carries a high risk of lymph node metastasis.

The most popular incision for total laryngectomy is the apron incision. When needed, additional lateral incisions may be used for neck dissection. The skin flaps are elevated deep to the platysma muscle to a level above the hyoid bone. Neck dissection is performed according to the clinical scenario. The strap muscles are then sectioned at the level of the thyroid isthmus, exposing the thyroid gland. For tumors with extensive subglottic involvement, the thyroid lobe on the side of the lesion should be included in the resection. The thyroid cartilage is fully exposed and skeletonized, cutting the insertions of the inferior pharyngeal constrictor muscle at the posterior border of the thyroid cartilage. The superior laryngeal vessels are then identified and ligated. The suprahyoid musculature is divided above the hyoid bone with the electrocautery. In a hyoid preserving approach, this cut is made below the hyoid bone, dividing the strap muscles from its hyoid insertions. The larynx may now be removed from below upwards or from above downwards, depending on tumor location and extension. Excessive removal of hypopharyngeal mucosa should be avoided during laryngectomy. Putting a finger into the pharyngeal opening helps the identification of tumor margins and allows a safe and adequate removal of the larynx preserving the mucosa of the uninvolved piriform sinus.

The type of pharyngeal closure employed depends on the amount of mucosa remaining after tumor resection. Usually a T-shaped closure, with either a continuous or interrupted suture, is performed and a feeding tube is maintained during the first postoperative days. In patients with sufficient remaining hypopharyngeal mucosa we prefer a 'tobacco pouch' closure using two parallel continuous sutures around the pharyngeal defect.[22] The first stitch runs 2–3 mm lateral to the circular opening of the hypopharynx. The second suture is placed 5 mm lateral and parallel to the first suture. No feeding tube is inserted and oral feeding is resumed by the third postoperative day. A carefully made 'tobacco pouch' suture is seldom associated with pharyngocutaneous fistula.

Results

Statistical comparisons of the results with different treatment options for glottic cancer can be done in several ways. Actuarial survival, local control with the first treatment, overall recurrence rates, morbidity, and even cost can be used as parameters for evaluation. For a comparison to be adequate, the procedures examined must be evaluated using the same criteria, something that is frequently overlooked in the literature. The result is a highly controversial field with an enormous amount of misleading figures. In addition, a general principle states that every author has the right to quote the references that are more favorable to his or her position, thus contributing to darken the already obscure domain of the results.

Oncologic results

T1 glottic cancer

Control rates for T1 glottic lesions with the three major options – partial laryngectomy, radiation therapy and transoral removal – are said to be similar and over 90%. However, this assertion deserves some comments.

Control rates using radiation therapy for T1 glottic lesions are unanimously reported as 90%.[10,20,30] This magic figure has been referred to as the '90% myth' because it hides some statistical skewing. It is widely recognized that a percentage of patients who undergo cordectomy for very small glottic lesions do not have cancer in the surgical specimen after laryngoscopic biopsy. In our experience that percentage is 13% and it may be as high as 20%.[12] It is likely that a similar percentage of patients treated with radiotherapy after biopsy do not have cancer at the beginning of their treatment. Radiation therapy, however, will be considered responsible for their cure when actually these cancers have been removed at the biopsy before the start of radiation therapy.

Another misleading factor is reporting together the results of first treatment and salvage treatment, assuming that partial laryngectomy is usually possible after radiation failures. In practice, conservation surgery is seldom feasible in patients previously irradiated because failures are often recognized too late. The concept that most radiation failures can be salvaged by partial laryngectomy[75] is not supported in our experience. In addition, planned radiotherapy plus salvage surgery results in a higher number of treatments when compared to surgery alone. We also know that approximately 10–15% of patients with glottic cancer who survive the first treatment will develop a second upper aerodigestive system cancer. Since most patients with T1 glottic lesions will be cured regardless of the treatment option, the possibilities of later disease must be considered, and our treatment options should not be exhausted.

Voice quality is the argument most frequently used in favor of radiation therapy for early glottic cancer, although few scientific studies have compared voice parameters between surgically treated and irradiated patients. In addition, there is great confusion among radiotherapists regarding the voice quality of different partial laryngectomies. The results of hemilaryngectomy are frequently mixed up with those of a simple cordectomy with the subsequent deterioration of voice quality in the analysis of the surgical group. It must be emphasized that hemilaryngectomy represents excessive treatment for T1 glottic cancers. Finally, the evaluation of the quality of life of our patients treated for laryngeal cancer indicate that radiation therapy may have a greater impact than voice on the overall adjustment of the patients after treatment.[4]

Surgical options have another advantage over radiation therapy: they produce a surgical specimen for pathologic examination. This is essential for accurate staging purposes, which is the basis for treatment comparisons between alternatives. Some clinically T1 glottic tumors may invade the anterior commissure, the thyroid cartilage, or the conus elasticus. These are actually histologic and biologic T3 cancers, which can be only accurately staged after surgical removal. For T1 glottic cancer involving the anterior commissure, frontolateral and anterior frontal partial laryngectomies offer better control of the disease than does radiation.[40]

The issue of cost is also raised when comparing treatment options for T1 glottic cancer. As a general rule, the cost of partial laryngectomy and radiotherapy are about the same, whereas transoral removal is considerably less expensive.[53] However, most studies do not include in the evaluation of the cost, the not negligible economic impact of patients not being able to work during a prolonged course of radiotherapy. In addition, the surgical procedure used for comparison is usually the hemilaryngectomy with tracheostomy and prolonged hospital stay. We already know that there are operations less expensive and more appropriate for the surgical treatment of T1 glottic lesions.

Between January 1984 and December 1994, 184 conventional partial operations were performed at the

Table 44.3 Surgical procedures for laryngeal cancer performed at La Paz Hospital between January 1984 and October 1994

Procedure	Number
Vertical partial laryngectomy	102
Cordectomy	70
Frontolateral laryngectomy	11
Anterior frontal laryngectomy	3
Hemilaryngectomy	18
Supraglottic laryngectomy	82
Subtotal operations	75
Total laryngectomy	322
Total	581

Department of Otolaryngology of La Paz Hospital. Of these, 102 were vertical procedures and 82 were supraglottic laryngectomies (see Table 44.3). Seventy patients with T1 glottic tumors were treated with laryngofissure and cordectomy without tracheostomy, 11 patients underwent frontolateral laryngectomy and three patients were treated with anterior frontal laryngectomy. All patients have a minimum follow-up of 3 years. Seven local recurrences (8.3%) occurred: five in cordectomy patients and two in frontolateral laryngectomy. The recurrences were managed with total laryngectomy plus radiotherapy (six patients) and near-total laryngectomy (one patient). Two patients died in spite of salvage treatment (one of them was the only patient with cordectomy as a salvage operation for radiation failure). Two more patients developed regional failure and were unsuccessfully treated with neck dissection and radiotherapy. Overall, 95.2% of the patients were cured and 95% of them retained a normal voice (in one case by means of a near-total laryngectomy).

T2 glottic cancer

Overall control rates for T2 lesions are less satisfactory, especially when there is impaired vocal cord mobility. The status of cord mobility affects the radiation therapy results more than the surgical results.[8] Local control with first treatment using radiation therapy for T2 lesions with mobile cord have been reported in the range of 70%.[27,34] Vocal cord mobility impairment deteriorates the local control rates with radiotherapy. The same has been reported with ventricular involvement.[8] After salvage treatment, about 70% of T2 patients may retain a functional larynx, although more than one treatment is required in more than 30% of the patients.[35]

Surgical treatment for T2 glottic tumors shows higher local control with the first treatment and fewer retreatments than radiation therapy, although long-term survival is very similar. In our practice, hemilaryngectomy for T2 glottic tumors yields a local control rate with first treatment of 87.5%. After surgical salvage for local-regional recurrences, 81.2% of the treated patients retained a normal larynx. Overall, 87.5% of the patients were cured of their primary tumor and only 18.7% of the patients required more than one treatment. This compares favorably with the results of patients initially treated with radiation therapy.

Advanced glottic cancer

The local control rates for T3 lesions by radiation therapy alone are in the range of 30–40%.[5,38,64,74] When transglottic cancers are excluded, local control may improve to approximately 50%.[28] The survivorship at 5 years, after surgical salvage, is about 55%, with more than 50% local recurrences. In other words, more than half of patients primarily treated with radiotherapy also undergo an operation.

When these figures are compared with the results of surgery for the same group of patients, the difference becomes evident. The 5-year survival reported by DeSanto[11] for T3 glottic tumors was 25% greater, with 50% higher local control and 37% fewer recurrences overall. Only in larynges preserved was there a difference favorable to radiation therapy. It seems that by looking only at the patients who survive and the larynges retained we fail to appreciate fully all the problems of the issue. One-third of the voices should not be preserved at the expense of the remaining two-thirds of the patients. In addition, voice-preserving operations are now available as an alternative to total laryngectomy or radiation therapy for advanced glottic tumors. The most useful are the supracricoid partial laryngectomy with CHEP and the near-total laryngectomy. The oncologic results of these operations are comparable to those of the total laryngectomy, with the advantage of excellent functional results in a high percentage of patients.[26,60,72] Also, the classic hemilaryngectomy may be safe for a few early T3 glottic cancers.[45]

Planned combined surgery and radiotherapy have also been proposed for advanced glottic tumors in an effort to increase local-regional control and survival. However, there is no evidence demonstrating a definite superiority of combined therapy over surgery alone for advanced glottic tumors. The actuarial or disease-free survival rates for patients treated with combined therapy have not been significantly increased over those obtained with a single modality in any randomized well-controlled study.[63] Postoperative radiotherapy may increase local control rates, although it does not improve survival.[65]

Functional results

The degree of voice alteration produced by cordectomy and its variations depends on the extent of the resection. In most cases the quality of the voice is somewhere between near-normal and poor, with all patients having a perfectly useful voice. These operations do not interfere with breathing or swallowing. Frontolateral laryngectomy and anterior frontal laryngectomy usually require a transient tracheostomy.

From a functional standpoint, hemilaryngectomy is the most disturbing conventional partial vertical operation. Most patients have some degree of glottic incompetence manifested by a whispery voice, although aspiration is seldom a serious problem. A tracheostomy tube is used during the first postoperative days. In addition, the patient is fed by a nasogastric tube for approximately 8 days.

Supracricoid subtotal laryngectomy with CHEP permits a physiologic voice without the need for a permanent tracheostomy. Objective analysis showed that the average fundamental frequency characteristics of speech after the operation were comparable to normal voice whereas other parameters were less efficient.[44] As for other partial operations, early removal of the tracheostomy tube is recommended. Swallowing rehabilitation is initiated after closure of the tracheostomy. The nasogastric feeding tube is removed when the patient is able to eat without much trouble. When successful swallowing is not achieved within the first postoperative month, a temporary percutaneous gastrostomy should be performed.

Successful speech rehabilitation is obtained in about 80% of patients treated with near-total laryngectomy.[26,46,58] While the speech results of near-total laryngectomy are comparable to those of tracheoesophageal puncture from a clinical standpoint, the near-total operation does not have the disadvantages of prosthetic rehabilitation. An important number of patients in our environment develop a permanent link with the hospital through the voice prosthesis, persisting even after they are cured of the disease. This results in a high rate of prosthesis withdrawal in the long term. With the near-total operation this is not a problem, because the shunt does not need to be cleaned or replaced. An additional advantage of the near-total operation is the high rate of patients who are able to speak without finger occlusion of the tracheostoma by using the Blom–Singer valve and the Barton button.[26] This could be attributed to the physiologic speech mechanisms involved in near-total laryngectomy voice production. Since the patient's own innervated vocal cord is what produces the sound, less pressure is needed and the tracheostoma valve is more easily adapted.

Finally, a number of different methods have been designed for the restoration of speech after total laryngectomy. These are addressed in a different chapter of this book and are not repeated here.

References

1. Baatenburg de Jong RJ, Rongen RJ, Laméris JS, Harthoorn M, Verwoerd CDA, Knegt P. Metastatic neck disease. Palpation vs ultrasound examination. *Arch Otolaryngol Head Neck Surg* 1989; **115**: 689–90.
2. Bailey BJ. Glottic carcinoma. In: Bailey BJ, Biller HF, eds. *Surgery of the Larynx*. Philadelphia: Saunders, 1985: 257–78.
3. Batsakis JG. *Tumors of the Head and Neck*, 2nd edn. Baltimore: Williams Wilkins, 1979.
4. Bermejo S, Caballos D, García F, García E, Martín L. Calidad de vida en pacientes operados de cáncer de laringe. In: *X Jornadas de Medicina Preventiva*. Madrid: UAM, 1997.
5. Brandenburg JH, Rutter SW. Residual carcinoma of the larynx. *Laryngoscope* 1977; **87**: 224–36.
6. Bridger GP. Staging the glottis and subglottis. In: Smee R, Bridger GP, eds. *Laryngeal Cancer*. Amsterdam: Elsevier, 1994: 253–61.
7. Bridger GP, Nassar VH. Cancer spread in the larynx. *Arch Otolaryngol* 1972; **95**: 497–505.
8. Bridger GP, Smee R. Glottic cancer, radiotherapy or conservation surgery. In: Shah JP, Johnson JT, eds. *Head and Neck Cancer. Vol IV. Proceedings at the Fourth International Head and Neck Oncology Conference (Toronto Meeting)*. Madison: Omnipress, 1996: 26–36.
9. Broyles EN. The anterior commissure tendon. *Ann Otol* 1943; **52**: 342–5.
10. Constable WC, White RL, El Mahdi AM, Fitz Hugh GS. Radiotherapeutic management of the cancer of the glottis, University of Virginia, 1956–1971. *Laryngoscope* 1975; **85**: 1494–503.
11. DeSanto LW. T3 glottic cancer: options and consequences of the options. *Laryngoscope* 1984; **94**: 1311–15.
12. DeSanto LW. Controversy in the management of laryngeal tumors: surgical perspective. In: Thawley SE, Panje WR, Batsakis JG, Lindberg RD, eds. *Comprehensive Management of Head and Neck Tumors*. Philadelphia: Saunders, 1987: 1029–39.
13. DeSanto LW. Early carcinoma of the larynx. In: Johnson J, Blitzer A, Ossoff RH, Thomas JR, eds. *Instructional Courses*. St Louis: Mosby, 1988: 353–9.
14. DeSanto LW, Pearson BW. Initial treatment of laryngeal cancer: principles of selection. *Minn Med* 1981; **64**: 691–8.
15. DeSanto LW, Beahrs OH, Holt JJ, O'Fallon WM. Neck dissection and combined therapy. Study of effectiveness. *Arch Otolaryngol* 1985; **111**: 366–70.
16. DeSanto LW, Olsen KD, Perry WC, Rohe DE, Keith RL. Quality of life after surgical treatment of cancer of the larynx. *Ann Otol Rhinol Laryngol* 1995; **104**: 763–9.
17. Feinmesser R, Freeman JL, Feinmesser M, Noyek AM, Mullen BM. Role of modern imaging in decision-making for elective neck dissection. *Head Neck* 1992; **14**: 173–6.
18. Ferlito A, Harrison DFN, Bailey BJ, DeSanto LW. Are clinical classifications for laryngeal cancer satisfactory? *Ann Otol Rhinol Laryngol* 1995; **104**: 741–7.
19. Ferlito A, Carbone A, DeSanto LW *et al.* Early cancer of the larynx: the concept as defined by clinicians, pathologists, and biologists. *Ann Otol Rhinol Laryngol* 1996; **105**: 245–50.
20. Fletcher GH, Lindberg RD, Hamberger A, Horiot JC. Reasons for irradiation failure in squamous cell carcinoma of the larynx. *Laryngoscope* 1975; **85**: 987–1003.
21. Gavilán C, Gavilán J. Nuevas tendencias en el tratamiento del cáncer de cabeza y cuello. In: González Barón M, ed. *Avances en Cáncer de Cabeza y Cuello*. Madrid: SMAR, 1992: 189–96.
22. Gavilán C, Cerdeira MA, Gavilán J. Pharyngeal closure following total laryngectomy: the 'tobacco pouch' technique. *Oper Tech Otolaryngol Head Neck Surg* 1993; **4**: 299–302.

23. Gavilán J, Cerdeira MA, Gavilán C. Laryngofissure and cordectomy without tracheostomy. *Oper Tech Otolaryngol Head Neck Surg* 1993; **4:** 262–70.
24. Gavilán J, Moñux A, Gavilán C. Extended hemilaryngectomy with epiglottic reconstruction. *Oper Tech Otolaryngol Head Neck Surg* 1993; **4:** 286–90.
25. Gavilán J, Herranz González J, Mañós M, Galindo N. Laringuectomma casi total. In: Alvarez Vicent JJ, Sacristán T, eds. *Cáncer de Laringe.* Madrid: Farma-Cusi, 1996: 283–90.
26. Gavilán J, Herranz González J, Prim P, Rabanal I. Speech results and complications of near-total laryngectomy. *Ann Otol Rhinol Laryngol* 1996; **105:** 729–33.
27. Goffinet DR, Eltringham JR, Glatstein E, Bagshaw MA. Carcinoma of the larynx. Results of radiation therapy in 213 patients. *Am J Roentgenol Radium Ther Nucl Med* 1973; **117:** 553–64.
28. Harwood AR, Bryce DP, Rider WD. Management of T3 glottic cancer. *Arch Otolaryngol* 1980; **106:** 697–9.
29. Hawkins NV. The treatment of glottic carcinoma: an analysis of 800 cases. *Laryngoscope* 1975; **85:** 1485–93.
30. Hendrickson FR. Radiation therapy treatment of larynx cancers. *Cancer* 1985; **55:** 2058–61.
31. Herranz González J, Martínez Vidal J, Gavilán J. Horizontal supraglottic laryngectomy: modifications to Alonso's technique. *Oper Tech Otolaryngol Head Neck Surg* 1993; **4:** 252–7.
32. Herranz González J, Gavilán J, Martínez Vidal J, Gavilán C. Supraglottic laryngectomy: functional and oncologic results. *Ann Otol Rhinol Laryngol* 1996; **105:** 18–22.
33. Hillsamer PJ, Schuller DE, McGhee RB, Chakeres D, Young DC. Improving diagnostic accuracy of cervical metastases with computed tomography and magnetic resonance imaging. *Arch Otolaryngol Head Neck Surg* 1990; **116:** 1297–301.
34. Horiot JC, Fletcher GH, Ballantyne AJ, Lindberg RD. Analysis of failures in early vocal cord cancer. *Radiology* 1972; **103:** 663–5.
35. Howell Burke D, Peters LJ, Goepfert H, Oswald MJ. T2 glottic cancer: recurrence, salvage, and survival after definitive radiotherapy. *Arch Otolaryngol Head Neck Surg* 1990; **116:** 830–5.
36. Jacobs C, Goffinet DR, Goffinet L, Kohler M, Fee WE. Chemotherapy as a substitute for surgery in the treatment of advanced resectable head and neck cancer. *Cancer* 1987; **60:** 1178–83.
37. Jacobs JJ, Ahmad K, Casiano R *et al.* Implications of positive surgical margins. *Laryngoscope* 1993; **103:** 64–8.
38. Karim ABMF, Snow GB, Hasman A, Chang SC, Keilholtz A, Hoekstra F. Dose response in radiotherapy for glottic carcinoma. *Cancer* 1978; **41:** 1728–32.
39. Kirchner JA. One hundred laryngeal cancers studied by serial section. *Ann Otol* 1969; **78:** 689–709.
40. Kirchner JA. Cancer at the anterior commissure of the larynx: results with radiotherapy. *Arch Otolaryngol* 1970; **91:** 524–5.
41. Kirchner JA, Som ML. Clinical significance of fixed vocal cord. *Laryngoscope* 1971; **81:** 1029–44.
42. Krespi YP, Meltzer CJ. Laser surgery for vocal cord carcinoma involving the anterior commissure. *Ann Otol Rhinol Laryngol* 1989; **98:** 105–9.
43. Laccourreye H, Laccourreye O, Weinstein G, Menard M, Brasnu D. Supracricoid laryngectomy with cricohyoidoepiglottopexy: a partial laryngeal procedure for glottic carcinoma. *Ann Otol Rhinol Laryngol* 1990; **99:** 421–6.
44. Laccourreye O, Crevier Buchman L, Weinstein G, Biacabe B, Laccourreye H, Brasnu D. Duration and frequency characteristics of speech and voice following supracricoid partial laryngectomy. *Ann Otol Rhinol Laryngol* 1995; **104:** 516–21.
45. Lesinski SG, Bauer WC, Ogura JH. Hemilaryngectomy for T3 (fixed cord) epidermoid carcinoma of the larynx. *Laryngoscope* 1976; **86:** 1563–71.
46. Levine PA, Debo RF, Reibel JF. Pearson near-total laryngectomy: a reproducible speaking shunt. *Head Neck* 1994; **16:** 323–5.
47. Looser KG, Shah JP, Strong EW. The significance of positive margins in surgically resected epidermoid carcinomas. *Head Neck Surg* 1978; **1:** 107–11.
48. Lynch RC. Intrinsic carcinoma of the larynx, with a second report of the cases operated on by suspension and dissection. *Trans Am Laryngol Assoc* 1920; **42:** 119–26.
49. Majer EH, Rieder W. Technique de laryngectomie permettant de conserver la perméabilité respiratoire. *Ann Otolaryngol Chir Cervicofac* 1959; **76:** 677–81.
50. McNeil BJ, Weichselbaum R, Pauker SG. Speech and survival: tradeoffs between quality and quantity of life in laryngeal cancer. *N Engl J Med* 1981; **305:** 982–7.
51. Micheau C, Luboinski B, Sancho H, Cachin Y. Modes of invasion of cancer of the larynx. A statistical, histological, and radioclinical analysis of 120 cases. *Cancer* 1976; **38:** 346–60.
52. Moñux A, Rabanal I, Cabra J, García-Polo J, Gavilán J. An easier technique for near total laryngectomy. *Laryngoscope* 1996; **106:** 235–8.
53. Myers EN, Wagner RL, Johnson JT. Microlaryngoscopic surgery for T1 glottic lesions: a cost-effective option. *Ann Otol Rhinol Laryngol* 1994; **103:** 28–30.
54. Olsen KD, DeSanto LW, Pearson BW. Positive Delphian lymph node: clinical significance in laryngeal cancer. *Laryngoscope* 1987; **97:** 1033–7.
55. Ossoff RH, Sisson GA, Shapshay SM. Endoscopic management of selected early vocal cord carcinoma. *Ann Otol Rhinol Laryngol* 1985; **94:** 560–4.
56. Pearson BW. Laryngeal microcirculation and pathways of cancer spread. *Laryngoscope* 1975; **85:** 700–13.
57. Pearson BW. Management of the primary site: larynx and hypopharynx. In: Pillsbury HC, Goldsmith MM, eds. *Operative Challenges in Otolaryngology Head and Neck Surgery.* Chicago: Year Book Medical Publishers, 1990: 346–76.
58. Pearson BW, DeSanto LW, Olsen KD. The functional and oncologic results of near-total laryngectomy. *Third International Conference on Head and Neck Cancer, San Francisco,* 1992.
59. Pearson BW, Woods RD, Hartman DE. Extended hemilaryngectomy for T3 glottic carcinoma with preservation of speech and swallowing. *Laryngoscope* 1980; **90:** 1950–61.
60. Piquet JJ, Chevalier D. Subtotal laryngectomy with crico-hyoido-epiglotto-pexy for the treatment of extended glottic carcinomas. *Am J Surg* 1991; **162:** 357–61.

61. Piquet JJ, Desaulty A, Decroix G. La crico-hyoïdo-épiglotto-pexie. Technique opératoire et résultats fonctionnels. *Ann Otolaryngol Chir Cervicofac* 1974; **91:** 681–6.
62. Robbins KT, Fontanesi J, Wong FSH *et al.* A novel organ preservation protocol for advanced carcinoma of the larynx and pharynx. *Arch Otolaryngol Head Neck Surg* 1996; **122:** 853–7.
63. Silverman CL, Marks JE. Radiation therapy of laryngeal tumors: planned combined radiotherapy and surgery. In: Thawley SE, Panje WR, Batsakis JG, Lindberg RD, eds. *Comprehensive Management of Head and Neck Tumors.* Philadelphia: Saunders, 1987: 919–28.
64. Skolnik EM, Martin L, Yee KF, Wheatley MA. Radiation failures in cancer of the larynx. *Ann Otol* 1975; **84:** 804–11.
65. Snow JB, Gelber RD, Kramer S, Davis LW, Marcial VA, Lowry LD. Comparison of preoperative and postoperative radiation therapy for patients with carcinoma of the head and neck. *Acta Otolaryngol (Stockh)* 1981; **91:** 611–26.
66. Soo KC, Shah JP, Gopinath KS, Jaques DP, Gerold FP, Strong EW. Analysis of prognostic variables and results after vertical partial laryngectomy. *Am J Surg* 1988; **156:** 264–8.
67. Steiner W, Ambrosch P. CO_2 laser microsurgery for hypopharyngeal carcinoma. In: Smee R, Bridger GP, eds. *Laryngeal Cancer.* Amsterdam: Elsevier, 1994: 606–9.
68. The Department of Veterans Affairs Laryngeal Study Group. Induction chemotherapy plus radiation compared with surgery plus radiation in patients with advanced laryngeal cancer. *N Engl J Med* 1991; **324:** 1685–90.
69. Thomas JV, Olsen KD, Neel HB, DeSanto LW, Suman VJ. Recurrences after endoscopic management of early (T1) glottic carcinoma. *Laryngoscope* 1994; **104:** 1099–104.
70. Tucker GF, Smith HR. A histological demonstration of the development of laryngeal connective tissue compartments. *Trans Am Acad Ophthalmol Otolaryngol* 1962; **66:** 308–18.
71. Tucker GF Jr, Alonso WA, Cowan M, Tucker JA, Druck N. The anterior commissure revisited. *Ann Otol* 1973; **82:** 625–36.
72. Tucker HM. Near-total laryngectomy with epiglottic reconstruction. *Oper Tech Otolaryngol Head Neck Surg* 1990; **1:** 17–20.
73. van den Brekel MWM, Castelijns JA, Stel HV *et al.* Occult metastatic neck disease: detection with US and US-guided fine-needle aspiration cytology. *Radiology* 1991; **180:** 457–61.
74. Vermund H. Role of radiotherapy in cancer of the larynx as related to the TNM system of staging: a review. *Cancer* 1970; **25:** 485–504.
75. Wang CC. Radiation therapy of laryngeal tumors: curative radiation therapy: In: Thawley SE, Panje WR, Batsakis JG, Lindberg RD, eds. *Comprehensive Management of Head and Neck Tumors.* Philadelphia: Saunders, 1987: 906–18.
76. Wolfensberger M, Dort JC. Endoscopic laser surgery for early glottic carcinoma: a clinical and experimental study. *Laryngoscope* 1990; **100:** 1100–5.

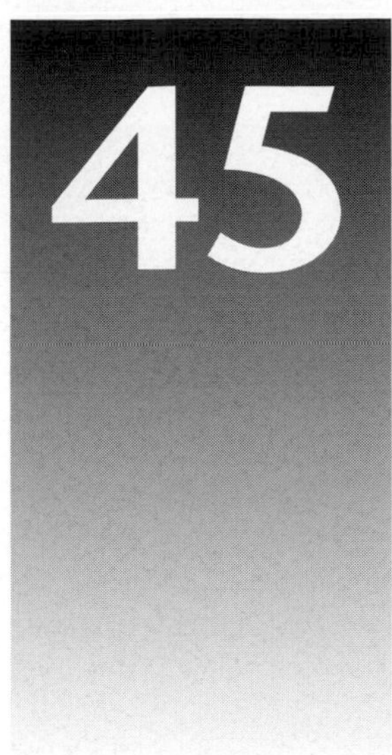

Cancer of the subglottis

Juan Bartual-Pastor

Subglottic cancer was first reported as a clinical entity in the latter part of the nineteenth century. The particular characteristics of this lesion account for it being the object of separate study. Incidence is highly variable, depending on geographic area, climate, eating habits, gender and race. Diagnosis is usually late unless phonation is initially affected. It is often difficult to distinguish whether the lesion is primary subglottic cancer, cancer of the vocal cords or a subglottic extension of a glottic tumor. This lesion requires special management and is not yet amenable to curative treatment by endoscopy with CO_2 laser and minimally invasive surgery.

Primary subglottic cancer is uncommon, with an estimated incidence of 0.8% in homogenous series.[9]

Spread patterns

Subglottic tumors can arise unilaterally on the lateral wall of the subglottic space and extend through the conus elasticus or below it and reach new pathways of spread. If a subglottic tumor spreads more than 1 cm anteriorly or more than 0.5 cm outwards posteriorly it will reach the cricothyroid membrane ventrad and the cricoid cartilage dorsad. This increases the risk of lymphatic spread to Poirier's prelaryngeal ganglia, the paratracheal and upper mediastinal nodes and the paralaryngeal spaces and has an impact on the prognosis and management of subglottic cancer.

Subglottic tumors usually extend toward the trachea[8] with practically no cephalad growth (Fig 45.1). According to other reports,[7,16,18] subglottic cancer is characterized by circumferential growth extending beneath the anterior commissure (Fig 45.2), early invasion of the cricoid cartilage and extralaryngeal spread. Olofsson[16] reported that primary subglottic tumors extend through the conus elasticus and involve the vocal cord, submucosally

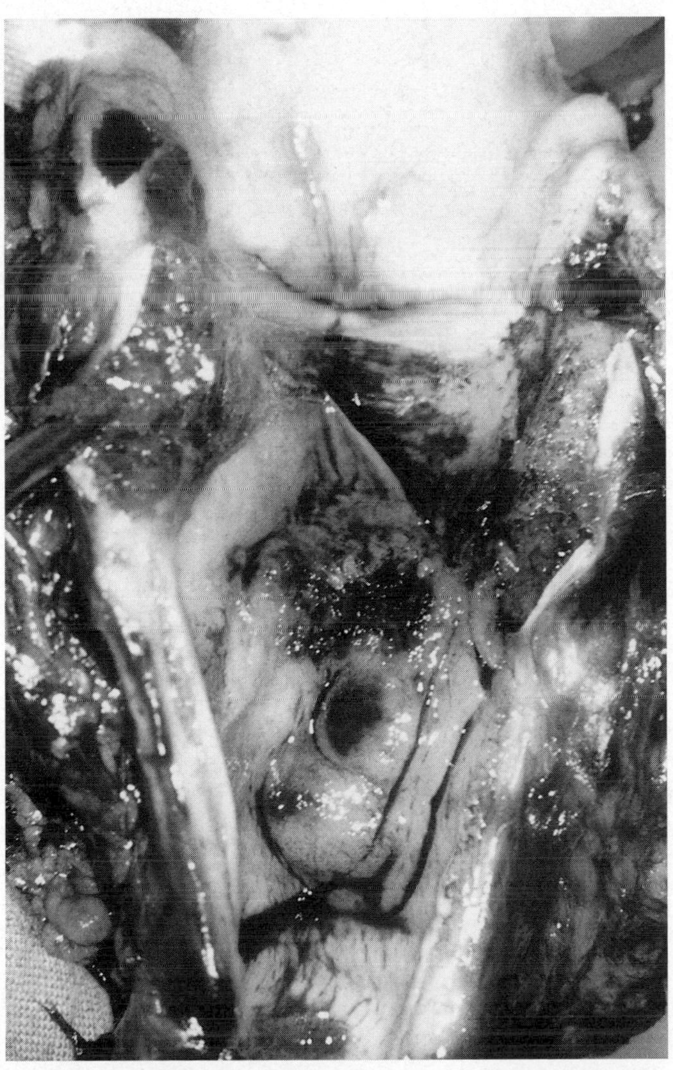

Figure 45.1 *Subglottic cancer with extension toward trachea.*

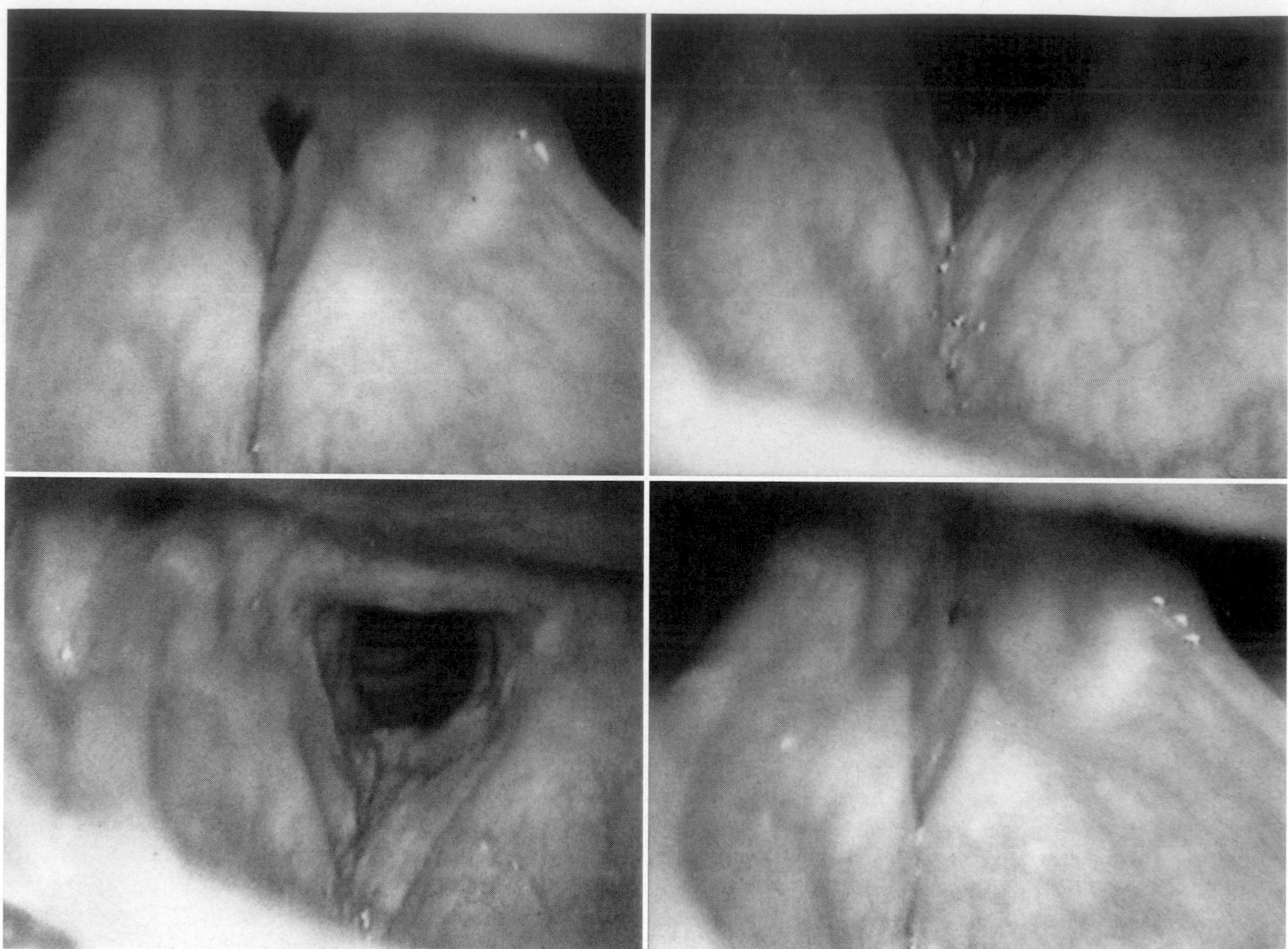

Figure 45.2 *Subglottic cancer with circumferential growth.*

invading muscles. The cricoid cartilage is involved in half of primary subglottic tumors (2/4) and spread outside the larynx is even more frequent (3/4). Posterior spread toward the hypopharynx and the esophagus above the posterior commissure or below the cricoid cartilage has also been reported.[3,7,8,11,12,16,18]

The incidence of lymphatic metastases in regional nodes is reported to be under 10%. Stell and Tobin[18] found the incidence of metastasis in primary subglottic cancer to be 16% and in secondary tumors with subglottic extension 5.5%. Pietrantoni *et al.*[17] reported an incidence of 9.25% nodal metastases in subglottic tumors and Harrison[11] considers metastasis in the paratracheal lymph nodes to be clinically undetectable, but histologically present in 50% of primary subglottic carcinomas examined by serial section. We found histologically an incidence of 32.35% nodal metastases in primary subglottic cancer.

This discrepancy is due to the different lymphatic chains examined in these series. A study by Welsh[20] shows that the subglottic region drains via three lymphatic pedicles. The anterior pedicle penetrates the cricothyroid membrane to drain to the prelaryngeal and pretracheal lymph nodes. The posterior pedicles penetrate the crico-tracheal membrane and end in the recurrent and the superior mediastinal lymph nodes. That is why the internal jugular chain should be considered a secondary site of lymphatic spread for subglottic cancers.[15]

Symptomatology

Initial symptoms are variable depending on whether the lesion is primary subglottic carcinoma or glottic cancer with secondary subglottic extension. The former presents with nonspecific symptoms among which paresthesia with foreign-body sensation and hoarseness prevail.

Invasive tumors with surface and deep growth may involve the vocal cord early and therefore be diagnosed as primary subglottic cancer. But most primary subglottic tumors are asymptomatic at onset and are found when there is considerable extension, particularly if growth is circumferential or spreads inferiorly toward the trachea (Figs 45.1 and 45.2).

The first symptom may be dysphonia due to vocal cord paralysis, apparently caused by a lesion of the recurrent laryngeal nerve. The patient presents a bitonal voice impairment and shortened maximum phonation time (MPh T). The primary lesion is difficult or impossible to assess by indirect laryngoscopy or even with a von Stuckrad loupe from above, since the free margin of the vocal cord conceals what lies below. The lesion grows unseen and all that can be assessed is unilateral recurrent laryngeal nerve paralysis.

When tumor growth is exophytic, paresthesia, dysphonia and stridor occur rapidly. Progressive dyspnea appears subsequently and diagnosis is possible at first examination by indirect laryngoscopy or with a von Stuckrad loupe. A red or grayish uni- or bilateral lesion, with an occasionally papillomatous appearance, can be seen protruding below the cords and reducing the laryngeal lumen. This symptomatology was present in 30% of the subglottic cancers reported by Stell and Tobin.[18]

If the predominant lesion is a subglottic edema, which may be ulcerated, a concentric narrowing of the region occurs causing progressive dyspnea, stridor, severe phonasthenia and shortened (MPh T), so that by speaking the patient has to inspirate frequently, giving an impression of fatigue.

A primary subglottic tumor is occasionally found on investigating the origin of a low cervical or tracheal adenopathy.

When primary subglottic cancer begins on the inner surface of the cricoid ring, early invasion of the perichondrium and cartilage may occur, causing neoplastic perichondritis and involving the thyroid isthmus and even the prelaryngeal node. This lesion may be mistaken for thyroid cancer or chronic thyroiditis.

The incidence of thyroid involvement in primary subglottic cancer varies from 20%[11] to 6.30%.[18] Unfortunately, the symptomatology of subglottic cancer may be the result of invasion by an adjacent malignant tumor, usually thyroid cancer. Dyspnea and impairment of vocalization in these cases are caused by extrinsic tracheal compression or early invasion of the recurrent nerves. Thus, bilateral recurrent laryngeal nerve paralysis at aperture (Ziemsen's syndrome) with aphonia, aspiration to the lower tract, dry cough and repeated bronchitis may be due to primary subglottic cancer, thyroid cancer or cancer of the cervical esophagus. A very thorough examination is therefore mandatory.

Diagnosis

Diagnosing primary subglottic cancer can be very difficult due to the aforementioned reasons. A suspected subglottic lesion or a recurrent laryngeal nerve paralysis of doubtful etiology requires endoscopic examination with a flexible fiberscope or direct microlaryngoscopy and simultaneous use of rigid telescopes with different angles (0°, 30°, 50° and 90°) according to the technique reported by Andréa and Dias.[2]

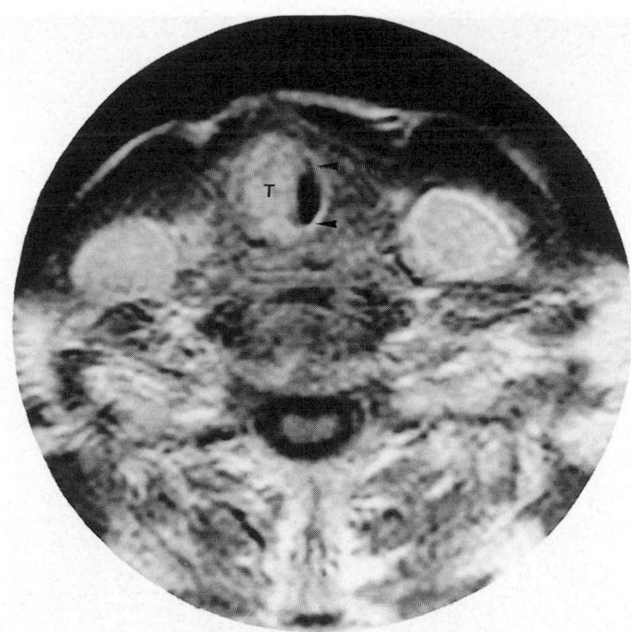

Figure 45.3 *Subglottic carcinoma. Axial MRI with intravenous contrast and fat suppression. T, subglottic tumor. (By courtesy of C R Guirado.)*

The examination must be completed with a CT and MRI imaging study, which can often detect the presence of primary subglottic lesions. However, these examinations help mainly to assess the subglottic extension of a glottic tumor or the spread of a subglottic cancer into the paraglottic or paralaryngeal space or into the cartilaginous skeleton. According to Guirado *et al.*,[10] MRI is the best current technique for diagnosis because the coronal view shows inferior extension below the free margin of the cord. Precise assessment of whether the tumor reaches the upper margin of the cricoid ring and involves the internal cortex of the cartilage has a strong bearing on management of the disease. MRI is very sensitive for detecting neoplastic invasion of ossified hyaline cartilage. The T1 sequences show that bone marrow, which appears with a strong signal due to its fat content, is replaced by tissue with a medium signal pertaining to the tumor (Fig 45.3).

CT provides high-resolution images of the deep anatomy of the larynx and respiratory tract. It enables us to examine the paraglottic and paralaryngeal spaces and enhances manual examination of cervical adenopathy, which is not very amenable to palpation in subglottic cancer. CT and MRI are used to evaluate the degree of local invasion and possible extralaryngeal spread of the tumor, show submucosal extension, estimate tumor volume and detect cervical and mediastinal lymph node metastases measuring 6 mm or more. Subclinical lymphatic metastases are particularly frequent and the CT scan must include the mediastinum and thorax as well as the neck.[6]

The examination is completed with a biopsy to confirm the nature of the tumor. If the result is negative or the

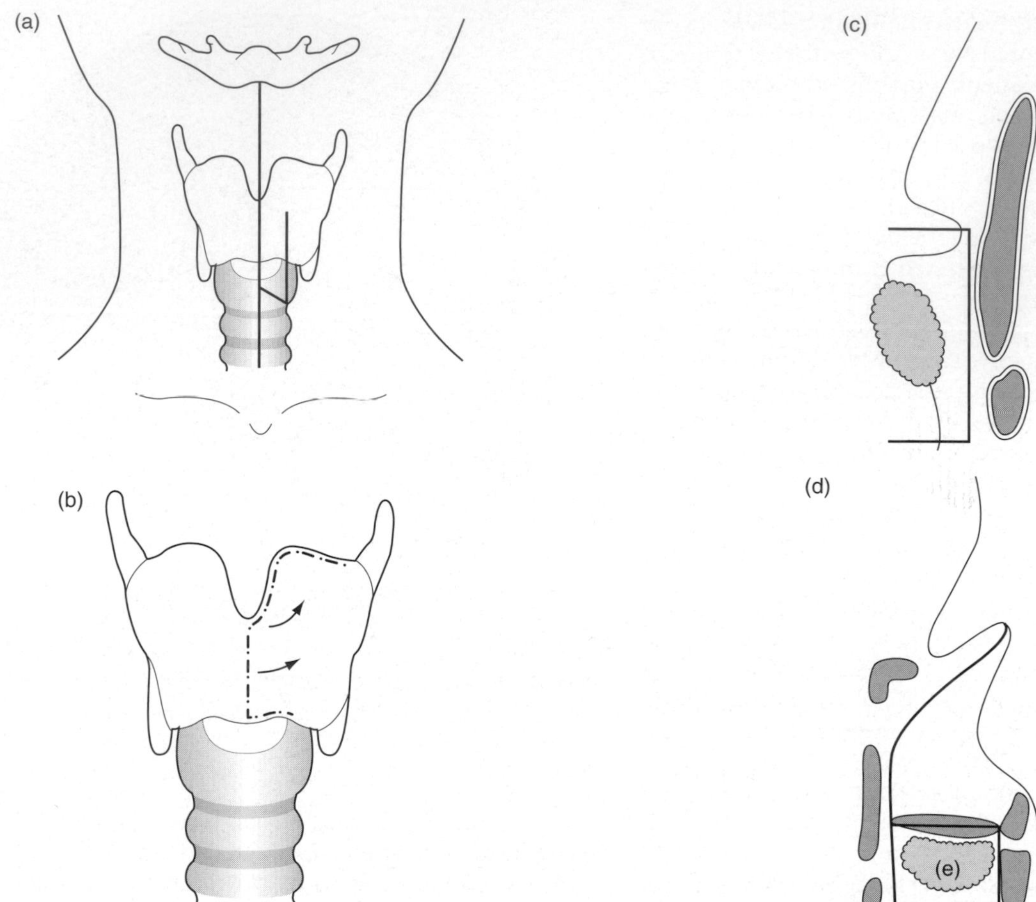

Figure 45.4 *Diagram of Torrens' technique for subglottic partial hemilaryngectomy. (a) Vertical and median cervical incision forming a precervical flap to cover the exposed area after excision. (b) Incision in the external perichondrium of the thyroid ala and separation on the side of the incision. (c) Frontal cut representing the excision that conserves the internal perichondrium. (d) Sagittal cut indicating the limits of the excision. (e) Tumor location and staging in Torrens' technique.*

nature and origin of the tumor doubtful, differential diagnosis must be performed in primary thyroid tumors by means of a fine-needle biopsy, T3, T4 and TSH, scintigraphy, ultrasonography and antithyroglobulin antibodies. Clinical examination, endoscopy and imaging studies are the basis for tumor staging (TNM) and for planning treatment.

Treatment

The management of subglottic cancer depends on multiple factors including age, local and general state of the patient, histologic type and potential radiosensitivity of the tumor, initial site and progression and the presence of regional or distant lymphatic metastases. Suzuki *et al.*[19] report a 5-year survival rate of 50% in subglottic cancer treated with exclusive radiotherapy in stages I and II.

We prefer surgical treatment in stages I and II and radiosurgical treatment in stages III and IV.

In certain circumstances (old age, high blood pressure and cardiopathy, diabetes mellitus, COPD, potential radiosensitivity of the tumor, etc.) primary radiotherapy may be advisable, including the cervical and recurrent lymphatic chains, even in stages I and II. The same is applicable to patients who refuse surgery. Patients treated with primary radiotherapy received a tumor dose of 66 Gy and 45 Gy on the lymphatic chains. Postoperative complementary irradiation covers the surgical field and the lymphatic chains in a 44 Gy dose, and treatment is continued with irradiation of the volume until reaching a total dose of 60 Gy in 6 weeks.

In stage IV, with tumor invasion into the perilaryngeal spaces, we perform total laryngectomy with total or partial excision of the thyroid gland and uni- or bilateral surgical removal of the recurrent and low cervical lymphatic chains. Treatment is completed with postoperative radiotherapy.

Depending on the initial site and staging of the tumor, in less advanced lesions the following surgical techniques can be conducted.

Partial subglottic hemilaryngectomy (Torrens' technique)

This technique is indicated for Tis and T1 tumors in the lateral subglottic wall which are histologically well differentiated, potentially radioresistant and strictly unilateral with normal mobility. It is essential for this technique that the anterior commissure and the arytenoid cartilage are not involved and that there is no invasion into the thyroid or cricoid cartilage or the laryngeal ventricle or spread into the trachea.

The surgical stages are as follows:

- vertical and median incision, preparing a flap to cover the exposed area;
- low preventive tracheotomy, initial or following endotracheal intubation and general anesthesia;
- classic laryngofissure and exposure of lesion;
- subperichondrial excision, preferably with a binocular microscope, of the entire vocal cord with its subglottic aspect to the level of the superior border of the cricoid ring;
- covering of the exposed area with the prelaryngeal skin flap, which must include subcutaneous tissue and platysma; and
- removal of prelaryngeal, recurrent and ipsilateral supraclavicular nodes (Fig 45.4).

Partial hemilaryngectomy with window surgery (Som's technique)

This technique is very similar to that of Torrens and can be performed in strictly unilateral primary subglottic T2N0M0 and T3N0M0 cancers of the lateral wall with cord fixation. Together with the vocal cord, resection must include the internal perichondrium of the thyroid ala, the relevant portion of the thyroid cartilage, the laryngeal ventricle and the free border of the ventricular band (Fig 45.5).

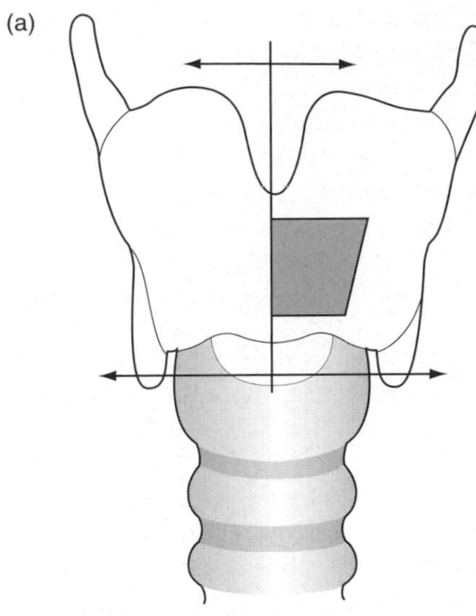

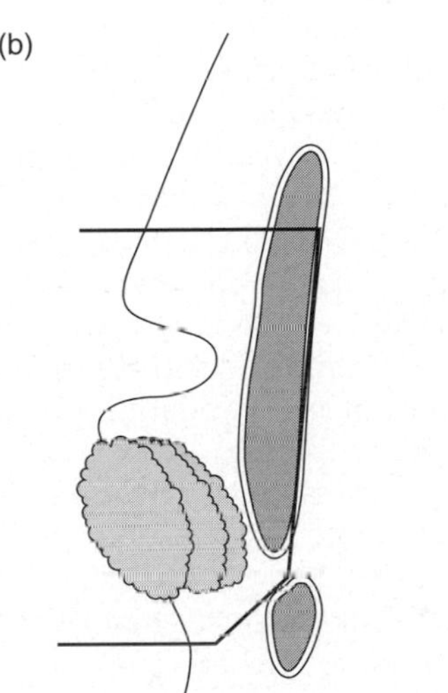

Figure 45.5 *Diagram of Som's technique. (a) Removal of perichondrium and window surgery in thyroid wing. (b) Frontal cut delimiting the extension of the excision, which includes the relevant portion of the thyroid ala and the internal perichondrium.*

Infravestibular horizontal partial laryngectomy (Bartual's technique)

This subtotal laryngectomy technique[1,4,5] can be performed in subglottic T2 cancers with their initial site in the anterior and/or posterior walls and no skeletal invasion, in primary lateral wall T1b tumors extending beyond the midline and into the opposite hemilarynx and in T3 tumors not extending beyond the first tracheal ring and not involving the anterior commissure and the cartilaginous skeleton. This technique can also be applied in glottic cancers, especially vocal cord tumors with cord fixation, even when they have spread to the arytenoid cartilage and posterior commissure and there is subglottic extension, provided there is no laryngeal skeleton invasion. The technique can be used in cancer of the vocal cords following relapse after laryngofissure provided the tumor is not exteriorized.

A similar technique was reported in 1950 by Hofmann Saguez[13,14] although this author conserved the cricoid cartilage and removed the anterior three-quarters of the thyroid cartilage, performing reconstruction with an acrylic mould. This conservative subtotal laryngectomy was used in a glottic cancer with extension into the subglottic space. In 1974, Algaba *et al.*[1] and Bartual and Portela[4] presented this method of subtotal laryngectomy for subglottic cancer, simultaneously but with technical differences, at the Annual Meeting of the SEORL.

Infravestibular horizontal partial laryngectomy is the reverse of the technique by Alonso for supraglottic tumors and has similar anatomic, embryologic, physiologic and oncologic bases which are common to horizontal surgery.

The supraglottic space and the upper respiratory tract are derived from the buccopharyngeal primordium, and the glottis and subglottis from the tracheobronchial primordium. This accounts for the larynx having two oncologically different regions. The dividing line runs along the lateral wall of the ventricle and over the vocal cord. This boundary is rarely crossed by primary vestibular tumors growing downward or glottic and subglottic tumors growing upward. The latter grow down and forward and rarely extend into the vestibule.

As a result of embryologic development, there are likewise two separate lymphatic territories, as mentioned above.

Consequently, if it is technically viable and oncologically beneficial to excise the upper half of the larynx, the same should be true for the lower half. Removal of the lower half of the larynx with the vocal cords can be partially compensated for by the vicarious hypertrophy of the ventricular bands and by all the pharyngolaryngeal musculature. If part of the thyroid skeleton is also conserved to maintain the laryngeal lumen patent and to support the aforementioned musculature, the main functions of the larynx can be conserved provided continuity with the trachea is reestablished.

The technique by Alonso showed that the epiglottis and the upper sphincter of the larynx could be removed with no serious effects on laryngeal functions. The same may be expected regarding removal of the lower half and the vocal cords. The physiology of the larynx will undergo a severe change, but will be conserved sufficiently to ensure the main functions and enable respiration, vocalization and swallowing to occur via natural paths.[5]

The objectives of infravestibular horizontal partial laryngectomy are as follows:

- total tumor removal with the lower half of the larynx and including one or more tracheal rings, according to caudad spread;
- conservation of the supraglottic half of the larynx and its thyroid skeleton to maintain the laryngeal lumen patent and favor decannulation; and
- restoration of main laryngeal functions, due to conservation of the epiglottis, the bands and on occasions the arytenoids.

Operative technique

- Low tracheotomy and endotracheal intubation.
- Classic Glück–Tapia incision which can be completed with a lateral discharge incision towards the supraclavicular fossa in order to remove the lymph nodes (neck dissection) if necessary. Exposure of the prelaryngeal musculature and sectioning of the hyoid insertions of the muscles, retracting the sectioned muscles downwards.
- Transverse incision of the external perichondrium at the level of the inferior border of both thyroid alae, lifting it upwards until Gurr's point.
- Transverse section of the thyroid cartilage 3.5–6 mm below the vertex of the incisura thyroidea depending on the size of the larynx. The bands are inserted in the upper part of the angle of the thyroid cartilage. The vocal cords and the thyroarytenoid ligaments are inserted about 3 mm below the bands. The distance between the pomum Adami and the thyroarytenoid ligament ranges in males from 3.5 to 6 mm and in females from 3 to 5 mm. The insertion of the vocal cords is usually indicated by a small depression (Gurr's point) beneath the angle formed by the confluence of both thyroid laminae, which is a valuable reference point to locate the level of the cartilaginous section. Thus, a third of the thyroid alae remains above the section together with its external and internal perichondrium, the bands and the epiglottis.
- Transverse section of the mucosa and opening of the larynx between the anterior band and vocal cord insertions. The cut is made with scissors paralleling the superior border of both cords until reaching the arytenoids. The pharyngeal mucosa is sectioned transversely at the level of the posterior border of the aditus laryngis. In some cases it is possible to conserve the arytenoid cartilage on one or both sides.
- Tracheal section below the first ring until reaching the anterior wall of the hypopharynx. Excision of the lower half of the larynx is completed, retracting submucosally the posterior surface of the cricoid cartilage as far as its upper limit, the site of the incision in the pharyngolaryngeal mucosa.
- The hypopharyngeal mucosa is sutured to the posterior wall and to the free edge of the remaining trachea, and the tracheal ring is sutured by means of two lateral stitches to the thyroid cartilage on both sides and one median stitch around the thyroid incisure. To prevent the cartilage breaking we make two drill holes with a reamer.
- The perichondrium is sutured to the trachea as a reinforcement. Musculature is replaced and sutured. Closure in layers (Fig 45.6). With the appropriate incision the lymphatic chains can be dissected in the same surgical intervention.

Results

Between 1977 and 1991 we have treated and monitored a total of 34 patients with primary subglottic cancer, excluding those with cord cancer and secondary subglottic extension.

The results are shown in Table 45.1. The 5-year survival rate of subglottic cancer is, on the whole, considering all forms of treatment, 64.71% (22/34). The 5-year survival rate for cases treated with infravestibular partial laryngectomy is 62.5% (15/24), with preservation of the laryngeal voice. Decannulation was possible in 40% (6/15) of the patients and swallowing was satisfactory in 93.33% (14/15) and bad in 6.6% (1/15). This patient required total laryngectomy for functional reasons (Fig 45.7).

The mucosa of the anterior wall of the pharynx that is sutured to the posterior wall of the trachea and to the dorsal end of the bands, or the arytenoid cartilage if

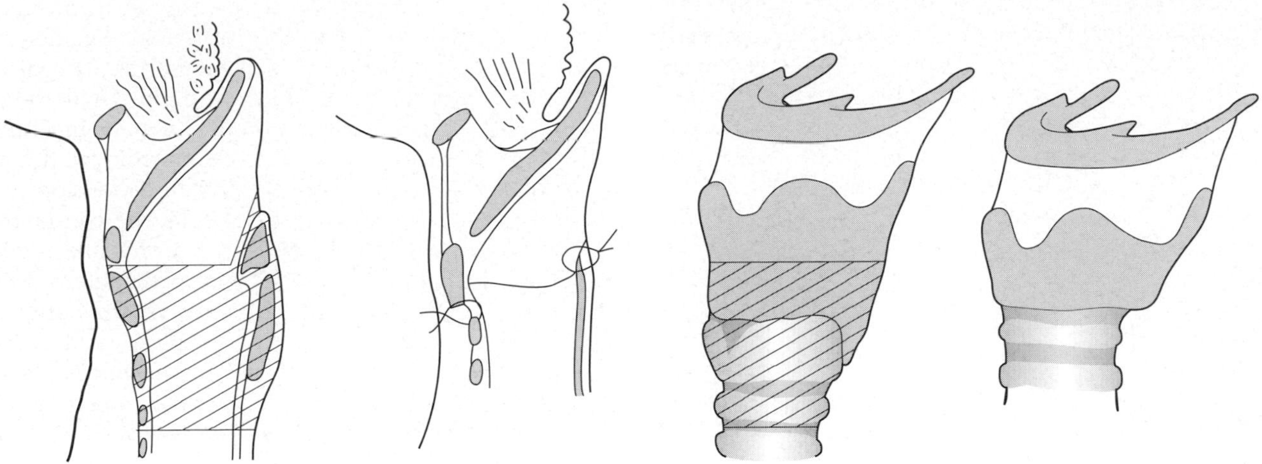

Figure 45.6 *Diagram of infravestibular horizontal partial laryngectomy by Bartual.[3] In the left part of this figure the shadowed areas show the parts of the larynx that have been removed; in the right part of the figure, diagrams show laryngeal reconstruction after tracheal ascension.*

Table 45.1 Five-year survival rate of the subglottic cancer

TNM stage	*Cases*	*Surgical technique*	*Radiotherapy (primary or complementary)*	*Local recurrence*	*Decannulation larynx voice*	*5-Year survival*	*Salvaged laryngectomy*	*Exitus laetalis*
pT1N0	2	Torrens	–	–	2/2	2/2	–	–
pT2N0$_0$	2	Som	–	–	2/2	2/2	–	–
pT3N0	1	Som	1		1/1	1/1	–	–
pT3N0	18	Bartual	–	4/18	5/13	13/18	4/18	5/18
pT3N1	4	Bartual	4	2/4	1/4	2/4	2/4	2/4
pT3N3	2	Bartual	2	–	–	0/2	–	2/2
pT4N1	2	Total laryng	2	1/2	–	1/2	–	1/2
pT4N2	3	Total laryng	3	2/3	–	1/3	–	2/3

Total laryng, total laryngectomy.

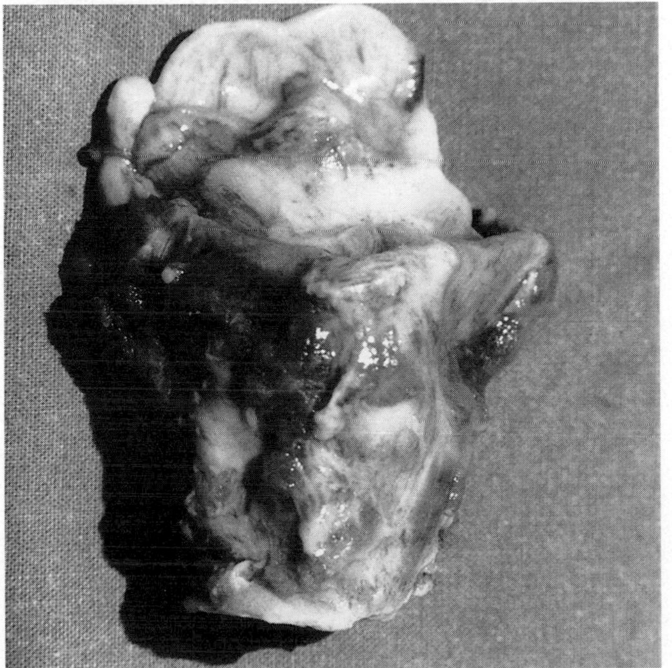

Figure 45.7 *Neolarynx following the Bartual technique, excised in one patient due to deglutition failure.*

conserved, forms a flap which, by way of an operculum or valve, closes the laryngeal lumen during swallowing and inspiration. This is the reason why most patients cannot be decannulated but can swallow. This valve vibrates during phonation, as do the bands that come toward the midline, producing much better phonation than in Serafini laryngectomies or in any type of fistuloplasty (Fig 45.8).

Decannulation is only possible when the thyroid skeleton conserves a patent laryngeal lumen and the bands are capable of abduction during inspiration.

The technique has very few indications but in certain cases may be the best solution for the patient.

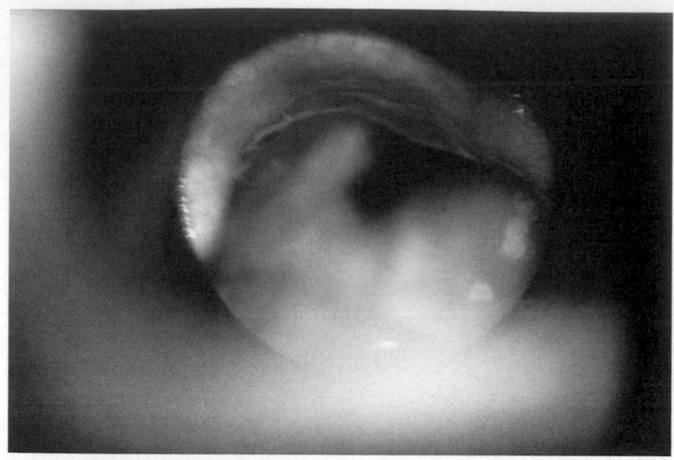

(a)

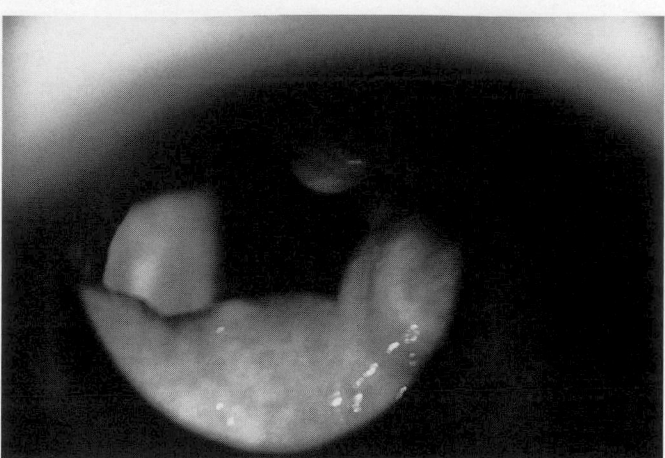

(b)

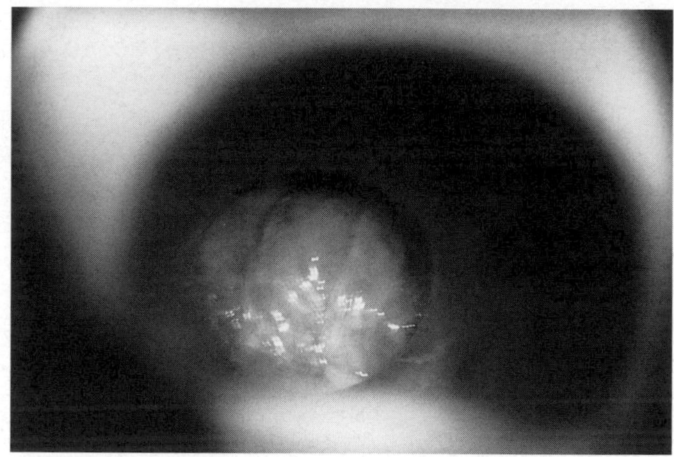

(c)

Figure 45.8 *Endoscopic views of patient with neolarynx following infravestibular horizontal laryngectomy. (a) Epiglottis and mucosal flap from hypopharynx; (b) Laryngeal lumen before decannulation; (c) Flap of hypopharyngeal mucosa protecting the lower airways during swallowing.*

Nowadays an ever-increasing number of laryngeal tumors are managed with minimally invasive surgery using suspension microlaryngoscopy and CO_2 laser. The results have been good in glottic and supraglottic cancer, but disappointing in anterior commissure and subglottic cancer. It is impossible to gain access with the microscope and other instruments to certain areas in subglottic tumors, especially the posterior area. For this reason we continue to recommend conventional open surgery and primary and/or complementary radiotherapy in management of the subglottic region.

References

1. Algaba J, Infantes E, Vergez A, Castillo F. Nueva técnica quirúrgica de laringectomia conservadora. Laringectomia horizontal transventricular. *Acta Otorrinolaringol Esp* 1974; **25:** 121–8.
2. Andréa M, Dias O. Endoscopia rígida y de contacto asociada a microcirugía laringea. In: Alvarez Vicent JJ, Sacristán Alonso T, eds. *Cáncer de cuerda vocal. Ponencia Oficial de la XXXII Reunión Anual de S.E.O.R.L.* Madrid: Jarpyo, 1995: 140–9.
3. Bartual J. Tratamiento quirúrgico de los cánceres subglóticos. In: Alvarez Vicent JJ, Sacristán Alonso T, eds. *Cáncer de laringe. Ponencia Oficial XVI Congr Nac S.E.O.R.L.* Madrid: Jarpyo, 1996: 193–9.
4. Bartual J, Portela J. Laringectomia parcial horizontal infravestibular. Indicaciones y técnica. *Acta Otorrinolaringol Esp* 1974; **25:** 81–94.
5. Bartual J, Roquette J. Infravestibular horizontal partial laryngectomy. A new surgical method. *Arch Otorhinolaryngol* 1978; **220:** 213–20.
6. Collins SL. Controversies in management of cancers of the neck. In: Thawley SE, Panje WR, Batsakis JG, Lindberg RD, eds. *Comprehensive Management of Head and Neck Tumors.* Philadelphia: Saunders, 1987: 1386–443.
7. Ehab YNA. Subglottic cancer. *Am J Otolaryngol* 1994; **15:** 322–8.
8. Ferlito A, Friedmann I. Squamous cell carcinoma. In: Ferlito A, ed. *Neoplasms of the Larynx.* Edinburgh: Churchill Livingstone, 1993: 113–33.
9. Ferlito A, Rinaldo A. The pathology and management of subglottic cancer. *Eur Arch Otorhinolaryngol* 2000; **257:** 168–73.
10. Guirado C, Martinez Pardo P, Salmeron J, Traserra J. Diagnostico por la imagen en el cáncer de laringe.

Resonancia magnetica. In: Alvarez Vicent JJ, Sacristán Alonso T, eds. *Cáncer de laringe. Ponencia Oficial XVI Congr Nac S.E.O.R.L.* Madrid: Jarpyo, 1996: 91–104.

11. Harrison DFN. The pathology and management of subglottic cancer. *Ann Otol* 1971; **80:** 6–12.
12. Harrison DFN. Laryngectomy for subglottic lesions. *Laryngoscope* 1975; **85:** 1208–10.
13. Hofmann Saguez MR. Laryngectomie subtotale conservatrice. *Soc Laryngol Hopitaux Paris* 1950: 811–16.
14. Hofmann Saguez MR. Nouveau cas de laryngectomie subtotale. *Soc Laryngol Hopitaux Paris* 1951: 736–7.
15. Johnson JT, Myers EN. Cervical lymph node disease in laryngeal cancer. In: Silver CE, ed. *Laryngeal Cancer.* New York: Thieme, 1991: 22–6.
16. Olofsson J. Specific features of laryngeal carcinoma involving the anterior commissure and the subglottic region. In: Alberti PW, Bryce DP, eds. *Workshops from the Centennial Conference on Laryngeal Cancer.* East Norwalk: Appleton-Century-Crofts, 1976: 626–44.
17. Pietrantoni L, Agazzi C, Fior R. Indications for surgical treatment of cervical lymph nodes in cancer of the larynx and hypopharynx. *Laryngoscope* 1962; **72:** 1511–27.
18. Stell BM, Tobin KE. The behaviour of cancer affecting the subglottic space. *Can J Otolaryngol* 1975; **4:** 612–17.
19. Suzuki H, Hasegawa T, Sano R, Kim Y. Results of treatment of laryngeal cancer. *Acta Otolaryngol Suppl (Stockh)* 1994; **511:** 186–91.
20. Welsh LW. The normal human laryngeal lymphatics. *Ann Otol* 1964; **73:** 569–82.

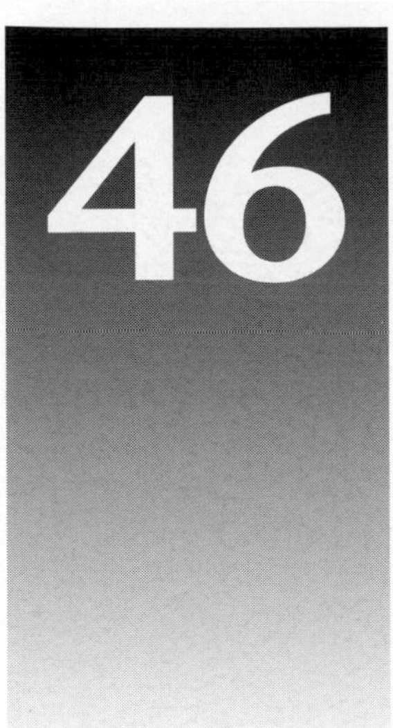

Cancer of the hypopharynx

Jatin P Shah and Dennis Lim

Squamous carcinoma of the hypopharynx has the worst prognosis of all sites in the upper aerodigestive tract.[35] Despite the increased knowledge of genetic alterations and pathogenesis of the disease and the use of multimodality treatment, the prognosis has not changed significantly in the past 20 years. Patients with hypopharyngeal malignancies tend to present late because the tumor is symptomatically silent in its early stages. It is frequently associated with clinically inapparent submucosal spread and a high incidence of field cancerization. The rich network of lymphatic channels of the pharynx leads to early involvement of the regional lymphatics. Treatment in the majority of cases usually consists of partial or total pharyngectomy with partial or total laryngectomy with neck dissection, some form of reconstruction and adjuvant irradiation. Laryngeal preservation protocols with induction chemotherapy and irradiation are showing some promise in randomized trials amongst responders with increased frequency of organ preservation, but no improvement in overall survival. Although the ability to achieve locoregional control has improved, the rising incidence of distant metastases as well as second primary tumors remains a therapeutic challenge.

Epidemiology

About 3000 new cases of hypopharyngeal carcinomas are reported each year in the USA, with an incidence of an age standardized rate (ASR) of 1.1 per 100 000 per year.[35] Elsewhere in the world the incidence varies greatly, from 15.2 per 100 000 per year in Bas Rhin, France; 11.9 per 100 000 per year in the black population in Bermuda; 10.8 per 100 000 per year in Ahmedabad, India; to 0.1 per 100 000 per year recorded in Shanghai, China.[44] The difference in the reported incidence reflects geographic variance, racial prevalence, exposure to risk factors as well as accuracy of the reporting agency. However, it drives home the role of environmental factors in the pathogenesis of this disease. With the exception of postcricoid carcinoma, which was more common in women, all other hypopharyngeal carcinomas are more common in men. In most reported series, 80–85% are males, usually between the ages of 55 and 70 years. In women the reversed ratio has been felt to be due to the Plummer–Vinson syndrome.

When anatomic subsites of the hypopharynx, according to ICD-9, are examined, there are regional differences. Pyriform sinus is the most commonly involved site, as a percentage of all hypopharyngeal cancers, ranging from 55.8% reported in England to 86.8% in Switzerland. Postcricoid cancer occurred in 38.3% in England and is not found in the Eurocare report on hypopharyngeal cancer in Switzerland.[6]

Etiology

An association exists between carcinoma of the upper aerodigestive tract, including hypopharyngeal carcinoma, and excessive tobacco use and alcohol consumption. There is agreement among most authors with regard to the important role played by tobacco in the development of precancerous lesions and carcinoma of the larynx and hypopharynx. Stell[37] found fewer nonsmokers and more heavy smokers amongst 190 laryngeal cancer patients than among controls. Burch *et al.*,[9] in a survey of 204 laryngeal patients and controls, found a marked association between laryngeal cancer, the male sex, and the abuse of tobacco and alcohol. Similarly, Müller and Krohn,[31] in a study of 148 autopsies, found severe dysplasia and carcinoma in situ in 47.2% of heavy smokers, 22.9% of average smokers, 12.5% of light smokers and in 4.2% of nonsmokers. Conversely, they found normal epithelium in only 30.6% of heavy smokers and 83.3% of light smokers. McCoy *et al.*[27] found a relation between smoking and alcohol with upper aerodigestive tract cancer, and surmised that alcohol abuse might lead to a secondary deficiency in important nutrients and thence exert an influence on detoxifying the enzyme system. Statistically, there is moderate synergy between alcohol and tobacco in increasing the risk of laryngeal and hypopharyngeal cancer, in that exposure to both increased the risk by about 50% more than the predicted additive effect.[18]

Vitamin A and its analogs, such as *cis*-retinoic acid, promote the normal maturation of squamous epithelium. The absence of adequate vitamin A in the diet may contribute to the persistence of a more primitive basal cell type and play a role in the etiology of carcinoma in the affected area.[11]

There is a remarkable correlation between the Plummer–Vinson, Patterson–Kelly syndrome or sideropenic dysphagia and carcinoma of the postcricoid region. Nearly 95% of all cases of this syndrome affect women in middle or old age. The disease is characterized by glossitis with papillary atrophy, dysphagia as a result of concentric stricture of the cervical esophagus and the development of webs in the postcricoid region. The progressive difficulty in swallowing leads patients to eat only small, well-chewed bites of food, causing a low body weight to be a common finding. Histologic examination showed hyperplasia, and atrophy of the squamous epithelium in the postcricoid area; often severe dysplasia was found on a background of chronic inflammation.[28] Kelly was the first to describe the combination of anemia and postcricoid carcinoma. Up to 90% of women and 10% of men with postcricoid carcinoma showed sideropenic dysphagia. Various estimates have found that 10–30% of patients with Plummer–Vinson syndrome developed postcricoid carcinoma.[28] Early detection and treatment of these patients with bougienage, iron replacement and vitamin B can reverse this disease process.[21]

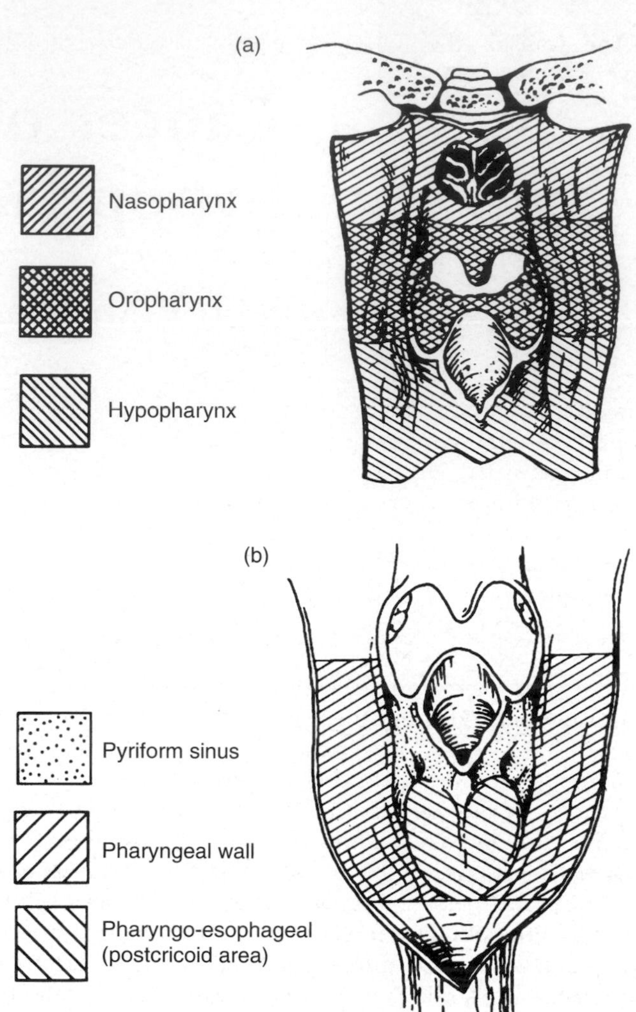

Figure 46.1 *(a) Anatomy of the pharynx. (b) Subsites of the hypopharynx.*

Anatomy

The hypopharynx, as defined by the UICC and the American Joint Committee on clinical staging, is a triangular area of the upper aerodigestive tract extending from the tip of the epiglottis to a plane through the lower border of the cricoid cartilage. It is divided into three anatomic subsites: the pyriform sinuses, the postcricoid area and the posterior pharyngeal wall (Fig 46.1). However, the anatomic boundaries of these subsites are not well defined and not clearly discernible in the living patient. There also appears to be considerable overlap of tumors from one subsite to another, making it often difficult to determine the exact site of origin.

The pyriform sinus forms an inverted pyramid of pharyngeal mucosa bounded by the lateral glossoepiglottic folds superiorly, the apex of the pyriform sinus inferiorly, the thyroid cartilage laterally, and the aryepiglottic and the arytenoid cartilage medially. Its lateral wall is contiguous with the posterior pharyngeal wall and its medial wall is contiguous with the postcricoid area. The transition between the supraglottic larynx and the pyriform sinus occurs at the aryepiglottic folds.

The posterior pharyngeal wall consists of the pharyngeal mucosa from the plane of the tip of the epiglottis down to the cricopharyngeus muscle. Its lateral wall is considered to be the posterior border of the lateral wall of the pyriform sinus.

The postcricoid area consists of mucosa covering the posterior surface of the cricoid cartilage, extending from the arytenoids superiorly to the lower border of the cricoid cartilage inferiorly. Its lateral walls are contiguous with the posterior margins of the medial wall of the pyriform sinus. The mucosa of all three subsites are contiguous with that of the cervical esophagus inferiorly, and oropharynx superiorly.

The wall of the hypopharynx is composed of four layers:

- an inner mucosa of stratified squamous epithelium over a loose stroma;
- a fibrous layer of pharyngeal aponeurosis;
- a muscular layer formed by the inferior constrictor of the pharynx and distal portion of the middle constrictor; and
- an outer layer of fascia derived from the buccopharyngeal fascia.

The hypopharynx and the cervical esophagus is richly supplied with lymphatics. Major lymphatic channels terminate in the lymph nodes along the jugular chain.[17] The first echelon of drainage is to the subdigastric, upper and mid-jugular nodes. Significant lymphatic drainage from the posterior pharyngeal wall drains to the retropharyngeal lymph nodes and to the node of Rouviere at the skull base.[2] The lymphatic channels draining the pyriform sinus runs along the recurrent laryngeal nerve through the cricothyroid membrane; these, together with the paratracheal lymph nodes, are the sentinel nodes to the inferior portion of the hypopharynx and the cervical esophagus.

Field cancerization

Epithelial changes are commonly observed in mucosa adjacent to laryngeal and hypopharyngeal tumors. These changes may be precancerous or frankly invasive. Not infrequently further carcinomatous foci can be observed at other sites. These second cancers are more frequent in patients with oral, pharyngeal and esophageal carcinoma than would be expected on the basis of chance alone. Slaughter *et al.*[36] termed this increased disposition for further cancer 'field cancerization' and the at-risk mucosa 'condemned mucosa'. In his examination of carcinoma of the oral mucosa, separate carcinomatous foci were found in 11.2% of the cases. This observation supports the assumption that in the carcinogenesis of squamous epithelium, no strictly localized process is involved, but rather the entire mucosa is subjected to synchronous or metachronous cancerization owing to the same etiologic factors at work. Squamous metaplasia, squamous hyperplasia with various grades of epithelial dysplasia, carcinoma in situ and multiple invasive carcinoma are often associated with an established carcinoma of the larynx. The whole organ system, like the respiratory tract, can be involved in the course of multicentric cancerization. Multiple primary cancers are found in about 5% of cancer patients,[41] and in patients with cancer of the upper respiratory tract, a second tumor is reported in 8.9% of cases.[8] Because of the high incidence of multifocal carcinomas, it is essential to look for another tumor in the upper aerodigestive tract during the initial investigation of laryngeal and hypopharyngeal cancer.

Tobacco and alcohol certainly contribute to the development of multiple carcinomas. The more a patient smokes before he develops the first carcinoma, the greater is the probability of developing a second cancer. If the patient continues to use tobacco and drink alcohol after the treatment of the first carcinoma, the probability of developing a second cancer increases significantly.[45]

In addition to these unicentric, circumscribed, and usually keratinizing carcinomas and field cancerization of the upper aerodigestive tract, there are also tumors, usually nonkeratinizing, that arise from a large epithelial surface and grow deeply over a wide front. Areas of in situ carcinoma alternating with sections of microinvasive carcinoma or with foci of frank invasion may be present over a large epithelial field. This type of squamous cell carcinoma is termed superficial spreading carcinoma. There is a broad spectrum from the common, relatively well-circumscribed squamous cell carcinoma at one extreme, to a 'carpet cancer', which can extend widely in the larynx and hypopharynx at the other. Carbone *et al.*[13] found 10% of 242 hypopharyngeal carcinomas to be of the superficially extending type, usually with microinvasive patterns, and half the cases had already metastasized. Many of these tumors extended over several regions of the hypopharynx.

Patterns of local spread

Pyriform sinus tumors may spread medially, displacing and fixing the lateral wall of the larynx, by extension into the paraglottic space. In addition, vocal cord fixation may occur by direct invasion of the cricoarytenoid joint or cricoarytenoid muscle, or the recurrent laryngeal nerve may also be directly invaded.[20] Larger tumors may extend along the lateral and posterior pharyngeal wall to involve the contralateral pyriform sinus. Pyriform sinus cancers that extend laterally frequently destroy the posterolateral portion of the thyroid cartilage. Direct extension into the thyroid gland is not rare,[20] but invasion of the cricoid cartilage is.

Posterior pharyngeal wall cancers usually attain a large size before becoming symptomatic; nevertheless, their invasion into the prevertebral fascia occurs late in the course of the disease. Superior extension to the tonsillar fossae and the oropharynx and inferior extension to the cervical esophagus occur frequently.

Postcricoid cancer tends to grow circumferentially, invading the cricoid cartilage and the cervical esophagus.

Patterns of lymphatic spread

The lymphatic drainage of the hypopharynx, especially the pyriform sinus, is profuse. The distribution of metastases from hypopharyngeal cancer is primarily to the jugular chain with secondary involvement of the accessory chain of lymph nodes in the posterior triangle of the neck. The risk of retropharyngeal node involvement is significant, especially when there are extensive neck nodes and spread of the primary lesion into the oropharynx.

Regional lymph node metastases are present in 60% of patients with posterior pharyngeal wall cancer, and they are frequently bilateral.[16] Retropharyngeal nodal metastases are present in 44% of patients with pharyngeal wall cancer.[3]

Patients with pyriform sinus cancer have a 75% incidence of lymph node metastases, whereas 40% of patients with postcricoid cancer will have regional disease.[24] Paratracheal lymph nodes are also frequently involved with metastases from postcricoid tumors.[43] Occult metastases are reported in 50–80% of patients who have primary cancer in the hypopharynx.[10] Different subsites within the pyriform sinus have different risks of occult contralateral neck node metastases: patients with medial wall cancer have a 14% risk of contralateral neck metastases, whereas those with lateral wall cancer have a much lower risk of 5%.[19]

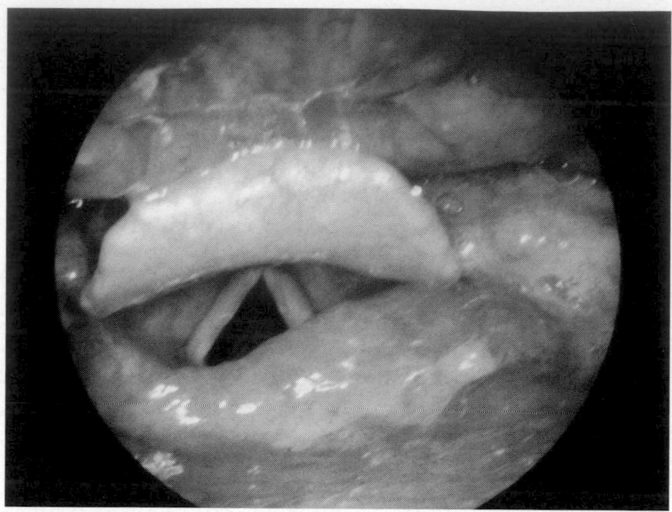

Figure 46.2 *Endoscopic appearance of a postcricoid carcinoma.*

Clinical presentation

The hypopharynx is a clinically 'silent' area in the upper aerodigestive tract. Early lesions have no associated symptoms. Advanced lesions produce a characteristic triad of odynophagia, referred otalgia and dysphagia.

Vague throat pain, usually unilateral and persistent, is indicative of an early lesion. Careful questioning may reveal frequent clearing of the throat and a sensation of a foreign body in the throat. Referred otalgia caused by a tumor in the pyriform sinus is carried by fibers in the internal branch of the superior laryngeal nerve, which synapses in the jugular ganglion, where the sensory fibers of the external acoustic meatus carried by Arnold's nerve also synapse. Hoarseness may be due to direct invasion of the arytenoid cartilage as well as the cricoarytenoid and interarytenoid musculature by a tumor of the medial wall of the pyriform sinus, or, it may be due to involvement of the recurrent laryngeal nerve by a tumor arising in the postcricoid region or cervical esophagus. Hemoptysis is present in some patients with large fungating or ulcerated lesions.

Weight loss is common in patients with this cancer and is more pronounced in patients with a circumferential lesion. It is usually additive to the patient's underlying malnutrition from an inadequate diet and excessive alcohol intake. Ptyalism, usually blood-tinged, is seen with ulcerated lesions.

Nearly two-thirds of the patients with hypopharyngeal carcinoma have a palpable lump in the neck, representing a metastatic cervical lymph node.

Tumors of the posterior pharyngeal wall and the upper pyriform sinus are usually seen easily by indirect mirror examination, whereas tumors of the apex of the pyriform sinus and of the postcricoid area produce indirect physical findings like pooling of saliva, edema and erythema, especially near the arytenoid (Fig 46.2). Direct extension into the soft tissue of the neck may be difficult to distinguish from adjacent lymph node metastases.

The fiberoptic laryngoscope is a critical tool in the evaluation of the hypopharynx. Valsalva maneuver during the examination is useful in delineating the mucosal extent of the disease.

Imaging

Current imaging techniques such as computed tomography (CT) and magnetic resonance imaging (MRI) have largely supplanted older methods such as soft tissue films of the neck, contrast laryngogram and laryngeal tomograms. The barium swallow remains a useful tool for evaluating the inferior extent of involvement, particularly for postcricoid cancer and to rule out the presence of a synchronous tumor in the esophagus.

The CT scan is very useful in the assessment of tumor thickness and invasion of contiguous structures such as the laryngeal framework, the paraglottic space, and the parapharyngeal and prevertebral spaces (Fig 46.3). It is important that the CT scan be performed with contrast and before excessive manipulation of the tumor occurs, as

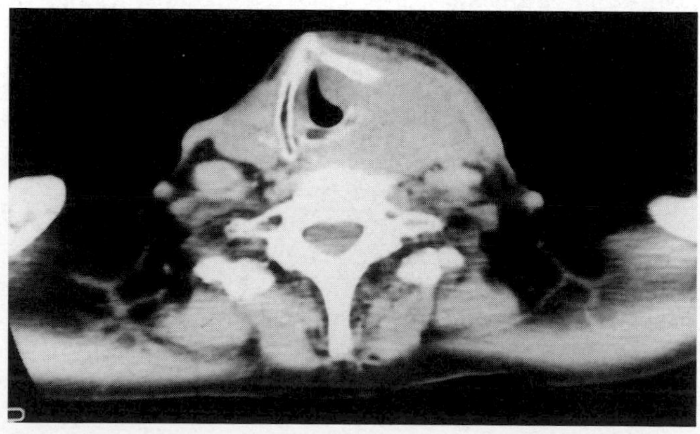

Figure 46.3 *Axial CT scan with contrast showing a large pyriform sinus carcinoma.*

postbiopsy edema can be difficult to distinguish from tumor spread. CT scan is very effective in detecting lymph node metastases; these are usually greater than 1.5 cm and have central necrosis with rim enhancement.[26] Enlarged retropharyngeal lymph nodes are readily visualized on CT scans.

MRI is superior in the examination of soft tissue details and fat planes. It can differentiate between tissue edema and tumor extension, but it is susceptible to motion artifact due to its long scan time of 30–45 minutes. The capabilities and limitations of MRI are currently being studied, and further correlative studies are required to clarify its role in the imaging of hypopharyngeal carcinomas.

Positron emission tomography (PET) scans provide useful information regarding the viability of a tumor. The images reflect the activity of glucose metabolism in the neoplastic cells. Currently its role in identifying residual or recurrent tumor following radiotherapy is under investigation.

Staging

The UICC and the American Joint Committee staging system for hypopharyngeal carcinoma, published in 1997, is shown in Table 46.1. The staging is clinical but may be supported by radiographic and endoscopic findings. Post-treatment staging with pathologic data and staging for recurrent tumors are described with suffixes of 'p' and 'r'.

Table 46.1 The UICC and American Joint Committee staging system for hypopharyngeal carcinoma

Primary tumor (T)

Tx	Primary tumor cannot be assessed
T0	No evidence of primary tumor
T1	Tumor limited to one subsite of the hypopharynx
T2	Tumor invades more than one subsite of the hypopharynx or an adjacent site, without fixation of the hemilarynx
T3	Tumor invades more than one subsite of the hypopharynx or an adjacent site with fixation of the hemilarynx
T4	Tumor invades adjacent structures (e.g. cartilage or soft tissues of the neck)

Lymph nodes (N)

Nx	Regional lymph nodes cannot be assessed
N0	No regional lymph node metastasis
N1	Metastasis in a single ipsilateral lymph node 3 cm or less in greatest dimension
N2	Metastasis in a single ipsilateral lymph node, >3 cm but <6 cm in greatest dimension, or in bilateral or contralateral lymph nodes, none >6 cm in greatest dimension
	N2a: metastasis in a single ipsilateral lymph node, >3 cm but <6 cm in greatest dimension
	N2b: metastases in multiple ipsilateral lymph nodes, none >6 cm in greatest dimension
	N2c: metastases in bilateral or contralateral lymph nodes, none >6 cm in greatest dimension
N3	Metastasis in a lymph node >6 cm in greatest dimension

Distant metastasis (M)

Mx	Presence of distance metastasis cannot be assessed
M0	No distant metastasis
M1	Distant metastasis

Stage grouping

Stage 0	Tis	N0	M0
Stage I	T1	N0	M0
Stage II	T2	N0	M0
Stage III	T3	N0	M0
	T1–3	N1	M0
Stage IV	T4	N0, 1	M0
	AnyT	N2, 3	M0
	AnyT	AnyN	M1

Factors affecting choice of treatment

Standard therapeutic modalities for cancer of the hypopharynx are surgery and radiotherapy, employed alone or in combination. Recently, induction chemotherapy in combination with radiation and surgery has been used in an attempt to increase locoregional control, decrease systemic metastases and prolong survival while preserving a functioning larynx. The main factors affecting the choice of the therapy can be broadly grouped into tumor factors, patient factors and health care provider factors.

Tumor factors play a key role in the choice of treatment modality. A large pyriform sinus tumor involving the arytenoid musculature medially and the thyroid gland and cartilage laterally is clearly not amenable to conservation (larynx-sparing) surgery, just as it is unlikely to respond completely to radiation alone or in combination with induction chemotherapy in an effort to preserve the larynx. On the other hand, a small tumor of the posterior pharyngeal wall, not involving the prevertebral fascia, can be treated with equal success by surgery alone or radiation alone. It is the large intermediate group of tumors between these extremes that require detailed assessment to determine the best treatment option. When larynx-sparing conservation surgery is considered, the following tumor factors are critically important:

- the tumor must be confined to its anatomical site of origin;
- the apex of the pyriform sinus must not be involved;
- there should not be extension to the base of the tongue;
- the ipsilateral hemilarynx must be mobile; and
- there must not be laryngeal involvement in a transglottic fashion.

T1 and low-volume, exophytic T2 hypopharyngeal cancers can be very effectively treated with radiation alone.[29] For the selected patients in whom the primary tumor is small and amenable to definitive irradiation but bulky metastases are present, bimodal therapy may be employed. This requires curative radiation for the primary and the neck accompanied by planned neck dissection, preferably prior to radiotherapy.[29] For most large tumors of the hypopharynx that present with lymph node metastases, the treatment is total laryngectomy with partial or total pharyngectomy, comprehensive neck dissection, appropriate reconstruction and adjuvant postoperative irradiation.

All treatment decisions in hypopharyngeal cancer require patient participation, but some more so than others. It is vitally important that the patients requiring laryngectomy as part of the surgical treatment have strong social and family support and are literate, as on average only about half of patients who undergo total laryngectomy and only a quarter of patients who undergo total laryngopharyngectomy end up with a satisfactory esophageal voice.[23] In conservation (larynx-sparing) surgery for hypopharyngeal cancer it is important that the patient is able to understand the nature of the treatment and has the capability to participate in a vigorous postoperative recovery effort in terms of pulmonary clearance of aspirated secretions. Good pulmonary function is crucial in tolerating small amounts of chronic aspiration. A treatment regimen consisting of induction chemotherapy and radiation, or concurrent chemo/radiotherapy for laryngeal preservation, requires a patient who is committed to frequent treatment and follow-up visits, tolerant of significant toxicity and fully aware of the possibility of a salvage laryngectomy should he fail locoregionally later or have persistent disease. Not every patient's psychosocial makeup is suitable for such a rigorous regimen.

The health care provider or surgeon factors are more than just the ability to perform the actual surgery. It includes the availability and expertise of other members of the 'Head and Neck Team', such as the reconstructive surgeon, a medical and radiation oncologist interested in head and neck cancer, the specially trained head and neck nursing staff, speech and swallowing therapist, social worker, etc. The physical facilities, e.g. the availability of a good imaging center, radiation treatment facility, multidisciplinary follow-up clinics, etc., all play a role in the selection of treatment.

Treatment trends

In order to understand the evolution of the current treatment preferences, it is first necessary to review the treatment trends over the past 30 years.

In the 1960s, surgery was the primary treatment modality for all hypopharyngeal carcinomas. Indications for unresectability were fixed cervical nodes involving the carotid artery, extension into and fixation to the vertebral column, extension into the cervical esophagus and any evidence of distant metastatic disease. These unresectable patients were offered palliative irradiation, with anticipated poor outcome. The success of surgery in the 1960s was limited by the available reconstructive techniques. Planned pharyngostomies with multistaged reconstruction using tubed skin pedicles was the state-of-the-art. With the development of regional pedicled flaps, like the medially-based deltopectoral flap popularized by Bakamjian,[1] the limits of resection were expanded and total laryngopharyngectomy was possible with a secure reconstruction.

Partial pharyngectomy was first described by Trotter in 1932 for the resection and primary closure of limited lesions of the hypopharynx and the postcricoid area.[39] Other authors, most notably Ogura *et al.*, later reported on their extensive experience with partial pharyngectomy.[33]

Preoperative radiation combined with surgical resection was the most common treatment for advanced hypopharyngeal carcinoma during the late 1960s and early 1970s. This is because early results with 2000–4500 cGy delivered over 1–4 weeks followed by planned surgery suggested improved tumor control.[7] It was observed, however, that the complications of surgery increased with increasing dose of preoperative radiotherapy. Therefore, in the late 1970s, postoperative radiotherapy became popular. It was believed that surgical complications would be lessened and doses of 6000 cGy could be safely given after the incision had healed and the pathologic specimen carefully studied.

Surgery combined with postoperative radiation yielded results that were still unsatisfactory, but the patterns of failure changed with an increase in distant metastases and failure in the opposite neck with decreased locoregional recurrence. Chemotherapy came into consideration with the availability of methotrexate, bleomycin and cisplatin showing good response in the treatment of unresectable and recurrent head and neck cancer. The expectations from neoadjuvant chemotherapy were to preserve the larynx, reduce distant metastases and improve overall survival. Prospective trials showed that response rate was significant and larynx preservation was possible in some selected cases showing complete response to induction chemotherapy. Despite the very encouraging results in phase III trials, no randomized trial has ever demonstrated improved survival after induction chemotherapy in squamous cell carcinoma of the head and neck. Only one trial had shown improved survival for inoperable stage III and IV carcinoma,[34] whereas others report no improvement in survival but a lower incidence of distant metastases.

Surgical treatment of hypopharyngeal cancer

Before embarking on a surgical option for hypopharyngeal carcinoma, it is crucial that the full extent of the tumor be appreciated. A detailed head and neck examination with appropriate fiberoptic and rigid scopes in the office should be supplemented by imaging studies and a final clinical and endoscopic examination under anesthesia just prior to the surgical procedure. Due to the tendency of hypopharyngeal cancer to spread in the submucosa beyond what is apparent clinically, frozen section examination for margins is imperative.

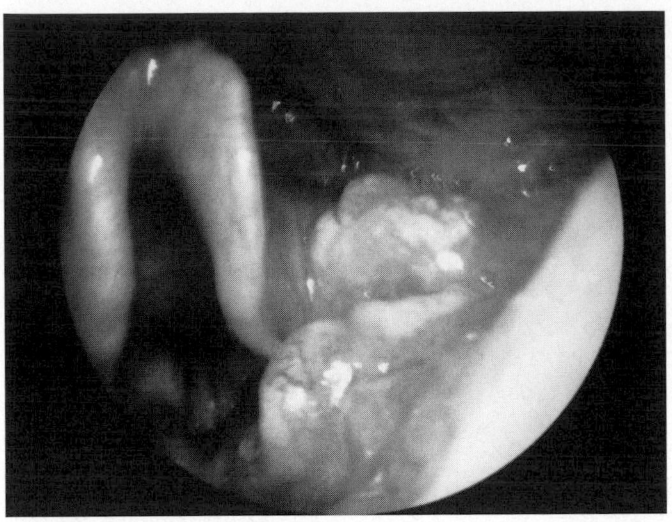

Figure 46.4 *Endoscopic appearance of a pyriform sinus carcinoma suitable for partial laryngopharyngectomy.*

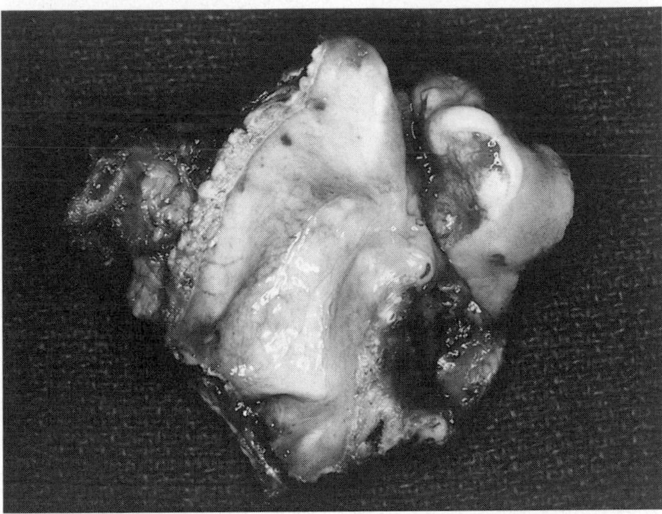

Figure 46.5 *Resected pyriform sinus carcinoma after partial laryngopharyngectomy.*

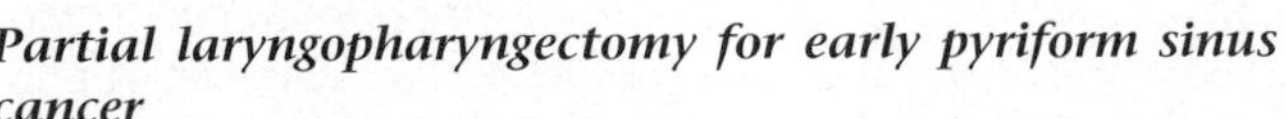

Partial laryngopharyngectomy for early pyriform sinus cancer

A small tumor of the pyriform sinus that is confined to its anatomic site of origin, not involving the apex, the base of tongue, and with a mobile hemilarynx is amenable to conservation surgery (Fig 46.4).

A preliminary tracheotomy, performed under local anesthesia, is preferred to translaryngeal endotracheal intubation as it minimizes trauma to the lesion, does not obstruct endoscopic evaluation and surgical manipulation. A transverse incision at the level of the thyrohyoid membrane is employed for the exposure of the supraglottic larynx and the hypopharynx. There are then many surgical approaches to the pyriform sinus; the transhyoid, lateral pharyngotomy, and horizontal or vertical thyrotomy with partial laryngectomy are the more common ones. The aim is to enter the hypopharynx away from the clinically evident and suspicious mucosa, permit surgical exposure of the lesion, while preserving as much pharyngeal wall as possible for subsequent reconstruction. The extent of laryngeal resection depends on the degree of involvement by the pyriform sinus primary, and may range from the resection of an arytenoid and the common wall to a hemilaryngectomy (Figs 46.5 and 46.6). Ogura *et al.* reported a series of 85 patients with supraglottic and pyriform sinus cancer treated with conservation surgery. Their 3-year actuarial survival was 59%, overall local control rate with pyriform sinus was 47%, and more than 50% of patients were able to retain a functioning larynx.[33]

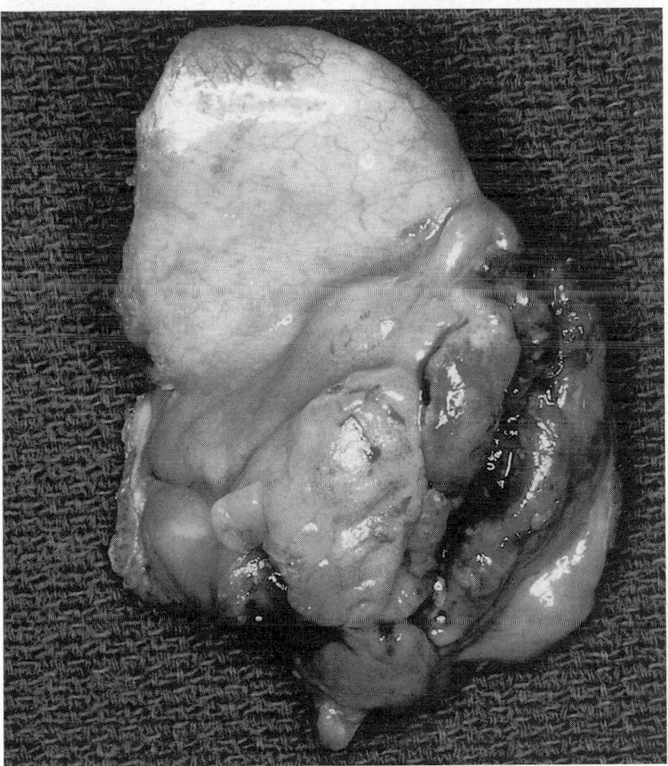

Figure 46.6 *Another hypopharyngeal carcinoma resected by conservative surgery.*

Resection of carcinoma of the posterior pharyngeal wall

Tumors of the posterior pharyngeal wall of limited extent are amenable to surgical resection via several routes, depending on their mucosal extent, depth of infiltration and location on the posterior pharyngeal wall. A small superficial tumor of the upper posterior pharyngeal wall that extends into the oropharynx can be excised through the open mouth. A similar small tumor lower down in the posterior pharyngeal wall can be approached through a transhyoid pharyngotomy. The surgical defect following

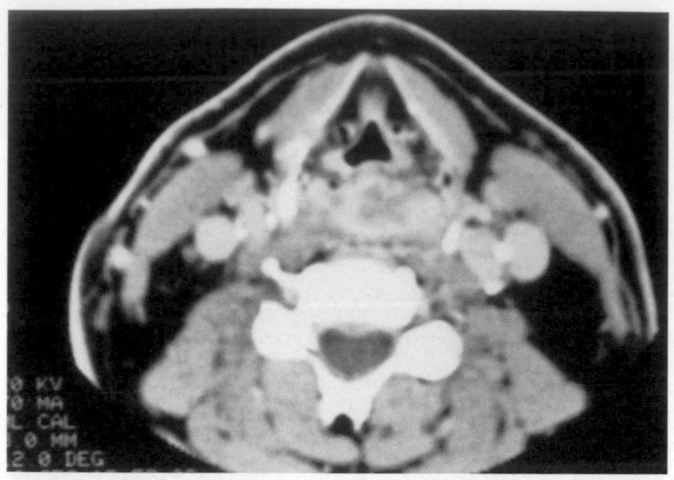

(a)

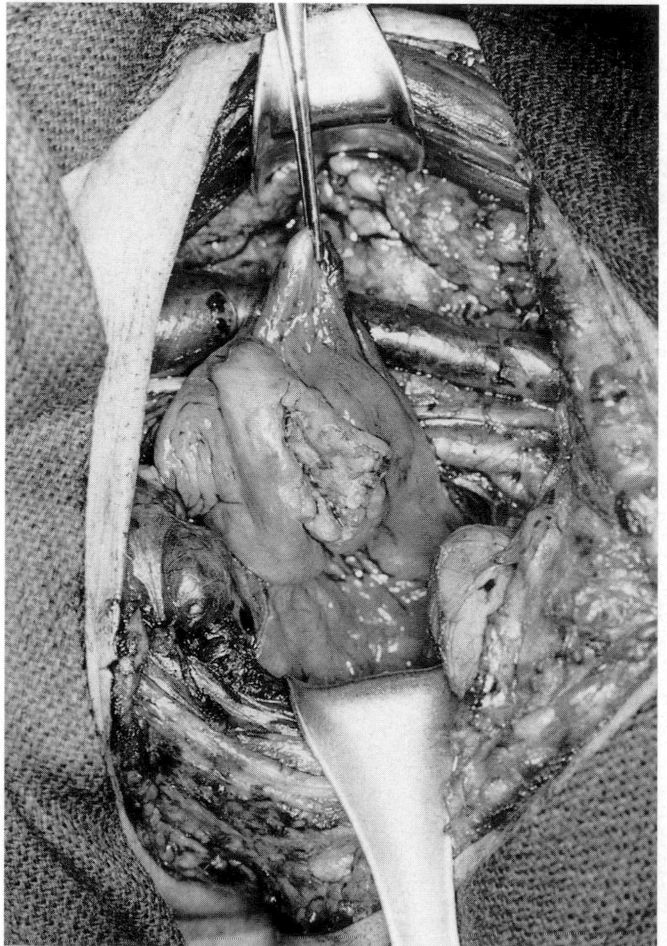

(b)

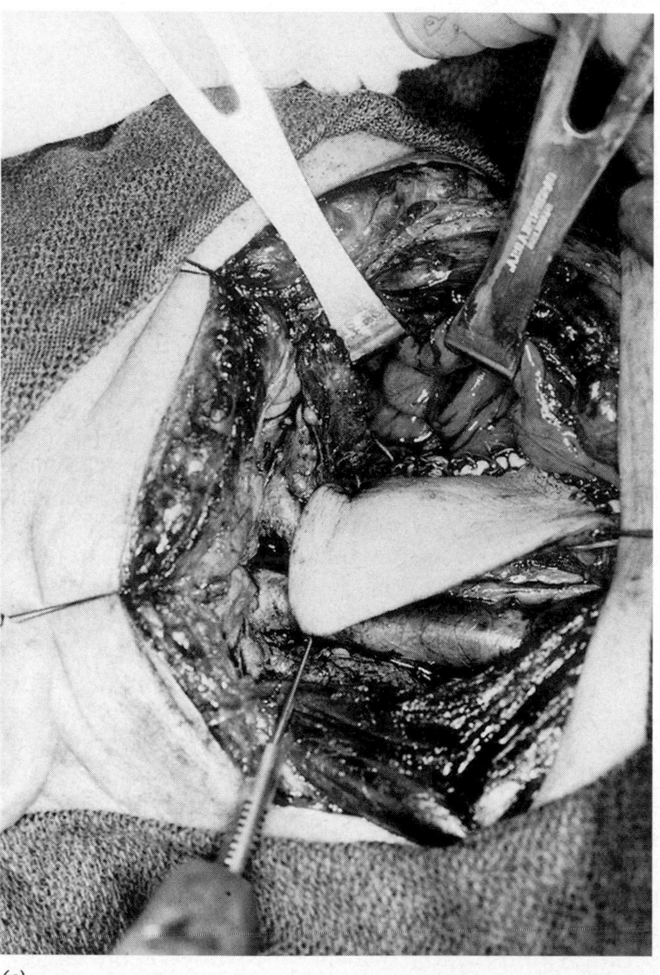

(c)

Figure 46.7 *(a) Axial CT scan of a posterior pharyngeal wall carcinoma. (b) Intraoperative appearance. (c) Reconstruction with a radial forearm free flap, shown here* in situ.

such limited excisions may be left open to granulate and heal by secondary intention, or may be repaired with a split thickness skin graft.

Larger resections of the posterior pharyngeal wall, extending from the lateral wall of one pyriform sinus to that of the other, while still preserving the larynx, can be undertaken, but a more elaborate reconstruction is required. The ideal choice in this setting would be a radial forearm microvascular free flap (Fig 46.7).

Total laryngectomy with partial pharyngectomy

The vast majority of patients with hypopharyngeal cancer present with an advanced pyriform sinus tumor.

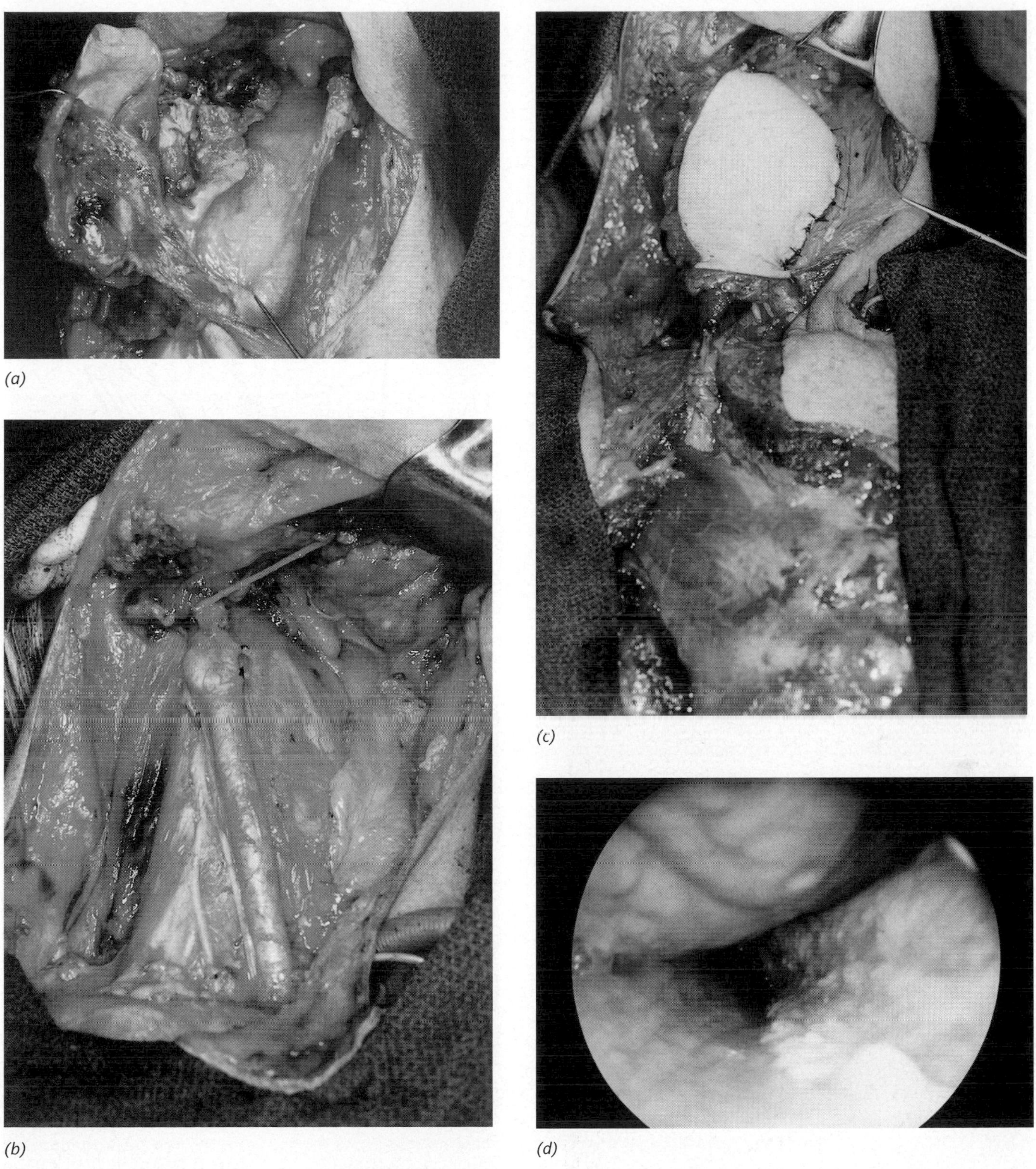

(a) (b) (c) (d)

Figure 46.8 *(a) Intraoperative appearance of a large pyriform sinus carcinoma. (b) Surgical defect after a total laryngectomy with partial pharyngectomy. (c) Reconstruction with a pedicled pectoralis major mucocutaneous flap. (d) Postoperative endoscopic appearance.*

Surgical management of these patients generally requires total laryngectomy and partial pharyngectomy. Indications for this procedure include involvement of the apex of the pyriform sinus, postcricoid mucosa, cartilaginous framework of the larynx or a paralysed hemilarynx. After a total laryngectomy with partial pharyngectomy, if

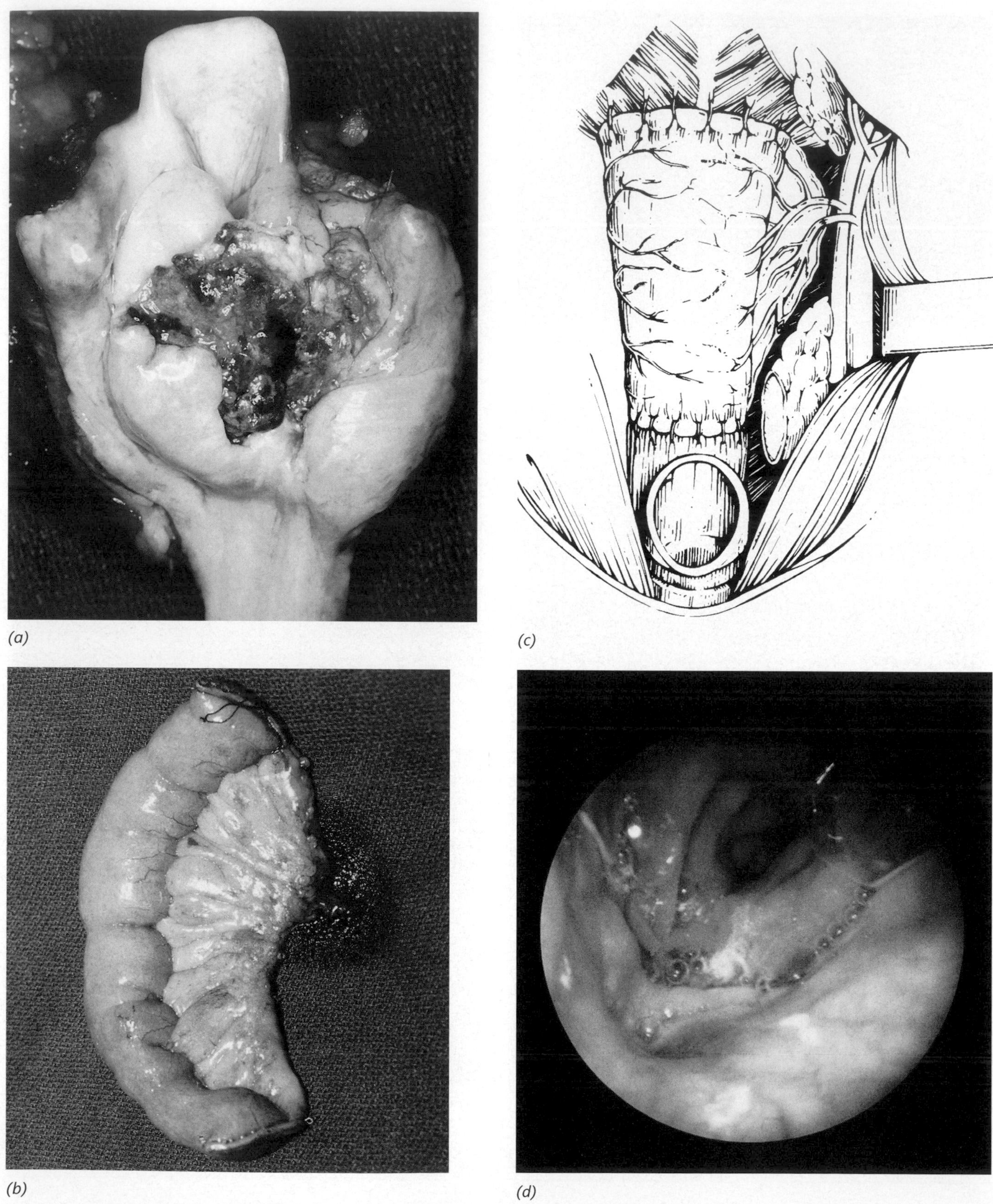

Figure 46.9 *(a) Large hypopharyngeal carcinoma with involvement of the pyriform sinus and the postcricoid region. (b) A jejunal segment harvested for reconstruction after total laryngectomy and total pharyngectomy. (c) Jejunal free flap* in situ. *(d) Endoscopic appearance postoperatively.*

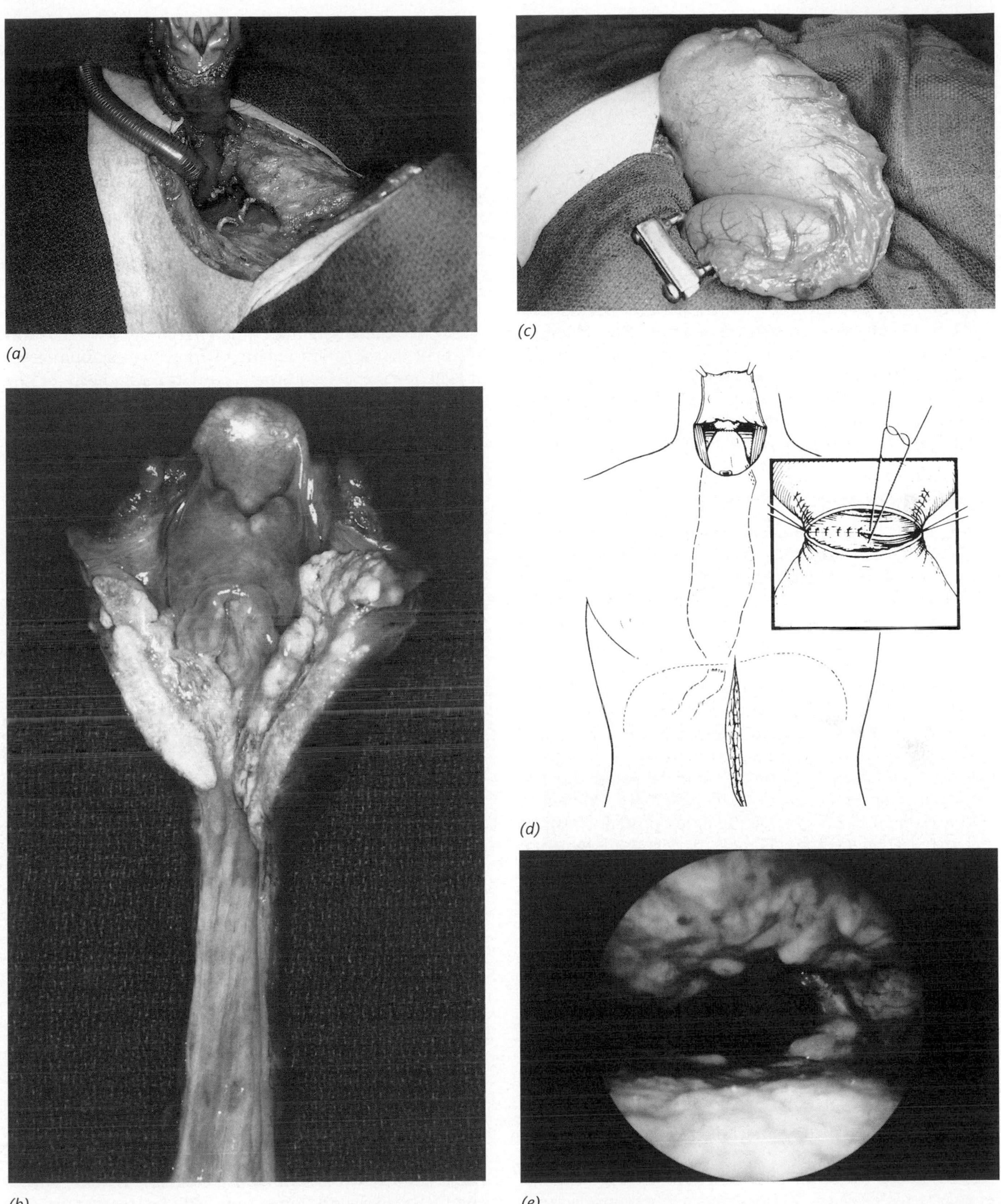

Figure 46.10 *(a) Intraoperative appearance of total laryngopharyngectomy for hypopharyngeal carcinoma with significant cervical esophagus involvement. (b) Resected specimen. (c) Mobilized stomach to be used for reconstruction. (d) Substernal transposition and pharyngogastric anastomosis. (e) Postoperative endoscopic appearance.*

the pharyngeal defect is less than one-third of the circumference of the pharynx, primary closure is feasible. If the pharyngeal defect is 50% or more of the circumference, then appropriate reconstruction with a radial forearm free flap or pectoralis major myocutaneous flap is indicated (Fig 46.8).

Total laryngopharyngectomy

The need for a total pharyngeal resection in addition to a total laryngectomy is based on the circumferential extent of the tumor and its inferior extent towards the cervical esophagus. The shape of the hypopharynx is like a funnel with a larger upper circumference that narrows down to the pharyngoesophageal junction. Hence, lesions of the cervical esophagus and the postcricoid region require a circumferential resection. The surgical defect thus created requires a tubular replacement to restore alimentary continuity. A free segment of jejunum is ideal, but a tubed radial forearm flap can also be used (Fig 46.9).

Total laryngopharyngoesophagectomy

When the primary lesion extends to involve the lower part of the cervical esophagus or upper thoracic esophagus, then a total laryngopharyngoesophagectomy is warranted. This operation, of necessity, requires the mobilization of the stomach and its transthoracic transposition into the neck to restore the continuity of the alimentary tract with a pharyngogastrostomy. Two surgical teams working almost simultaneously are ideal for this procedure. The head and neck team works on the resection of the primary tumor and mobilization of the upper esophagus in the superior mediastinum, and the abdominal team mobilizes the stomach and the lower thoracic esophagus. Key technical points include careful dissection of the esophagus off the membranous posterior wall of the trachea, meticulous hemostasis of the segmental blood supply of the esophagus, adequate kocherization of the duodenum, pyloromyotomy and hemostatic pharyngogastrostomy, without tension on the suture line (Fig 46.10).

Reconstruction

When pharyngeal resection requires laryngectomy, special consideration must be given to the closure of the pharynx. For a lesion that requires resection of less than one-third of the circumference of the pharynx, primary tension-free closure is all that is needed. A single-layer transverse closure with interrupted absorbable sutures provides adequate repair.

In instances where 33–70% of the pharyngeal circumference is resected, the optimal reconstruction is accomplished with a pectoralis major myocutaneous flap. This 'work horse' of the head and neck region is easily raised in the same surgical field, is reliable in most hands and provides a large skin island. Extreme care should be exercised during rotation of the flap to avoid twisting or kinking of its skeletonized vascular pedicle over the clavicle. However, the flap is occasionally too bulky and leaves an unsightly donor site scar if a lot of skin is taken. This flap is clearly too bulky in women, and leaves an unacceptable breast distortion on the chest wall. A radial forearm free flap, which is thinner and more pliable in most people, can be used instead of the pectoralis major flap to avoid the donor site deformity, especially in women. It requires microvascular expertise and equipment, but is a more satisfying functional and cosmetic reconstruction.

When the remnant pharyngeal mucosa after resection is only a narrow posterior strip, it is preferred to convert it to a circumferential pharyngectomy. Such short segment defect is best repaired with a free jejunum graft. It will require a laparotomy, and reanastomosis of the jejunum, preferably done by a second surgical team, and microvascular expertise is again required. The jejunum can be split at its antimesenteric border at the upper end to match the larger pharyngeal circumference.

When a hypopharyngeal cancer involves the cervical esophagus and the resection extends to include the upper thoracic esophagus, then a gastric transposition is the ideal reconstruction after laryngopharyngoesophagectomy. If the stomach has been previously resected or is unsuitable for whatever reason, a pedicled transverse colon can be used for interposition.

These reconstructive methods have all been proven to be effective in many large studies; however, it remains for the surgeon to individualize the best reconstruction for each patient's disease.

Management of the neck

Once appropriate treatment of the squamous carcinoma of the hypopharynx has been determined, the management of the neck must be considered in the overall treatment plan. As noted in many series, the incidence of occult metastases is as high as 30–40%, hence N0 neck needs to be addressed in most instances.

In patients with clinically N-positive neck, the treatment should be a comprehensive neck dissection, with the possible modification of preserving the spinal accessory nerve (XI) if it is not directly involved by metastatic disease. Candela *et al.* reviewed the patterns of lymph node metastases in hypopharyngeal cancer,[12] and found that for pyriform sinus tumors with clinically N0 necks, levels II and III were most frequently involved with occult metastases; however for N-positive necks, all levels were at risk of involvement. They concluded that for patients with N0 neck, a selective neck dissection clearing levels II, III and IV would be considered appropriate, but a comprehensive neck dissection will be needed in any patient with clinically positive neck.

Postoperative irradiation of the dissected neck for better regional control seems logical in patients with multiple positive nodes and for patients with extracapsular spread on pathologic examination. Many retrospective publications[4,22] support the use of postoperative radiotherapy for improved regional control.

The management of the clinically N0 neck depends very much on the chosen treatment modality for the primary tumor. If radiotherapy is chosen for the treatment of the primary tumor, then the radiation portals are designed to include the N0 neck at risk. To control the N0 neck a minimum of 5000 cGy is required.

There is considerable difference in the reported incidence of occult lymph node metastases in the contralateral neck. Murakami *et al.* found histologically positive nodes in the contralateral neck in 30% of their cases,[32] leading the authors to advise bilateral neck dissection in all patients with hypopharyngeal cancer except those with well differentiated T1 or T2 lesions. Johnson *et al.*[19] found increased incidence of nodal recurrence in the unoperated contralateral neck in patients with lesions of the medial wall of the pyriform sinus, and recommended bilateral neck dissections for cancer involving the medial wall of the pyriform sinus, in addition to tumor that crosses the midline.

The majority of studies, however, suggested that when postoperative radiotherapy is given, control of microscopic disease in the contralateral neck can be obtained with doses in the range of 6000 cGy.

Role of radiotherapy in hypopharyngeal cancer

Radiation therapy, whether employed alone or in combination with surgery or chemotherapy, is the keystone for treatment of hypopharyngeal carcinoma. When employed alone it is effective for superficial lesions confined to the pyriform sinus with normal cord mobility. Local control for this group of patients can be expected in up to 90% of patients.[30] Radiotherapy is preferred for such patients since it leaves them with nearly normal swallowing and speech. The neck is usually prophylactically treated. For T1 and small T2 lesions, up to 6500 cGy is given over 7 weeks and up to 7000 cGy in 8 weeks is given for larger T2 and T3 lesions.

Posterior pharyngeal wall tumors can also be treated by radiation alone with good results. As these lesions tend to show significant submucosal spread and skip lesions, the whole posterior pharyngeal wall is treated together with the jugular chain, spinal accessory and retropharyngeal lymph nodes.

Except for selected cases described above, radiation therapy is usually utilized in conjunction with surgery. The rationale for combination therapy in the treatment of large tumors was based on the fact that disease-free margins were difficult to obtain at surgery, and that even with microscopically free margins, recurrence was not infrequent and was attributed to field cancerization or residual microscopic disease. In addition, surgical treatment of cervical lymph nodes would not address retropharyngeal lymph nodes, which can easily be covered by radiotherapy. On the other hand, radiation alone cannot eradicate large tumor volume, hence combination of surgery and radiation therapy is recommended for advanced-stage tumors.[15]

The sequencing of treatment, however, has been debated for a long time. A randomized prospective trial, comparing preoperative and postoperative radiation in the treatment of hypopharyngeal cancer, was carried out by Vandenbrouck *et al.*[40] The first group (n = 259) was treated with preoperative radiation of 50 Gy to the tumor bed and lymph node basin, followed 2 weeks later with total laryngopharyngectomy and radical neck dissection. The second group had surgery followed by postoperative radiation of 55 Gy within 4 weeks. There were five cases of fatal carotid hemorrhage in the preoperative radiation group compared with one in the postoperative treatment group. The 5-year survival was 36% in the preoperative radiation group but was 56% in the postoperative radiation group. This and other studies suggest that postoperative radiation yields better locoregional control, is associated with a lower complication rate and allows full histologic evaluation of the untreated lesion.

Multimodality therapy

Although conservation surgery and radiation are effective in the control of smaller hypopharyngeal cancers, the recurrence rate in the more advanced disease is very significant. The effectiveness of cisplatin-based chemotherapy has been shown in a palliative setting with significant response rates in head and neck squamous carcinoma, hence its role in an induction or neoadjuvant setting needs further study. Several uncontrolled trials of induction chemotherapy for untreated head and neck cancer reported complete response (CR) rates of up to 60% in patients treated with two to three cycles of cisplatin-based chemotherapy.[14,42] Up to 70% of these patients with CR were found to have no pathologic evidence of residual tumor on subsequent biopsy or resected specimen.

To date, however, no reported trials of induction chemotherapy have demonstrated improved survival over conventional treatment of surgery and postoperative radiotherapy.

Even though the survival rate was not improved, the encouraging response rate led to a new era of laryngeal preservation with induction chemotherapy. In a trial comparing immediate laryngectomy and radiation with induction chemotherapy and radiation for locally advanced laryngeal cancer, the VA study group showed the feasibility of laryngeal preservation with no adverse impact on survival.[38]

A large randomized EORTC trial of advanced resectable hypopharyngeal carcinoma, compared standard treatment of surgery and postoperative radiation to a larynx-preserving protocol of induction chemotherapy plus definitive radiation in complete responders and salvage surgery in non-responders. Lefebvre *et al.*[25] reported that the treatment failure at local, regional sites and the frequency of a second primary are similar in both arms of the study. But the rate of distant metastases was lower in the larynx-preservation/induction chemotherapy group (25% vs 36%, *P* <0.041). The median survival was equivalent in both arms, and the 3- and 5-year estimates of retaining a functional larynx were 42% and 35%, respectively. The authors concluded that larynx preservation without jeopardizing survival appears feasible in patients with hypopharyngeal carcinoma. On the other hand, Beauvillian *et al.*, in a trial comparing induction chemotherapy and radiotherapy with induction chemotherapy, surgery and radiotherapy for locally advanced but resectable hypopharyngeal carcinoma, after a mean follow-up of 92 months, found that local control rate and overall survival rate were significantly poorer in the group treated with induction chemotherapy and radiation. Five-year local control rate was 63% versus 39%, *P* <0.01. The poor response rate has been attributed to the chemotherapeutic selection of resistant cells that are 'leaner and meaner'.[5]

References

1. Bakamjian VY. A two stage method for pharyngo-esophageal reconstruction with primary pectoral skin flap. *Plast Reconstr Surg* 1965; **36:** 173–9.
2. Ballantyne AJ. Significance of retropharyngeal nodes in cancer of the head and neck. *Am J Surg* 1964; **108:** 500–4.
3. Ballantyne AJ. Methods of repair after surgery for cancer of the pharyngeal wall, postcricoid area and the cervical esophagus. *Am J Surg* 1971; **122:** 482–6.
4. Barkley HT Jr, Fletcher GH, Jesse RH, Lindberg RD. Management of cervical lymph node metastases in squamous cell carcinoma of the tonsillar fossa, base of tongue, supraglottic larynx and hypopharynx. *Am J Surg* 1972; **124:** 462–7.
5. Beauvillian C, Mahe M, Boudin S, Penvrel P. Final result of a randomized trial comparing chemotherapy plus radiation with chemotherapy plus surgery plus radiation in locally advanced but resectable hypopharyngeal cancer. *Laryngoscope* 1997; **107:** 648–53.
6. Berrino F, Sant M, Verdecchia A, Capocaccia R, Hakulinen T, Esteve J. *Survival of Cancer Patients in Europe: the EUROCARE Study.* Lyon: IARC Scientific Publications, 1995.
7. Biller HF, Ogura JH, Davis WH, Powers WE. Planned pre-operative irradiation for cancer of the larynx and hypopharynx treated by total or partial laryngectomy. *Laryngoscope* 1969; **79:** 1387–95.
8. Black RJ, Gluckman JL, Shumrick DA. Multiple primary tumors of the upper aerodigestive tract. *Clin Otolaryngol* 1983; **8:** 277–81.
9. Burch JD, Howe GR, Miller AB, Semenciw R. Tobacco, alcohol, asbestos and nickel in the etiology of the cancer of the larynx: a case controlled study. *J Natl Cancer Inst* 1981; **67:** 1219–24.
10. Byers RM, Wolf PF, Ballantyne AJ. Rationale for elective modified neck dissection. *Head Neck* 1988; **10:** 160–7.
11. Cameron E, Pauling L, Leibovitz B. Ascorbic acid and cancer: a review. *Cancer Res* 1979; **39:** 663–8.
12. Candela FC, Kothari K, Shah JP. Pattern of lymph node metastases from squamous carcinoma of the oropharynx and hypopharynx. *Head Neck* 1990; **12:** 197–203.
13. Carbone A, Micheau C, Bosq J, Caillaud J-M, Vandenbrouck C. Superficial extending carcinoma of the hypopharynx: report of 26 cases of an underestimated carcinoma. *Laryngoscope* 1983; **93:** 1600–6.
14. Ervin TJ, Clark JR, Weichselbaum RR *et al.* An analysis of induction and adjuvant chemotherapy in the multidisciplinary treatment of squamous cell carcinoma of the head and neck. *J Clin Oncol* 1987; **5:** 10–20.
15. Fletcher GH, Jesse FH. The place of irradiation in the management of the primary lesion in head and neck cancer. *Cancer* 1977; **39:** 862–7.
16. Guillamondegui OM, Meoz R, Jesse RH. Surgical treatment of squamous cell carcinoma of the pharyngeal walls. *Am J Surg* 1978; **136:** 474–6.
17. Haagensen CD, Feind CR, Herter FP. The lymphatics in cancer. In: Haagensen CD, Feind CR, Herter FP, Slanetz CA Jr, Weinberg JA, eds. *The Head and Neck.* Philadelphia: Saunders, 1972.
18. Herity B, Moriaty M, Daly L, Dunn J, Bourke GJ. The role of alcohol and tobacco in the etiology of lung and larynx cancer. *Br J Cancer* 1982; **46:** 961–4.
19. Johnson JT, Bacon GW, Myers EN. Medial vs lateral wall pyriform sinus carcinoma: implication for management of regional lymphatics. *Head Neck* 1994; **16:** 401–5.
20. Kirchner JA. Pyriform sinus cancer: a clinical and laboratory study. *Ann Otol Rhinol Laryngol* 1975; **84:** 793–803.
21. Larsson LG, Sandstrom A, Westling P. Relationship of Plummer–Vinson disease to cancer of the upper alimentary tract in Sweden. *Cancer Res* 1975; **35:** 3308–16.
22. Leemans CR, Tiwari R, van der Waal I, Karim AB, Nauta JJ, Snow GB. The efficacy of comprehensive neck dissection with or without post-operative radiotherapy in nodal metastases of squamous cell carcinoma of the upper respiratory and digestive tract. *Laryngoscope* 1990; **100:** 1194–8.
23. Lefebvre JL, Bonneterre J. Current status of larynx preservation trials. *Curr Opin Oncol* 1996; **8:** 209–14.
24. Lefebvre JL, Castelain B, De La Torre JC, Delobelle Deroide A, Vankemmel B. Lymph node invasion in hypopharynx and lateral epilarynx carcinoma: a prognostic factor. *Head Neck Surg* 1987; **10:** 14–18.
25. Lefebvre JL, Chevalier D, Luboinski B, Kirkpatrick A, Collette L, Sahmoud T. Larynx preservation in pyriform sinus cancer: preliminary results of a European Organization for Research and Treatment of Cancer phase III trial. *J Natl Cancer Inst* 1996; **88:** 890–9.
26. Mancuso AA, Maceri D, Rice D. CT of cervical lymph node cancer. *AJR Am J Roentogenol* 1981; **136:** 381–5.
27. McCoy GD, Hecht TS, Wynder EL. The roles of tobacco, alcohol and diet in the etiology of upper alimentary and respiratory tract cancers. *Prev Med* 1980; **9:** 622–9.
28. McNab J, Jones RF. The Paterson–Kelly–Brown syndrome. Its relationship with iron deficiency and postcricoid carcinoma. *J Laryngol Otol* 1961; **75:** 529–43.
29. Mendenhall WM, Parson JT, Devine JW, Cassisi NJ, Million RR. Squamous cell carcinoma of the pyriform sinus treated with surgery and/or radiotherapy. *Head Neck* 1987; **10:** 88–92.

30. Million RR, Cassisi NJ. Radical irradiation for carcinoma of the pyriform sinus. *Laryngoscope* 1981; **91:** 439–50.
31. Müller KM, Krohn BR. Smoking habits and their relationship to precancerous lesions of the larynx. *J Cancer Res Clin Oncol* 1980; **96:** 211–17.
32. Murakami Y, Ikari T, Haraguchi S, Maruyama T, Saito S. Excision level and indication for contralateral neck dissection in hypopharyngeal cancer surgery. *Auris Nasus Larynx* 1985; **12:** 36–40.
33. Ogura JH, Marks JE, Freeman RB. Results of conservation surgery for cancer of the supraglottis and pyriform sinus. *Laryngoscope* 1980; **90:** 591–600.
34. Paccagnella A, Orlando A, Marchiori C *et al.* Phase III trial of initial chemotherapy in stage III or IV head and neck cancers: a study by the Gruppo di Studio sui Tumori della Testa e del Collo. *J Natl Cancer Inst* 1994; **86:** 265–72.
35. Ries LAG, Miller BA, Haskay BF. *SEER Cancer Statistic Review, 1973–1991: Tables and Graphs, National Cancer Institute.* NIH Pub. No 94-2789 (1994).
36. Slaughter DP, Southwick HW, Smejkal W. 'Field cancerization' in oral stratified squamous epithelium. *Cancer* 1953; **5:** 963–8.
37. Stell PM. Smoking and laryngeal cancer. *Lancet* 1972; **1:** 617–18.
38. The Department of Veterans Affairs Laryngeal Cancer Study Group. Induction chemotherapy plus radiation compared with surgery plus radiation in patients with advanced laryngeal cancer. *N Engl J Med* 1991; **324:** 1685–90.
39. Trotter W. Malignant disease of the hypopharynx and its treatment by excision. *Br Med J* 1932; **1:** 510–18.
40. Vandenbrouck C, Sancho H, Le Fur R, Richard JM, Cachin Y. Results of a randomized clinical trial of preoperative irradiation versus postoperative in treatment of tumors of the hypopharynx. *Cancer* 1977; **39:** 1445–9.
41. Wallace AF. Multiple malignant primary neoplasms. *Br J Surg* 1962; **45:** 165–9.
42. Weaver A, Flemming S, Kish J *et al.* Cis-platin and 5-flurouracil as induction therapy in advanced head and neck cancer. *Am J Surg* 1982; **144:** 445–8.
43. Weber RS, Marvel J, Smith P, Hankins P, Wolf P, Goepfert H. Paratracheal lymph node dissections for carcinoma of the larynx, hypopharynx and cervical esophagus. *Otolaryngol Head Neck Surg* 1993; **108:** 11–17.
44. Whelan SL, Parkin DM, Masuyer E, Smans M. *Patterns of Cancer in Five Continents.* Vol. XVIII. No. 102. Lyon: IARC Scientific Publications, 1990.
45. Wynder EL, Mushinski MH, Spivak JC. Tobacco and alcohol consumption in relation to the development of multiple primary cancers. *Cancer* 1977; **40:** 1872–8.

47 Treatment of the neck in squamous carcinoma of the larynx

Jesus E Medina

Anatomy of the lymphatic drainage

The lymphatics of the larynx originate in the mucosa where they constitute a continuous network. This network, which is located in the superficial layers of the submucosa, must be studied separately for the supraglottic, glottic and subglottic regions of the larynx.

In the supraglottic region, the lymphatic network covers the entire laryngeal surface of the epiglottis, the false cords and the aryepiglottic folds without discontinuity.[48] This feature of the supraglottic lymphatic drainage has important therapeutic implications; because of its continuous nature, all areas of the supraglottic mucosa have the potential to drain to the lymph nodes of both sides of the neck. This has been demonstrated by Welsh, who used injections of radioactive tracers to define laryngeal lymphatic drainage. After lateralized injection in the supraglottic region, the tracer could be found primarily in the ipsilateral upper and mid-jugular lymph nodes; however, small amounts of tracer were also found in the contralateral lymph nodes.[57] The supraglottic lymphatics also communicate superiorly with the lymphatic network of the base of the tongue and, posteriorly around the arytenoids, with the hypopharyngeal network. The superficial supraglottic lymphatic network converges onto three to four lymphatic trunks on each side (the superior lymphatic pedicle of Roubaud), which, following the direction of the superior laryngeal vessels, pierce the thyrohyoid membrane and drain into the upper jugular or level II lymph nodes (Fig 47.1).[48]

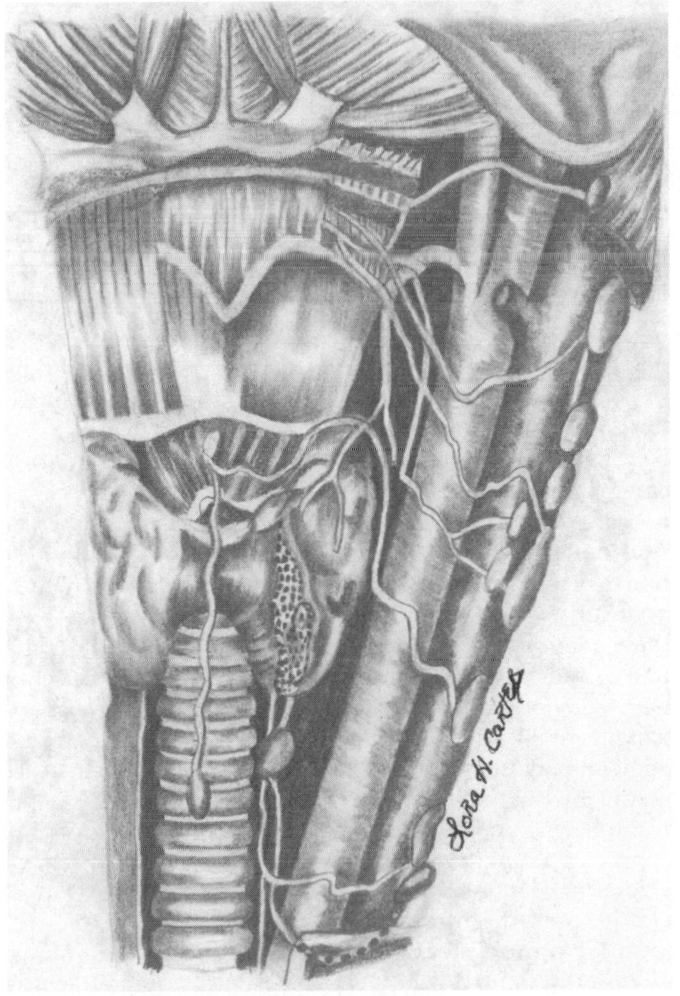

Figure 47.1 *Anatomy of the lymphatics of the larynx.*

In the subglottic region, the lymphatic network is also well developed, although not as much as in the preceding region. Superiorly it appears to end abruptly at the free border of the vocal cord, whereas inferiorly it blends in with the tracheal lymphatics. The anterior portion of this network drains, through small trunks that pierce the cricothyroid membrane near the midline, into the prelaryngeal lymph nodes. The efferents from the prelaryngeal nodes follow two directions: laterally toward the mid-jugular lymph nodes (level III) and medially towards the pretracheal lymph nodes. The posterior subglottic lymphatics drain through small trunks that traverse the cricotracheal ligament, near the membranous portion of the trachea, and drain into the paratracheal lymph nodes located alongside the recurrent laryngeal nerve. The efferents from these nodes drain towards the lower jugular/supraclavicular nodes.

In the glottic region, the lymphatics are notably scarce. They communicate upward with the supraglottic network and downward with the subglottic lymphatics.

Distribution of lymph node metastases

The majority of metastases from laryngeal squamous cell carcinomas are found in lymph nodes located in levels II, III and IV.[11] In a recent study of 93 patients with advanced (T3–T4) laryngeal cancer who underwent comprehensive neck dissection, Moe *et al.* found that no patients with glottic cancer had level I or V involvement, whereas no level V involvement was seen in patients with supraglottic cancer with N0 necks.[32] Other authors have reported almost identical observations in supraglottic cancers.[16,42]

The findings reported by Li *et al.* in 1996 are typical. They studied retrospectively 384 radical neck dissection specimens of patients with squamous cell carcinoma of the upper aerodigestive tract. There were 73 patients with carcinoma of the larynx. Of these, 48 underwent therapeutic and 25 elective radical neck dissections. Metastases were confirmed histologically in 43 specimens. Level I nodes were involved in one patient (2%) and level V nodes were involved in four (9%).[25] It is noteworthy that in some studies metastases were found in level V in 1% or less of the cases.[16,42]

In addition to the nodes in the lateral compartment of the neck, metastases from laryngeal squamous cell carcinoma can occur to the paratracheal lymph nodes. In a study of 91 selected patients with squamous cell carcinoma of the larynx who underwent paratracheal lymph node dissection, Weber *et al.* found that metastases to these lymph nodes occurred primarily in patients with transglottic tumors, but they also occurred in patients with subglottic tumors.[56] In a prospective study of 45 patients with advanced glottic cancers, who underwent bilateral paratracheal node dissection as part of their treatment, Shenoy *et al.* found metastases in the ipsilateral paratracheal nodes in 9% of the 22 positive necks and contralateral metastases in 4.5%.[45] Interestingly, Weber *et al.* found 'paratracheal node' metastases in three supraglottic tumors. Unfortunately, they did not describe the location of these metastases, apparently because the study did not discriminate between paratracheal and pretracheal or prelaryngeal nodes.[56]

The risk of 'contralateral' bilateral lymph node metastases is an important consideration in cancers of the supraglottic larynx. In a series of 846 patients retrospectively studied by Marks *et al.*, contralateral lymph node metastases were identified at presentation or developed later in 26% of patients with glossoepiglottic tumors (suprahyoid epiglottis, vallecula, base of the tongue), 14% with marginal supraglottic tumors, 7% with central supraglottic tumors, 4% of transglottic tumors and in 13% of patients with pyriform sinus cancers. The authors caution that the incidence of contralateral metastases is probably higher than they report since most of the patients in their series received variable doses of radiation.[27] Myers and Alvi have reported similar observations in a series of 103 patients treated for supraglottic carcinoma at the University of Pittsburgh. Among the 14 patients who had recurrence in the neck, five (36%) occurred in the 'contralateral' side of the neck.[34]

It is clear from this review of the recent literature that the incidence of occult metastases from laryngeal squamous cell carcinomas to lymph node levels I and V is insignificant, that bilateral lymph node metastases are a distinct hazard in supraglottic cancers and that the possibility of metastases to the paratracheal nodes needs to be kept in mind in advanced glottic, transglottic and subglottic tumors; however, studies are needed to determine their frequency.

Frequency of lymph node metastases

Although the ability to detect occult cervical lymph node metastases has improved with the advent of modern imaging techniques, particularly when combined with fine-needle aspiration biopsy, a considerable number of such metastases remain undetectable without histopathologic examination of the lymph nodes. Currently, therapeutic decisions for patients with laryngeal cancer and stage N0 neck are, for the most part, based on the probability of lymph node metastases for a given tumor. For many years, clinicians have used the stage of the primary tumor and its site of origin to estimate the probability of lymph node metastases.

The predictive value of the tumor site of origin and stage leaves a lot to be desired – thus, the need for the identification of factors related to the primary tumor, the host, or both that would enhance the physician's ability to predict the presence or absence of metastases in the lymph nodes. In this regard, McGavran *et al.* have studied the relationship between various characteristics of the primary tumor and the probability of lymph node metastases in a homogenous series of 96 patients, who underwent *en bloc* laryngectomy and radical neck dissection. They found that the incidence of lymph node metastases was significantly higher in patients whose tumors measured >2 cm in diameter, or were poorly differentiated, or exhibited an infiltrating rather than a pushing margin or perineural invasion.[30] Unfortunately these authors did not perform a multivariate analysis. More recently, Kowalski *et al.* performed a similar study of 103 patients with laryngeal carcinoma who underwent either unilateral or bilateral comprehensive neck dissection. Interestingly, a logistic regression analysis demonstrated that tumor site (supraglottic origin) and poor histologic differentiation were the only predictors of nodal metastases. When they consider only cases staged N0, the probability of occult lymph node metastases was influenced significantly only by a supraglottic origin of the primary tumor.[23] In studies of advanced laryngeal cancer, the highest incidence of cervical lymph node metastases is associated with supraglottic tumors (65%), whilst metastases are found in only 20–22% of advanced glottic tumors.[32,47]

A number of other putative predictive factors have been studied. For instance, some investigators have found a correlation between DNA index and lymph node status in laryngeal carcinomas, with a higher incidence of neck node metastases in patients with high DNA content in tumor cells.[58] Expression of epidermal growth factor (EGF) is another potentially useful biological marker. A significant correlation between expression of EGF and the risk of lymph node metastases was recently observed by Maurizi *et al.*, in a study of 140 cases of laryngeal carcinoma.[29]

Treatment of the N0 neck

When managing patients with laryngeal squamous cell carcinoma who do not have clinical or radiographic evidence of lymph node metastases (stage N0), the clinician must confront the following issues:

- is elective treatment of the regional nodes beneficial?
- should the lymph nodes be removed surgically or treated electively with radiation?
- if surgery is performed, how extensive should the dissection of the lymph nodes be?

Unfortunately, none of these issues has been resolved scientifically. Therefore, the answers to these questions can not be dogmatic. Furthermore, the management of the N0 neck in larynx cancer patients varies with institutional policies and resources, with the medical, psychological and social characteristics of the patient, and with the choice of therapy for the primary tumor. What follows is a discussion of the options that may be considered suitable for the management of the N0 neck.

Observation with therapeutic neck dissection when needed

The value of elective treatment of the neck is not universally accepted. The notion of watching the neck and treating it only when metastases become clinically apparent is allegedly supported by two prospective randomized studies involving cancers of the oral cavity.[10,51] In both studies the survival of patients who underwent 'elective' neck dissection was not significantly better than the survival of patients who underwent a delayed therapeutic neck dissection. Unfortunately, these studies have not resolved the controversy; in fact, they have been criticized because the number of patients studied was insufficient to be conclusive.

The efficacy of elective treatment of the neck in patients with laryngeal squamous cell carcinoma has been recently compared to that of therapeutic neck dissection at the time metastases become clinically apparent, in an interesting retrospective study by Gallo *et al.*[16] From a population of 1808 patients with cancer of the larynx treated at the University of Florence, two groups of patients were selected for comparison. The first group of 54 patients had clinically an N0 neck, underwent elective neck dissection and were found to have histologically positive nodes. The second group consisted of 96 patients who were initially staged N0, but subsequently developed lymph node metastases and underwent therapeutic neck dissection. Postoperative radiation to the neck was given to 11% of the patients in the first group and to 20.8 % in the second group (P = 0.178). The criteria used to determine when patients were selected for one group or the other were not established *a priori*. However, the authors state that patients were 'usually' selected to undergo elective neck dissection when they had an advanced tumor (T3–T4), a fat, short or muscular neck that was not easy to evaluate clinically, a low educational level and when poor follow-up was anticipated. In this study, there was not a statistically significant difference for the two groups of patients in overall, determinant and actuarial survival rates, with a minimum follow-up of 5 years. This is surprising since patients who underwent delayed therapeutic neck dissection had a significantly higher incidence of distant metastases, multiple positive nodes and extracapsular tumor spread.[16] Other retrospective studies have found that elective neck dissection decreases the neck recurrence rates significantly in patients treated for N0 supraglottic carcinoma.[41]

Self-examination by the patient and reliable follow-up are essential for watchful waiting to succeed in the management of the N0 neck. Unfortunately, a significant number of the patients who do not undergo elective neck dissection can not be salvaged later, when they present with palpable metastases, because the disease is too far advanced.[10] In a review of 122 patients with T3–T4N0 cancers of the larynx who were treated by total laryngectomy and observation of the neck at the University of Hong Kong, 36% of the patients who later presented with palpable metastases had inoperable disease, amenable to palliative treatment only. Furthermore, of the patients that were operable, 42% eventually died of a neck recurrence. These observations, in combination with the idiosyncrasies of character and social background of many larynx cancer patients, are the reasons why most head and neck surgeons prefer to treat the neck electively, even though the impact of this decision on patient survival remains controversial.[59]

An alternative to this all or none approach has been offered by van den Brekel *et al.*[50] Using ultrasound examination of the neck and fine-needle aspiration biopsy, dissection is performed only when the nodes are histologically positive. Whilst this approach is clearly a step in the right direction, the reported sensitivity of it is only between 44% and 73%. Furthermore, in a study of 92 patients who were N0 and cytologically negative, who were followed for 1–3 years, 19 (21%) subsequently developed a neck node metastasis. Six of these 19 patients (32%) died of distant metastases or locoregional recurrence.[49]

Another alternative has been advocated by the surgeons at the Gustave Roussy Institute and by other authors. It consists of performing intraoperative frozen sections of jugulodigastric lymph nodes. If the presence of metastasis is demonstrated, neck dissection is performed.[44,46]

Elective treatment of the neck

Indications

Glottic cancer

Given the low probability of occult lymph node metastases, elective treatment of the regional lymph nodes is not indicated in patients with T1 and T2 glottic tumors. However, according to Olsen *et al.*, when a positive delphian node is found in the course of performing a partial laryngectomy for a T1–T2 glottic cancer, an ipsilateral neck dissection is indicated, based on the high rate (40%) of subsequent lateral neck metastases observed in these patients.[36] Likewise, ipsilateral neck dissection may be considered in recurrent T1–T2 tumors, because of the reported risk of occult metastases (20–22%).[40] Whilst some surgeons believe that elective treatment of the lymph nodes is not indicated in patients with T3 glottic tumors, others have observed lymph node metastases in 17–22% of the cases and recommend elective treatment of the neck.[18,47] The incidence of lymph node metastases in patients with T4 tumors is sufficiently high to warrant elective treatment.[45]

Supraglottic cancer

The probability of occult metastases when the primary tumor is located in the supraglottic larynx is sufficiently high, regardless of the tumor stage, that elective treatment is warranted. A possible exception to this may be T1 tumors of the suprahyoid epiglottis. Because 'as many as 75% of cervical failures occur in the undissected' contralateral side of the neck, elective treatment of the neck in supraglottic cancers should include the lymph nodes at risk on both sides of the neck.[40]

Subglottic cancer

In the absence of adequate information, it is difficult to make recommendations about elective treatment of the cervical lymph nodes in true subglottic cancers. However, because of our knowledge about the distribution of lymph node metastases in these cases, it seems prudent to treat the lymph nodes of the anterior compartment of the neck. On the other hand, elective treatment of the lateral compartments of the neck does not seem necessary, since the reported incidence of metastases to these nodes is relatively low (10%).[24,28]

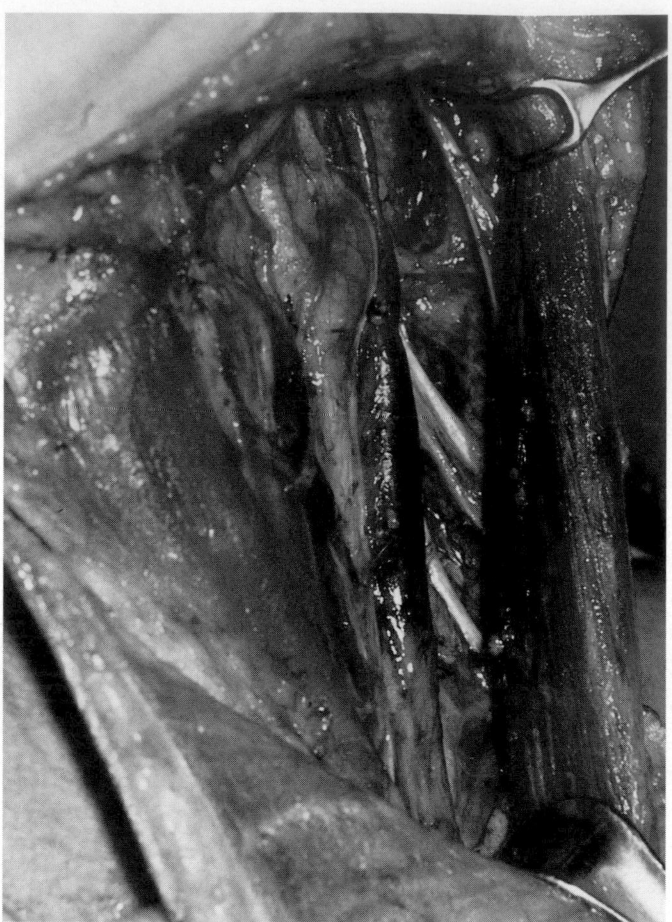

Figure 47.2 *Lateral neck dissection. Intraoperative photography illustrating the posterior extent of the dissection, beyond the jugular vein up to the level of posterior border of the sternocleidomastoid muscle. Note the cutaneous branches of the cervical plexus.*

Elective lymph node dissection

In general, when surgery is selected as the treatment modality for the primary tumor and elective treatment of the lymph nodes is indicated, a neck dissection is performed. Elective surgical treatment of the neck in patients with laryngeal squamous cell carcinoma should consist of a lateral neck dissection[20] (Fig 47.2) or a modified radical neck dissection type III ('functional neck dissection'), which removes lymph node levels I, II, III, IV and V and preserves the sternocleidomastoid muscle, the internal jugular vein and the spinal accessory nerve. In addition, ipsilateral paratracheal node dissection may be beneficial for 'transglottic' tumors and for tumors that exhibit subglottic extension.

The rationale to include level V in elective neck dissections for patients with cancer of the larynx has to be questioned, in light of the results of recent studies of functional neck dissection specimens from patients with larynx cancer. These studies have shown that the lymph nodes of the posterior triangle of the neck are seldom involved in these patients.[16,42] Interestingly, Steiner *et al.* (cf. Ambrosch *et al.*[1]) advocate dissecting levels II and III only. They have reported very low recurrence rates in level IV or anywhere in the neck using this approach.[1]

Houck and Medina report that the recurrence rate in the neck following lateral neck dissection is 0% when the lymph nodes removed are histologically negative.[19] Comparably, the recurrence rates observed following 'functional' neck dissection vary between 0 and 16.5%.[3,6,17,22,26,33] It should be emphasized that the lateral neck dissection does not consist of removal of nodes immediately surrounding the internal jugular vein or the fibrofatty tissue medial to the jugular vein, as is suggested by the term interjugular dissection.[12] Rather, it consists of removal of the tissue containing lymph nodes in the lateral compartment of the neck, underlying the sternocleidomastoid muscle. The dissection extends beyond the level of the internal jugular vein, up to the posterior border of the sternocleidomastoid muscle. The posterior extent of the dissection is marked by the cutaneous branches of the cervical plexus (Fig 47.2).

Depending upon the results of the histopathologic examination of the lymph nodes, postoperative radiation therapy may be indicated. Most surgeons today would prescribe radiation therapy when there are more than two or three histologically positive nodes, particularly when they are located in multiple levels of the neck and when there is evidence of extracapsular spread of tumor.[40]

In patients in whom the need for postoperative radiation is anticipated based on the characteristics of the primary tumor, as is frequently the case in T4 tumors, the neck could be left undisturbed at the time of the surgical treatment of the primary tumor and treated electively with radiation. The Kidwai Memorial Institute of Oncology recently reported a series of 45 patients with advanced glottic (T3–T4) cancers, who were treated with total laryngectomy, ipsilateral/bilateral thyroid lobectomy, bilateral paratracheal clearance, and bilateral clearance of lymph node levels II, III and IV. Postoperative radiation was prescribed when the primary tumor was staged T4 , there was significant subglottic extension or jugular/paratracheal metastatic deposits were found. Interestingly, 91% of the cases (41/45) qualified for postoperative radiation. It can be argued that the neck was overtreated in most of these patients, and that it could have been treated instead with elective radiation after laryngectomy.[45]

Bilateral neck dissection is indicated in the surgical management of supraglottic squamous cell carcinoma.[55] Perhaps past hesitancy to recommend bilateral elective treatment of the neck in these patients, was due to the morbidity associated with bilateral radical neck dissections, when this was the only operation used for the treatment of the neck. With the use of selective neck dissection, the issue of postoperative morbidity has been reduced significantly. In a recent review of the clinical course of 76 patients undergoing excision of supraglottic squamous carcinoma combined with bilateral neck dissection, a decrease in neck recurrences from 20% to 9% was attributed to the use of bilateral neck dissection.[55]

Elective neck irradiation

If a laryngeal cancer is treated with radiation, the lymph nodes at high risk are also treated with radiation. Following elective neck irradiation, the risk of developing clinically positive nodes in an N0 neck is about 5%.[14,31] In a recent study, isolated neck failure was observed in 1% of 413 patients with larynx cancer treated by elective neck irradiation at the Institute Gustave Roussy.[44] This compares favorably with a 2.9% rate of recurrence in the neck in 328 cases treated at the same institution with selective neck dissection, extended to a modified radical neck dissection if positive at frozen section.

Treatment of the N+ neck

When palpable cervical lymph node metastases are present in patients with laryngeal squamous cell carcinoma, a neck dissection is the mainstay of treatment. The extent of the dissection to be performed depends on the extent of the disease in the neck. In some instances it is necessary to resect structures not routinely removed during neck dissection (e.g. the hypoglossal nerve, the carotid, the overlying skin). In other instances, the metastases in the neck can be adequately removed while preserving the spinal accessory nerve, the internal jugular vein or the sternocleidomastoid muscle. In the case of N+ disease, selective lateral neck dissection can be as valid as modified radical neck dissection, providing patients have only limited metastatic disease.[13,38] The combination of judicious surgery and radiation therapy affords excellent tumor control in the neck while preserving function and cosmesis.[5]

The rates of tumor control in the neck reported with the modified radical neck dissection with preservation of the spinal accessory nerve vary between 5 and 20%.[2,4,7,9,37,43] Interestingly, similar results (3.4–30.4%) have been reported for the 'functional' neck dissection.[3,6,17,22,26,33]

Numerous studies suggest that the rate of tumor recurrence in the neck is decreased by the addition of radiation, when multiple nodes are involved at multiple levels of the neck, and when extracapsular spread (ECS) of tumor is found.[8,21,35,54] The dose of postoperative radiation therapy is essential to achieve optimal results. Daily fractions of 1.8 Gy to a total dose of 57.6 Gy to the entire operative bed is currently recommended. Sites of increased risk for recurrence, such as areas of the neck where ECS of tumor was found, should be boosted to

63 Gy.[39] Timing of the initiation of radiotherapy is also important; delays beyond 6 weeks may compromise tumor control.[54]

In cases with advanced neck metastases (>3 cm in diameter) with a small primary tumor in the larynx, in which the neck has to be treated with surgery whilst the primary can be successfully treated with radiation alone, Verschuur *et al.* have performed a neck dissection first, followed within 4 weeks by radiotherapy to the primary and to the neck. In a group of 15 patients treated in this manner, no recurrence in the neck was observed at 5 years.[53] Using a similar treatment approach in 65 patients with tumors of the larynx and hypopharynx, the French Head and Study Group observed a rate of recurrence in the neck of 4.6%.[15]

Therapeutic radiation

Cases of squamous cell carcinoma larynx with clinically positive neck nodes up to 1 cm can be treated with radical radiotherapy to the primary as well as the lymph node metastases.[52]

A multivariate analysis of various factors in relationship to outcome of treatment of the positive neck with radiation resulted in a model with node size <1 cm as the most important predictor of neck node control (P <0.01).[52]

References

1. Ambrosch P, Freudenberg L, Kron M, Steiner W. Selective neck dissection in the management of squamous cell carcinoma of the upper digestive tract. *Eur Arch Otorhinolaryngol* 1996; **253:** 329–35.
2. Andersen PE, Shah JP, Cambronero E, Spiro RH. The role of comprehensive neck dissection with preservation of the spinal accessory nerve in the clinically positive neck. *Am J Surg* 1994; **168:** 499–502.
3. Bocca E, Pignataro O, Oldini C, Cappa C. Functional neck dissection: an evaluation and review of 843 cases. *Laryngoscope* 1984; **94:** 942–5.
4. Brandenburg JH, Lee CY. The eleventh nerve in radical neck surgery. *Laryngoscope* 1981; **91:** 1851–9.
5. Byers RM. Modified neck dissection. A study of 967 cases from 1970 to 1980. *Am J Surg* 1985; **150:** 414–21.
6. Calearo CV, Teatini G. Functional neck dissection. Anatomical grounds, surgical technique, clinical observations. *Ann Otol Rhinol Laryngol* 1983; **92:** 215–22.
7. Carenfelt C, Eliasson K. Cervical metastases following radical neck dissection that preserved the spinal accessory nerve. *Head Neck Surg* 1980; **2:** 181–4.
8. Carter RL, Barr LC, O'Brien CJ, Soo KC, Shaw HJ. Transcapsular spread of metastatic squamous cell carcinoma from cervical lymph nodes. *Am J Surg* 1985; **150:** 495–9.
9. Chu W, Strawitz JG. Results in suprahyoid, modified radical, and standard radical neck dissections for metastatic squamous cell carcinoma: recurrence and survival. *Am J Surg* 1978; **136:** 512–15.
10. Fakih AR, Rao RS, Borges AM, Patel AR. Elective versus therapeutic neck dissection in early carcinoma of the oral tongue. *Am J Surg* 1989; **158:** 309–13.
11. Ferlito A, Rinaldo A. Level I dissection for laryngeal and hypopharyngeal cancer: is it indicated? *J Laryngol Otol* 1998; **112:** 438–40.
12. Ferlito A, Rinaldo A. Selective lateral neck dissection for laryngeal cancer in the clinically negative neck: is it justified? *J Laryngol Otol* 1998; **112:** 921–4.
13. Ferlito A, Rinaldo A. Selective lateral neck dissection for laryngeal cancer with limited metastatic disease: is it indicated? *J Laryngol Otol* 1998; **112:** 1031–3.
14. Fletcher GH. Elective irradiation of subclinical disease in cancers of the head and neck. *Cancer* 1972; **29:** 1450–4.
15. French Head and Neck Study Group (GETTEC). Early pharyngolaryngeal carcinomas with palpable nodes. *Am J Surg* 1991; **162:** 377–80.
16. Gallo O, Boddi V, Bottai GV, Parrella F, Fini Storchi O. Treatment of the clinically negative neck in laryngeal cancer patients. *Head Neck* 1996; **18:** 566–72.
17. Gavilan C, Gavilan J. Five-year results of functional neck dissection for cancer of the larynx. *Arch Otolaryngol Head Neck Surg* 1989; **115:** 1193–6.
18. Hao SP, Myers EN, Johnson JT. T3 glottic carcinoma revisited. Transglottic vs. pure glottic carcinoma. *Arch Otolaryngol Head Neck Surg* 1995; **121:** 166–70.
19. Houck JR, Medina JE. Management of cervical lymph nodes in squamous carcinomas of the head and neck. *Semin Surg Oncol* 1995; **11:** 228–39.
20. Johnson JT. Carcinoma of the larynx: selective approach to the management of cervical lymphatics. *Ear Nose Throat J* 1994; **73:** 303–5.
21. Johnson JT, Myers EN, Bedetti CD, Barnes EL. Cervical lymph node metastases. *Arch Otolaryngol Head Neck Surg* 1985; **111:** 534–7.
22. Joseph CA, Gregor RT, Davidge-Pitts KJ. The role of functional neck dissection in the management of advanced tumours of the upper aerodigestive tract. *S Afr J Surg* 1985; **23:** 83–7.
23. Kowalski LP, Franco EL, De Andrade Sobrinho J. Factors influencing regional lymph node metastasis from laryngeal carcinoma. *Ann Otol Rhinol Laryngol* 1995; **104:** 442–7.
24. Lederman M. Cancer of the larynx – Part 1: Natural history in relation to treatment. *Br J Radiol* 1971; **44:** 569–78.
25. Li XM, Wei WI, Guo XF, Yuen PW, Lam LK. Cervical lymph node metastatic patterns of squamous carcinomas in the upper aerodigestive tract. *J Laryngol Otol* 1996; **110:** 937–41.
26. Lingeman RE, Stephens R, Helmus C, Ulm J. Neck dissection: radical or conservative. *Ann Otol* 1977; **86:** 737–44.
27. Marks JE, Devineni VR, Harvey J, Sessions DG. The risk of contralateral lymphatic metastases for cancers of the larynx and pharynx. *Am J Otolaryngol* 1992; **13:** 34–9.
28. Mårtensson B, Fluur E, Jacobsson F. Aspects on treatment of cancer of the larynx. *Ann Otol* 1967; **76:** 313–29.
29. Maurizi M, Almadori G, Cadoni J *et al.* EGFR expression in primary laryngeal cancer patients: an independent prognostic factor for lymph node metastasis. *Br J Cancer* 1998; **77(Suppl 1):** Abstract 1.37a.

30. McGavran MH, Bauer WC, Ogura JH. The incidence of cervical lymph node metastases from epidermoid carcinoma of the larynx and their relationship to certain characteristics of the primary tumor. *Cancer* 1961; **14:** 55–66.
31. Mendenhall WM, Million RR, Cassisi NJ. Elective neck irradiation in squamous-cell carcinoma of the head and neck. *Head Neck Surg* 1980; **3:** 15–20.
32. Moe K, Wolf GT, Fisher SG, Hong WK. Regional metastases in patients with advanced laryngeal cancer. *Arch Otolaryngol Head Neck Surg* 1996; **122:** 644–8.
33. Molinari R, Chiesa F, Cantu G, Grandi C. Retrospective comparison of conservative and radical neck dissection in laryngeal cancer. *Ann Otol* 1980; **89:** 578–81.
34. Myers EN, Alvi A. Management of carcinoma of the supraglottic larynx: evolution, current concepts and future trends. *Laryngoscope* 1996; **106(5 Pt 1):** 559–67.
35. O'Brien CJ, Smith JW, Soong SJ, Urist MM, Maddox WA. Neck dissection with and without radiotherapy: prognostic factors, patterns of recurrence and survival. *Am J Surg* 1986; **152:** 456–63.
36. Olsen KD, DeSanto LW, Pearson BW. Positive delphian node: clinical significance in laryngeal cancer. *Laryngoscope* 1987; **97:** 1033–7.
37. Pearlman NW, Meyers AD, Sullivan WG. Modified radical neck dissection for squamous carcinoma of the head and neck. *Surg Gynecol Obstet* 1982; **154:** 214–16.
38. Pellitteri PK, Robbins KT, Neuman T. Expanded application of selective neck dissection with regard to nodal status. *Head Neck* 1997; **19:** 260–5.
39. Peters LJ, Goepfert H, Kian Ang K *et al.* Evaluation of the dose for postoperative radiation therapy of head and neck cancer: first report of a prospective randomized trial. *Int J Radiat Oncol Biol Phys* 1993; **26:** 3–11.
40. Pillsbury HC III, Clark M. A rationale for therapy of the N0 neck. *Laryngoscope* 1997; **107:** 1294–315.
41. Ramadan HH, Allen GC. The influence of elective neck dissection on neck relapse in N0 supraglottic carcinoma. *Am J Otolaryngol* 1993; **14:** 278–81.
42. Redaelli de Zinis LO, Nicolai P, Barezzani MG, Tomenzoli D, Antonelli AR. Incidence and distribution of lymph node metastases in supraglottic squamous cell carcinoma: therapeutic implications. *Acta Otorhinolaryngol Ital* 1994; **14:** 19–27.
43. Roy PH, Beahrs OH. Spinal accessory nerve in radical neck dissections. *Am J Surg* 1969; **118:** 800–4.
44. Schwaab G, Luboinski B, Julieron M, Bourhis J, Richard JM. Management and results of N0 neck in laryngeal cancers: experience of the Gustave Roussy Institute 1975–1984. *2nd World Congress on Laryngeal Cancer, Sydney, Australia.* Abstract.
45. Shenoy AM, Nanjundappa A, Kumar P *et al.* Interjugular neck dissection and post-operative irradiation for neck control in advanced glottic cancers – are we justified? *J Laryngol Otol* 1994; **108:** 26–9.
46. Sun X, Guo Z, Lu C. Clinical significance of intraoperative frozen biopsy of cervical lymph node for laryngeal cancer. *Chin J Otorhinolaryngol* 1994; **29:** 104–6.
47. Terhaard C, Hordijk G, van den Broek P *et al.* T3 laryngeal cancer: a retrospective study of the Dutch head and neck oncology cooperative group: study design and general results. *Clin Otolaryngol* 1992; **17:** 393–402.
48. Testut L, Latarjet A. Aparato de la respiracion y fonacion: In: Testut L, Latarjet A, eds. *Tratado de Anatomia Humana.* Barcelona: Salvat Editores, 1959: 925–6.
49. van den Brekel MWM, Reitsma LC, Snow GB, Castelijns JA. The outcome of a wait and see policy for the neck after negative ultrasound guided cytology results and follow-up with ultrasound guided cytology. *Br J Cancer* 1998; **77(Suppl 1):** Abstract 4.11.
50. van den Brekel MWM, Castelijns JA, Stel HV, Golding RP, Meyer CJL, Snow GB. Modern imaging techniques and ultrasound-guided aspiration cytology for the assessment of neck node metastases: a prospective comparative study. *Eur Arch Otorhinolaryngol* 1993; **250:** 11–17.
51. Vandenbrouck C, Sancho-Garnier H, Chassagne D, Saravane D, Cachin Y, Micheau C. Elective versus therapeutic radical neck dissection in epidermoid carcinoma of the oral cavity. Results of a randomized clinical trial. *Cancer* 1980; **46:** 386–90.
52. Varghese C, Sankaranarayanan R, Nair B, Nair MK. Predictors of neck node control in radically irradiated squamous cell carcinoma of the oropharynx and laryngopharynx. *Head Neck* 1993; **15:** 105–8.
53. Verschuur HP, Keus RB, Hilgers FJM, Balm AJM, Gregor RT. Preservation of function by radiotherapy of small primary carcinomas preceded by neck dissection for extensive nodal metastases of the head and neck. *Head Neck* 1996; **18:** 277–82.
54. Vikram B, Strong EW, Shah JP, Spiro R. Failure in the neck following multimodality treatment for advanced head and neck cancer. *Head Neck Surg* 1984; **6:** 724–9.
55. Weber PC, Johnson JT, Myers EN. The impact of bilateral neck dissection on pattern of recurrence and survival in supraglottic carcinoma. *Arch Otolaryngol Head Neck Surg* 1994; **120:** 703–6.
56. Weber RS, Marvel J, Smith P, Hankins P, Wolf P, Goepfert H. Paratracheal lymph node dissection for carcinoma of the larynx, hypopharynx and cervical esophagus. *Otolaryngol Head Neck Surg* 1993; **108:** 11–17.
57. Welsh L. The normal human laryngeal lymphatics. *Ann Otol* 1964; **73:** 569–81.
58. Wolf GT, Fisher SG, Truelson JM, Beals TF. Department of Veterans Affairs Laryngeal Study Group. DNA content and regional metastases in patients with advanced laryngeal squamous carcinoma. *Laryngoscope* 1994; **104:** 479–83.
59. Yuen A, Wei W, Wong S. Critical appraisal of watchful waiting policy in the management of N0 neck of advanced laryngeal carcinoma. *Arch Otolaryngol Head Neck Surg* 1996; **122:** 742–5.

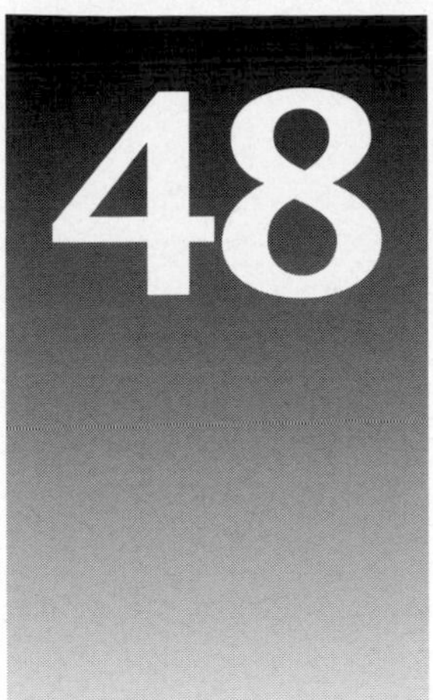

Treatment of the N0 neck in non-conventional squamous carcinoma of the larynx*

Alfio Ferlito, Alessandra Rinaldo, Kenneth O. Devaney and Antonino Carbone

There is evidence that the optimal approach to the evaluation of 'clinically' negative nodes is yet to be defined. At present, we are unable to establish lymph node involvement accurately using noninvasive methods (computed tomography, magnetic resonance imaging, ultrasound, ultrasound-guided fine-needle aspiration cytology, ultrasound-guided fine-needle aspiration biopsy, single photon emission computed tomography, positron emission tomography, radioimmunoscintigraphy).[5,7,17,29,35,38,40,48–51,53,54,56–59,64]

In general, the primary histologic diagnosis in a patient with a laryngeal mass clinically suggestive of a malignancy will be presumed initially to be a squamous cell carcinoma until biopsy results are available; however, it should be borne in mind that approximately 10% of malignant neoplasms of the larynx ultimately prove to be tumors of a different histology. If the tumor is not a squamous cell carcinoma, what kind of neck treatment should be applied when it is stage N0?

The designation N0 neck is generally assumed to refer to the clinically negative neck in cases of primary squamous cell cancer. In its broadest sense, however, 'cancer' is a word which may be employed to describe many different histologic tumor types with a different prognosis and distinct impact on patient survival.[27] Discussions of cervical metastases often do not consider different types of laryngeal cancer, despite the fact that each histologic type of laryngeal cancer possesses its own distinctive natural history. This chapter discusses the treatment of the N0 neck in a variety of uncommon primary malignancies of the larynx (including both uncommon epithelial tumors as well as mesenchymal tumors), considering the biologic behavior and propensity to metastasize to regional lymph nodes of different epithelial and mesenchymal neoplasms.

Verrucous carcinoma

This tumor is characterized by slow growth and a relatively indolent course. Regional lymph node and distant metastases from laryngeal verrucous carcinoma have not been reported to date.[4,16] Any kind of neck dissection is therefore not indicated, even when enlarged and tender lymph nodes can be palpated. In fact, histologic examination of these nodes has revealed only an inflammatory reaction.[13,37] Radiotherapy is far less effective than surgery because this tumor, though not

*This chapter has been recently published as an article review and has been reproduced with minor changes and with the permission of the Editor of the *Journal of Laryngology and Otology*.

radio-resistant, is less radio-sensitive than conventional squamous carcinoma.[22] The prognosis is excellent.[44]

Papillary squamous cell carcinoma

This tumor is an uncommon, distinct and little-recognized variant of squamous cell carcinoma. It generally has a better prognosis than that of conventional squamous cell carcinoma.[55] Ishiyama *et al.*[33] believe that patients with lesions in stage T3 or greater should undergo a prophylactic neck dissection, in consideration of the high rate of neck metastasis.

Spindle cell carcinoma

There is no significant difference in clinical behavior between laryngeal spindle cell carcinoma and conventional squamous cell carcinoma.[32,43] Considering that the same treatment policy is advocated for both lesions, there is consensus to treat surgically the N0 neck in laryngeal spindle cell carcinoma, if the primary lesion is surgically treated.

Basaloid squamous cell carcinoma

This tumor has an aggressive biologic behavior and neck dissection is recommended because of the high likelihood of cervical lymph node metastases.[23]

Lymphoepithelial carcinoma

The tumor is radio-responsive and radiotherapy is appropriate initial locoregional therapy for patients with this disease.[28] Neck dissection is not indicated. Surgery should be reserved for patients who have persistent lymph node disease 6 weeks after completing radiotherapy.[9]

Carcinoid tumor

Neck dissection is not indicated since the likelihood of metastases is very low.[11,25]

Atypical carcinoid

Neck dissection is advisable in all cases of atypical carcinoid because of the high likelihood of cervical lymph node metastases, as well as the high incidence of regional node involvement during the course of this disease.[25,30,39]

Small cell neuroendocrine carcinoma

Neck dissection does not appear necessary, in view of the fact that the treatment of choice is the combination of chemotherapy and radiotherapy.[12]

Paraganglioma

Any kind of neck dissection is not indicated in laryngeal paraganglioma because this tumor is almost always benign.[25] Essentially, all reported cases of aggressive and metastasizing malignant paraganglioma of the larynx were actually atypical carcinoids.[2,19] The presence of a neck mass might be indicative of a metachronous carotid body paraganglioma. The possibility of multicentric paraganglioma should be considered before concluding that a given tumor has metastasized.[26]

Melanoma

Neck dissection is not usually recommended for malignant melanoma[10] because the incidence of cervical lymph node metastases is considered low.[46] Therapeutic neck dissection is indicated for involved lymph nodes in patients with no evidence of distant metastatic disease. Lymph node metastases usually indicate an advanced and uncontrolled or uncontrollable neoplasm[13] and the presence of metastatic disease generally portends a rapidly fatal outcome.[60]

Mucoepidermoid carcinoma

The tumor may metastasize to cervical lymph nodes and visceral metastases may also occur, particularly in the lung. Neck dissection is indicated in particular in high-grade mucoepidermoid carcinomas.

Adenoid cystic carcinoma

Any kind of neck dissection is not indicated in this tumor because regional metastases to the cervical lymph nodes are extremely rare. Ferlito *et al.*[18] consider that the lymph nodes are reached by direct extension of the lesion and that true embolic lymph node metastases are exceptional. Conversely, distant metastases may be detected (in the lung, liver, bones, brain) in the terminal stage. A cervical mass is not always a lymph node secondary, as it may be a recurrence or persistence of the primary tumor.[15,18] Occasionally, a metastasis from a basaloid squamous cell carcinoma may be mistaken for an adenoid cystic carcinoma.[23]

Adenosquamous carcinoma

This tumor is considered as a highly malignant neoplasm and neck dissection is indicated because of the high frequency of regional metastases.

Fibrosarcoma

The bloodstream is the usual route for the spread for fibrosarcomas, which are much less commonly encountered tumor types than were once thought.[20] Examples of pure laryngeal fibrosarcoma are exceedingly rare[14] and regional lymph node metastases are rarer still, making any kind of neck dissection unnecessary.[20]

Malignant fibrous histiocytoma

Neck dissection is not justified, considering that lymph node metastases are rare in this condition.[24]

Liposarcoma

To date, none of the reported liposarcomas of the larynx has metastasized to the lymph nodes,[36a,61] so any kind of neck dissection is not indicated.

Leiomyosarcoma

Neck dissection is not indicated because metastases from this tumor are almost always hematogenous and usually go to the lungs, followed in order of frequency by the liver and skeleton,[3] whereas the incidence of metastases to cervical lymph nodes is low.[36]

Rhabdomyosarcoma

All histologic variants of rhabdomyosarcoma (embryonal, botryoid, alveolar and pleomorphic) have been described in the larynx,[3] but about 65–75% are of embryonal and/or botryoid type. Multimodality regimens with a combination of non-radical surgery, radiation and multi-agent chemotherapy have markedly improved the survival of patients with embryonal, botryoid and alveolar rhabdomyosarcomas. In these cases, elective neck dissection is not indicated because of the low incidence of cervical metastases, and because of the fact that regional control is excellent with adjuvant chemotherapy and radiation.[62] Neck dissection is not indicated for pleomorphic rhabdomyosarcoma either, since this would represent an overtreatment.[6] In fact, metastatic lymph node involvement has only been reported in one case.[63]

Hemangiopericytoma

Any kind of neck dissection does not appear indicated because metastasis in laryngeal hemangiopericytoma has only been reported in one case and the secondary site was not specified.[52]

Synovial sarcoma

No lymph node metastases have been described in any of the reported cases of laryngeal synovial sarcoma and is quite exceptional in hypopharyngeal lesions so any kind of neck dissection is unnecessary.[1,8]

Chondrosarcoma

Approximately 600 cases of chondrosarcomas of the larynx have been documented to date[47] and only 13 of the patients had neck metastases.[42,47] Cervical metastases are rare, and neck dissection is not consequently mandatory, except when clinically suspicious lymph nodes are present.[31,41]

Lymphomas

Radiotherapy is considered to be the treatment of choice when the lesion has not involved extranodal sites (solitary laryngeal lymphomas). Neck dissection is not indicated.[34]

Table 48.1 Indications for neck dissection according to oncotype in the treatment of the 'clinically negative' neck in unusual laryngeal tumors

Laryngeal tumor	*Is neck dissection indicated?*
Verrucous squamous cell carcinoma	No
Papillary squamous cell carcinoma	Yes
Spindle cell carcinoma	Yes
Basaloid squamous cell carcinoma	Yes
Lymphoepithelial carcinoma	No
Carcinoid tumor	No
Atypical carcinoid	Yes
Small cell neuroendocrine carcinoma	No
Paraganglioma	No
Melanoma	No
Mucoepidermoid carcinoma	Yes
Adenoid cystic carcinoma	No
Adenosquamous carcinoma	Yes
Fibrosarcoma	No
Malignant fibrous histiocytoma	No
Liposarcoma	No
Leiomyosarcoma	No
Rhabdomyosarcoma	No
Hemangiopericytoma	No
Synovial sarcoma	No
Chondrosarcoma	No
Lymphomas	No

Other malignant tumors have been reported in the larynx, i.e. salivary duct carcinoma, epithelial-myoepithelial carcinoma, clear cell carcinoma, acinic cell carcinoma, carcinoma in pleomorphic adenoma, adenoid squamous cell carcinoma, sebaceous carcinoma, giant cell carcinoma, malignant myoepithelioma, osteosarcoma, angiosarcoma, Kaposi sarcoma, Ewing sarcoma, primitive neuroectodermal tumor, malignant granular cell tumor, malignant mesenchymoma, malignant nerve sheath tumor, etc. The behavior of these neoplasms in this particular location is difficult to assess accurately in view of their rarity.

Before performing a neck dissection, it is important to understand the natural history of a specific phenotype, so that any kind of neck dissection is not performed in cancers which never metastasize to cervical lymph nodes (i.e. verrucous squamous cell carcinoma, etc.), but rather will be held in reserve for use in those cancers with a well established propensity for regional spread (i.e. basaloid squamous cell carcinoma, atypical carcinoid, etc.).

Table 48.1 summarizes the indications for neck dissection in the treatment of the clinically negative neck in unusual tumors of the larynx.

Cervical lymphadenopathy may be etiologically unrelated to metastatic disease in laryngeal cancer patients[17] and the clinician should always consider this possibility. Dual lymph node pathologies sometimes exist.[21,45]

References

1. Amble FR, Olsen KD, Nascimento AG, Foote RL. Head and neck synovial cell sarcoma. *Otolaryngol Head Neck Surg* 1992; **107:** 631–7.
2. Barnes L. Paraganglioma of the larynx. A critical review of the literature. *ORL J Otorhinolaryngol Relat Spec* 1991; **53:** 220–34.
3. Barnes L, Ferlito A. Soft tissue neoplasms. In: Ferlito A, ed. *Neoplasms of the Larynx*. Edinburgh: Churchill Livingstone, 1993: 265–304.
4. Becker M, Moulin G, Kurt A-M *et al.* Atypical squamous cell carcinoma of the larynx and hypopharynx: radiologic features and pathological correlation. *Eur Radiol* 1998; **8:** 1541–51.
5. Braams JW, Pruim J, Freling NJM *et al.* Detection of lymph node metastases of squamous-cell cancer of the head and neck with FDG-PET and MRI. *J Nucl Med* 1995; **36:** 211–16.
6. Da Mosto MC, Marchiori C, Rinaldo A, Ferlito A. Laryngeal pleomorphic rhabdomyosarcoma. A critical review of the literature. *Ann Otol Rhinol Laryngol* 1996; **105:** 289–94.
7. de Bree R, Roos JC, Quak JJ *et al.* Clinical imaging of head and neck cancer with technetium-99m-labelled monoclonal antibody E48 IgG or F(ab')2. *J Nucl Med* 1994; **35:** 775–83.
8. Dei Tos A, Dal Cin P, Sciot R *et al.* Synovial sarcoma of the larynx and hypopharynx. *Ann Otol Rhinol Laryngol* 1998; **107:** 1080–5.
9. Dubey P, Ha CS, Ang KK *et al.* Nonnasopharyngeal lymphoepithelioma of the head and neck. *Cancer* 1998; **82:** 1556–62.
10. Duwel V, Michielssen P. Primary malignant melanoma of the larynx. A case report. *Acta Otorhinolaryngol Belg* 1996; **50:** 47–9.
11. El-Naggar AK, Batsakis JG. Carcinoid tumor of the larynx. A critical review of the literature. *ORL J Otorhinolaryngol Relat Spec* 1991; **53:** 188–93.
12. Ferlito A. Diagnosis and treatment of small cell carcinoma of the larynx: a critical review. *Ann Otol Rhinol Laryngol* 1986; **95:** 590–600.
13. Ferlito A. Malignant laryngeal epithelial tumors and lymph node involvement: therapeutic and prognostic considerations. *Ann Otol Rhinol Laryngol* 1987; **96:** 542–8.
14. Ferlito A. Laryngeal fibrosarcoma: an over-diagnosed tumor. *ORL J Otorhinolaryngol Relat Spec* 1990; **52:** 194–5.
15. Ferlito A, Caruso G. Biological behaviour of laryngeal adenoid cystic carcinoma. Therapeutic considerations. *ORL J Otorhinolaryngol Relat Spec* 1983; **45:** 245–56.
16. Ferlito A, Recher G. Ackerman's tumor (or verrucous carcinoma) of the larynx. A clinicopathological study of 77 cases. *Cancer* 1980; **46:** 1617–30.
17. Ferlito A, Silver CE. Neck dissection. In: Silver CE, Ferlito A, eds. *Surgery for Cancer of the Larynx and Related Structures*, 2nd edn. Philadelphia: Saunders, 1996: 299–324.
18. Ferlito A, Barnes L, Myers EN. Neck dissection for laryngeal adenoid cystic carcinoma: is it indicated? *Ann Otol Rhinol Laryngol* 1990; **99:** 277–80.
19. Ferlito A, Barnes L, Wenig BM. Identification, classification, treatment, and prognosis of laryngeal paraganglioma. Review of the literature and eight new cases. *Ann Otol Rhinol Laryngol* 1994; **103:** 525–36.
20. Ferlito A, Nicolai P, Barion U. Critical comments on laryngeal fibrosarcoma. *Acta Otorhinolaryngol Belg* 1983; **37:** 918–25.
21. Ferlito A, Recher G, Visonà A. Laryngeal cancer metastatic to lymph nodes with lymphocytic leukaemia. *J Laryngol Otol* 1986; **100:** 233–7.
22. Ferlito A, Rinaldo A, Mannarà GM. Is primary radiotherapy an appropriate option for the treatment of verrucous carcinoma of the head and neck? *J Laryngol Otol* 1998; **112:** 132–9.
23. Ferlito A, Altavilla G, Rinaldo A, Doglioni C. Basaloid squamous cell carcinoma of the larynx and hypopharynx. *Ann Otol Rhinol Laryngol* 1997; **106:** 1024–35.
24. Ferlito A, Nicolai P, Recher G, Narne S. Primary laryngeal malignant fibrous histiocytoma. Review of the literature and report of seven cases. *Laryngoscope* 1983; **93:** 1351–8.
25. Ferlito A, Barnes L, Rinaldo A, Gnepp DR, Milroy CM. A review of neuroendocrine neoplasms of the larynx: update on diagnosis and treatment. *J Laryngol Otol* 1998; **112:** 827–34.
26. Ferlito A, Milroy CM, Wenig BM, Barnes L, Silver CE. Laryngeal paraganglioma versus atypical carcinoid tumor. *Ann Otol Rhinol Laryngol* 1995; **104:** 78–83.
27. Ferlito A, Rinaldo A, Devaney KO, Devaney SL, Milroy CM. Impact of phenotype on treatment and prognosis of laryngeal malignancies. *J Laryngol Otol* 1998; **112:** 710–14.
28. Ferlito A, Weiss LM, Rinaldo A *et al.* Lympho-epithelial carcinoma of the larynx, hypopharynx, and trachea. *Ann Otol Rhinol Laryngol* 1997; **106:** 437–44.
29. Fielding LP. Prognostic factor development. An important caution from a small study. *Cancer* 1997; **80:** 1363–5.
30. Goldman NC, Katibah GM, Medina J. Carcinoid tumors of the larynx. *Ear Nose Throat J* 1985; **64:** 130–4.
31. Gripp S, Pape H, Schmitt G. Chondrosarcoma of the larynx. The role of radiotherapy revisited – a case report and review of the literature. *Cancer* 1998; **82:** 108–15.
32. Hellquist HH, Olofsson J. Spindle cell carcinoma of the larynx. *APMIS* 1989; **97:** 1103–13.
33. Ishiyama A, Eversole LR, Ross DA *et al.* Papillary squamous neoplasms of the head and neck. *Laryngoscope* 1994; **104:** 1446–52.
34. Kato S, Sakura M, Takooda S, Sakurai M, Izumo T. Primary non-Hodgkin's lymphoma of the larynx. *J Laryngol Otol* 1997; **111:** 571–4.
35. Lenz M, Kersting-Sommerhoff B, Gross M. Diagnosis and treatment of the N0 neck in carcinomas of the upper aerodigestive tract: current status of diagnostic procedures. *Eur Arch Otorhinolaryngol* 1993; **250:** 432–8.
36. Lippert BM, Schlüter E, Claassen H, Werner JA. Leiomyosarcoma of the larynx. *Eur Arch Otorhinolaryngol* 1997; **254:** 466–9.

36a. Mandell DL, Brandwein MS, Woo P, Som PM, Biller HF, Urken ML. Upper aerodigestive tract liposarcoma: report on four cases and literature review. *Laryngoscope* 1999; **109:** 1245–52.

37. McCaffrey TV, Witte M, Ferguson MT. Verrucous carcinoma of the larynx. *Ann Otol Rhinol Laryngol* 1998; **107:** 391–5.
38. Mendelsohn MS, Shulman HS, Noyek AM. Diagnostic imaging. In: Ferlito A, ed. *Neoplasms of the Larynx.* Edinburgh: Churchill Livingstone, 1993: 401–23.
39. Moisa II, Silver CE. Treatment of neuroendocrine neoplasms of the larynx. *ORL J Otorhinolaryngol Relat Spec* 1991; **53:** 259–64.
40. Myers LL, Wax MK, Nabi H, Simpson GT, Lamonica D. Positron emission tomography in the evaluation of the N0 neck. *Laryngoscope* 1998; **108:** 232–6.
41. Nicolai P, Ferlito A, Sasaki CT, Kirchner JA. Laryngeal chondrosarcoma: incidence, pathology, biological behavior, and treatment. *Ann Otol Rhinol Laryngol* 1990; **99:** 515–23.
42. Nicolai P, Caruso G, Redaelli de Zinis LO *et al.* Regional and distant metastases in laryngeal and hypopharyngeal sarcomas. *Ann Otol Rhinol Laryngol* 1998; **107:** 540–6.
43. Olsen KD, Lewis JE, Suman VJ. Spindle cell carcinoma of the larynx and hypopharynx. *Otolaryngol Head Neck Surg* 1997; **116:** 47–52.
44. Orvidas LJ, Olsen KD, Lewis JE, Suman VJ. Verrucous carcinoma of the larynx: a review of 53 patients. *Head Neck* 1998; **20:** 197–203.
45. Pacheco-Ojeda L, Micheau C, Luboinski B *et al.* Squamous cell carcinoma of the upper aerodigestive tract associated with well-differentiated carcinoma of the thyroid gland. *Laryngoscope* 1991; **101:** 421–4.
46. Panje WJ, Moran WJ. Melanoma of the upper aerodigestive tract. A review of 21 cases. *Head Neck Surg* 1986; **8:** 309–12.
47. Rinaldo A, Howard DJ, Ferlito A. Laryngeal chondrosarcoma: a 24-year experience at The Royal National Throat, Nose and Ear Hospital. *Acta Otolaryngol (Stockh)* 2000; in press.
48. Schuller DE, Bier-Laning CM. Laryngeal carcinoma nodal metastases and their management. *Otolaryngol Clin North Am* 1997; **30:** 167–77.
49. Snow GB, Patel P, Leemans CR, Tiwari R. Management of cervical lymph nodes in patients with head and neck cancer. *Eur Arch Otorhinolaryngol* 1992; **249:** 187–94.
50. Steiner W, Hommerich CP. Diagnosis and treatment of the N0 neck of carcinomas of the upper aerodigestive tract. Report of an International Symposium, Göttingen, Germany, 1992. *Eur Arch Otorhinolaryngol* 1993; **250:** 450–6.
51. Stern WBR, Silver CE, Zeifer BA, Persky MS, Heller KS. Computed tomography of the clinically negative neck. *Head Neck* 1990; **12:** 109–13.
52. Stout AP. Tumors featuring pericytes: glomus tumor and hemangiopericytoma. *Lab Invest* 1956; **5:** 217–33.
53. Takes RP, Baatenburg de Jong RJ, Schuuring E *et al.* Markers for assessment of nodal metastasis in laryngeal carcinoma. *Arch Otolaryngol Head Neck Surg* 1997; **123:** 412–19.
54. Takes RP, Knegt P, Manni JJ *et al.* Regional metastasis in head and neck squamous cell cancer: the value of ultrasound with UGFNAB revised. *Fourth International Conference on Head and Neck Cancer, Toronto* 1996: Abstract no. 307, p. 135.
55. Thompson LDR, Wenig BM, Heffner DK, Gnepp DR. Exophytic and papillary squamous cell carcinomas of the larynx: a clinicopathologic series of 104 cases. *Otolaryngol Head Neck Surg* 1999; **120:** 718–24.
56. van den Brekel MWM, Stel HV, Castelijns JA, Croll GA, Snow GB. Lymph node staging in patients with clinically negative neck examinations by ultrasound and ultrasound-guided aspiration cytology. *Am J Surg* 1991; **162:** 362–6.
57. van den Brekel MWM, Stel HV, van der Valk P, van der Waal I, Meyer CJLM, Snow GB. Micrometastases from squamous cell carcinoma in neck dissection specimens. *Eur Arch Otorhinolaryngol* 1992; **249:** 349–53.
58. van den Brekel MWM, van der Waal I, Meijer CJLM, Freeman JL, Castelijns JA, Snow GB. The incidence of micrometastases in neck dissection specimens obtained from elective neck dissections. *Laryngoscope* 1996; **106:** 987–91.
59. van den Brekel MWM, Stel HV, Castelijns JA *et al.* Cervical lymph node metastasis: assessment of radiologic criteria. *Radiology* 1990; **177:** 379–84.
60. Wenig BM. Laryngeal mucosal malignant melanoma. A clinicopathologic, immunohistochemical, and ultrastructural study of four patients and a review of the literature. *Cancer* 1995; **75:** 1568–77.
61. Wenig BM, Nakayama M. Adipose tissue neoplasms. In: Ferlito A, ed. *Surgical Pathology of Laryngeal Neoplasms.* London: Chapman and Hall, 1996: 375–92.
62. Wharam MD, Beltangady MS, Heyn RM *et al.* Pediatric orofacial and laryngopharyngeal rhabdomyosarcoma. An intergroup rhabdomyosarcoma study report. *Arch Otolaryngol Head Neck Surg* 1987; **113:** 1225–7.
63. Wilhelm H-J, Dietz R, Schätzle W. Primäre maligne mesenchymale Tumoren im Kopf-Hals-Bereich. Zur Problematik ihrer Diagnose und Therapie. *Laryngorhinootologie* 1980; **59:** 211–20.
64. Yamamoto N, Kato Y, Yanagisawa A, Ohta H, Takahashi T, Kitagawa T. Predictive value of genetic diagnosis for cancer micrometastasis. Histologic and experimental appraisal. *Cancer* 1997; **80:** 1393–8.

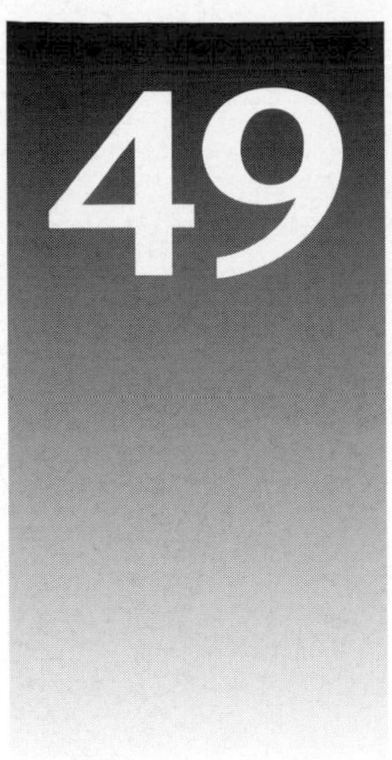

Laser surgery in laryngeal diseases

Lou Reinisch, C Gaelyn Garrett
and Robert H Ossoff

Introduction

History of the laser

In 1917, Einstein's (Fig 49.1) paper in the *Physikalische Zeit*, 'Zur Quanten Theorie der Strahlung' was the first discussion of the basic principle of the laser, stimulated emission.[32] Yet it was not until 1954 that the first microwave laser, a maser, was built.[104] In May of 1960, Theodore Maiman at Hughes Aircraft Co. made the first visible light laser.[63] He used a ruby as the laser medium and the laser produced pulses of light in the red region of the spectrum at 694 nm. Lasers quickly moved from a laboratory instrument to the clinic. In 1962, Leon Goldman consulted with Zaret to study the occupational hazards of the laser.[42,133] At the same time, Zweng *et al.* were using ruby lasers on human patients for eye care.[134] In 1964, Leon Goldman developed a medical laser laboratory to look not only at the hazards of the laser, but also to consider the potential uses of the laser in medicine.

Otolaryngologists–head and neck surgeons realized the potential of the laser very early. In fact, in the early 1960s they considered different methods to use pulsed laser systems in the middle ear and labyrinth.[48,103] At approximately the same time, Geza Jako began studying the effects of laser energy on human vocal folds.[49] His first attempts at tissue ablation were made with the neodymium doped glass laser, with a wavelength of 1.06 µm. The absorption characteristics of the tissue were not suitable for precise excision with this wavelength of light. In 1965, Strully and Yahr tried to enhance the absorption of the tissue by painting the tissue with a copper sulfate solution.[119] The results were still unsatisfactory. They still needed higher intensity levels, could produce only small lesions, and were left with significant destruction of the tissue next to the lesion.

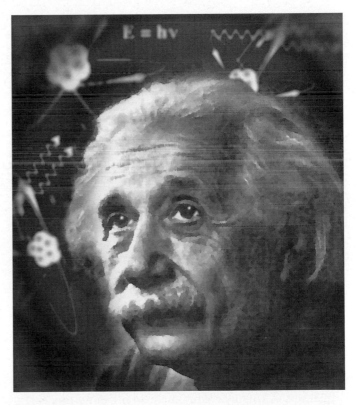

Figure 49.1 *Albert Einstein; his theory of stimulated emission is the basis of the laser.*

In 1965, the carbon dioxide (CO_2) laser was developed. Two years later, in 1967, Polanyi tested the CO_2 laser in human cadaver larynges and was encouraged by the ability to produce discrete wounds. These results spurred the development of an endoscopic delivery system so the laser could be tested *in vivo*.[14,15,95] Additional refinements

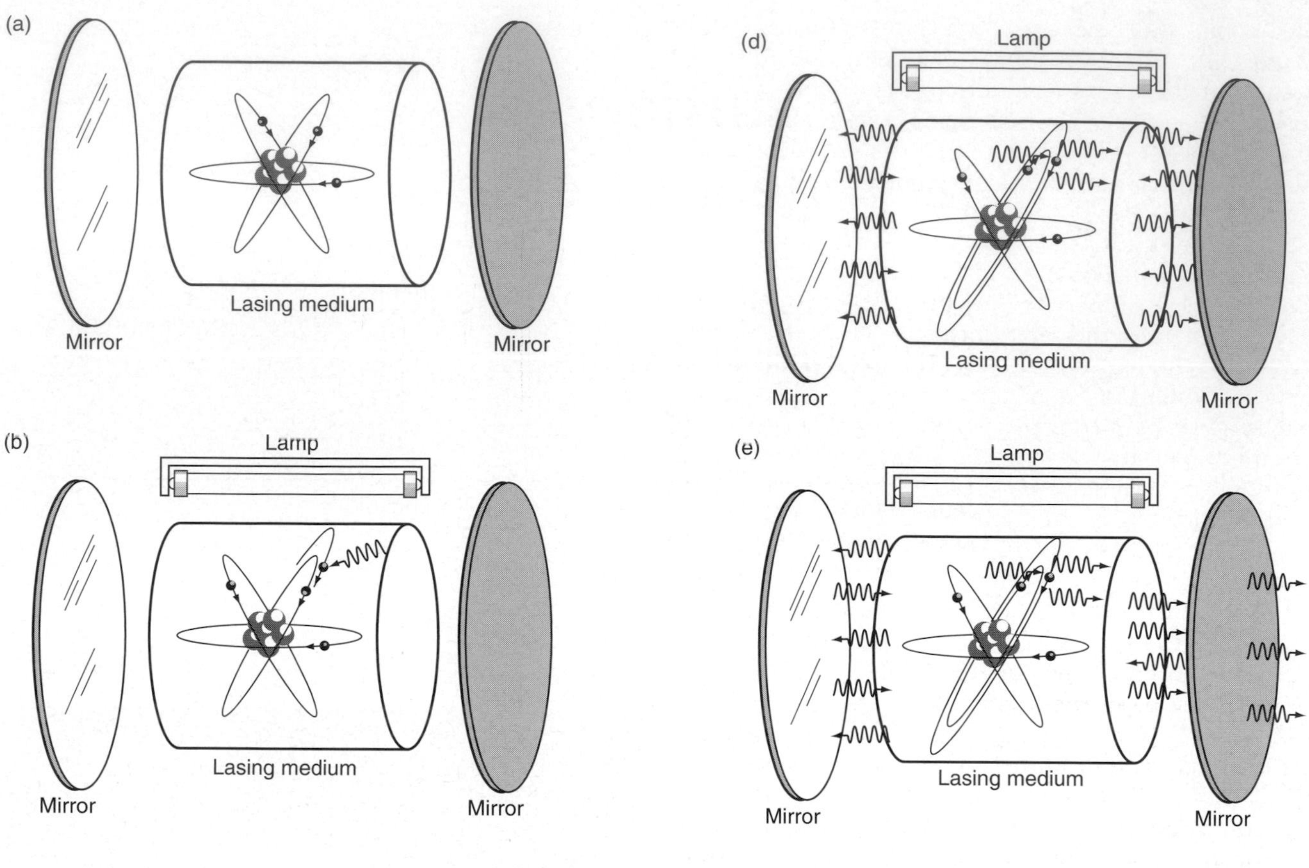

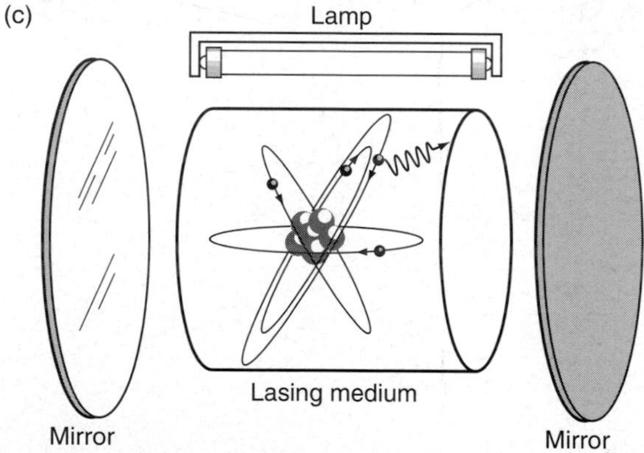

Figure 49.2 *(a) The lasing medium placed between two parallel mirrors. The atoms of the medium are schematically shown in the low energy state. (b) The lasing medium being excited by the lamp. The atoms of the medium are schematically shown absorbing a wave of light and the electron moving to a higher energy level. (c) The lasing medium spontaneously decaying from the higher energy state to the lower energy state. Light is emitted in random directions during this process. (d) The lasing medium with stimulated emission. The light trapped between the mirrors can cause atoms in the excited state to decay to the lower energy state and emit light. (e) The light is emitted from the laser cavity by making one of the mirrors partially reflecting.*

lead to the development of an endoscopic delivery system designed to be coupled with the binocular microscope for binocular microlaryngoscopy. In 1972, Jako reported the initial use of this new equipment in a canine model.[49,116] The first human use of the CO_2 laser in otolaryngology was to ablate vocal fold papillomatosis.[94,112] It was from this point that lasers were used in otolaryngology–head and neck surgery, and the use has continued to spread.

Description of the laser

Laser is an acronym that stands for '*l*ight *a*mplification by the *s*timulated *e*mission of *r*adiation'. The acronym describes the operation of the lasers. There are three essential elements to a laser.[38] The first element is the lasing medium. In the first laser, the lasing medium was a ruby crystal.[63] There also needs to be an excitation source. In the first laser made, the excitation source was a flash lamp, similar to the flash from a camera. Finally, one needs two mirrors to provide the optical feedback.

What happens in the lasing process can be explained in the following series of steps as shown in Fig 49.2. First the lasing medium (e.g. a ruby crystal) is placed in a resonant cavity (see Fig 49.2a). The resonant cavity can be two mirrors precisely aligned parallel to one another. The atoms or molecules in the lasing medium are in a low energy state. Once the lasing medium is in place, it is excited. Lasers can be excited with flash lamps, continuous lamps, other lasers, or electrical current. The atoms or molecules in the lasing medium are excited to a higher energy state (see Fig 49.2b). The atoms or molecules in the excited state can decay back to the lower energy state in a process termed 'spontaneous emission' (see Fig 49.2c). When the atom or molecule decays to the ground state, it emits or gives up the energy that it absorbed. This emitted energy can be light. The emission is at random and is in all directions and some of the emission can be reflected back into the laser medium. When the light reflected by the mirror reenters the laser medium, it stimulates additional radiation. As the light travels through the lasing medium, when it finds a molecule or an atom in an excited state it will tickle or stimulate that atom to release its energy and make the transition to the ground state (see Fig 49.2d). So one wave of light becomes two waves of light. Both of these waves of light continue to propagate through the lasing medium. If the light waves are incident upon additional atoms in the lasing medium, there is additional stimulated emission. To achieve a net amplification of the light, more atoms or molecules must be in the excited state than those in the ground state. This is termed a 'population inversion'.

The laser light is transmitted out of the resonant cavity by making one of the mirrors partially reflecting (see Fig 49.2e). A fraction of the light leaks out of the laser cavity while the remaining fraction of the light stays in the cavity to maintain the lasing process. The lasing process continues in the resonant cavity as long as the excitation source keeps the molecules or atoms in the laser medium excited.

Laser properties

Monochromatic

What makes a laser a laser and distinct from a flashlight? Laser light has four intrinsic properties. The first property is the light is monochromatic. First consider a tungsten lamp, for instance, a typical desk lamp. When the light from the lamp is put through a prism and incident on the wall, one sees a beautiful rainbow with each of the colors of the spectrum (see Fig 49.3a). On the other hand, if a laser light passes through a prism, there would not be a rainbow of colors projected on the wall. Instead, one or a few separate, distinct lines would appear on the wall. Each line is a single, different color.

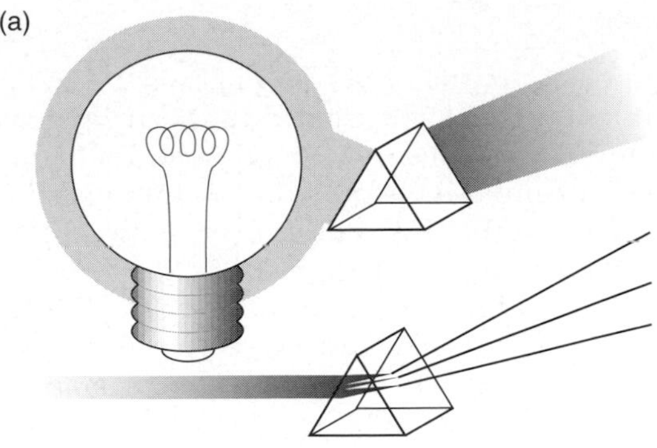

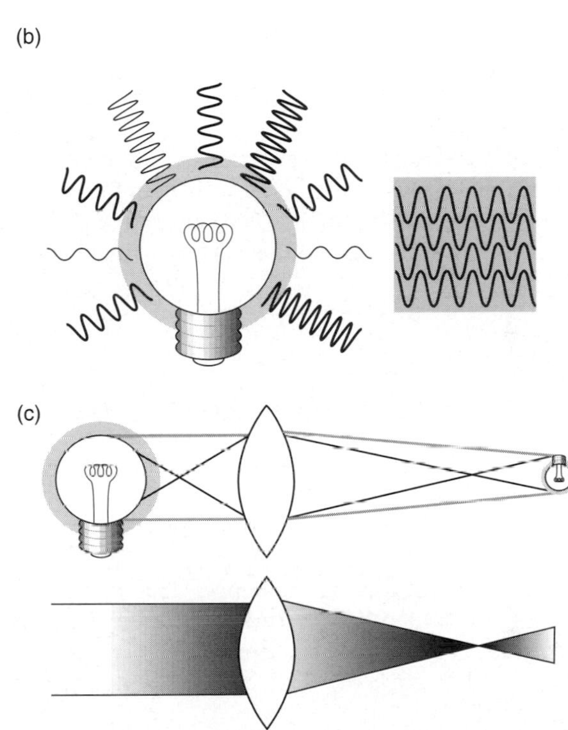

Figure 49.3 *(a) The light from a tungsten lamp will show a continuous spectrum of colors after being passed through a prism. A laser, on the other hand, will show separate, discrete colors after passing through a prism. (b) The light emitted from a tungsten lamp has a variety of wavelengths traveling in different directions. Laser light is single wavelengths, all traveling in the same direction, and all moving up and down in phase. (c) The light from the tungsten lamp can be focused to an image of the bulb.*

Coherent

Laser light is coherent. This property is used very often in physics and chemistry and not very often in medicine. The coherence of laser light means that all the waves 'march in step'. In other words, all the waves go up and down at the same time. The coherence is due to the stimulated emission process. Not only is the light stimulated to be emitted in the same direction and with the same wavelength, but it also is emitted in phase with all the other light (see Fig 49.3b). There are experimental measurements of the tympanic membrane motion or motion of the vocal folds using interferometric techniques (G Gardner, personal communication).[23] These novel applications do make use of the coherence property of laser light.

Collimated

The third characteristic of the laser light is the collimated nature of the light. Light from a tungsten light bulb is emitted in all directions. If a lens is used, the light from the tungsten lamp can be focused to an image of the bulb (see Fig 49.3c). If the lens is placed very close to the light bulb to collect a large fraction of the light, the image will be very large. To focus the light to a very small image (or small spot size), the lens must be very far from the light bulb. With the lens very far from the light bulb, only a small fraction of the light emitted from the bulb is collected by the lens. On the other hand, a laser produces a pencil beam of light that is very nearly parallel. If the parallel laser light is focused through a lens, it will focus down to a 'diffraction limited spot' – or the smallest possible spot. Also, no matter how far the lens is placed from the laser, it is relatively easy to collect all the parallel laser beam with the lens.

The collimated nature of laser light is the crucial aspect of lasers that is used in medicine. It is being able to focus the light to the minimum spot size and have the highest energy density that allows the surgeon to ablate tissue with light.

High power

The last characteristic of laser light is the high power of the light. When dealing with power, one should always remember to use power density or irradiance, which is the intensity of the laser divided by the area of the beam. The normal units for irradiance are watts per square centimeter (W/cm^2). Besides the irradiance, one needs to know the energy density or the laser fluence. The fluence is the irradiance multiplied by the exposure time. The units of fluence are typically watts times seconds per square centimeter ($W\ s/cm^2$) or, equivalently, joules per square centimeter (J/cm^2).

$$\text{Irradiance} = \text{intensity/area} : W/cm^2$$

$$\text{Fluence} = (\text{intensity} \times \text{time})/\text{area} : W\ s/cm^2 = J/cm^2$$

The large irradiance possible with laser light is important in medicine, because it is the large irradiance that allows the surgeon to use the laser for ablation. However, one should be mindful that the absolute intensity (typically tens of watts) from the laser is not that large. It is the ability to focus the laser beam to a small point and achieve a large irradiance that is important.

Other parameters

There are still many aspects that can vary with each laser. Laser light can either be continuous wave (CW) or can be pulsed. There also are various materials used in lasers. Each laser material emits at specific wavelength(s). There are solid materials, such as the ruby, that lases in the red part of the spectrum, 0.694 microns (μm, or 694 nm), the neodymium doped yttrium-aluminum-garnet crystal (Nd:YAG) at 1.064 μm in the near-infrared, the holmium doped YAG (Ho:YAG) at about 2.1 μm and the erbium doped YAG (Er:YAG) at 2.94 μm. There are also gas lasers. An example of a gas laser is the CO_2 laser at 10.6 μm in the mid-infrared part of the spectrum. There are also the argon ion (Ar^+) laser in the blue-green region of the spectrum with strong lines at 0.514 and 0.488 μm (or 514 and 488 nm), the krypton ion (Kr^+) in the orange region of the spectrum with a strong line at 0.647 μm (647 nm), the helium-neon (HeNe) aiming laser at 0.633 μm (633 nm), and the excimer lasers, such as the krypton fluoride at 0.248 μm (248 nm) and the argon fluoride laser at 0.193 μm (193 nm). Both these excimer lasers are in the ultraviolet region of the spectrum. In addition, there are other laser materials, such as gallium-arsenide (the material in diode lasers). The diode lasers are commonly used in laser pointers and emit in the red to near-infrared region of the spectrum (0.650–0.980 μm). There are also laser dyes. There are many different dyes, and they can be tuned throughout the visible and near ultraviolet region of the spectrum.

Laser light delivery

Light can be delivered by a number of different mechanisms. In this section, each of the mechanisms will be reviewed.

Hand-held lasers

The first mechanism is hand-held lasers. This is becoming more feasible as laser technology is producing smaller and lighter weight lasers, and probably there will be hand-held lasers used routinely in surgery in the very near future.

Articulated arms

Laser light can be delivered by articulated arms. The articulated arm is a very simple but elegant device. There are mirrors placed at 45° to tubes carrying the laser light. The tubes can rotate about the normal axis of the mirrors. The articulated arm is typically used with the CO_2 laser. The arm does have some disadvantages for surgery. Due to the circular hinges, one often must move in an arc to move from point A to point B.

Optical fibers

Laser light can be delivered by an optical fiber. Optical fibers are frequently used with near-infrared and visible lasers. The light is trapped in the glass and propagates down through the fiber in a process called 'total internal reflection'. Optical fibers can be very small and light in weight. They can be tens of microns in diameter or greater than hundreds of microns in diameter. They transmit high intensities of light with almost no loss. They have two disadvantages:

- The beam is no longer collimated when emitted from the fiber; and
- The light emitted from the fiber is no longer coherent.

Nonetheless, optical fibers are the preferred method for laser light delivery. There has been a push for many years to come up with optical fibers to work in the infrared and that can deliver both the Er:YAG laser and the CO_2 laser light. Some of these fibers are now commercially available.

Transport patient

The fourth method for delivering laser light to the patient is to bring the patient up to the laser. The ophthalmologist has been doing this for quite some time.

Beam profiles

Most commercial lasers produce a beam with a Gaussian profile (see Fig 49.4). This profile is termed the fundamental mode or the TEM_{00} mode of the laser. Manufacturers work very hard to produce the fundamental mode. A laser beam does not have a constant intensity across the beam diameter; instead the intensity peaks at the center of the beam. The peak intensity then falls off with a normal type (or Gaussian type) of distribution. This particular mode of lasing gives the smallest focal point when the beam is focused through a lens.

One can work both in and out of the focal plane of the laser beam. When working with the light in focus, one gets a more direct incision. When working out of the focal plane, one has more of a surface removal of tissue. In diagrams of light being focused by lens, one frequently sees pictures of a cone of light focused down to an infinitely small spot (see, for instance, Fig 49.3c). In reality, light does not focus to an infinitely small spot. This focus to a minimum size, or what is called a 'beam waist', is determined by the focal length of the lens, the laser beam diameter and the wavelength of light. For large focal length lenses, such as the 400 mm objective lens on the surgical microscope for microlaryngeal surgery, the beam waist is quite large (it can be 0.8 mm in diameter). When one uses a hand piece with a 100 mm focal length, there is a much smaller spot size or beam waist (0.1 mm). There is an advantage to a large beam waist. If one has a very large beam waist, the beam is in focus for a relatively large distance. So, the laryngeal surgeon finds the focal length is a bit 'forgiving'. Using a hand piece, on the other hand, one must be extremely careful to keep the laser beam in focus to preserve a specific irradiance.

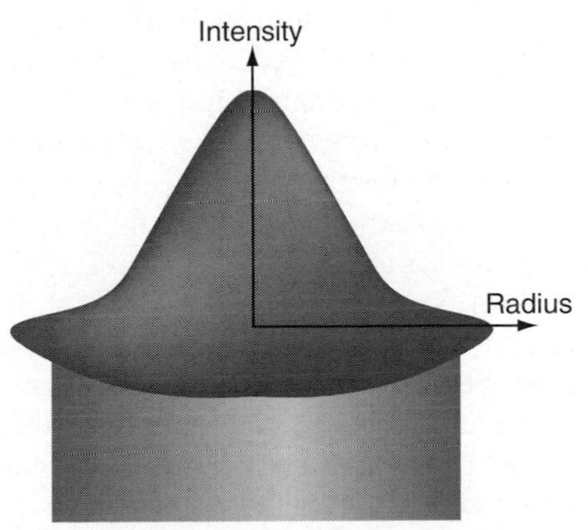

Figure 49.4 *The intensity is not uniform across the diameter of the laser beam. Instead, the intensity follows a normal distribution with a peak at the center.*

Temporal profiles

Lasers can be continuous wave (CW) or pulsed. In pulse duration, the variability is great. Most surgical lasers are CW lasers with shutters. The shutters allow for pulses of 0.01 seconds or longer. Shorter pulses have not been typically used in surgery. However, there is research that indicates lasers with pulses approximately 10 μs long might have an advantage for laser surgery (unpublished data).

Light and tissue interactions

The actual tissue effects produced by the radiant energy of a laser vary with the specific wavelength of the laser used. The interaction of laser energy with living tissue can result from three different processes. First, the laser energy can be absorbed by chromophores within the tissue. The resulting effect can be the production of heat. This is the thermal effect seen in most conventional laser systems in use today. Second, the radiant energy of a laser can stimulate or react with specific molecules within a cell. This reaction can cause a chemical change to occur within the cell. This effect is termed photochemical. An example is the reaction that occurs with injection of a photosensitizing drug into tissue and the biochemical effect that is produced when the drug is activated by the stimulating effect of radiant laser energy. Third, the use of short pulses of high wattage laser energy can disrupt cellular architecture because of the production of sound waves or photoacoustic shock waves.[27] This mechanical disruption of tissue is an example of a nonthermal tissue effect.

Light can interact with tissue in four different mechanisms: transmission, reflection, absorption and scatter. Light is transmitted through tissues with little or no absorption. Some light reflects off the surface of all tissue. The greater the angle of incidence or larger the glancing angle that the light hits the surface, the greater the amount of light that reflects from a surface. The chromophores in tissue will absorb the laser light. Most of the laser energy is then transformed into heat. This increasing heat in the tissue leads to the vaporization of water and then to the ablation of tissue. The scattering does two things:

- It spreads out the beam of light or defocuses a spot of light. This translates into the irradiation of a larger area than anticipated.
- Scattering also limits the depth of penetration by scattering the light backwards as well as in the forward direction.

The ablation process

Photothermal ablation, the most common mechanism of laser incisions, is a straightforward process. The energy of the laser is absorbed by the tissue and changed to heat energy. The tissue heats, and once the temperature passes above 100°C, the water in the tissue starts to vaporize. Once sufficient energy has been added to change the water from a liquid to steam, the tissue is torn open by the expansion of the steam.

In the center of the wound created by a CO_2 laser a volume of tissue is vaporized. Here just a few flakes of carbon debris are noted. Immediately next to this volume is a zone of thermal necrosis measuring approximately 100 μm wide. Next is a volume of thermal conductivity and repair, usually 300–500 μm wide. Small vessels, nerves, and lymphatics are sealed in the zone of thermal necrosis; the minimal operative trauma combined with the vascular seal probably account for the notable absence of postoperative edema characteristic of laser wounds.[72]

Additional damage near the bottom of the crater can be from forward scattered light. The damage around the mouth of the crater can be from the edges of the focused beam with sub-ablation fluence. The nearly isotropic damage is typically from thermal diffusion. In addition, blood vessels can transport heat away from the ablation site, creating cooler locations or locations with less thermal damage.

When the laser beam is focused, it incises tissue in a fashion similar to a sharp blade but with improved hemostasis.[77] Lateral thermal damage from scattered light can be reduced by using infrared lasers. To decrease lateral thermal damage from thermal diffusion, one must ablate the tissue with a very short pulse of light.

There are negative consequences to short laser pulses. If the pulses are too short, the extremely high intensities of the laser can initiate many nonlinear processes, photobleach the sample, and cause damage from the photoacoustic signal that is created when the light is absorbed.

Use of laser in otolaryngology

In otolaryngology–head and neck surgery, the most common use of medical laser is for tissue ablation. The CO_2 laser energy can create intense localized heating sufficient to vaporize both extra- and intracellular water, producing a coagulative necrosis.[35,43,67] Advantages of the laser include:

- The laser can interact remotely with the tissue. It is only necessary to have a line of site (or optical conduit) between the laser and the tissue.
- The laser is gentle in its interaction with tissue when compared to the hammer, mallet, saw or drill. Due to the minimal damage to tissue adjacent to the ablation site, the CO_2 laser is often the laser of choice.

In 1984, Beamis and Shapshay reported on the use of the Nd:YAG laser at 1.06 μm for malignant and vascular lesions in the tracheobronchial tree.[10] Applications of the argon laser, and later yellow pulsed dye lasers to vascular cutaneus lesions have permitted the successful treatment of port-wine stains.[17,92,122] Finally, the argon dye laser for use in photodynamic therapy offers exciting possibilities in the treatment of early or superficially spreading cancers.

Not only has the choice of lasers and the best wavelength for a given application been carefully considered, but the optimal delivery system for each laser and application has also been investigated. The drive for new and better laser delivery systems comes, in part, from the fact that all medical systems have their limitations. The potential for increased morbidity and mortality is due, to some extent, to these limitations. For instance, in otolaryngology–head and neck surgery, the CO_2 laser is commonly used in microlaryngeal surgery. Vocal fold fibrosis results from prolonged or high-intensity exposure to the laser. The excess heat in the larynx can leave a scarred vocal fold when vaporizing normal vocalis muscle.[80]

Type of lasers used in otolaryngology

The Nd:YAG laser

The Nd:YAG laser emits light at 1.06 μm, and this laser has the deepest penetration of the surgical lasers. This laser incision is accompanied by a homogenous zone of thermal coagulation and necrosis that may extend 4 mm from the impact site. The CW light can be delivered through optical fibers. The laser normally does not have any special power requirements and does not need external cooling water.

The primary applications for the Nd:YAG laser in otolaryngology–head and neck surgery include palliation of obstructing tracheobronchial lesions,[11,28,107,124] palliation of obstructing esophageal lesions,[34] photocoagulation of vascular lesions of the head and neck,[97,106] and photocoagulation of lymphatic malformations.[5] Hemorrhage is the most frequent and dangerous complication associated with laser bronchoscopy, and its control is extremely important. Control of hemorrhage is more secure with the Nd:YAG laser because of the deep penetration into tissue. Nd:YAG laser can be used through an open, rigid bronchoscope. Used in this fashion, it allows for multiple distal suction capabilities with concurrent laser application. The rapid removal of tumor fragments and debris helps to prevent hypoxemia. Use of the Nd:YAG laser with a rigid bronchoscope permits ventilatory control of a compromised airway, palpation of the tumor to cartilage interface, use of the bronchoscope tip as a 'cookie cutter', and use of the bronchoscope tip to compress a bleeding tumor bed for temporary hemostasis. The flexible fiberoptic bronchoscope is often used through the open, rigid scope to provide pulmonary toilet and more distal laser application after the major airway is secure.

The Nd:YAG laser has a limited application in intralaryngeal use. Specifically, the increased depth of penetration makes this laser ideal for the treatment of vascular lesions, such as cavernous hemangiomas, where hemostasis and vessel coagulation are the treatment goals.

Due to the penetration depth of the light at 1.06 µm, the Nd:YAG laser is used primarily to photocoagulate tumor masses rapidly at power settings in the upper and lower aerodigestive tract of 15–20 W, exposures of 0.1–1.0 seconds. The laser beam is always applied parallel to the wall of the tracheobronchial tree, whenever possible. The rigid tip of the bronchoscope is used mechanically to separate the devascularized tumor mass from the wall of the tracheobronchial tree.

The selection of patients for Nd:YAG laser bronchoscopy should include a flexible fiberoptic bronchoscopic examination of the tracheobronchial tree and tracheal polytomography or computerized tomography. Patients in whom extrinsic compression of the airway can be demonstrated should be excluded from bronchoscopic laser surgery.

The KTP laser

The potassium titanyl phosphate (KTP or KTP/532) laser emits light at 532 nm (green light) in a quasi-CW mode and can be delivered through optical fibers. The single wavelength of this KTP laser is centered on a moderately strong hemoglobin absorption band. The laser normally does not have any special power requirements and does not require external water to cool the laser. The lasing source is an Nd:YAG laser at 1.06 µm. The Nd:YAG laser rod is continuously pumped with a krypton arc lamp and Q-switched. The 1.06 µm light is frequency doubled by a nonlinear optical process in the potassium titanyl phosphate crystal yielding the 532 nm green light.

The radiant energy from the KTP laser is transmitted through clear aqueous tissues. Certain tissue pigments, such as melanin and hemoglobin, absorb the KTP laser light effectively. The power density chosen for a given application determines the tissue interaction. When low levels of green laser light interact with highly pigmented tissues, a localized coagulation takes place within these tissues. The KTP laser can be selected for procedures requiring precise surgical excision with minimal damage to surrounding tissue, vaporization, or photocoagulation.

The KTP laser light is normally delivered through an optical fiber, which can be used in association with a micromanipulator attached to an operating microscope or free-hand in association with various hand-held delivery probes having several different tip angles. These hand-held probes facilitate use of the KTP laser for functional endoscopic sinus surgery and other intranasal applications,[59] otologic applications[123] and microlaryngeal applications.[7] The optical fiber delivery of the 532 nm laser light can be manipulated through a rigid pediatric bronchoscope as small as 3.0 mm, facilitating lower tracheal and endobronchial lesion treatment in infants and neonates.[126] Examples of hand-held KTP laser applications include tonsillectomy,[51,56,57,61,120] stapedectomy,[9,121] excision of acoustic neuroma[66] and excision of benign and malignant laryngeal lesions.[6] The KTP laser can also be used as an automatic scanning device to treat areas of pigmented dermal lesions, such as port wine stains.[3,64,65]

Special wavelength-specific safety glasses must be worn by the surgeon and all personnel in the operating room. The visible green light from the KTP laser can penetrate into the eye and cause retinal damage. Also, the eyes of the patient must be protected during a laser procedure. Specific protocols for the protection for the patient is covered later in this chapter.

The Ho:YAG laser

In the near-infrared, the holmium:YAG (Ho:YAG) lases at 2.1 µm. This is a newer laser that interacts with tissue in a more precise manner than the Nd:YAG or KTP lasers. The 2.1 µm wavelength can propagate through conventional optical fibers. The technology for these lasers is still evolving. The current lasers normally require 220 V and are air cooled.

The short penetration depth of the laser and the pulse structure has shown great promise in orthopedic surgery. In otolaryngology–head and neck surgery, the Ho:YAG has been considered for facial nerve decompression.[98] Yet, large temperature transients still preclude this procedure. The future applications of this laser will probably involve cartilage reshaping.

Other lasers

Other lasers include the flash-lamp excited dye laser (FEDL). This laser emits light at 585 nm in a pulsed mode. Each pulse is approximately 0.4 ms long. The parameters have been optimized for the selective treatment of vascular lesions with minimal damage to the dermis. The light is delivered through an optical fiber bundle. The laser normally requires 220 V and cooling water.

Recent investigations have considered the diode laser. These lasers operate in the red to near-infrared region of the spectrum (800–980 nm). They are small and require no water for cooling. The lasers operate CW and the light is delivered through an optical fiber. They have been investigated for photodynamic therapy and tissue welding.[70,115]

The CO_2 laser

The work-horse of laser surgery, the CO_2 laser, emits light at 10.6 µm. The invisible laser beam has a coaxial helium-neon laser beam to act as an aiming beam. The light from a CO_2 laser is strongly absorbed by water. Therefore, its energy is well absorbed by all soft tissues that are high in water content. The mid-infrared light at 10.6 μm cannot propagate through glass optical fibers and is normally delivered through an articulated arm. Silver halide optical fibers for the CO_2 laser as well as waveguides have recently been introduced to the market.[2,52,69] The laser energy can be delivered to tissue either through a handpiece for macroscopic surgery or adapted to an operating microscope for microscopic surgery. The universal endoscopic coupler allows for delivery of the laser energy through a rigid bronchoscope.[84,90] Transmission through rigid endoscopes facilitates use of the CO_2 laser for bronchoscopy, laparoscopy and arthroscopy. This laser does not have special electrical requirements and is air-cooled.

The CO_2 laser has become the laser of choice for most microlaryngoscopic applications. The advantages of microscopic control and decreased postoperative edema have made this the instrument of choice for many benign laryngeal diseases, such as for removal of recurrent respiratory papillomatosis. Other applications include subglottic stenosis, webs, granuloma and capillary hemangiomas. Surgery for other benign laryngeal disease processes, such as polyps, nodules, leukoplakia and cysts, may also be performed with the CO_2 laser; however, cold knife excision has been shown to produce equal, if not improved, postoperative results. Surgery in the pediatric group for webs, subglottic stenosis and capillary hemangiomas have all been significantly improved by decreased postoperative edema associated with the CO_2 laser. The decreased postoperative edema is more important in pediatric patients, secondary to a smaller airway.

Microscopic applications

All the laser wavelengths previously discussed may be adapted for use with the binocular operating microscope. The KTP and Nd:YAG lasers may be used with fiberoptic delivery probes that are fed through a suction catheter and used in either a contact or noncontact mode. The CO_2 and KTP laser have the added ability of being delivered by an optical system with a micromanipulator. This allows precise, noncontact delivery at a predetermined focal length.

The current micromanipulators deliver the laser colinear with the optical axis with no parallax error.[88] These micromanipulators have also reduced the spot size from 800 μm to 250–300 μm with a 400 mm focal length lens.[111] As the thermal effects of laser applications have become better understood, the desirability of using a smaller spot size for tissue interaction has become evident.

The helium-neon laser acting as an aiming beam may occasionally be difficult to visualize or perfectly align with the CO_2 laser. This shortcoming has been rectified in the KTP laser, which uses the same aiming and treatment beam, with the aiming beam attenuated by several orders of magnitude.

Specific pathologies

Recurrent respiratory papillomatosis

The CO_2 laser has become the standard treatment modality for patients with recurrent respiratory papillomatosis. Although successful treatment of recurrent respiratory papillomatosis has been reported with the KTP laser, the less predictable depth of penetration and increased potential for thermal injury in surrounding normal tissue make the KTP laser less than ideal for this application.[118] Though the CO_2 laser cannot cure the disease, it is effective in preserving normal laryngeal structures and maintaining an airway.

Recurrent respiratory papillomatosis is a virally mediated disease affecting the upper aerodigestive tract. The virus induces the formation of papillary-like projections that interfere with vocal and respiratory function. It is a mucosal process without deep invasion. Treatment is aimed at removal of the mucosal lesion with minimal injury to the surrounding tissue. The CO_2 laser is well suited to the treatment of this disease. Difficulty, however, arises secondary to the recurrent nature of the disease process. Studies by Pignatari *et al.* have shown that the viral particle is frequently identified in asymptomatic tissue surrounding the symptomatic lesions.[93] This makes ablation of all viral particles impossible and leads to the recurrent nature of the disease.

When treating recurrent respiratory papillomatosis, the first CO_2 laser treatment should be directed at removing as much papilloma from one vocal fold as possible and then as much as possible from the other. Involvement of the anterior commissure precludes complete excision, as 2–3 mm of untreated mucosa should be left on one vocal fold to prevent webbing. The papilloma overlying the true vocal fold should be vaporized or excised to the vocal ligament. Following the initial CO_2 laser removal of papilloma, a planned repeat operation should be considered in approximately 6 weeks. Superficial spreading of recurrent respiratory papillomatosis cannot always be seen in an office clinical examination. The complication rate has dramatically decreased with time. In 1985, a complication rate of 45% was reported.[129] In 1987, a reported complication rate had dropped to 28.7%.[21] In a series reported in 1991, 22 patients underwent 105 excisions with the CO_2 laser. The intraoperative soft tissue complication rate was zero. The delayed soft tissue complication rate, consisting of two patients with slight true vocal fold scarring and one patient with a small posterior web, was down to 13.6%.[85]

Tracheal and bronchial disease require treatment with the CO_2 endoscopic coupler for the bronchoscope. Inspection of the trachea and main bronchi may be initially performed with a 0° or 30° endoscope. Lesions are biopsied or vaporized starting at the most distal portion of the most distal lesion. Care must be taken not to circumferentially denude tracheal or bronchial mucosa. This will result in cicatricial scarring and airway stenosis.

Fortunately, the majority of symptomatic lesions are not confluent and areas of mucosa can be spared between lesions to lessen the chance for scar formation. Deep removal will also promote scarring.

Multiple staged endoscopies are required for surveillance and palliation. As was mentioned with laryngeal disease, a planned second look should be considered at 6 weeks. This is continued until good disease control has been achieved. Interval endoscopic evaluations can then be lengthened to 3–6 months depending on the rate of viral expression.

Substantial attention has been given to the possible detection of papilloma virus in the laser plume. Conflicting reports exist on both sides of the issue.[1,40] We have treated both surgeons and anesthesiologists for the disease that was manifest only after clinical exposure. Current recommendations to lessen the potential risk of exposure include the use of adequate smoke evacuation and high-filtration face masks.

Stenosis

The management of laryngotracheal stenosis is a difficult problem. The first decision, whether open management is necessary or if endoscopic techniques alone are adequate, is probably the most demanding. Patients with laryngotracheal stenosis first need staging direct laryngoscopy and bronchoscopy to determine the extent and degree of stenosis. It is advisable to have the laser readily available during this staging laryngoscopy. With the laser, scarring can be easily removed or incised. Supplemental dilation with the bronchoscope or stent placement may then be beneficial in further management of the stenotic area.[100]

The addition of the CO_2 laser to the endoscopic treatment of tracheal stenosis is a logical application of laser technology. Tissue interaction principles of the laser can be used to facilitate hemostasis in excision or vaporization of endoluminal scar.

The etiology of tracheal stenosis is varied. However, a review of multiple small series of patients indicates that acquired tracheal stenosis from prior endotracheal intubation is probably the most common etiology.[8,50,55,108,110,117] The second most common etiology is prior tracheal surgery. This includes both tracheostomy and tracheal resection.[55,108,110,117] This is followed by congenital lesions.

Stenotic lesions appropriate for endoscopic management have certain features in common.[112] First, all lesions treated with endoscopic techniques must have intact external cartilaginous support. Attempted endoscopic incision or excision of areas of tracheomalacia can have disastrous results if surrounding structures are perforated. Second, lesions appropriate for endoscopic management have a vertical length that is usually less than 1 cm. Combined with prolonged stenting, favorable results have been reported for lesions up to 3 cm long.[108,131] Finally, total cervical tracheal or subglottic stenosis does not usually respond well to endoscopic management. Again, prolonged stenting has produced successful case reports.[108]

Treatment of tracheal stenosis by endoscopic CO_2 laser bronchoscopy has resulted in a 34%,[108] to 77%[55] success rate. This has led surgeons to try to identify factors that are associated with a favorable endoscopic treatment prognosis. Simpson *et al.* found that scarring with cicatricial contraction, scarring wider than 1 cm in vertical dimension, previous history of severe bacterial infection and tracheomalacia with loss of cartilaginous support were associated with poor outcome after attempted endoscopic management.[112] Ossoff *et al.* confirmed these observations and added carinal involvement to the list of poor prognostic indicators.[90]

Preoperative assessments consisting of history, physical examination, flexible office endoscopy and radiographic evaluation are imperative before initiation of treatment. Radiographic evaluation with computerized tomography or magnetic resonance imaging will help to identify the condition or involvement of the tracheal cartilage. The endoscopic approach is only appropriate for lesions consisting of endoluminal scar tissue.

Endoscopic management of laryngotracheal stenosis relies on mucosal preservation. The two techniques advocated for this task are radial incision with the micro-trapdoor flap[13,24,29,30,128] and bronchoscopic dilation.[108] The micro-trapdoor flap technique uses the CO_2 laser to make a horizontal incision in the mucosa overlying the stenosis. The laser is then used to vaporize the underlying scar tissue. Either microscissors or the laser can then be used to incise the lateral portions of the inferiorly based flap to permit redraping of the preserved mucosa. The mucosal flap should be thin, yet with intact microcirculation. During creation of the lateral incisions the flap usually contracts so that a U-shaped uncovered area is created. This, however, is smaller than the area that would be created if the entire flap was excised and usually remucosalizes rapidly. The micro-trapdoor flap has been used in a sequential, staged manner on circumferential stenosis with fair to good results.[13,128]

It is more common to treat laryngotracheal stenosis with radial incisions and dilation. In bronchoscopic dilation the laser is used to make a radial incision, like the spokes of a wheel, in the stenotic area (see Fig 49.5a). A laryngoscope, subglottiscope or bronchoscope is then passed through the incised area of stenosis and rotated 90° from maximal dilation (see Fig 49.5b). The incision is carried on until the mucoperichondrium is exposed. Care should be use to avoid the exposure of cartilage. Often multiple procedures are required for maintenance of the airway lumen. Using this technique, Shapshay *et al.* were successful in treating five patients with moderate to severe subglottic and tracheal stenosis.[108] Three of these patients required more than one endoscopic procedure. Ossoff *et al.* were also successful in treating four of four patients with web-like tracheal stenosis.[90] They required an average of two procedures per patient.

The development of the microsubglottiscope facilitates the use of the CO_2 laser in the subglottis and cervical trachea. This specially designed endoscope fits through

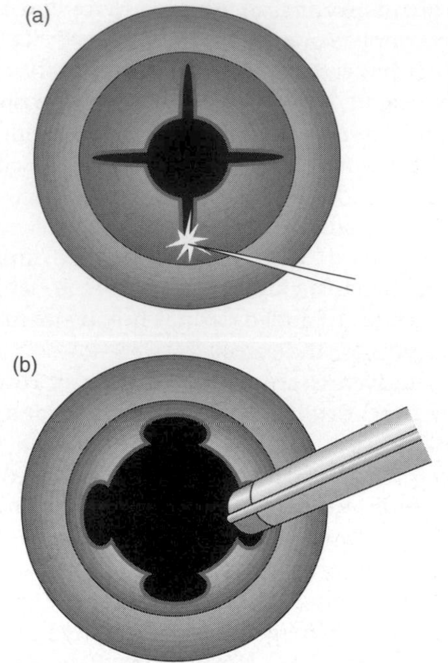

Figure 49.5 *(a) Radial incisions are made in the subglottic stenosis with the laser. (b) The airway is dilated using the bronchoscope.*

the vocal folds and permits binocular vision of the entire subglottis and upper cervical trachea. The CO_2 laser can then be attached to the operating microscope through a micromanipulator and lesions can be approached through a microlaryngoscopic technique as opposed to a bronchoscopic technique. Both adult[82] and pediatric sizes are available.[127] The use of the CO_2 laser is further facilitated by the addition of a smoke evacuation channel and a port for jet Venturi ventilation.

Whilst the CO_2 laser appears to be the most useful laser for the management of laryngotracheal stenosis, several surgeons are reporting favorable results in lesions treated with the Nd:YAG laser.[68,108] The Nd:YAG laser has the advantage of a fiberoptic delivery system that facilitates its use in otherwise difficult to expose subglottic or cervical tracheal lesions. Secondary to the somewhat unpredictable depth of penetration, however, care must be taken not to produce thermal injury in the underlying cartilage. Also, extreme care should be taken in the bronchi and at the carina to avoid injury to the great vessels. This is best avoided by using low-power settings with short pulse duration.

Finally, the Ho:YAG laser with a wavelength of 2.1 μm has been used to incise cricoid cartilage in animal models. The endoscopic technique is being explored as an alternative to traditional open cricoid splitting in neonatal and pediatric subglottic stenosis.[4]

Polypoid degeneration

For extensive polypoid degeneration that does not resolve with conservative measures, surgical excision is indicated. In this case, the preferred technique involves the elevation of a laryngeal microflap.[19] Gentle medial traction is placed on the polypoid tissue. An incision is made using the CO_2 laser or, more commonly, with a microsickle knife on the superior surface of the true vocal fold just medial to the laryngeal ventricle. A flap of epithelium is elevated from lateral to medial with specialized microsurgical instrumentation, and the mucoid material is suctioned. The redundant epithelium is removed using microscissors. The remaining epithelium is placed over the true vocal fold. A breathy voice will be present for 6–8 weeks postoperatively. Both true vocal folds can be treated with this technique at the same operation if care is taken to preserve a 2–3 mm cuff of epithelium over one true vocal fold at the anterior commissure.

Granulomas

Vocal process granuloma that persists after treating for gastric reflux, and after speech therapy, becomes a potential candidate for surgical excision. If, additionally, dysphonia or airway compromise is present, then surgical excision is indicated. The posterior commissure should be exposed using a posterior commissure laryngoscope or other appropriate laryngoscope.[83] The granuloma is grasped, and a large portion is excised using the CO_2 laser. The small bit of granuloma that remains should be vaporized carefully until the granuloma matrix is encountered. This represents the deep level of the dissection and prevents exposure of the underlying vocal process. Care should be taken to debride the charred, carbonaceous debris.[31] Benjamin and Croxson have noted no difference in recurrence rates when granulomas are excised by conventional microlaryngeal or laser techniques.[12]

Granulation tissue

Tracheal obstruction caused by granulation tissue is amenable to CO_2 laser bronchoscopic resection. Granulation tissue, a reaction to inflammation, is a mass of chronic inflammatory cells with a fibrous matrix. The inciting process can be induced by the tip of the endotracheal tube, tracheotomy tube, from over-vigorous suctioning through an endotracheal tube or from over-inflation of an endotracheal tube cuff. Over-inflation produces a shearing force on the tracheal mucosa during movement and can lead to mucosal membrane necrosis or disruption.[75]

The chronic inflammation induced by membrane disruption and localized bacterial overgrowth often progresses to perichondritis. This results in perichondrial inflammation with disruption of the blood supply to the cartilage, cartilage resorption and tracheal collapse. Tracheal granulation tissue should therefore be treated promptly with antibiotics. Failure to achieve a response with antibiotic therapy or progression of the granulation tissue to respiratory compromise may necessitate endoscopy for the removal of the obstructing lesion.

Endoscopy is aimed at excision of the lesion with relief of tracheal obstruction. Work by Healy suggests improved results in the treatment of tracheal or subglottic stenosis can be achieved when antibiotics are used prophylactically.[44]

As in papilloma, during the excision of granulation tissue by CO_2 laser bronchoscopy, the endoscope is inserted to the most distal portion of the most distal lesion. Excision and/or vaporization is undertaken in a retrograde fashion. Again, care must be taken to avoid circumferential mucosal excision as this will result in cicatricial scar formation and stenosis. Often, staged excisions are necessary to prevent cicatricial scarring. These can be performed at intervals of 2–4 weeks with intervening dilations as necessary to maintain an airway. If possible, tracheostomy should be avoided as this will increase the likelihood of bacterial colonization, and may increase the rate of perichondritis and eventual tracheomalacia.[102] Tracheostomy, however, was not found to be a significant limiting factor to the successful treatment of tracheal stenosis by Ossoff *et al.*[90] They found the laser to be particularly useful in the treatment of tracheal granulation tissue and were successful in the treatment of four of four lesions by endoscopic methods. The patients each underwent an average of 1.5 procedures. Beamis *et al.* also found the CO_2 laser particularly useful for the excision of tracheal granulation tissue because it is an excellent cutting tool and vaporizes tissue adequately.[11]

Nodules

Excision of the nodule may become necessary for fibrotic nodules and compliant patients who do not improve with voice therapy. Microsurgical, cold knife, excision techniques are the time-tested treatment of choice for this disease. The CO_2 laser can be used with an increased risk of potential scarring from thermal injury to surrounding tissue. When used, the CO_2 laser should be set at the lowest power density necessary to vaporize the nodule. An excisional biopsy should be performed when there is a question of pathology. The preferred laser technique involves shaving the nodule with half the laser beam and allowing the other half to fall on the suction platform.

Bilateral true vocal fold immobility

When true vocal fold immobility is bilateral, treatment is aimed at widening the glottis. Multiple procedures, both open and endoscopic, have been employed, and all have met with variable success. Currently accepted techniques, both open and endoscopic, are aimed at widening the posterior glottis and preserving the integrity of the membranous glottis for voice. Microlaryngoscopic techniques and the CO_2 laser are well suited for this task.[89] Total unilateral arytenoidectomy remains the gold standard technique. Success, however, has been reported with other procedures including posterior cordotomy[25,53] and medial arytenoidectomy.[22]

The technique of laser arytenoidectomy is as follows. Use of the posterior commissure laryngoscope aids in exposing the arytenoid cartilage. The mucoperichondrium overlying the corniculate cartilage is vaporized, exposing the underlying cartilage. Next, the mucoperichondrium overlying the apex and upper body of the arytenoid cartilage is vaporized, followed by the vaporization of the apex and upper body. Thereafter, the mucoperichondrium overlying the lower body of the arytenoid is ablated, followed by the vaporization of the lower body of the arytenoid itself. The lateral ligament is transected, and the cricoid cartilage is exposed. Next, the mucoperichondrium over the vocal process and most of the remaining muscular process are vaporized. Then the vocal process with an adjacent portion of vocalis muscle and the muscular process up to, but not including, the attachment of the arytenoideus muscle is vaporized. The mucosa of the interarytenoid cleft must not be injured. Following this step, a small area lateral to the vocalis muscle is vaporized to help in lateralization of the vocal fold during the healing by secondary intention.

The CO_2 or KTP laser can be used to incise the vocal fold at the junction of the vocal process as a simple cordotomy or shave the medical surface of the arytenoid body as a medial arytenoidectomy, respectively. These techniques can be employed either unilaterally or bilaterally to gain an adequate airway. Their use does not preclude eventual arytenoidectomy if later required to further improve the glottic airway. Any procedure designed to statically open the glottis to improve airflow will also adversely affect the voice, most commonly with increased breathiness. Rehabilitation of the glottis for air passage is a compromise accepted to eliminate the need for tracheostomy in these patients.

Malignant laryngeal disease

Endoscopic management of malignant laryngeal disease is not a new idea. In 1920, Lynch reported 39 patients with early glottic cancers that he successfully treated with transoral excision.[62] New and Dorton in 1941 reported a 90% cure rate with transoral excision and diathermy.[78] Lillie and DeSanto in 1973 reported 98 patients with early glottic carcinoma who were treated with transoral excision; all were cured, although five of these patients required further treatment.[60] These five patients did develop recurrent or second primary tumors. Four were successfully retreated by endoscopic excision, and the fifth patient had a laryngectomy 8 years after the initial endoscopic excision.

Transoral treatment of squamous cell carcinoma of the larynx using the CO_2 laser is therefore an obvious extension of the application of this surgical instrument.[54,100,130] The advantages of precision, hemostasis and decreased postoperative edema allow the laryngologist to perform exquisitely accurate and relatively bloodless endoscopic surgery of the larynx. The laser has facilitated a renaissance in the endoscopic management of early vocal fold carcinomas.[74,98]

Our current treatment plan for the endoscopic management of T1 vocal fold carcinoma includes an excisional biopsy with the CO_2 laser or with cold steel microflap techniques.[84] Supravital staining with toluidine blue can be performed as a diagnostic aid before biopsy. The surgical specimen is labeled and sent for frozen section examination. Any questionable margins are controlled by frozen section. If the tumor is T3 or T4, the patient is later treated by conventional surgical techniques (partial or total laryngectomy).

The endoscopic CO_2 laser excision of mid-cordal cancer can be curative, with rates equal to both radiation therapy and laryngofissure with cordectomy. The major advantage of CO_2 laser excision is the ability to differentiate deeply invasive 'early mid-cordal' T1 glottic cancers from those that are truly superficial in nature. Currently, worrisome lesions are biopsied with a cold knife technique. If frozen section shows severe dysplasia, carcinoma in situ or carcinoma with microinvasion, then a cold knife microflap technique is used to excise the involved mucosa with a 2 mm margin. The deep and lateral margins are inspected. If they are free of disease, then the laser can be used on low power settings to vaporize the deeper layers of Reinke's space. If the deep margins are involved with disease, then the laser can be used in a focused mode to excise a portion of the vocal ligament and underlying vocalis muscle for a deep margin. This technique can be used for lesions involving the membranous vocal folds. However, when invasive lesions are present near the anterior commissure or encroaching in the vocal process, then partial laryngectomy or radiation therapy is recommended secondary to enhanced lymphatic drainage from these areas and anatomic difficulty in obtaining adequate margins. The need for further treatment then will be apparent in cases with deep cancer invasion. The CO_2 laser excisional biopsy can be used repeatedly and does not interfere with further treatment.

Obstructing tracheal malignancy

The treatment of obstructing endobronchial malignant lesions poses a challenge to the bronchologist. The disease is often recurrent and the patient's pulmonary and medical condition is typically poor. Yet, the symptoms of tracheal bronchial obstruction are severe and palliation to prevent death from suffocation is necessary. Bronchoscopic therapy provides an excellent option for relief of obstruction with relatively minimal morbidity.

Shapshay *et al.* compared their experience in the endoscopic treatment of tracheal and bronchial malignancies with the CO_2 and Nd:YAG lasers.[109] Of 506 operations performed on 273 patients, they found the Nd:YAG laser to be preferable to the CO_2 laser secondary to improved hemorrhage control. In addition, they were able to use telescopic visualization with the Nd:YAG laser through a rigid bronchoscope, whereas this was not possible with the closed CO_2 laser system. It is worthy of mention that they often used the flexible fiberoptic bronchoscope through the open rigid bronchoscope. The open scope served as a conduit for both the laser and the telescope. It also served as a port for the removal of necrotic and excised tumor. Nd:YAG laser bronchoscopy is currently the treatment of choice for the palliation of malignant lesions.

Complications of laser laryngoscopy

Laser surgery of the larynx can be highly efficacious and safe as demonstrated by Healy *et al.*[45] A complication rate of 0.2% (9 complications in a total of 4416 patients) can be expected when the appropriate precautions are taken. A similar low complication rate has been reported by Ossoff *et al.*[87] They reported 12 complications in 204 patients involving all types of CO_2 laser surgery. None of the untoward events was life-threatening; they consisted of six problems related to the use of the laser and two minor injuries to OR staff and the remaining complications related to the laryngeal suspension system. Of the six patient injuries that were related to the use of the laser, one was secondary to retained metallic tape in the oropharynx, one was secondary to perichondritis with posterior laryngeal web formation, one involved a laser burn of a tooth and there were two instances of postoperative airway obstruction (one due to edema and one due to a retained pharyngeal pack).

Strong and Jako[116] and later Snow *et al.*[113] warned of the possible complications associated with laser surgery of the upper aerodigestive tract including the risks of endotracheal tube fires and tissue damage from reflection of the laser beam. Following these early warnings, several reports of complications uniquely attributable to the use of the CO_2 laser appeared in the literature.[16] Fried reported on complications from a large survey in 1984.[36] A total of 229 questionnaires were mailed with a response rate of 92. Of the physicians who responded, 49% had used the laser without complications. An additional 27% did not use the laser at all at the time of the survey. The remaining 49 physicians had a total of 81 complications. The most frequent was endotracheal explosion, with facial burns being the next most common occurrence. Five cases of pneumothorax and two of subcutaneous emphysema also were reported. Facial burns occurred nine times, and laryngeal subglottic or tracheal stenoses were reported in eight patients. Moreover, it was noted that increased experience with the laser did not necessarily guarantee fewer complications. The greater the number of cases performed, the more likely a complication is to occur.

The most serious laser complication is the ignition of the endotracheal tube.[20,36,46,47,71,105,113,125] This can occur when the laser acts on the external surface of an unprotected tube or in the dehiscence of a poorly wrapped tube. Combustible items such as a dry cottonoid can be ignited as well. Perforation of the airway with a pneumothorax and subcutaneous emphysema also has been experienced.[39]

Inadvertent CO_2 laser beam irradiation of the tissues of the perioperative field can lead to additional complications. The anterior commissure of the larynx must be respected with the laser just as it must be with conventional microlaryngeal techniques. Failure to preserve the mucosa on one side of the commissure will lead to an acquired glottic web. Fried reported 15 cases of laryngeal webs in his survey.[36] Subglottic stenosis secondary to laser treatment of subglottic capillary hemangioma has recently been reported by Cotton and Tewfik.[18] Vocal fold fibrosis is a distinct possibility following laser surgery. The mechanism of injury involves too much power for too long being delivered to the true vocal fold; this results in the vaporization of normal vocalis muscle, leaving a scarred vocal fold as a permanent reminder of the inappropriate radiant exposure that was delivered to the larynx. The CO_2 laser should not be used in the continuous mode when working on the larynx except in very rare instances. The pulsed mode is the preferred method of delivery of laser energy to the larynx.

Granulomas following laser surgery have been reported by Fried[36] in his survey and by Feder.[33] At the conclusion of the laser case, attempts should be made to remove all the black carbonaceous debris from the operative wound. This is best done with microsuction, irrigation and gentle rubbing with saline-saturated cottonoids.

Limitations of laser laryngoscopy

Before any surgical procedure, the surgeon must consider whether the laser is the best method to treat a particular laryngeal disorder. Although the laser is a highly precise instrument when used in conjunction with the operating microscope, thermal injury and carbonaceous debris may stimulate submucosal fibrosis that may be unacceptable in certain types of patients, as in the professional voice user. Newer microlaryngeal techniques with delicate instruments many times offer improved healing over laser techniques for benign vocal fold lesions. Moreover, the surgeon must be aware that the laser may not be functional on the particular day of surgery, and alternative plans should be available.

If indeed the laser is felt to be the optimal method of treatment, limitations may be imposed by the patient's particular anatomic configuration. Mandible size and position as well as spinal column flexibility may limit the type of laryngoscope that can be used and thereby affect visualization of the larynx. Patients with cervical arthritis, retrognathia, prominent teeth, or hypertrophy of the base of the tongue may be difficult candidates for endoscopy. Patients with ischemic cardiovascular disease may not withstand the prolonged laryngoscopic suspension that stimulates the vagus nerve and may produce subsequent cardiac arrhythmias as well as silent myocardial infarctions. Even in ideal circumstances, laser laryngoscopy may require more time to complete than other surgical techniques. For example, the patient with unstable cardiac disease suspected of having a laryngeal tumor may well best be treated with operative visualization and biopsy by conventional techniques rather than with use of the laser.[37]

Patients with chronic obstructive or restrictive pulmonary disease may be difficult to ventilate. In such situations, an endotracheal tube may be mandatory and by its presence may limit laryngeal visualization and access.

Prevention of complications

Exposure to some type of formal laser education program has to be a prerequisite to the use of this technology. If the surgeon has not received adequate training in laser surgery during residency, they should attend one of the many excellent hands-on training courses in laser surgery. The curriculum should include lectures on laser biophysics, tissue interaction, clinical applications, safety precautions, and supervised hands-on training with laboratory animals. It is suggested that the surgeon plan to further increase these newly acquired skills with the laser by working on cadaver or animal specimens before progressing to the simpler procedures on patients.

Each hospital performing laser surgery should appoint a laser safety officer and form a laser safety committee; the membership of this committee should include the laser safety officer, two or three physician-laser users, one or two nurses from the operating room, a hospital administrator, and a biomedical engineer. The purpose of this committee is to develop policies and procedures for the safe use of lasers in the hospital; these protocols will vary with each specialty using the laser. Other functions of this important committee include recommendations regarding the appropriate credentialing mechanisms required for physicians and nurses to become involved with each type of laser in the hospital. Policies regarding laser education for surgeons, anesthesiologists and nurses working with the laser should be developed. Other responsibilities of the laser safety committee include the accumulation of laser patient data when investigational lasers are used, and a periodic review of all complications related to the use of the laser.

The successful development of an effective safety protocol that stresses compliance and meticulous attention to detail by the surgeon, anesthesiologist and operating room nurse (laser surgery team) is probably the single most important reason this potentially dangerous surgical technology can be used so safely in treating patients with diseases of the head and neck.[81] General considerations concern the provision for protection of the patient's and operating room personnel's eyes and skin, and the provision for adequate smoke (laser plume) evacuation from the operative field. Other precautions include the choice of anesthetic techniques, the choice and protection of endotracheal tubes, and the selection of proper instruments, including bronchoscopes.

The best method of prevention is adequate preparation. It is imperative that all members of the surgical team, including nurses and the anesthesiologist, be familiar with the laser and contingency plans if complications should occur (e.g. endotracheal tube ignition). Equipment should be checked, and the aiming and CO_2 laser beams should be aligned at the outset of each case. The endotracheal tube and its wrapping should be tested. Steroids should be administered to prevent laryngeal edema. All members of the OR staff as well as the patient should have adequate eye protection. The all-metal endotracheal tube with saline placed in the distal cuff has been very safe for both CO_2 and KTP laser procedures. Other laser-specific endotracheal tubes are available and should be used in lieu of physician-wrapped tubes.

The surgeon should use binocular vision whenever possible and keep the laser in the center of the operative field. This avoids reflection off the side of the laryngoscope and allows for increased surgical precision. If, however, the surgical field must encompass more than what is visualized with the laryngoscope, both the laser and endoscope should be repositioned before the procedure is continued. Protection should be afforded to the vocal fold not being operated on. This can be done with vocal fold protectors that are commercially available and prevent the complication of anterior commissure webbing.

Smoke evacuation

All laser cases should be equipped with two separate suction setups; one provides for adequate smoke and steam evacuation from the operative field, whilst the second is connected to the surgical suction tip for the aspiration of blood and mucus from the operative wound.[114] Constant suctioning is required to remove laser-induced smoke from the operative field when performing laser surgery with a closed anesthetic system. Suctioning should be limited to an intermittent basis to maintain the partial pressure of oxygen at a safe level when working with an open anesthetic system or with a jet ventilation system. Laryngoscopes, bronchoscopes, operating platforms, mirrors, and anterior commissure and ventricle retractors with built-in smoke evacuating channels simplify removal of smoke from the operative field.[79] Filters in the suction lines should be used to prevent clogging by the black carbonaceous smoke debris created by the laser.[73]

Eye protection

Certain precautions must be followed to reduce the risk of ocular damage during cases involving the laser. A sign must be placed on the operating room door warning all persons entering the room to wear the appropriate protective glasses because the laser is in use. The doors to the operating room should remain closed during laser surgery. Protection of the eyes of the patient, surgeon and operating room personnel must be provided, with the actual protective device varying according to the wavelength of the laser used.

A double layer of saline-moistened eye pads is placed over the patient's eyes when using the CO_2 laser. When working with the Ho:YAG, Nd:YAG, KTP, or FEDL, the patient's eyes should be protected by a double layer of saline-moistened eye pads covered by aluminum foil; a pair of wavelength-specific glasses is placed on the patient along with the previously mentioned eye pads and foil. Eye shields have been developed for the patient's eyes and consist of a sandwich of polymethylmethacrylate and metal foil.[76] These shields have been tested with the Nd:YAG and CO_2 lasers. The shields are said to be safe, comfortable and easy to clean.

All operating room personnel must wear wavelength-specific protective glasses. Broadband protective glasses are necessary when using the KTP laser to protect at 532 nm and the Nd:YAG output at 1.064 μm. The surgeon need not wear protective glasses with the CO_2 laser only if he is using the operating microscope.[87]

Although it may appear that the beam direction and point of interaction of the laser and tissue are confined within the endoscope and optical fiber, inadvertent deflection of the beam may occur due to a faulty contact, a break in the fiber, or accidental disconnection between the fiber and endoscope. Therefore, strict compliance with this portion of the safety protocol is necessary. A detailed radiometric analysis of the output from a frosted tip surgical probe of a 30 W Nd:YAG laser shows that a 'nominal hazard zone' extends 1.3 m in all directions from the frosted probe.[99] All personnel within the 1.3 m range must wear standard protective eye wear.

Skin protection

A double layer of saline-saturated surgical sponges, towels, or lap pads is used to protect all exposed skin and mucous membranes of the patient outside the surgical field. Teeth in the operative field also need to be protected; this is usually accomplished by using saline-saturated Telfa, surgical sponges or specially constructed metal dental impression trays. Because it is possible for the beam to reflect off the proximal rim of the laryngoscope when performing microlaryngeal laser surgery, the patient's face is completely draped with saline-saturated surgical towels, exposing only the proximal lumen of the laryngoscope. For all laser cases, the meticulous attention that is paid to the protective draping procedures at the beginning of the case should be displayed throughout the case.

Anesthetic considerations

Anesthetic management of the patient undergoing laser surgery of the head and neck must include attention to the safety of the patient, the hazards of the equipment, and the requirements of the surgeon. The surgeon and anesthesiologist are the two principal members of the surgical team and as such should be completely familiar with the equipment being used, the patient being treated, and the anticipated outcome and potential complications. A discussion of the various possible techniques should occur before the operation.[80] The final decision for the particular technique must be compatible with the anesthesiologist's need to ventilate the patient as well as the surgeon's goals so that both can be accomplished readily.

Most patients will require general anesthesia and any of the nonflammable anesthetic agents is suitable; halothane and enflurane are most often used. Because of the risk of fire associated with laser surgery under general endotracheal anesthesia, the inspired concentration of oxygen, a potent oxidizing gas, is important. Mixtures of helium plus oxygen should be used to maintain the fractional volume of oxygen around but not above 40% and insure that the patient is adequately oxygenated.[91]

The Venturi anesthetic system removes the possibility of endotracheal tube combustion. The injector system may be placed either proximally or distally in the laryngoscope or through a metal endotracheal tube.[41,101,132] When the insufflation device is placed distally, it may impair the surgeon's visibility. Since this is a cuffless system, patients with restrictive pulmonary disease may be difficult to ventilate. Moreover, if a tear is produced in the mucosa and a high-pressure system is used, particularly when placed distally, the anesthetic agent may dissect outside the airway, causing subcutaneous emphysema, pneumomediastinum, or pneumothorax.[39]

Usually when esophagoscopy and bronchoscopy are to be performed at the time of laryngoscopy, such as in the staging of new pharyngeal cancers, the Venturi technique cannot be used throughout the procedure. Some surgeons prefer to have an endotracheal tube placed at the outset and then switch to Venturi insufflation for the laser portion of the procedure. If an endotracheal tube is to be used during laser surgery the cuff should be protected by moist cottonoids and filled with saline, which acts as a heat sink should the laser impact on the cuff and cause disruption.[58]

A continuous dialogue should occur throughout the operation between the surgeon and anesthesiologist concerning the status of ventilation, the amount of bleeding encountered, the motion of vocal folds, and the timing of laser use in conjunction with respiration. This latter is particularly important when the Venturi system is used.

Endotracheal tube ignition must be avoided and strict compliance to the laser safety protocol is mandatory. Protection of the endotracheal tube from either direct or reflected laser beam irradiation is extremely important. Should the laser beam strike an unprotected endotracheal tube carrying oxygen, ignition of the tube could result in a catastrophic, intraluminal, blowtorch-type endotracheal tube fire.[86] The cuff should be inflated with methylene blue-colored saline and saline-saturated cottonoids need to be placed above the cuff in the subglottic larynx to protect the cuff.[87] The cottonoids must be kept moistened during the laser procedure; they could flare up when dry. Should the cuff become deflated from an errant hit of the laser beam, the already saturated cottonoids would turn blue to warn the surgeon of impending danger.

There are courses designed for anesthesiologists that focus on the precautions that must be taken when lasers are used. These courses are highly recommended to ensure an informed and coherent laser surgery team. A new journal course for nurse anesthetists, covering several aspects of the laser in medicine, has been written.[26]

Conclusions

The laser is a unique tool. The monochromatic beam of light can be focused to irradiate small volumes of tissue and effect ablation. The thermal ablation process can be used to incise or excise tissue, as necessary. Many different materials can be used to create a laser. Each material emits characteristic wavelengths of light. The most common lasers in laryngeal surgery include the Nd:YAG, the Ho:YAG, the KTP, the FEDL, the diode laser and the CO_2 laser.

Lasers have been used for many applications in laryngeal surgery. The strong absorption of the 10.6 μm light emitted from the CO_2 laser make it well suited for many of the applications. In general, the CO_2 laser provides adequate hemostasis and minimal thermal damage to the surrounding tissue.

In the past three decades of laser use in otolaryngology, the delivery systems have improved and smaller focal spots are achieved. We expect the future changes will permit substantially shorter pulse durations (in the order of microseconds) to further limit collateral thermal damage.

It should be remembered that the laser is, for the most part, an additional cutting tool for the otolaryngologist. Many of the procedures that can be performed with the laser can be performed as well with cold knife microsurgical techniques. The laser does have an advantage when attempting to coagulate vascular malformations or treating telangiectatic vessels.

Certain precautions must be followed when using the laser. These include the use of protective eye wear, shielding the patient from misdirected laser exposure, and utmost care with anesthesia. Studies have shown that when safety protocols are followed, the laser is a safe and effective tool for otolaryngology.

References

1. Abramson AL, DiLorenzo TP, Steinberg BM. Is papillomavirus detectable in the plume of laser-treated laryngeal papilloma? *Arch Otolaryngol Head Neck Surg* 1990; **116:** 604–7.
2. Absten GT. Physics of light and lasers. *Obstet Gynecol Clin North Am* 1991; **18:** 407–27.
3. Apfelberg DB, Smoller B. Preliminary analysis of histological results of Hexascan device with continuous tunable dye laser at 514 (argon) and 577 nm (yellow). *Lasers Surg Med* 1993; **13:** 106–12.
4. April MM, Rebeiz EE, Aretz HT, Shapshay SM. Endoscopic holmium laser laryngotracheoplasty in animal models. *Ann Otol Rhinol Laryngol* 1991; **100:** 503–7.

5. April MM, Rebeiz EE, Friedman EM, Healy GB, Shapshay SM. Laser therapy for lymphatic malformations of the upper aerodigestive tract. An evolving experience. *Arch Otolaryngol Head Neck Surg* 1992; **118**: 205–8.
6. Atiyah RA. The KTP/532 laser in laryngeal surgery. *KTP/532 Clinical Update*. San Jose, CA: Laserscope, 1988: No. 21.
7. Atiyah RA, Friedman CD, Sisson GA. The KTP/532 laser in glossal surgery. *KTP/532 Clinical Update*. San Jose, CA: Laserscope, 1988: No. 22.
8. Bagwell CE, Marchildon MB, Pratt LL. Anterior cricoid split for subglottic stenosis. *J Pediatr Surg* 1987; **22**: 740–2.
9. Bartels LJ. KTP laser stapedotomy: is it safe? *Otolaryngol Head Neck Surg* 1990; **103**: 685–92.
10. Beamis JF Jr, Shapshay SM. Nd-YAG laser therapy for tracheobronchial disorders. *Postgrad Med* 1984; **75**: 173–80.
11. Beamis JF Jr, Vergos K, Rebeiz EE, Shapshay SM. Endoscopic laser therapy for obstructing tracheobronchial lesions. *Ann Otol Rhinol Laryngol* 1991; **100**: 413–19.
12. Benjamin B, Croxson G. Vocal cord granulomas. *Ann Otol Rhinol Laryngol* 1985; **94**: 538–41.
13. Beste DJ, Toohill RJ. Microtrapdoor flap repair of laryngeal and tracheal stenosis. *Ann Otol Rhinol Laryngol* 1991; **100**: 420–3.
14. Bredemeier HC. Laser accessory for surgical applications. U.S. Patent No. 3.659.613. 1969, issued 1972.
15. Bredemeier HC. Stereo laser endoscope. U.S. Patent No. 3.796.220. 1973, issued 1974.
16. Burgess GE, LeJeune FE. Endotracheal tube ignition during laser surgery of the larynx. *Arch Otolaryngol* 1979; **105**: 561–2.
17. Cosman B. Experience in the argon laser therapy for port-wine stains. *Plast Reconstr Surg* 1980; **65**: 119–29.
18. Cotton RT, Tewfik TL. Laryngeal stenosis following carbon dioxide laser in subglottic hemangioma. Report of three cases. *Ann Otol Rhinol Laryngol* 1985; **94**: 494–7.
19. Courey MS, Garrett CG, Ossoff RH. Medial microflap for excision of benign vocal fold lesions. *Laryngoscope* 1997; **107**: 340–4.
20. Cozine K, Rosenbaum LM, Askanazi J, Rosenbaum JH. Laser-induced endotracheal tube fire. *Anesthesiology* 1981; **55**: 583–5.
21. Crockett DM, McCabe BF, Shive CJ. Complications of laser surgery for recurrent respiratory papillomatosis. *Ann Otol Rhinol Laryngol* 1987; **96**: 639–44.
22. Crumley RL. Endoscopic laser medical arytenoidectomy for airway management in bilateral laryngeal paralysis. *Ann Otol Rhinol Laryngol* 1993; **102**: 81–4.
23. Decraemer WF, Dirckx JJ, Funnell WR. Shape and derived geometrical parameters of the adult, human tympanic membrane measured with a phase-shift moiré interferometer. *Hear Res* 1991; **51**: 107–21.
24. Dedo HH, Sooy CD. Endoscopic laser repair of posterior glottic, subglottic and tracheal stenosis by division or micro-trapdoor flap. *Laryngoscope* 1984; **94**: 445–50.
25. Dennis DP, Kashima H. Carbon dioxide laser posterior cordectomy for treatment of bilateral vocal cord paralysis. *Ann Otol Rhinol Laryngol* 1989; **98**: 930–4.
26. De Vane GG. AANA journal course. New technologies in anesthesia: update for nurse anesthetists-lasers. *AANA J* 1990; **58**: 313–19.
27. Doukas AG, McAuliffe DJ, Flotte TJ. Biological effects of laser-induced shock waves: structural and functional cell damage *in vitro*. *Ultrasound Med Biol* 1993; **19**: 137–46.
28. Dumon JF, Reboud E, Garbe L, Aucomte F, Meric B. Treatment of tracheobronchial lesions by laser photoresection. *Chest* 1982; **81**: 278–84.
29. Duncavage JA, Ossoff RH, Toohill RJ. Laryngotracheal reconstruction with composite nasal septal cartilage grafts. *Ann Otol Rhinol Laryngol* 1989; **98**: 581–5.
30. Duncavage JA, Piazza LS, Ossoff RH, Toohill RJ. Microtrapdoor technique for the management of laryngeal stenosis. *Laryngoscope* 1987; **97**: 825–8.
31. Durkin GE, Duncavage JA, Toohill RJ, Tieu TM, Caya JG. Wound healing of true vocal cord squamous epithelium following CO_2 laser ablation and cup forceps stripping. *Otolaryngol Head Neck Surg* 1986; **95**: 273–7.
32. Einstein A. Zur quanten theorie der strahlung. *Physikalishe Zeit* 1917; **18**: 121–3.
33. Feder RJ. Laryngeal granuloma as a complication of the CO_2 laser. *Laryngoscope* 1983; **93**: 944–5.
34. Fleischer D. Endoscopic laser therapy for gastrointestinal neoplasms. *Otolaryngol Clin North Am* 1984; **64**: 947–53.
35. Fox JL. The use of laser radiation as a surgical 'light knife'. *J Surg Res* 1969; **9**: 199–205.
36. Fried MP. Limitations of laser laryngoscopy. *Otolaryngol Clin North Am* 1984; **17**: 199–207.
37. Fried MP, Kelly JH, Strome M. *Complications of Laser Surgery of the Head and Neck*. Chicago: Year Book Medical Publishers, 1986.
38. Fuller TA. The physics of surgical lasers. *Lasers Surg Med* 1980; **1**: 5–14.
39. Ganfield RA, Chapin JW. Pneumothorax with upper airway laser surgery. *Anesthesiology* 1982; **56**: 398–9.
40. Garden JM, O'Banion MK, Shelnitz LS *et al.* Papillomavirus in the vapor of carbon dioxide laser-treated verrucae. *JAMA* 1988; **259**: 1199–202.
41. Gofarth AJ, Cooke JE, Putney FJ. An anesthesia technique for laser surgery of the larynx. *Laryngoscope* 1983; **93**: 822–3.
42. Goldman L, Blaney D, Kindel DJ Jr, Richfield D, Franke EK. Pathology of the effect of the laser beam on the skin. *Nature* 1963; **197**: 912–14.
43. Hall RR. The healing of tissues incised by carbon-dioxide laser. *Br J Surg* 1971; **58**: 222–5.
44. Healy GB. An experimental model for the endoscopic correction of subglottic stenosis with clinical applications. *Laryngoscope* 1982; **92**: 1103–15.
45. Healy GB, Strong MS, Shapshay S, Vaughan C, Jako G. Complication of CO_2 laser surgery of the aerodigestive tract: experience of 4416 cases. *Otolaryngol Head Neck Surg* 1984; **92**: 13–18.
46. Hirshman CA, Leon D. Ignition of an endotracheal tube during laser microsurgery. *Anesthesiology* 1980; **53**: 177.
47. Hirshman CA, Smith J. Indirect ignition of the endotracheal tube during carbon dioxide laser surgery. *Arch Otolaryngol* 1980; **106**: 639–41.
48. Högberg L, Stahle J, Vogel K. The transmission of high-

power ruby laser beam through bone. *Acta Soc Med Ups* 1967; **72:** 223–8.

49. Jako GJ. Laser surgery of the vocal cords: an experimental study with carbon dioxide laser on dogs. *Laryngoscope* 1972; **82:** 2204–16.
50. Johnson DG, Stewart DR. Management of acquired tracheal obstructions in infancy. *J Pediatr Surg* 1975; **10:** 709–17.
51. Joseph M, Reardon E, Goodman M. Lingual tonsillectomy: a treatment for inflammatory lesions of the lingual tonsil. *Laryngoscope* 1984; **94:** 179–84.
52. Kao MC. Video endoscopic sympathectomy using a fiberoptic CO_2 laser to treat palmar hyperhidrosis. *Neurosurgery* 1992; **30:** 131–5.
53. Kashima HK. Bilateral vocal fold motion impairment: pathophysiology and management by transverse cordotomy. *Ann Otol Rhinol Laryngol* 1991; **100:** 717–21.
54. Koufman JA. The endoscopic management of early squamous carcinoma of the vocal cord with the carbon dioxide surgical laser: clinical experience and a proposed subclassification. *Otolaryngol Head Neck Surg* 1986; **95:** 531–7.
55. Koufman JA, Thompson JN, Kohut RI. Endoscopic management of subglottic stenosis with the CO_2 surgical laser. *Otolaryngol Head Neck Surg* 1981; **89:** 215–20.
56. Krespi YP, Har-El G, Levine TM, Ossoff RH, Wurster CF, Paulsen JW. Laser laryngeal tonsillectomy. *Laryngoscope* 1989; **99:** 131–5.
57. Kuhn F. The KTP/532 laser in tonsillectomy. *KTP/532 Clinical Update*. San Jose, CA: Laserscope, 1988: No. 06.
58. LeJeune FE Jr, Guice C, LeTard F, Marice H. Heat sink protection against lasering endotracheal cuffs. *Ann Otol Rhinol Laryngol* 1982; **91:** 606–7.
59. Levine HL. Endoscopy and the KTP/532 laser for nasal sinus disease. *Ann Otol Rhinol Laryngol* 1989; **98:** 46–51.
60. Lillie JC, DeSanto LW. Transoral surgery of early cordal carcinoma. *Trans Am Acad Ophthalmol Otolaryngol* 1973; **77:** 92–6.
61. Linden BE, Gross CW, Long TE, Lazar RH. Morbidity in pediatric tonsillectomy. *Laryngoscope* 1990; **100:** 120–4.
62. Lynch RC. Intrinsic carcinoma of the larynx with a second report of the cases operated on by suspension and dissection. *Trans Am Laryngol Assoc* 1920; **42:** 119.
63. Maiman TH. Stimulated optical radiation in ruby. *Nature* 1960; **187:** 493.
64. McDaniel DH. Clinical usefulness of the Hexascan. Treatment of cutaneus vascular and melanocytic disorders. *J Dermatol Surg Oncol* 1993; **19:** 312–19.
65. McDaniel DH, Mordon S. Hexascan: a new robotized scanning laser handpiece. *Cutis* 1990; **45:** 300–5.
66. McGee TM. The KTP/532 laser in otology. *KTP/532 Clinical Update*. San Jose, CA: Laserscope, 1988: No. 08.
67. McKenzie AL. How far does thermal damage extend beneath the surface of CO_2 laser incisions? *Phys Med Biol* 1983; **28:** 905–12.
68. Mehta AC, Lee FY, Cordasco EM, Kirby T, Eliachar I, De Boer G. Concentric tracheal and subglottic stenosis. Management using the Nd-YAG laser for mucosal sparing followed by gentle dilatation. *Chest* 1993; **104:** 673–7.
69. Merberg GN. Current status of infrared fiber optics for medical laser power delivery. *Lasers Surg Med* 1993; **13:** 572–6.
70. Merguerian PA, Seremetis G, Becher MW. Hypospadias repair using laser welding of ventral skin flap in rabbits: comparison with sutured repair. *J Urol* 1992; **148:** 667–71.
71. Meyers A. Complication of CO_2 laser surgery of the larynx. *Ann Otol* 1981; **90:** 132–4.
72. Mihashi S, Jako GJ, Incze J, Strong MS. Laser surgery in otolaryngology: interaction of the CO_2 laser in soft tissue. *Ann N Y Acad Sci* 1976; **267:** 263–94.
73. Mohr RM, McDonnell BC, Unger M, Mauer TP. Safety considerations and safety protocol for laser surgery. *Surg Clin North Am* 1984; **64:** 851–9.
74. Myers EN, Wagner RL, Johnson JT. Microlaryngoscopic surgery for T1 glottic lesions: a cost-effective option. *Ann Otol Rhinol Laryngol* 1994; **103:** 28–30.
75. Nagaraj HS, Shott R, Fellows R, Yacoub U. Recurrent lobar atelectasis due to acquired bronchial stenosis in neonates. *J Pediatr Surg* 1980; **15:** 411–15.
76. Nelson CC, Pasyk KA, Dootz GL. Eye shield for patients undergoing laser treatment. *Am J Ophthalmol* 1990; **110:** 39–43.
77. Nemeth AJ. Lasers and wound healing. *Dermatol Clin* 1993; **11:** 183–9.
78. New GB, Dorton HE. Suspension laryngoscopy and the treatment of malignant disease of the hypopharynx and larynx. *Mayo Clin Proc* 1941; **16:** 411.
79. Ossoff RH, Karlan MS. Instrumentation for micro-laryngeal laser surgery. *Otolaryngol Head Neck Surg* 1983; **91:** 456–60.
80. Ossoff RH, Reinisch L. Complications of laser surgery. In: Eisele DW, ed. *Complications in Head and Neck Surgery*. Philadelphia: BC Decker, 1993: 306–16.
81. Ossoff RH, Reinisch L. Laser surgery in otolaryngology: basic principles and safety considerations. In: Cummings CW, Frederickson JM, Harker LA, Krause CJ, Schuller DE, eds. *Otolaryngology–Head and Neck Surgery*, 2nd edn. St Louis: Mosby, 1993: 199–213.
82. Ossoff RH, Duncavage JA, Dere H. Microsubglottoscopy: an expansion of operative microlaryngoscopy. *Otolaryngol Head Neck Surg* 1991; **104:** 842–8.
83. Ossoff RH, Karlan MS, Sisson GA. Posterior commissure laryngoscope for carbon dioxide laser surgery. *Ann Otol Rhinol Laryngol* 1983; **92:** 361.
84. Ossoff RH, Sisson GA, Shapshay SM. Endoscopic management of selected early vocal cord carcinoma. *Ann Otol Rhinol Laryngol* 1985; **94:** 560–4.
85. Ossoff RH, Werkhaven JA, Dere H. Soft-tissue complications of laser surgery for recurrent respiratory papillomatosis. *Laryngoscope* 1991; **101:** 1162–6.
86. Ossoff RH, Duncavage J, Eisenman TE, Karlan MS. Comparison of tracheal damage from laser ignited endotracheal tube fires. *Ann Otol Rhinol Laryngol* 1983; **92:** 333–6.
87. Ossoff RH, Hotaling AJ, Karlan MS, Sisson GA. CO_2 laser in otolaryngology head and neck surgery: a retrospective analysis of complications. *Laryngoscope* 1983; **93:** 1287–9.
88. Ossoff RH, Herkhaven JA, Raif J, Abraham M. Advanced microspot microslad for the CO_2 laser. *Otolaryngol Head Neck Surg* 1991; **105:** 411–14.

89. Ossoff RH, Sisson GA, Duncavage JA, Moselle HI, Andrews PE, McMillan WI. Endoscopic laser arytenoidectomy for the treatment of bilateral vocal cord paralysis. *Laryngoscope* 1984; **94:** 1293–7.
90. Ossoff RH, Duncavage JA, Gluckman JL *et al.* The universal endoscopic coupler bronchoscopic carbon dioxide laser surgery: a multi-institutional clinical trial. *Otolaryngol Head Neck Surg* 1985; **93:** 824–30.
91. Pashayan AG, Gravenstein JS. Helium retards endotracheal tube fires from CO_2 lasers. *Anesthesiology* 1985; **62:** 274–7.
92. Pickering JW, Butler PH, Ring BJ, Walker EP. Computed temperature distributions around ectatic capillaries exposed to yellow (578 nm) laser light. *Phys Med Biol* 1989; **34:** 1247–58.
93. Pignatari S, Smith EM, Gray SD, Shive C, Turek LP. Detection of human papillomavirus infection in diseased and nondiseased sites of the respiratory tract in recurrent respiratory papillomatosis patients by DNA hybridization. *Ann Otol Rhinol Laryngol* 1992; **101:** 408–12.
94. Polanyi TG. Laser physics. *Otolaryngol Clin North Am* 1983; **16:** 753–74.
95. Polanyi TG, Bredemeier HC, Davis TW Jr. A CO_2 laser for surgical research. *Med Biol Eng* 1970; **8:** 541–8.
96. Qadir R, Kennedy D. Use of the holmium:yttrium aluminum garnet (Ho:YAG) laser for cranial nerve decompression: an in vivo study using the rabbit model. *Laryngoscope* 1993; **103:** 631–6.
97. Rebeiz E, April MM, Bohigian RK, Shapshay SM. Nd-YAG laser treatment of venous malformations of the head and neck: an update. *Otolaryngol Head Neck Surg* 1991; **105:** 655–61.
98. Rice DH, Wetmore SJ, Singer M. Recurrent squamous cell carcinoma of the true vocal cord. *Head Neck* 1991; **13:** 549–52.
99. Rockwell RJ Jr, Moss CE. Hazard zones and eye protection requirements for a frosted surgical probe used with an Nd:YAG laser. *Lasers Surg Med* 1989; **9:** 45–9.
100. Rothfield RE, Myers EN, Johnson JT. Carcinoma in situ and microinvasive squamous cell carcinoma of the vocal cords. *Ann Otol Rhinol Laryngol* 1991; **100:** 793–6.
101. Ruder CB, Rapheal NL, Abramson AL, Oliverio RM Jr. Anesthesia for carbon dioxide laser microsurgery of the larynx. *Otolaryngol Head Neck Surg* 1981; **89:** 732–7.
102. Sasaki CT, Horiuchi M, Koss N. Tracheostomy-related subglottic stenosis: bacteriologic pathogenesis. *Laryngoscope* 1979; **89:** 857–65.
103. Sataloff J. Experimental use of laser in otosclerotic stapes. *Arch Otolaryngol* 1967; **85:** 614–16.
104. Schawlow AL, Townes CH. Infrared and optical masers. *Physical Rev* 1958; **112:** 1940–1.
105. Schramm VL Jr, Mattox DE, Stool SE. Acute management of laser-ignited intracheal explosion. *Laryngoscope* 1981; **91:** 1417–26.
106. Shapshay SM, Oliver P. Treatment of hereditary hemorrhagic telangiectasia by Nd-YAG laser photocoagulation. *Laryngoscope* 1984; **94:** 1554–6.
107. Shapshay SM, Simpson GT. Lasers in bronchology. *Otolaryngol Clin North Am* 1983; **16:** 879–86.
108. Shapshay SM, Beamis JF Jr, Dumon JF. Total cervical tracheal stenosis: treatment by laser, dilation, and stenting. *Ann Otol Rhinol Laryngol* 1989; **98:** 890–5.
109. Shapshay SM, Dumon JF, Beamis JF Jr. Endoscopic treatment of tracheobronchial malignancy. Experience with Nd-YAG and CO_2 lasers in 506 operations. *Otolaryngol Head Neck Surg* 1985; **93:** 205–10.
110. Shapshay SM, Beamis JF Jr, Hybels RL, Bohigian RK. Endoscopic treatment of subglottic and tracheal stenosis by radial laser incision and dilation. *Ann Otol Rhinol Laryngol* 1987; **96:** 661–4.
111. Shapshay SM, Wallace RA, Kveton JF, Hybels RL, Setzer SE. New microspot micromanipulator for CO_2 laser application in otolaryngology–head and neck surgery. *Otolaryngol Head Neck Surg* 1988; **98:** 179–81.
112. Simpson GT, Polanyi TG. History of the carbon dioxide laser in otolaryngologic surgery. *Otolaryngol Clin North Am* 1983; **16:** 739–52.
113. Snow JC, Norton ML, Saluja TS, Estanislao AF. Fire hazard during CO_2 laser microsurgery on the larynx and trachea. *Anesth Analg* 1976; **55:** 146–7.
114. Spilman LS. Nursing precautions for CO_2 laser surgery. Symposium Proceedings. *Laser Inst Am* 1983; **37:** 63–4.
115. Spitzer M, Krumholz BA. Photodynamic therapy in gynecology. *Obstet Gynecol Clin North Am* 1991; **18:** 649–59.
116. Strong MS, Jako GJ. Laser surgery in the larynx. Early clinical experience with continuous CO_2 laser. *Ann Otol* 1972; **81:** 791–8.
117. Strong MS, Healy GB, Vaughan CW, Fried MP, Shapshay S. Endoscopic management of laryngeal stenosis. *Otolaryngol Clin North Am* 1979; **12:** 797–805.
118. Strong MS, Vaughan CW, Cooperband SR, Healy GB, Clemente MA. Recurrent respiratory papillomatosis: management with the CO_2 laser. *Ann Otol* 1976; **85:** 508–16.
119. Strully KJ, Yahr W. Biological effects of laser radiation enhancements by selective stains. *Fed Proc* 1965; **24:** S81.
120. Strunk CL, Nichols ML. A comparison of the KTP/532-laser tonsillectomy vs. traditional dissection/snare tonsillectomy. *Otolaryngol Head Neck Surg* 1990; **103:** 966–71.
121. Strunk CL, Quinn FB Jr, Bailey BJ. Stapedectomy techniques in residency training. *Laryngoscope* 1992; **102:** 121–4.
122. Tan OT, Carney JM, Margolis R *et al.* Histologic responses of port-wine stains treated by argon, carbon dioxide, and tunable dye lasers. A preliminary report. *Arch Dermatol* 1986; **122:** 1016–22.
123. Thedinger BS. Applications of the KTP laser in chronic ear surgery. *Am J Otol* 1990; **11:** 79–84.
124. Toty A, Personne C, Colchen A, Vourch G. Bronchoscopic management of tracheal lesions using the Nd:YAG laser. *Thorax* 1981; **36:** 175–8.
125. Vourch G, Tannieres M, Freche G. Ignition of a tracheal tube during laryngeal laser surgery. *Anaesthesia* 1979; **34:** 685.
126. Ward RF. Treatment of tracheal and endobronchial lesions with the potassium titanyl phosphate laser. *Ann Otol Rhinol Laryngol* 1992; **101:** 205–8.

127. Ward RF, Arnold JE, Healy GB. Flexible minibronchoscopy in children. *Ann Otol Rhinol Laryngol* 1987; **96:** 645–9.

128. Werkhaven JA, Weed DT, Ossoff RH. Carbon dioxide laser serial microtrapdoor flap excision of subglottic stenosis. *Arch Otolaryngol Head Neck Surg* 1993; **119:** 676–9.

129. Wetmore SJ, Key JM, Suen JY. Complications of laser surgery for laryngeal papillomatosis. *Laryngoscope* 1985; **95:** 798–801.

130. Wetmore SJ, Key JM, Suen JY. Laser therapy for T1 glottic carcinoma of the larynx. *Arch Otolaryngol Head Neck Surg* 1986; **112:** 853–5.

131. Whitehead E, Salam MA. Use of the carbon dioxide laser with the Montgomery T-tube in the management of extensive subglottic stenosis. *J Laryngol Otol* 1992; **106:** 829–31.

132. Woo P, Strong MS. Venturi jet ventilation through the metal endotracheal tube: a nonflammable system. *Ann Otol Rhinol Laryngol* 1983; **92:** 405–7.

133. Zaret M, Ripps H, Siegel IM, Breinin GM. Biomedical experimentation with optical lasers. *J Opt Soc Am* 1962; **52:** 607–9.

134. Zweng HC, Flocks M, Kapany NS, Silbertrust N, Peppers NA. Experimental laser photocoagulation. *Am J Ophthalmol* 1964; **58:** 353–62.

Radiobiology of larynx cancer and its treatment

Thomas J Keane

Larynx cancer has been seen by many authors as the ideal cancer to treat with radiation. The reason for this is threefold. Local eradication of cancer is attained in a high proportion of cases. This is usually associated with long-term cure and maintenance of laryngeal function in a high proportion of cases. This combination of cure with organ preservation and function is a most desirable outcome for patients.

Successful radiation treatment of laryngeal cancer requires careful attention to radiation treatment delivery such that the required dose is accurately delivered to the tumor target volume and the dose to critical normal tissues is kept to a minimum. As the physical aspect of treatment is beyond the scope of this chapter, it will be assumed to be optimized in the discussion of the radiobiological principles underlying radiation treatment.

The concept of therapeutic ratio

In theory, radiation treatment, if delivered in sufficient dose, can eradicate all clonogenic tumor cells in a particular tumor. It is important to understand that it is the clonogenic cells, i.e. those so-called stem cells capable of unlimited reproduction, that are the target if cure is desired. The actual number of clonogenic cells in a particular tumor is generally a small proportion of the total cells in a tumor. The remaining cells are either differentiated nonclonogenic cells or stromal elements, which are radiobiologically irrelevant to radiocurability. The concept of therapeutic ratio applied to successful cancer treatment requires that the treatment must induce greater net clonogenic cell killing in the tumor relative to radiation damage sustained by the normal tissues. As a result, it is the normal tissue tolerance that limits the total dose of radiation that can be delivered to a tumor and is therefore the limiting factor to eradicating the cancer completely. In general, human normal tissue responses to radiation are much more predictable and homogenous than what is observed for human tumors.

Damage to normal tissue in the case of larynx cancer treatment can be described as either acute, late or consequential. Each will be described briefly, as an understanding of the differences is crucial to reducing serious treatment toxicity. Acute toxicity is seen in rapidly proliferating normal tissues, which in the case of the larynx are mucosa and skin epithelium. This desquamating effect is generally self-limiting and transient and due to a temporary reduction in the stem cell component responsible for replacing the mucosal or skin epithelial surface. Homeostatic proliferative responses occur in these tissues such that mucosal and skin reactions usually heal rapidly and completely after completion of radiation treatment. Late normal tissue toxicity in the form of damage to late reacting tissues such as bone, cartilage and blood vessels and spinal cord is the most feared complication of radiation therapy. Years of experience have yielded very accurate estimates of the dose thresholds for these effects with conventional daily fractionation. Most conventional dosage schemes are designed to limit risks of late damage to 1–5% within 5 years. As the dose–response curve is steep for these complications, most radiation oncologists allow a margin of safety in their dose prescription such that these complications can generally be reduced to a very low probability of occurrence. The final form of injury, known as consequential late injury, is relatively recent in description. It occurs when acute toxicity is so severe that healing will not occur. This type of injury has been observed with the more accelerated fractionation schedules where high doses are delivered in very short treatment times.[19] Radiobiologically, it is similar to an acute injury that fails to heal.

The understanding of normal tissue effects has resulted in a number of strategies to exploit biological differences

Table 50.1 Radiobiologic-based strategies to improve therapeutic ratio

Strategy	*Rationale*
Fractionation	
Standard daily	Exploits recovery of normal tissues and tumor reoxygenation
Hyperfractionation	Exploits differential repair of radiation damage between tumor cells and late-reacting normal tissues
Accelerated fractionation	Advantageous in treating rapidly proliferating tumors
Anti-hypoxia strategies	
Hyperbaric oxygen therapy	Increased O_2 delivery to tumor
Hypoxic cell drugs sensitizers	Oxygen mimetic drugs
Hypoxic cell cytotoxins	Target hypoxic tumor cells specifically
Vasoactive agents	Enhance tumor blood flow
Radiation and chemotherapy	Sensitization effect of some chemotherapeutic agents Additive cytoreduction

between tumors and normal tissues in order to improve therapeutic ratio. Table 50.1 summarizes the major strategies that have been considered to improve the therapeutic ratio in the treatment of larynx cancer. Each of these strategies will be considered separately.

Fractionation

The earliest observation by the French school of radiation therapy that normal tissues were relatively protected by giving radiation daily over many weeks rather than in a few large single treatments was the earliest strategy to improve therapeutic ratio. Whilst the initial emphasis was on the diminution of acute effects such as radiation mucositis, it became clear that fractionation also led to a decrease in the incidence of what were called late effects, in particular laryngeal cartilage necrosis. In more recent times, the potential advantage of allowing reoxygenation of tumors associated with fractionation over several weeks was also recognized. The benefits of fractionation led to the concept of hyperfractionation. This is defined as the delivery of higher than conventional total doses of radiation by increasing the number of treatments and reducing the dose per treatment while keeping the overall treatment time the same by treating more than once daily. Mathematical calculations from experimental data suggested that for total doses in the clinical range, a doubling of the number of fractions would allow 10–15% more dose to be delivered without an increase in late normal tissue effects such as fibrosis or necrosis. Experience over the past 20 years has confirmed this prediction of the relative sparing of late-reacting normal tissues by reducing the dose per fraction. The relative degree of improvement in tumor control when total dose is increased is still debated but the available evidence suggests that the benefits in terms of improved tumor control in a population of human tumors are directly proportional to the increment in the total dose, i.e. for each 1% increase in total dose at the 50% control level, a corresponding increase of 1% (median) in tumor control is observed.[15] This relatively flat dose–response curve has significant implications for clinical trial design, requiring the recruitment of large numbers of patients to demonstrate the benefits of dose escalation on tumor control. The concept of hyperfractionation as defined earlier is quite different from the concept of accelerated fractionation even though both regimens employ multiple fractions per day. In this situation, the goal is to significantly reduce the overall treatment time while keeping the total dose at or near the levels used in conventional fractionation. The best examples of this in the treatment of a variety of head and neck cancers, including larynx cancer, have been recently published.[5,12] The absence of a demonstrable benefit with these regimens to date may be due to the significant reductions in total dose in the case of the CHART trial[5] or the fact that rapid proliferation may be the cure-limiting factor in only a subset of patients.

An important feature of fractionation related to the effect of overall treatment time has been extensively studied in the past decade.[2,14,18] Interruption or prolongation of treatment, usually to minimize or as a consequence of acute normal tissue reactions, has been repeatedly demonstrated to reduce the probability of tumor control. The magnitude of this effect in larynx cancer appears to be much larger than originally thought, resulting in a measurable decrease in tumor control in the order of 1–3% per day of prolongation without dose adjustment.[6] The message from these data is clear. Treatment interruption or prolongation should be avoided if at all possible. Adjusting total dose to compensate for such interruptions may be hazardous, particularly in the case of split course therapy. This was confirmed in the study by Overgaard *et al.*[17] where a split course dosage increment to achieve tumor control comparable with conventional fractionation led to a dramatic increase in severe postradiation laryngeal edema. This finding confirmed experimental data that late normal tissue effects such as necrosis and late laryngeal edema are time independent and are closely correlated with total dose and dose per treatment. In other words, reductions in acute toxicity can be achieved with treatment prolongation or interruption as total dose is increased. This strategy will not, however, similarly prevent late normal tissue toxicity as total doses are increased.

Antihypoxic strategies

The response of cells to radiation is strongly dependent on the presence of oxygen.[7] This effect and the observation that oxygen gradients occur within experimental and human tumors has focused attention on the relative radioresistance of hypoxic cells as a possible cause of treatment failure following curative radiation. Experimental data have demonstrated that the oxygen effect is only observed when oxygen is present during irradiation or within a few milliseconds of radiation being completed.[11] The effect is believed to be due to the fixation of radiation damage by the binding of oxygen with free radicals in cells such that the chemical composition of the target within the DNA molecule is altered. In the absence of oxygen, such fixation of damage is much less likely to occur and the biologic effect of radiation is less. The magnitude of the oxygen effect is such that the enhancing effect of oxygen on cell killing may be increased threefold when compared to that observed for hypoxic cells.

Initial concepts of tumor hypoxia focused on chronic hypoxia of tumor cells at the limit of the distance diffused by oxygen in poorly vascularized tumors. More recently, the presence of acute hypoxia due to the temporary closing of small vessels within tumors has been demonstrated.[10] It seems likely that both acute and chronic hypoxia are operative in producing the hypoxic state. The strategies to deal with both acute and chronic hypoxia are, however, very different.

The magnitude and potential of the oxygen effect led to a variety of approaches to increase the oxygen status of tumors thought to be chronically hypoxic. The observation that many tumors will reoxygenate as they reduce in size during a fractionated course of radiation is still an important justification for fractionating radiation treatment over 4–6 weeks. It is possible that additional acute effects of radiation on blood flow and cellular respiration may also contribute to improved oxygenation within hours of radiation treatment.

Improving oxygen delivery by increasing the amount of oxygen delivered to tumors was tested clinically in randomized trials by Henk[8,9] who treated patients with a variety of head and neck cancers with hyperbaric oxygen therapy (HBO) as an adjuvant to radiation treatment. These studies demonstrated a significant enhancement in tumor control in patients receiving HBO. Unfortunately, the technical difficulties associated with delivering radiation in a hyperbaric setting and limitations on patient eligibility limited the development of this approach.

The next major approach was the development and clinical testing of drugs with oxygen mimetic characteristics. The major class of these compounds, nitroimidazoles, were subjected to extensive clinical trials in many tumor sites including the head and neck and larynx. A meta-analysis[16] of hypoxic cell sensitizer studies in the radiation treatment of head and neck cancer including the larynx suggested a significant improvement in local control. This effect appeared more striking for supraglottic than glottic carcinoma. Unfortunately, for many of these studies, particularly with the drug misonidazole, peripheral neuropathy was a significant drug-related toxicity.

The failure of these trials to convince many radiation oncologists of the benefits of this approach led to a general reduction in interest in anti-hypoxia strategies in head and neck cancer. Despite this, there would appear to be sufficient evidence to believe that counteracting tumor hypoxia may be beneficial. In this respect, there is a new interest in exploiting tumor hypoxia by selectively targeting hypoxic cells with hypoxic cell cytotoxins which are preferentially metabolized under anaerobic conditions.[1] Trials of drugs in this class possibly combined with agents that temporarily enhance tumor hypoxia are currently being considered.

Whilst most of the studies described in this section have focused on the correction of the chronic hypoxic state, there has been a significant recent interest in the possibility of combating acute hypoxia by delivering vasoactive agents to improve tumor blood flow. Clinical trials of this approach are awaited in head and neck and larynx cancer.

Radiation and chemotherapy

The possibility that combinations of radiation and chemotherapy would improve the therapeutic ratio has been the subject of many clinical studies in larynx cancer. Many of these studies have been pragmatic, i.e. combining chemotherapeutic agents that appear to be active against squamous carcinoma with radiation delivered in a concurrent or neoadjuvant manner. The majority of studies of concurrent chemotherapy demonstrated improved response rates though improved local control was not consistently demonstrated.[13] Unfortunately, therapeutic ratio was often not improved as the increases in acute toxicity in many cases compromised either the patient outcome or the radiation treatment to the extent that radiation treatment was never completed at the planned dose, or the treatment schedule was prolonged such that tumor repopulation may have counteracted any gain achieved with the added cell killing achieved with chemotherapy. A definitive trial comparing chemotherapy with cisplatin and 5-fluorouracil (5-FU) combined with radiation either concurrently or sequentially compared with radiation therapy alone is nearing completion in the USA. The failure of neoadjuvant chemotherapy to improve therapeutic ratio compared to radiation alone has been very disappointing, particularly with the high initial response rates observed with the platinum-containing combinations.

A critical review of the role of chemotherapy in combination with radiation in head and neck cancer by Jassem and Bartelink[13] is recommended to readers wishing more detailed information.

Heterogeneity of tumor response

The preceding discussions will, I hope, make it apparent that there are many biologic reasons why tumors may fail to be cured with radiation. Just as there are many possible causes of treatment failure, there are equally many strategies which, when applied clinically, may have positive or negative consequences. It is, for example, quite possible that an intense accelerated course of radiation therapy such as CHART[5] may be advantageous in killing tumors that are rapidly proliferating but may compromise reoxygenation in chronically hypoxic tumors that would optimally reoxygenate over a longer period of 6 weeks. In any population of patients with larynx cancer it is highly likely that multiple causes of treatment failure may exist in the population under study and even in individual patients. As an example, consider a group of patients subjected in clinical trial to a very effective anti-hypoxia strategy. The clinical trial may be negative, as the power of the trial will be weakened by the presence in the study of many patients who do not have hypoxia as the reason for failure and therefore cannot benefit from the strategy under test. This reality must be confronted by clinicians designing clinical trials of new approaches. The biologic rationale, be it hypoxia, countering repopulation, etc., must be directed at those patients most likely to benefit from the approach. If such an approach is not taken, trials will likely be negative and little new information obtained. What is needed is appropriate screening methods to assess underlying biologic characteristics and to match these patients to appropriate interventions. The recent clinical application of oxygen measurements using the tumor-directed probes,[4] or assays for predicting proliferation kinetics of individual tumors[3] will be a step in the right direction in selecting patients for future studies.

Future radiobiology

Our understanding of the biological basis for current approaches to improving therapeutic ratio in the radiation treatment of larynx cancer is undergoing dramatic change as the cellular mechanism which impacts on the traditional four 'R's of radiobiology – repair, redistribution, reoxygenation and repopulation – are elucidated. In addition, the response of tumor cells to stresses such as radiation and hypoxia may be understood and manipulated for therapeutic benefit. It can reasonably be anticipated that the next millennium will build on today's radiobiologic information and create new opportunities to improve the therapeutic ratio of the treatment of larynx cancer with radiation.

References

1. Adams G, Stratford I. Hypoxia selective bioreductive drugs. In: Peckham M, Piredo H, Veronesi U, eds. *Oxford Textbook of Oncology*. Vol 1. Oxford: Oxford Medical Publications, 1995: 785–95.
2. Barton MB, Keane TJ, Gadalla T, Maki E. The effect of treatment time and treatment interruption on tumour control following radical radiotherapy of laryngeal cancer. *Radiother Oncol* 1992; **23:** 137–43.
3. Beggs AC, McNally NJ, Shrieve DC, Kärcher H. A method to measure the duration of DNA synthesis and the potential doubling time from a single sample. *Cytometry* 1985; **6:** 620–6.
4. Brizel DM, Sibley GS, Prosnitz LR, Scher RL, Dewhirst MW. Tumor hypoxia adversely affects the prognosis of carcinoma of the head and neck. *Int J Radiat Oncol Biol Phys* 1997; **38:** 285–9.
5. Dische S, Saunders M, Barrett A, Harvey A, Gibson D, Parmar M. A randomized multicentre trial of CHART versus conventional radiotherapy in head and neck cancer. *Radiother Oncol* 1997; **44:** 123–36.
6. Fowler JF, Lindstrom MJ. Loss of local control with prolongation in radiotherapy. *Int J Radiat Oncol Biol Phys* 1992; **23:** 457–67.
7. Gray L, Conger A, Ibert B. The concentration of oxygen dissolved in tissues at the time of irradiation as a factor in radiotherapy. *Br J Radiol* 1953; **26:** 638–48.
8. Henk JM. Late results of a trial of hyperbaric oxygen and radiotherapy in head and neck cancer: a rationale for hypoxic cell sensitizers? *Int J Radiat Oncol Biol Phys* 1986; **12:** 1339–41.
9. Henk JM, James KM. Comparative trial of large and small fractions in the radiotherapy of head and neck cancer. *Clin Radiol* 1978; **29:** 611–16.
10. Horsman MR, Overgaard J. Overcoming tumor radiation resistance resulting from acute hypoxia. *Eur J Cancer* 1992; **28:** 717–18.
11. Howard-Flanders P, Moore D. The time interval after pulsed irradiation within which injury in bacteria can be modified by dissolved oxygen. *Radiat Res* 1958; **9:** 422–37.
12. Jackson SM, Weir LM, Hay JH, Tsang VH, Durham JS. A randomized trial of accelerated versus conventional radiotherapy in head and neck cancer. *Radiother Oncol* 1997; **43:** 39–46.
13. Jassem J, Bartelink H. Chemotherapy in locally advanced head and neck cancer: a critical reappraisal. *Cancer Treat Rev* 1995; **21:** 447–62.
14. Maciejewski B, Preuss-Bayer G, Trott KR. The influence of the number of fractions and of overall treatment time on local control and late complication rate in squamous cell carcinoma of larynx cancer. *Int J Radiat Oncol Biol Phys* 1983; **9:** 321–8.
15. Okunieff P, Morgan D, Niemierko A, Suit HD. Radiation dose-response of human tumors. *Int J Radiat Oncol Biol Phys* 1995; **32:** 1227–37.
16. Overgaard J, Horsman M. Overcoming hypoxic cell radioresistance. In: Steel G, ed. *Oxford Textbook of Oncology*. Vol 1. London: Arnold, 1993: 163–72.
17. Overgaard J, Hjelm-Hansen M, Johansen L, Andersen AP. Comparison of conventional and split-course radiotherapy as primary treatment in carcinoma of the larynx. *Acta Oncol* 1988; **27:** 147–52.
18. Withers HR, Taylor JM, Maciejewski B. The clinical hazard from accelerated tumor clonogen repopulation during radiotherapy. *Acta Oncol* 1988; **27:** 131–46.
19. Withers HR, Peter LJ, Taylor JM *et al.* Late normal tissue sequelae from radiation therapy for carcinoma of the tonsil: patterns of fractionation study of radiobiology. *Int J Radiat Oncol Biol Phys* 1995; **33:** 563–8.

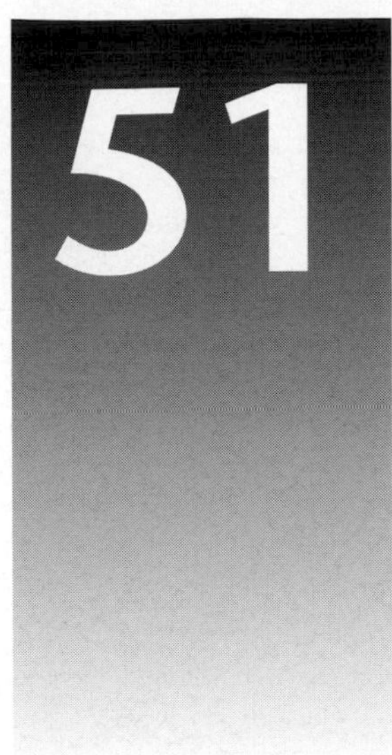

Radiotherapy for laryngeal cancer

François Eschwège and Olivier Dupuis

Historical perspective

Radiotherapy in the cancer of the larynx was born in Europe, but before 1922 no large series have been reported. The first publications have been written by Coutard, Regaud and Hautant who were, respectively, radio-oncologist, radiobiologist and surgeon at the Institut du Radium in Paris (Institut Curie nowadays).

Before Coutard, some investigators had delivered radiotherapy using radon seeds, radium interstitial puncture, irradiation of the larynx through a thyrotomy wound or external irradiation with radium, without evidence of an improvement in local control and/or survival. Coutard first reported on six patients with advanced diseases (including one with tumor causing skin ulceration) treated with fractionated radiotherapy in 1921 and showed that all of them were alive 1 year and some even 15 years after the irradiation.[16] This first experience allowed Coutard to continue his work and 32 patients with larynx carcinoma had been treated by 1922 and 77 patients by 1926. Coutard, in cooperation with Baclesse, continued to treat laryngeal cancer with irradiation in the early 1930s and they published on 142 cases, reporting a 5-year survival rate of 27%.[17] These authors emphasized the effects of protraction of the treatment and dose fractionation on normal tissue tolerance and tumor control. Among their results, the same authors also noted the variability of the response between exophytic and infiltrative tumors, and the necessity of a homogenous irradiation for high-dose treatments. Following this, many teams began to experience such treatment during the next two decades.[31] After those pioneers, technical advances and the use of cobalt-60 units since the 1950s definitely established the role of radiotherapy alone in selected cases or in association with surgery.[68,75,120] The more recent availability of accurate contention systems, simulators and computerized dosimetry have improved the quality of radiation delivery whilst the main goal of the first authors, who wished to cure their patient without a total laryngectomy, remains true for the present radio-oncologist.

Radiation therapy planning

Preparation of the patient

Because the treatment of laryngeal cancers by radiation therapy can be a source of some acute toxicity, the patient should be fully informed about the anticipated reactions and reassured that proper measures will be taken to help him. More specifically, nutritional support and pain control are very important during and following the radiotherapy course. The medical staff must also try to convince the patient to stop smoking (and drinking alcohol), not only because of the risk of second primaries but because it has been shown that smoking could decrease the probability of control and the quality of functional results.[8,112] The patient should also be aware of the detrimental effect on the probability of cure of any treatment interruption to reinforce his compliance.

Even in the case of glottis irradiation, dental preparation is necessary. Decayed teeth must be extracted before radiation therapy begins but this should not delay the onset of the treatment since these teeth are always out of the radiation fields. When the submaxillary and/or the parotid regions are included in the fields, fluoride trays should be prepared and the patient motivated to use them every day.

Positioning of the patient

The supine position is more widely used because of its good reproducibility. The patient's neck should be in relative hyperextension to keep the submandibular region and oropharyngeal mucosa out of the irradiated volume and to straighten the spinal column. Nevertheless, the patient must be sufficiently comfortable to ensure he can keep the same position during all the treatment. Elevation of the head or even of the chest can be useful to allow an adjustment of the spine curvature. Utilization of a head support, which fits to the posterior surface of the head and neck, can help the patient to maintain the position. These devices can be standard or can be made from foaming agents that form a customized mold around the patient's head and shoulders. Lateral decubitus is used in some institutions for early vocal cord cancer because the limits of the thyroid cartilage are clinically easier to determine.

Immobilization of the patient

Immobilization is crucial in head and neck radiotherapy because the treatment position is very difficult to maintain and may even be altered by swallowing and respiration. Modern and effective techniques have been described, some of which can be adapted in most departments at a reasonable cost. A standard chin support may be fixed to the treatment couch to prevent the patient from lowering his head (Fig 51.1); two lateral disks can also be tightened at both sides of the patient's head to keep it straight. The bite-block system usually consists in a piece of dental impression material attached to a horizontal graduated bar, which is in turn fixed to the patient's head support. The dental material is softened in hot water and placed in the patient's mouth and then the treatment position is decided. The graduation of the bar is recorded to assure precise reproduction of this position. Facial masks made of thermoplastic materials allow very tight immobilization and are now very easy and rapid to use. This material becomes pliable when placed in hot water and can be applied over the patient's face. It hardens in a few minutes and is then fixed to the patient's head support with anchor points (Fig 51.2).

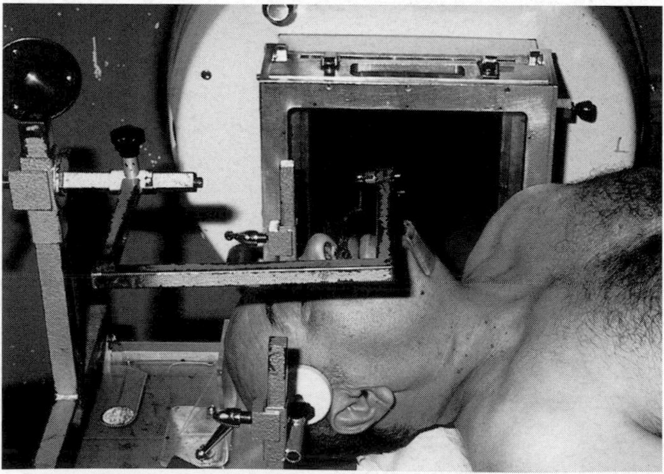

Figure 51.1 *An immobilization system consisting of a chin support fixed to an arm and two lateral disks.*

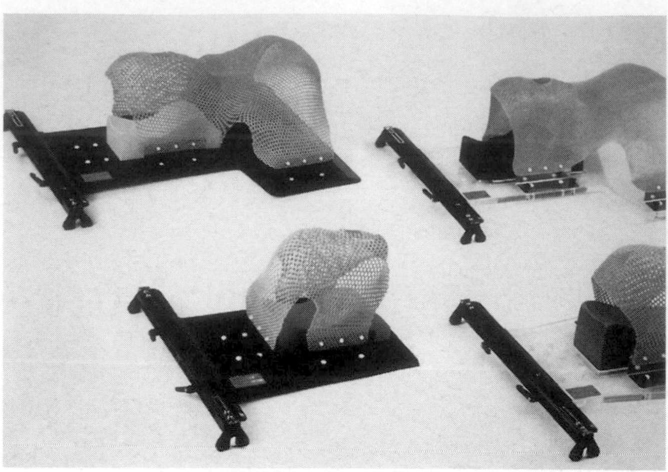

Figure 51.2 *Customized thermoformed plastic masks with different head supports.*

Treatment technique

Arrangement of fields

When regional lymphatic irradiation is necessary, two lateral opposed fields are generally used, encompassing the primary tumor and the superior and mid-jugular cervical lymph nodes. A third anterior field is used if the bilateral supraclavicular lymph nodes must be treated. When the spinal cord tolerance dose is reached (42–45 Gy), the lateral fields are reduced off the cord and a higher dose is delivered in the primary tumor and anterior neck. This field reduction can be performed by using a block or by shifting the beam axis and reducing the size of the collimator. The median part of the anterior field is also shielded at this moment if a higher dose is prescribed to the lower region of the neck; otherwise this field can be discontinued. A second field reduction is frequently performed in the lateral field to deliver the highest dose in the primary tumor only. Should the posterior cervical nodes be treated beyond a prophylactic dose, lateral electron fields are used, selecting their energy to prevent spinal cord overdosage (generally 8–12 MeV electrons). The depth of the spinal cord and the percentage depth dose of the electrons must then be known. If electrons are not available, the posterior neck is treated via two oblique beams. Special attention must be made to eliminate the overlapping of the anterior with the two lateral fields. Because lateral fields diverge caudally into the anterior field, which in turn diverge cephalad into the lateral fields, there is a risk of delivering very high dose to the spinal cord. Several techniques are used to resolve such a problem. The simplest method is to allow a sufficient margin between the cephalad limit of the supraclavicular field and the caudal limits of the lateral fields (0.5 cm at

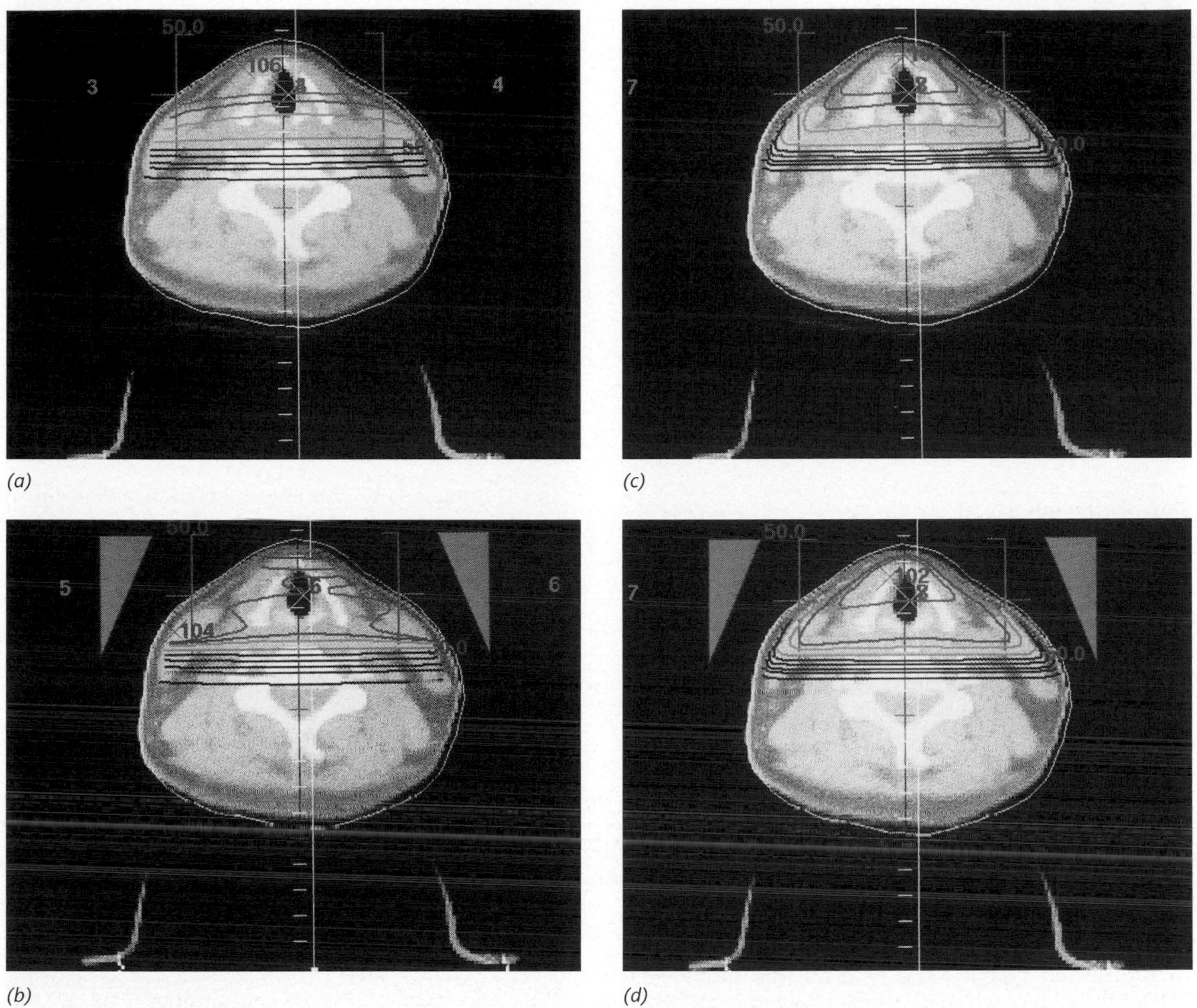

Figure 51.3 *Isodose distribution using opposed lateral fields to treat an early glottic cancer: dose distribution using Cobalt 60-rays without wedges (a) or 33° wedges (b); dose distribution using 6 MV x-rays without wedges (c) and 30° wedges (d).*

skin level has been demonstrated sufficient[7]). Another technique consists of inserting a block in the lateral fields to shield the caudal part of the spinal cord; conversely, shielding the cephalad part of the cord in the anterior field is rarely appropriate in the case of laryngeal cancer since it could result in protecting part of the tumor.

Treatment simulation

Usually, the determination of the size of the fields and their arrangement is decided during a simulation procedure during which the patient is in the treatment position. Radiopaque markers are used to indicate palpable nodes and surgical scars. Radiographs are made and will serve to delimit the margins of the treatment fields and to decide the position of the personalized blocks. Generally, blocks are inserted in the lateral fields to protect the buccal mucosa and the anterior part of the oropharynx as well as the occipital region. If an anterior field is used, blocks are placed below the clavicles to protect the apex of the lung.

Beam energy

The beam energy should be γ-rays from cobalt-60 or 4 MV x-rays from linear accelerators. Theoretically, the use of higher energy photons can be detrimental because the dose distribution tends to be less adequate in the posterior part of the field and in the soft tissues of the neck due to a lack of ionization buildup. Moreover, the presence of an air cavity near the surface of the vocal cord can result in an underdosage as high as 18% of some parts of the mucosa as has been demonstrated with 6 MV x-rays.[92]

Dose prescription and calculation

Dose prescription should be done on the central axis at the midplane of the patient for opposed fields and on the central axis at a precise depth (approximately 3 cm) for the anterior supraclavicular field according to Report 50 of the ICRU.[52] Because a difference in thickness between the cephalad and the caudal part of the neck, as well as between its anterior and posterior aspects, is frequent, the dose effectively delivered in the larynx may be higher than the central axis dose and adjustment must be made, if necessary. A representation of the dose distribution in the sagittal plane and in particular axial planes can therefore be useful to determine if tissue compensators or wedges are advantageous (Fig 51.3).

Dose fractionation

In western continental Europe and in the USA, treatment is generally delivered in five daily fractions of 2 Gy each week, without any interruption until the prescribed dose is reached. Each field should be treated each day to limit late reactions. Usual total doses are 65–70 Gy in 6.5–7 weeks to the primary tumor and involved lymph nodes and 45–50 Gy in prophylactically treated sites.

Treatment

Radical radiotherapy

Cancer of the glottis

For T1 lesions, the treated volume is limited to the larynx because lymph node involvement is very rare (Fig 51.4). At the Institut Gustave Roussy (IGR), the treatment is delivered through two small lateral opposed fields (5 × 5 to 6 × 6 cm) flashing over the anterior skin to prevent anterior commissure underdosage and whose limits are:

- upper limit of the thyroid cartilage;
- anterior border of the vertebral bodies or anterior border of the arytenoid cartilage for anterior tumors; and
- inferior limit of the cricoid cartilage.

A posterior reduction may be performed to exclude the arytenoids after 55–60 Gy when the tumor is located in the anterior third of the cord. Wedges are frequently used to improve the dose homogeneity unless the tumor is localized to the anterior commissure/anterior third of the cord where a 'hot spot' may be useful. Because the treated volume is small and the larynx mobile, regular checking of the position of the fields is performed at the IGR as in other institutions, using weekly portal films and daily clinical examination during the treatment. This precaution is probably more important than any other sophisticated immobilization device.

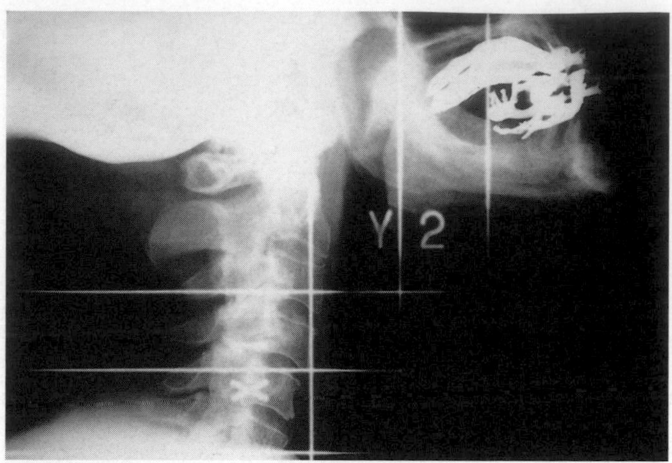

Figure 51.4 *Treatment fields for an early glottic tumor.*

In T2 tumors, the subclinical nodal involvement is considered very rare (<5%) and the ports are often basically the same as for T1, with margins adapted to the supraglottic or the subglottic extension of the tumor.[5,81,95,96,104]

When the larynx is fixed, subdigastric/mid-jugular lymph nodes are treated prophylactically in most institutions by using larger lateral fields which are reduced to the primary tumor when the spinal cord tolerance dose is reached (Fig 51.5). These fields are limited by the level of

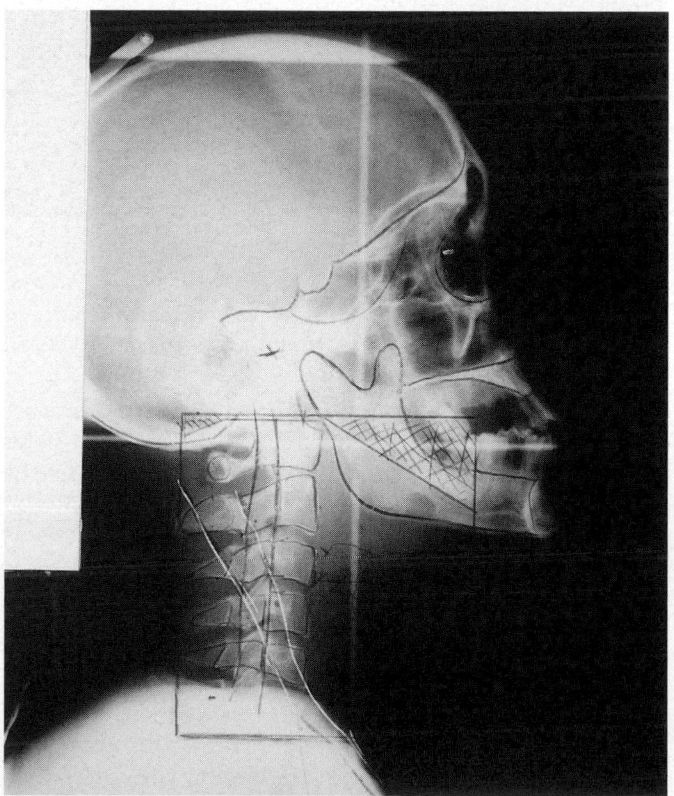

Figure 51.5 *Treatment fields after total laryngectomy for a T4 glottic carcinoma.*

the mandibular angle and posteriorly by the spinous process of the vertebra (a smaller posterior limit may not encompass the whole internal jugular chain[3]). The inferior limit is under the cricoid cartilage or lower in cases of subglottis extension.

In more advanced cases, the treatment volume is tailored to the extension of the tumor and of the clinical nodal disease (Fig 51.6). Usually, two lateral fields encompassing the primary tumor, the bilateral upper mid-jugular nodes and the posterior cervical chains and one anterior bilateral supraclavicular field are used.

Cancer of the supraglottis

The treated volume should include the primary tumor and the bilateral jugular chains and supraclavicular areas because even small supraglottis tumors can spread to the lymph nodes. When the neck disease is not extensive, a first off-cord field reduction is accomplished at 42–45 Gy and a further field reduction may be made after 50–55 Gy to give the higher dose in the primary tumor only.

Cancer of the subglottis

For this rare location, the treated volume is adapted to the tumor extension. Because there is a possibility of lymphatic involvement through the recurrent chain, anterior and posterior fields are frequently used to treat the primary tumor, lower cervical and upper mediastinal lymph nodes (caudal limit at the carina level). Following a dose of 40–45 Gy, field arrangement must be modified to protect the spinal cord and oblique anterior or lateral opposed fields may be used. Nevertheless, experience without such a prophylactic irradiation of the upper mediastinum does not show any detrimental effect of this omission for early tumors.[44]

Postoperative radiotherapy

After partial laryngectomy

The target volume is usually limited to the lymphatic drainage to keep the remaining larynx functional and the treatment is delivered through anterior or anterior/posterior fields with a block shielding the buccal region and the larynx. When surgical margins are positive at the level of the vallecula or base of tongue, two lateral fields are used to treat the upper neck and the lower part of the oropharynx and an anterior field is used to treat the lower neck with a block protecting the larynx.

After total laryngectomy

The target volume comprises the tumor bed and bilateral cervical lymph nodes. If surgical margins are safe, the total dose will be limited to 50 Gy. Following this, a boost dose of 10–15 Gy using electron beams of appropriate energy (8–10 MeV) is delivered at the sites of lymph node capsular rupture. Special attention must be paid to the risk of recurrence around the tracheostomy, which is about 10%, especially in cases of subglottis involvement, soft tissue spread, extensive cervical lymph node metastasis or when a tracheostomy has been performed days or weeks before the radical surgery. Because the dose delivered at this site through the anterior supraclavicular field is limited to 45 Gy by the spinal cord tolerance, a bolus material may be placed over the stoma to increase the superficial dose and a boost dose may be delivered with an electron beam.

The role of radiotherapy in the treatment of laryngeal carcinomas

Indications

The place of radiation therapy in the treatment of laryngeal carcinoma should not only be evaluated based on local regional control and survival results but also taking into consideration the possibility of preserving a functional larynx.

There is no widely accepted consensus about treatment of laryngeal squamous cell carcinoma throughout the world.[93] Early glottic and supraglottic tumors are generally treated with partial surgery or radiotherapy alone and no direct comparison between these two modalities has been attempted. In more advanced diseases, most teams before mid-1980 (predominantly head and neck surgeons) have chosen surgery as the primary treatment followed by postoperative radiotherapy guided on histopathologic findings. In other institutions in Canada, the UK and Western Europe, radiotherapy with salvage surgery in reserve has been selected. Here also, no direct comparisons have been documented. Since the mid-1980s, induction chemotherapy has been used in many cases followed by radiotherapy in patients showing good or complete response.

Early glottic tumors

Early cancers limited to the vocal cord (T1) or with minimal subglottic or supraglottic extension (T2a) are considered highly curable with conventional radiotherapy, leaving no place for unorthodox techniques.

T2b glottic tumors

Impairment of the vocal cord mobility significantly reduces the probability of definitive control with conventional radiotherapy, the results of which must be compared with those of partial surgery. This is probably due to the spread to a rich capillary network but also to the higher tumor volume of these cancers. The dose used in conventional radiotherapy (65–70 Gy in 6.5–7 weeks in most western Europe and USA institutions) may be insufficient to sterilize high-volume tumors and thus justifies the use of hyperfractionated and/or accelerated regimens in other institutions.[86,122] To date, no randomized trials have been published to confirm the superiority of these altered fractionation schemes in laryngeal cancer. In other teams, T2b tumors are considered eligible for so-called 'organ preservation' protocols and have even been included in the Veterans Affairs trial although a partial or subtotal laryngectomy may have been feasible.[21]

T3 glottic tumors

Fixation of a vocal cord and invasion of the cartilaginous framework of the larynx is considered by many authors as a contraindication for radical irradiation. In fact, histopathologic studies after total laryngectomy in T2 glottic carcinomas have frequently shown at least a microscopic cartilage infiltration.[18] More recently, CT studies have demonstrated such an involvement in tumors that would have been clinically classified as T2, suggesting that subgroups of T3 tumors could be effectively treated with radiotherapy. The choice of the treatment varies in different countries of the world and strongly depends on institution, skills, habits and speciality of the attending physician (head and neck surgeon or radiation oncologist). However, favorable results in these tumors with primary radiotherapy needs experienced teams to select appropriate cases and to allow early salvage surgery when necessary.

In those T3 glottic carcinomas, many strategies have been tested in order to enhance the radiosensitivity of the tumor cells. Hyperbaric oxygen, although showing positive results, is not a practical technique for routine therapy;[46] radiosensitizers,[37] and neutrons[25] have been used without evidence of an improvement. More recently, hyperfractionation with or without acceleration have been found of particular interest in phase II[34,84] and in one phase III trial.[24] Finally, the role of induction chemotherapy in selecting patients suitable for definitive radiation therapy has not been definitively established by the recent organ preservation randomized trials since response to chemotherapy appeared as a poor marker of radiocurability.[57,106,127] Concomitant chemotherapy and radiotherapy is a promising strategy and is under evaluation in recently activated randomized trials in the USA and in Europe.

Another issue which may become an important guide in the choice of the primary treatment is its overall cost.[64,127] For example, Laramore calculated that in the USA, the treatment of 100 T3N0M0 patients with radiotherapy and salvage surgery, surgery with postoperative radiotherapy or a larynx preservation protocol would cost 4.2, 6.2 and 6.4 million US$, respectively.[64]

Supraglottic carcinoma

Radiotherapy remains the standard treatment of small exophytic cancers of the supraglottic larynx without neck involvement. Infiltrative or bulky tumors with or without impaired vocal cord mobility, tumors associated with nodes larger than 2–3 cm are more suitable for partial or total laryngectomy with cervical lymph node dissection. Postoperative radiotherapy is recommended for tumors with extralaryngeal extension, positive margins and/or N+ disease.

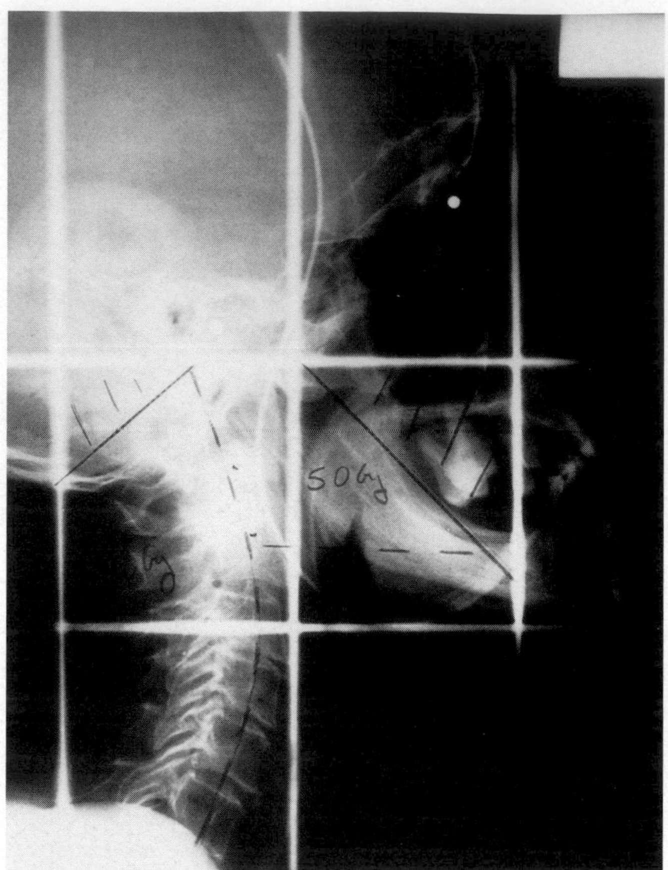

Figure 51.6 *Treatment fields for a large supraglottic cancer. A first reduction is made after 42 Gy to protect the spinal cord and a second after 50 Gy to treat the primary and the palpable nodes only.*

The cases in between have been the subject of intense discussion in the literature. Predictive factors of radiotherapy failure are weakly represented by the T classification of the UICC. In particular, tumors classified as T3 because of a minimal extension of the pre-epiglottic space on a CT scan or spread to the medial wall of the pyriform sinus may have a similar control rate to a T2. When neck involvement is present, radiotherapy with planned neck dissection for residual disease is probably a promising option for laryngeal preservation.[82,126]

Advanced laryngeal cancer

Radiotherapy is rarely considered as the primary treatment of operable cases although fair results have been shown in cases of minimal extension to the oropharynx or to the thyroid cartilage with clinically negative neck.[40,61,98] Regression after a dose of 50–55 Gy could even help to select radiocurable patients and this criteria has been used in trained teams.[56,111] The role of postoperative radiotherapy has been well defined in the last decades.[2,4,89,116] It is

Table 51.1 Results of radiotherapy in T1N0 glottic cancer

Author(s) (period)	*n*	*Radiotherapy schedule (dose/time)*	*Local control (% 5 years)*	*Survival (%)*	*Surgical salvage* (%)*	*Adverse prognostic factors (when studied)*
Inoue *et al.*[50] (1967–82)	274	60–66 Gy/6–6.5 weeks	T1a: 80; T1b: 90	65 (10 years)	37/55 (67)	No tumor regression at 40 Gy
Lusinchi *et al.*[73] (1970–83)	197	65 Gy/6.5 weeks	85.7	65 (10 years)	16/38 (42)	Tumor extension, bulky aspect, suspicion of T2
Terhaard *et al.*[112] (1975–85)	194	66 Gy/6.5 weeks	89	91 (cs)	15/21 (71)	Tumor extension, continue smoking†
Mendenhall *et al.*[81] (1964–84)	171	56–67 Gy/5–6.5 weeks	T1a: 94; T1b: 93	NA	7/12 (58)	NA
Cellai *et al.*[14] (1972–83)	155	60–64 Gy/6–6.5 weeks	T1a: 88; T1b: 75	87	16/31 (51.5)	T1b, number of subsites involved†
Akine *et al.*[1] (1967–83)	154	67 Gy/6.5–7 weeks	89	87	17/18 (94)	Anterior commissure (P = 0.06)
Olszewski *et al.*[91] (1966–80)	137	56–70 Gy/6–7.5 weeks	80	NA	22/27 (82)	Anterior commissure involvement, poorly differentiated, size of field when Co-60 used
Pellitteri *et al.*[95] (1969–84)	113	66 Gy/6 weeks	93	NA	6/8 (75)	NA
Robson *et al.*[98] (1966–83)	107	57.5 Gy/5.5 weeks	T1a: 95; T1b: 84	94; 79	6/6 (100)	NA
Fein *et al.*[27,30] (1980–91)	93	66 Gy/6.5 weeks	85	NA	NA	Hemoglobin <13 g/dl†
Rudoltz *et al.*[99] (1966–89)	91	64 Gy/6.5 weeks	80	92	13/18 (72)	Prolonged treatment time†
Sinha[104] (1971–83)	74	66 Gy/6–8 weeks	T1a: 86; T1b: 75	91	(54)	Continue smoking
Benninger *et al.*[5] (1974–84)	48	60–70 Gy/6–8 weeks	81	NA	NA	Continue smoking

Survival: 5 years overall survival unless specified (cs, corrected survival). NA, data not available.
*Number of patients controlled with salvage surgery/number of local failures.
†Multivariate analysis.

now recommended in cases of positive surgical margins, invasion of subcutaneous tissues, pericapsular spread and when a tracheostomy has been performed several days before the laryngectomy.

When the patient is not operable for medical or locoregional reasons or when he refuses surgery, non-conventional treatment should probably be used if cure is intended. In this setting, accelerated regimens or concomitant chemoradiotherapy may be the best choice in the medically fit patient although the risk of severe acute and/or late complication is most probably enhanced.

Acute reactions

Radiation therapy for early glottic cancer is very well tolerated in most cases because of the small mucosal volume treated. The voice may improve during the first 2 weeks of the treatment and then the hoarseness frequently increases with a mild dysphagia, which rarely requires analgesics. Voice returns frequently to normal in a few months and dysphonia very infrequently impairs normal activity.[73,81] For more advanced lesions, as well as for supralaryngeal cancer, acute reactions are more important and may require more intensive care, especially in older patients. Daily steam inhalations, analgesics and corticosteroids may be useful, as well as nutritional support. As a whole, at our institution, less than 10% of the treatments must be postponed for 1–2 weeks.

Results

Early and moderately advanced glottic cancer

Numerous studies have been published concerning the results of treatment in tumors limited to the vocal cords without mobility impairment (i.e. T1). Radiotherapy is frequently considered as the treatment of choice because local results are equal to, and functional results are better than, cordectomy.[93,103] Surgical treatment is reserved for relapse although it is favored when follow-up may be difficult and in young patients. Five-year local control rates are between 80 and 93% with a total dose of 60–65 Gy in 6–6.5 weeks (see Table 51.1). It is noticeable that in series where very long follow-up is reported, late relapse

Table 51.2 Results of radiotherapy in T2N0 glottic cancer

Author(s) (period)	*n*	*Radiotherapy schedule (dose/time)*	*Local control (% 5 years)*	*Survival (%)*	*Surgical salvage* (%)*	*Adverse prognostic factors (when studied)*
Harwood *et al.*[39] (1965–77)	244	50 Gy/4–5 weeks to 55 Gy/5 weeks	All: 69; T2a: 80; T2b: 52	67	45/75 (60)	Mobility impaired
Slevin *et al.*[105] (1970–84)	242	55 Gy/3 weeks	82	64	19/54 (35)	Mobility impaired†
Wang[122] (1952–78)	190	65–67 Gy/6.5–7 weeks	All: 71; T2a: 79; T2b: 61	NA	26/55 (47)	Mobility impaired, male
Turesson *et al.*[117] (1963–83)	132	Various schedules	T2a: 76; T2b: 60	96 cs; 79 cs	15/19 (79); 19/32(60)	Mobility impaired
Fein *et al.*[27] (1977–89)	115	63–67.5 Gy/6 weeks or HFRT	All: 83; T2a: 87; T2b: 76	NA	14/18 (78)	Mobility impaired†
Howell-Burke *et al.*[49] (1970–85)	114	65–78 Gy/6–8 weeks	67.5	92 dfs	28/37 (75.5)	Subglottis extension (nonsignificant in multivariate analysis)
Schwaab *et al.*[101] (1974–84)	68	70 Gy/7 weeks	All: 66; T2a: 64; T2b: 75	T2a: 71; T2b: 41	12/19 (63); 0/3	NA
Van den Bogaert *et al.*[118] (1962–77)	61	40–70 Gy/4–7 weeks	63	48	7/20 (35)	Long overall treatment time
Pellitteri *et al.*[95] (1969–84)	48	64–70 Gy/6–7 weeks	All: 73; T2a: 80; T2b: 57	NA	9/13 (69)	Both cord and anterior commissure involvement

Survival: 5 years overall unless specified (cs, corrected survival; dfs, disease-free survival). HFRT, hyperfractionated radiotherapy (1.2 Gy b.i.d.); NA, data not available.
*Number of patients controlled with salvage surgery/number of locoregional failures.
†Multivariate analysis.

(>5 years) is not rare and not discernible from second laryngeal primaries.[50,73] In cases of relapse, 50–82% of the patients are successfully salvaged with surgery. This surgical salvage frequently necessitates a total laryngectomy but recent experiences show that partial or subtotal laryngectomy may be effective in selected cases.[90,101] Reported 5- and 10-year survival rates are around 80 and 65%, respectively, with most of the deaths due to second primaries or intercurrent diseases.[77] Predictive factors of local relapse have been mainly studied with univariate analysis (see Table 51.1). Patients who continue smoking are at higher risk of recurrence, as shown in several series.[5,104,112] Tumor extension to the whole cord and/or large tumor size is frequently associated with lower control rates[73,81,112] but the value of distinguishing between T1a and T1b tumors and the effect of anterior commissure involvement are much more controversial. The patient's hemoglobin level has recently been reported of prognostic significance in one study using multivariate analysis[30] but this was not found in another study.[117] Actually, an optimal radiotherapy technique is probably most important to assure the highest local control rate as is shown by the improvement of the results in most of the institutions during the past decades.[74] For example, Wang noted that results for the tumors with posterior third involvement were better after the introduction of wedge filters in the Massachussetts General Hospital.[121] In addition, the beam energy may be critical since the local control was reported much lower with 6, 8 or 10 MV x-rays than with Co-60 or 4 MV x-rays in retrospective studies.[23,54] Nevertheless, an 89% local control rate is reported using 6 MV x-rays for T1N0 glottic carcinoma in one report.[1] Even in these small tumors, prolongation of the treatment has been shown to be detrimental by some authors[97,99] although others do not find this influence,[123] or find a lower control rate only when the dose per fraction is lower than 2 Gy.[12]

Carcinoma in situ of the vocal cord has been treated by radiation therapy in many institutions with control rates superior to 80%.[29] This management may be useful when a recurrence occurs after a vocal cord stripping or a laser treatment and especially when surveillance of the patient is difficult.

Stage T2 glottic cancer comprises a heterogenous group of tumors that are frequently subclassified as T2a (supra and/or subglottic extension) and T2b (impairment of the vocal cord mobility). Local control rates are around 80% for T2a, very close to the results of T1, but when the cord mobility is impaired the results are less satisfying, with 52–76% of patients controlled with radiation alone (see Table 51.2). Nevertheless, results may probably be enhanced when the overall treatment time is optimal and/or the total dose increased as shown by the results of hyperfractionated regimens.[27] Even in institutions where lymph nodes are not irradiated, the neck recurrence rate is between 2 and 5% when the tumor is locally controlled.[28,49,83,95,117] When a recurrence occurs, 25–35% of the patients are inoperable because of the extension of the

Table 51.3 Results of radiotherapy in T3N0 glottic cancer

Author(s) (period)	*n*	*Radiotherapy schedule (dose/time)*	*Locoregional control (%)*	*Survival (% 5-yr)*	*Surgical salvage* (%)*	*Adverse prognostic factors*
Harwood *et al.*[41] (1963–77)	112	50–55 Gy/4–5 weeks	51	NA	32/55 (57)	LC = 60% if optimal dose (55 Gy/5 weeks)
Mendenhall *et al.*[84] (1966–94)	75†	60–75 Gy/6–8 weeks or HFRT	58	78 ds; 54 os	15/25 (60)	Tumor volume >3.5 cm^3 (local control), tracheostomy before treatment (survival)
Wang[122] (1952–78)	70	65–67 Gy/6.5–7 weeks	36	NA	15/45 (33)	Male
Bryant *et al.*[10] (1961–89)	55	50–70 Gy/5–7 weeks	42	NA	NA	Tracheostomy before treatment
Sandberg *et al.*[100] (1963–83)	19	55–70 Gy/5–7 weeks	39	NA	NA	LC = 70% if XRT ≥70 Gy
Mills[87] (1968–75)	18	56–60 Gy/8–9 weeks (split course)	44.5	NA	6/10 (60)	Moderately and poorly differentiated tumors

HFRT, hyperfractionated radiotherapy 74–79.2 Gy in two daily fractions of 1.2–1.4 Gy; ds, disease-specific survival; os, overall survival; NA, data not available.
*Number of patients controlled with salvage surgery/number of local-regional relapses.
†21% patients were clinically N+.

Table 51.4 Results of radiotherapy in supraglottic cancer

Author(s) (period)	*n & stage*	*Radiotherapy schedule (dose/time)*	*Locoregional control (%)*	*Survival (% 5-yr)*	*Surgical salvage* (%)*	*Adverse prognostic factors (when studied)*
Glinski *et al.*[33] (1979–89)	250, stage I–II	66–76 Gy/6–7.5 weeks	NA	Stage I: 83 dfs; stage II: 70 dfs	15/49 (30.5)	Stage II, lower supraglottis
Inoue *et al.*[51] (1967–82)	100, stage I–II	56–76 Gy/6–7.5 weeks	68	NA	15/29 (52)	Tumor of the false cord, no response at 40 Gy
Cailleux[13] (1970–84)	166 T1–2, N0: 81%	65–76 Gy/6–8 weeks	T1: 73; T2: 71	N0: 61 cs; N1–2: 37 cs; N3: 41 cs	18/47 (38)	Number of subsites, epiglottis involvement
Wendt *et al.*[125] (1970–81)	98 T2–3, N0: 70%	70 Gy/7 weeks	63	45 os	NA	NA
Robson *et al.*[98] (1966–83)	44 T3–4N0	57 Gy/5 weeks	T3: 56; T4: 62	T3: 52 dfs; T4: 52 dfs	4/18 (22)	NA
Spaulding *et al.*[107] (1968–81)	83 T1–4 N0–1	60–65 Gy/5–6.5 weeks	T1N0–1: 88; T2N0–1: 65; T3N0–1: 22; T4N0–1: 28	NA	T1N0–1 & T2N0–1: 4/10 (40); T3N0–1 & T4N0–1: 2/10 (20)	Number of subsites, transglottic tumor, N2–3
Harwood *et al.*[43] (1960–79)	410 all stages	50–55 Gy/4–5 weeks	T1–4N0: 62	N0: 73 cs; N+: 46 cs	NA	Nodal disease, T3–4 (UICC 79)
Mendenhall *et al.*[82] (1964–92)	209 all stages		Stages: I: 90; II: 83; III: 64; IVA: 63; IVB: 50	100 cs; 90 cs; 80 cs; 53 cs; 40 cs	I–II: 3/7 (43); III: 9/19 (47); IV: 7/36 (19)	T stage, impaired mobility, tumor volume >6 cm^3
Levendag *et al.*[71] (1965–79)	203 all stages	60–70 Gy/7–12 weeks	T1–2: 57; T3–4: 45	T1: 71 dfs; T2: 53 dfs; T3: 52 dfs; T4: 39 dfs	40/95 (42)	T stage, long overall treatment time
Issa[53] (1963–81)	76, all	65–78 Gy/5.5–7 weeks	Stages: I: 90; II: 100	I: 90 os; II: 93 os	0	NA

os, overall survival; cs, corrected survival; dfs, disease-free survival; NA, data not available.
*Number of patients controlled with salvage surgery/number of locoregional failures.

Table 51.5 Results of radiotherapy in subglottis cancer

Author(s) (period)	*n*	*Radiotherapy schedule (dose/time)*	*Local control (%)*	*Survival (%)*	*Surgical salvage* (%)*
Haylock and Deutsch[44] (1976–90)	23	66 Gy/6.5 weeks	T1–2: 92; T3: 43; T4: 33	All: 68 dfs; All: 58 os	2/7 (28)
Warde *et al.*[124] (1971–82)	22	50–55 Gy/4–5 weeks	T1–3: 100; T4: 36	All: 61 cs; All: 26 os	1/7 (14)
Guedea *et al.*[36] (1964–85)	6	61–75 Gy/ 6–7 weeks	Tis: 1/1; T2: 1/2; T4: 2/3	All: 4/6 cs; All: 2/6 os	0/2

os, overall survival; cs, corrected survival; dfs, disease-free survival.
*Number of patients controlled with salvage surgery/number of local failures.

disease and/or poor medical status. As a whole, more than half the patients can be effectively salvaged with surgery. This surgery must be a total laryngectomy in most cases although a partial vertical or a subtotal laryngectomy may be suitable in selected cases.[90,101] Although the disease-free survival is high with radiation plus surgical salvage, many patients die from tobacco-related disease and overall 5-year survival is around 50–60%.

Stage T3N0 glottic cancer is a rare presentation (<10%) but has been the subject of many reports concerning the possibility of tumor control with voice preservation using primary radiotherapy (see Table 51.3). Because most series report on relatively few patients treated over long periods, definitive conclusions are difficult to make. Reported local control rates are between 39 and 53% with conventional radiotherapy but seem better when dose/time factors are optimal[42,100] or when hyperfractionation is used to increase the dose.[61,84] Unilateral exophytic lesions without airway compromise are probably more suitable for primary radiotherapy. Accurate staging using CT scan is also probably very useful to select tumors that are at high risk of recurrence following radiotherapy, as shown in a recent study at the university of Florida:[94] tumor volume >3.5 cm^3, extension to the paraglottic space at the level of false cords or to the arytenoid face/interarytenoid region, arytenoid and cricoid cartilage sclerosis were associated with lower local control rates. When patients are adequately followed, a surgical salvage of local recurrence is effective in 33–70%. On the whole, disease-specific survival is frequently in the range of the reported results with surgery with or without postoperative radiation,[10,84] although a real comparison is precluded by the fact that patient selection is very different in surgical and radiotherapy series.

Early supraglottic cancer

Stage I and II supraglottic tumors may be effectively treated with radiotherapy allowing voice preservation in more than two-thirds of patients. It also permits the treatment of patients who are not eligible for functional surgery due to their medical status. Most series report local control rates above 80% for T1 and above 70% for T2 (see Table 51.4). In the experience of the IGR, as well as in others, surgical salvage is more difficult than for early glottic cancer with reported control of 0–52% and a poor outcome when lymph nodes are involved at the time of recurrence (B. Luboinski, personal communication and reference 71). Neck relapse is more frequent than for glottic tumors, thus justifying elective neck irradiation: relapse rates above 25% are reported when the lymphatic chains are not irradiated[42,71] and are between 3 and 14% when large fields are used.[13,51,70,107] In these early tumors, few prognostic factors have been recognized because most studies mix both early and more advanced tumors. The adverse prognostic significance of an infiltrative or ulcerative aspect is well known. Tumors arising from the lateral epilarynx are often considered of worst prognosis because their invasion pattern mimics hypopharyngeal cancer,[13,108] although opposite results have been reported in recent series.[33,51,82]

Subglottic cancer

Because tumors arising in the subglottic larynx are very rare, representing 1%[35,102,124] to 8%[44,85] of all the laryngeal carcinomas, data are very scarce about the role of radiation therapy (see Table 51.5). In a review of 20 articles published before 1970, Vermund[120] reported a 5-year survival of 36% for 127 patients treated with irradiation alone. More recent experiences confirm the high curability of early subglottis cancer with radiotherapy.[44,124] The results in T3 tumors are more controversial with good control in some series[85,124] contrasting with high failure rates in other experiences.[44] In more advanced tumors, the risk of local recurrence is 50–60% and salvage surgery is infrequently possible. When surgery is used first, postoperative radiotherapy should be given for T3–T4 and/or N+ tumors. Special attention must then be paid to treat adequately the stoma, which is a common site of recurrence, rarely salvageable.[67]

Advanced laryngeal cancer

Radiotherapy is not the primary treatment for advanced laryngeal cancers, which are treated with surgery (mainly total laryngectomy) and postoperative radiotherapy in most institutions.[93] Nevertheless, some authors defend a

Table 51.6 Results of primary radiotherapy in advanced laryngeal cancer

Author(s) (period)	*n & stage*	*Radiotherapy schedule (dose/time)*	*Locoregional control (%)*	*Survival (% 5-yr)*	*Surgical salvage* (%)*	*Adverse prognostic factors (when studied)*
Lindelov and Hansen[72] (1965–86)	584, stage III–IV	67 Gy/ 6–7 weeks	Stage III: 35;* stage IV: 30*	29 os	NA	Size ≥40 mm, T3–4
Meredith *et al.*[85] (1969–78)	150, T3–4	NA	NA	Stage III: 59 cs; T4N0: 25 cs; stage IV: 8 cs	NA	Supraglottis, N stage, poorly differentiated
Karim *et al.*[61] (1974–84)	137, T3–4	72–78 Gy/7–8 weeks or HFRT	67	40	21/44 (48)	Stage N2–3, total dose
Davidson *et al.*††[19] (1982–86)	129	50 Gy/4 weeks or 50 Gy/8 weeks + chemotherapy	53	NA	15/60 (25)	NA
Terhaard *et al.*[113] (1975–84)	104, T3N0–3	66 Gy/7 weeks or HF + split course	53	NA	24/45 (53)	N stage
Robson *et al.*[98] (1966–83)	97, T3–4N0	57.5 Gy/4.5 weeks	58	50.5 dfs	12/42 (28.5)	NA
Harwood *et al.*[42] (1965–77)	72, T4, glottic	50–55 Gy/4–5 weeks	T4N0: 56; T4N+: 12.5	NA	4/24 (17); 1/14 (7)	N stage, hypo-pharyngeal extension vs cartilaginous invasion
Eschwège *et al.*[26] (1978–84)	51, T3–4	70 Gy/7 weeks	43	38 os; 62 cs	3/29 (10)	NA
Van den Bogaert *et al.*[119] (1962–77)	35, T3–4, glottic	40–70 Gy + split course	23	22 os	5/27 (18.5)	NA

HFRT, hyperfractionated radiotherapy; os, overall survival; cs, corrected survival; dfs, disease-free survival.
*All sites unless specified.
†Number of patients controlled with salvage surgery/number of local failures.
††Randomized study, no difference between the two treatment arms.

Table 51.7 Results of surgery + postoperative radiotherapy in advanced laryngeal cancer

Institution (period)	*n & stage*	*Treatment*	*Locoregional control (%)*	*Survival (%)*	*Adverse prognostic factors (when studied)*
MD Anderson[128] (1959–79)	242, T3–4	Surgery alone (192); surgery + XRT (50)	T3: 82; T4: 68; T3: 90; T4: 95	80 dfs; 63 dfs; 89 dfs; 94 dfs	NA
IGR (1975–84)	236, stage III–IV	Postop. XRT	86	NA	Insufficient margins, N+, N+R+
RTOG†[116] (1973–79)	118, T3–4	Preop XRT; Postop XRT	58 (P = 0.007); 80	32 os (P = 0.18); 42 os	NA
FNCLCC[89] (1980–85)	116, T2–4 (N+: 68%)	Postop. XRT	78	76 dfs	T4, N+R+, positive surgical margins*

IGR, Institut Gustave Roussy (Villejuif), F. Eschwège personal data; FNCLCC, Fédération française des centres de lutte contre le cancer; RTOG, Radiation therapy oncology group; os, overall survival; dfs, disease-free survival; NA, data not available.
*Multivariate analysis.
†Randomized study.

strategy of primary radiotherapy with surgical salvage in reserve for selected cases[40,42,56,82,111] or even as a standard attitude.[61,85,98] Adverse prognostic factors indicating poor local control with radiotherapy alone are tumor size[72] or volume,[82] and extension to the hypopharynx.[42] Nodal disease is widely accepted as a major factor affecting survival but also local control.[40,42,61,85,113] When conventional radiotherapy is given, reported locoregional control

Table 51.8 Results of larynx-preservation randomized trials

Series	*n, tumor site & T stage*	*Median follow-up (months)*	*Locoregional control (%)*	*Salvage laryngectomy (%)*	*Alive with larynx (%)*	*Survival (%)*	*Distant failure (%)*
VALCSG[21]	332, supraglottis, glottis, T2–4	60	C+RT: 80; S±RT: 93	35; –	52/79 (66); –	C+RT: 53.3; S±RT: 55.9	11; 17
EORTC[65]	202, pyr. sinus, aryep. fold, T2–4	36	C+RT: 71; S±RT: 73	43 + 8 tracheostomies; –	28/100 (28); –	C+RT: 57; S±RT: 43	25; 36
GETTEC (unpublished)	68, glottis, T3	60	NA	NA	23; –	C+RT: 30.5; S±RT: 65†	NA
Depondt *et al.**[22]	115, larynx, hypopharynx, T2–4	36	57; 57	NA	NA	NA	NA

C+RT, induction chemotherapy arm; S±RT, conventional surgical arm; NA, data not available; VALCSG, Veterans Affairs laryngeal cancer study group; GETTEC, Groupe d'étude des tumeurs de la tête et du cou; EORTC, European organization for research and treatment of cancer.
*Study comprising all head and neck sites, no analysis by subsite.
†Difference is significant.

rates range between 23 and 56%, mainly depending on the selection of patients (see Table 51.6). Time/dose factors are also probably important to explain these differences with poor results of split course radiotherapy[119] and better control when accelerated (hypofractionated)[19,40,42,62,98] or hyperfractionated radiotherapy[61,82,84] is used. Surgical salvage is less effective than in early tumors and approximately one-third (range 17–53% in Table 51.6) of the patients may be cured at recurrence.[19] Survival is highly influenced by N stage and the disease-free survival of T3–T4N0 is roughly 50–80% compared with 25–50% for T3–T4N1–N3. Finally, the addition of resection of the residual neck disease 3–4 months after the completion of the radiotherapy probably enhances the possibility of cure while preserving the larynx.[82,126]

Results of surgery with postoperative radiotherapy are frequently better (see Table 51.7) although true comparison is difficult: surgical cases are often more advanced tumors but some patients in the radiotherapy series are inoperable for locoregional or medical reasons. The addition of a postoperative irradiation improves the results, especially when neck disease is present, in T4 tumors and when a preoperative tracheostomy has been performed.[4,67,128] Preoperative radiotherapy is probably less effective as shown in supraglottic cancer in a randomized study.[116] Widely recognized prognostic factors for both locoregional control and survival are node metastasis, even more if capsular rupture is present, and positive resection margins.[2,4,88]

Radiotherapy and chemotherapy in laryngeal cancer

When the dramatic response in inoperable head and neck carcinomas were first reported using cisplatin combinations, induction chemotherapy protocols were designed to enhance the results of local treatment and reduce the distant failure rate with the hope of improving the poor survival rates obtained with surgery and radiotherapy. Unfortunately, although the high initial response rates were confirmed in randomized studies, no improvement in survival was found. Nevertheless, subset analysis showed that the patients who did respond to chemotherapy but refused surgery and were irradiated had a survival similar to those operated on. Some authors then investigated the possibility of substituting radiotherapy for surgery in patients responding to induction chemotherapy.[55] These first experiences confirmed that survival of the irradiated patients was similar to those who were operated after insufficient response to chemotherapy. It was also shown that histologic complete response to chemotherapy was not necessary and that a very good clinical response was sufficient to select patients for radical radiotherapy. Finally, the response to chemotherapy was considered as a predictive factor of the response to radiotherapy. In the mid-1980s, multicentric randomized studies were initiated, including somewhat different groups of patients. The Department of Veterans Affairs study[21] concerned patients with T2–T3 supraglottic or glottic cancers while the European Organization for Research and Treatment of Cancer (EORTC) trial studied patients with aryepiglottic fold or mainly hypopharyngeal tumors.[65] The GETTEC (Groupe d'Etude des Tumeurs de la Tête et du Cou) included only endolaryngeal T3N0 tumors (B. Luboinsky and F. Eschwège, unpublished data) and the data concerning the larynx preservation in the second French study are barely analyzable[22] (see Table 51.8). Patients were randomized to surgery and postoperative radiotherapy (conventional arm) or to receive two or three cycles of chemotherapy followed by radiotherapy for responders or surgery with postoperative radiotherapy for nonresponders (experimental arm). Response to chemotherapy was considered sufficient if it was

Table 51.9 Experiences with hyperfractionated and/or accelerated regimens in laryngeal cancer

Author(s) (period)	*n, site, extension*	*Radiotherapy*	*Locoregional control (%)*	*Survival (%)*	*Surgical salvage**	*Complications (%)*
Karim *et al.*[61] (1974–84)	52 SG, G, T3–4	HF: 67.5–72.5 Gy/ 60–65 f/5.5–6 weeks	73	NA	NA	NA
Garden *et al.*[32] (1984–92)	236 SG, H, O, T2–4	HF: 76.8 Gy/ 60–70 f/6.5–7 weeks	75	70 os	29/60 (48)	Feeding tube: 16; weight loss >10%: 5; severe late sequelae: 9[c]
Mendenhall *et al.*[82] (1980–94)	48 SG, T1–4	HF: 74–79.2 Gy/ 60–65 f/6–6.5 weeks	65	NA	12/17 (70.5)	Severe late sequelae: 6
Bujko *et al.*[11] (1988–89)	65 SG, 21 N+	Concomitant boost[a] = 66 Gy/6 weeks	T1–2: 68; T3–4: 54	78 os; 44 os	NA	Grade 2–3 dysphagia: 50; severe late sequelae: 12
Johnson *et al.*[59] (1981–88)	13 L, T1–4	Concomitant boost[a] = 70.2 Gy/6.5 weeks	100	NA	NA	Temporary tracheotomy: 7.5; laryngectomy: 7.5
Corvo *et al.*[15] (1989–92)	19 L, H, T3–4	Concomitant boost[a] = 72–75 Gy/6 weeks	48	NA	NA	Feeding tube for acute mucositis: 13; severe late sequelae: 10.5
Glover *et al.*[34] (1986–89)	18 SG, G, T2–4	CHART[b] = 54 Gy/ 36 f/12 d	67	78 cs; 39 os	3/6 (50)	No severe complication

NA, data not available; HF, hyperfractionation. Sites: O, oropharynx; L, larynx; SG, supraglottis; G, glottis; H, hypopharynx.
*Number of patients controlled with salvage surgery/number of local failures.
[a]Large volume fraction = 1.8 Gy; boost volume fraction 1.4–1.5 Gy beginning at week 5.
[b]Continuous hyperfractionated accelerated radiotherapy (CHART): results of a pilot study.
[c]Significantly fewer sequelae when interfraction interval was increased from 4 to 6 hours and fraction dose decreased from 1.2 to 1.1 Gy.

complete[22,65] or even partial in the GETTEC and the Veterans studies.[21] These trials confirmed that approximately one third of the patients may be cured while retaining their larynges (23–39%), the best conservative results being obtained in small volume tumors.[106] In studies where hypopharyngeal or supraglottic tumors were included, the overall survival was the same in the experimental arm as in the surgical arm and the distant failure was decreased or delayed.[21,65] Nevertheless, in the GETTEC study, where only endolaryngeal tumors were studied, the 5-year disease-free and overall survival rates were significantly lower in the conservative arm than in the surgical arm. General conclusions are difficult to make from these data but this conservative approach should not be considered as standard for all the patients with laryngeal cancers. The design of a recently activated Intergroup trial supports this view in randomizing patients in a first arm with induction chemotherapy with local treatment depending on the response, a second arm with radiotherapy alone and a third arm with radiotherapy with concurrent cisplatin. Since in the Veterans study, patients with only partial response who were irradiated had a lower survival than the poor responders who were laryngectomized, one can consider that response is not a very sensitive prognostic factor for radiocurability. Even more, induction chemotherapy could induce accelerated repopulation of surviving tumor cells, resulting in a lower control with conventional radiotherapy.[6] Some biologic factors such as DNA content or histologic patterns could help in the future to identify the patients who really benefit from induction chemotherapy.[35,106,114]

Altered fractionation schemes

Evidence continues to emerge to question whether conventional fractionation (i.e. 60–70 Gy in 2 Gy daily fractions over 6–7 weeks) is an optimal treatment for every patient with laryngeal cancer. Hyperfractionation uses two or more small fractions a day in order to increase the total dose, while keeping the late reactions constant. In laryngeal cancer, hyperfractionation is commonly used in some institutions with improved results compared to historical control for supraglottic or advanced laryngeal tumors[32,61,82] (see Table 51.9). Although there is no randomized study in laryngeal cancers, this fractionation scheme has been demonstrated to improve both local control and survival in T3 oropharyngeal squamous cell carcinomas.[48] Doses up to 74–79 Gy may be delivered without increasing the rate of late complications, using two daily 1.1 or 1.2 Gy fractions with a minimal interval of 6 hours between them.[32,82] Of note, the use of the smallest fractions (i.e 1.1 Gy), although reducing both acute and late reactions, was associated with a higher failure rate in the more advanced tumors.[32] Acceleration of the radiotherapy is designed to reduce the overall treatment time and compensate the accelerated repopulation of the surviving clonogenic cells, which probably occurs 2–3 weeks after the onset of the treatment.[115] Besides the long experience of institutions using hypofractionation, which results in short overall time but low total dose, this acceleration may be obtained with two or three daily fractions delivered during the whole treatment time (continuous acceleration) or with a second daily fraction delivered in a small volume during the second half of the treatment time (concomitant boost). The concomitant boost technique was first designed in Houston to treat oro- and nasopharyngeal primaries.[63] This schedule was not extended to treat laryngeal primaries in this institution because hyperfractionation was preferred in order to reduce the late reactions.[32] In other institutions, a similar schedule was found feasible and safe[11,15,59,60] (see Table 51.9). Continuous accelerated radiotherapy was explored in two randomized studies including laryngeal primaries.[24,47] Local control was enhanced in the EORTC study although late complications were excessive, owing to a too short interfraction interval.[47] In the CHART trial, an advantage was found only in the more advanced cases and laryngeal primaries.[24] The limiting toxicity of these accelerated regimens is the enhanced acute mucous membrane reactions, which may in turn induce nonreparable late injuries. Hence, very accelerated schedules may not be the better way to improve the local regional control with preservation of a functional larynx in advanced hypopharyngeal or laryngeal primaries.

Functional results

An accurate knowledge of the functional results after treatment for laryngeal cancer is a major issue when selecting the therapeutic modality. In early tumors, this concern is of primary importance because oncologic results are sufficiently good with surgery or radiotherapy alone. In more advanced cases, survival is considered the major problem although one study has pointed out that some people would risk a decreased probability of cure to retain a functional larynx.[79] Even if this study may be flawed by the fact that only healthy individuals were interviewed, informed patient choice is now emerging as a guide to decision-making in oncology.

The vast majority of patients with early laryngeal cancer experience an improvement of their voice after radiotherapy although most of them report the persistence of some difficulties (voice volume, vocal fatigue). In a study of 223 patients with T1 or T2 tumors, Stoicheff reported that although 83% had subjective normal or minimally impaired voice, 80% of the patients complained about some vocal problem.[109] Evaluation using objective tests confirms these abnormalities.[66] Nevertheless, very few patients experience such a vocal deterioration as to induce social and/or professional consequences. Harwood and Rawlinson reported that only 3% of their patients were forced to retire and 4% had to change employment after radiotherapy.[38] In a study of 197 patients with early glottic cancer, Lusinchi stated that 2.5% had dysphonia only marked or substantially impairing normal activity.[73] Similar results are shown in supraglottic larynx: at the IGR, only 7 of 127 patients (5.5%) with T1–T2 had a severe dysphonia whereas 88 (69%) had no or only intermittent dysphonia.[13] Reported factors predicting a poor functional outcome have been continuation of smoking[5,112] and extensive pretreatment biopsy.[5] Very hypofractionated schemes are expected to produce more late reactions with consequential alteration of the quality of voice but are in fact well tolerated when small fields are used.[45,96]

In more advanced cases, effect of treatment on quality of life is frequently more important although it is probably less than for pharyngeal tumors.[58] Vocal problems were self-reported by 37% of the patients in a study of moderately advanced laryngeal tumors.[58] Professional disability was reported by 15% of the patients in this later study and in 21% of patients with T3–T4 tumors studied by Harwood and Rawlinson.[38] Deglutition impairment is rare, affecting 11% of the patients in the study by Jensen *et al.*[58]

Complications of therapy

Xerostomia is unusual although a sensation of throat dryness may be reported by one-third of patients.[38] It may be more prevalent when the whole internal jugular chain must be irradiated up to the base of the skull because of an extensive nodal involvement. Severe complications of radiotherapy are most feared because they can result in loss of the larynx. Although larynx edema is frequent after radiation therapy, it is rarely symptomatic: in 159 evaluable patients, 57 (36%) had edema at inspection but only 8 (5%) had some clinical problem.[73] Severe edema or stenosis, cartilage or mucosal necrosis can necessitate a temporary or definitive tracheotomy or a total laryngectomy. These major complications are reported in 1.7–4.1% in series including early-stage glottic cancer[73,81,105] but may probably be less than 1%.[69,80,110] In more advanced tumors, the risk is higher although the real incidence is difficult to estimate from the literature. Irradiation for supraglottic primaries is more at risk because the fields are frequently larger than for glottic tumors.[110] In a study of 157 supraglottic cancers from the Institut Curie in Paris, severe morbidity was reported in 25% of the deceased patients and 6% in those alive at 3 years.[9] Late reactions are increased when high fractional doses (>2.5 Gy) are used[20,76,105,110] or when high total doses are delivered.[53,112] It must, nevertheless, be kept in mind that in institutions used to relative hypofractionation, total dose is low and fields are frequently of limited size with no attempt to encompass the lymphatic drainage, resulting in lower late morbidity than expected.[45,87,96,105] The influence of acceleration of the radiotherapy on late complications is theoretically low when the interfraction interval is >6–8 hours. However, more extended follow-up is needed for such regimens because the enhanced acute reactions could result in more late sequelae: in reports of concomitant boost irradiation, severe reactions seem to be more frequent for laryngeal sites than for oropharyngeal or oral cavity primaries.[15,59] Severe postoperative morbidity is frequently said to be increased when radiotherapy is given to full dose but recent reports do not support this point of view.[19,90,101] Salvage partial laryngectomy may even be used for failure of early-stage tumors.[90,101] In patients receiving induction chemotherapy, the rate of postoperative complications does not seem to be increased[65,106] although they were said to be more severe in the Veterans study.[127] One of the difficulties when late reactions are present is to determine if they predict a local recurrence. Severe complications are considerably more frequent in patients who ultimately show local relapse.[9,87] By contrast, the histology of the specimen after laryngectomy for recurrence sometimes only reveals necrosis.[81] A conservative treatment should therefore be attempted during 2–6 weeks before planning the surgery, using corticosteroids, antibiotics and in more severe cases hyperbaric oxygen, tube feeding and temporary tracheotomy.[78] Methods of differential diagnosis include biopsy (which may nevertheless enhance a radionecrosis) and PET scan using fluorodeoxyglucose; MRI and CT scan can barely distinguish tumor from necrosis.[78]

Conclusions

Radiotherapy has an important role in the treatment of laryngeal cancer. Whilst it is one of the major therapeutic options in early glottic or supraglottic tumors, radiation therapy is extensively used in the postoperative setting in advanced cancer. In selected T3 and T4 patients, exclusive radiotherapy may permit organ preservation.

The definitive role of accelerated or hyperfractionated radiotherapy needs more follow-up, as does concomitant chemoradiotherapy. New trials including data on biologic prognostic factors are in progress. In the future, besides the survival and locoregional control end points, the quality of life and the economic issues of the different options will have to be specifically studied.

References

1. Akine Y, Tokita N, Ogino T *et al.* Radiotherapy of T1 glottic cancer with 6 MeV X-rays. *Int J Radiat Oncol Biol Phys* 1991; **20**: 1215–18.
2. Amdur RJ, Parsons JT, Mendenhall WM, Million RR, Stringer SP, Cassisi NJ. Postoperative irradiation for squamous cell carcinoma of the head and neck: an analysis of treatment results and complications. *Int J Radiat Oncol Biol Phys* 1989; **16**: 25–36.
3. Aref A, Gross M, Fontanesi J, Devi S, Kopel C, Thornton D. Adequate irradiation of the internal jugular lymph node chain: technical considerations. *Int J Radiat Oncol Biol Phys* 1997; **37**: 269–73.
4. Arriagada R, Eschwège F, Cachin Y, Richard JM. The value of combining radiotherapy with surgery in the treatment of hypopharyngeal and laryngeal cancers. *Cancer* 1983; **51**: 1819–25.
5. Benninger MS, Gillen J, Thieme P, Jacobson B, Dragovich J. Factors associated with recurrence and voice quality following radiation therapy for T1 and T2 glottic carcinomas. *Laryngoscope* 1994; **104**: 294–8.
6. Bourhis J, Wilson G, Wibault P *et al.* Rapid tumor proliferation after induction chemotherapy in oropharyngeal cancer. *Laryngoscope* 1994; **104**: 468–72.
7. Bridier A, Wibault P, Chavaudra J, Houlard JP, Eschwège F. Amélioration de la méthode utilisée à l'IGR pour l'établissement des plans de traitement en radiothérapie ORL. *Bull Cancer Radiother* 1991; **78**: 55–8.
8. Browman GP, Wong G, Hodson I *et al.* Influence of cigarette smoking on the efficacy of radiation therapy in head and neck cancer. *N Engl J Med* 1993; **328**: 159–63.
9. Brugère J, Bataini P, Jaulerry C, Brunin F. Les complications de la radiothérapie des cancers du sinus piriforme et de la margelle laryngée latérale. In: Leroux-Robert J, Guerrier Y, eds. *Complications et Séquelles de l'Irradiation des Tumeurs Cervico-Faciales.* Paris: Masson, 1981: 104–8.
10. Bryant GP, Poulsen MG, Tripcony L, Dickie GJ. Treatment decision in T3N0M0 glottic carcinoma. *Int J Radiat Oncol Biol Phys* 1995; **31**: 285–93.
11. Bujko K, Skoczylas JZ, Bentzen SM *et al.* A feasibility study of concomitant boost radiotherapy for patients with cancer of the supraglottic larynx. *Acta Oncol* 1993; **32**: 637–40.
12. Burke LS, Greven KM, McGuirt WT, Case D, Hoen HM, Raben M. Definitive radiotherapy for early glottic carcinoma: prognostic factors and implications for treatment. *Int J Radiat Oncol Biol Phys* 1997; **38**: 37–42.
13. Cailleux PE. Cancers limités du vestibule laryngé: étude de 166 cas traités à l'Institut Gustave Roussy par radiothérapie exclusive de 1970 à 1983. *Mémoire.* Paris: Université de Paris Sud, 1987.
14. Cellai E, Chiavacci A, Olmi P. Causes of failure of curative radiation therapy in 205 early glottic cancers. *Int J Radiat Oncol Biol Phys* 1990; **19**: 1139–42.
15. Corvò R, Sanguineti G, Scala M *et al.* Primary site as a predictive factor for local control in advanced head and neck tumors treated by concomitant boost accelerated radiotherapy. *Tumori* 1994; **80**: 135–8.
16. Coutard H. Roentgenthérapie des épithéliomas de la région amygdalienne, de l'hypopharynx et du larynx au cours des années 1920 à 1926. *Radiophys Radiother* 1932; **2**: 541–75.
17. Coutard H, Baclesse F. Roentgen diagnosis during course of roentgen therapy of epitheliomas of larynx and hypopharynx. *Am J Roentgenol* 1932; **28**: 293–312.
18. Cummings BJ. Definitive radiation therapy for glottic cancer. In: Smee R, Bridger GP, eds. *Laryngeal Cancer.* Amsterdam: Elsevier Science, 1994: 9–13.
19. Davidson J, Briant D, Gullane P, Keane T, Rawlinson E. The role of surgery following radiotherapy failure for advanced laryngopharyngeal cancer. *Arch Otolaryngol Head Neck Surg* 1994; **120**: 269–76.
20. Deore SM, Supe SJ, Sharma V, Dinshaw KA. The predictive

role of bioeffect dose models in radiation-induced late effects in glottic cancers. *Int J Radiat Oncol Biol Phys* 1992; **23**: 281–4.
21. Department of Veterans Affairs Laryngeal Cancer Study Group. Induction chemotherapy plus radiation compared with surgery plus radiation in patients with advanced laryngeal cancer. *N Engl J Med* 1991; **324**: 1685–90.
22. Depondt J, Gehanno P, Martin M *et al.* Neoadjuvant chemotherapy with carboplatin/5-fluorouracil in head and neck cancer. *Oncology* 1993; **50**: S23–7.
23. Devineni VR, King K, Perez C, Mittal B, Simpson J, Emami B. Early glottic carcinoma treated with radiotherapy: impact of treatment energy on success rate. *Int J Radiat Oncol Biol Phys* 1992; **24**: S186–7.
24. Dische S, Saunders MI, Barrett A, Harvey A, Gibson D, Parmar M. A randomised multicentre trial of CHART versus conventional radiotherapy in head and neck cancer. *Radiother Oncol* 1997; **44**: 123–36.
25. Duncan W, Arnott SJ, Batterman JJ, Orr JA, Schmitt G, Kerr GR. Fast neutrons in the treatment of head and neck cancers: the results of a multi-centre randomly controlled trial. *Radiother Oncol* 1984; **2**: 271–9.
26. Eschwège F, Ghilezan M, Mamelle G, Wibault P, Lusinchi A, Luboinski B. Results of T3, T4 laryngeal cancers treated by exclusive external radiotherapy. Experience of the Institute Gustave Roussy (IGR). In: Smee R, Bridger GP, eds. *Laryngeal Cancer.* Amsterdam: Elsevier Science, 1994: 536–8.
27. Fein DA, Mendenhall WM, Parsons JT, Million RR. T1–T2 squamous cell carcinoma of the glottic larynx treated with radiotherapy: a multivariate analysis of the variables potentially influencing local control. *Int J Radiat Oncol Biol Phys* 1993; **25**: 605–11.
28. Fein DA, Hanlon AL, Lee WR, Ridge JA, Coia LR. Neck failure in T2N0 squamous cell carcinoma of the true vocal cords: the Fox Chase experience and review of the literature. *Am J Clin Oncol* 1997; **20**: 154–7.
29. Fein DA, Mendenhall WM, Parsons JT, Stringer SP, Cassisi NJ, Million RR. Carcinoma in situ of the glottic larynx: the role of radiotherapy. *Int J Radiat Oncol Biol Phys* 1993; **27**: 379–84.
30. Fein DA, Lee RW, Hanlon AL *et al.* Pretreatment hemoglobin level influences local control and survival of T1–T2 squamous cell carcinomas of the glottic larynx. *J Clin Oncol* 1995; **13**: 2077–83.
31. Fletcher GH. History of irradiation in squamous cell carcinomas of the larynx and hypopharynx. *Int J Radiat Oncol Biol Phys* 1986; **12**: 2019–24.
32. Garden AS, Morrison WH, Ang KK, Peters LJ. Hyperfractionated radiation in the treatment of squamous cell carcinomas of the head and neck: a comparison of two fractionation schedules. *Int J Radiat Oncol Biol Phys* 1995; **31**: 493–502.
33. Glinsky B, Reinfuss M, Walasek T, Skolyszewski J. Radiothérapie exclusive de 250 cancers du larynx susglottique stade I–II. *Bull Cancer Radiother* 1996; **83**: 177–9.
34. Glover GW, Saunders MI, Dische S. CHART (continuous hyperfractionated accelerated radiotherapy) with laryngectomy for failure in carcinoma of the larynx. In: Smee R, Bridger GP, eds. *Laryngeal Cancer.* Amsterdam: Elsevier Science, 1994: 553–5.
35. Gregg CM, Beals TE, Fisher SG, Wolf GT. DNA content and tumor response to induction chemotherapy in patients with advanced laryngeal squamous cell carcinoma. *Otolaryngol Head Neck Surg* 1993; **108**: 731–7.
36. Guedea F, Parsons JT, Mendenhall WM, Million RR, Stringer SP, Cassisi NJ. Primary subglottic cancer: results of radical radiation therapy. *Int J Radiat Oncol Biol Phys* 1991; **21**: 1607–11.
37. Guichard M, Lartigau E. New trends for improving radiation sensitivity by counteracting chronic and acute hypoxia. *Adv Radiat Biol* 1994; **18**: 123–47.
38. Harwood AR, Rawlinson E. The quality of life of patients following treatment for laryngeal cancer. *Int J Radiat Oncol Biol Phys* 1983; **9**: 335–8.
39. Harwood AR, Beale FA, Cummings BJ, Keane TJ, Rider WD. T2 glottic cancer: an analysis of dose-time volume factors. *Int J Radiat Oncol Biol Phys* 1981; **7**: 1501–5.
40. Harwood AR, Hawkins NV, Beale FA, Rider WD, Bryce DP. Management of advanced glottic cancer. A 10 year review of the Toronto experience. *Int J Radiat Oncol Biol Phys* 1979; **5**: 899–904.
41. Harwood AR, Beale FA, Cummings BJ, Hawkins NV, Keane TJ, Rider WD. T3 glottic cancer: an analysis of dose time-volume factors. *Int J Radiat Oncol Biol Phys* 1980; **6**: 675–80.
42. Harwood AR, Beale FA, Cummings BJ, Keane TJ, Payne D, Rider WD. T4N0M0 glottic cancer: an analysis of dose-time volume factors. *Int J Radiat Oncol Biol Phys* 1981; **7**: 1507–12.
43. Harwood AR, Beale FA, Cummings BJ *et al.* Supraglottic laryngeal carcinoma: an analysis of dose-time-volume factors in 410 patients. *Int J Radiat Oncol Biol Phys* 1983; **9**: 311–19.
44. Haylock BJ, Deutsch GP. Primary radiotherapy for subglottic carcinoma. *Clin Oncol* 1993; **5**: 143–6.
45. Henk JM, James KW. Comparative trial of large and small fractions in the radiotherapy of head and neck cancer. *Clin Radiol* 1976; **29**: 611–16.
46. Henk JM, Smith KW. Radiotherapy and hyperbaric oxygen in head and neck cancer. Interim report of second clinical trial. *Lancet* 1977; **2**: 104–5.
47. Horiot JC, Bontemps P, van den Bogaert W *et al.* Accelerated fractionation (AF) compared to conventional fractionation (CF) improves loco-regional control in the radiotherapy of advanced head and neck cancers: results of the EORTC 22851 randomized trial. *Radiother Oncol* 1997; **44**: 111–21.
48. Horiot JC, Le Fur R, N'Guyen T *et al.* Hyperfractionation versus conventional fractionation in oropharyngeal carcinoma: final analysis of a randomized trial of the EORTC cooperative group of radiotherapy. *Radiother Oncol* 1992; **25**: 231–41.
49. Howell-Burke D, Peters LJ, Goepfert H, Oswald MJ. T2 glottic cancer. *Arch Otolaryngol Head Neck Surg* 1990; **116**: 830–5.
50. Inoue T, Inoue T, Ikeda H, Teshima T, Murayama S. Prognostic factor of telecobalt therapy for early glottic carcinoma. *Cancer* 1992; **70**: 2797–801.
51. Inoue T, Matayoshi Y, Inoue T, Ikeda H, Teshima T, Murayama S. Prognostic factors in telecobalt therapy for early supraglottic carcinoma. *Cancer* 1993; **72**: 57–61.

52. International Commission on Radiation Units and Measurements. Prescribing, recording, and reporting photon beam therapy. *ICRU Report 50* Bethesda: ICRU, 1993.
53. Issa PY. Cancer of the supraglottic larynx treated by radiotherapy exclusively. *Int J Radiat Oncol Biol Phys* 1988; **15:** 843–50.
54. Izuno I, Sone S, Oguchi M, Kiyono K, Takei K. Treatment of early vocal cord carcinoma with ^{60}Co gamma rays, 8/10 MV X-rays, or 4 MV X-rays. Are the results different? *Acta Oncol* 1990; **29:** 637–9.
55. Jacobs C, Goffinet DR, Goffinet L, Kohler M, Fee WE. Chemotherapy as a substitute for surgery in the treatment of advanced resectable head and neck cancer. A report from the Northern California Oncology Group. *Cancer* 1987; **60:** 1178–83.
56. Jaulerry C, Dubray B, Brunin F *et al.* Prognostic value of tumor regression during radiotherapy for head and neck cancer: a prospective study. *Int J Radiat Oncol Biol Phys* 1995; **33:** 271–9.
57. Jaulerry C, Rodriguez J, Brunin F *et al.* Induction chemotherapy in advanced head and neck tumors: results of two randomized trials. *Int J Radiat Oncol Biol Phys* 1992; **23:** 483–9.
58. Jensen AB, Hansen O, Jorgensen K, Bastholt L. Influence of late side-effects upon daily life after radiotherapy for laryngeal and pharyngeal cancer. *Acta Oncol* 1994; **33:** 487–91.
59. Johnson CR, Schmidt-Ullrich RK, Wazer DE. Concomitant boost technique using superfractionated radiation therapy for advanced squamous cell carcinoma of the head and neck. *Cancer* 1992; **69:** 2749–54.
60. Kaanders JHAM, van Daal WAJ, Hoogenraad WJ, van der Kogel AJ. Accelerated fractionation radiotherapy for laryngeal cancer, acute, and late toxicity. *Int J Radiat Oncol Biol Phys* 1992; **24:** 497–503.
61. Karim AB, Kralendonk JH, Njo KH, Tierie AH, Hasman A. Radiation therapy for advanced (T3T4N0–N3M0) laryngeal carcinoma: the need for a change of strategy: a radiotherapeutic viewpoint. *Int J Radiat Oncol Biol Phys* 1987; **13:** 1625–33.
62. Keane TJ, Cummings BJ, O'Sullivan B *et al.* A randomized trial or radiation therapy compared to split course radiation therapy combined with mitomycin C and 5-fluorouracil as initial treatment for advanced laryngeal and hypopharyngeal squamous carcinoma. *Int J Radiat Oncol Biol Phys* 1993; **25:** 613–18.
63. Knee R, Fields RS, Peters LJ. Concomitant boost radiotherapy for advanced squamous cell carcinoma of the head and neck. *Radiother Oncol* 1985; **4:** 1–7.
64. Laramore GE. T3N0M0 glottic cancer: are more treatment modalities necessarily better? *Int J Radiat Oncol Biol Phys* 1995; **31:** 423–5.
65. Lefebvre JL, Chevalier D, Luboinski B, Kirkpatrick A, Collette L, Sahmoud T. Larynx preservation in pyriform sinus cancer: preliminary results of a European Organization for Research and Treatment of Cancer phase III trial. *J Natl Cancer Inst* 1996; **88:** 890–9.
66. Lehman JJ, Bless DM, Brandenburg JH. An objective assessment of voice production after radiation therapy for stage I squamous cell carcinoma of the glottis. *Otolaryngol Head Neck Surg* 1988; **98:** 121–9.
67. Leon X, Quer M, Burgués J, Abello P, Vega M, de Andrés L. Prevention of stomal recurrence. *Head Neck* 1996; **18:** 54–9.
68. Leroux-Robert J, Ennuyer A. Résultats de l'association chirurgie-roentgenthérapie ou de la chirurgie seule dans les épithéliomas du larynx. *Otolaryngol Chir Cervicofac* 1956; **73:** 521–45.
69. Lesnicar H, Smid L, Zakotnik B. Early glottic cancer: the influence of primary treatment on voice preservation. *Int J Radiat Oncol Biol Phys* 1996; **36:** 1025–32.
70. Levendag P, Vikram B. The problem of neck relapse in early stage supraglottic cancer. Results of different treatment modalities for clinically negative neck. *Int J Radiat Oncol Biol Phys* 1987; **13:** 1621–4.
71. Levendag PC, Hoekstra CJM, Eukenboom WMH, Reichgelt BA, Van Putten WLJ. Supraglottic larynx cancer, T1–4 N0, treated by radical radiation therapy. *Acta Oncol* 1988; **27:** 253–60.
72. Lindelov B, Hansen HS. Advanced squamous cell carcinoma of the larynx. *Acta Oncol* 1990; **29:** 505–8.
73. Lusinchi A, Dube P, Wibault P, Kunkler I, Luboinski B, Eschwège F. Radiation therapy in the treatment of early glottic carcinoma: the experience of Villejuif. *Radiother Oncol* 1989; **15:** 313–19.
74. Lustig RA, Krall JM, Curran WJ, Hanks GE. Improvements observed in care and outcome in carcinoma of the larynx. *Int J Radiat Oncol Biol Phys* 1991; **20:** 101–4.
75. MacComb WS, Fletcher GH. *Policy of Treatment – Cancer of the Larynx.* University of Texas, Houston: MD Anderson Hospital and Tumor Institute, 1957.
76. Maciejewski B, Taylor JMG, Withers HR. Alpha/beta value and the importance of size of dose per fraction for late complications in the supraglottic larynx. *Radiother Oncol* 1986; **7:** 323–6.
77. McDonald S, Haie C, Rubin P, Nelson D, Divers LD. Second malignant tumors in patients with laryngeal carcinoma: diagnosis, treatment, and prevention. *Int J Radiat Oncol Biol Phys* 1989; **17:** 457–65.
78. McGuirt WF. Laryngeal radionecrosis versus recurrent cancer. *Otolaryngol Clin North Am* 1997; **30:** 243–50.
79. McNeil BJ, Weichselbaum R, Pauker SG. Speech and survival. *N Engl J Med* 1981; **305:** 982–7.
80. Medini E, Medini A, Gapany M, Levitt SH. Radiation therapy in early carcinoma of the glottic larynx T1N0M0. *Int J Radiat Oncol Biol Phys* 1996; **36:** 1211–13.
81. Mendenhall WM, Parsons JT, Million RR, Fletcher GH. T1–T2 squamous cell carcinoma of the glottic larynx treated with radiation therapy: relationship of dose-fractionation factors to local control and complications. *Int J Radiat Oncol Biol Phys* 1988; **15:** 1267–73.
82. Mendenhall WM, Parsons JT, Mancuso AA, Stringer SP, Cassisi NJ. Radiotherapy for squamous cell carcinoma of the supraglottic larynx: an alternative to surgery. *Head Neck* 1996; **18:** 24–35.
83. Mendenhall WM, Parsons JT, Brant TA, Stringer SP, Cassisi NJ, Million RR. Is elective neck treatment indicated for T2N0 squamous cell carcinoma of the glottic larynx? *Radiother Oncol* 1989; **14:** 199–202.
84. Mendenhall WM, Parsons JT, Mancuso AA, Pameijer FJ, Stringer SP, Cassisi NJ. Definitive radiotherapy for T3

squamous cell carcinoma of the glottic larynx. *J Clin Oncol* 1997; **15**: 2394–402.

85. Meredith APD'E, Randall CJ, Shaw HJ. Advanced laryngeal cancer: a management perspective. *J Laryngol Otol* 1987; **101**: 1046–54.
86. Million RR. The larynx...so to speak: everything I wanted to know about laryngeal cancer I learned in the last 32 years. *Int J Radiat Oncol Biol Phys* 1992; **23**: 691–704.
87. Mills EED. Early glottic carcinoma: factors affecting radiation failure, results of treatment and sequelae. *Int J Radiat Oncol Biol Phys* 1979; **5**: 811–17.
88. Naudé J, Dobrowsky W. Postoperative irradiation of laryngeal carcinoma. The prognostic value of tumour-free surgical margins. *Acta Oncol* 1997; **36**: 273–7.
89. Nguyen TD, Malissard L, Théobald S *et al.* Advanced carcinoma of the larynx: results of surgery and radiotherapy without induction chemotherapy (1980–1985): a multivariate analysis. *Int J Radiat Oncol Biol Phys* 1996; **36**: 1013–18.
90. Nibu K, Kamata S, Kawabata K, Nakamizo M, Nigauri T, Hoki K. Partial laryngectomy in the treatment of radiation-failure of early glottic carcinoma. *Head Neck* 1997; **19**: 116–20.
91. Olszewski SJ, Vaeth JM, Green JP, Schroeder AF, Chauser B. The influence of field size, treatment modality, commissure involvement and histology in the treatment of early vocal cord cancer with irradiation. *Int J Radiat Oncol Biol Phys* 1985; **11**: 1333–7.
92. Ostwald PM, Kron T, Hamilton CS. Assessment of mucosal underdosing in larynx irradiation. *Int J Radiat Oncol Biol Phys* 1996; **36**: 181–7.
93. O'Sullivan B, Mackillop W, Gilbert R *et al.* Controversies in the management of laryngeal cancer: results of an international survey of pattern of care. *Radiother Oncol* 1994; **31**: 23–32.
94. Pameijer FA, Mancuso AA, Mendenhall WM, Parsons JT, Kubilis PS. Can pretreatment computed tomography predict local control in T3 squamous cell carcinoma of the glottic larynx treated with definitive radiotherapy? *Int J Radiat Oncol Biol Phys* 1997; **37**: 1011–21.
95. Pellitteri PK, Kennedy TL, Vrabec DP, Beiler D, Hellstrom M. Radiotherapy. The mainstay in the treatment of early glottic carcinoma. *Arch Otolaryngol Head Neck Surg* 1991; **117**: 297–301.
96. Randall ME, Springer DJ, Raben M. T1–T2 carcinoma of the glottis: relative hypofractionation. *Radiology* 1991; **179**: 569–71.
97. Robertson AG, Robertson C, Boyle P, Symonds RP, Wheldon TE. The effect of differing radiotherapeutic schedules on the response of glottic carcinoma of the larynx. *Eur J Cancer* 1993; **29**: 501–10.
98. Robson NL, Oswal VH, Flood LM. Radiation therapy of laryngeal cancer: a twenty year experience. *J Laryngol Otol* 1990; **104**: 699–703.
99. Rudoltz MS, Benammar A, Mohiuddin M. Prognostic factors for local control and survival in T1 squamous cell carcinoma of the glottis. *Int J Radiat Oncol Biol Phys* 1993; **26**: 767–72.
100. Sandberg N, Mercke C, Turesson I. Glottic laryngeal carcinoma with fixed vocal cord treated with full-dose radiation, total laryngectomy or combined treatment. *Acta Oncol* 1990; **29**: 509–11.
101. Schwaab G, Mamelle G, Lartigau E, Parise O Jr, Wibault P, Luboinski B. Surgical salvage treatment of T1/T2 glottic carcinoma after failure of radiotherapy. *Am J Surg* 1994; **168**: 474–5.
102. Sessions DG, Ogura JH, Fried MP. Carcinoma of the subglottic area. *Laryngoscope* 1975; **85(9)**: 1417–23.
103. Simpson CB, Postma GN, Stone RE, Ossoff RH. Speech outcomes after laryngeal cancer management. *Otolaryngol Clin North Am* 1997; **30**: 189–205.
104. Sinha PP. Radiation therapy in early carcinoma of the true vocal cords (stage I and II). *Int J Radiat Oncol Biol Phys* 1987; **13**: 1635–40.
105. Slevin NJ, Vasanthan S, Dougal M. Relative influence of tumor dose versus dose per fraction on the occurrence of late normal tissue morbidity following larynx radiotherapy. *Int J Radiat Oncol Biol Phys* 1992; **25**: 23–8.
106. Spaulding MB, Fischer SG, Wolf GT and the Department of Veterans Affairs Cooperative Laryngeal Cancer Study Group. Tumor response, toxicity, and survival after neoadjuvant organ-preserving chemotherapy for advanced laryngeal carcinoma. *J Clin Oncol* 1994; **12**: 1592–9.
107. Spaulding CA, Krochak RJ, Hahn SS, Constable WC. Radiotherapeutic management of cancer of the supraglottis. *Cancer* 1986; **57**: 1292–8.
108. Spector JG, Sessions DG, Emami B, Simpson J, Haughey B, Fredrickson JM. Squamous cell carcinomas of the aryepiglottic fold: therapeutic results and long-term follow-up. *Laryngoscope* 1995; **105**: 734–46.
109. Stoicheff ML. Voice following radiotherapy. *Laryngoscope* 1975; **85**: 608–18.
110. Taylor JMG, Mendenhall WM, Lavey RS. Dose, time and fraction size issues for late effects in head and neck cancers. *Int J Radiat Oncol Biol Phys* 1992; **22**: 3–11.
111. Terhaard CHJ, Wiggenraad RG, Hordjik GJ, Ravasz LA. Regression after 50 Gy as a selection for therapy in advanced laryngeal cancer. *Int J Radiat Oncol Biol Phys* 1988; **15**: 591–7.
112. Terhaard CHJ, Snippe K, Ravasz LA, van der Tweel I, Hordjik GJ. Radiotherapy in T1 laryngeal cancer: prognostic factors for locoregional control and survival, uni- and multivariate analysis. *Int J Radiat Oncol Biol Phys* 1991; **21**: 1179–86.
113. Terhaard CHJ, Karim ABMF, Hoogenraad WJ *et al.* Local control in T3 laryngeal cancer treated with radical radiotherapy, time dose relationship: the concept of nominal standard dose and linear quadratic model. *Int J Radiat Oncol Biol Phys* 1991; **20**: 1207–14.
114. Truelson JM, Fisher SG, Beals TE, McClatchey KD, Wolf GT. DNA content and histologic growth pattern correlate with prognosis in patients with advanced squamous cell carcinoma of the larynx. *Cancer* 1992; **70**: 56–62.
115. Tubiana M, Dutreix J, Wambersie A. *Radiobiologie*. Paris: Hermann, 1986.
116. Tupchong L, Scott CB, Blitzer PH *et al.* Randomized study of preoperative versus postoperative radiation

therapy in advanced head and neck carcinoma: long-term follow-up of RTOG study 73–03. *Int J Radiat Oncol Biol Phys* 1991; **20:** 21–8.

117. Turesson I, Sandberg N, Mercke C, Johansson KA, Sandin I, Wallgren A. Primary radiotherapy for glottic laryngeal carcinoma stage I and II. *Acta Oncol* 1991; **30:** 357–62.
118. van den Bogaert W, Ostyn F, van der Schueren E The significance of extension and impaired mobility in cancer of the vocal cord. *Int J Radiat Oncol Biol Phys* 1983; **9:** 181–4.
119. van den Bogaert W, Ostyn F, van der Schueren E. The primary treatment of advanced vocal cord cancer: laryngectomy or radiotherapy? *Int J Radiat Oncol Biol Phys* 1983; **9:** 329–34.
120. Vermund H. Role of radiotherapy in cancer of the larynx as related to the TNM system of staging. A review. *Cancer* 1970; **25:** 485–504.
121. Wang CC. Treatment of glottic carcinoma by megavoltage radiation therapy and results. *Am J Roentgenol* 1974; **120:** 157–63.
122. Wang CC. Factors influencing the success of radiation therapy for T2 and T3 glottic carcinomas. *Am J Clin Oncol* 1986; **9:** 517–20.
123. Wang CC, Efird JT. Does prolonged treatment course adversely affect local control of carcinoma of the larynx? *Int J Radiat Oncol Biol Phys* 1994; **29:** 657–60.
124. Warde P, Harwood AR, Keane T. Carcinoma of the subglottis. Results of initial radical radiation. *Arch Otolaryngol Head Neck Surg* 1987; **113:** 1228–9.
125. Wendt CD, Peters LJ, Ang KK *et al.* Hyperfractionated radiotherapy in the treatment of squamous cell of the supraglottic larynx. *Int J Radiat Oncol Biol Phys* 1989; **17:** 1057–62.
126. Wolf GT, Fisher SG. Effectiveness of salvage neck dissection for advanced regional metastases when induction chemotherapy and radiation are used for organ preservation. *Laryngoscope* 1992; **102:** 934–9.
127. Wolf GT, Hong WK. Induction chemotherapy for organ preservation in advanced laryngeal cancer: is there a role? *Head Neck* 1995; **17:** 279–83.
128. Yuen A, Medina JE, Goepfert H, Fletcher G. Management of stage T3 and T4 glottic carcinomas. *Am J Surg* 1984; **148:** 467–72.

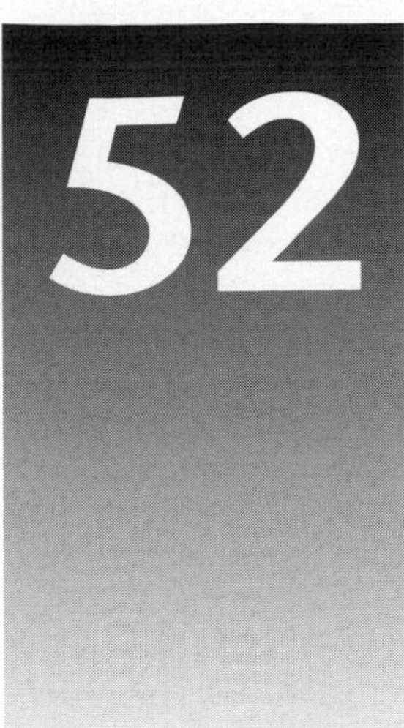

Chemotherapy for laryngeal cancer

Gregory T Wolf

The management of patients with laryngeal cancer is at the forefront of an evolution in oncologic philosophy in the treatment of head and neck squamous carcinoma. Over the last 25 years, changes in treatment approaches for cancers of the larynx have challenged traditional principles of oncologic surgical management. This is reflected in an increasing emphasis on limited resections for disease of moderate extent and more intensive, multimodality treatment for advanced disease with innovative integrations of surgery, radiation and chemotherapy. These approaches have been stimulated by a better appreciation of a tumor's metastatic capability, increased reliance on precise radiographic imaging techniques, better understanding of local patterns of cancer spread, improved prognostic factors and a renewed emphasis on quality of life issues for patients with cancer of the larynx.

The introduction of chemotherapy into the management of head and neck cancers has been a major factor in this evolution. Perhaps more for the larynx than other head and neck sites, a patient's perceptions of surgical treatment and the morbidity of losing a larynx, together with the physician's bias against laryngectomy, have pushed the boundaries of partial laryngectomy and led to exploration of nonsurgical treatment approaches using radiation or chemotherapy. This chapter reviews the progress made in chemotherapy for larynx cancer and looks to the future where more specific patient selection criteria for chemotherapy or radiation may be available through a better understanding of the genetic and biologic characteristics of a particular cancer, and where genetic manipulations of a cancer could become therapeutically useful.

The use of chemotherapy as an adjuvant to conventional surgery or radiation in patients with potentially curable disease is largely experimental and remains controversial. There exists strong rationale for exploring the use of adjuvant chemotherapy (Table 52.1). The list of agents active against squamous cell carcinoma is extensive (Table 52.2). Increased interest in the use of chemotherapy has been stimulated by the recent development of highly active agents such as cisplatin, paclitaxel and gemcitabine that can be safely combined with other drugs and that may be synergistic with radiation. These newer drugs have opened the way for more effective combination drug regimens. With such regimens, higher rates of clinical and often histologic complete tumor regressions have been achieved. These results have been most notable in previously untreated patients. High rates of complete response have traditionally been the hallmark of progress in the chemotherapy of neoplasia.

Up until the early 1980s, the use of chemotherapy in patients with head and neck cancer was relegated to a palliative role. Chemotherapy treatment of potentially

Table 52.1 Rationale for adjuvant chemotherapy in head and neck squamous carcinoma

- Large numbers of active chemotherapeutic drugs
- High rate of distant metastases in advanced disease
- Effectiveness of adjuvant chemotherapy in Wilms' tumor, rhabdomyosarcoma
- Effectiveness of systemic chemotherapy in leukemias
- Potential impact on local/regional control
- Poor overall survival in advanced disease

Table 52.2 Cumulative response rates with single-drug chemotherapy in head and neck squamous carcinoma

Drug	*Evaluable patients*	*Response rate (%)*
Methotrexate	998	31
Bleomycin	347	21
Cisplatin	288	28
Carboplatin	115	26
5-Fluorouracil	118	15
Cyclophosphamide	86	36
Hydroxyurea	38	32
Vinblastine	35	29
Adriamycin	34	23
Paclitaxel	30	40
Docetaxel	60	32
Gemcitabine	54	13

curable, previously untreated patients remained largely investigational except for sites such as the larynx, where combined induction chemotherapy, radiation and salvage surgery treatment programs were used for larynx preservation. Data from a multitude of randomized trials, however, have failed to demonstrate improved survival when chemotherapy has been combined with surgery and radiation therapy.

The interpretations of the results of prior chemotherapy studies is confounded by the heterogeneity of treatments and tumor sites, inaccurate tumor staging, variations in drug regimens and the ways chemotherapy was integrated into treatment. Although some studies have suggested an impact of chemotherapy on distant metastases, few have combined drugs in an adjuvant fashion in sufficient dose or duration to expect an impact that would be likely to affect survival rates.

Randomized trials of chemotherapy

Because the results of individual clinical trials have not defined a precise role for chemotherapy, several meta-analyses of randomized trials of adjuvant chemotherapy in head and neck cancer have been published.[7,65,75,94,95] Despite the large number of individual trials that have been conducted, most contain too few patients and have insufficient statistical power to detect meaningful treatment differences. Few centers see large enough numbers of patients with advanced head and neck cancers to conduct single institution randomized trials and multi-institutional studies have been difficult and expensive to undertake. Combining the results of many small, randomized trials through meta-analysis has provided an alternative method to try to assess benefit. Unfortunately, even the results of meta-analyses are not clear (Table 52.3).[7,65,75,94,95]

Stell and Rawson's[95] analysis using 23 trials was only able to demonstrate a non-significant improvement in cancer mortality of 0.5% with the addition of chemotherapy. Deaths at 2 years were analyzed and in many trials, the number of deaths was estimated from published survival curves. However, they cautioned that in nine trials in which they had toxicity data, the mortality rate from chemotherapy was 6.5%. Munro[75] analyzed results from 52 trials. He reported an overall improvement in survival of 6.5% with chemotherapy that was associated with an odds ratio of only 1.37. Subset analysis indicated that single-agent chemotherapy combined with radiation appeared better than neoadjuvant chemotherapy.

The results of the largest meta-analysis (MACH-NC) have recently been presented.[7] This analysis is of particular interest because it was performed using individual patient data obtained from the original trial investigators and included both published and unpublished trials. This technique tends to minimize a potentially serious bias in survival analysis when literature-based data are used.

The MACH-NC analysis covered an extended period (1965–93) using updated patient data from 63 trials. A total of 10 717 patients were included and locoregional treatment was compared to the same treatment plus chemotherapy. A small (4%) but significant improvement in survival with chemotherapy was detected. As with the Munro analysis, a significant interaction with timing of chemotherapy was noted. The only significant improvement in survival was seen with concomitant chemotherapy/radiation trials. All of these meta-analyses, however, suffer from significant heterogeneity in trial design, treat-

Table 52.3 Meta-analyses of randomized clinical trials of chemotherapy for head and neck cancer

Author(s)	*No. trials*	*No. patients*	*Effect of chemotherapy on survival*	*P value*	*Odds ratio (95% confidence interval)*
Stell and Rawson[95]	23	3398	↑ 0.5% (2 year)	NS	1.02 (0.89–11.17)
Stell[94]	28	3977	↑ 2.8%	NS	–
Munro[75]	52	7443	↑ 6.5%	$<10^{-10}$	1.37 (1.24–1.5)
Bourhis *et al.*[7]	63	10 717	↑ 4% (5 year)	<0.001	0.91 (0.85–0.94)
Lefebvre *et al.**[65]	3	602	↓ 6% (5 year)	NS	1.19 (0.97–1.47)

NS, not significant.
*Three trials of organ preservation using chemotherapy and radiation for advanced cancer of the larynx and hypopharynx. Overall slight decrease in survival with chemotherapy ($P = 0.1$).

ment regimens and patients treated such that they are most helpful in only suggesting future directions for clinical research.

A subset meta-analysis of the large MACH-NC meta-analysis was reported for three randomized trials of neoadjuvant chemotherapy combined with radiation as part of an organ preservation strategy for patients with advanced cancers of the larynx and laryngopharynx.[65] Neither disease-free nor overall survival was improved with the experimental treatment (Table 52.3);[7,65,75,94,95] however, functional larynx preservation was 67% and 58% among patients alive at 3 and 5 years respectively.

Defining the use of chemotherapy in laryngeal cancer is frustrated by the dilemma of having extraordinarily powerful drugs and drug combinations yet failing to achieve significant survival benefit when chemotherapy is combined with conventional therapies. The interpretation of data from individual clinical trials and even large meta-analyses is confounded by the heterogeneity of treatments and patients. Despite this, a number of factors will be discussed in this chapter that assure a future role for chemotherapy in the treatment of laryngeal cancer. These include the consistent observations in all trials of the prolonged survival of chemotherapy responders compared to non-responders. Also, the use of chemotherapy to select patients for organ preserving radiation therapy as a legitimate alternative to laryngectomy has been proven. A decrease in distant metastases has been suggested and most recently, an increased understanding of genetic factors that might predict chemotherapy response offers the possibility that future treatment based on tumor histology may be more selective and effective. The need for further work and continued clinical trials is compelling and promising.

Why has so much effort been expended to explore the use of chemotherapy? The reasons go beyond the simple rationale of reducing tumor bulk and include an increasing appreciation by oncologists that most cancers are systemic derangements of host homeostasis in which cell growth regulation is consistently and permanently altered. In a growing tumor, increased tumor size is due to an imbalance between the cancer's cellular growth rate and the effects of natural and immune-mediated cytolysis, including programmed cell death. Local systemic drugs that increase cytolysis should be of benefit. Factors controlling distant cancer dissemination and growth are equally complex and not readily addressed by advances in surgery or radiation. Tumor regressions with modern chemotherapy regimens are dramatic in the speed and volume of cytoreduction. The availability of such therapeutic tools that can be combined with local treatment in feasible ways assures that an important role for chemotherapy will be defined in the future.

Drugs, drug regimens and toxicity

Chemotherapy-related toxicities are common in the treatment of patients with advanced head and neck cancers. Poor nutrition, swallowing difficulties, general debilitation, anemia and problems with aspiration are commonly associated features that predispose laryngeal cancer patients to enhanced toxicity. The most frequent and dose-limiting toxicities are myelosuppression, mucositis and the gastrointestinal and neurotoxicities associated with cisplatin. Because chemotherapy is often combined with radiation, mucositis is particularly problematic and can lead to treatment interruptions and late sequelae such as laryngeal and pharyngeal stenosis. Strategies to try to limit therapy-induced mucositis include use of anti-inflammatory agents, oral rinses containing sucralfate, antifungals or antibiotics and the liberal use of agents to reduce gastroesophageal reflux.

Cisplatin

Toxicities associated with cisplatin are primarily renal, otologic, neurologic and gastrointestinal. Most can be largely reduced by substituting the platinum analogue, carboplatin.[108] Most oncologists, however, believe the activity of cisplatin is slightly greater than that of carboplatin and tend to prefer cisplatin for use when renal impairment is not an issue or when myelosuppression is a concern. The major disadvantage of cisplatin is severe nausea and vomiting, which is best controlled through concurrent use of specific serotonin receptor antagonists.

Cisplatin is usually administered in an intermittent single dose bolus schedule (80–120 mg/m^2 every 3–4 weeks). A less toxic schedule of 20 mg/m^2/day for 5 days has been suggested to have similar activity.[86] Higher doses of cisplatin have been studied with response rates over 70% and responses have been reported in patients failing standard-dose cisplatin. Several investigators have utilized high-dose cisplatin intra-arterially to try and achieve even higher tissue levels with less systemic toxicity.[31,32,74,84] For laryngeal cancers, intra-arterial therapy poses vascular access problems to isolate vessels that adequately perfuse the tumor and nodes. To address this issue, Robbins *et al.*[84] have proposed using supraselective arteriography and have recently used this approach as part of an organ-preservation strategy combined with radiation.

Carboplatin

Carboplatin is often preferred over cisplatin for outpatient administration. Bolus carboplatin has pharmacokinetic and toxicity profiles similar to continuous-infusion cisplatin and significantly less renal, otologic, neurologic or gastrointestinal toxicity than bolus cisplatin. Reversible myelosuppression (primarily thrombocytopenia) is the dose-limiting toxicity for carboplatin. Carboplatin is usually given in monthly bolus (400 mg/m^2) or fractionated (80 mg/m^2/day for 5 days) schedules. In the presence of renal impairment, reduced-dose schedules of carboplatin are administered according to a standardized Egorin formula.[25] Because of myelosuppression, combinations of carboplatin with other myelosuppressive drugs such as methotrexate are challenging and dangerous.

Methotrexate

Methotrexate has been the standard chemotherapy agent to which other drugs have been compared for activity and toxicity. Myelosuppression and hepatotoxicity are dose-limiting toxicities. Because methotrexate is excreted by the kidneys, combinations of cisplatin and methotrexate have been hazardous due to platinum-induced renal impairment. Standard dose and schedule for palliative treatment is 40 mg/m^2/week IV or IM with dose escalations to toxicity or tumor response. At these dose levels, methotrexate is convenient, inexpensive, relatively non-toxic and can be easily administered to outpatients. Moderately increased and even higher doses (up to 100-fold increases) have been used with leucovorin 'rescue' of myelosuppression. Randomized studies, however, have failed to confirm superiority over conventional dose levels.[12] Likewise, direct comparison of methotrexate with cisplatin have shown similar response rates, 25–30% as single agents in patients with advanced disease (Table 52.2).[48]

Bleomycin

Bleomycin has a spectrum of toxicity that is distinctive. It causes dose-related mucositis and skin toxicity, but because of a lack of myelosuppression has been frequently combined with methotrexate and cisplatin. The most feared toxicity is pulmonary fibrosis. Because many head and neck cancer patients also suffer from smoking-induced pulmonary disease, Al-Sarraf substituted 5-fluorouracil for bleomycin in combination with cisplatin.[2] This led to development of one of the most active current drug combinations in head and neck cancer. The most commonly used combination regimen administers cisplatin 80–120 mg/m^2 day 1 followed by a 5-day continuous infusion of 5-fluorouracil, 1000 mg/m^2/day.

5-Fluorouracil (5-FU)

5-FU is less active as a single agent than cisplatin, methotrexate or bleomycin. Dose-limiting toxicity with bolus administration is myelosuppression. Prolonged administration (common when combined with cisplatin) results in mucositis, diarrhea and cutaneous erythema. Although widely used as a 5-day infusion following bolus cisplatin, the schedule dependency of 5-FU has received little study. Because combinations of cisplatin and 5-FU have achieved response rates approaching 90% in previously untreated patients, and objective responses in up to 78% of patients with recurrent disease,[2,56] this regimen has become the work horse of the head and neck oncologist. Higher response rates are achieved with the combination compared to either single agent alone[52] and these are associated with well understood and manageable toxicities. The combination of carboplatin and 5-FU produces similar results with more myelosuppression and less nausea. Unfortunately, improved response rates with multi-agent drug regimens have not yet translated into superior survival differences. This may be due principally to the far advanced nature of the disease in patients entered into drug evaluation studies where chemotherapy may have little overall benefit on survival.

New drugs

A number of promising new drugs with high activity against squamous carcinoma have recently been introduced. Drug development has also included studies of analogues of methotrexate (e.g. trimetrexate, piritrexim and edatrexate) and increased dosage and chemical modifications designed to alter the pharmacokinetics or toxicity (primarily 5-FU) of existing agents. The most exciting new drugs with promise in head and neck cancer include paclitaxel, docetaxel and gemcitabine.

Paclitaxel (Taxol)

The taxoid class of agents were originally extracted from the bark of the Pacific yew (*Taxis brevifolia*). Paclitaxel, a taxane derivative is a new agent that has a novel mechanism of action. The effects of paclitaxel are directed at microtubules where it binds to β-tubulin and prevents depolymerization of tubulin and promotes stabilization of spindle microtubules resulting in a G_2-M block. In interphase cells, paclitaxel induces formation of microtubule bundles inhibiting DNA synthesis and inducing apoptosis. Significant clinical activity has been reported in ovarian, breast and lung cancers. The effects of paclitaxel have also been studied extensively in squamous carcinoma cell lines,[36] including laryngeal cancer cell lines.[27] DNA synthesis was blocked at concentrations 100-fold less than typical serum levels achieved after a single-dose of 200 mg/m^2. Phase II studies at 250 mg/m^2 as a 24-hour infusion have demonstrated a 40% response rate.[30,33] The initial development of taxol was limited because of hypersensitivity reactions, but these have since been limited by slow, low-dose infusions or administration of steroids, diphenhydramine and H2-receptor antagonists. The major toxicities with paclitaxel are neutropenia, peripheral neuropathy and arthralgias/myalgias.

The recent emphasis in clinical research for the taxoids is now focused on developing multidrug combinations with cisplatin, carboplatin, methotrexate, ifosfamide, 5-FU and combinations with radiation therapy.[34,85] Paclitaxel has shown activity as a radiation sensitizing agent in cancers of the lung, cervix and bladder.[107] It is also particularly attractive to combine with radiation, since mucositis is not a common toxicity with the taxoids. Studies are underway in head and neck cancers at doses of 50–100 mg/m^2 weekly to tri-weekly during radiation. As with most chemoradiation regimens, significant mucosal toxicity has been reported.[100] A large study of various dose schedules showed that toxicities and activity were similar when paclitaxel at either 200 mg/m^2 or 135 mg/m^2 as a 24-hour infusion was combined with cisplatin (75 mg/m^2

on day 2). The major toxicities were grade 3 or 4 neutropenia in 76% of patients and febrile neutropenia in 40%. Treatment was stopped because of toxicity in 32% of patients. More complete responses were seen at the lower dose level. Overall 1-year survival in this group of advanced patients was nearly 30%.[34]

Docetaxel

Docetaxel is a semisynthetic analog of paclitaxel that is more potent than paclitaxel against human tumor cell lines and has important biologic and chemical differences that affect the formation of stable non-functional microtubule bundles and the drug's affinity for binding sites. This may explain the lack of cross-resistance between these agents in clinical studies.[109] Docetaxel toxicity is most common in patients with poor liver function because of reduced drug clearance by the liver. Doses should be reduced if liver enzymes are elevated. Problematic toxicities include hypersensitivity and skin reactions and fluid retention. Many of these can be minimized by steroid premedication. Fluid retention seems related to cumulative dose and is uncommon at cumulative doses <400 mg/m^2. A phase II study at 60 mg/m^2 by brief infusion every 3–4 weeks in 74 patients showed a response rate of 30%. Major toxicities included neutropenia in 83% of patients, alopecia (87%), anorexia (58%) and general fatigue (54%). No febrile neutropenia or hypersensitivity reactions occurred despite not using premedication.[24] Others have reported higher response rates at higher doses.[106] Docetaxel has recently been added to cisplatin and 5-FU as an induction regimen and resulted in a 100% response rate with a 67% complete response (CR) rate. All CRs were histologically negative on biopsy. Toxicity was formidable, but with the added efficacy might be justified in selected patients as part of an organ preservation approach.[82] Further studies of differing schedules and combinations with radiation are needed.

Gemcitabine

Gemcitabine is a nucleoside analog and an antimetabolite that has shown clinical activity against a variety of solid malignancies. Its cytotoxicity is related to rapid intracellular phosphorylation to gemcitabine triphosphate, which inhibits ribonucleotide reductase and serves as both an inhibitor and a substrate for DNA synthesis.[90] In head and neck cancer, patients treated at dose levels of 800–1250 mg/m^2/week, a response rate of 13% was observed.[13] Hematologic toxicity was low. Most common toxicities were hepatocellular and malaise.

Gemcitabine has been shown to be a potent radiosensitizer for head and neck cancer cell lines, even at noncytotoxic concentrations.[90,91] Phase I studies in eight patients treated with concurrent low dose gemcitabine (300 mg/m^2/weekly) with standard radiation showed significant skin and mucosal toxicity with an 88% local regional control rate and no significant hematologic toxicity. An additional 12 patients were treated after reducing the dose to 150 mg/m^2/week and acute mucositis was effectively reduced, but late complete pharyngeal stenosis occurred in two patients and partial stenosis in six. The complete response rate was 83%. Cellular levels of phosphorylated gemcitabine in tumor biopsies were similar at all levels.[26] The potency of this combination in patients with very large, advanced cancers is impressive. The ability to achieve significant radiosensitizing levels of intracellular drugs at reduced dosage suggests that even lower dose levels should achieve similar efficacy at reduced toxicity. Developing strategies for managing acute and late toxicities should allow even more effective combinations of non-cross-resistant drugs and radiation.

Adjuvant chemotherapy

Over the past 20 years, the emphasis in the development of adjuvant chemotherapy in laryngeal cancer has been on induction or neoadjuvant regimens. This was predicated on the higher response rates achieved in untreated patients, better nutritional and performance status of such patients, better tumor vascularity and the ability to monitor the effects of treatment on the tumor. This approach was relatively unique for treatment of solid cancers since most adjuvant approaches concentrated on adding chemotherapy during or after conventional treatment in an attempt to kill disseminated cancer cells.

The precise role of chemotherapy in the routine management of patients with head and neck cancer is, however, unclear. For patients with potentially curable disease, the use of chemotherapy is reported with both enthusiasm[22] and skepticism.[96] For patients with incurable or widely metastatic disease, routine use of systemic single or multidrug chemotherapy alone or combined with palliative radiation is well accepted. The frequency of tumor response to drugs in this setting is generally less than 50%, duration of response is short and prolongation of survival is unlikely unless a significant or complete clinical regression of tumor is achieved. Despite this, the palliative use of chemotherapy can bring significant temporary symptomatic relief to the patient in terms of decreases in pain, bleeding from the tumor, dysphagia and other symptoms related to tumor bulk. Unfortunately, these limited benefits are sometimes accompanied by severe and potentially lethal drug toxicities. Most toxicities are dose- and schedule-dependent and therefore can be ameliorated by somewhat lower and less effective dosage. Patient debilitation and a desire to maximize quality of life are also potential limiting factors in the use of palliative chemotherapy.

The major expected effects of neoadjuvant chemotherapy that might, in theory, support its use include tumor regressions of sufficient magnitude to allow a reduction in the extent of subsequent surgery. In addition, chemotherapy response data could then be used to select subsequent adjuvant chemotherapy that would have

Table 52.4 Largest randomized trials of neoadjuvant (induction) chemotherapy for head and neck cancer

Author(s)	*n*	*Standard therapy*	*Induction (no. cycles)*	*Results (years)*
HNCP-178[45]	462	S + RT	DDP, BLM (1)	No survival difference (5)
Schuller *et al.*[88]	158	S + RT	DDP, BLM, VCR (3)	No survival difference (5)
Paccagnella *et al.*[79]	221	S + RT	DDP, 5-FU (4)	No difference DFS
Gehanno *et al.*[38]	219	S + RT or RT	CP, 5-FU (3)	No survival difference, 30% reduction in S (2)
Jaulerry *et al.*[53]	208	RT	DDP, BLM, V Mito (2) or DDP, 5-FU (3)	No survival difference, fewer DM with chemotherapy (5)
Martin *et al.*[68]	107	S + RT or RT	DDP, 5-FU, BLM, MTX (3)	No survival difference (1)
Kun *et al.*[60]	83	RT ± S	BLM, MTX, 5-FU, CTX (2)	Better survival standard (2)
Toohill *et al.*[102]	60	RT ± S	DDP, 5-FU (3)	Better survival standard (1.5)

Abbreviations: BLM, bleomycin; CP, carboplatin; DDP, cisplatin; DFS, disease-free survival; DM, distant metastases; 5-FU, 5-fluorouracil; Mito, Mitomycin C; MTX, methotrexate; RT, radiation therapy; S, surgery; V, vindisine; VCR, vincristine.

known effectiveness and could potentially kill microscopic tumor and enhance local and disseminated microscopic disease control. In 1975, the feasibility of neoadjuvant chemotherapy in head and neck cancer was first demonstrated by Tarpley *et al.*[97] using preoperative, moderate dose methotrexate. This led to widespread investigation in large randomized clinical trials (Table 52.4).[38,45,53,60,68,79,88,102]

The final results of the initial randomized trials were consistent in that they failed to show a significant survival benefit with the addition of neoadjuvant therapy. The first and largest of these trials, termed the Head and Neck Contracts Program, was initiated in 1978.[45] This three-arm study compared a single course of preoperative cisplatin and bleomycin combined with conventional surgery and postoperative radiation therapy to the same treatment followed by six cycles of monthly cisplatin and to conventional treatment alone in patients with stage III/IV cancer of the oral cavity, larynx or hypopharynx. A total of 462 patients were entered on this study. A major trial limitation was a low overall complete response rate (3%) to the neoadjuvant chemotherapy regimen. No benefit was demonstrated with neoadjuvant chemotherapy, although detailed analysis of various subsets of patients suggested that induction chemotherapy plus maintenance may have had a beneficial effect in patients with oral cavity cancer, small primaries (T1–T2) or neck disease (N1–N2).[50] In addition, the group of patients receiving maintenance chemotherapy showed a delay in the appearance of distant metastases.[50] Over the years, this observation has been cited as suggestive evidence for an impact of adjuvant chemotherapy on disseminated disease. However, careful analysis of the trial data shows that these results could be attributed to the method of analysis. Only patients disease-free after surgery were included in the distant metastases analysis. Substantially more patients who were randomized to the maintenance arm had gross residual disease at the time of surgery and were excluded from analysis compared to the other treatment arms. When all patients were included in analysis, there was no difference in time to distant disease. Other confounding factors include the fact that the analysis was performed based on the site of *first* tumor relapse and only 27% of patients received three or more cycles of maintenance chemotherapy and nearly half never received any. It is probably unreasonable to expect much benefit on the overall rate of distant disease from such limited adjuvant therapy. This trial and others that followed demonstrated how difficult it was to deliver maintenance chemotherapy to patients with head and neck cancer. Patients were unreliable, compliance was problematic and the rigors of conventional treatment resulted in such debility that long-term chemotherapy was frequently not feasible.

The Head and Neck Contracts Program and others that followed did demonstrate some important findings which led to the next generation of neoadjuvant chemotherapy trials. The studies were consistent in demonstrating that patients achieving a complete regression of cancer after neoadjuvant chemotherapy enjoyed a survival advantage. Also, response to chemotherapy tended to predict a favorable overall response after subsequent radiation therapy.[28,39,47,53] Jacobs *et al.*[51] and Karp *et al.*[54] were the first to incorporate these observations into a treatment paradigm that used chemotherapy to select patients for treatment that might avoid mutilating surgery. Others[81,104] rapidly confirmed the feasibility of this new approach. This led to the first large, prospective, randomized trial combining neoadjuvant chemotherapy with radiation as an alternative treatment for patients who traditionally were felt to require surgical resection for optimal management. Advanced cancer of the larynx was the site first studied by a group of investigators from the Department of Veterans Affairs.[20] This site was selected because of the long-term morbidity of total laryngectomy, the proven effectiveness of radiation on small laryngeal cancers and the fact that some surgeons and patients would accept treatment with radiation alone as an alternative to laryngectomy, even if it meant risking lower survival rates.

The design of the Department of Veterans Affairs Cooperative Study (VA CSP 268) of neoadjuvant

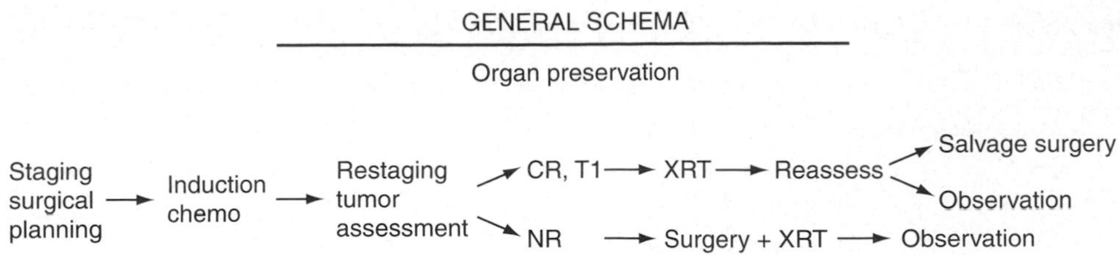

Figure 52.1 *General schema of the treatment paradigm for organ preservation in advanced laryngeal cancer using induction chemotherapy and radiation. After two or three cycles of induction chemotherapy, patients down-staged to either T1 or complete response (CR) at the primary site are treated with definitive radiation therapy. Non-responders (NR) to chemotherapy undergo surgery and postoperative radiation.*

chemotherapy for patients with laryngeal cancer has become the prototype for organ preservation trials (Fig 52.1). Only patients with previously untreated stage III or IV (AJC 1988) squamous carcinoma of the larynx were eligible for this study. A total of 332 patients were entered with 166 randomly assigned to one of two treatment strategies. The experimental treatment arm included three cycles of induction chemotherapy consisting of cisplatin 100 mg/m^2 on day 1 and 5-fluorouracil 1000 mg/m^2/day over 24 hours for 5 continuous days. Responders to chemotherapy received definitive radiation. Surgical salvage was an integral part of the trial design. Three clinical response assessments were performed. The first assessment was performed after two cycles of induction chemotherapy. If there was not at least a 50% reduction in primary tumor size and at least stable disease in the neck, chemotherapy treatment was stopped and salvage surgery was performed, followed by postoperative radiation. If at least a partial response (>50%) was noted after two cycles, patients received a third cycle of induction chemotherapy followed by a second tumor assessment and primary site biopsy. This was followed by definitive radiation (66–76 Gy). Twelve weeks after the completion of radiation, a third tumor assessment by direct laryngoscopy was performed. If biopsy-proven cancer was found, a salvage laryngectomy was performed. If not, the patient entered a standardized common follow-up schedule. The control group in this trial was treated with total laryngectomy and modified radical or radical neck dissection followed by postoperative radiation. The results of this trial were analyzed on an intention to treat basis and all patients were included on the treatment arm to which they had been randomized.

The results of this study have been extensively analyzed.[10,41,46,73,93,113,114,116] At the 5-year follow-up, there were no significant differences in survival rates between the treatment arms. The 5-year rate for the surgery group was 46% and it was 42% for patients randomized to initial chemotherapy. The rate of larynx preservation was 62% among patients randomized to induction chemotherapy. Of surviving patients, 66% retained a functioning larynx, although this group represented only 31% of the total 166 patients initially randomized to chemotherapy. At 10 years, only 93 (28%) patients were alive, 51 in the group randomized to surgery and 42 in the group of patients randomized to chemotherapy (P = 0.34 log rank). At 12 years, 23% of patients were still alive and 61% of the survivors randomized to initial chemotherapy had successful organ preservation (Fig 52.2). These long-term results confirm that an approach in which response to initial chemotherapy is used to determine whether laryngectomy is required is feasible. Larynx preservation rates are sustained long term and overall long-term survival rates are achieved that are similar to initial laryngectomy.

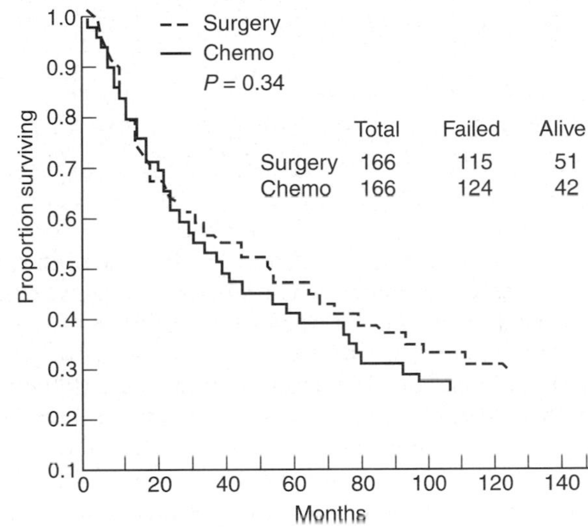

Figure 52.2 *Overall survival of patients with advanced laryngeal cancer entered in the Department of Veterans Affairs Laryngeal Cancer Study (VA CSP 268). Long-term follow-up survival data were obtained from the National Death Index. Survival for the entire cohort is 28% at 10 years; 30% for the group randomized to surgery; and 25% for the group randomized to chemotherapy (P = 0.34, log rank test, power estimate to detect a 15% difference in survival rates is >0.90).*

What the VA CSP 268 study did not prove was whether chemotherapy added significant benefit compared to radiation alone. The study design did not contain a radiation alone arm. This was because the trial was not designed to compare surgery to radiation therapy, but rather to test whether radiation delivered to cancers

Table 52.5 Larynx preservation in selected (limited) advanced laryngeal cancer patients: radiation with surgical salvage

Authors	*Site*	*Extent*	*n*	*% Alive (5 years)*	*% Organ preservation in survivors*
Goepfert *et al.*[40]	Supraglottic	III, IV	59	55 (deter.)	64*
Harwood *et al.*[43]	Glottic	T3N0	68	49	65
Harwood *et al.*[42]	Glottic	T3N0	112	49	60
Harwood *et al.*[44]	Supraglottic	T3,4N0	265	51	64
Croll *et al.*[18]	Glottic/supraglottic	T3,4	55	51	73

*Percentage of total, alive and dead.

Table 52.6 Larynx preservation in selected (extensive) advanced laryngeal cancer patients: radiation with surgical salvage

Authors	*Site*	*Extent*	*n*	*% Alive (5 years)*	*% Organ preservation in survivors*
Harwood *et al.*[43]	Glottic	T4N0	39	38	90
Harwood *et al.*[44]	Supraglottic	N+	145	24	39
Meredith *et al.*[71]	Glottic/supraglottic	T3,4 (73% N0)	150	41	44

reduced to small or microscopic size by chemotherapy could cure as many patients as immediate surgery. Other nonrandomized studies of radiation alone with surgery salvage have achieved survival rates and organ preservation rates similar to the VA study without the addition of induction chemotherapy (Table 52.5).[18,40,42–44] However, those studies consisted of highly selected patients with predominately T3N0 or limited T4N0 tumors. Survival rates and successful organ preservation rates were significantly lower in patients with more advanced tumors and in patients with regional metastases (Table 52.6).[43,44,71] In the VA study, there was no selection bias for earlier disease. Of 479 patients screened for entry, 70% were randomized. Exclusions were primarily due to poor medical status (14%) or patient refusal (13%). Nearly 46% had regional metastases and of those, 60% had advanced N2 or N3 neck disease. Further, there were no imbalances between treatment groups with respect to known prognostic variables. Several other pilot studies of organ preservation using induction chemotherapy for stage III and IV larynx cancer have also reported similar 2-year survival rates of 58–71% with 69–85% rates of organ preservation.[17,81]

A recent update of the Toronto experience with hyperfractionated radiation and salvage surgery for advanced laryngopharyngeal cancers failed to show any improvement over conventional radiation therapy.[19] Of 133 patients treated for larynx cancer, salvage laryngectomy was performed in 38 (29%). However, for the entire cohort of treated patients (larynx, hypopharynx and oropharynx), the 5-year survival rates were only 33% and only 18% in those undergoing salvage surgery. Positive surgical margins were reported in 25% and had the strongest negative correlation with survival. It should be noted that locoregional recurrences occurred in 48% of the entire cohort of patients and one third of those were not able to undergo potentially curative surgery. Half of those were due to unresectability, one-quarter because of patient refusal and the rest because of medical reasons or death due to other causes.[19] Other investigators have also indicated high rates (35%) of positive margins for salvage laryngectomy that are also even higher for pharyngeal primaries (47%) compared to larynx (18%).[58]

Whether radiation alone with surgery salvage is superior to laryngectomy or to a treatment strategy that includes induction chemotherapy may be answered by a second randomized organ preservation clinical trial that is currently underway in the USA. It is a three-arm trial sponsored by the Radiation Therapy Oncology Group (Fig 52.3) and compares a regimen similar to the VA Study to two different radiation treatment arms, one using conventional radiation doses and fractionation and the other using cisplatin 100 mg/m^2 on days 1, 22 and 43, administered concurrent with radiation therapy. The radiation on each arm is 70 Gy/35 fractions over 7 weeks. Eligibility criteria in this study are limited to those patients with T2, T3 or early T4 cancers. Patient accrual on this study

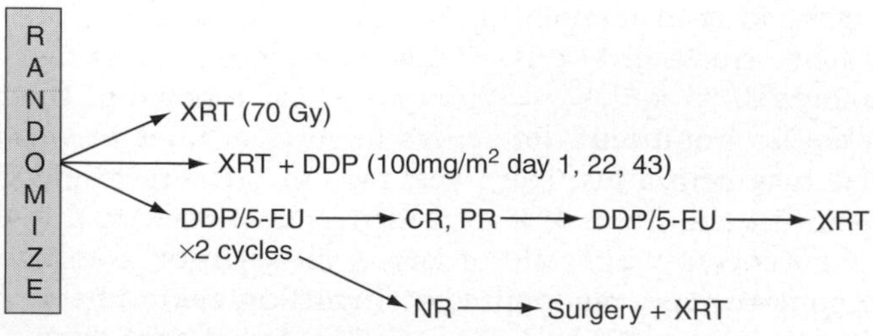

Figure 52.3 *Intergroup Organ Preservation Study (RTOG 91-11) for patients with advanced laryngeal cancer. No. of patients required = 546.*

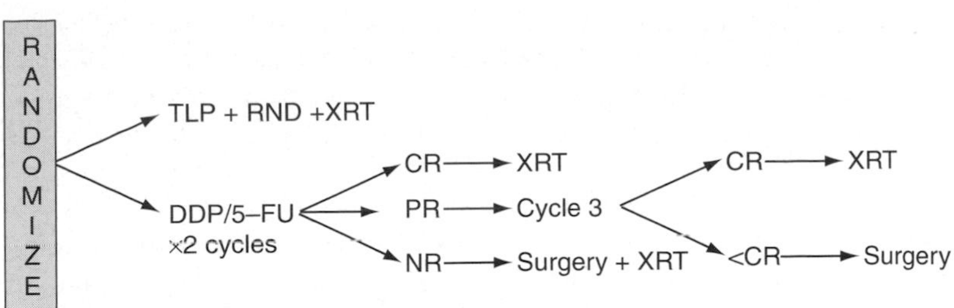

Figure 52.4 *Schema for organ preservation in hypopharyngeal carcinoma (EORTC 24-891).*

requires 546 patients in order to test the hypothesis that one arm is superior. Unless chemotherapy is detrimental to the success of radiation, it is hard to conceive that the radiation-alone treatment arm could be superior to the other two. The trial will also address the issue of whether concurrent or sequential chemotherapy is a better treatment approach for larynx preservation.

It is worth noting that theoretical concern has been expressed by some investigators that induction chemotherapy may contribute to the development of radiation resistance through a mechanism of accelerated repopulation.[8,23,80,111] Although such an effect has never been proven in the clinical setting, experimental evidence supports the concept and provides rationale for integrating chemotherapy in a simultaneous fashion into radiation fractionation schedules rather than as a pre-radiation, sequential modality. At least one reported randomized trial indicated no overall difference in overall survival with induction chemotherapy followed by radiation compared to radiation alone, but did identify a significant decrease in distant metastases.[53] Several other clinical trials have suggested that concurrent or alternating chemotherapy and radiation is superior to either radiation alone or to induction chemotherapy followed by radiation.[1,3,72,89] However, acute mucositis is usually increased with simultaneous drug and radiation administration. This is particularly true when multidrug regimens are used and can result in potentially detrimental interruptions of treatment[23] or reductions in radiation dose. Optimal drug combinations, dose, schedule and sequence remain to be determined. Basic science investigations into the mechanisms of chemotherapy and radiation resistance may provide important clues to the future design of optimal regimens.

Induction chemotherapy for organ preservation has not been studied extensively for sites other than larynx cancer. Some investigators have conducted pilot studies in oral cavity and oral pharynx[81,104,115] with encouraging preliminary results, but most emphasis has been on sites such as tongue base and hypopharynx where standardized surgical treatment often entails total laryngectomy.

A second important randomized trial of combined chemotherapy/radiation for organ preservation was conducted in Europe by the EORTC in patients with advanced hypopharyngeal cancer (Fig 52.4).[64] A total of 202 patients were randomly assigned to receive either surgery (total laryngectomy with partial pharyngectomy and neck dissection) and postoperative radiation (50–79 Gy) or induction chemotherapy (cisplatin and 5-fluorouracil). Complete responders to induction chemotherapy after either two or three cycles were treated with definitive radiation. Those not responding completely to chemotherapy underwent planned surgery and postoperative radiation. Salvage surgery for the primary tumor or neck metastases was performed for recurrences after chemotherapy and radiation. With a median follow-up of 51 months, actuarial survival was similar for both treatment groups with a longer median survival for the chemotherapy group (44 months vs 25 months). Analysis of patterns of relapse showed similar recurrence rates for local, regional or second primary tumor in the treatment groups, but a lower rate of distant relapse in the chemotherapy group, which was of borderline statistical significance. Unfortunately, the overall 3-year disease-free survival rates remained dismal for both groups of patients (surgery group, 31%; chemotherapy group, 43%). At 3 years, 40% of patients randomized to chemotherapy were alive, disease-free with an intact larynx and without tracheostomy or feeding tube. Long-term follow-up (personal communication with J L Lefebvre) indicates similar overall survival rates between the two groups.

These results are particularly important because they confirm that an organ preservation approach combining chemotherapy and radiation can be successful even for a non-laryngeal tumor site that historically has poor survival rates with radiation alone. That an approach incorporating surgical salvage can be effective for the hypopharynx is particularly compelling, since surgical salvage is difficult for radiation failures where extensive submucosal spread can be present. Furthermore, the hypopharynx is a site where the lymphatic supply is abundant and regional or distant metastases are more common than for larynx cancer. That surgical salvage is part of planned treatment for chemotherapy non-responders may be critical to maintain survival rates. A recent small European study in which patients were randomized to either laryngopharyngectomy or radiation after induction chemotherapy, regardless of chemotherapy response, demonstrated significantly poorer local control and survival rates for patients treated with radiation alone for their hypopharynx cancer.[5] By contrast, it is interesting to note that in the VA Laryngeal Cancer Study, salvage surgery was highly effective with survival rates as good as

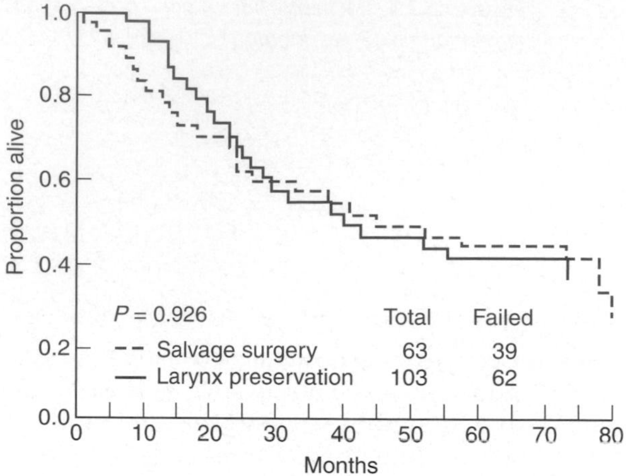

Figure 52.5 *Comparison of overall actuarial survival among 166 patients randomized to chemotherapy on VA CSP 268 who underwent salvage laryngectomy compared to the group of patients who had successful larynx preservation (P = 0.926 log rank test).*

the group of patients achieving organ preservation and similar to those treated with immediate laryngectomy (Fig 52.5).

Management guidelines for organ preservation

The combined experience of prior investigators has elucidated a number of management guidelines that are important for the safe and optimal integration of chemotherapy in organ-preserving approaches for patients with advanced laryngeal cancer. These guidelines all center on a team approach utilizing the specialized skills of surgical, medical and radiation oncologists. Specialized support from speech pathology, dentistry, prosthodontics, dietetics, psychology, social services and nursing are also often important, but not unique to the needs of laryngeal cancer patients undergoing chemotherapy.

Since *surgical salvage* is such an important part of the success of the approach, proper staging and pretreatment assessment of tumor extent, planning for potential surgical resection and tattooing of potential resection margins is critical. Many patients will benefit from pretreatment CT or MRI, particularly to delineate extent of tumor in pre-epiglottic and paraglottic spaces. For some patients with deeply invasive or submucosal tumors, these radiologic images become the best method to measure tumor response, since surface measurements in such situations are often unreliable.

Clinical surveillance for tumor recurrence and for tumor response assessments is also critical. This relies heavily on the skill and experience of the surgeon and cannot be relegated to medical or radiation oncologists or to radiologic imaging alone. Important observations derived from early studies include the finding that fixed vocal cords often remain fixed, even after tumor eradication. Areas of gross tumor are replaced by scarred and fibrotic tissue and thus restoration of normal phonation is less likely the larger the size of the tumor. Aspiration following major tumor regression is uncommon. This may be due to the slow disappearance of tissue bulk during tumor regression, allowing patients to adapt their protective swallowing mechanisms to such slow changes in laryngeal anatomy. In the VA Larynx Trial, no patients required permanent tracheostomy because of aspiration and only 4 of 166 required permanent tracheostomy because of chronic laryngeal fibrosis, edema or chondritis. Three other patients with permanent tracheostomy were never rendered disease free and died of cancer within 6 months of diagnosis (unpublished data).

Surgical guidelines for chemotherapy/radiation organ-preservation protocols

Perhaps one of the most important observations arising out of the VA study was the importance of *optimal management of regional metastases.* Because clinical responses after chemotherapy for the primary tumor and any regional metastases were assessed separately in the VA study, it was found that differences in response of primary and nodal disease (mixed responses) occurred over 50% of the time. The neck node response was less than the primary tumor response 28% of the time and the neck node response was greater than that of the primary tumor 24% of the time. When success of treatment and the need for salvage surgery were analyzed according to response of the clinically palpable neck nodes to induction chemotherapy, it was found that even large nodes (N2, N3) that disappeared completely after chemotherapy were usually controlled by radiation therapy.[113] These data have been confirmed by investigators in Boston[15] and New York.[4] However, if palpable neck disease persisted post-induction chemotherapy, radiation frequently failed. In a group of 42 patients with N2 or N3 disease randomized to chemotherapy on the VA study, only 30% were cured if less than a complete response occurred in the neck, compared to 67% survival if the neck nodes disappeared after chemotherapy. Of those with less than a complete response, 68% required subsequent salvage surgery. Many of the patients needing salvage surgery were found to be inoperable in the neck.[113] This led to change in treatment approach in subsequent studies in which planned neck dissections were performed in any patient with persistent neck disease after induction chemotherapy. The feasibility of performing neck dissections in the interval between chemotherapy and radiation without resecting the primary site was demonstrated by Thomas *et al.*[99] in a series of 60 patients treated with induction chemotherapy as part of an organ-preservation strategy. Twenty patients underwent planned interval neck dissections. Control rates were significantly improved compared to the VA study and survival increased to 50%. There were no differences in regional recurrence or patterns of recurrence compared to patients with N0 disease. Also, overall survival and control of neck disease was similar to a group of 19 patients who achieved a complete response in the neck after chemotherapy and who did not undergo neck dissection. Complications were minimal. Other investigators have recommended planned neck dissections after radiation therapy for all patients with initial N2 or N3 disease.[62,63] Rationale for this approach is based on poor overall survival rates in patients with N3 disease and a high incidence of microscopic residual disease found in the neck after radiation therapy. Optimal timing for postradiation neck dissection has not been established, but generally surgery is planned between 4 and 10 weeks after radiation. Higher complication rates can be expected with neck dissections after completion of radiation. Long-term results with such an approach have not been prospectively compared to earlier planned neck dissections performed immediately after chemotherapy. As increasing numbers of investigators adopt combination regimens incorporating concurrent radiation and chemotherapy for organ preservation, most planned neck dissections will, by necessity, be performed following radiation. What is clear is that even in the presence of fairly massive regional metastases, tumors that are readily sensitive to and disappear after chemotherapy are often controlled with radiation even when such tumors would rarely be expected to be controlled with radiation alone. These observations argue that some demonstrable benefit exists for chemotherapy added to radiation if appropriate patients could be identified.

Several authors have cited increased *complication rates* for surgery following radiation and chemotherapy. Most reports suggest that surgery can be safely performed following chemotherapy without an increase in morbidity. However, increased complication rates following radiation are well known and even higher rates have been reported after chemotherapy/radiation.[63,76,87]

An analysis of major wound complications following organ preservation with chemotherapy and radiation indicated that complication rates are increased in cases of salvage surgery.[87] In such situations, major complications occurred in over 60% of cases and were more common when the pharynx was resected than if just a neck dissection was performed. Major wound complications were more common with early salvage surgery performed within 12 months of radiation compared to later salvage procedures. The severity of complications such as fistulae and neck skin slough was also felt to be increased after chemotherapy/radiation. Salvage surgery in such settings poses unique challenges that require careful surgical planning, appropriate incisions, judicious nutritional and metabolic assessment, liberal use of modern, well-vascularized soft tissue reconstructions and a thorough knowledge of pathways of cancer spread.

Recurrences following chemotherapy/radiation are often insidious. Extensive submucosal disease can be present. Wide resections that encompass at least the original extent of tumor are mandatory.[66] This need reinforces the importance of good pretreatment planning and consistent follow-up by the head and neck surgical oncologist. Meticulous tissue handling and hemostasis are important. Although blood transfusion has been implicated as a negative prognostic factor, the analysis of the VA data failed to demonstrate that transfusion requirement was an independent negative prognostic variable.[70] Regardless, risk of hepatitis, AIDS and potential immune suppression argue for very judicious transfusion decisions. In situations of early salvage laryngectomy when neck tissues are indurated and inflamed, it may be advisable to postpone voice restoration with primary tracheoesophageal puncture to a secondary procedure after the patient is well healed from his laryngectomy.

Quality of life after larynx preservation

A detailed analysis of vocal function, speech and swallowing following chemotherapy and radiation in the VA study has now been completed.[46] At 2-year follow-up, patients randomized to chemotherapy had significantly better speech intelligibility and communication profile scores than the surgery group. Self-reported swallowing behavior scores were similar among both groups.[46]

A *quality of life* survey of 46 long-term survivors (12-year follow-up) on the VA Larynx Study has recently been completed.[98] The preliminary analysis indicates that 62% of patients randomized to chemotherapy continue to maintain their larynx intact and have better SF-36 scores and head and neck quality of life scores than patients randomized to surgery. The differences are most significant for mental health and pain. There was surprisingly little difference in self-reported speech scores. This is in contrast to objective speech quality assessments made by trained observers at 2 years.[46] Thus, a patient's perception of how the quality of speech affects his quality of life may not be accurately reflected in objective measures of intelligibility and communication ability.

When analyzed according to whether or not the patient underwent laryngectomy, the organ-preservation group had similar scores in all domains of the SF-36 compared to healthy US males, ages 55–64, except for bodily pain, which was worse for the cancer group. The group of long-term laryngectomy patients had significantly lower scores in all domains compared to normal US males. The results of this analysis are particularly important because the groups of cancer patients had similar survival rates, thus eliminating confounding factors of 'trade-offs' between quality and quantity of life.

Thus, it becomes necessary to consider all of these variables in assessing the overall wisdom and effectiveness of induction chemotherapy in treating larynx cancer. Are the improvements in quality of life for most patients sufficient to offset increased morbidity, cost and risk of adding some therapeutic redundancy to the percentage of patients who fail to respond to nonsurgical management? It is unknown whether a patient's perceptions of quality of life are the same as the treating physician. A study from the Mayo Clinic[21] indicated that living with a stoma was the biggest quality of life issue for laryngectomee patients, rather than loss of voice. Our own analysis of quality of life measures in long-term survivors after either surgery or organ preservation approaches indicated no major differences in the speech domains of the assessment instrument despite significant differences in terms of mental health, pain and depression compared to laryngectomy patients.[98]

Current trials

There are currently three ongoing randomized trials of chemotherapy and organ preservation for patients with advanced laryngeal or hypopharyngeal cancer. The US trial (RTOG 91-11) was initiated in 1991 and designed with three arms. Eligible patients with T2 or T3 larynx cancer and N0–N3 are randomized to compare conventional radiation to concomitant radiation and three cycles of cisplatin to induction chemotherapy with radiation only to chemoresponders and surgery for non-responders (Fig 52.3). Two European trials are underway. The first (EORTC 22-954) compares conventional radiation to radiation and concurrent cisplatin. Only patients with advanced larynx or hypopharynx cancers are eligible. The second European trial (EORTC 24-954) compares induction chemotherapy with two cycles of cisplatin and 5-FU followed by radiation and concurrent chemotherapy for responders (surgery for non-responders) to concomitant cisplatin and 5-FU alternating with radiation therapy. In this treatment group, there is an option for surgery salvage if less than a partial response is achieved after week 6 of therapy. Each of these randomized trials has accrual expectations of over 500 patients. The results of these various trials will be important in establishing whether chemotherapy added to radiation is superior to radiation alone. They should also provide insight into whether concurrent, alternating or sequential schedules for integrating chemotherapy with radiation are better. A potentially critical variable that is not well controlled in these studies is the role of salvage surgery. If timely, appropriate and radical surgery for non-responders or for salvage of locoregional recurrence is necessary to achieve survival rates with chemotherapy/radiation that are similar to standard laryngectomy, then decreases in survival associated with variable surgical salvage may occur and not be appreciated in the comparison of treatment arms. This is because a surgical control arm is not included. Many investigators still consider surgery the 'gold standard' for treatment of advanced laryngeal cancer, since no other therapy has ever been shown to achieve better overall survival rates.

Future trials

The field of chemotherapy in laryngeal cancer is actively evolving. The expected results with induction chemotherapy combined with radiation are now established because the long-term results from randomized trials are known. However, increasing evidence indicates that concurrent radiation and chemotherapy may be better than radiation alone. Although toxicity with concurrent therapy is generally greater, local control rates are clearly better and there is some indication that survival may even be improved.[1,3,7,72] Whether sequential chemotherapy is better than concurrent chemotherapy when combined with radiation is yet unknown. Most investigators, however, favor concurrent therapy.

Some laryngeal cancers will be intrinsically resistant to radiation and will require salvage surgery after concurrent radiation and chemotherapy. Tumor surveillance and subsequent surgery after concurrent therapy can be very difficult. Identification of such 'non-responding' patients prior to therapy would be optimal, but methods to do so are currently lacking. One experimental approach adopted at the University of Michigan builds on past results that indicate that a major tumor regression (>50%) after a single cycle of induction chemotherapy correlates with and predicts subsequent successful larynx preservation.[110] After tumor response is assessed following a single cycle of cisplatin/5-fluorouracil, a decision is made for surgery or for concurrent cisplatin/radiation therapy followed by two cycles of adjuvant cisplatin/5-FU. Patients exhibiting less than a 50% tumor reduction after a single cycle of induction therapy are subjected to immediate salvage surgery. Results with this approach in 16 patients with advanced stage III and IV larynx cancer show 94% survival at a median follow-up of 2 years (range 6–33 months). Larynx preservation has been achieved in 75% of patients and 69% are alive with an intact larynx. Until the results of randomized trials are available or accurate biologic predictive factors are discovered, differing combinations and treatment paradigms will be developed at many institutions.

Biologic markers

The concept that biology of a tumor can influence the response to therapy is well accepted by cancer investigators. Considerable effort has been expended to try and define the biologic basis of chemotherapy resistance and the existence of genes that modify radiation sensitivity. It is axiomatic that the definition of biologic characteristics that relate to a tumor's radiation or chemotherapy sensitivity would be beneficial by allowing better selection of patients for therapy and potentially allow design of experimental approaches which would modify a tumor's biology to enhance therapeutic efficacy.

Considerable recent attention has been focused on cell cycle regulators and response to therapy, particularly radiation and chemotherapy. A number of factors have been variably suggested as prognostically important in larynx cancer in general. These have included DNA content, proliferating cellular nuclear antigen (PCNA), expression, histologic growth pattern and expression of epidermal growth factor (EGF) and other cell surface receptors.[6,29,41,49,55,69,101,103,110,112] Specific factors that might predict chemotherapy response have included expression of p53 and PCNA (cyclin D).[10,11,67] These and other regulators of cell cycle proliferation and apoptosis have also been implicated in radiation sensitivity.[57,59] In particular, the *bcl-2* family of genes (*bcl-x, bax, bad*) and the ICE family of proteases are thought to be important.[83,92] Results from the VA CSP 268 trial suggested that immunohistologic expression of p53 and PCNA were predictive of successful organ preservation in logistic regression analysis.[9] Work is currently underway to determine the relevance of *bcl-2, bcl-x* and *bax* genes in determining chemotherapy response and organ preservation with chemotherapy/radiation combinations.[105] Important to the interpretation of such work is the possibility that factors which predict chemotherapy response may differ from those which predict radiosensitivity. Also, differences may exist between tumors of different sites and histologies. We and others have already observed that prognostic factors differ depending on the therapy used to treat a head and neck cancer.[37,103] Thus, a pretreatment biologic factor that correlates with favorable prognosis after surgery may very well be different from one that predicts favorable outcome after chemotherapy. It is therefore important that clinical studies testing biologic markers be homogenous for tumor site, stage and histology and treatment modality.

An exciting outgrowth of our increasing knowledge of factors regulating cell growth has been the feasibility of introducing genes into tumors in order to induce apoptosis or modify the effectiveness of chemotherapeutic agents.[16,77,117] This work has been limited to intratumoral injections of various genes including p53, E1A, E1B and herpes thymidine kinase in patients with incurable disease. Other approaches to increase the effectiveness of chemotherapy that are being investigated include the use of monoclonal antibodies to target specific cellular antigens or enzymes [e.g. EGF receptor (EGFR), retinoid receptors, protein kinase C] that influence cellular proliferation. Biologic response modifiers such as the interleukins, the interferons, retinoids, antiangiogenesis factors and prostaglandins are also exciting candidates for combination therapy with cytotoxic chemotherapeutic drugs.[14,35,78,118]

Conclusions

The future prospects for chemotherapy in laryngeal cancer are bright. Neoadjuvant chemotherapy has not yet been shown to be effective and is not recommended outside of clinical trial settings. However, neoadjuvant chemotherapy combined with radiation as an alternative to laryngectomy has been shown to be clinically useful and could be offered to patients where skilled multidisciplinary treatment teams are available. Such approaches are being expanded to cancers of the base of tongue and hypopharynx that would also normally require laryngectomy. Candidates for this use of neoadjuvant chemotherapy should be limited to those whose tumors require total laryngectomy. The number of patients requiring total laryngectomy continues to decrease as more patients with earlier cancers are diagnosed and the scope of subtotal partial laryngectomy procedures expands. Some recent clinical studies have even reported successful treatment of small laryngeal cancers with chemotherapy alone.[61]

The role of chemotherapy combined with radiation has even greater promise. Evidence that combined concurrent therapy is superior to radiation alone is increasing. The development of newer regimens will undoubtedly focus on improved results with less toxicity. The role of systemic adjuvant chemotherapy, particularly in patients at high risk for distant metastases (i.e. advanced neck nodes, extracapsular spread, resectable recurrent cancers), has not been adequately explored. Until randomized trials are designed and completed and better methods to ameliorate the side effects of long-term adjuvant chemotherapy are developed, it is unlikely that significant improvements in long-term survival for advanced laryngeal cancer patients will be achieved.

The experience gained with induction chemotherapy in cancer of the larynx has identified many important new questions. The most critical of these are largely philosophical, i.e. does chemotherapy really add benefit? It is obvious that some tumors disappear rapidly with drug therapy. These patients seem to exhibit favorable prognostic characteristics. If drug treatments were equally effective on small tumor burdens, some eradication of micro-disseminated disease might be expected and this certainly could have potential benefit since we have no effective therapy for distant metastases. The optimal timing, duration and type of patient suitable for chemotherapy are unknown. But, if one could select those patients with responsive tumors, either radiation alone, or radiation combined with or followed by chemotherapy would seem desirable for patients with advanced disease. Immunotherapy, gene therapy and biologic treatments with other regulatory factors (e.g. anti-EGFR combined with chemotherapy) remain largely untested. Future treatment protocols will hopefully address issues of patient selection so that more custom-tailored protocols can be used that minimize morbidity and maximize both cure rates and quality of life. Testing of these treatment protocols will require large numbers of patients and will demand a level of inter-institutional and international cooperation never before achieved.

References

1. Adelstein DJ, Sharan VM, Earle AS *et al.* Simultaneous versus sequential combined technique therapy for squamous cell head and neck cancer. *Cancer* 1990; **65:** 1685–91.
2. Al-Sarraf M. Chemotherapeutic management of head and neck cancer. *Cancer Metastasis Rev* 1987; **6:** 181–98.
3. Al-Sarraf M, LeBlanc M, Giri PG *et al.* Chemoradiotherapy versus radiotherapy in patients with advanced nasopharyngeal cancer: phase III randomized Intergroup Study 0099. *J Clin Oncol* 1998; **16:** 1310–17.

4. Armstrong J, Pfister D, Strong E *et al.* The management of the clinically positive neck as part of a larynx preservation approach. *Int J Radiat Oncol Biol Phys* 1993; **26:** 759–65.
5. Beauvillain C, Mahé M, Bourdin S *et al.* Final results of a randomized trial comparing chemotherapy plus radiotherapy with chemotherapy plus surgery plus radiotherapy in locally advanced resectable hypopharyngeal carcinomas. *Laryngoscope* 1997; **107:** 648–53.
6. Bier H, Hoffman T, Knecht R *et al.* Clinical trial with escalating doses of the anti-epidermal growth factor receptor (EGFR) humanized monoclonal antibody EDM 72000 in patients with head and neck cancer: a multiple administration study. *Head Neck* 1998; **20:** 447.
7. Bourhis J, Pignon JP, Designe L, Luboinsk M, Guerin S, Domenge C and The MACH-NC Collaborative Group. Meta-analysis of chemotherapy in head and neck cancer. *Proc Am Soc Clin Oncol* 1998: 386.
8. Bourhis J, Wilson G, Wibault P *et al.* Rapid tumor cell proliferation after induction chemotherapy in oropharyngeal cancer. *Laryngoscope* 1994; **104:** 468–72.
9. Bradford CR, Wolf GT, Zhu S *et al.* Predictive markers for chemotherapy response and organ preservation in advanced laryngeal carcinoma. *Otolaryngol Head Neck Surg* 1998; **119:** 80.
10. Bradford CR, Zhu S, Poore J *et al.* p53 mutation as a prognostic marker in advanced laryngeal carcinoma. *Arch Otolaryngol Head Neck Surg* 1997; **123:** 605–9.
11. Bradford CR, Zhu S, Wolf GT *et al.* Overexpression of p53 predicts organ preservation using induction chemotherapy and radiation in patients with advanced laryngeal cancer. *Otolaryngol Head Neck Surg* 1995; **113:** 408–12.
12. Browman GP, Goodyear MD, Levine MN, Russell R, Archibald SD, Young JE. Modulation of the antitumor effect of methotrexate by low-dose leucovorin in squamous cell head and neck cancer: a randomized placebo-controlled clinical trial. *J Clin Oncol* 1990; **8:** 203–8.
13. Catimel G, Vermorken JB, Clavel M *et al.* A phase II study of gemcitabine (LY188011) in patients with advanced squamous cell carcinoma of the head and neck. EORTC Early Clinical Trials Group. *Ann Oncol* 1994; **5:** 543–7.
14. Chang EH. p53-mediated, tumor-targeted sensitization of SCCHN to radiotherapy and chemotherapy. *Head Neck* 1998; **20:** 449.
15. Clark JR, Busse PM, Norris CM Jr *et al.* Induction chemotherapy with cisplatin, flurouracil and high dose leucovorin for squamous cell carcinoma of the head and neck: long term results. *J Clin Oncol* 1997; **15:** 3100–10.
16. Clayman GL, El-Naggar AK, Roth JA *et al.* In vivo molecular therapy with p53 adenovirus for microscopic residual head and neck squamous carcinoma. *Cancer Res* 1995; **55:** 1–6.
17. Clayman GL, Weber RS, Guillamondegui O *et al.* Laryngeal preservation for advanced laryngeal and hypopharyngeal cancers. *Arch Otolaryngol Head Neck Surg* 1995; **121:** 219–23.
18. Croll GA, Gerritsen GJ, Tiwari RM, Snow GB. Primary radiotherapy with surgery in reserve for advanced laryngeal carcinoma. Results and complications. *Eur J Surg Oncol* 1989; **15:** 350–6.
19. Davidson J, Keane T, Brown D *et al.* Surgical salvage after radiotherapy for advanced laryngopharyngeal carcinoma. *Arch Otolaryngol Head Neck Surg* 1997; **123:** 420–4.
20. Department of Veterans Affairs Laryngeal Cancer Study Group. Induction chemotherapy plus radiation compared with surgery plus radiation in patients with advanced laryngeal cancer. *N Engl J Med* 1991; **324:** 1685–90.
21. DeSanto LW, Olsen KD, Perry WC, Rohe DE, Keith RL. Quality of life after surgical treatment of cancer of the larynx. *Ann Otol Rhinol Laryngol* 1995; **104:** 763–9.
22. Dimery IW, Hong WK. Overview of combined modality therapies for head and neck cancer. *J Natl Cancer Inst* 1993; **85:** 95–111.
23. Duncan W, MacDougall RH, Kerr GR, Downing D. Adverse effects of treatment gaps in the outcome of radiotherapy for laryngeal cancer. *Radiother Oncol* 1996; **41:** 203–7.
24. Ebihara S, Fujii H, Sasaki Y, Inuyama Y. A late phase II study of docetaxel (Taxotere) in patients with head and neck cancer. *Proc Annu Meet Am Soc Clin Oncol* 1997; **16:** A1425.
25. Egorin MJ, Van Echo DA, Olman EA, Whitacre MY, Forrest A, Aisner J. Prospective validation of a pharmacologically based dosing scheme for the cis-diammedichloro platinum analogue diammino-cyclobutane-dicarboxylato-platinum. *Cancer* 1985; **45:** 6502–6.
26. Eisbruch A, Shewach DS, Bradford CR *et al.* Radiation concurrent with low dose gemcitabine for head and neck cancer: interim results of a Phase I study. *Proc Am Soc Clin Oncol* 1998: 405a.
27. Elomaa L, Joensuu H, Kulmala T, Klemi P, Grenman R. Squamous cell carcinoma is highly sensitive to Taxol, a possible new radiation sensitizer. *Acta Otolaryngol (Stockh)* 1995; **115:** 340–4.
28. Ensley JF, Jacobs JR, Weaver A *et al.* Correlation between response to cisplatinum-combination chemotherapy and subsequent radiotherapy in previously untreated patients with advanced squamous cell cancers of the head and neck. *Cancer* 1984; **54:** 811–14.
29. Ensley JF, Maciorowski Z, Hassan M *et al.* Cellular DNA content parameters in untreated and recurrent squamous cell cancers of the head and neck. *Cytometry* 1989; **10:** 334–8.
30. Forastiere AA. Paclitaxel (Taxol) for the treatment of head and neck cancer. *Semin Oncol* 1994; **21:** 49–52.
31. Forastiere AA, Baker SR, Wheeler R, Medvec BR. Intra-arterial cisplatin and FUDR in advanced malignancies confined to the head and neck. *J Clin Oncol* 1987; **5:** 1601–6.
32. Forastiere AA, Takasugi BJ, Baker SR, Wolf GT, Kudla-Hatch V. High-dose cisplatin in advanced head and neck cancer. *Cancer Chemother Pharmacol* 1987; **19:** 155–8.
33. Forastiere AA, Shank D, Neuberg D, Taylor SG IV, DeConti RC, Adams G. Final report of a phase II evaluation of paclitaxel in patients with advanced squamous cell carcinomas of the head and neck: an Eastern Cooperative Group trial. *Cancer* 1998; **82:** 2270–4.
34. Forastiere AA, Leong T, Murphy B *et al.* A phase III trial of high-dose paclitaxel + cisplatin + G-CSF versus low-dose paclitaxel + cisplatin in patients with advanced

squamous cell carcinoma of the head and neck: an Eastern Cooperative Oncology Group trial. *Proc Annu Meet Am Soc Clin Oncol* 1997; **16:** A1367.

35. Frederick MJ, Holton PR, Hudson M, Wang M, Clayman GL. Expression of apoptosis-related genes in human head and neck squamous cell carcinomas undergoing p53-mediated programmed cell death. *Head Neck* 1998; **20:** 453.
36. Gan Y, Wientjes MG, Schuller DE, Au JL. Pharmacodynamics of Taxol in human head and neck tumors. *Cancer Res* 1996; **56:** 2086–93.
37. Gasparini G, Bevilacqua P, Bonoldi E *et al.* Predictive and prognostic markers in a series of patients with head and neck squamous cell invasive carcinoma treated with concurrent chemo-radiation-therapy. *Clin Cancer Res* 1995; **1:** 1375–83.
38. Gehanno P, Depondt J, Peynegre R *et al.* Neoadjuvant combination of carboplatin and 5-FU in head and neck cancer: a randomized study. *Ann Oncol* 1992; **3:** S43–6.
39. Glick JH, Marcial V, Richter M, Velez Garcia E. The adjuvant treatment of inoperable stage III and IV epidermoid carcinoma of the head and neck with platinum and bleomycin infusions prior to definitive radiotherapy: an RTOG pilot study. *Cancer* 1980; **46:** 1919–24.
40. Goepfert H, Jesse RH, Fletcher GH, Hamberger A. Optimal treatment for the technically resectable squamous cell carcinoma of the supraglottic larynx. *Laryngoscope* 1975; **85:** 14–32.
41. Gregg CM, Beals TE, McClatchy KM, Fisher SG, Wolf GT. DNA content and tumor response to induction chemotherapy in patients with advanced laryngeal squamous cell carcinoma. *Otolaryngol Head Neck Surg* 1993; **108:** 731–7.
42. Harwood AR, Bryce DP, Rider WD. Management of T3 glottic cancer. *Arch Otolaryngol* 1980; **106:** 697–9.
43. Harwood AR, Hawkins NV, Beale FA, Rider WD, Bryce DP. Management of advanced glottic cancer. A 10 year review of the Toronto experience. *Int J Radiat Oncol Biol Phys* 1979; **5:** 899–904.
44. Harwood AR, Beale FA, Cummings BJ *et al.* Supraglottic laryngeal carcinoma: an analysis of dose-time-volume factors in 410 patients. *Int J Radiat Oncol Biol Phys* 1983; **9:** 311–19.
45. Head and Neck Contracts Program. Adjuvant chemotherapy for advanced head and neck squamous carcinoma. Final report. *Cancer* 1987; **60:** 301–11.
46. Hillman RE, Walsh MJ, Wolf GT, Fisher SG, Hong WK. Functional outcomes following treatment for advanced laryngeal cancer. Part I: voice preservation in advanced laryngeal cancer. Part II: laryngectomy rehabilitation: the state of the art in the VA System. *Ann Otol Rhinol Laryngol* 1998; **107:** S1–27.
47. Hong WK, Bromer R, Amato DA *et al.* Patterns of relapse in locally advanced head and neck cancer patients who achieved complete remission after combined modality therapy. *Cancer* 1985; **56:** 1242–5.
48. Hong WK, Schaefer S, Issell B *et al.* A prospective randomized trial of methotrexate versus cisplatin in the treatment of recurrent squamous cell carcinoma of the head and neck. *Cancer* 1983; **52:** 206–10.
49. Huang SM, Harari PM. Anti-EGF receptor monoclonal antibody (C225) inhibits proliferation and enhances radiation sensitivity in human squamous cell carcinoma of the head and neck. *Head Neck* 1998; **20:** 457.
50. Jacobs C, Makuch R. Efficacy of adjuvant chemotherapy for patients with resectable head and neck cancer: a subset analysis of the Head and Neck Contracts Program. *J Clin Oncol* 1990; **8:** 838–47.
51. Jacobs C, Goffinet DR, Goffinet L, Kohler M, Fee WE. Chemotherapy as a substitute for surgery in the treatment advanced resectable head and neck cancer. A report from the Northern California Oncology Group. *Cancer* 1987; **60:** 1178–83.
52. Jacobs C, Lyman G, Velez Garcia E *et al.* A phase III randomized study comparing cisplatin and fluorouracil as single agents and in combination for advanced squamous cell carcinoma of the head and neck. *J Clin Oncol* 1992; **10:** 257–63.
53. Jaulerry C, Rodriguez J, Brunin F *et al.* Induction chemotherapy in advanced head and neck tumors: results of two randomized trials. *Int J Radiat Oncol Biol Phys* 1992; **23:** 483–9.
54. Karp DD, Vaughan CW, Carter R *et al.* Larynx preservation using induction chemotherapy plus radiation as an alternative to laryngectomy in advanced head and neck cancer: a long term follow-up report. *Am J Clin Oncol* 1991; **14:** 273–9.
55. Kearsley JH, Bryson G, Battistutta D, Collins RJ. Prognostic importance of cellular DNA content in head and neck squamous cell cancers. A comparison of retrospective and prospective series. *Int J Cancer* 1991; **47:** 31–7.
56. Kish JA, Weaver A, Jacobs J, Cummings G, Al-Sarraf M. Cisplatin and 5-flurouracil infusion in patients with recurrent and disseminated epidermoid cancer of the head and neck. *Cancer* 1984; **53:** 1819–24.
57. Kokoska MS, Piccirillo JF, el Mofty SK, Emami B, Haughey BH, Schoinick SB. Prognostic significance of clinical factors and p53 expression in patients with glottic carcinoma treated with radiation therapy. *Cancer* 1996; **78:** 1693–700.
58. Kraus DH, Pfister DG, Harrison LB *et al.* Salvage laryngectomy for unsuccessful larynx preservation therapy. *Ann Otol Rhinol Laryngol* 1995; **104:** 936–41.
59. Kropveld A, Slootweg PJ, van Mansfeld ADM, Blankenstein MA, Hordijk GJ. Radioresistance and p53 status of T2 laryngeal carcinoma. Analysis by immunohistochemistry and denaturing gradient gel electrophoresis. *Cancer* 1996; **78:** 991–7.
60. Kun LE, Toohill RJ, Holoye PY *et al.* A randomized study of adjuvant chemotherapy for cancer of the upper aerodigestive tract. *Int J Radiat Oncol Biol Phys* 1986; **12:** 173–8.
61. Laccourreye O, Brasnu D, Bassot V, Ménard M, Khayat D, Laccourreye H. Cisplatin-fluorouracil exclusive chemotherapy for T1–T3N0 glottic squamous cell carcinoma complete clinical responders: five-year results. *J Clin Oncol* 1996; **14:** 2331–6.
62. Lavertu P, Adelstein DJ, Saxton JP *et al.* Management of the neck in a randomized trial comparing concurrent chemotherapy and radiotherapy with radiotherapy alone

in resectable stage II and IV squamous cell head and neck cancer. *Head Neck* 1997; **19:** 559–66.

63. Lavertu P, Bonafede JP, Adelstein DJ *et al.* Comparison of surgical complications after organ-preservation therapy in patients with stage III or IV squamous cell head and neck cancer. *Arch Otolaryngol Head Neck Surg* 1998; **124:** 401–6.
64. Lefebvre JL, Chevalier D, Luboinski B, Kirkpatrick A, Collette L, Sahmoud T. Larynx preservation in pyriform sinus cancer: preliminary results of an EORTC phase III trial. *J Natl Cancer Inst* 1996; **88:** 890–9.
65. Lefebvre JL, Wolf G, Luboinski B *et al.* Meta-analysis of chemotherapy in head and neck cancer: larynx preservation using neoadjuvant chemotherapy in laryngeal and hypopharyngeal carcinoma. *Proc Am Soc Clin Oncol* 1998: 382a.
66. Loré JM Jr, Diaz Ordaz E, Spaulding M *et al.* Improved survival with preoperative chemotherapy followed by resection uncompromised by tumor response for advanced squamous cell carcinoma of the head and neck. *Am J Surg* 1995; **170:** 506–11.
67. Lowe SW, Ruley HE, Jacks T, Housman DE. p53-dependent apoptosis modulates the cytotoxicity of anticancer agents. *Cell* 1993; **74:** 957–67.
68. Mazeron JJ, Martin M, Brun B *et al.* Induction chemotherapy in head and neck cancer: results of a phase III trial. *Head Neck* 1992; **14:** 85–91.
69. Maurizi M, Almadori G, Ferrandina G *et al.* Prognostic significance of epidermal growth factor receptor in laryngeal squamous cell carcinoma. *Br J Cancer* 1996; **74:** 1253–7.
70. McCulloch TM, Van Daele DJ, Hillel A. Blood transfusion as a risk factor for death in stage III and IV operative laryngeal cancer. *Arch Otolaryngol Head Neck Surg* 1995; **121:** 1227–35.
71. Meredith AP, Randall CJ, Shaw HJ. Advanced laryngeal cancer: a management perspective. *J Laryngol Otol* 1987; **101:** 1046–54.
72. Merlano M, Rosso R, Sertoli M *et al.* Randomized comparison of two chemotherapy, radiotherapy schemes for stage III and IV unresectable squamous cell carcinoma of the head and neck. *Laryngoscope* 1990; **100:** 531–5.
73. Moe K, Wolf GT, Fisher SG, Hong WK. Regional metastases in patients with advanced laryngeal cancer. *Arch Otolaryngol Head Neck Surg* 1996; **122:** 644–8.
74. Mortimer JE, Taylor ME, Schulman S, Cummings C, Weymuller E Jr, Laramore G. Feasibility and efficacy of weekly intraarterial cisplatin in locally advanced (stage III and IV) head and neck cancers. *J Clin Oncol* 1988; **6:** 969–75.
75. Munro AJ. An overview of randomized controlled trials of adjuvant chemotherapy in head and neck cancer. *Br J Cancer* 1995; **71:** 83–91.
76. Newman JP, Terris DJ, Pinto HA, Fee WE Jr, Goode RL, Goffinet DR. Surgical morbidity of neck dissection after chemoradiotherapy in advanced head and neck cancer. *Ann Otol Rhinol Laryngol* 1997; **106:** 117–22.
77. O'Malley BW, Lope KA, Chen SH, Li D, Schwarta MR, Woo SL. Combination gene therapy for oral cancer in a murine model. *Cancer Res* 1996; **56:** 1737–41.
78. Osman I, Sherman EJ, Venkatraman E *et al.* p53 gene expression and impact on treatment outcomes in patients with squamous cell carcinoma of the head and neck treated with larynx preservation intent. *Head Neck* 1998; **20:** 469.
79. Paccagnella A, Orlando A, Marchiori C *et al.* Phase III trial of initial chemotherapy in stage III or IV head and neck cancers: a study by the Gruppo di Studio sui Tumori della Testa e del Collo. *J Natl Cancer Inst* 1994; **86:** 265–72.
80. Peters LJ, Withers HR. Applying radiobiological principles to combined modality treatment of head and neck cancer: the time factor. *Int J Radiat Oncol Biol Phys* 1997; **39:** 831–6.
81. Pfister DG, Strong E, Harrison L *et al.* Larynx preservation with combined chemotherapy and radiation in advanced but resectable head and neck cancer. *J Clin Oncol* 1991; **9:** 850–9.
82. Posner M, Noris C, Colevas A *et al.* Phase I/II trial of docetaxel, cisplatin, 5-flurouracil and leucovorin for curable, locally advanced squamous cell cancer of the head and neck. *Proc Am Soc Clin Oncol* 1997; **16:** 387a.
83. Reed JC. Bcl-2 and the regulation of programmed cell death. *J Cell Biol* 1994; **124:** 1–6.
84. Robbins KT, Fontanesi J, Wong FS *et al.* A novel organ preservation protocol for advanced carcinoma of the larynx and pharynx. *Arch Otolaryngol Head Neck Surg* 1996; **122:** 853–7.
85. Robbins KT, Kumar P, Regine WF *et al.* Efficacy of targeted supradose cisplatin and concomitant radiation therapy for advanced head and neck cancer: the Memphis experience. *Int J Radiat Oncol Biol Phys* 1997; **38:** 263–71.
86. Sako K, Razack MS, Kalnins I. Chemotherapy for advanced and recurrent squamous cell carcinoma of the head and neck with high and low dose cis-diaminedichloroplatinum. *Am J Surg* 1978; **136:** 529–33.
87. Sassler AM, Esclamado RM, Wolf GT. Surgery after organ preservation therapy. Analysis of wound complications. *Arch Otolaryngol Head Neck Surg* 1995; **121:** 162–5.
88. Schuller DE, Metch B, Stein DW, Mattox D, McCraken JD. Preoperative chemotherapy in advanced resectable head and neck cancer: final report of the Southwest Oncology Group. *Laryngoscope* 1988; **98:** 1205–11.
89. Shanta V, Krishnamurthi S. Combined bleomycin and radiotherapy in oral cancer. *Clin Radiol* 1980; **31:** 617–20.
90. Shewach DS, Lawrence TS. Gemcitabine and radiosensitization in human tumor cells. *Invest New Drugs* 1996; **14:** 257–63.
91. Shewach DS, Hahn TM, Chang E, Hertel LW, Lawrence TS. Metabolism of 2',2'-difluoro-2'-deoxycytidine and radiation sensitization of human colon carcinoma cells. *Cancer Res* 1994; **54:** 3218–23.
92. Spafford MF, Koeppe J, Pan Z, Archer PG, Meyers AD, Franklin WA. Correlation of tumor markers p53, *bcl-2*, CD34, CD44H, CD44v6 and Ki-67 with survival and metastasis in laryngeal squamous cell carcinoma. *Arch Otolaryngol Head Neck Surg* 1996; **122:** 627–32.
93. Spaulding MB, Fisher SG, Wolf GT. Tumor response, toxicity and survival after neo-adjuvant organ preserving chemotherapy for advanced laryngeal carcinoma. *J Clin Oncol* 1994; **12:** 1592–9.

94. Stell PM. Adjuvant chemotherapy for head and neck cancer. *Semin Radiat Oncol* 1992; **2:** 195–205.
95. Stell PM, Rawson NS. Adjuvant chemotherapy in head and neck cancer. *Br J Cancer* 1990; **61:** 779–87.
96. Tannock IF, Bromer GP. Lack of evidence for a role of chemotherapy in the routine management of locally advanced head and neck cancer. *J Clin Oncol* 1986; **4:** 1121–6.
97. Tarpley JL, Chretien PB, Alexander JC Jr, Hoye RC, Block JB, Ketcham AS. High dose methotrexate as a preoperative adjuvant in the treatment of epidermoid carcinoma of the head and neck. A feasibility study and clinical trial. *Am J Surg* 1975; **130:** 481–6.
98. Terrell JE, Fisher SG, Wolf GT. Long-term quality of life after treatment for laryngeal cancer. *Arch Otolaryngol Head Neck Surg* 1998; **124:** 964–71.
99. Thomas GR, Greenberg J, Wu KT *et al.* Planned early neck dissection before radiation for persistent neck nodes after induction chemotherapy. *Laryngoscope* 1997; **107:** 1129–37.
100. Tishler RB, Busse PM, Norris CM *et al.* Concomitant paclitaxel and once daily radiotherapy in the treatment of head and neck cancer. *Proc Am Soc Clin Oncol* 1997; **16:** 386.
101. Tomasino RM, Daniele E, Bazan V *et al.* Prognostic significance of cell kinetics in laryngeal squamous cell carcinoma: clinicopathological associations. *Cancer Res* 1995; **55:** 6103–8.
102. Toohill RJ, Duncavage JA, Grossmam TW *et al.* The effects of delay in standard treatment due to induction chemotherapy in two randomized prospective studies. *Laryngoscope* 1987; **97:** 407–12.
103. Truelson JM, Fisher SG, Beals TF, McClatchey KD, Wolf GT. DNA content and histologic growth pattern correlate with prognosis in patients with advanced squamous cell carcinoma of the larynx. *Cancer* 1992; **70:** 56–62.
104. Urba S, Forastiere AA, Wolf GT, Esclamado RM, McLaughlin PW, Thornton AF. Intensive induction chemotherapy and radiation for organ preservation in patients with advanced resectable head and neck carcinoma. *J Clin Oncol* 1994; **12:** 946.
105. Urba S, Wolf GT, Eisbruch A *et al.* Chemoradiation for larynx preservation in patients with advanced, resectable laryngeal carcinoma. *Head Neck* 1998; **20:** 481.
106. Verweij J, Catimel G, Sulkes A *et al.* Phase II studies of docetaxel in the treatment of various solid tumours. EORTC Early Clinical Trials Group and the EORTC Soft Tissue and Bone Sarcoma Group. *Eur J Cancer* 1995; **31:** S21–4.
107. Vogt HG, Martin T, Kolotas C, Schneider L, Strassmann G, Zamboglou N. Simultaneous paclitaxel and radiotherapy: initial clinical experience in lung cancer and other malignancies. *Semin Oncol* 1997; **24:** S101–5.
108. Von Hoff DD. Whither carboplatin? A replacement for or an alternative to cisplatin? *J Clin Oncol* 1987; **5:** 169–71.
109. Von Hoff DD. The taxoids: same roots, different drugs. *Semin Oncol* 1997; **24:** S3–10.
110. Welkoborsky HJ, Hinni M, Dienes HP, Mann WJ. Predicting recurrence and survival in patients with laryngeal cancer by means of DNA cytometry, tumor front grading, and proliferation markers. *Ann Otol Rhinol Laryngol* 1995; **104:** 503–10.
111. Withers HR, Maciejewski B, Taylor JM, Hliniak A. Accelerated repopulation in head and neck cancer. *Front Radiat Ther Oncol* 1988; **22:** 105–10.
112. Wolf GT, Carey TE. Tumor antigen phenotype, biologic staging, and prognosis in head and neck squamous carcinoma. *J Natl Cancer Inst Monogr* 1992; **13:** 67–74.
113. Wolf GT, Fisher SG. Effectiveness of salvage neck dissection for advanced regional metastases when induction chemotherapy and radiation are used for organ preservation. *Laryngoscope* 1992; **102:** 934–9.
114. Wolf GT, Hong WK, Fisher SG. Neoadjuvant chemotherapy for organ preservation: current status. In: Shah JP, Johnson JT, eds. *Proceedings of the Fourth International Head and Neck Oncology Conference (Toronto Meeting).* Madison: Omnipress, 1996: 89–97.
115. Wolf GT, Urba S, Hazuka M. Induction chemotherapy for organ preservation in advanced squamous cell carcinoma of the oral cavity and oropharynx. *Recent Results Cancer Res* 1994; **134:** 133–43.
116. Wolf GT, Fisher SG, Truelson JM, Beals TF. DNA content and regional metastases in patients with advanced laryngeal squamous carcinoma. *Laryngoscope* 1994; **104:** 479–83.
117. Yoo GH, Ensley J, Jacobs J *et al.* Intratumoral E1A gene therapy for patients with unresectable and recurrent head and neck cancer. *Proc Am Assoc Cancer Res* 1998; **39:** 322.
118. Zhu S, Trask DK, Wolf GT, Carey TE, Wicha M, Bradford CR. Bcl-x_S transfer increases the chemosensitivity of laryngeal carcinoma cells *in vitro. Head Neck* 1998; **20:** 485.

Management of recurrent laryngeal cancer

Amy Y Chen and Helmuth Goepfert

In 1997, it was estimated that cancer of the larynx would strike approximately 1900 people in the USA, most of whom would be men.[2] The larynx is the most common site of cancer in the upper aerodigestive tract. More than 90% of laryngeal cancers are squamous cell carcinomas. In this chapter we discuss the general principles of primary treatment for cancer of the glottic and supraglottic larynx, as practiced at the University of Texas MD Anderson Cancer Center, and we outline the diagnostic steps and treatment alternatives for laryngeal cancer recurrence after definitive therapy. Our recent experience, as well as a literature survey of the management of recurrent laryngeal cancer, are discussed.

Glottic larynx

The glottis encompasses the true vocal cords, including the anterior and posterior commissures. Tumors of the glottis initially remain confined to the site of origin primarily because of four anatomic barriers: the vocal ligament, the anterior commissure ligament, the thyroglottic ligament, and the conus elasticus.

Initially, tumors are confined to Reinke's space. The vocal ligament is an effective barrier that forces cancer cells to spread along the mucosal surface rather than to deeply invade. At the anterior commissure, Broyles' ligament prevents cancer spread as well, although, when breakthrough occurs at this region, there is usually invasion into the thyroid cartilage. The thyroglottic ligament superiorly and the conus elasticus inferiorly are dense connective tissue barriers that delay cancer invasion. Glottic cancers rarely produce lymph node metastasis before presentation (in less than 4% of patients). If glottic cancer metastasizes, it will do so to levels II and III and, in the case of subglottic extension, into the parathyroidal and paratracheal lymph nodes.

Because cancer affects the function of the vocal cords, tumors in this area show symptoms (hoarseness) earlier than cancers in the supraglottic larynx. The mobility of the vocal cords and arytenoid cartilage is important information that should be obtained before the initiation of treatment and in the follow-up examination of patients treated with conservation therapy, especially radiation therapy. Vocal cord mobility is an important variable to observe in the follow-up of patients treated by radiation therapy because progressive fixation may indicate submucosal tumor relapse.

Supraglottic larynx

The supraglottic larynx comprises of several adjoining areas – the suprahyoid epiglottis (lingual and laryngeal surfaces), infrahyoid epiglottis, arytenoepiglottic folds, arytenoid cartilage, and ventricular bands or false cords. Conventionally, the inferior border of the supraglottis is drawn about a horizontal plane through the apex of the laryngeal ventricle and along the upper surface of the vocal fold. An argument arises in a situation where the ventricle bulges up lateral to the false cord.

Most cancers in the supraglottic larynx arise on the epiglottis and specifically in the infrahyoid portion. The pattern of the spread of supraglottic laryngeal carcinoma depends on where the cancer arises and the contiguous sites that are involved in tumor progression. The anatomy of the epiglottic cartilage allows tumors in the inferior portion of the epiglottis and ventricular bands to penetrate the pre-epiglottic space. The lymphatic spread of supraglottic laryngeal cancer often occurs early and moves bilaterally because the submucosa is permeated by a rich plexus of interconnecting lymphatic vessels with efferent channels to both sides. The efferent lymphatics drain into lymph nodes located about the carotid bifurcation and the mid-jugular and low jugular lymph nodes (levels II, III and IV).

Patients with supraglottic laryngeal cancer tend to present later in the course of the disease with dysphagia, hoarseness and frequently with a neck mass. The incidence of lymph node metastasis of this cancer varies significantly depending on the subsite involved and is highest for lesions arising or invading the aryepiglottic folds and the mucosa of the arytenoid cartilage.

Cancer originating in the suprahyoid epiglottis usually appears as an exophytic growth and is seldom infiltrating or ulcerative. By contrast, cancer about the infrahyoid epiglottis tends to be invasive, reaching easily into the pre-epiglottic space and progressing into the false cord and even into the upper paraglottic space as it extends in a caudal direction. It is important to determine the extent of invasion in the pre-epiglottic space. The vallecula can be involved either by superficial extension of the cancer from the epiglottic rim or by deep penetration through the pre-epiglottic space. Cancer arising on the false cords or in the laryngeal ventricle has easy access into the paraglottic and pre-epiglottic spaces and through the submucosal tissue planes into the pyriform sinus. Cancer arising in the aryepiglottic folds can extend laterally into the pyriform sinus, where it may be difficult to differentiate from a primary tumor.

Transglottic cancers bridge the laryngeal ventricle and invade the mucosa of the glottic and supraglottic regions.

Table 53.1 Local control rates (%) of treatment modalities (radiation, surgery) on glottic laryngeal primaries

	Radiation	*Surgery*
T1	93–100*	98†
T2	81–85*	84†
T3	62††	79†
T4	38††	38†

*Mendenhall *et al.*[21]
†Johnson *et al.*[16]
††Mendenhall *et al.*[23]

Table 53.2 Local control rates (%) of treatment modalities (radiation, surgery) on supraglottic laryngeal primaries

	Radiation	*Surgery ± radiation*
T1	100*	100†
T2	81*	80†
T3	61*	94†
T4	33*	83†

*Mendenhall *et al.*[22]
†Weems *et al.*[43]

Primary treatment

Two main options are available for treatment of early glottic and supraglottic cancer: surgery and radiation therapy.[38] The goals of treatment of laryngeal cancer are eradication of the disease in a prompt and cost-efficient manner; preservation of organ function and, if lost, optimal voice rehabilitation; and prevention of second primary tumors that occur frequently in patients with squamous carcinoma of the larynx. The preferred treatment of laryngeal cancer varies greatly depending on the training and experience of the individual practitioner or treatment team. Tables 53.1 and 53.2, respectively, summarize the results of various types of therapy for glottic and supraglottic cancers. Most reports of large series give comparable results for these various respective treatment modalities.[17,24] The surgical excision of early laryngeal cancer includes endoscopic procedures (laser and non-laser), thyrotomy with cordectomy,[27] vertical hemilaryngectomy,[26] horizontal laryngectomy, supracricoid laryngectomy,[19] and near-total laryngectomy. The details of radiation therapy vary by site and stage of cancer and are beyond the scope of this chapter. Chemotherapy is being used with increasing frequency either as a neoadjuvant or as a concomitant treatment with radiation therapy with the goal of organ preservation.

The incidence of complications resulting from radiation therapy should be below 2%.[21] The principal sequelae of radiation therapy are fibrosis to the dermis, submucosa, and soft tissues of the neck, laryngeal edema, and possibly perichondritis and cartilage necrosis. When cancer invasion has destroyed laryngeal structure, the treatment may often result in an organ with poor function. This has been especially noticeable after some chemotherapy induction or chemotherapy/radiation therapy combination protocols. Complications resulting from radiation with or without chemotherapy and delayed sequelae from treatment are often underreported. A recurrent or persistent tumor after radiation therapy may be difficult to diagnose because of the presence of sequelae from treatment, such as a persistent edema. The main sequelae of conservation surgery of the larynx are aspiration, hoarseness and stridor that can be the result of normal wound healing after the surgical procedure. Except for laser excision of early glottic cancer confined to the membranous middle third of the vocal cord, we at UT MD Anderson Cancer Center do not practice conservation surgery for early staged untreated glottic cancer.

For supraglottic laryngeal cancer it has been our practice to treat most stage T1, T2 and selected T3 cancers by radiation therapy. More advanced lesions are treated on clinical protocols of radiotherapy with and without chemotherapy or by conservation surgery followed by radiation therapy if this is indicated.

Diagnosis of tumor recurrence

Patients who have had treatment for laryngeal cancer often ignore the new symptoms of disease for too long and present with massive tumor recurrence and respiratory distress that requires demanding urgent attention for respiratory distress.

Certain information must be available and certain diagnostic procedures are required before salvage therapy can be started for recurrent laryngeal cancer. The site and TNM stage of the initial lesion, must be noted as well as the details of the treatment given, including the size of field, dose and timing for radiotherapy. This information should be reviewed in all cases before any surgery is performed. If the patient was treated initially by conservation surgery, the operative details should be reviewed. Time elapsed since treatment for the initial cancer is important. Generally, a rapid recurrence after adequate therapy denotes a more aggressive tumor. A possible second primary cancer may be suspected when, after the initial cancer treatment for a specific location in the larynx, the patient is reevaluated and found to have a tumor in a new location within the larynx. Under these circumstances, it is important to determine whether this is a recurrent or new primary cancer.

Keep in mind that prior cancer treatment will alter the lymphatic pathways, so the search for lymph node metastasis must be extended beyond the classical sentinel lymph node groups. Comorbid factors, including pulmonary reserve and cardiovascular status, should be assessed, especially in cases where conservation salvage surgery is a possibility.

The methods for diagnosis have improved considerably in the last few years, especially the availability of videoscopic recording with or without stroboscopy. Imaging studies [computed tomography (CT), magnetic resonance imaging (MRI) and positron emission tomography (PET)] must be used judiciously.[5] The prior treatment may have produced significant tissue alteration that will make interpretation of diagnostic imaging difficult. An experienced radiologist can be a significant asset under these circumstances. If a biopsy is needed, it should be done after adequate inspection of the organ and before any imaging studies are done.

If a patient has been treated for laryngeal cancer and develops new symptoms, or if old symptoms recur, then regrowth of the tumor should be suspected until proved otherwise. The signs and symptoms of persistent or recurrent tumor include the reappearance of hoarseness, stridor, pain, dysphagia, laryngeal edema, airway obstruction, fixation of the larynx and aspiration.

Laryngeal edema

Laryngeal edema after radiation therapy is a result of increased vascular permeability, lymphatic obstruction, infection, and sometimes, perichondritis, especially if ulcerations are present. Laryngeal edema is unusual after radiation therapy to treat glottic cancer, but it is common after radiation therapy for supraglottic cancer, especially if the arytenoid cartilage is included in the field of treatment. Factors contributing to persistent edema include continued smoking, excessive use of alcohol, and gastroesophageal reflux disease. In the absence of any irritants, the edema from radiation therapy should subside within 4–6 months with conservative management. All patients treated with radiotherapy should avoid voice abuse, alcohol consumption and smoking. The treatment of gastroesophageal reflux disease is imperative.

Persistent laryngeal edema, especially if progressive, can indicate recurrent disease. The incidence of laryngeal edema lasting longer than 3 months after treatment is about 15%.[12] In the report by Fu *et al.*,[12] laryngeal edema was associated with persistent or recurrent cancer in 45% of patients. However, only one-quarter of the patients with uncontrolled cancer have laryngeal edema. O'Brien[31] reported that 50% of patients with edema, or necrosis of the larynx, or both, have recurrent cancer. Others in general recommend that laryngeal biopsy be performed to document recurrent disease if the edema is progressive and unresponsive to conservative management.[3,11,12,21,31,42] Nevertheless, if edema is mild and stable and no signs of recurrence are visible, then a biopsy should be deferred because it may induce necrosis. Most authors warn that any biopsy of an irradiated larynx should be done judiciously because trauma may aggravate edema and precipitate necrosis, chondritis and even laryngeal obstruction.

Perichondritis and chondritis

The prevalence of perichondritis and chondritis after radiotherapy has been reported to be about 15%.[25] The criteria for diagnosis of perichondritis have been defined as:

- progressive laryngeal edema requiring intensive medical therapy (with antibiotics and corticosteroids) or a tracheostomy to provide an adequate airway;
- persistent pain, dysphagia, and laryngeal tenderness;
- ulceration of the larynx and exposed laryngeal cartilage; and
- development of a laryngocutaneous fistula.[25]

Mintz *et al.*[25] report a 50% incidence of residual or recurrent carcinomas in patients with clinical signs of perichondritis and osteoradionecrosis about the larynx. Based on the authors' experience, an aggressive approach is recommended when chondritis is present, with close follow-up and, if necessary, frequent biopsies.

The factors predisposing to the development of perichondritis are:

- high total dose of radiation therapy given: with a dose below 64 Gy, the incidence of perichondritis is below 14%, and with a dose above 65 Gy the incidence is 30%;
- the type of radiation therapy and the technique used;
- uncontrolled infection;
- mechanical injury during biopsy or surgery; and

- impaired tissue resistance due to an intercurrent disease such as diabetes.

Patients who continue to smoke increase their chances of developing necrosis and perichondritis.[18,20] If the perichondrium remains intact and has not been penetrated by cancer, higher doses of radiation therapy can be tolerated. Age, sex, partial laryngeal surgery, prior tracheostomy, and the histologic grade of the tumor do not appear to be important factors in the development of significant histologic chondronecrosis or osteomyelitis.[11]

Keene *et al.*,[18] in 1982, studied whole-organ histologic sections of 265 specimens to determine the incidence and location of what they called osteomyelitis and chondronecrosis in laryngeal carcinoma. Chondronecrosis was present in 1 of 41 T1 and T2 lesions and in 39 of 143 more advanced tumors. The arytenoid cartilage was the most frequent site of chondronecrosis. Early effects of radiation therapy on capillary endothelium and lymphatics were obliteration, atrophy and fibrosis. The subintimal fibrosis and hyalinization appeared to be more marked in veins than in arteries, and this was an important factor in the development of postirradiation edema. When chondronecrosis develops, it is clinically difficult to distinguish between tumor invasion and the results of radiation therapy on the basis of simple clinical examination and imaging studies. In the Keene *et al.*[18] study of 265 specimens, 248 revealed residual carcinoma at the primary site.

Use of imaging to diagnose tumor

Imaging studies assist the clinician in determining recurrence and should be obtained before biopsy. Computed tomography (CT) is useful to evaluate carcinoma at presentation, and is probably as effective as magnetic resonance imaging (MRI). However, after previous radiation therapy, CT is less accurate in detecting recurrence. MRI, especially with gadolinium enhancement, offers some additional accuracy.[5] Positron emission tomography (PET) with fluorodeoxyglucose is a promising technique. Greven *et al.*[13] suggested that PET scanning was useful to distinguish cancer from benign changes following treatment of laryngeal cancer. Although the study sample was small (n = 11), the five patients with positive isotope uptake in the larynx had cancer in the subsequent laryngectomy specimen. Although PET is advantageous because it is noninvasive, it does have drawbacks. False-positive results can occur, such as with an increased pooling of saliva in the vallecula and the lack of resolution of PET scanning is notorious in lesions of <1 cm in diameter.

Use of biopsy to diagnose tumor recurrence

There is little argument that recurrent cancer must be documented by biopsy. However, the timing of such intervention after prior treatment is important. We recommend that, after completion of radiation therapy, the clinician refrains from biopsy if there is no clear clinical evidence of persistent cancer. During the first 3 months after completion of irradiation, biopsies may cause significant necrosis and complicate the patient's recovery. Evidence of residual tumor in the larynx should be absent within 120 days from the completion of radiotherapy.

Viani *et al.*[40] state that the sensitivity and specificity of preoperative histologic diagnosis are 97% and 25%, respectively. Crellin *et al.*[6] established a surgeon's subjective ability to determine recurrence with the sensitivity at 98% and the specificity at 46%. These studies suggest that the experience of a clinician is important to detect recurrence. The value of experience in evaluating patients after radiation therapy should not be underestimated. The more time that elapses after treatment, the more significant are laryngeal findings in making the diagnosis of recurrence. This is especially if the abnormalities are progressive and no other factors explain an abnormal appearing organ.

Management of tumor recurrence

It is accepted that 10–20% of early carcinomas and 50–60% of advanced laryngeal cancer recur after radiation therapy.[44] After the diagnosis of recurrent cancer has been established, there are several treatment options. In general, if treatment with radiotherapy fails, surgery is the only remaining option, although repeat irradiation is sometimes possible. If the recurrent lesion is small, the cancer may be removed by endoscopic means, especially with the use of a carbon dioxide laser. There is little documentation in the literature about the use of this technique to treat recurrent laryngeal cancer or cancer appearing in the irradiated larynx. We have had success using endoscopy with a carbon dioxide laser in ten patients (up to 1997). Some cases may require serial endoscopic excisions performed over several months until the organ is free of recurrent disease.

Partial laryngectomy is possible in about 20–25% of patients with recurrent glottic cancer.[7,28–30,35,37,39] It is safe to assume that total laryngectomy is most often the only option for recurrent laryngeal cancer after prior conservation treatment. The indications for laryngectomy include a positive biopsy, or a high clinical suspicion of recurrence in an organ whose function is severely impaired, and significant symptoms and signs of chondronecrosis. The results of salvage surgery are usually more favorable for recurrent glottic than supraglottic cancer. A partial laryngectomy is seldom possible after radiotherapy for recurrent supraglottic cancer.

Although total laryngectomy is most often performed, partial laryngectomy is feasible for selected patients whose cancer recurred after radiation therapy. Vertical hemilaryngectomy can be performed when one cord is involved and minimal crossover at the anterior commissure has occurred. Vertical partial laryngectomy after radiation therapy is not an option when:

Table 53.3 Literature review of efficacy of salvage surgery

Authors	*Stage/site*	*XRT failures (%)*	*Salvage surgery*	*Ultimate control of disease (%)*
Harwood *et al.*[14]	T3 GL	76/144 (53)	PL & TL	55
Fisher *et al.*[10]	T1–2 GL	24/212 (11)	TL	76 T1, 96 T2
Croll *et al.*[8]	T3–4 GL, SGL	19/55 (35)	TL/PL	20/55 (36)
Howell-Burke *et al.*[15]	T2 GL	37/114 (32)	Majority TL	92
Alcock *et al.*[1]	T1–4 larynx, HP	320/734 (43)	151 TL (47%)	Not specified
Schwaab *et al.*[34]	T1–2 GL	50/259 (19)	TL/PL	82
Parsons *et al.*[32]	T1–4 SGL	46/206 (22)	PL & TL	29 (of those who developed failure)
Kanonier *et al.*[17]	T1 GL	3/46 (6)	PL	100
		27/33 (81)	PL & TL	82
Davidson *et al.*[9]	T3–4 larynx, HP, OP	191/336 (56)	Majority TL	22% (for surgical patients)

GL, glottic; HP, hypopharynx; OP, oropharynx; SGL, supraglottic; PL, partial laryngectomy; TL, total laryngectomy.

- the true vocal cords are immobile or fixed;
- the arytenoid cartilage and its mucosa are directly involved by tumor;
- tumor involves more than the anterior one-third of the opposite vocal cord;
- there is evidence of perichondritis or significant transglottic spread of the disease.

Laccourreye *et al.*[19] have suggested that supracricoid laryngectomy with cricohyoidopexy is a possible salvage procedure for postradiation recurrence of both glottic and supraglottic cancers, especially if both cords are involved and at least one arytenoid cartilage is free of cancer. We have done this procedure for recurrent glottic cancer with increasing frequency during the last year; the results are encouraging with good functional outcome, albeit a breathy voice. One of five patients has experienced local relapse and was deemed inoperable after salvage supracricoid laryngectomy and cricohyoidopexy failure.

In Table 53.3 we have tabulated the results of salvage surgery for disease recurrence after radiation therapy. Data derived from a review of the literature are difficult to compare because of the wide range in variables, methods and results reported. Whereas some investigators specifically refer to glottic cancer, others may group data on recurrences for glottic, supraglottic and even hypopharyngeal primary cancers. In addition, how the outcome of surgical salvage is reported varies. The references reviewed in Table 53.4 were selected according to the availability of results for the number of recurrences after radiation therapy, the method of salvage surgery, and the final cancer control rates.

At The University of Texas MD Anderson Cancer Center, 72 salvage laryngectomies were performed between 1985–95 to treat the recurrence of laryngeal cancer after radiation. Sixty-seven (90%) of these procedures were for initially staged T1 and T2 lesions. The median time between the first treatment and recurrence was 13 months (range 3–130 months). Forty-four (61%) patients underwent a total laryngectomy, seventeen (24%) underwent hemilaryngectomy, and six (9%) underwent laser vaporization of recurrent cancer. At last contact, 41 (57%) patients were living and had no evidence of recurrent disease.

Table 53.4 Complications of salvage surgery

Authors	*Fistula rate*	*Overall complication rate*
Harwood *et al.*[14]	Not reported	Not reported
Fisher *et al.*[10]	3/22 (14%)	Not reported
Croll *et al.*[8]	6/16 (38%)	9/16 (56%)
Howell-Burke *et al.*[15]	None reported	5/37 (14%)
Alcock *et al.*[1]	Not reported	Not reported
Schwaab *et al.*[34]	Not reported	41% local wound problems
Parsons *et al.*[32]	20%	37%
Kanonier *et al.*[17]	Not reported	Not reported
Davidson *et al.*[9]	13/108 (12%)	29%

The complication rates of salvage surgery are reported to be as high as 40% as shown in Table 53.4. Complications include serious wound infection, pharyngocutaneous fistula, need for permanent tracheostomy or persistent aspiration after partial laryngectomy, and significant bleeding caused by the necrosis of a major vessel.

Management of cervical lymph node metastasis

The management of cervical lymph node metastasis in recurrent laryngeal cancer deserves special attention. If no lymph node metastases are clinically apparent and no suspicious nodes are found on the imaging studies, a neck dissection may not be necessary, especially if no lymph node metastasis was present at the time of the original treatment. Yuen *et al.*[44] showed that node-positive patients have a significantly higher recurrence rate from distant metastasis than node-negative patients, despite adequate locoregional tumor control. Elective therapy to cervical lymphatics is important in supraglottic larynx cancer, but it is less important in primary glottic cancers. If salvage surgery for recurrence at the primary site is needed, we recommend that neck dissection be done at levels II, III and IV and the paratracheal nodes. Radical neck dissection can be avoided, provided lymph node metastases were not clinically present at the time of the initial therapy or at the time of relapse. If surgery is done for recurrent supraglottic larynx cancer, we dissect at least levels II, III and IV and the paratracheal nodes on both sides. For glottic cancer in cases of total laryngectomy, we recommend dissections of levels II, III and IV, the paratracheal nodes and the thyroid lobe on the side of the lesion. In case of significant subglottic extension of the disease, a generous cuff of trachea (two to four rings beyond the tumor) should be included. The presence of any palpable nodes will dictate the extent of neck dissection. The skin incisions should be planned carefully to obtain adequate exposure of the operative site and prevent the exposure of major blood vessels in the event of postoperative wound breakdown. When patients are operated upon for recurrent carcinoma following radiation therapy for glottic cancer, the presence of significant subglottic extension of the disease and lymph node metastases, especially of multiple lymph nodes or extracapsular spread, may require the use of postoperative radiation therapy. It is important to have information on the fields of radiotherapy used to treat the initial cancer to avoid excessive irradiation over the previous field and to decrease the risk of tissue necrosis. To control wound breakdown, we have performed a 'controlled' pharyngocutaneous fistula at the time of wound closure following total laryngectomy. This fistula can be closed 3–5 weeks later under local anesthesia. Local and regional muscle flaps can be used over the pharyngeal mucosal suture line as a technique to prevent fistula formation.

Other management modalities

There are isolated reports on the use of hyperfractionation,[4,36] interstitial radiation,[33] and re-irradiation,[41] for the management of recurrent laryngeal cancer after prior radiation therapy. Unfortunately, there is little information about the results of these treatments, specifically their effects on the larynx.

Conclusions

Most early glottic cancers (T1, T2) respond well to conservation treatment, and in our experience the preferred treatment is radiation therapy. For supraglottic laryngeal cancer, radiation therapy is a good option for most T1 and T2 and some T3 stage primary lesions. The complications and sequelae include damage to skin, edema of the larynx, perichondritis and cartilage tissue necrosis. It is often difficult to differentiate cancer recurrence from perichondritis and cartilage or bone necrosis. In general, if edema persists longer than 6 months and is resistant to appropriate conservative treatment a laryngoscopy and biopsy should be done, especially if the symptoms are progressive. If clinical suspicion for recurrence is high or if the larynx is nonfunctional, surgery is indicated. In patients with recurrence after radiation therapy, salvage surgery is more effective for glottic than for supraglottic cancer and more effective in node-negative than node-positive patients. Other modalities of treatment for recurrence include hyperfractionation and conventional re-irradiation. Prospective studies are needed to delineate further the role of salvage surgery for glottic and supraglottic cancers and the effect of such salvage surgery on survival based on initial staging of the primary cancer. Chemotherapy is of limited benefit in treating the recurrence of laryngeal cancer at the primary site.

References

1. Alcock CJ, Fowler JF, Haybittle JL, Hopewell JW, Rezvani M, Wiernik G. Salvage surgery following irradiation with different fractionation regimes in the treatment of carcinoma of the laryngo-pharynx: experience gained from a British Institute of Radiology study. *J Laryngol Otol* 1992; **106**: 147–53.
2. American Cancer Society. *Cancer J for Clinicians* 1997; **47**: 5–12.
3. Bahadur S, Amayta RC, Kacker SK. The enigma of post-radiation edema and residual or recurrent carcinoma of the larynx and pyriform fossa. *J Laryngol Otol* 1985; **99**: 763–5.
4. Benchalal M, Bachaud JM, François P *et al.* Hyperfractionation in the reirradiation of head and neck cancers. Result of a pilot study. *Radiother Oncol* 1995; **36**: 203–10.
5. Castelijns JA, van den Brekel MWM, Smit EMT *et al.* Predictive value of MR imaging-dependent and non-MR imaging-dependent parameters for recurrence of laryngeal cancer after radiation therapy. *Radiology* 1995; **196**: 735–9.
6. Crellin RP, Gaze MN, White A, Maran AGD, MacDougall RH. Salvage laryngectomy after radical radiotherapy for laryngeal carcinoma. *Clin Otolaryngol* 1992; **17**: 449–51.
7. Croll GA, Broek PVD, Tiwari RM, Manni JJ, Snow GB. Vertical partial laryngectomy for recurrent glottic carcinoma after irradiation. *Head Neck Surg* 1985; **7**: 390–3.
8. Croll GA, Gerritsen GJ, Rammohan M, Snow T, Snow GB. Primary radiotherapy with surgery in reserve for advanced laryngeal carcinoma. *Eur J Surg Oncol* 1989; **15**: 350–6.
9. Davidson J, Keane T, Brown D *et al.* Surgical salvage after radiotherapy for advanced laryngopharyngeal carcinoma. *Arch Otolaryngol Head Neck Surg* 1997; **123**: 420–4.
10. Fisher AJ, Caldarelli DD, Chacko DC, Holinger LD. Glottic cancer. *Arch Otolaryngol Head Neck Surg* 1986; **112**: 519–21.
11. Flood LM, Brightwell AP. Clinical assessment of the irradiated larynx. *J Laryngol Otol* 1984; **98**: 493–8.
12. Fu KK, Woodhouse RJ, Quivey JM, Phillips TL, Dedo HH. The significance of laryngeal edema following radiotherapy of carcinoma of the vocal cord. *Cancer* 1982; **49**: 655–8.

13. Greven KM, Williams DW III, Keyes JW Jr *et al.* Distinguishing tumor recurrence from irradiation sequelae with positron emission tomography in patients treated for larynx cancer. *Int J Radiat Oncol Biol Phys* 1994; **29:** 841–5.
14. Harwood AR, Bryce DP, Rider WD. Management of T3 glottic cancer. *Arch Otolaryngol* 1980; **106:** 697–9.
15. Howell-Burke D, Peters LJ, Goepfert H, Oswald MJ. T2 glottic cancer: recurrence, salvage and survival after definitive radiotherapy. *Arch Otolaryngol Head Neck Surg* 1990; **116:** 830–5.
16. Johnson JT, Myers EN, Hao SP, Wagner RL. Outcome of open surgical therapy for glottic carcinoma. *Ann Otol Rhinol Laryngol* 1993; **102:** 752–5.
17. Kanonier G, Rainer T, Fritsch E, Thumfart WF. Radiotherapy in early glottic carcinoma. *Ann Otol Rhinol Laryngol* 1996; **105:** 759–63.
18. Keene M, Harwood AR, Bryce DP, Van Nostrand AWP. Histopathological study of radionecrosis in laryngeal carcinoma. *Laryngoscope* 1982; **92:** 173–80.
19. Laccourreye O, Weinstein G, Naudo P, Cauchois R, Laccourreye H, Brasnu D. Supracricoid partial laryngectomy after failed laryngeal radiation therapy. *Laryngoscope* 1996; **106:** 495–8.
20. McGovern FH, Fitz-Hugh JS, Constable W. Post-radiation perichondritis and cartilage necrosis of the larynx. *Laryngoscope* 1973; **83:** 808–15.
21. Mendenhall WM, Parsons JT, Million RR, Fletcher GH. T1–T2 squamous cell carcinoma of the glottic larynx treated with radiation therapy: relationship of dose-fractionation factors to local control and complications. *Int J Radiat Oncol Biol Phys* 1988; **15:** 1267–73.
22. Mendenhall WM, Parsons JT, Stringer SP, Cassisi NJ, Million RR. Carcinoma of the supraglottic larynx: a basis for comparing the results of radiotherapy and surgery. *Head Neck* 1990; **12:** 204–9.
23. Mendenhall WM, Parsons JT, Stringer SP, Cassisi NJ, Million RR. Stage T3 squamous cell carcinoma of the glottic larynx: a comparison of laryngectomy and irradiation. *Int J Radiat Oncol Biol Phys* 1992; **23:** 725–32.
24. Million RR, Cassisi NJ, Parsons JT, Mendenhall WM. Radiation therapy in the management of carcinoma of the larynx. In: Fried MP, ed. *The Larynx: a Multidisciplinary Approach*, 2nd edn. St Louis: Mosby, 1996: 571–96.
25. Mintz DR, Gullane PJ, Thomson DH, Ruby RRF. Perichondritis of the larynx following radiation. *Otolaryngol Head Neck Surg* 1981; **89:** 550–4.
26. Mohr RM, Quenelle DJ, Shumrick DA. Vertico-frontolateral laryngectomy (hemilaryngectomy). *Arch Otolaryngol* 1983; **109:** 384–95.
27. Neel HB III, Devine KD, DeSanto LW. Laryngofissure and cordectomy for early cordal carcinoma: outcome in 182 patients. *Otolaryngol Head Neck Surg* 1980; **88:** 79–84.
28. Nichols RD, Mickelson SA. Partial laryngectomy after irradiation failure. *Ann Otol Rhinol Laryngol* 1991; **100:** 176–80.
29. Nichols RD, Stine PH, Greenawlard KJ. Partial laryngectomy after radiation failure. *Laryngoscope* 1980; **90:** 1324–8.
30. Norris CM, Peale AR. Partial laryngectomy for irradiation failure. *Arch Otolaryngol* 1966; **84:** 558–62.
31. O'Brien PC. Tumor recurrence or treatment sequelae following radiotherapy for larynx cancer. *J Surg Oncol* 1996; **63:** 130–5.
32. Parsons JT, Mendenhall WM, Stringer SP, Cassisi NJ, Million RR. Salvage surgery following radiation failure in squamous cell carcinoma of the supraglottic larynx. *Int J Radiat Oncol Biol Phys* 1995; **32:** 605–9.
33. Puthawala AA, Syed AMN. Interstitial re-irradiation for recurrent and/or persistent head and neck cancers. *Int J Radiat Oncol Biol Phys* 1987; **13:** 1113–14.
34. Schwaab G, Mamelle G, Lartigau E, Parise O Jr, Wibault P, Luboinski B. Surgical salvage treatment of T1/T2 glottic carcinoma after failure of radiotherapy. *Am J Surg* 1994; **168:** 474–5.
35. Shah JP, Loree TR, Kowalsky L. Conservation surgery for radiation-failure carcinoma of the glottic larynx. *Head Neck* 1990; **12:** 326–31.
36. Skolyszewski J, Korzeniowski S. Re-irradiation of recurrent head and neck cancer with fast neutrons. *Br J Radiol* 1988; **61:** 527–8.
37. Sorensen H, Hansen HS, Thomsen KA. Partial laryngectomy following irradiation. *Laryngoscope* 1980; **90:** 1344–9.
38. Stewart JG, Brown JR, Palmer MK, Cooper A. The management of glottic carcinoma by primary irradiation with surgery in reserve. *Laryngoscope* 1975; **85:** 1477–84.
39. Strauss M. Hemilaryngectomy rescue surgery for radiation failure in early glottic carcinoma. *Laryngoscope* 1988; **98:** 317–20.
40. Viani L, Stell PM, Dalby JE. Recurrence after radiotherapy for glottic carcinoma. *Cancer* 1991; **67:** 577–84.
41. Wang CC, McIntyre J. Re-irradiation of laryngeal carcinoma – techniques and results. *Int J Radiat Oncol Biol Phys* 1993; **26:** 783–5.
42. Ward PH, Calcaterra TC, Kagan AR. The enigma of post-radiation edema and recurrent or residual carcinoma of the larynx. *Laryngoscope* 1975; **85:** 522–9.
43. Weems DH, Mendenhall WM, Parsons JT, Cassisi NJ, Million RR. Squamous cell carcinoma of the supraglottic larynx treated with surgery and/ or radiation therapy. *Int J Radiat Oncol Biol Phys* 1987; **13:** 1483–7.
44. Yuen APW, Wei WI, Ho CM. Results of surgical salvage for radiation failures of laryngeal carcinoma. *Otolaryngol Head Neck Surg* 1995; **112:** 405–9.

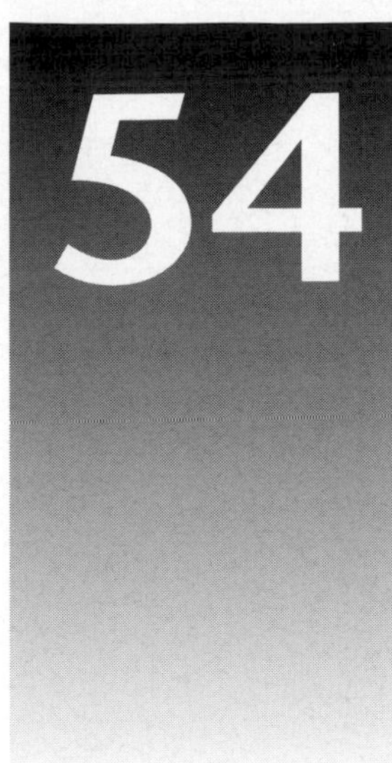

Peristomal cancer

Alfio Ferlito, Carl E Silver,
Alessandra Rinaldo and Helen Kim

Presence of cancer at the trachea stoma, frequently termed 'stomal recurrence', is usually a devastating sequela to total laryngectomy and often carries a dismal prognosis. Stomal recurrence is most often associated with advanced cancer of the larynx and hypopharynx, although it occasionally has been reported after surgery for cancers developing in other areas of the head and neck. Squamous cell carcinoma is the most frequent type of tumor found in stomal recurrences, but verrucous squamous cell carcinoma,[28,36,60] spindle cell carcinoma,[28] basaloid squamous cell carcinoma,[31,46] malignant fibrous histiocytoma[30] and chondrosarcoma[27] have all been shown to occur in the peristomal area. Stomal recurrence is considered the most lethal complication of laryngeal cancer. It occurs rarely following treatment for non-laryngeal or non-hypopharyngeal tumors.

Definition

Stomal recurrence can be defined as the neoplastic infiltration of the junction of the resected trachea and the skin[41] and may present as a single or multiple nodules.

Incidence

The incidence of stomal recurrence reported in the literature varies from 1.7%[26] to 24%.[25] We have calculated the overall incidence of stomal recurrence to be 5.2% in a comprehensive review of 48 references encompassing 14 426 patients (see Table 54.1).[1,2,6,8,9,11–15,17,19,20,22,25,26,28,32,34,39,41–45,47–52,54,55,57,58,60,61,63–66,76,77,80,81,84–86] Ninety-four percent of all stomal recurrences occur within 2 years[64] and 80% or more occur within 6–12 months.[72]

Risk factors

The precise pathogenesis of stomal recurrence is unknown and several mechanisms have been proposed:

- persistence of cancer in the trachea after incomplete surgical removal;
- neoplastic cell implantation into the surgical wound during surgical treatment;
- residual cancer in unresected thyroid tissue;
- neoplastic involvement of the prelaryngeal, pretracheal and paratracheal lymph nodes; and
- development of a second primary cancer in the trachea.

The pre-resection tracheostomy, referred to in the literature as 'prior' tracheostomy or 'preoperative' tracheostomy, is the most frequently discussed and controversial risk factor mentioned in the literature and has been thought to be associated with an increased incidence of peristomal recurrence and reduced survival. Keim *et al.*,[41] in 1965 implicated the pre-resection tracheostomy as the major factor in peristomal recurrence. This has led to the use of emergency laryngectomy[5,34,51,61,82] to decrease the chance of tumor cell implantation in the stoma. More recently, in 1996, Fagan and Loock[29] examined the association between pre-resection tracheostomy, as an independent variable, and peristomal recurrence in patients treated by a combination of total laryngectomy and radiotherapy. The authors concluded that tracheostomy does not cause peristomal recurrence.

Another consideration regarding predisposition to peristomal cancer is the fact that patients treated with high-dose radiotherapy followed by salvage laryngectomy have

Table 54.1 Literature summary of the presence of cancer at the trachea stoma

Author(s)	*Year*	*No. patients*	*No. stomal recurrences*	*Percent*
Latella[47]	1952	240	8	3.3
Mounier-Kuhn *et al.*[57]	1959	210	8	3.8
Norris[63]	1959	181	7	3.9
Boccuzzi and Tomasetti[11]	1961	290	15	5.2
Bauer *et al.*[8]	1962	86	6	7
Debain *et al.*[25]	1965	50	12	24
Keim *et al.*[41]	1965	116	17	14.6
Bolla and Scolari[12]	1967	167	8	4.8
Burnam and Hudson[15]	1967	109	13	11.9
Molinari and Milanesi[55]	1967	1842	63	3.4
Loewy and Laker[49]	1968	138	4	2.9
Condon[22]	1969	110	6	5.4
de Jong[26]	1969	114	2	1.7
Modlin and Ogura[54]*	1969	243	12	4.9
Kuehn and Tennant[43]	1971	124	9	7.2
Stell and Van Den Broek[77]†	1971	196	8	4.1
Bonneau and Lehman[13]	1975	92	11	11.9
Schneider *et al.*[66]	1975	246	31	12.6
Myers and Ogura[60]††	1979	452	33	7.3
Weisman *et al.*[81]	1979	251	14	5.6
Calzavara *et al.*[17]	1980	388	32	8.2
Mantravadi *et al.*[50]	1981	507	26	5.1
Bignardi *et al.*[9]	1983	681	17	2.5
Fini-Storchi *et al.*[32]	1983	1515	58	3.8
Antonelli *et al.*[2]	1984	305	18	5.9
Cervellera *et al.*[20]	1984	372	28	7.5
Komiyama *et al.*[42]	1984	112	11	9.8
Amatsu *et al.*[1]	1985	340	20	5.9
Griebie and Adams[34]	1987	281	10	3.5
Breneman *et al.*[14]	1988	18	2	11.1
Lahoz *et al.*[45]	1989	349	10	2.9
Snow and Balm[76]	1989	220	10	4.5
Barr *et al.*[6]	1990	106	14	13.2
Rubin *et al.*[65]	1990	444	15	3.4
Castro *et al.*[19]	1991	350	20	5.7
McCombe and Stell[51]	1991	233	14	6
Rockley *et al.*[64]	1991	91	12	13.2
Esteban *et al.*[28]§	1993	209	17	8.1
Hosal *et al.*[39]	1993	488	13	2.7
Murakami[58]	1993	667	38	5.7
Narula *et al.*[61]	1993	13	2	15.4
Weber *et al.*[80]	1993	141	6	4.2
Kuratomi *et al.*[44]	1994	112	11	9.8
León *et al.*[48]	1996	296	6	2
Yotakis *et al.*[84]	1996	352	21	6
Yuen *et al.*[85]	1996	322	17	5.3
Zbären *et al.*[86]	1996	130	13	10
Metternich and Brusis[52]	1997	127	10	7.9
Total		14 426	758	

*Ten additional cases of stomal recurrence reported by the authors have not been included in the table because they were incidental cases and not evaluated from overall surgical series.
†The authors did not list another case of stomal recurrence in a patient who underwent total maxillectomy for carcinoma of the maxillary antrum.
††The authors included in their series three cases of stomal recurrence in patients treated for cancers of the oral cavity.
§Five cases were verrucous carcinoma and one spindle cell carcinoma.

Table 54.2 Peristomal presence of cancer following treatment for non-laryngeal or non-hypopharyngeal tumors

Author(s)	*Year*	*No. patients*	*Site of lesion*
Stell and Van Den Broek[77]	1971	1	Maxillary antrum
Myers and Ogura[60]	1979	3	Oral cavity NOS
Molinari *et al.*[56]	1991	5	Floor of mouth (2); tonsil (1); tongue (1); palatoglossal area (1)
Armstrong and Price[3]	1992	1	Tongue
Clayman *et al.*[21]	1993	2	Tongue; tongue and tonsil
Murakami[58]	1993	1	Tongue
Sesenna *et al.*[67]	1995	1	Tongue
Campbell *et al.*[18]	1999	2	Floor of mouth; mandibular gingiva

NOS, not otherwise specified.

stomal recurrence more often than those treated by primary laryngectomy and the difference is statistically significant.[86]

Rubin *et al.*[65] believe that the lack of correlation between stomal recurrence and pre-resection tracheotomy as well as the low incidence of stomal recurrence in patients previously treated with conservation surgery make implantation of neoplastic cells a less likely pathogenic mode. The autotransplantation or implantation of cancer cells is a rare, but the only theoretically possible, mechanism to explain the rare cases of peristomal recurrence developing in patients with cancer remote from the larynx and hypopharynx who have undergone composite resections with tracheostomies (see Table 54.2).[3,18,21,56,58,60,67,77]

Spread of tumor through the thyroid gland plays an important role in the development of stomal cancer. Secondary involvement of thyroid isthmus must be suspected in the presence of transglottic or advanced anterior commissure cancers. In such cases, the risk of residual cancer is so high as to warrant partial thyroidectomy.[37]

Submucosal subglottic spread at the margin of the resection and metastases to paratracheal lymph nodes appear plausible as pathogenic mechanisms.

Subglottic extension of glottic cancer or persistent cancer from incomplete resection are statistically the most important risk factors associated with peristomal cancer.[50] Involvement of prelaryngeal, pretracheal and paratracheal lymph nodes is also an important factor in the development of stomal recurrence in laryngeal carcinomas with aggressive biologic behavior. In these cases stomal recurrence can be simply considered one of the expressions associated with more advanced disease prior to laryngectomy. The pathogenetic mechanism of metastases to the prelaryngeal, pretracheal and paratracheal lymph nodes does not account for the occasional stomal recurrence associated with verrucous carcinoma,[28] a tumor that does not metastasize.

The development of a secondary primary cancer of the trachea may, on rare occasions, account for peristomal cancer.[38] The presence of a primary tracheal malignancy was found in only 1 of 20 stomal recurrences studied by Batsakis *et al.*[7] and in some observations and specimens of stomal recurrence made by Michaels.[53]

Thus the etiology of peristomal recurrence is a complex matter to determine and probably it is multifactorial.

Classification

The classification system of Sisson *et al.*[74] for staging stomal recurrence is of paramount importance for therapeutic and prognostic implications. They describe four types of recurrent stomal tumor in relation to the location and the extent of involvement (see Fig 54.1):

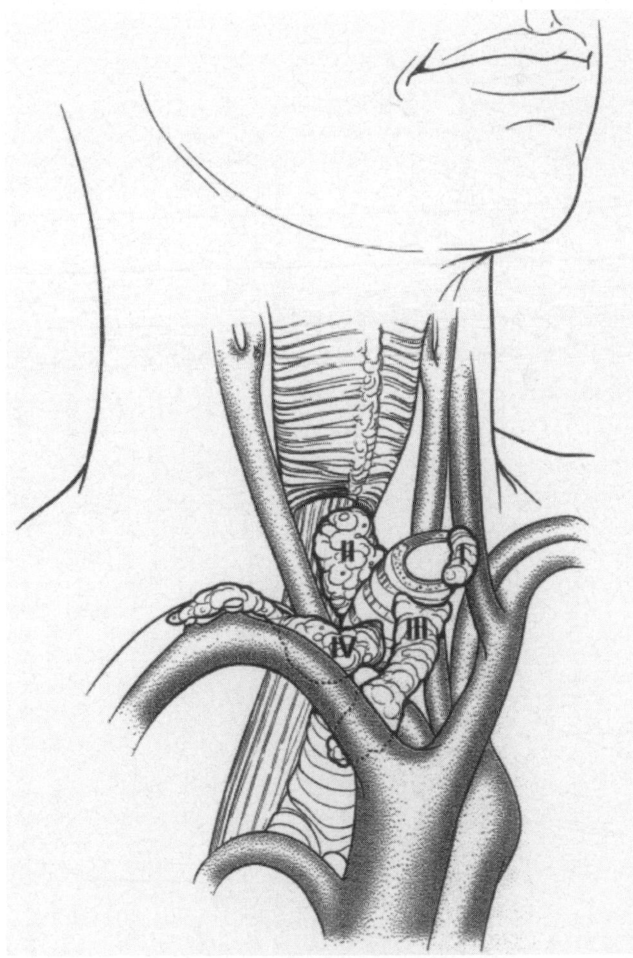

Figure 54.1 *Types of tracheal stomal recurrence of cancer. (Reproduced with permission from Silver CE, Ferlito A.* Surgery for Cancer of the Larynx and Related Structures, *2nd edn. Philadelphia: Saunders, 1996.)*

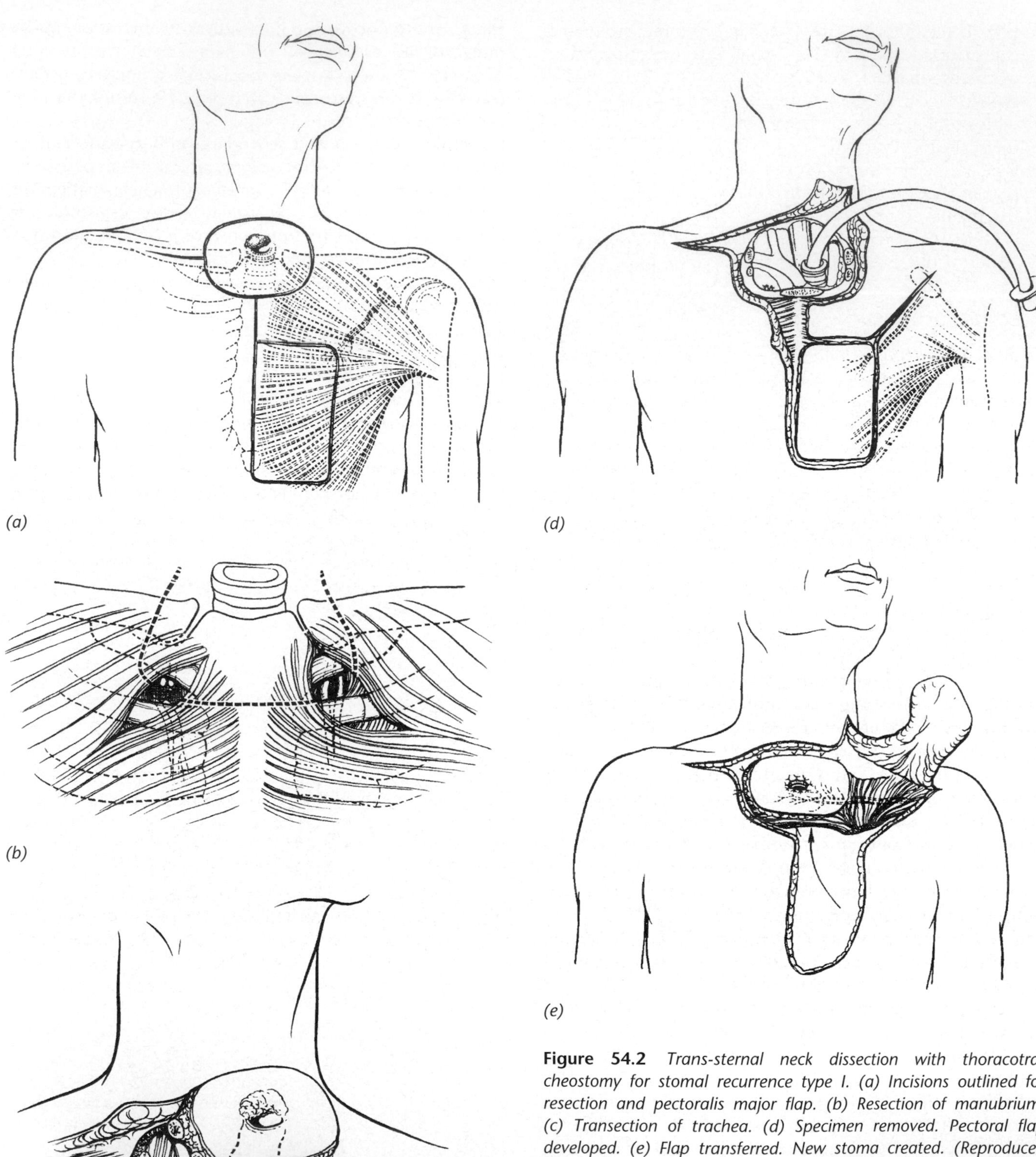

Figure 54.2 *Trans-sternal neck dissection with thoracotracheostomy for stomal recurrence type I. (a) Incisions outlined for resection and pectoralis major flap. (b) Resection of manubrium. (c) Transection of trachea. (d) Specimen removed. Pectoral flap developed. (e) Flap transferred. New stoma created. (Reproduced with permission from Silver CE.* Surgery for Cancer of the Larynx. *New York: Churchill Livingstone, 1981.)*

- type I: recurrence is localized as a discrete nodule in the superior aspect of the stoma (without involvement of the esophagus);
- type II: recurrence is localized superior to the stoma with esophageal involvement but no inferior involvement of the stoma;
- type III: recurrence is always localized in the inferior part of the stoma and usually has direct extension into the mediastinum; and
- type IV: recurrence extends laterally and often under either of the clavicles.

Preoperative evaluation

Staging evaluation is mandatory for therapeutic reasons and should include physical examination, tracheoscopy, bronchoscopy, esophagoscopy, high-resolution computed tomography (CT) and/or magnetic resonance imaging (MRI) and mediastinoscopy. In selected cases, i.e. in those patients in whom conventional studies are not confirmatory, the thoracoscopy, a procedure in which mediastinal contents can be directly visualized and tissue biopsied, may provide additional information in judging the surgical resectability of patients with stomal recurrence.[79]

Treatment

The highest cure rate is achieved by an aggressive radical surgical approach with wide excision of the skin, the manubrium, the trachea and the mediastinum lymphatics. Modern methods of soft tissue reconstruction have eliminated much of the morbidity previously associated with postoperative exposure of great vessels in the mediastinum. Silver[68] and Silver and Rodriguez[69] have reported on the pectoral myocutaneous flap for the reconstruction of the deficit that has been used successfully by many surgeons since the late 1970s. More recently, free revascularized flaps provide the surgeon with many options for safe reconstruction of the resected area after wide, aggressive and complete surgical resection. Cordeiro *et al.*[23] recently reported successful use of radial forearm fasciocutaneous flaps for this purpose.

Only types I and II lesions are considered resectable, whilst nonsurgical treatment is suggested for types III and IV lesions.

Surgical procedures for tracheal stomal recurrence

The major steps in resection of a type I tracheal stomal recurrence are demonstrated in Fig 54.2. The overlying skin is widely excised *en bloc* with the manubrium, distal trachea and lymph nodes of the superior mediastinum. The resulting defect is covered by rotating a pectoralis major myocutaneous flap from the adjacent portion of the chest. A new tracheostome (thoracotracheostomy) is created through an appropriate incision in the skin paddle. The thick healthy myocutaneous flap provides excellent protection for the great vessels of the superior mediastinum.

The technique of trans-sternal neck dissection with thoracotracheostomy and esophagectomy for stomal recurrence type II and repair by greater pectoral muscle myocutaneous flap and gastric transposition is demonstrated in Fig 54.3. The skin, sternum and trachea are mobilized in continuity with the esophagus, and blunt digital extraction of the esophagus with gastric transposition is performed from cervical and abdominal approaches. A pharyngogastrostomy is constructed to restore alimentary continuity, and the mediastinal defect is covered with a pectoralis myocutaneous flap. A thoracotracheostomy is constructed through the flap.

Complications

The mediastinum is one of the most challenging areas for the head and neck surgeon, in terms of resection and reconstruction. The complications seen after operations for stomal cancer are largely related to the danger of exposing or contaminating the great vessels that lie under the sternum, surrounding the lower trachea.[40,59] In 1991, Josephson and Krespi divided the relevant complications into three categories: immediate intraoperative, immediate postoperative, and late complications.[40]

Intraoperative complications

The most frequent and usual fatal complication is an injury to the great blood vessels (carotid, subclavian and brachiocephalic arteries and veins) that causes massive hemorrhage that may be difficult to control. Meticulous digital or blunt dissection is suggested.[58] Air embolism, which may result from venous injury, is a second acute complication. Damage to the pleura may occur and pneumothorax is an acute dangerous complication, either from mediastinal dissection or from blunt esophagectomy, that requires immediate diagnosis and resolution. Chyle leaks may occur, most commonly on the left side. The leak should be sutured at the time of surgery with nonabsorbable material to avoid formation of a postoperative chyle fistula or chyloma.[40,69]

Immediate postoperative complications

The first 5 days after surgery comprise the immediate postoperative period and the most frequent complications are mediastinitis, airway obstruction and pneumothorax. Mediastinitis may occur secondary to an infected hematoma, seroma or leaky suture line.[40]

Late postoperative complications

These may appear after the fifth postoperative day and the arterial erosion of a major vessel (in particular the brachiocephalic or the left common carotid artery) is possible with the tracheostoma in a lower position. This

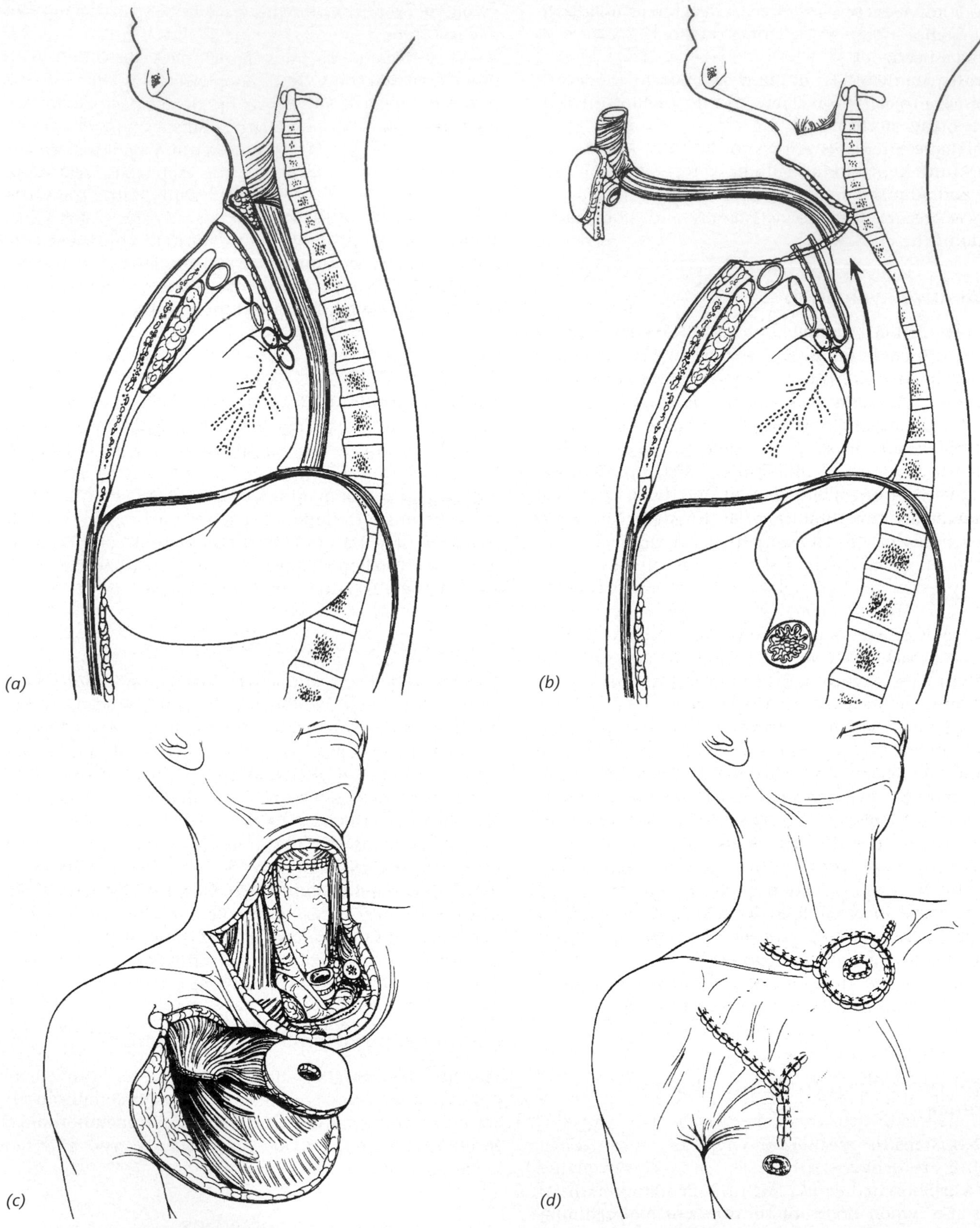

Figure 54.3 *Trans-sternal neck dissection with thoracotracheostomy and esophagectomy for stomal recurrence type II. (a) Relations of the tumor involving posterior wall of stoma and adjacent esophagus are shown. (b) The peristomal skin, stoma, manubrium and attached esophagus are mobilized with blunt extraction of the thoracic esophagus and transposition of the entire stomach to replace the thoracic and cervical esophagus. (c) Pharyngogastrostomy is constructed, and pectoralis myocutaneous flap rotated to cover the mediastinal defect. (d) Tracheostome created and incision closed. (Reproduced with permission from Silver CE, Ferlito A.* Surgery for Cancer of the Larynx and Related Structures, *2nd edn. Philadelphia: Saunders, 1996.)*

complication may result from tracheocutaneous separation or from tracheal necrosis caused by pressure from an overinflated cuff.[59] Infection of the wound is also possible and subsequently aspiration pneumonia may occur.[40] Flap necrosis has been reported, but whilst major flap loss is now rare, the incidence of minor flap necrosis is about 10% of patients.[83] Pharyngocutaneous fistula, hypothyroidism and hypoparathyroidism may occur. Pneumothorax and pulmonary collapse are also fatal postoperative complications, in particular in patients in poor general condition.[58]

Results

In the past, stomal recurrence was invariably fatal. Sisson *et al.* in 1962 introduced the technique of mediastinal dissection in six patients but the survival was low and the immediate morbidity was high.[75] In 1970, Sisson[70] reported 17% median survival at 2.3 years. In 1985, he reported 35% survival at 42 months for all cases compiled over a 30-year span.[71] By 1985, Sisson agreed that mediastinal dissection, utilizing the gastric pull-up and pectoralis major myocutaneous flap for closure, was the treatment of choice for stomal recurrence.

Gluckman *et al.*[33] reported that the overall 2-year survival for operated patients was 16% with a 24% determinate survival. Further analysis revealed a 45% 5-year survival with type I and type II lesions and 9% survival with type III and type IV lesions. These data suggest that early lesions (type I and type II) can be treated successfully with surgery, whereas in more advanced lesions (type III and type IV), and in particular in type IV, surgery has an unacceptably high perioperative morbidity with appalling prognosis. Sisson, in the 1989 Ogura Memorial Lecture, reported the survival rate had increased to 45% (50% of which were 2.5–5 years).[72] The risk should be evaluated in relation to possible benefit.[69] Nevertheless, extensive surgery offers the best chance of cure at the present time.

Radiotherapy is often used as a palliative therapy.[50] Gunn, in 1965,[35] reported 12 cases of stomal recurrences treated with radiation therapy (in every instance approximated or exceeded 40 Gy in 4 weeks) and 11 of them underwent moderate to marked regression. They concluded that in nearly all cases temporary palliation of pain or bleeding can be afforded with accompanying regression of tumor masses. Rockley *et al.*[64] reported 12 patients with stomal recurrence and all except one patient died. None was treated with surgery. León *et al.*[48] reported six patients treated with radiotherapy or chemotherapy and all six died within the first year as a consequence of tumor. Furthermore, many patients have already had full courses of radiation after surgical treatment of the primary cancer and are not candidates to receive further therapeutic doses. Synchronous combinations of chemotherapy (vincristin sulfate, bleomycin and methotrexate) and radiotherapy have been used in small groups of patients with favorable long-term results.[4] In five of eight patients, complete local remission was achieved with the survival varying from 8 months to 7 years after treatment. Of the three patients who died, only one had recurrent disease around the tracheostoma. The other two patients were free of disease in the neck when they died 6 and 16 months after treatment of, respectively, lung metastases and a second primary tumor in the lung. Encouraging results in two cases were also obtained with induction chemotherapy by Davis and Shapshay[24] but the number of patients is too small. Recently, Nikolaou *et al.*[62] treated with 13-*cis*-retinoic acid and interferon-α patients with unresectable recurrent head and neck carcinoma, eight of whom had stomal recurrence, and the results were not encouraging. All patients died after a survival of 3–17 months. There were four cases with progressive disease, three cases of stable disease and only one case of partial response.

Silver and Rodriguez[69] believe that in many cases supervoltage radiation therapy or aggressive chemotherapy may produce symptomatic relief and survival comparable to that obtainable by extensive surgery.

Prevention

The best treatment is prevention. Planned postoperative radiation to the peristoma has been shown to be of benefit in patients considered to be at risk of developing stomal recurrence,[78] such as those having subglottic tumor extension and locally advanced cancers.[64] Also the pretracheal and paratracheal lymph node dissection should be performed in all laryngeal cancers with subglottic extension. Hosal *et al.*[39] emphasize the importance of pretracheal, paratracheal and retrosternal dissection in patients with subglottic cancer of the larynx (primarily or secondarily) and postoperative radiotherapy if positive nodes are found. The incidence of peristomal recurrence decreased in their series from 11.5% to 2.7% using these therapeutic modalities.

Thorough irrigation of the whole wound with saline solution after all larynx resections is indicated,[1] as tumor cell implantation has proved to be a mechanism.[28] It is prudent to avoid the re-use of instruments that have been in direct contact with tumor surfaces.[21] The use of emergency laryngectomy to prevent peristomal recurrence is questionable.[29] Rockley *et al.*[64] believe that there is no evidence that emergency laryngectomy reduces the incidence of stomal recurrence and therefore this procedure is unnecessary.

Komiyama *et al.*[42] suggest the preoperative FAR (a combination of 5-FU, vitamin A and radiation) therapy against stomal recurrence after emergency tracheostomy. Postoperative pharyngoperistomal fistula may represent a risk factor.[86]

Conclusions

The results of surgical salvage for patients at earlier stages have been evolving, and patients with type I and type II lesions are often salvaged by early aggressive surgical intervention. Trans-sternal mediastinal dissection, employment of myocutaneous flaps,[10,16,73] availability of reliable methods for esophageal replacement and appropriate postoperative support have led to successful control of these tumors. Patients with lesions too advanced (type III and type IV lesions) should be treated palliatively with nonsurgical methods.[69]

References

1. Amatsu M, Makino K, Kinishi M. Stomal recurrence – etiological factor and prevention. *Auris Nasus Larynx* 1985; **12:** 103–10.
2. Antonelli A, Oldini C, Leonardelli GB, Ghidoni P. La recidiva postoperatoria stomale/peristomale del cancro laringeo. Studio anatomo-clinico di 18 osservazioni. *Otorinolaringologia* 1984; **34:** 41–6.
3. Armstrong M Jr, Price JC. Tumor implantation in a tracheotomy. *Otolaryngol Head Neck Surg* 1992; **106:** 400–3.
4. Balm AJM, Snow GB, Karim ABMF, Versluis RJJ, Njo KH, Tiwari RM. Long-term results of concurrent polychemotherapy and radiotherapy in patients with stomal recurrence after total laryngectomy. *Ann Otol Rhinol Laryngol* 1986; **95:** 572–5.
5. Baluyot ST, Shumrick DA, Everts EC. 'Emergency' laryngectomy. *Arch Otolaryngol* 1971; **94:** 414–17.
6. Barr GD, Robertson AG, Liu KC. Stomal recurrence: a separate entity? *J Surg Oncol* 1990; **44:** 176–9.
7. Batsakis JG, Hybels R, Rice DH. Laryngeal carcinoma: stomal recurrences and distant metastases. *Can J Otolaryngol* 1975; **4:** 906–14.
8. Bauer WC, Edwards DL, McGavran MH. A critical analysis of laryngectomy in the treatment of epidermoid carcinoma of larynx. *Cancer* 1962; **15:** 263–70.
9. Bignardi L, Gavioli C, Staffieri A. Tracheostomal recurrences after laryngectomy. *Arch Otorhinolaryngol* 1983; **238:** 107–13.
10. Biller HF, Krespi YP, Lawson W, Baek S. A one-stage flap reconstruction following resection for stomal recurrence. *Otolaryngol Head Neck Surg* 1980; **88:** 357–60.
11. Boccuzzi V, Tomasetti L. Sulle recidive reali ed apparenti della stomia tracheale dopo laringectomia totale. *Boll Mal Orec Gola Naso* 1961; **79:** 179–89.
12. Bolla A, Scolari R. Le recidive peristomali del cancro laringeo. *Minerva Otorinolaringol* 1967; **17:** 157–60.
13. Bonneau RA, Lehman RH. Stomal recurrence following laryngectomy. *Arch Otolaryngol* 1975; **101:** 408–12.
14. Breneman JC, Bradshaw A, Gluckman J, Aron BS. Prevention of stomal recurrence in patients requiring emergency tracheostomy for advanced laryngeal and pharyngeal tumors. *Cancer* 1988; **62:** 802–5.
15. Burnam JA, Hudson WR. Stomal recurrence of malignancy: an evaluation and its significance in post-laryngectomy patient. *South Med J* 1967; **60:** 823–6.
16. Burnstein FD, Calcaterra TC. The pectoral major myocutaneous flap. Use in surgery of the lower neck and superior mediastinum. *Arch Otolaryngol Head Neck Surg* 1987; **113:** 773–7.
17. Calzavara F, Pizzi GB, Corti L, Zorat PL, Sotti G. Localizzazioni secondarie sul tracheostoma dopo laringectomia e radioterapia nel cancro della laringe. *Atti Riunioni Integrate di Oncologia, Fiera del Levante, Bari* 1980: 160.
18. Campbell AC, Gleich LL, Barrett WL, Gluckman JL. Cancerous seeding of the tracheostomy site in patients with upper aerodigestive tract squamous cell carcinoma. *Otolaryngol Head Neck Surg* 1999; **120:** 601–3.
19. Castro A, Ostos P, Mellado R, Cantillo E, López-Villarejo P. Nuestra experiencia en recidiva estomal de laringuectomizados con traqueostomia previa. *An Otorrinolaringol Ibero Am* 1991; **6:** 57–60.
20. Cervellera G, Fiorella R, Petrone D. Tracheotomia e recidiva neoplastica peristomale. *Acta Otorhinolaryngol Ital* 1984; **4:** 231–8.
21. Clayman G, Cohen JI, Adams GL. Neoplastic seeding of squamous cell carcinoma of the oropharynx. *Head Neck* 1993; **15:** 245–8.
22. Condon HA. Postlaryngectomy stomal recurrence: the influence of endotracheal anaesthesia. *Br J Anaesth* 1969; **41:** 531–3.
23. Cordeiro PG, Mastorakos DP, Shaha AR. The radial forearm fasciocutaneous free-tissue transfer for tracheotomy reconstruction. *Plast Reconstr Surg* 1996; **98:** 354–7.
24. Davis RK, Shapshay SM. Peristomal recurrence: pathophysiology, prevention, treatment. *Otolaryngol Clin North Am* 1980; **13:** 499–507.
25. Debain JJ, Siardet J, Andrieu-Guitrancourt J. Les récidives péritrachéales après laryngectomie totale. *Ann Otolaryngol Chir Cervicofac* 1965; **82:** 382–4.
26. de Jong PC. Intubation and tumour implantation in laryngeal carcinoma. *Practica Otorhinolaryngol* 1969; **31:** 119–21.
27. Escher A, Escher F, Zimmermann A. Zur Klinik und Pathologie chondromatoser Tumoren des Larynx. *HNO* 1984; **32:** 269–85.
28. Esteban F, Moreno JA, Delgado-Rodriguez M, Mochon A. Risk factors involved in stomal recurrence following laryngectomy. *J Laryngol Otol* 1993; **107:** 527–31.
29. Fagan JJ, Loock JW. Tracheostomy and peristomal recurrence. *Clin Otolaryngol* 1996; **21:** 328–30.
30. Ferlito A. Histiocytic tumors of the larynx. A clinicopathological study with review of the literature. *Cancer* 1978; **42:** 611–22.
31. Ferlito A, Altavilla G, Rinaldo A, Doglioni C. Basaloid squamous cell carcinoma of the larynx and hypopharynx. *Ann Otol Rhinol Laryngol* 1997; **106:** 1024–35.
32. Fini-Storchi O, Rucci L, Fiorentino G. Sull'importanza di una pregressa tracheotomia nelle recidive alla stomia tracheale dopo laringectomia totale. *Otorinolaringologia* 1983; **33:** 9–13.
33. Gluckman JL, Hamaker RC, Schuller DE, Weissler MC, Charles GA. Surgical salvage for stomal recurrence: a multi-institutional experience. *Laryngoscope* 1987; **97:** 1025–9.
34. Griebie MS, Adams GL. 'Emergency' laryngectomy and stomal recurrence. *Laryngoscope* 1987; **97:** 1020–4.
35. Gunn WG. Treatment of cancer recurrent at the tracheostome. *Cancer* 1965; **18:** 1261–4.

36. Hagen P, Lyons GD, Haindel C. Verrucous carcinoma of the larynx: role of human papillomavirus, radiation, and surgery. *Laryngoscope* 1993; **103:** 253–7.
37. Harrison DFN. Thyroid gland in the management of laryngopharyngeal cancer. *Arch Otolaryngol* 1973; **97:** 301–2.
38. Heffner DK. Diseases of the trachea. In: Barnes L, ed. *Surgical Pathology of the Head and Neck.* Vol I. New York: Marcel Dekker, 1985: 487–531.
39. Hosal IN, Önerci M, Turan E. Peristomal recurrence. *Am J Otolaryngol* 1993; **14:** 206–8.
40. Josephson JS, Krespi YP. Management of stomal recurrence. In: Silver CE, ed. *Laryngeal Cancer.* New York: Thieme, 1991: 240–5.
41. Keim WF, Shapiro MJ, Rosin HD. Study of postlaryngectomy stomal recurrence. *Arch Otolaryngol* 1965; **81:** 183–6.
42. Komiyama S, Watanabe H, Yanagita T, Kuwano M, Hiroto I. Inhibition of stomal recurrence in laryngectomy with preoperative FAR therapy – a statistical evaluation. *Auris Nasus Larynx* 1984; **11:** 43–9.
43. Kuehn PG, Tennant R. Surgical treatment of stomal recurrences in cancer of larynx. *Am J Surg* 1971; **122:** 445–50.
44. Kuratomi Y, Tomita K, Inokuchi A, Komiyama S. Stomal recurrence in laryngectomy with preoperative combination therapy of 5-FU, vitamin A, and radiation (FAR therapy). *Second World Congress on Laryngeal Cancer, Sydney* 1994: Abstract no. P213.
45. Lahoz T, Faubel M, Campos JJ. Las recidivas periestomales tras, laringuectomía total. *An Otorrinolaringol Ibero Am* 1989; **26:** 649–57.
46. Larner JM, Malcolm RH, Mills SE, Frierson HF, Banks ER, Levine PA. Radiotherapy for basaloid squamous cell carcinoma of the head and neck. *Head Neck* 1993; **15:** 249–52.
47. Latella PD. An analysis of 240 cases of cancer of the larynx, with respect to the terminal phases and death. *Ann Otol* 1952; **61:** 266–75.
48. León X, Quer M, Burgués J, Abelló P, Vega M, de Andrés L. Prevention of stomal recurrence. *Head Neck* 1996; **18:** 54–9.
49. Loewy A, Laker HI. Tracheal stoma problems. *Arch Otolaryngol* 1968; **87:** 477–83.
50. Mantravadi R, Katz AM, Skolnik EM, Becker S, Freehling DJ, Friedman M. Stomal recurrence. A critical analysis of risk factors. *Arch Otolaryngol* 1981; **107:** 735–8.
51. McCombe A, Stell PM. Emergency laryngectomy. *J Laryngol Otol* 1991; **105:** 463–5.
52. Metternich FU, Brusis T. Parastomale Tumoren nach Laryngektomie: Ätiologie und Therapie. *Laryngorhinootologie* 1997; **76:** 88–95.
53. Michaels L. *Pathology of the Larynx.* Berlin: Springer-Verlag, 1984: 213–17.
54. Modlin B, Ogura JH. Post-laryngectomy tracheal stomal recurrences. *Laryngoscope* 1969; **79:** 239–50.
55. Molinari R, Milanesi I. Interpretazione patogenetica delle recidive al tracheostoma in laringectomizzati per carcinoma. *Tumori* 1967; **53:** 299–313.
56. Molinari R, Garramone R, Chiesa F, Costa L, Mattavelli F, Sala L. Le cosiddette recidive stomali. Patogenesi e terapia. In: Serafini I, ed. *Il Carcinoma Glottico e Sottoglottico.* Padova: Piccin, 1991: 213–27.
57. Mounier-Kuhn P, Gaillard J, Bonnefoy J, Fontvieille J. Les recidives peri-canulaires apres laryngectomie donnees therapeutiques. *J Fr Otorhinolaryngol* 1959; **8:** 519–22.
58. Murakami Y. Stomal recurrence after total laryngectomy. In: Ferlito A, ed. *Neoplasms of the Larynx.* Edinburgh: Churchill Livingstone, 1993: 545–57.
59. Myers EM. Complications in surgery for stomal recurrences. *Laryngoscope* 1983; **93:** 285–8.
60. Myers EM, Ogura JH. Stomal recurrences: a clinicopathological analysis and protocol for future management. *Laryngoscope* 1979; **89:** 1121–8.
61. Narula AA, Sheppard IJ, West K, Bradley PJ. Is emergency laryngectomy a waste of time? *Am J Otolaryngol* 1993; **14:** 21–3.
62. Nikolaou AC, Fountzilas G, Danilidis I. Treatment of unresectable recurrent head and neck carcinoma with 13-cis-retinoic acid and interferon-α. A phase II study. *J Laryngol Otol* 1996; **110:** 857–61.
63. Norris CM. Causes of failure in surgical treatment of malignant tumors of the larynx. *Ann Otol* 1959; **68:** 487–508.
64. Rockley TJ, Powell J, Robin PE, Reid AP. Post-laryngectomy stomal recurrence: tumour implantation or paratracheal lymphatic metastasis? *Clin Otolaryngol* 1991; **16:** 43–7.
65. Rubin J, Johnson JT, Myers EN. Stomal recurrence after laryngectomy: interrelated risk factor study. *Otolaryngol Head Neck Surg* 1990; **103:** 805–12.
66. Schneider JJ, Lindberg RD, Jesse RH. Prevention of tracheal stoma recurrences after total laryngectomy by postoperative irradiation. *J Surg Oncol* 1975; **7:** 187–90.
67. Sesenna E, Ferrari S, De Riu G. Insemenzamento neoplastico di carcinoma squamoso della lingua in sede di tracheotomia. *Acta Otorhinolaryngol Ital* 1995; **15:** 47–50.
68. Silver CE. *Surgery for Cancer of the Larynx and Related Structures.* New York: Churchill Livingstone, 1981: 55–81.
69. Silver CE, Rodriguez E. Tracheal stomal stenosis and recurrence. In: Silver CE, Ferlito A, eds. *Surgery for Cancer of the Larynx and Related Structures,* 2nd edn. Philadelphia: Saunders, 1996: 339–59.
70. Sisson GA. Mediastinal dissection for recurrent cancer after laryngectomy. *Trans Am Acad Ophthalmol Otolaryngol* 1970; **74:** 767–77.
71. Sisson GA. Mediastinal dissection – resectability and curability of stomal recurrence after total laryngectomy. *Auris Nasus Larynx* 1985; **12:** 61–6.
72. Sisson GA, Sr. Ogura Memorial Lecture: mediastinal dissection. *Laryngoscope* 1989; **99:** 1262–6.
73. Sisson GA, Goldman ME. Pectoral myocutaneous island flap for reconstruction of stomal recurrence. *Arch Otolaryngol Head Neck Surg* 1981; **107:** 446–9.
74. Sisson GA, Bytell DE, Becker SP. Mediastinal dissection – 1976: indications and newer techniques. *Laryngoscope* 1977; **87:** 751–9.
75. Sisson GA, Straehly CJ, Johnson NE. Mediastinal dissection for recurrent cancer after laryngectomy. *Laryngoscope* 1962; **72:** 1064–77.
76. Snow GB, Balm AJM. Il ruolo della chemioterapia nel

carcinoma squamoso della laringe. In: Carlon G, Serafini I, eds. *Il Carcinoma Sovraglottico*. Padova: Piccin, 1989: 245–56.

77. Stell PM, Van Den Broek P. Stomal recurrence after laryngectomy: aetiology and management. *J Laryngol Otol* 1971; **85:** 131–40.
78. Tong D, Moss WT, Stevens KR Jr. Elective irradiation of the lower cervical region in patients at high risk for recurrent cancer at the tracheal stoma. *Radiology* 1977; **124:** 809–11.
79. Wax MK, Garnett JD, Graeber G. Thoracoscopic staging of stomal recurrence. *Head Neck* 1995; **17:** 409–13.
80. Weber RS, Marvel J, Smith P, Hankins P, Wolf P, Goepfert H. Paratracheal lymph node dissection for carcinoma of the larynx, hypopharynx, and cervical esophagus. *Otolaryngol Head Neck Surg* 1993; **108:** 11–17.
81. Weisman RA, Colman M, Ward PH. Stomal recurrence following laryngectomy. A critical evaluation. *Ann Otol* 1979; **88:** 855–60.
82. Wickham MH, Narula AA, Barton RP, Bradley PJ. Emergency laryngectomy. *Clin Otolaryngol* 1990; **15:** 35–8.
83. Withers EH, Davis L, Lynch JB. Anterior mediastinal tracheostomy with a pectoralis major musculocutaneous flap. *Plast Reconstr Surg* 1981; **67:** 381–4.
84. Yotakis J, Davris S, Kontozoglou T, Adamopoulos G. Evaluation of risk factors for stomal recurrence after total laryngectomy. *Clin Otolaryngol* 1996; **21:** 135–8.
85. Yuen APW, Wei WI, Ho WK, Hui Y. Risk factors of tracheostomal recurrence after laryngectomy for laryngeal carcinoma. *Am J Surg* 1996; **172:** 263–6.
86. Zbären P, Greiner R, Kengelbacher M. Stoma recurrence after laryngectomy: an analysis of risk factors. *Otolaryngol Head Neck Surg* 1996; **114:** 569–75.

Managing complications of surgical laryngeal intervention

Yasushi Murakami

For the management of laryngeal diseases, especially of laryngeal carcinomas, surgical treatment is selected in many cases as the first choice or as a revision surgery. Many kinds of complication, major or minor, may occur during the surgical procedure or in postoperative period, and the management of these complications is an important task for head and neck surgeons.

Complications of endoscopic surgery

Web formation

No matter what kind of method is utilized, such as excision by forceps or laser vaporization, web formation in the anterior commissure is a well documented complication after laryngomicrosurgery. For this reason, T1b glottic carcinoma is not a good candidate for complete excision by, for example, endoscopic laser surgery, but radiotherapy may alternatively be selected providing almost the same result of 5-year survival. Hoarseness is a prominent symptom in the patient with cicatricial web, and surgical management is often mandatory. Endoscopic incision in the midline and the use of a Kiel, such as an indwelling silicone plate for 3 weeks, may be the treatment of choice.[15]

Perichondritis and chondronecrosis

In patients with recurrent glottic carcinoma who have been irradiated with more than 60 Gy, and especially are diabetic, laser vaporization deep into the paraglottic space or into the anterior commissure may result in perichondritis and chondronecrosis of the thyroid cartilage.[3] The use of antibiotics and steroids is recommended to prevent an infection of causative bacilli such as *Staphylococcus aureus*, *Proteus vulgaris*, *Haemophilus influenzae*, and so on. Chondronecrosis is usually progressive, emitting a characteristic fetor throughout the room. It may be debrided and the sequestrum may be removed. In many cases, however, a total laryngectomy is indicated as a surgical salvage for this hazardous condition.

Pyogenic granuloma

Pyogenic granuloma in the cartilaginous portion of the vocal cord is also a well known complication after laser surgery for T1 or T2 glottic carcinomas that extend into the mucosa over the arytenoid cartilage. An injury on the surface of the arytenoid cartilage by laser vaporization may often result in the development of this granuloma. Surgical extirpation of the pyogenic granuloma with the use of curet forceps or laser vaporization may often fail, resulting in repeated recurrences, whilst it has been reported that the inhalation of beclomethasone dipropionate, four to five times a day and for about 2–3 months, may give an excellent result.[8]

Subglottic granuloma

A huge granuloma may be seen in the subglottic space, which is thought to originate from mucosal wound by the cuff of an intubation tube for general anesthesia, which may disappear spontaneously in many instances without any active treatment. However, when it is obstructive to the airway and causes dyspnea, a low tracheotomy is necessary. Surgical removal of the granuloma can be done by cutting into the cavity through an inter-cricotracheal incision under general anesthesia. The incision is applied just at the level between the cricoid cartilage and the first tracheal ring, providing an excellent view of the subglottic

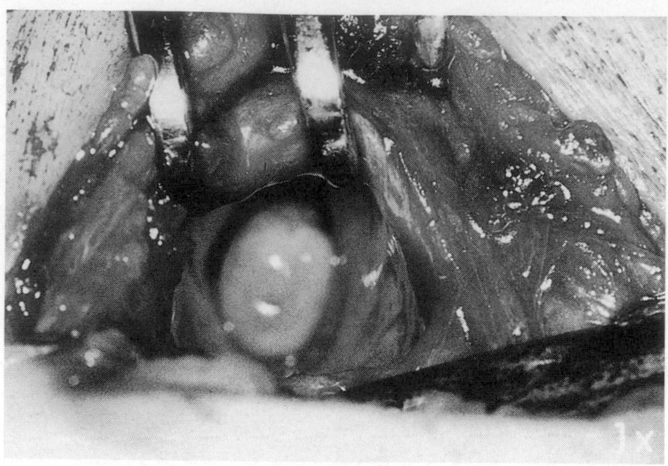

Figure 55.1 *Post-intubation granuloma in the subglottic space seen through an inter-cricotracheal incision.*

space (Fig 55.1). The wound can be closed primarily without using a stent.

Recurrent laryngeal nerve paralysis

Recurrent laryngeal nerve paralysis is also a complication after intubation anesthesia, which is usually seen in the left side and is considered a functional damage of the nerve due to hypoxia by an excessive pressure of the cuff for more than 3 hours. Spontaneous recovery can be expected within 6 months, otherwise the surgical mobilization of the paralyzed vocal cord into median position by the thyroplasty type I is indicated in order to prevent the aspiration of foods and dysphonia.

Complications of partial laryngectomy and tracheotomy

In partial laryngectomies, vertical or horizontal, a tracheotomy should be done and a tracheal cannula is utilized. Complications of these surgical procedures have been well documented.

Arterial bleeding

Though rare, arterial bleeding may occur from the carotid artery, superior or inferior thyroid arteries during partial laryngectomies. The innominate artery crosses the anterior wall of the trachea high at the level just inferior to the thyroid isthmus in elderly patients with atherosclerosis, and it is certainly in danger of injury by accident during a tracheotomy.[14] The thyroid arteries and the external carotid artery may be safely ligated. However, if a laceration of the common or internal carotid artery or of the innominate artery has occurred, they may not be ligated and repair of the laceration by sutures is preferred. Prior to final closure of the laceration, a temporary release of the distal end of the arterial occlusion, promoting back bleeding, should be applied to remove intra-arterial air.

Venous bleeding, air embolism

Bleeding may occur from an inadvertent laceration of the internal jugular vein or its tributaries. The distal portion of the internal jugular vein is potentially a dangerous site of injury to promote air embolism, resulting in pulmonary infarction that is often fatal if not properly managed. Every effort should be made to promptly detect the injury by the identification of mill wheel murmurs and to effectively respond to the situation. Inadvertent use of a hemostat may worsen the laceration, and a calm approach with compression of the vein by a finger followed by ligature sutures is highly recommended.[7] During a tracheotomy, bleeding from the thyroid ima vein is often encountered.

Nerve injury

The recurrent laryngeal nerve may be injured unintentionally during a dissection of paratracheal nodes, and care should be exercised in identifying the nerve. Hemostasis by electrocautery should be avoided in this area. Since the nerve invariably lies close to the trachea in the left side, it is at risk during tracheotomy by excessive incision of the tracheal wall. Some return of tonus in paralyzed vocal cords may be anticipated if a neurorrhaphy is accomplished at the time of injury. It is uncertain, however, as to how much clinical value this may have, since a reasonable recovery of the vocal cord function can never be expected.

The internal branch of the superior laryngeal nerve is well known to play an important part in the laryngopharyngeal phase of the swallowing, and should be preserved at least unilaterally in partial laryngectomies. Bilateral loss of function of the nerve, however, may occur during a supraglottic laryngectomy, and inevitably results in severe crippling of the swallowing function with aspiration of foods. On the other hand, the cut end of the nerve should be ligated when it is sacrificed, otherwise an amputation neuroma may be developed, producing an irritant pain, tenderness and hazardous cough by pressure or simple tapping on it. In such a case, excision of the neuroma is the best form of treatment.

Hematoma

Hematoma formation is a common postoperative complication in partial laryngectomies with neck dissection, and it may cause hazardous problems such as wound infection, skin necrosis, pharyngocutaneous fistula and carotid artery rupture. Meticulous hemostasis of the wound and the use of a continuous suction drainage with a compression dressing have been proved to be most important in avoiding hematoma formation. Whenever a hematoma is recognized by signs of a painful swelling of the wound and dark red color of the skin, the wound should be reopened immediately in the operating room under general anesthesia and the hematoma evacuated under sterile conditions. Bleeding vessels can be identified and carefully ligated by suture ligatures. Hematomas treated by early operative intervention may heal primarily without increase of morbidity or prolonged hospitalization of the patients.

Wound infection

Inadequate closure of the laryngopharyngeal wounds and a disruption of the suture line may lead to salivary leak and wound infection. Salivary secretions are usually polymicrobial, and contain oral flora including Gram-positive anaerobic and Gram-negative aerobic bacteria.[1] Poor nutritional status with hypoproteinemia, anemia, diabetes mellitus, and previous history of radiotherapy are the factors most clearly identified with delayed healing of the wound followed by infection and necrosis. Fever, erythema and induration with tenderness, leukocytosis and an increase in CRP may indicate the wound infection. When a collection of purulent exudate is encountered either through needle aspiration or reopening a part of the wound, the diagnosis of wound infection can be established. Effective induction of purulent fluid by applying an adequate drain is the key to avoid further development of infectious debris with progressive venous thrombosis and ischemic necrosis of adjacent tissues. Necrotic tissue should be debrided to prevent a life-threatening complication of carotid artery necrosis and rupture. The use of a vascularized skin flap to cover the desiccated carotid artery and to create a new and fresh pharyngocutaneous fistula is a recommended life-saving technique. This technique of surgical intervention is discussed in the part in the section on salivary fistula after total laryngectomy (page 748).

Complications of tracheotomy wound

Infection of the tracheotomy wound may lead to necrosis and exhaust of tracheal cartilage, resulting in stenosis of the cervical trachea. A tracheal cannula with a low-pressure cuff should be used to avoid pressure necrosis of the tracheal wall and the resultant stenosis. Tracheal mucosa may be injured by a high-pressure cuff, and the pressure should be kept at the level of the minimum requirement, as low as 20–25 mmHg.[6] It has been reported that the cilia of the tracheal mucosa are destroyed by the mildest pressure of the inflatable cuff, and this may involve the mucosa, the submucosal structures, the capillaries and venules and then progress into the stroma and, finally, the tracheal cartilage.[2] Stenting a Silastic T-tube has been used for successful rehabilitation of the stenosed trachea. In cases of annular stenosis due to cicatricial fibrosis, end-to-end anastomosis of the trachea after removing the involved part is a well established technique.

The most dangerous complication of a tracheotomy is massive bleeding from the innominate artery. This complication is almost always fatal from asphyxiation, when it occurs unexpectedly in the ward. Gauze packing into the tracheotomized wound can never control the bleeding. Innominate artery rupture is usually associated with an improper size and shape of the tracheal cannula or with a very low tracheotomy (Fig 55.2). Improper high pressure of the cuff also contributes to a necrosis of the tracheal wall and, then, of the innominate artery.

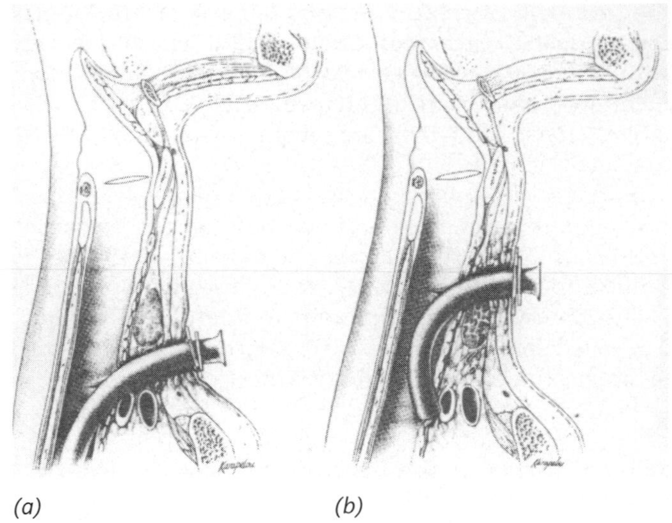

(a) (b)

Figure 55.2 *Innominate artery rupture may be associated with a very low tracheotomy (a), or with improper size and shape of tracheal cannula (b). (Reproduced with permission from Conley JJ.* Complications of Head and Neck Surgery. *Philadelphia: Saunders, 1979: 288.)*

The innominate artery rupture usually occurs 10–14 days after tracheotomy but may occur earlier in previously irradiated patients. A warning sign with a sentinel bleed of a small amount of bright arterial blood usually heralds this exsanguinating bleeding. Careful investigation of this prodromal sign may give the surgeon the only chance to rescue the patient. If erosion of the innominate artery is suspected, even to the slightest degree, by an endoscopic inspection of the necrotic finding of the anterior tracheal wall, a prophylactic ligation of the innominate artery under general anesthesia in the operating room should be considered immediately. Removal of the sternal manubrium offers much better exposure of the innominate artery so that consideration can be given to artery repair by sutures or the creation of a bypass.

Considerable improvements have been made in the surgical management of a necrotic innominate artery. However, we should realize that this complication still remains fatal in the majority of instances, and should be attentive to its prevention by careful surgical procedures and by the use of an appropriate tracheal cannula with well matching shape and size.

Complications after total laryngectomy

In the treatment of advanced laryngeal carcinoma, a total laryngectomy with or without radical neck dissection is the treatment of choice. It is also done as salvage surgery for residual or recurrent carcinomas after radiotherapy with more than 60 Gy. Most of the complications mentioned above may also happen during or after a total laryngectomy, and they are frequently seen in heavily irradiated patients.

Among them, pharyngocutaneous salivary fistula is a troublesome complication, since it is always associated with tissue necrosis that may result in carotid artery rupture and massive bleeding. A life-threatening bleeding is also observed in the innominate artery, that certainly originated from the necrosis of the tracheal wall caused by application of an ill-suited tracheal cannula.

Salivary fistula, tissue necrosis and carotid artery rupture

Salivary fistula after total laryngectomy is usually seen low in the neck just superior to the tracheostoma at the weakest point of suture line of the pharyngeal mucosa, whereas in other patients it is seen high in the neck at the three-point junction of bilateral pharyngeal mucosa to the base of the tongue. The frequency and factors thought to increase the likelihood of salivary fistula have been mentioned in several articles.[4,5,9,12] There is no doubt that the direct factor to all salivary fistulae is a breakdown in the suture line of the pharyngeal mucosa, which is often ascribed to the previous radiotherapy. It has been reported that complications of any kind were observed in more than 70% of patients who underwent total laryngectomy as a salvation surgery after radiotherapy with more than a full dose, and that the salivary fistula was seen in more than 40% of these patients.[11]

Combined diseases such as diabetes mellitus, anemia with bone marrow suppression, and hypoproteinemia due to chemotherapy are well documented factors for the development of salivary fistula.

Saliva from a minute fistula causes tissue infection and micro-venous thrombosis that results in actual loss of tissue due to partial slough of the mucosa. This micronecrosis with infection usually occurs in 5–7 postoperative days, and the salivary fistula is very small at this stage. The patient's temperature rises unexpectedly with marked leukocytosis and an increase of CRP. The neck skin onto the salivary fistula becomes tender and discolors slightly into dark red. These findings are reliable indicators for the development of salivary fistula accompanied by infection and tissue necrosis.

Repair of the salivary fistula is often difficult, particularly if the local area is scarred and irradiated. It can never be a good idea to watch and wait for a spontaneous closure by draining the involved field through a small incision of the affected skin simply by the use of a drain and a pressure dressing around the neck or by cauterizing the salivary fistula with a silver nitrate stick.[18] If possible, it would take a long time, more than a month, prolonging the patient's stay in hospital, and in the majority of cases may leave a difficulty in swallowing due to fibrous stenosis.[10]

Removal of necrotic tissues

The necrosis is really problematic because it often progresses, involving the surrounding tissues with infection by anaerobic organisms. In order to prevent the necrosis extending to surrounding tissues, the salivary fistula should be exteriorized widely enough to drain the field and all necrotic tissues should be debrided completely. A clean wound without infection can be obtained by repeated removal of necrotic tissues with utmost attention not to injure the carotid artery, and a healthy mucocutaneous junction can be expected in no later than a month. The operation to close the fistula is performed at this time.

Creation of clean salivary fistula and carotid artery protection

In severe patients who are diabetic and have a history of radiotherapy, the necrosis may affect the carotid artery. The protection of the carotid artery by covering it with healthy tissue is an urgent task for the surgeon, otherwise a fatal rupture would be feasible.

Necrotic tissues with discolored cervical skin are carefully elevated along the carotid artery and just at the surface of the prevertebral fascia under general anesthesia, and completely removed. Necrotic tissues that surround the fistula are excised sharply by scissors, leaving an intact part of pharyngeal mucosa. A pedicled skin flap is raised in the anterior chest wall so as to contain the second and third perforators of the internal thoracic artery and the concomitant veins. The flap is rotated about 90° into the neck and the fresh wound, after the removal of necrotic tissue, is covered with this skin flap. The neck skin between the wound and the flap is separated by a longitudinal incision, and the pedicle of the rotation flap is sutured to both edges of the separated neck skin. A new salivary fistula that has a clean mucocutaneous junction is created by suturing the flap to the viable part of pharyngeal mucosa. This is useful to exteriorize the salivary stream more effectively. The exposed carotid artery can well be covered with this skin flap, and is protected safely and effectively. The donor defect on the anterior chest is closed simply by suturing both edges of the defect. For adequate rotation of the flap and advancement of surrounding skin, it is mandatory to undermine the skin as far as possible, taking the utmost care not to injure the perforating vessels for the flap (Figs 55.3 and 55.4).

Closure of salivary fistula

After the inevitable period of waiting for 3–4 weeks until a good mucocutaneous junction is completed, an operation to close the fistula is performed. Many surgical methods to close the salivary fistula have been

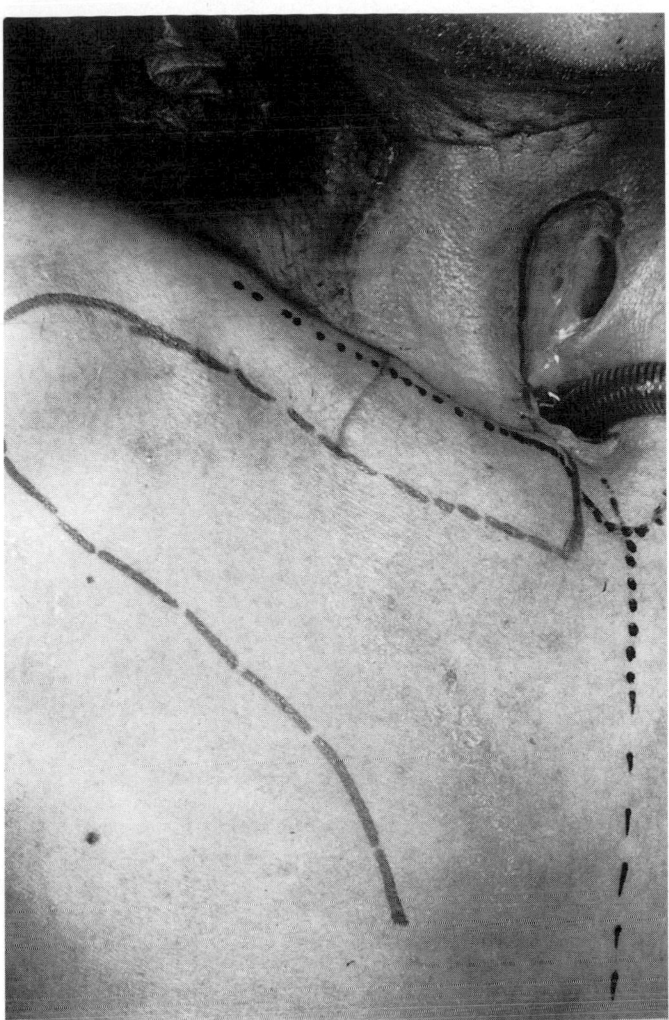

Figure 55.3 *Design of skin incision for a rotation flap to cover the carotid artery and to create a new and clean pharyngocutaneous fistula.*

reported,[13,17,19,20] but the principles of providing two epithelial surfaces are the same: one to provide an internal lining closing the pharyngeal cavity and the other to provide an external lining. A simple closure using two local skin flaps that surround the fistula is not successful, certainly because of hypovascularity of these flaps.

The author has experience with many successful repairs by a combined use of two kinds of pedicled skin flap – a small hinge flap of the surrounding cervical skin and a pedicled skin flap obtained from the anterior aspect of the chest. This combination is reliable for patients who have not been irradiated. In heavily irradiated patients, however, whose cervical skin has deteriorated in its biologic character, the success rate of this combination is not always satisfactory, and further reinforcement with a pedicled pectoralis major muscle flap is preferable, producing much better results.[16]

A small hinge flap is designed in the neck using a piece of skin that surrounds the fistula. The fistula is closed

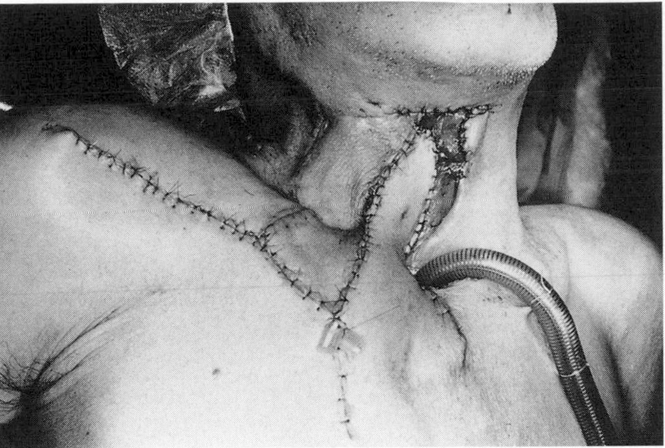

Figure 55.4 *The carotid artery can well be protected with the rotation flap. The donor defect on the anterior chest is closed simply by suturing both edges of the defect. A new fistula works effectively to exteriorize the salivary stream.*

primarily with this small hinge flap, providing the internal lining of the fistula. Irradiated and hypovascular cervical skin can be utilized as an internal lining only when it is covered with an external lining using viable, nonirradiated distant flaps such as an anterior chest skin flap. The hinge flap can be raised from the skin that has already been rotated into the neck for the carotid artery protection. A new skin flap can be harvested from the other side of the chest. The width of this skin flap is about

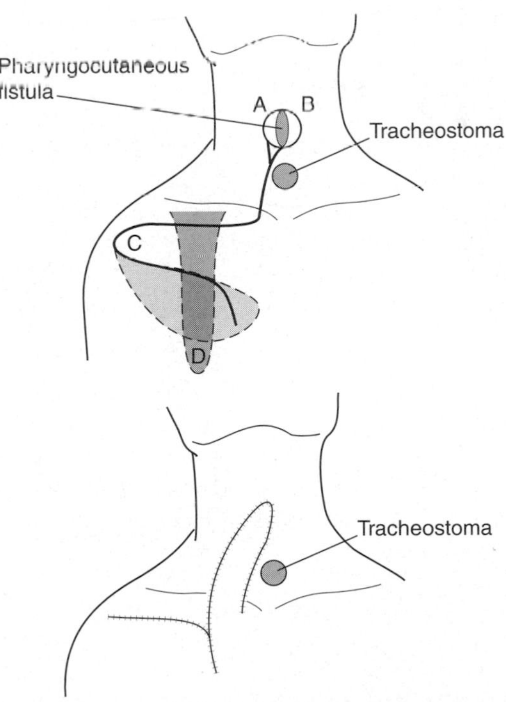

Figure 55.5 *Schema of surgical procedures to close pharyngocutaneous fistula by a combined use of three kinds of pedicled flaps; hinge flap next to the fistula (A, B), rotation flap on the anterior chest (C), and a superiorly based pectoralis major muscle flap (D).*

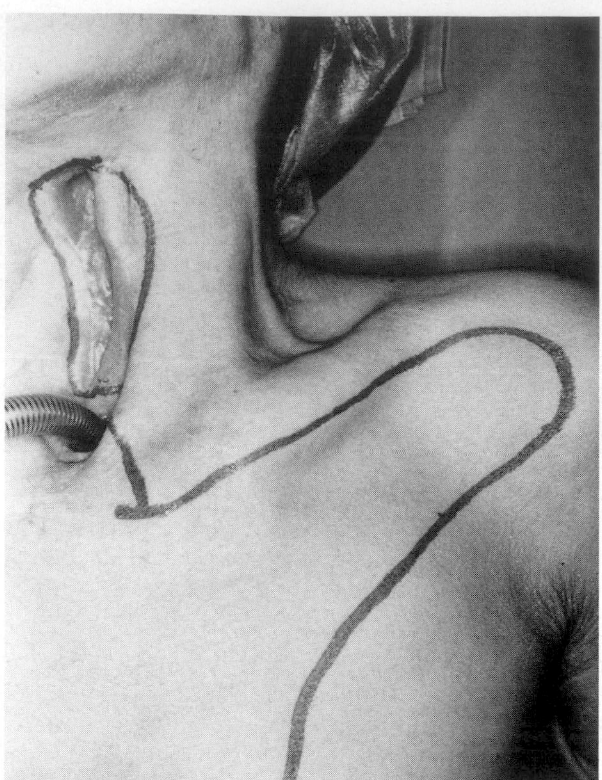

Figure 55.6 *Design of skin incisions for a rotation flap to close a large pharyngocutaneous fistula of the same patient as in Figs 55.3 and 55.4.*

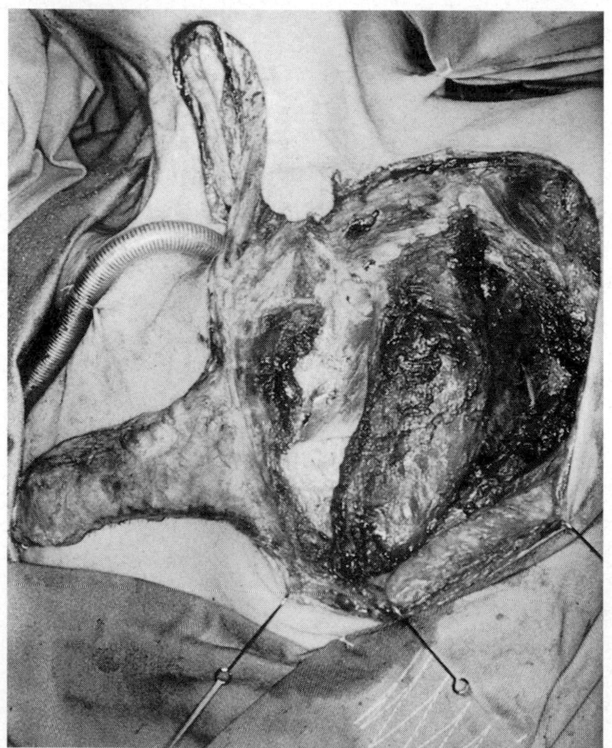

Figure 55.7 *A hinge flap in the neck and a rotation flap on the anterior chest are elevated, and a superiorly based pectoralis major muscle flap is ready for the combined use with these skin flaps.*

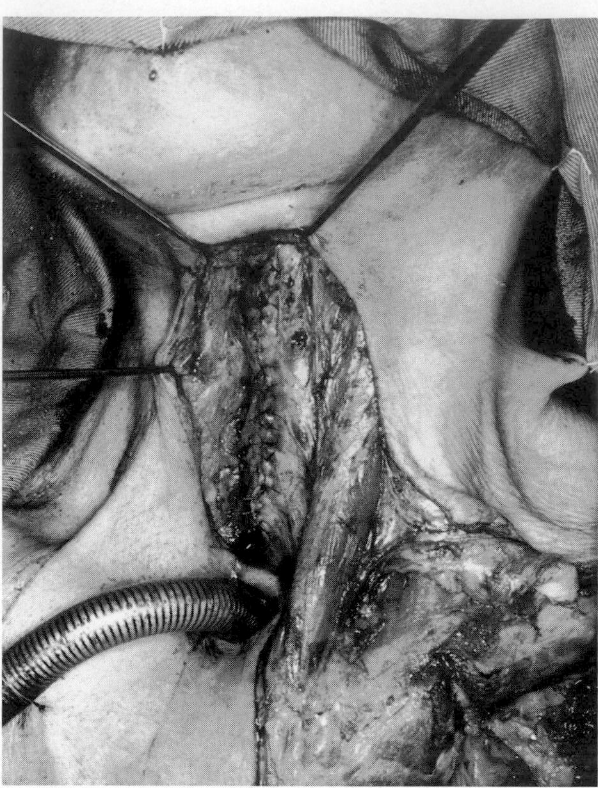

Figure 55.8 *Fistula is closed primarily with a hinge flap providing the internal lining of the fistula.*

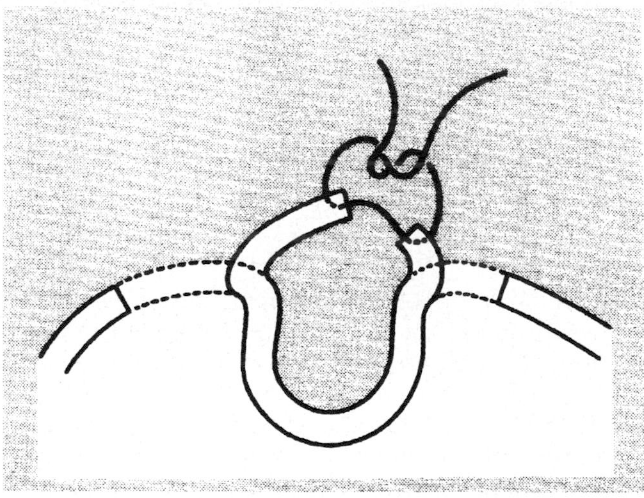

Figure 55.9 *Schema of how to suture the skin flaps.*

5 cm and its length is about 10–12 cm, which may diverge in each case depending on how far the fistula is located from the base of the flap. After raising this skin flap, the chest skin is undermined downward to the level of the nipple and laterally to expose the pectoralis major muscle as extensively as possible. After being divided from the pectoralis minor, a longitudinal pectoralis major muscle flap that measures about 5 × 10 cm is raised upward to

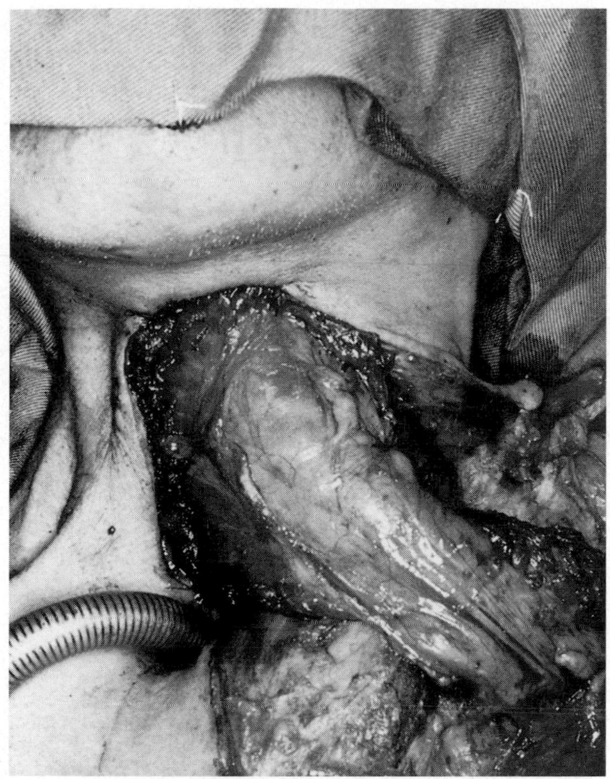

Figure 55.10 *The wound of internal lining of the fistula is covered and satisfactorily reinforced with the muscle flap.*

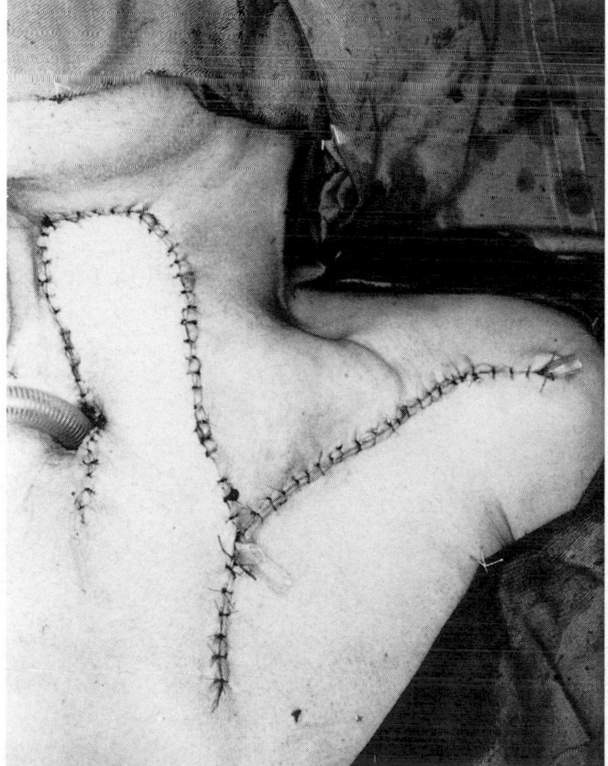

Figure 55.11 *A rotation flap on the anterior chest is sutured over the muscle flap as an external lining of the fistula. The donor defect can be closed simply.*

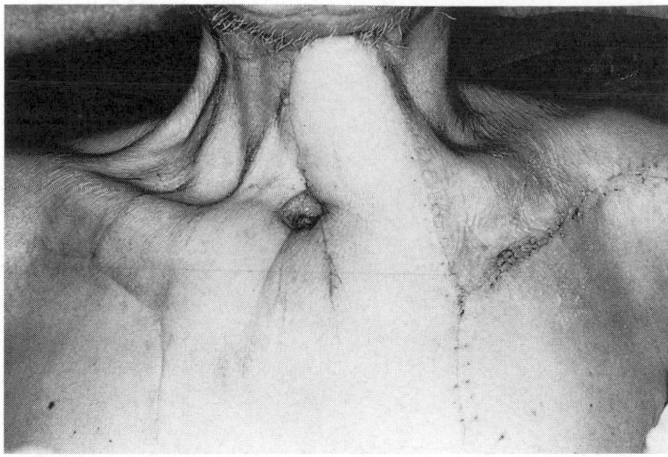

Figure 55.12 *Repair of the salivary fistula with severe necrosis has been completed by the use of bilateral rotation flaps on the anterior chest: right side for protecting the carotid artery in the first stage and the left side for closing the fistula in the second stage. The patient began to swallow foods 2 weeks after the second stage without difficulty.*

the clavicle so as to contain the nutrient thoracoacromial artery and its concomitant veins. By detaching muscle insertions to the clavicle, the muscle flap is mobilized as a superiorly based and vascular pedicled flap, and can be rotated over the clavicle and into the neck without difficulty. The wound of internal lining of the fistula is covered and satisfactorily reinforced with this muscle flap. The anterior chest skin flap, rotated about 90° into the neck, is sutured over the muscle flap as an external lining of the fistula (Figs 55.5–55.12).

The pectoralis major myocutaneous flap is utilized in many cases of head and neck reconstruction, but is not a good candidate for the repair of a small salivary fistula near the tracheostoma because of the thickness of the tissue complex being transferred. The muscle flap, on the other hand, can well be utilized in most cases since it does not contain a thick subcutaneous fat layer, and can easily be harvested through a relatively small skin incision for the anterior chest skin flap.

Necrosis of trachea and innominate artery rupture

Necrosis of the tracheal wall that may provoke a life-threatening bleeding from the innominate artery is observed as a complication of a tracheotomy, as mentioned above. However, we should realize that the incidence of this hazardous complication is much higher in patients after total laryngectomy, if a tracheal cannula with an improper size and shape is used inadvertently.

In cases where a tracheostoma is skillfully created and a continuous suction drainage works well in a completely closed wound, the use of a tracheal cannula is not always necessary for the patients after simple laryngectomy. It is, however, usually adopted for about 7–10 postoperative

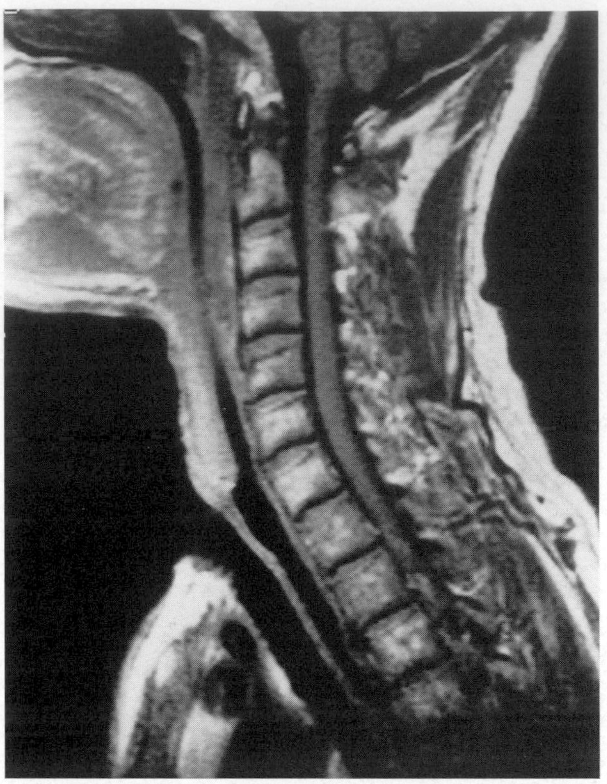

Figure 55.13 *MRI demonstrates flexion of the trachea of a laryngectomized patient, that is almost straight with only a very slight curvature.*

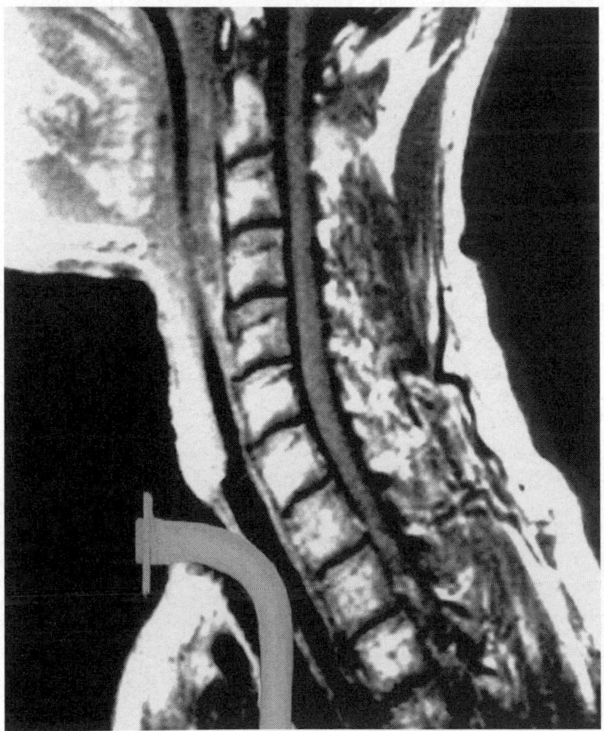

Figure 55.14 *Pressure necrosis of the posterior wall of the trachea is feasible, if a tracheal cannula with an improper flexion is used. The tip of the cannula may injure the anterior wall of the trachea and, then, the innominate artery, resulting in massive bleeding.*

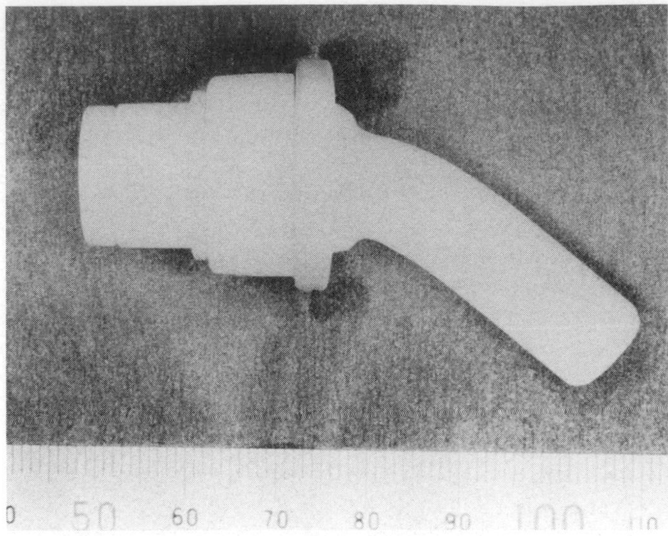

Figure 55.15 *A newly developed tracheal cannula is almost straight with only a very slight curvature.*

days when a total laryngectomy is accomplished together with radical neck dissection, extended resection of paratracheal nodes and unilateral thyroidectomy. This is because combined use of a continuous suction drainage with a tracheal cannula and sterilized gauzes for a mild pressure dressing is good enough to eliminate a dead space that may occur just lateral to or behind the tracheostoma. For the patients who are connected to a respirator, the use of a cuff of the tracheal cannula is also mandatory.

We should realize that the flexion of tracheal cannulas available as commercial products is too sharp and can not harmonize with the trachea after total laryngectomy, because the trachea is actually almost straight, down to the carina, showing only a very mild curvature, which is clearly demonstrated in MRI of laryngectomized patients (Fig 55.13). Necrosis of the posterior wall of the trachea

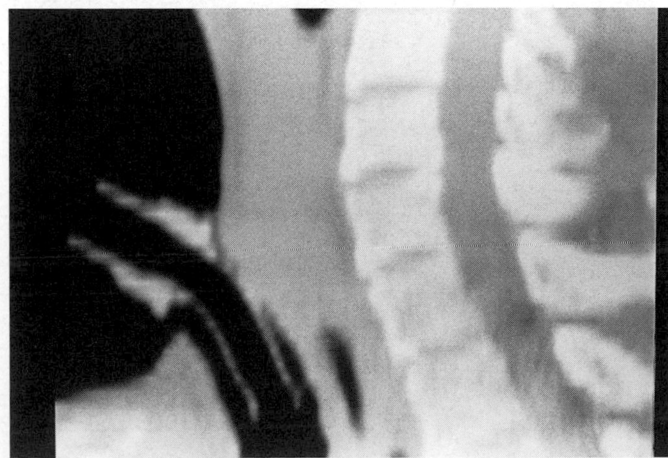

Figure 55.16 *MRI shows a new cannula fits well to the trachea of a laryngectomized patient.*

is feasible, if the pressure of an improperly shaped cannula disturbs the microcirculation of the tracheal mucosa. The anterior wall of the trachea is susceptible to a pressure necrosis by the tip of the cannula, which may progressively injure the innominate artery, resulting in massive bleeding (Fig 55.14). This exsanguinating bleeding from the innominate artery is almost always fatal when it occurs unexpectedly in the ward, and we should be attentive to its prevention. A new tracheal cannula has been developed for this purpose, which is almost straight with only a very mild curvature and fits well to the trachea of laryngectomized patients (Figs 55.15 and 55.16).

References

1. Becker GD, Parell GJ, Busch DF, Finegold SM, Acquarelli MJ. Anaerobic and aerobic bacteriology in head and neck cancer surgery. *Arch Otolaryngol* 1978; **104:** 591–4.
2. Conley JJ. Tracheostomy complications. In: Conley JJ, ed. *Complications of Head and Neck Surgery.* Philadelphia: Saunders, 1979: 274–92.
3. Crockett DM, McCabe BF, Shive CJ. Complications of laser surgery for recurrent respiratory papillomatosis. *Ann Otol Rhinol Laryngol* 1987; **96:** 639–44.
4. Dedo DD, Alonso WA, Ogura JH. Incidence, predisposing factors and outcome of pharyngocutaneous fistulas complicating head and neck surgery. *Ann Otol* 1975; **84:** 833–40.
5. Dejong PC, Struber WH. Pharyngeal fistula after laryngectomy. *J Laryngol Otol* 1970; **84:** 897–903.
6. Grillo HC, Cooper JD, Geffin B, Pontoppidan H. A low-pressure cuff for tracheostomy tubes to minimize tracheal injury. A comparative clinical trial. *J Thorac Cardiovasc Surg* 1971; **62:** 898–907.
7. Johnson JT, Myers EN. Management of complications of head and neck surgery. In: Myers EN, Suen JY, eds. *Cancer of the Head and Neck,* 3rd edn. Philadelphia: Saunders, 1996: 693–711.
8. Kawaida M, Fukuda H, Kawasaki J. Conservative therapy for nonspecific laryngeal granuloma. *Jpn J Phoniatr Logoped* 1991; **32:** 11–17.
9. Kent SE, Liu KC, Das Gupta AR. Postlaryngectomy pharyngocutaneous fistulae. *J Laryngol Otol* 1985; **99:** 1005–8.
10. Kirchner JA, Scatliff JH. Disabilities resulting from healed salivary fistula. *Arch Otolaryngol* 1962; **75:** 46–9.
11. Kraus DH, Pfister DG, Harrison LB *et al.* Salvage laryngectomy for unsuccessful larynx preservation therapy. *Ann Otol Rhinol Laryngol* 1995; **104:** 936–41.
12. Lavelle RJ, Maw AR. The etiology of post laryngectomy pharyngo-cutaneous fistula. *J Laryngol Otol* 1972; **86:** 785–93.
13. Maisel RH, Liston SL. Combined pectoralis major myocutaneous flap with medially based deltopectoral flap for closure of large pharyngocutaneous fistulas. *Ann Otol* 1982; **91:** 98–100.
14. Miller DR, Bergstrom L. Vascular complications of head and neck surgery. *Arch Otolaryngol* 1974; **100:** 136–40.
15. Montgomery WW. *Surgery of the Upper Respitatory System.* Vol 2. Philadelphia: Lea & Febiger, 1973.
16. Murakami Y, Ikari T, Haraguchi S, Okada K, Maruyama T, Tateno H. Repair of salivary fistula after reconstruction of pharyngoesophagus. *Arch Otolaryngol Head Neck Surg* 1988; **114:** 770–4.
17. Parnes SM, Goldstein JC. Closure of pharyngocutaneous fistulae with the rhomboid flap. *Laryngoscope* 1985; **95:** 224–5.
18. Raman R, Ariayanayagam C. Closure of orocutaneous and pharyngocutaneous fistulas. *Plast Reconstr Surg* 1987; **79:** 310. [Letter]
19. Sawyer R, Papavasiliou A. Repair of large pharyngeal defects: new application of split-thickness skin graft. *J Laryngol Otol* 1982; **96:** 125–34.
20. Shanmugham MS. Repair of pharyngocutaneous fistula using bipedicled tubed flap. *J Laryngol Otol* 1986; **100:** 493–6.

Evaluation and management of chronic aspiration

Andrew Blitzer

Aspiration is contamination of the airway with saliva, secretions or food material and may produce life-threatening pulmonary disease. Intermittent or persistent aspiration may cause symptoms including cough, intermittent fever, recurrent tracheobronchitis, atelectases, pneumonia and/or empyema. The pulmonary disease may be associated with weight loss, cachexia and dehydration. Aspiration causes approximately 50 000 deaths in stroke patients alone per year. Laryngeal dysfunction may cause aspiration, allowing pulmonary contamination with swallowed material. In other cases it is related to dysfunction of the oral, pharyngeal, or esophageal phases of swallowing. In other cases it is a combination of laryngeal and swallowing dysfunction. Elderly patients are more prone to aspiration due to muscle weakness with mechanical disability and neurologic impairment. With an ever-increasing aging of our population, these disabilities will be on the rise. The management of these disorders should be based on an evaluation and understanding of the underlying functional impairment.

Pulmonary consequences of aspiration

Small amounts of secretions may be aspirated in normal individuals, during sleep, but they are easily able to clear their airway. Viral infections, ethanol ingestion and altered states of consciousness may increase the amount of the aspirate, decrease the response and therefore increase the severity of the tracheobronchial and pulmonary response. The quantity and frequency of aspiration increases with mechanical impairment of the larynx and pharynx, neurologic impairment and decreasing levels of consciousness.[9,15,37,59] Therefore, the consequences of the aspiration are more severe in these patients.

The pulmonary response to small quantities of aspirated material may vary according to the amount of aspirate, the pH of the aspirate and the underlying status of the pulmonary, cardiovascular and immune systems. Larger amounts of aspirated material, especially with a low pH, usually produce an intense bronchospasm as well as severe injury to the pulmonary capillary endothelium and the epithelium of the distal airway (Mendelson's syndrome).[53] The result of this severe injury is hypotension, hypoxia, hypercapnia and pulmonary edema and in many cases, death. Aspiration of small solid particles may obstruct bronchi, causing a secondary pneumonia and possible empyema. Larger particles may completely obstruct the airway, causing asphyxia and death. A chest radiograph of patients who chronically aspirate often shows scattered irregular densities or occluded segment, mostly the right lower lobes. The upper lobes are often involved in patients who remain supine.[1,7,21,36]

Aspiration related to neurologic dysfunction

Central nervous system disorders may result in significant dysfunction of the larynx and pharynx, producing swallowing disorders. Elderly patients are more likely to develop disorders of the neuromuscular system related to vascular or degenerative diseases.

Changes in the cortex, including stroke, drug-induced changes, seizure disorders, infection, tumors, and/or trauma, often lead to laryngeal dysfunction, swallowing disorders and consequent aspiration. More diffuse brain lesions can cause increased intracranial pressure that may produce altered levels of consciousness, stupor or coma, and therefore a diminished response to the aspirate. Diffuse CNS processes include:

- neoplasia, hematoma, abscess, massive infarction; meningitis, encephalitis, cerebritis;
- degenerative diseases including Jacob–Creutzfeldt disease or adrenoleukodystrophy;
- excess ingestion of alcohol, narcotics or barbiturates; and
- increased or decreased serum calcium, sodium or glucose.

Aspiration may also be seen in the extrapyramidal syndromes of Parkinson's disease, Huntington's disease, myoclonus and tardive dyskinesia. The motor neuron disorders, including progressive spinal muscle atrophy (PSMA), progressive bulbar palsy (PBP), amyotrophic lateral sclerosis (ALS) and poliomyelitis, tend to produce severe laryngeal and pharyngeal dysfunction. Disorders of transmission at the neuromuscular junction such as myasthenia gravis and the Eaton–Lambert syndrome, peripheral nerve disorders, such as Guillain–Barré syndrome, or primary muscle disorders such as muscular dystrophy, poliomyelitis, or metabolic myopathies may also cause aspiration or swallowing disorders.[16]

Normal swallowing physiology

Swallowing is a synchronized, coordinated system of muscular contractions and relaxation of voluntary and involuntary activity which results in the movement of a bolus of material from the oral cavity, through the pharynx, past the laryngeal inlet, and then into the esophagus. When these events are disordered, aspiration, choking, nasal reflux or regurgitation may occur.

The oral phase of swallowing, which is voluntary, consists of the tongue preparing the bolus for swallowing. Food is mixed with saliva and big particles are sorted out to be chewed again. The tongue then compresses the bolus against the palate, shaping it and coating it with mucus, and squeezes the bolus into the oropharynx. The soft palate is then elevated, separating the nasopharynx from the oropharynx, preventing nasal reflux. When the bolus reaches the vallecula, the larynx is elevated, and the pharyngeal phase or involuntary portion of the swallow is initiated.[30]

During this phase, respiration is inhibited. Once the bolus reaches the oropharynx, the tongue base first moves posteriorly, the epiglottis is tipped posteroinferiorly, and the larynx is raised by the supraglottic musculature. The bolus is diverted posterolaterally, by the epiglottis, away from the airway. The bolus descends into the hypopharynx, with the airway raised and protected by the epiglottis, the aryepiglottic folds, false cords, and closure of the true vocal cords.[1,4,30,60]

Once the bolus passes through the upper esophageal sphincter, the esophageal phase begins. If the upper esophageal sphincter (the cricopharyngeus muscle) fails to open, or the esophagus fails to contract, swallowing will be impaired and aspiration may occur.[40,80,88] After the pharyngeal phase of swallowing, the cricopharyngeus muscle must relax, allowing passage of the bolus, and then contracts to a pressure equal to or greater than the resting pressure.

The nerve fibers supplying the cricopharyngeus arise in the vagal nuclei and pass without synapse to the motor end plates via the vagus nerve. The motor end plates are cholinergically mediated through nicotinic junctions. The tonic contraction is neurogenic, whilst central inhibition is responsible for the relaxation during swallowing.[25] The cricopharyngeus normally exerts a pharyngeal pressure of 15–23 mmHg and must be overcome by the hypopharynx to induce the opening of the upper esophageal sphincter. Conditions that damage vagal fibers and interfere with the relaxation of the cricopharyngeus, such as basilar artery thrombosis, may cause cricopharyngeal spasm or achalasia. Neuropathic and myopathic processes may also produce a relative cricopharyngeal achalasia, dyssynchrony and dysphagia.

Evaluation of swallowing function

In order to decipher the cause of dysphagia, each phase of swallowing must be evaluated. The evaluation should include a thorough history and physical examination. A fiberoptic laryngoscopy during the swallow can identify any defects in the larynx or pharynx, pooling of secretions in the vallecula or hypopharynx, or a mass lesion which may produce obstruction.

Salivary analysis may be useful in patients who have oral-phase problems, identifying problems or quantity or composition of saliva.[77] The most definitive analysis is a modified barium swallow or 'cookie swallow' in which a video tape is produced and can be replayed at various speeds to identify subtle changes within the phases of the swallow. The patient is kept in an upright position and given small amounts of barium of different consistencies. This best assesses the oral and pharyngeal phases of the swallow, observing for adynamic areas, relative or true obstructions, and dyssynchrony. Assessment of aspiration related to the consistency of the bolus, the position of the patient, and any other associated dysfunction can also be made during this study. The best head position can easily be determined during the swallow which may benefit planned swallowing therapy.[49,50]

Multiple port manometry, in which simultaneous pressure measurement can be taken in the pharynx, cricopharyngeus and esophagus, is a useful way of identifying subtle failures of pressure generation or hyperfunction of the sphincter. Manometry does not, however, yield any information about aspiration. McConnel[52] has shown that the combination of manometry and videofluoroscopy may more accurately diagnose the site of dysfunction.

Ultrasonography has been used to help in assessing the oral phase of swallowing, but cannot be used for the pharyngeal or esophageal phases due to interference of the cervical spine. This study is noninvasive and safe and can be repeated on regular intervals without harm to the patient.[71,74] Radionuclide scans have also been found useful to document aspiration in the evaluation of the patients who have dysphagia. A radioactive bolus, usually composed of ^{99}Tc sulfur colloid, is fed to the patient. The swallow is recorded with a gamma scintillation camera as the bolus passes from the oropharynx to the esophagus. The pharyngeal transit time, clearance rate, and degree of aspiration can easily be quantified.[74] CT and MRI scans can be used to detect brainstem or cortical lesions which may be the etiology of a neurologic dysfunction producing dysphagia.

Laryngopharyngeal sensory testing is a new avenue for evaluating the causes of aspiration. The sensory apparatus can be tested utilizing a pressure- and duration-controlled puff of air delivered to the anterior wall of the pyriform sinus (the area innervated by the superior laryngeal nerve). The air puff is delivered from an internal port of a flexible fiberoptic laryngoscope made especially for this purpose (Pentax Precision Instrument Corporation, Orangeburg, New York). To determine an individual's sensory pressure threshold, air pressure is varied according to the psychophysical method of limits while the duration of the air puff is held constant at 50 milliseconds (ms).[5]

The testing is done via a flexible laryngoscope with an operative channel hooked to the air puff generator. Testing begins by orienting the subject to the supraglottic stimulus with a suprathreshold stream of air for 5 seconds. After a 15-second rest period, presentation of air puffs begins. Six blocks of stimulus administration trials are given in which a threshold is obtained for each block. The mean of the lowest detected pressures from the six blocks is used as that subject's sensory threshold. Both the right and left sides of the pharynx and supraglottic larynx are studied. Sensory decrease and consequent decreased reflexes may lead to aspiration.[5]

Treatment for swallowing disorders

The management of swallowing disorders should address the underlying defect and/or to help provide compensatory activity. In some patients, swallowing therapy addressing consistency, temperature, quantity of food, as well as head position can be of benefit, whilst others may need gavage feedings to bypass the oral phase.[49] Patients with rhinolalia and nasal reflux from velopharyngeal insufficiency may benefit from a prosthetic appliance that will elevate the soft palate, soft palate or posterior pharyngeal wall augmentation, or pharyngeal flaps.

The epiglottis is useful in swallowing, but not crucial as is evidenced by the swallowing abilities of patients after epiglottectomy or supraglottic laryngectomy. Treatment of a combined oral and pharyngeal phase defect in swallowing may include gavage or nasogastric tube feedings. Some patients with nasogastric tubes continue to aspirate a reflux of material around the tube. These patients may need a gastrostomy, and/or tracheostomy, and/or other laryngeal and pharyngeal procedures to prevent life-threatening aspiration.[49,50,72]

Some patients with oral deficits, paralysis, or other dysfunction may be addressed with the use of dental prostheses, such as obturators or guide bar appliances. These can direct food away from nonfunctional areas of the mouth, and allow the more functional areas to deal with the ingested food material. The construction of such an appliance is based upon the functional deficits detected on clinical examination and the modified barium swallow. The benefit of such an appliance can be documented on a repeat modified barium swallow. Adjustments to the appliance can be performed based on this follow-up study.[24,86]

The management of disabilities of the pharyngeal phase of swallowing is usually related to cricopharyngeal muscle dysfunction. True cricopharyngeal achalasia or relative cricopharyngeal achalasia is often aided with a cricopharyngeal myotomy. The myotomy is not, however, a cure-all for dysphagia attributable to a variety of neurologic conditions. Patients who have difficulty in all phases of swallowing from generalized mechanical failure related to such conditions as ALS, brainstem stroke, or myopathies have limited or no benefit from cricopharyngeal myotomy.[3,10,20,44,55,58,64,69,75,84]

Esophageal dysmotility may cause dysphagia, pooling in the hypopharynx, or true regurgitation. Peristalsis is mediated through vagal cholinergic fibers and can be abolished with curare and succinylcholine in the proximal esophagus and by atropine in the distal esophagus. Two agents commonly used to increase contractility of the esophagus are bethanechol (which increases esophageal contractility, but also increases the production of gastric acid) and metoclopramide (a potent antiemetic which has been found additionally to increase contractility without increasing gastric acidity).[29,68] The effect of these or other agents on the upper esophagus and upper esophageal sphincter are still not precisely known. In patients who have diffuse esophageal spasm, the use of histamine blockers in conjunction with calcium channel blockers such as nifedipine or diltiazem (although not FDA approved for this purpose) has been shown to be effective in some cases.[19]

Patients with Parkinson's disease may also present with swallowing disorders. These patients have been found to have:

- a lengthened oral phase of swallowing related to lingual dysmotility;
- a lengthened pharyngeal phase with vallecular stasis; and
- a lengthened esophageal phase due to dysmotility.

These finding are not seen in patients with essential tremor. Poor motility and decreased sphincter pressure is also commonly found in diabetic patients.[68]

Severe esophageal dysmotility may also be found in patients who have acute and chronic changes from caustic ingestion. Caustic agents may also lead to aspiration due to decreased sensation and fibrosis. These changes may be irreversible and difficult to treat. In severe cases, it may be necessary to bypass the esophagus with a gastric pull-up, or interposition of small or large bowel.

Laryngeal incompetence

Aspiration may take place with a normal functioning larynx, if at the end of the swallow, material is left in the hypopharynx. The larynx descends, and as the vocal cords open, retained material may run into the airway, producing a cough or soilage of the airway.

One cause of laryngeal dysfunction is diminished or absent supraglottic sensation which will fail to produce a necessary laryngeal closure. In the normal larynx, unilateral sensory stimulation will evoke reflex adduction of the vocal cords. The sensory signal is carried via the superior laryngeal nerve, and the bilateral motor response is carried via the recurrent laryngeal nerves. Without laryngeal closure, swallowed material may spill through the glottis until it is detected by sensory fibers of the recurrent laryngeal nerve, which provides sensation of the undersurface of the vocal cord and subglottis. If the vagal sensory fibers are also disabled, a cough may not be initiated, and the foreign material will descend into the tracheobronchial tree, until it provokes a response from the vagal tracheal fibers which have considerable cross-over.

Mechanical or neuromuscular impairment of the vocal cords may also lead to aspiration. When a unilateral vocal cord paralysis prevents complete glottic closure, the airway may become soiled during a swallow. The cough reflex is also diminished since it becomes much harder to build up an adequate subglottic pressure without lateralizing the paralyzed cord. Mechanical disabilities such as congenital abnormalities, anatomic changes due to trauma, or deficiencies due to surgery or loss of vocal cord volume may leave an open glottis and lead to aspiration. Traumatic dislocation of the cricoarytenoid joint may also predispose a patient to aspiration when the vocal cord is fixed in a relatively open position.[48,70]

Evaluation of laryngeal dysfunction

Indirect laryngoscopy and fiberoptic laryngoscopy should be performed at rest and during function, in patients who have an open glottic chink, hoarseness, and intermittent aspiration, to determine the etiology. The movement (including tremors, twitches and other unusual movements) and the coordination of the vocal cord activity can be evaluated visually. In addition, the use of a stroboscope will slow the motion to allow for evaluation of very rapid, unusual or uncoordinated movements. This examination can be combined with feeding the patient material with bright green food coloring to observe for clearance, pooling and laryngeal penetration.

Electromyography of the larynx will provide electrical evidence of early neuromuscular change such as patterns of denervation, reinnervation, tremor, myoclonus and myopathy.[14]

Electroglottography and photoglottography have also been used to study characteristics of the vocal cord movement. Electroglottography is based on the change in electrical potential from the motion of the vocal cords, as measured by surface electrodes. Photoglottography is based on the change of transglottic transmission of light by the opening and closing of the vocal cords. In cases where a brainstem or central etiology for the laryngeal dysfunction is being considered, electroencephalography, brainstem-evoked response audiometry, CT and MRI scans are often essential.[35]

Treatment of aspiration and laryngeal incompetence

Once the etiologic evaluation is complete, and a presumptive diagnosis has been made, a treatment plan can be made. The therapeutic plan should be based on the patient's underlying disease, the likelihood for recovery, general medical status, quality of life issues, severity of aspiration, and laryngeal incompetence.

Patients who chronically aspirate copious secretions may warrant a separation of the airway and food passages. Tracheotomy is the most commonly used method of providing this separation. The airway can be secured utilizing a tracheotomy tube with a cuff. The tracheotomy tube cuff will keep secretions or food substances from entering the airway. It will also provide access for good pulmonary toilet. Suctioning of secretions above the cuff is necessary to prevent soilage of the airway upon cuff deflation. Tracheotomy is only a short-term solution, since with time, pressure from the cuff will produce tracheomalacia, and an inability to obtain an effective seal, allowing continued airway soilage. Therefore, other solutions are necessary for long-term disability.[18,32,51]

Glottic prosthesis

A glottic stent is an attempt to separate the food and air passages without the use of an inflated cuffed tracheotomy tube, much like a cork in a bottle. The prosthesis can be prefabricated or custom made and is placed in the larynx endoscopically, is usually held in place with transcutaneous sutures, and can be removed if the patient improves. The patient has a tracheotomy for an airway. The problems with this technique have been related to local inflammation, discomfort, scarring at the glottic level, and the leak of fluid around the prosthesis due to an ineffective seal.[83]

A new type of stent has recently been described by Eliachar *et al.*[31] It is made of a soft silicone material which minimizes local tissue inflammation, discomfort and scarring. It easily contours to prevent leakage around the stent. Since it is hollow and soft, it has a superior slit in it, which allows phonation through the tube while maintaining a seal in the glottic opening. The stent is placed through the tracheostomy over a Yankower suction tip, and is held in place by an external adjustable tab.

Vocal cord augmentation

The lateralized vocal cord due to anatomic deficiency, mechanical impairment, or a neuromuscular disability should be corrected if symptomatic. In 1911, Brunings[17] reported moving a paralyzed vocal cord toward the midline using an injection of paraffin, but it produced granulomas and was abandoned. Other materials were tested including glycerine, cartilage, bone dust, and tantalum. Tantalum and glycerine and then Teflon and glycerine were first used by Arnold,[2] in 1962. Other authors[46,63,67] have since reported successful treatment of vocal cord paralysis using Teflon injection. Teflon is injected into the larynx during a direct laryngoscopy using local anesthesia so that the airway and voice can be continuously assessed. Vocal cord injection of Teflon percutaneously has also been performed in selected patients via the cricothyroid membrane, as recently reported by Ward *et al.*[82] We are currently injecting Teflon with an oral injector, observing via a videofiberoptic laryngoscope.

Once injected, Teflon is difficult to remove from the larynx, therefore judicious use is imperative. Teflon accidentally placed in the vocalis muscle may provoke fibrosis and produce a change in the resonant characteristics of the vocal cord. In addition to medializing the paralyzed vocal cord, Teflon can be used to augment some vocal cord deficiencies. An alternative to Teflon is fat injection or autologous collagen, which is not permanent but can medialize the vocal cord for a year or more.[28,33,65,66]

In patients who have had recurrent laryngeal nerve trauma or brainstem stroke where there is a possibility of return of function, glycerine or Gelfoam injection can be used for medialization for a limited time until the material is resorbed.[67] If function does not return and the patient again becomes symptomatic, the vocal cord can be medialized with a more permanent material.

For patients with larger laryngeal defects, augmentation with autogenous costochondral, nasal, septal or thyroid cartilage, or alloplastic materials may be safer and more effective. Meurmann, in 1952,[54] first described a technique in which cartilage was placed submucosally through a midline thyrotomy. This technique was later refined by others.[45,54,62,73,81] Isshiki described several different procedures for modifying the laryngeal framework, including a medialization laryngoplasty (type I) for voice improvement and correcting glottic incompetency to avoid aspiration in cases of a vocal cord paralysis.[38,39] In this procedure a window is created in the thyroid ala, and the paralyzed vocal cord is medialized using cartilage or alloplastic material inserted via the window. Other authors have devised their own modifications of this technique, achieving good results.[27,41,61]

The implant procedure can be combined with a vocal fold adduction procedure, as described by Isshiki, to provide good posterior laryngeal closure.[38] Woodson[85] recently described a modification of Isshiki's technique which improves the exposure of the postcricoid area during surgery and allows for a simultaneous cricopharyngeal myotomy.

Glottic and supraglottic laryngeal closure

Surgical closure of the larynx will allow adequate separation of the food and air passages. This avoids tracheal damage from a constantly inflated cuffed tracheotomy tube, and creates a potentially reversible situation if the patient recovers laryngeal and pharyngeal function.

A glottic closure procedure, which is performed through a median thyrotomy, was described by Montgomery in 1975.[57] The mucosa of the vocal cords is stripped bilaterally, and a figure-of-eight suture is placed to close the glottis, allowing fibrous union of the vocal cords. This technique allows adequate separation of the air and food passages with a permanent tracheotomy. The problems associated with this procedure are:

- the patient cannot phonate;
- the seal may pull apart before healing and leak posteriorly if the vocal cords are functional preoperatively; and
- the procedure is not easily reversed due to scarring of the vocal folds with poor vibration.

An alternative is closure of the supraglottis, a procedure that does not produce glottic webs or vocal fold scar. Habel and Murray, in 1972,[34] described a two-layered horizontal closure of the supraglottis via a pharyngotomy. The epiglottis, aryepiglottic folds, arytenoids and interarytenoid area are then incised and the tip of the epiglottis is then folded over the arytenoids and sutured in place. Patients cannot phonate, and breathe through a tracheotomy tube. The procedure is reversible as reported by Strome and Fried[76] in 1983. In some cases recurrent aspiration occurs, perhaps due to the suture line opening posteriorly from the spring of the epiglottic cartilage. Castellanos[23] recently described a procedure in which the supraglottis is closed using what he termed a petiole supraglottopexy. This procedure is approached via a thyrotomy. A wide pre-epiglottic dissection is performed to free the epiglottis from its ligamentous attachments. Once mobilized, the epiglottic petiole is sewn onto the incised interarytenoid mucosa to form a superior line closure. Then the false cords are approximated to form a second layer of supraglottic closure. The failures of supraglottic closure due to muscle tension pulling apart the suture line has recently been addressed by Thumfart *et al.*[78] He described using preoperative botulinum toxin injections to weaken the laryngeal muscles, thereby decreasing the muscle pull.

A vertical supraglottic closure was created to avoid the posterior opening and leave a small opening at the top by Biller *et al.* in 1983 for patients undergoing total glossectomy.[12] This procedure leaves an opening at the level of the tip of the epiglottis, aspiration doesn't occur, but phonation is possible in some patients. This author has used this closure, via a pharyngotomy, successfully in several patients with intractable aspiration. Once the pharynx is open and the supraglottis exposed, a continuous incision is made along the lateral borders of the epiglottis, onto the aryepiglottic folds, across the arytenoid mucosa and connected posteriorly in the interarytenoid mucosa. Dual mucosal flaps are then elevated, forming two separate layers for closure, with the formation of a vertical tube from these supraglottic structures. Patients often can again eat, and some can speak.

Laryngeal diversion

Lindeman,[47] in 1975, described a potentially reversible procedure to separate air and food passage. He separates the trachea at the third or fourth tracheal ring, with the distal portion of the trachea brought out and sewn to the neck skin. The proximal tracheal stump and larynx are sewn end to side to a small opening in the esophagus, allowing all swallowed material entering the larynx to exit into the esophagus; since the airway is separated, there is no chance of contamination. However, phonation is not possible due to airway separation. Lindeman[47] reported two such reversals of his procedure in patients who recover function and no longer need the airway separation. This author has used this technique many times with success.[13,87] Baron and Dedo[8] reported an alternative technique in which a blind end pouch is created from the proximal trachea, in patients who had high tracheostomies, with a relatively immobile segment. Another approach to the patient with a very high preliminary tracheostomy was described by Krespi *et al.*,[43] in which a superiorly based mucosal flap is created and there is resection of the cricoid cartilage and the first and second tracheal rings. An esophagotomy is made at the level of the first tracheal ring and the tracheal mucosal flap is sutured end to side to the esophagotomy. An alternative diversion technique in which both the proximal and distal trachea stumps are diverted to the anterior cervical skin was described by Tucker (double-barrelled tracheostoma).[79] The proximal trachea is brought out to the skin through a split in the sternocleidomastoid muscle, allowing compression of the trachea, minimizing leakage of aspirated material to the skin. This procedure has the obvious disadvantage of draining corrosive substances to the cervical skin.

Partial cricoid resection

Some patients who have head and neck cancer resections develop postoperative aspiration due to a narrowed hypopharyngeal inlet. Krespi and Sisson[42] described a submucosal dissection of the posterior aspect of the cricoid, followed by the removal of a large segment of the center of the posterior cricoid lamina. This resection in conjunction with a cricopharyngeal myotomy leaves a large hypopharyngeal portal for secretions and food, and decreases the anteroposterior diameter of the larynx. Patients may require a permanent tracheotomy, but phonatory capability remains. Another procedure for patients who have continued aspiration after supraglottic laryngectomy, was described by Biller and Urken.[11] Vertical cuts are made in half of the cricoid cartilage, allowing for a collapse of the hemilarynx., thereby decreasing the space available for airway soilage, and in some patients a functional airway is maintained. Cummings[26] described a subperichondrial cricoidotomy as an alternative to laryngectomy for patients with little chance of recovery of neurologic function. The cricoid cartilage is exposed and divided anteriorly. The inner and outer perichondrium are then closed as two layers and a sternohyoid muscle flap is interposed between the subglottis and the necessary tracheostomy.

Laryngectomy

The oldest treatment for life-threatening aspiration has been a total laryngectomy. Total laryngectomy provides a permanent cutaneous tracheostoma and a permanent separation of the airway and food passage, but eliminates phonation, or the possibility of reversal in patients who might recover some or all of their function.[56] Some suggest that laryngectomy, particularly a narrow-field laryngectomy, is still indicated in patients with poor prognoses or associated medical problems.[22]

New alternatives for management of aspiration due to muscle weakness or paralysis include nerve grafting. Aviv *et al.*[6] described sensory nerve grafting to restore supraglottic sensation, and thereby diminish the chance of aspiration. Motor nerve grafting has not returned normal function, but has returned some motor tone to weakened muscles.[90] Electrical pacing of weakened or paralyzed laryngeal muscles may also be useful in patients who aspirate. The pacers have been used with respiratory sensors to pace paralyzed abductor muscle for patients with bilateral vocal fold paralysis. The pacing system may also benefit the adductor muscles and pharynx when the appropriate sensors have been developed.[89]

Conclusions

Laryngeal dysfunction and swallowing disorders may produce chronic recurrent aspiration and become life-threatening. A thorough evaluation to identify which of the diverse etiologies is causing the disability is mandatory. Based on the etiology, there is an eclectic group of therapeutic modalities available to address the etiology or allow better laryngeal and swallowing function. Many innovative surgical procedures are available to compensate for some of the functional deficits. If the patient recovers from his/her underlying disability, some of the procedures can be reversed. In the future it may be possible to use more sophisticated nerve grafting or electronic microcomputerized laryngeal pacing to allow return of laryngeal and pharyngeal function. Continued research in these areas will allow physicians to better treat disorders leading to life-threatening aspiration.

References

1. Ardan GM, Kemp FH. The protection of laryngeal airway during swallowing. *Br J Radiol* 1952; **25**: 406–16.
2. Arnold GE. Vocal rehabilitation of paralytic dysphonia. *Arch Otolaryngol* 1962; **76**: 358–68.
3. Asherson N. Achalasia of the cricopharyngeal sphincter. *J Laryngol Otol* 1950; **64**: 747–58.
4. Atkinson M, Kramer P, Wyman SM, Ingelfinger FJ. The dynamics of swallowing. I. Normal pharyngeal mechanisms. *J Clin Invest* 1957; **36**: 581–8.
5. Aviv JE, Martin JH, Keen, MS, Debell M, Blitzer A. Air pulse quantification of supraglottic and pharyngeal sensation: a new technique. *Ann Otol Rhinol Laryngol* 1993; **102**: 777–80.
6. Aviv JE, Mohr JP, Blitzer A, Thomson JE, Close LG. Restoration of laryngopharyngeal sensation by neural anastomosis. *Arch Otolaryngol Head Neck Surg* 1997; **123**: 154–60.
7. Awe WC, Fletcher WS, Jacob SW. The pathophysiology of aspiration pneumonitis. *Surgery* 1966; **60**: 232–9.
8. Baron BS, Dedo HH. Separation of the larynx and trachea for intractable aspiration. *Laryngoscope* 1980; **90**: 1927–32.
9. Bartlett JG, Gorbach SL. The triple threat of aspiration pneumonia. *Chest* 1975; **68**: 560–6.
10. Begley MD. Cricopharyngeal achalasia. *J Coll Radiol* 1962; **6**: 138–41.
11. Biller HF, Urken M. Cricoid collapse. A new technique for management of glottic incompetence. *Arch Otolaryngol* 1985; **111**: 740–1.
12. Biller HF, Lawson W, Baek SM. Total glossectomy. A technique of reconstruction eliminating laryngectomy. *Arch Otolaryngol* 1983; **109**: 69–73.
13. Blitzer A. Evaluation and management of chronic aspiration. *N Y State J Med* 1987; **87**: 154–60.
14. Blitzer A, Lovelace RE, Brin MF, Fahn S, Fink ME. Electromyographic findings in focal laryngeal dystonia (spastic dysphonia). *Ann Otol Rhinol Laryngol* 1985; **94**: 591–4.
15. Bonano PC. Swallowing dysfunction after tracheostomy. *Ann Surg* 1970; **174**: 29–33.
16. Brin MF, Younger D. Neurologic disorders and aspiration. *Otolaryngol Clin North Am* 1988; **21**: 691–701.
17. Brunings W. Uber eine neue behandlungsmethode. *Verh Dtsch Laryngol* 1911; **18**: 93–151.
18. Bryant LR, Tinkle JK, Dubiler L. Tracheal damage from cuffed tracheostomy tubes. *JAMA* 1971; **215**: 625–8.
19. Buchin PJ. Swallowing disorders: diagnosis and medical treatment. *Otolaryngol Clin North Am* 1981; **21**: 663–7.
20. Calcaterra TC, Kadell BM, Ward PH. Dysphagia secondary to cricopharyngeal muscle dysfunction: surgical management. *Arch Otolaryngol* 1975; **101**: 726–9.
21. Cameron JL, Reynolds J, Zuidema GD. Aspiration in patients with tracheostomies. *Surg Gynecol Obstet* 1973; **136**: 68–70.
22. Cannon CR, McLean WC. Laryngectomy for chronic aspiration. *Am J Otolaryngol* 1982; **3**: 145–9.
23. Castellanos PF. Method and clinical results of a new transthyrotomy closure of the supraglottic larynx for the treatment of intractable aspiration. *Ann Otol Rhinol Laryngol* 1997; **106**: 451–60.
24. Chalian VA, Drane JB, Standish SM. *Maxillofacial Prosthetics: Multidisciplinary Approach*. Baltimore: Williams & Wilkins, 1971.
25. Christenson J. Innervation and function of the esophagus. In: Stipa S, Belsey RHR, Moraldi A, eds. *Medical and Surgical Problems of the Esophagus*. London: Academic Press, 1981: 14–16.
26. Cummings CW. Epiglottis sewdown (epiglottopexy) procedure. In: *Atlas of Laryngeal Surgery*. St Louis: Mosby, 1984: –.
27. Cummings CW, Purcell LL, Flint PW. Hydroxylapatite laryngeal implants for medialization: a retrospective analysis. *Ann Otol Rhinol Laryngol* 1993; **102**: 843–51.
28. Dedo HH, Urrea RD, Lawson L. Intracordal injection of Teflon in the treatment of 135 patients with dysphonia. *Ann Otol* 1973; **82**: 661–7.
29. Diamant NE. Normal esophageal physiology. In: Cohen S, Soloway RD, eds. *Diseases of the Esophagus*. New York: Churchill Livingstone, 1982: 1–33.
30. Didio LJA, Anderson MC. *The 'Sphincters' of the Digestive System*. Baltimore: Williams & Wilkins, 1968.
31. Eliachar I, Roberts JK, Hayes JD, Tucker HM. A vented laryngeal stent with phonatory and pressure relief capability. *Laryngoscope* 1987; **97**: 1264–8.
32. Fee WE Jr, Ward PH. Permanent tracheostomy: a new surgical technique. *Ann Otol* 1977; **86**: 635–8.
33. Ford CN. Laryngeal injection techniques. In: Ford CN, Bless DM, eds. *Phonosurgery: Assessment and Surgical Management of Voice Disorders*. New York: Raven Press, 1991: 123–41.
34. Habel MB, Murray JE. Surgical treatment of life endangering chronic aspiration pneumonia. *Plast Reconstr Surg* 1972; **49**: 305–11.
35. Hanson DG, Gerratt BR, Ward PH. Glottographic measurements of vocal dysfunction: a preliminary report. *Ann Otol Rhinol Laryngol* 1983; **92**: 413–20.
36. Hawkins DB. Noninfectious disorders of the lower respiratory tract. In: Bluestone CD, Stool SE, eds. *Pediatric Otolaryngology*. Philadelphia: Saunders, 1983: 1265–9.
37. Huxley EJ, Viroslav J, Gray WR, Pierce AK. Pharyngeal aspiration in normal adults and patients with depressed consciousness. *Am J Med* 1978; **64**: 564–8.
38. Isshiki N. Recent advances in phonosurgery. *Folia Phoniatr (Basel)* 1980; **32**: 119–54.
39. Isshiki N, Okamura H, Ishikawa T. Thyroplasty type I (lateral compression) for dysphonia due to vocal cord paralysis or atrophy. *Acta Otolaryngol (Stockh)* 1975; **80**: 465–73.
40. Kirchner JA. The motor activity of the cricopharyngeus muscle. *Laryngoscope* 1958; **68**: 1119–59.
41. Koufman JA. Laryngoplasty for vocal cord medialization: an alternative to Teflon. *Laryngoscope* 1986; **96**: 726–31.
42. Krespi Y, Sisson GA. Management of chronic aspiration by subtotal and submucosal cricoid resection. *Ann Otol Rhinol Laryngol* 1985; **94**: 580–3.

43. Krespi Y, Quatela VC, Sisson GA, Som ML. Modified tracheo-esophageal diversion for chronic aspiration. *Laryngoscope* 1984; **94:** 1298–301.
44. Lebo CP, Sang K, Norris FH. Cricopharyngeal myotomy in amyotrophic lateral sclerosis. *Laryngoscope* 1976; **86:** 862–8.
45. Levine HL, Tucker HM. Surgical management of the paralyzed larynx. In: Bailey B, Biller HF, eds. *Surgery of the Larynx.* Philadelphia: Saunders, 1985: 117–47.
46. Lewy RB. Glottic rehabilitation with Teflon injection the return of voice, cough, and laughter. *Acta Otolaryngol (Stockh)* 1964; **58:** 214–22.
47. Lindeman RA. Diverting the paralyzed larynx: a reversible procedure for intractable aspiration. *Laryngoscope* 1975; **85:** 157–80.
48. Litton WB, Leonard JR. Aspiration after partial laryngectomy: cineradiographic studies. *Laryngoscope* 1969; **79:** 887–907.
49. Logemann JA. *Evaluation and Treatment of Swallowing Disorders.* San Diego: College Hill, 1983.
50. Logemann JA, Bytell DE. Swallowing disorders in three types of head and neck surgical patients. *Cancer* 1979; **44:** 1095–105.
51. MacDonald RE, Smith C, Mitchell D. Airway problems in children following prolonged endotracheal intubation. *Ann Otol* 1966; **75:** 975–86.
52. McConnel FMS. Analysis of pressure generation and bolus transit during pharyngeal swallowing. *Laryngoscope* 1988; **98:** 71–8.
53. Mendelson CL. Aspiration of stomach contents into lungs during obstetrical anesthesia. *Am J Obstet Gynecol* 1946; **52:** 191–205.
54. Meurmann Y. Operative mediofixation of the vocal cord in complete unilateral paralysis. *Arch Otolaryngol* 1952; **55:** 544–53.
55. Mills CP. Dysphagia in pharyngeal paralysis treated by cricopharyngeal sphincterotomy. *Lancet* 1973; **1:** 455–7.
56. Montgomery WW. Total laryngectomy. In: Montgomery WW, ed. *Surgery of the Upper Respiratory System.* Philadelphia: Lea & Febiger, 1973: 484–96.
57. Montgomery WW. Surgical laryngeal closure to eliminate chronic aspiration. *N Engl J Med* 1975; **292:** 1390–1.
58. Montgomery WW, Lynch JP. Oculopharyngeal muscular dystrophy treated by inferior constrictor myotomy. *Trans Am Acad Ophthalmol Otolaryngol* 1971; **75:** 986–93.
59. Nahum AM, Harris JP, Davidson TM. The patient who aspirates – diagnosis and management. *J Otolaryngol* 1981; **10:** 10–16.
60. Negus JE. The second stage of swallowing. *Acta Otolaryngol Suppl (Stockh)* 1949; **78:** 78–82.
61. Netterville JL, Stone RE, Luken ES, Civantos FJ, Ossoff RH. Silastic medialization and arytenoid adduction: the Vanderbilt experience. A review of 116 phonosurgical procedures. *Ann Otol Rhinol Laryngol* 1993; **102:** 413–24.
62. Opheim O. Unilateral paralysis of the vocal cord. *Acta Otolaryngol (Stockh)* 1955; **45:** 226–30.
63. Rontal E, Rontal M, Morse G, Brown EM. Vocal cord injection in the treatment of acute and chronic aspiration. *Laryngoscope* 1976; **86:** 625–34.
64. Ross ER, Green R, Auslander MD, Biller HF. Cricopharyngeal myotomy: management of cervical dysphagia. *Otolaryngol Head Neck Surg* 1982; **90:** 434–41.
65. Rubin HJ. Intracordal injection of silicone in selected dysphonias. *Arch Otolaryngol* 1965; **81:** 604–7.
66. Rubin HJ. Misadventures with injectable polytef (Teflon). *Arch Otolaryngol* 1975; **101:** 114–16.
67. Schramm VL, May M, Lavorato AS. Gelfoam paste injection for vocal cord paralysis: temporary rehabilitation of glottic competence. *Laryngoscope* 1978; **88:** 1268–73.
68. Schulze-Delrieu K. Esophageal pharmacology. In: Cohen S, Soloway RD, eds. *Diseases of the Esophagus.* New York: Churchill Livingstone, 1982: 35–49.
69. Seaman WB. Cineroentgenographic observations of the cricopharyngeus. *Am J Roentgenol Radium Ther Nucl Med* 1966; **96:** 922–31.
70. Sessions DG, Ogura JH, Ciralsky RH. Late glottic insufficiency. *Laryngoscope* 1975; **85:** 950–9.
71. Shawker T, Sonies B, Stone M. Real-time ultrasound visualization of tongue movement during swallowing. *JCU J Clin Ultrasound* 1983; **11:** 485–90.
72. Shedd DP, Scatliff JA, Kirchner JA. A cineradiographic study of post-resectional alterations in oropharyngeal physiology. *Surg Gynecol Obstet* 1960; **110:** 69–89.
73. Smith GW. Aphonia due to vocal cord paralysis corrected by medial positioning of the affected vocal cord with a cartilage autograft. *Can J Otolaryngol* 1972; **1:** 295–8.
74. Sonies BC, Baum BJ. Evaluation of swallowing pathophysiology. *Otolaryngol Clin North Am* 1988; **21:** 637–48.
75. Stevens KM, Newell RC. Cricopharyngeal myotomy in dysphagia. *Laryngoscope* 1971; **81:** 1616–20.
76. Strome M, Fried MP. Rehabilitative surgery for aspiration. *Arch Otolaryngol* 1983; **109:** 809–11.
77. Stuchell RN, Mandel ID. Salivary gland dysfunction and swallowing disorders. *Otolaryngol Clin North Am* 1988; **21:** 649–61.
78. Thumfart WF, Pototschnig CA, Schneider I. Successful closure of the larynx for the treatment of chronic aspiration with the use of botulinum toxin A. *Ann Otol Rhinol Laryngol* 1996; **105:** 521–4.
79. Tucker HM. Management of the patient with an incompetent larynx. *Am J Otolaryngol* 1979; **1:** 47–56.
80. van Overbeck JJ, Betlem HC. Cricopharyngeal myotomy in pharyngeal paralysis. Cineradiographic and manometric indications. *Ann Otol* 1979; **88:** 596–602.
81. Waltner JG. Surgical rehabilitation of voice following laryngofissure. *Arch Otolaryngol* 1958; **67:** 99–101.
82. Ward PH, Hanson DG, Abemayor E. Transcutaneous Teflon injection of the paralyzed vocal cord: a new technique. *Laryngoscope* 1985; **95:** 644–9.
83. Weisberger EC, Huebsch SA. Endoscopic treatment of aspiration using a laryngeal stent. *Otolaryngol Head Neck Surg* 1982; **90:** 215–22.
84. Wilkins SA. Indications for the section of the cricopharyngeus muscle. *Am J Surg* 1964; **108:** 533–8.
85. Woodson G. Cricopharyngeal myotomy and arytenoid adduction in the management of combined laryngeal and pharyngeal paralysis. *Otolaryngol Head Neck Surg* 1997; **116:** 339–43.

86. Wurster CF, Krespi YP, Davis JW. Combined functional oral rehabilitation after radical cancer surgery. *Arch Otolaryngol* 1985; **111:** 530–3.
87. Yarington CT, Linderman RC, Sutton D. Clinical experience with the tracheoesophageal anastomosis for intractable aspiration. *Ann Otol* 1976; **85:** 609–12.
88. Yoshida Y, Miyazaki T, Hirano M, Shin T, Totoki T, Kanaseki T. Localization of efferent neurons innervating the pharyngeal constrictor muscles and the cervical esophagus muscle in the cat by means of horseradish peroxidase method. *Neurosci Lett* 1981; **22:** 91–5.
89. Zealear DL, Netterville JL, Ossoff RH. Electrical pacing of the human larynx. *Ann Otol Rhinol Laryngol* 1996; **105:** 689–93.
90. Zheng H, Li Z, Zhou S, Cuan Y, Wen W. Update: laryngeal reinnervation for unilateral vocal cord paralysis with the ansa cervicalis. *Laryngoscope* 1996; **106:** 1522–7.

Prognostic factors of laryngeal cancer

Alfio Ferlito and Byron J Bailey

Various indicators may predict the clinical course of malignant neoplasms of the larynx. These can be grouped into host factors, tumor factors and treatment factors.

Host factors include age, gender, nutritional status, general condition and immunologic response.

Tumor factors include T stage, N stage, M stage, oncotype (or histologic cell type), grade of malignancy, biologic attributes and the presence of another cancer (whether synchronous or metachronous).

Treatment factors include all available types of therapy and various combinations of these modalities.

Host factors

Age

Data in the literature are controversial concerning the effects of age on survival. Some authors think that prognosis is better in younger patients, whereas others claim it is better in the more elderly. Stell[90] showed that age and sex are not significant prognostic factors in patients with laryngeal cancer. Though statistical analysis shows that survival is significantly shorter in older versus younger patients,[41,45] this probably depends on the fact that older patients are also usually affected by other diseases.

A recent investigation concerning the role of age as a factor in cancer patient survival has been reported by Clayman *et al.*[15] from the MD Anderson Cancer Center. They studied 43 patients with head and neck squamous cell cancer who were 80 years of age and older. When they were computer-matched on the basis of TNM stage, site, gender and race with patients 22–65 years of age, no differences in postoperative complications or survival were found between the two groups. They concluded that in those patients for whom surgical management is deemed appropriate, advanced age should not be considered a negative factor.[15]

Several reports in the literature suggest that young patients with laryngeal cancer have a relatively poor survival rate compared with older patients. A study of 20 patients less than 40 years old with stage I–III laryngeal carcinoma revealed that, although a high percentage of these younger patients presented for treatment with advanced disease, the survival rate compared favorably with the survival in older patients. Shvero *et al.*[81] concluded that this observation supports the aggressive treatment of the initial lesion as well as any recurrence or second primary.

Gender

The site of laryngeal carcinoma differs widely according to gender. For males, the glottis is the commonest site, followed by the supraglottis and then the subglottis. Women are more likely to have cancer of the supraglottis than of the glottis.[93]

Nutritional status

This correlates closely with the host's immunocompetence. Patients in negative nitrogen balance have a worse general condition and respond less well to therapy.[90]

General condition

The patient's performance status is a factor in decisions as to the type of treatment to implement. General condition naturally deteriorates with increasing age.[92] The host's general condition is usually evaluated according to three different systems, as outlined below.

Host [American Joint Committee on Cancer (AJCC)][2]

- H: the physical state (performance scale) of the patient, considering all cofactors determined at the time of stage classification and subsequent follow-up examinations
- H0: normal activity
- H1: symptomatic and ambulatory; cares for self
- H2: ambulatory more than 50% of time; occasionally needs assistance
- H3: ambulatory 50% or less of time; nursing care needed
- H4: bedridden; may need hospitalization

Karnofsky scale: performance status (PS) criteria[44]

Able to carry on normal activity; requires no special care:

- 100: normal; no complaints; no evidence of disease
- 90: able to carry on normal activity; minor signs or symptoms of disease
- 80: able to carry on normal activity with effort; some signs or symptoms of disease

Unable to work; able to live at home and care for most personal needs; requires varying amount of assistance:

- 70: cares for self; unable to carry on normal activity or to do active work
- 60: requires occasional assistance but is able to care for most of own needs
- 50: requires considerable assistance and frequent medical care

Unable to care for self; requires equivalent of institutional or hospital care; disease may be progressing rapidly:

- 40: disabled; requires special care and assistance
- 30: severely disabled; hospitalization indicated although death not imminent
- 20: very sick; hospitalization necessary; active supportive treatment necessary
- 10: moribund, fatal processes progressing rapidly
- 0: dead

Eastern Cooperative Oncology Group Scale (ECOG)[105]

Grade:

- 0: fully active, able to carry on all predisease activities without restriction (Karnofsky 90–100)
- 1: restricted in physically strenuous activity but ambulatory and able to carry out work of a light or sedentary nature, for example light housework or office work (Karnofsky 70–80)
- 2: ambulatory and capable of all self-care but unable to carry out any work activities. Up and about more than 50% of waking hours (Karnofsky 50–60)
- 3: capable of only limited self-care, confined to bed or chair 50% or more of waking hours (Karnofsky 30–40)
- 4: completely disabled, cannot carry on any self-care, totally confined to bed or chair (Karnofsky 10–20)

Other systems are also used in oncology to measure the quality of life of cancer patients, e.g. the Performance Status Scale for Head and Neck Cancer Patients,[51] the Spitzer Quality of Life Index,[89] the Functional Assessment of Cancer Therapy – Head and Neck Version.[14] List *et al.*[52] suggest the use of the Functional Assessment of Cancer Therapy – Head and Neck Scale and the Performance Status Scale for Head and Neck Cancer Patients to describe performance status and quality of life of head and neck cancer patients. A longitudinal assessment of quality of life in laryngeal cancer patients has recently been published.[53]

The patient's performance status can affect not only prognosis but also the choice of treatments.[64] Patients with decreased functional capacity may be deemed 'too sick' for one treatment (e.g. surgery) and receive an alternative (e.g. irradiation).[64] Patients with cancer of the larynx often have other diseases and illnesses in addition to their cancer. These other conditions, which are generally referred to as comorbidities,[26] have a profound effect on treatment selection and prognosis.[65]

Piccirillo and Feinstein[64] have reminded us that the AJCC TNM system for cancer staging is more than 30 years old and is constrained in its ability to provide useful prognostic information. Tumor descriptive data is converted to four disease 'stages' which are associated with a statistical gradient, but this staging process is very limited in terms of its predictive utility. We need information beyond the gross and microscopic extent of the cancer to recommend optimal treatment regimens and to answer questions raised by our patients.

As our knowledge of tumor biology and molecular markers increases, we will be able to expand the number of significant variables available to predict tumor behavior, host resistance and the probability of a successful outcome. We have become more aware of the significance of comorbidity in planning treatment and predicting survival. Severe comorbidity, especially advanced pulmonary and cardiovascular disease predicts the following:

- Radiation therapy will be used alone rather than combined with surgery.
- Length of hospital stay will be increased when surgery is included.
- Prognosis for survival is worse for oral cavity, oropharyngeal and laryngeal cancers.

Immunologic response

Opinions on available immunologic parameters of prognostic relevance vary widely.[33] Many patients with cancer of the larynx have immune deficits or abnormal immune reactions,[57,77] but this altered immunologic condition could depend on multiple mechanisms (alcohol abuse, viruses, malnutrition, aging, etc.). Lymphocytes and plasma cell infiltration at the edge of the neoplasm can be regarded as an expression of the host's reactive potential against tumor cells.[74] However, the prognostic value of markers associated with the host's immune system has not been sufficiently evaluated to date.

Tumor factors

T stage

When the International Union Against Cancer (UICC) published the document *TNM Classification of Malignant Tumours* in 1987[95] and the AJCC followed suit with the same system in 1988,[2] there was agreement for the first time on the TNM classification for laryngeal cancer. The criticism of the new system that subsequently came from laryngologists around the world emphasizes the differences of opinion that are held concerning the prognostic importance of certain biologic, biochemical, histopathologic and clinical findings. It is important to recognize that the TNM laryngeal cancer classification provides only a standardized group of categories for patients with laryngeal cancer, i.e. the system allows us to stratify patients according to the severity of their illness.[4] Then we may share clinical observations from different parts of the world with confidence that we are comparing similar groups of patients. The TNM system provides information on the primary tumor's anatomic location and size and on the presence of regional and distant metastases.[42] Of course, this is useful in predicting survival and the tumor's precise location within the larynx is a relevant factor influencing prognosis. Patients with a supraglottic cancer usually have a worse prognosis than patients with a glottic cancer; in particular, cancers of the aryepiglottic folds present the worst clinical prognosis.[83] Considerable discrepancies can occur between pre therapeutic classification and the actual extension of the tumor, particularly in the case of the larger lesions. Despite recent advances in imaging techniques [computed tomography (CT) and magnetic resonance imaging (MRI)], the tumor's extension, and its depth of invasion in particular, are clinically very difficult to assess. Stell[91] stated that the T stage has very little impact on survival: 'Survival did fall dramatically with an increase in T stage, but this fall is almost entirely due to the increasing incidence of lymph node metastases.' When survival was analyzed by multifactorial methods using Cox's regression technique and taking interactions into account, only N status – not T stage – proved a significant prognostic indicator.[91]

N stage

Treatment and prognosis for patients with laryngeal cancer are mainly determined by nodal status. The most significant single prognostic indicator is the presence or absence of metastatic cancer in cervical lymph nodes. Neck node status is the only factor that significantly predicts length of survival in patients who die of their cancer.[91] Squamous cell carcinoma of the larynx tends to metastasize to the cervical lymph nodes in the form of emboli. Few lymph nodes are involved in the great majority of cases. The level of cervical lymph node involvement is also important: metastases to level 1 (submandibular) and 5 (supraclavicular) worsen the prognosis[60] and so does involvement of the prelaryngeal node.[68] Contralateral involvement, whether synchronous or occurring after primary treatment, is an ominous prognostic finding. Although the number, size and level of invaded nodes is clearly important, these factors are secondary to the overriding prognostic significance of extracapsular spread.[13,19,38,43,46,48,68,86,87,91] Errors in determining the presence and size of occult lymph node metastases have been reduced by the use of ultrasound, ultrasound-guided fine-needle aspiration biopsy, CT and MRI, which should be used for clinical staging. Application of the AJCC/UICC TNM system provides prognostic information. As observed in other organs, monoclonal antibodies can identify occult micrometastases to the cervical lymph nodes which go undetected by conventional light microscopy.[24] In conclusion, the extent of cervical lymph node metastatic distribution is clearly of paramount prognostic importance.

Prognostic information of great importance in laryngeal cancer can be obtained by careful histopathologic examination of cervical lymph nodes. Popella and Glanz.[66] analyzed 5581 lymph nodes from 167 patients with T2–T4 laryngeal cancers and found metastatic cancer in 397 nodes. They found positive nodes in the lower third of the neck in 16% of T2 tumors, 15% of T3 tumors and 19% of T4 tumors. In addition, they found extracapsular spread in 80% of the N3 cases, 41% of the N2 cases, 55% of the N1 cases and 16% of the N0 cases. The pN-5-year-survival rate showed that only 22% of the patients with metastases in the lower third of the neck or with capsular ruptures survived this observation period.

M stage

Distant metastases in squamous cell carcinoma are usually preceded by lymph node metastases. Blood-borne metastases are uncommon, but widespread dissemination to various viscera may occur in advanced stages of laryngeal cancer. The sites which appear to be most affected by distant metastatic spread are the mediastinal lymph nodes, lungs, liver, pleura, skeletal system, kidney, heart, spleen and pancreas.[4] The cavernous sinus and temporal bones are an unusual site for metastasis.[104] Naturally, distant metastases have been correlated with a poor prognosis.

Some tumors, particularly adenoid cystic carcinoma,[28] basaloid squamous cell carcinoma[29] and some sarcomas, may metastasize to several viscera without cervical lymph node metastases.

Histologic cell type

The oncotype, or histological cell type, provides a qualitative diagnosis of the disease. Approximately 90% of malignant neoplasms of the larynx are squamous cell carcinomas and can be graded as well (G1), moderately (G2), or poorly (G3) differentiated. Cancers other than squamous cell carcinoma are not considered for the purposes of this analysis, but about 10% of malignant laryngeal tumors do belong to other oncotypes, differing not only in histologic findings but also in clinical behavior. Biologic behavior varies from one type of cancer to another so only similar types are comparable for prognostic implications.

Survival is generally related to specific histologic types of laryngeal cancer. It is common knowledge that a laryngeal small cell neuroendocrine carcinoma metastasizes more frequently than a squamous cell carcinoma and that the latter is more malignant than a verrucous squamous cell carcinoma. Each malignant tumor has its own degree of intrinsic aggressiveness strictly correlated with the structure of the neoplasm.

Prognosis for such tumors consequently differs enormously (e.g. it is excellent for verrucous squamous cell carcinoma, generally fair for common squamous cell carcinoma and poor for small cell neuroendocrine carcinoma). Specifically, 5-year survivals are 95% for verrucous squamous cell carcinoma,[27] 90% for chondrosarcoma,[50] 80% for mucoepidermoid carcinoma,[39] 68% for squamous cell carcinoma,[84] 68% for spindle cell carcinoma,[62] 48% for atypical carcinoid tumor,[99] 20% for melanoma,[85] 17.5% for basaloid squamous cell carcinoma[29] and 5% for small cell neuroendocrine carcinoma of the larynx,[34] considering all stages of the disease. If we take squamous cell carcinoma as a standard for comparison with other specific histologic types of laryngeal cancer, the following are more favorable: verrucous squamous carcinomas, chondrosarcomas and most mucoepidermoid carcinomas.[31] The less favorable types include: small cell neuroendocrine carcinoma, basaloid squamous cell carcinoma, melanoma, atypical carcinoid tumor and spindle cell carcinoma. Moreover, the exact identification of the type of laryngeal tumor permits specific and individual tumor staging, according to the oncotype involved (tumor staging evaluation in verrucous squamous cell carcinomas is not the same as in neuroendocrine carcinomas or lymphomas). The oncotype should be considered as a guideline for selecting treatment.

Histologic grading of malignancy

The variability of a tumor's differentiation in separate areas of a laryngectomy specimen is generally acknowledged and invalidates the grading of biopsy specimens,[33] but the degree of a neoplasm's differentiation should not be confused with its histologic grading. Factors allowing for a better assessment of the histologic grading of malignancies include:

- degree of structural differentiation;
- cellular anaplasia or pleomorphism;
- mitotic activity index (frequency and abnormality of mitotic figures);
- expansive or infiltrative growth;
- inflammatory response to the tumor;
- necrosis;
- lymphatic and blood vessel invasion.

Poorly differentiated cancers usually have a higher rate of metastatic disease when compared with well differentiated cancers, but this correlation is not always valid.[18] Also, the degree of differentiation suffers from the subjectivity of interpretation by pathologists.

Some investigators found a correlation between perineural invasion at the primary site and cervical node metastasis, but others have not been able to confirm this correlation.

Tumor angiogenesis has been indicated as a prognostic factor and is correlated with lymph node metastasis in different sites, whilst various reports provide contradictory findings in predicting either aggressiveness or proclivity to metastasize in head and neck cancer.[20,58,80] Petruzzelli[63] believes that clinical pathologic studies correlating the angiogenesis of head and neck carcinomas with node metastasis, survival and recurrence rate are currently conflicting.

Contradictory prognostic results have also been reported in tumor-associated tissue eosinophilia in laryngeal cancer.[17,35,75]

Biologic attributes

There are now numerous emerging technologies which promise to provide much more prognostic information on neoplasms. Among the developing technologies are: immunohistochemistry [immunohistochemical detection of proliferation markers, such as the proliferating cell nuclear antigen (PCNA) and Ki-67 (MIB 1)], molecular biology (p53, c-*myc* and *ras*, EGFR and TGF-α), nucleolus organizer regions (NORs), the determination of clonality by molecular diagnostic techniques including the polymerase chain reaction (PCR), the use of *in situ* hybridization (ISH), DNA ploidy by flow cytometry or image analysis, TUNEL, cell cycle regulators (including p34cdc2 or CDK1, and the D family of cyclins), and so on.[18] To be realistic, the enthusiasm associated with the application of these new and special techniques has to be tempered: discrepancies in results are evident in the literature[6,10,11,16,21,23,25,36,37,55,56,59,61,67,68,70–72,76,82,88,94,96,101–103] and different and sensitive new methods in pathology have not always been found related to prognosis in neoplasms of the larynx.[39,55] All the present biologic parameters are often of 'unproven' prognostic value. Considering the current situation, it is impossible to define subgroups of patients with a different biologic behavior. Additional studies are needed to confirm these findings and compare the prognostic value of these and other markers with other parameters in large groups of patients, with the support of statistical studies. Many papers complete the discussion with an inconclusive remark, such as 'this marker could be of valid prognostic significance', but no acceptable marker of prognosis has been found so far for clinical application in patients with cancer of the larynx. The limitations of currently used biologic markers in predicting tumor behavior are well recognized in laryngeal oncology. Conversely, there are many diagnostic markers that are very useful to support the histologic diagnosis (such as neuroendocrine markers). However, having emphasized the need to consider the prognostic implications of the new technologies with caution, it is worth mentioning a few of the most promising findings reported to date.

It has been noted that chromosome 18 is often rearranged or lost in squamous cell cancer of the larynx. Carey *et al.*[12] reported at the Fourth International Conference on Head and Neck Cancer (Toronto) that all or part of chromosome 18 was lost in 26/40 tumors and that survival time was shorter in the patients concerned. Of the patients surviving at 3 years, only 25% had chromosome 18 loss, whereas 75% of those who had died had chromosome 18 loss. The authors proposed the loss of chromosome 18 as an independent prognostic indicator, probably because it is the site of one or more important tumor suppressor genes.

These observations were confirmed by Scholnick *et al.*[78] at the University of Washington, who examined specimens from a retrospectively assembled population of 59 laryngeal cancer patients, who all had squamous cell carcinoma of the supraglottic larynx, treated surgically with a view to cure, and had been followed up for more than 5 years unless they had died of their laryngeal cancer. They found three different tumor suppressor genes on chromosome 8, with the gene at 8p23 previously unreported. Statistical analysis suggests that loss of this new suppressor gene significantly correlates with poor disease-specific survival and that this is an independent predictor of survival in laryngeal cancer.

Molecular markers have been reported to have an important role in detecting occult neoplastic cells in the resection margins after head and neck cancer excision. The PCR and cloning can identify a single malignant cell among 10 000 normal cells when the primary tumor contains a p53 mutation. Brennan *et al.*[9] studied 25 patients with p53 mutation of their head and neck carcinomas and found one or more positive margins by means of this sensitive molecular probe. These findings proved of great value in a prognostic sense, in that the patients with negative margins by molecular analysis were observed to have a significantly increased survival. They also noted that there was a 'lack of response to primary radiation therapy in patients who have the p53 mutation' and suggested that alternative and more aggressive therapy might be more appropriate in this instance.

The UM-A9 monoclonal antibody will bind with most squamous cell carcinoma cell culture lines, suggesting that it displays tumor specificity (as it will not bind to fibroblasts, lymphocytes, red blood cells, melanomas or normal keratinocytes). Immunohistology has confirmed that most SCC tumors express this antigen and many tumors show high levels of the antigen at the growing edge of tumor nests and inside the tumor cells. Of the greatest importance in a prognostic sense is the finding that the disease-free survival decreases in head and neck SCC patients as the intensity of A9 antigen expression increases.[97]

Increased DNA content of laryngeal cancer cells as measured by the adjusted DNA index (aDI) appears to reflect an increased proliferative capacity and a greater frequency of cervical lymph node metastasis. Wolf *et al.*[98] studied 94 patients with stage III and stage IV laryngeal carcinoma and found that a shorter time to recurrence, higher number of positive nodes and generally worse prognosis correlates with higher levels of DNA content. Milroy *et al.*[59] believe that the role of DNA ploidy as an independent prognostic indicator has yet to be determined.

The presence of another cancer

Another important factor influencing survival is the presence of other, synchronous or metachronous primary cancers, whether in the head and neck or elsewhere, but especially in the esophagus, lung and oral cavity. Cancers of the larynx tend to have second primaries in the lung,[69] whereas neoplasms in the oral cavity tend to have second primaries in the esophagus. The presence of a previous or synchronous cancer halves survival.[91]

Treatment factors

An important factor in the management of cancer of the larynx is the determination of whether the carcinoma is in situ, early invasive[32] or frankly invasive. 'Minimal laryngeal cancer' defines carcinoma in situ and early invasive carcinoma and the prognosis is generally favorable. Invasive cancer of the larynx, left untreated, is inevitably a fatal disease: 90% of untreated patients die within 3 years.[79] Surgery and radiation therapy, either alone or in combination, are the conventional modalities for the management of malignant laryngeal tumors. Laser surgery is also a valid means of treatment for early squamous cell carcinoma and verrucous cancer of the glottis. Chemotherapy is also indicated in some rare, nonsquamous carcinomas, such as small cell neuroendocrine carcinomas, diffuse lymphomas, etc. In squamous cell carcinoma, the role of chemotherapy in conjunction with conventional treatment remains controversial and adjuvant chemotherapy does not usually improve the survival rate achieved by conventional surgery and radiotherapy.

Kowalski *et al.*[47] reported that in 145 consecutive patients with stage I and stage II glottic cancer, the rate of failure was higher after radiation therapy than in the group of patients treated surgically. Surgical salvage improved survival rates to a level equivalent to surgery, but total laryngectomy was required. The only prognostic factor found to be statistically significant in their analysis was extension of the carcinoma to involve the vocal process of the arytenoid cartilage. Arytenoid involvement predicted higher rates of recurrent carcinoma and a higher mortality.

The treatment of laryngeal cancer should be selected according to the histologic cell type, the stage of disease and the presence of comorbidities. The final decision regarding treatment may also be influenced by other factors, including the host's age, general condition and occupation, the physician's experience, the treatment centers available, etc. Of course, the choice of treatment is an important parameter influencing not only prognosis but also, more important, the patient's quality of life. Obviously, the prognosis is better if the most suitable therapy is implemented from the start.

Various reports provide contradictory findings on the effects of blood transfusions on prognosis[1,3,5,7,8,100] and although immune suppression due to perioperative transfusions has been implicated in a worse prognosis after laryngectomy, this remains to be demonstrated conclusively.[22] Recently, León *et al.*[49] reviewed the literature and concluded that homologous perioperative transfusion did not imply a significant risk regarding global control or survival in their laryngeal or hypopharyngeal cancer patients.

Stomal recurrence

Stomal recurrence, although relatively uncommon, carries a dismal prognosis for survival. Recent reports[40,73] have described the prognostic correlation between subglottic tumor extension and stomal recurrence, with one analysis indicating that 80% of these patients had tumors in the subglottis. The incidence of peristomal recurrence decreased from 11.5% to 2.7% in one series with the routine use of pretracheal, paratracheal and mediastinal node dissection in high-risk patients.

Considerations

The TNM system is only an anatomic means of classification which takes into account neither the biologic aggressiveness of various neoplasms, nor the host's immunologic response. It was not developed to serve as a specific guideline for the management of a particular patient, nor does the system have the ability to predict the outcome of individual patients. But whilst physicians are focused on the concept of optimal treatment, patients are interested in their prognosis and one of the most important tasks is to assess our present ability to predict the likely outcome for a particular patient with laryngeal cancer. Some surgeons feel that we are on the verge of major advances in our search for prognostic indicators, whereas others have observed that the growing body of scientific literature in the field of laryngeal cancer may represent nothing more than an 'encyclopedia of ignorance'.[54]

The various staging systems were examined along with a report on the outcome of an international survey on the applicability of the TNM system in relation to laryngeal neoplasms, promoted by The Laryngeal Cancer Association[30] which has promoted a worldwide survey to collect expert opinions on the applicability of the TNM system to cancer of the larynx.[4] Of those laryngologists who responded to the survey, only about 10% were entirely satisfied with its practical use. As a consequence, the Association appointed an International Committee on the Classification of Laryngeal Cancer consisting of Byron J Bailey, MD (Chairman, Galveston, Texas, USA), Lawrence W DeSanto, MD (Scottsdale, Arizona, USA), Alfio Ferlito, MD (Padua, Italy), Helmuth Goepfert, MD (Houston, Texas, USA), Michael E Johns, MD (Baltimore, Maryland, USA), Willy Lehmann, MD (Geneva, Switzerland), Jan Olofsson, MD (Bergen, Norway) and Philip M Stell, MD (Liverpool, Great Britain). This committee was asked to analyze the current TNM classification system and to explore the opportunities for its correlation with other prognostic features. One of the useful methods for approaching this type of analysis is to begin by determining the opinions of a specific set of field experts. We therefore devised a questionnaire that listed 38 positive prognostic factors and 55 negative prognostic factors that appear in the literature most frequently. This informal survey was circulated with a request that each member of the committee respond by indicating his current level of enthusiasm for each of these potential prognostic indicators. The overall purpose of the survey was to collect information from a laryngeal cancer study group and organize these opinions, drawing from many decades of clinical and research observation, to see if there is any level of consensus at the present time. This effort was exploratory and preliminary in nature and made no attempt to make far-reaching conclusions, but we found the responses interesting.

Each respondent was asked to indicate whether he strongly agreed, agreed, was neutral, disagreed or strongly disagreed that each of a series of individual features represents either a favorable or an unfavorable prognostic indicator. The results are summarized in Table 57.1. In analyzing the list of positive predictive factors, we used three of these factors as a 'gold standard' in terms of wide acceptance on the basis of inclusion in the TNM system. In general, the most unanimously agreed indicators of a favorable outcome were felt to be the absence of any metastasis, a low T stage and a low N stage. These responses reflect a general acceptance of the value of TNM staging, though it is important to emphasize once again that it is not the primary purpose of the TNM system to predict outcome or direct the treatment of individual patients.

The strongest consensus regarding a factor outside the TNM system was expressed in regard to the absence of extracapsular tumor spread. This is ranked as equivalent to a low T or a low N stage as a predictor of favorable outcome. Next in its predictive value is the clinical finding that a glottic primary is limited to the membranous portion of the true vocal cord. This is obviously related to T stage in that all such primaries would be T1 tumors. The high consensus of responders that this represents a predictor of favorable outcome could reflect such

Table 57.1 Laryngeal panel consensus regarding the most influential favorable and unfavorable prognostic features for laryngeal cancer (in diminishing order of importance)

Favorable features	*Unfavorable features*
No metastasis	Lymph nodes less movable to fixed
Low T	Recurrent disease
Low N	Tumor involves overlying skin
No extracapsular spread	Extracapsular spread
Glottic primary limited to membranous portion of true cord	Second malignant primary
Clear resection margins	Continued exposure to carcinogens
Normal vocal cord mobility	Tumor at resection margin
Ceased exposure to carcinogens	Transglottic lesions
Glottic primary	Airway obstruction and emergency tracheotomy
Highly differentiated histology	High tumor volume doubling time
Only unilateral or ipsilateral lymph nodes	Poor performance status
Lesser total tumor volume	Extension to posterior commissure
Lesser depth of invasion	Nerve sheath (perineural) invasion
Lymph nodes easily movable	Neuroendocrine tumors (atypical carcinoid and small cell neuroendocrine carcinoma)
Retain epithelial movement over the vocal ligament	Subglottic extension more than 1 cm
Exophytic growth pattern	Greater tumor volume
Good performance status	More depth of tumor invasion
Histological 'pushing' tumor margins	Lymph node metastasis in laryngectomy specimen
Smaller lymph nodes size within the range	Impaired vocal cord mobility
Host's good nutritional status	Microscopic vascular invasion
Fewer palpable lymph nodes within stage	'Burrowing' growth pattern
Primary tumor size less than 2 cm	Larger lymph nodes in N stage range
Low tumor volume doubling time	More lymph nodes in N stage

opinions as the better prognosis of glottic primaries as opposed to supraglottic or transglottic primaries. The response could also reflect the opinion that small primaries have a better prognosis, even within the T1 category range of tumor sizes and sites.

The next two features in terms of consensus are clear resection margins confirmed by histological assessment and normal true vocal cord mobility.

After that, there were three factors felt to be of considerable importance and these are cessation of exposure to carcinogens (a behavioral feature), glottic location of the primary (rather than supraglottic, subglottic or transglottic) and highly differentiated tumor histology. Thereafter, in descending order, were unilateral or ipsilateral lymph nodes, lesser total tumor volume and lesser depth of invasion.

The list of unfavorable prognostic features in regard to laryngeal cancer consists in some instances of the features opposite to those on the favorable prognosis list. Other examples of unfavorable features are distinct and independent negative factors on their own. The most unfavorable prognostic features according to the response to our questionnaire are the finding of lymph node(s) from less movable to fixed in nature. This feature is somewhat outside the TNM staging system but represents a distinction within an already lower-survival category (in that the patient must already have palpable nodes in order to have less movable to fixed nodes).

The second worst prognostic features were recurrent malignant disease and tumor involving the overlying skin.

Then came the presence of lymph node extracapsular spread, the detection of a second malignant primary tumor and the patient's continued exposure to carcinogens, followed by the presence of tumor at the resection margin.

Three features that tied for the next level of unfavorable prognosis were transglottic lesions, airway obstruction with the need for emergency tracheotomy and high tumor volume doubling time, as measured by cell cycle kinetics.

Next in order were poor performance status, extension to the posterior commissure of the larynx, nerve sheath (perineural) invasion and certain neuroendocrine carcinomas (atypical carcinoid tumor and small cell neuroendocrine carcinoma).

The development and application of molecular biology tools to analyze biopsy material may be predictive for the biologic behavior of laryngeal cancer in the near future.

References

1. Alun-Jones T, Clarke PJ, Morrissey S, Hill J. Blood transfusion and laryngeal cancer. *Clin Otolaryngol* 1991; **16:** 240–4.
2. American Joint Committee on Cancer (AJCC). *Manual for Staging of Cancer*, 3rd edn. Philadelphia: Lippincott, 1988.

3. Austin JR, Weber RS. Blood transfusions in head and neck surgery. *Curr Opin Otolaryngol Head Neck Surg* 1995; **3:** 89–94.
4. Bailey BJ. Beyond the 'new' TNM classification. *Arch Otolaryngol Head Neck Surg* 1991; **117:** 369–70.
5. Barra S, Barzan L, Maione A *et al*. Blood transfusion and other prognostic variables in the survival of patients with cancer of the head and neck. *Laryngoscope* 1994; **104:** 95–8.
6. Bellacosa A, Almadori G, Cavallo S *et al*. Cyclin D1 gene amplification in human laryngeal squamous cell carcinomas: prognostic significance and clinical implications. *Clin Cancer Res* 1996; **2:** 175–80.
7. Böck M, Grevers G, Koblitz M, Heim MU, Mempel W. Influence of blood transfusion on recurrence, survival and postoperative infections of laryngeal cancer. *Acta Otolaryngol (Stockh)* 1990; **110:** 155–60.
8. Bongioannini G, Vercellino M, Rugiu MG, Ferreri A, Succo G, Cortesina G. Influence of perioperative transfusion therapy on the recurrence potential of locally advanced laryngeal carcinoma. *ORL J Otorhinolaryngol Relat Spec* 1990; **52:** 260–4.
9. Brennan JA, Mao L, Hruban RH *et al*. Molecular assessment of histopathologic staging in squamous-cell carcinoma of the head and neck. *N Engl J Med* 1995; **332:** 429–35.
10. Cappiello J, Nicolai P, Antonelli AR *et al*. DNA index, cellular proliferative activity and nucleolar organizer regions in cancers of the larynx. *Eur Arch Otorhinolaryngol* 1995; **252:** 353–8.
11. Carey TE. Integrin signaling and expression in squamous cell carcinoma. In: Shah JP, Johnson JT, eds. *Proceedings of the Fourth International Conference on Head and Neck Cancer, Toronto*. Madison: Omnipress, 1996: 486–92.
12. Carey TE, Van Dyke DL, Worsham MJ *et al*. Chromosome 18 loss is a prognostic indicator in squamous cell carcinoma. *Fourth International Conference on Head and Neck Cancer, Toronto* 1996: Abstract no. 58, p. 73.
13. Carter RL, Bliss JM, Soo KC, O'Brien CJ. Radical neck dissections for squamous carcinomas: pathological findings and clinical implications with particular reference to transcapsular spread. *Int J Radiat Oncol Biol Phys* 1987; **13:** 825–32.
14. Cella DF, Tulsky DS, Gray G *et al*. The Functional Assessment of Cancer Therapy scale: development and validation of the general measure. *J Clin Oncol* 1993; **11:** 570–9.
15. Clayman GL, Callender DL, Razmpa E, Weber RS, Byers RM, Goepfert H. Surgical outcome in patients with squamous carcinoma of the upper aerodigestive tract 80 years of age and older. *Fourth International Conference on Head and Neck Cancer, Toronto* 1996: Abstract no. 350, p. 146.
16. Cooke L, Cooke T, Forster G, Helliwell T, Stell P. Cellular DNA content and prognosis in surgically treated squamous carcinoma of the larynx. *Br J Cancer* 1991; **63:** 1018–20.
17. Deron P, Goossens A, Halama AR. Tumour-associated tissue eosinophilia in head and neck squamous-cell carcinoma. *ORL J Otorhinolaryngol Relat Spec* 1996; **58:** 167–70.
18. Devaney KO, Hunter BC, Ferlito A, Rinaldo A. Pretreatment pathologic prognostic factors in head and neck squamous cell carcinoma. *Ann Otol Rhinol Laryngol* 1997; **106:** 983–8.
19. Devineni VR, Simpson R, Sessions D *et al*. Supraglottic carcinoma: impact of radiation therapy on outcome of patients with positive margins and extracapsular nodal disease. *Laryngoscope* 1991; **101:** 767–70.
20. Dray TG, Hardin NJ, Sofferman RA. Angiogenesis as a prognostic marker in early head and neck cancer. *Ann Otol Rhinol Laryngol* 1995; **104:** 724–9.
21. Dursun G, Sak SD, Akyol G *et al*. Overexpression of p53 in laryngeal carcinoma: clinicopathological implications. *Ear Nose Throat J* 1995; **74:** 645–8.
22. Ell SR, Stell PM. Blood transfusion and survival after laryngectomy for laryngeal carcinoma. *J Laryngol Otol* 1991; **105:** 293–4.
23. El Naggar AK, Lopez-Varela V, Luna MA, Weber R, Batsakis JG. Intratumoral DNA content heterogeneity in laryngeal squamous cell carcinoma. *Arch Otolaryngol Head Neck Surg* 1992; **118:** 169–73.
24. Farrell RWR, McKenna DM, Clegg RT. Micrometastases from laryngeal carcinoma in cervical lymph nodes: an immunohistochemical study (abstract). *Clin Otolaryngol* 1991; **16:** 519–20.
25. Feinmesser R, Freeman JL, Noyek A. Flow cytometric analysis of DNA content in laryngeal cancer. *J Laryngol Otol* 1990; **104:** 485–7.
26. Feinstein AR. The pre-therapeutic classification of co-morbidity in chronic disease. *J Chron Dis* 1970; **23:** 455–69.
27. Ferlito A. Atypical forms of squamous cell carcinoma. In: Ferlito A, ed. *Neoplasms of the Larynx*. Edinburgh: Churchill Livingstone, 1993: 135–67.
28. Ferlito A, Barnes L, Myers EN. Neck dissection for laryngeal adenoid cystic carcinoma: is it indicated? *Ann Otol Rhinol Laryngol* 1990; **99:** 277–80.
29. Ferlito A, Altavilla G, Rinaldo A, Doglioni C. Basaloid squamous cell carcinoma of the larynx and hypopharynx. *Ann Otol Rhinol Laryngol* 1997; **106:** 1024–35.
30. Ferlito A, Sir Harrison DFN, Bailey BJ, DeSanto LW. Are clinical classifications for laryngeal cancer satisfactory? *Ann Otol Rhinol Laryngol* 1995; **104:** 741–7.
31. Ferlito A, Rinaldo A, Devaney KO, Devaney SL, Milroy CM. Impact of phenotype on treatment and prognosis of laryngeal malignancies. *J Laryngol Otol* 1998; **112:** 710–14.
32. Ferlito A, Carbone A, DeSanto LW *et al*. 'Early' cancer of the larynx: the concept as defined by clinicians, pathologists and biologists. *Ann Otol Rhinol Laryngol* 1996; **105:** 245–50.
33. Friedmann I, Ferlito A. *Granulomas and Neoplasms of the Larynx*. Edinburgh: Churchill Livingstone, 1988.
34. Gnepp DR. Small cell neuroendocrine carcinoma of the larynx. A critical review of the literature. *ORL J Otorhinolaryngol Relat Spec* 1991; **53:** 210–19.
35. Goldsmith MM, Cresson DH, Askin FB. Part II. The prognostic significance of stromal eosinophilia in head and neck cancer. *Otolaryngol Head Neck Surg* 1987; **96:** 319–24.
36. Goldsmith MM, Cresson DH, Postma DS, Askin FB, Pillsbury HC. Significance of ploidy in laryngeal cancer. *Am J Surg* 1986; **152:** 396–402.
37. Goldsmith MM, Cresson DH, Arnold LA, Postma DS,

Askin FB, Pillsbury HC. Part I. DNA flow cytometry as a prognostic indicator in head and neck cancer. *Otolaryngol Head Neck Surg* 1987; **96:** 307–18.
38. Hirabayashi H, Koshii K, Uno K *et al.* Extracapsular spread of squamous cell carcinoma in neck lymph nodes: prognostic factor in laryngeal cancer. *Laryngoscope* 1991; **101:** 502–6.
39. Ho K-J, Jones JM, Herrera GA. Mucoepidermoid carcinoma of the larynx: a light and electron microscopic study with emphasis on histogenesis. *South Med J* 1984; **77:** 190–5.
40. Hosal IN, Önerci M, Turan E. Peristomal recurrence. *Am J Otolaryngol* 1993; **14:** 206–8.
41. Huygen PLM, Van Den Broek P, Kazem I. Age and mortality in laryngeal cancer. *Clin Otolaryngol* 1980; **5:** 129–37.
42. International Union Against Cancer. Sobin LH, Wittekind Ch, eds. *TNM Classification of Malignant Tumours*, 5th edn. New York: Wiley-Liss, 1997.
43. Johnson JT, Myers EN, Bedetti CD, Barnes EL, Schramm VL, Thearle PB. Cervical lymph node metastases. Incidence and implications of extracapsular carcinoma. *Arch Otolaryngol* 1985; **111:** 534–7.
44. Karnofsky DA, Abelman WH, Craver LF, Burchenal JH. The use of nitrogen mustard in the palliative treatment of carcinoma with particular reference to bronchogenic carcinoma. *Cancer* 1948; **1:** 634–9.
45. Katz AE. Immunobiologic staging of patients with carcinoma of the head and neck. *Laryngoscope* 1983; **93:** 445–63.
46. Kowalski LP, Franco EL, de Andrade Sobrinho J, Oliveira BV, Pontes PL. Prognostic factors in laryngeal cancer patients submitted to surgical treatment. *J Surg Oncol* 1991; **48:** 87–95.
47. Kowalski LP, Batista MBP, Santos CR *et al.* Prognostic factors in glottic carcinoma clinical stage I and II treated by surgery or radiotherapy. *Am J Otolaryngol* 1993; **14:** 122–7.
48. Lefebvre JL, Castelain B, de la Torre JC, Delobelle-Deroide A, Vankemmel B. Lymph node invasion in hypopharynx and lateral epilarynx carcinoma: a prognostic factor. *Head Neck Surg* 1987; **10:** 14–18.
49. León X, Quer M, Maestre L, Burgués J, Muñiz E, Madoz P. Blood transfusions in laryngeal cancer: effect on prognosis. *Head Neck* 1996; **18:** 218–24.
50. Lewis JE, Olsen KD, Inwards CY. Cartilaginous tumors of the larynx: clinicopathologic review of 47 cases. *Ann Otol Rhinol Laryngol* 1997; **106:** 94–100.
51. List MA, Ritter-Sterr CA, Lansky SB. A performance status for head and neck cancer patients. *Cancer* 1990; **66:** 564–9.
52. List MA, D'Antonio LL, Cella DF *et al.* The Performance Status Scale for Head and Neck Cancer Patients and the Functional Assessment of Cancer Therapy-Head and Neck Scale. A study of utility and validity. *Cancer* 1996; **77:** 2294–301.
53. List MA, Ritter-Sterr CA, Baker TM *et al.* Longitudinal assessment of quality of life in laryngeal cancer patients. *Head Neck* 1996; **18:** 1–10.
54. Maran AGD. Head and neck surgery: an encyclopaedia of ignorance. *J Laryngol Otol* 1990; **104:** 529–33.
55. Masuda M, Hirakawa N, Nakashima T, Kuratomi Y, Komiyama S. Cyclin D1 overexpression in primary hypopharyngeal carcinomas. *Cancer* 1996; **78:** 390–5.
56. Maurizi M, Scambia G, Benedetti Panici P *et al.* EGF receptor expression in primary squamous laryngeal cancer: correlation with clinico-pathological features and prognostic significance. *Int J Cancer* 1992; **52:** 862–6.
57. Mickel RA, Kessler DJ, Taylor JM, Lichtenstein A. Natural killer cell cytotoxicity in the peripheral blood, cervical lymph nodes, and tumor of head and neck cancer patients. *Cancer Res* 1988; **48:** 5017–22.
58. Mikami Y, Tsukuda M, Ito K, Arai Y, Ito T. Peritumoral angiogenesis in carcinomas of the head and neck. *Auris Nasus Larynx* 1996; **23:** 57–62.
59. Milroy CM, Ferlito A, Devaney KO, Rinaldo A. Role of DNA measurements of head and neck tumors. *Ann Otol Rhinol Laryngol* 1997; **106:** 801–4.
60. Moe K, Wolf GT, Fisher SG, Hong WK. Regional metastases in patients with advanced laryngeal cancer. *Arch Otolaryngol Head Neck Surg* 1996; **122:** 644–8.
61. Murakami Y, Yasuda N, Kawata R, Nakai S. Markers on metastatic spread of squamous cell carcinoma. In: Shah JP, Johnson JT, eds. *Proceedings of the Fourth International Conference on Head and Neck Cancer, Toronto.* Madison: Omnipress, 1996: 502–7.
62. Olsen KD, Lewis JE, Suman VJ. Spindle cell carcinoma of the larynx and hypopharynx. *Otolaryngol Head Neck Surg* 1997; **116:** 47–52.
63. Petruzzelli GJ. Tumor angiogenesis. *Head Neck* 1996; **18:** 283–91.
64. Piccirillo JF, Feinstein AR. Clinical symptoms and comorbidity: significance for prognostic classification of cancer. *Cancer* 1996; **77:** 834–42.
65. Piccirillo JF, Wells CK, Sasaki CT, Feinstein AR. New clinical severity staging system for cancer of the larynx. Five-year survival rates. *Ann Otol Rhinol Laryngol* 1994; **103:** 83–92.
66. Popella C, Glanz H. The prognostic significance of metastases according to their site in the neck and capsular rupture in patients with carcinoma of the larynx. *Fourth International Conference on Head and Neck Cancer, Toronto* 1996: Abstract no. 341, p. 144.
67. Resnick MJM, Uhlman D, Niehans GA *et al.* Cervical lymph node status and survival in laryngeal carcinoma: prognostic factors. *Ann Otol Rhinol Laryngol* 1995; **104:** 685–94.
68. Resta L, Micheau C, Cimmino A. Prognostic value of the prelaryngeal node in laryngeal and hypopharyngeal carcinoma. *Tumori* 1985; **71:** 361–5.
69. Rinaldo A, Marchiori C, Faggionato L, Saffiotti U, Ferlito A. The association of cancers of the larynx with cancers of the lung. *Eur Arch Otorhinolaryngol* 1996; **253:** 256–9.
70. Roland NJ, Caslin AW, Bowie GL, Jones AS. Has the cellular proliferation marker Ki67 any clinical relevance in squamous cell carcinoma of the head and neck? *Clin Otolaryngol* 1994; **19:** 13–18.
71. Ropka ME, Goodwin WJ, Levine PA, Sasaki CT, Kirchner JC, Cantrell RW. Effective head and neck tumor markers. The continuing quest. *Arch Otolaryngol Head Neck Surg* 1991; **117:** 1011–14.
72. Ruá S, Comino A, Fruttero A *et al.* Relationship between histologic features, DNA flow cytometry, and clinical behavior of squamous cell carcinomas of the larynx. *Cancer* 1991; **67:** 141–9.
73. Rubin J, Johnson JT, Myers EN. Stomal recurrence after laryngectomy: interrelated risk factor study. *Otolaryngol Head Neck Surg* 1990; **103:** 805–12.

74. Sala O, Ferlito A. Morphological observations of immunobiology of laryngeal cancer. Evaluation of the defensive activity of immunocompetent cells present in tumour stroma. *Acta Otolaryngol (Stockh)* 1976; **81:** 353–63.
75. Sassler AM, McClatchey KD, Wolf GT, Fisher SG. Eosinophilic infiltration in advanced laryngeal squamous cell carcinoma. *Laryngoscope* 1995; **105:** 413–16.
76. Schantz SP. The challenge of tumor markers. In: Shah JP, Johnson JT, eds. *Proceedings of the Fourth International Conference on Head and Neck Cancer, Toronto.* Madison: Omnipress, 1996: 479–85.
77. Schantz SP, Shillitoe EJ, Brown B, Campbell B. Natural killer cell activity and head and neck cancer: a clinical assessment. *J Natl Cancer Inst* 1986; **77:** 869–75.
78. Scholnick SB, Sunwoo JB, El-Mofty SK, Haughey BH. Allelic loss of chromosome Arm 8p and the prognosis of supraglottic laryngeal cancer patients. *Fourth International Conference on Head and Neck Cancer, Toronto* 1996: Abstract no. 60, p. 73.
79. Shimkin MB. Duration of life in untreated cancer. *Cancer* 1951; **4:** 1–8.
80. Shpitzer T, Chaimoff M, Gal R, Stern Y, Feinmesser R, Segal K. Tumor angiogenesis as a prognostic factor in early oral tongue cancer. *Arch Otolaryngol Head Neck Surg* 1996; **122:** 865–8.
81. Shvero J, Hadar T, Segal K, Abraham A, Sidi J. Laryngeal carcinoma in patients 40 years of age and younger. *Cancer* 1987; **60:** 3092–6.
82. Sidransky D. Molecular markers in head and neck cancer. In: Shah JP, Johnson JT, eds. *Proceedings of the Fourth International Conference on Head and Neck Cancer, Toronto.* Madison: Omnipress, 1996: 509–15.
83. Silvestri F, Bussani R, Stanta G, Cosatti C. Ferlito A. Supraglottic versus glottic laryngeal cancer: epidemiological and pathological aspects. *ORL J Othorinolaryngol Relat Spec* 1992; **54:** 43–8.
84. Sinard RJ, Netterville JL, Garrett CG, Ossoff RH. Cancer of the larynx. In: Myers EN, Suen JY, eds. *Cancer of the Head and Neck*, 3rd edn. Philadelphia: Saunders, 1996: 381–421.
85. Smith BC, Wenig BM. Neurogenic neoplasms including melanoma. In: Ferlito A, ed. *Surgical Pathology of Laryngeal Neoplasms.* London: Chapman & Hall, 1996: 195–247.
86. Snow GB, Annyas AA, van Slooten EA, Bartelink H, Hart AAM. Prognostic factors of neck node metastasis. *Clin Otolaryngol* 1982; **7:** 185–92.
87. Snyderman NL, Johnson JT, Schramm VL Jr, Myers EN, Bedetti CD, Thearle P. Extracapsular spread of carcinoma in cervical lymph nodes. Impact upon survival in patients with carcinoma of the supraglottic larynx. *Cancer* 1985; **56:** 1597–9.
88. Spafford MF, Koeppe J, Pan Z, Archer PG, Meyers AD, Franklin WA. Correlation of tumor markers p53, *bcl-2*, CD34, CD44H, CD44v6, and Ki-67 with survival and metastasis in laryngeal squamous cell carcinoma. *Arch Otolaryngol Head Neck Surg* 1996; **122:** 627–32.
89. Spitzer WO, Dobson AJ, Hall J *et al.* Measuring the quality of life of cancer patients. A concise QL-index for use by physicians. *J Chron Dis* 1981; **34:** 585–97.
90. Stell PM. Prognostic factors in laryngeal carcinoma. *Clin Otolaryngol* 1988; **13:** 399–409.
91. Stell PM. Prognosis in laryngeal carcinoma: tumour factors. *Clin Otolaryngol* 1990; **15:** 69–81.
92. Stell PM. Prognosis in laryngeal carcinoma: host factors. *Clin Otolaryngol* 1990; **15:** 111–19.
93. Stephenson WT, Barnes DE, Holmes FF, Norris CW. Gender influences subsite of origin of laryngeal carcinoma. *Arch Otolaryngol Head Neck Surg* 1991; **117:** 774–8.
94. Tamura K, Wada Y. Proliferating activity in the proliferating cell nuclear antigen of human laryngeal carcinoma. *Larynx Jpn* 1994; **6:** 1–5.
95. Union Internationale Contre le Cancer (International Union Against Cancer). *TNM Classification of Malignant Tumours*, 4th edn. Berlin: Springer-Verlag, 1987.
96. Wada Y, Nunomura S, Simada T, Ishitani Y, Koike Y. Valuation of proliferating activity of laryngeal carcinoma. Using anti proliferating cell nuclear antigen antibody. *Larynx Jpn* 1993; **5:** 55–8.
97. Wolf GT, Carey TE. Tumor antigen phenotype, biologic staging, and prognosis in head and neck squamous carcinoma. *JNCI Monograph* 1992; **13:** 67–74.
98. Wolf GT, Fisher SG, Truelson JM, Beals TF. DNA content and regional metastases in patients with advanced laryngeal squamous carcinoma. *Laryngoscope* 1994; **104:** 479–83.
99. Woodruff JM, Senie RT. Atypical carcinoid tumor of the larynx. A critical review of the literature. *ORL J Otorhinolaryngol Relat Spec* 1991; **53:** 194–209.
100. Woolley AL, Hogikyan ND, Gares GA, Haughey BH, Schechtman KB, Goldenberg JL. Effect of blood transfusion on recurrence of head and neck carcinoma. Retrospective review and meta-analysis. *Ann Otol Rhinol Laryngol* 1992; **101:** 724–30.
101. Yamamoto Y, Itoh T, Saka T, Sakakura A, Takahashi H. Estimation of proliferative activity of laryngeal carcinoma by AgNOR staining method and DNA cytofluorometry. *Larynx Jpn* 1993; **5:** 91–6.
102. Yamamoto Y, Itoh T, Saka T, Sakakura A, Takahashi H. Prognostic value of nucleolar organizer in supraglottic carcinoma. *Auris Nasus Larynx* 1997; **24:** 85–90.
103. Yano G, Nakashima T, Nomura Y. Prognostic significance of argyrophilic nucleolar organizer region in carcinomas of the larynx and hypopharynx. *Larynx Jpn* 1995; **7:** 31–4.
104. Zahra M, Tewfik HH, McCabe BF. Metastases to the cavernous sinus from primary carcinoma of the larynx. *J Surg Oncol* 1986; **31:** 69–70.
105. Zubrod CG, Schneiderman M, Frei E, Brindley C. Appraisal of methods for the study of chemotherapy in man: comparative therapeutic trial of nitrogen mustard and triethylene thiophosphoramide. *J Chron Dis* 1960; **11:** 7–33.

Chemoprevention of laryngeal cancer

Boudewijn J M Braakhuis and Gordon B Snow

Chemoprevention is defined as the use of specific natural or synthetic chemical agents to reverse, suppress or prevent carcinogenesis.[34] This approach has the potential to become an important treatment strategy, but as it is still in a developmental stage, many issues still have to be resolved before it can be applied in standard clinical practice. This review will focus on important aspects of chemoprevention: the background, the characteristics of clinical trials, results obtained until now and the future perspectives. These matters will be discussed in relation to cancer in general, but, if applicable, attention will be focused on head and neck squamous cell carcinoma (HNSCC) and laryngeal cancer in particular.

Background

Epidemiologic and animal studies form the basis for the concept of chemoprevention. In addition, the knowledge of the process of carcinogenesis has considerably increased during the last decade and this understanding has provided a firmer theoretical basis for the idea that cancer chemoprevention can be accomplished by interfering with these mechanisms.

Epidemiologic findings

Several epidemiologic studies indicate that a shortage of certain micronutrients is associated with a higher risk for respiratory and upper digestive tract (HNSCC, lung and esophagus) cancer. The frequent intake of vegetables and fruits, especially those containing carotenoids and vitamin E (tocopherol) is associated with a lower risk of cancer of the mouth, esophagus and larynx.[22,25,39] When analyzing blood plasma, it appeared that low levels of α- and β-carotene and γ-tocopherol were associated with an increased risk of upper aerodigestive tract cancer.[24,40] An inverse relationship between selenium plasma levels and cancer risk was suggested in lung and stomach cancer.[37] These epidemiologic data suggest that some micronutrients are involved in the etiology of upper aerodigestive tract cancer. It is not precisely known how the variety of micronutrients interact with carcinogens and which metabolic pathways are involved herein. It is postulated that these compounds inhibit carcinogenesis by their antioxidant activity (see below).

Animal models

Animal models have been used for a long time to study the effect of intervention on chemical carcinogenesis. In 1929 it was shown that dichlorethyl sulfide could inhibit the formation of tumors that were induced by tar on the skin of mice.[2] In general, animals are exposed to a certain carcinogen and the effect of the administration of an agent on the development of carcinomas is measured. The time scheduling between the administration of the chemopreventive drug and the carcinogen as well as the length of administration are important. When medication is administered before or concurrently with the carcinogen, the emphasis will lie on the effect in the early phase of carcinogenesis (the initiation phase), and when the chemopreventive drug is administered after the carcinogen, the later phases are studied. Tumor-specific animal models now play an important role in preclinical efficacy evaluation of promising new chemopreventive drugs. The Chemoprevention Branch of the Division of Cancer Prevention and Control of the National Cancer Institute (NCI) of the USA is using a panel involving, lung, colon, breast, mammary, skin and bladder cancer and these tumors are chemically induced in mouse, rat or hamster.[35] Based on the efficacy in these *in vivo* models, the decision is made as to which drugs to test in clinical trials.

For laryngeal cancer a specific model to test chemopreventive drugs is not available. The most widely used animal with relevance for HNSCC is the hamster. To study oral carcinogenesis the hamster cheek pouch model can be used.[12,31] 12-Dimethylbenz[*a*]anthracene (DMBA) is applied on the mucosa of the cheek or the tongue and this leads to the development of squamous cell carcinomas within 20 weeks. In addition, the NCI of the USA use hamsters in which tracheal squamous carcinomas are induced with *N*-methyl-*N*-nitrosourea (MNU) and lung adenocarcinomas with *N,N*-diethylnitrosamine (DEN).[35]

Mechanistic studies

During the last two decades the knowledge on the process of carcinogenesis has considerably expanded. This has direct consequences for the understanding of how chemopreventive drugs can interfere within the multistep process of carcinogenesis and how new strategies should be designed. Tumor initiation is the first process in carcinogenesis and involves the exposure of a cell to chemical or physical stress. Once a cell has obtained a genetic change, it exerts an altered responsiveness to intra- and extracellular stimuli. Tumor promotion results in proliferation and is associated with an increased number of additional genetic changes (progression), which make the tumor cell more and more independent of host control. This eventually leads to invasive growth and metastasis.

Classes of chemopreventive agents

Test systems have been developed to study the various aspects of carcinogenesis and how agents can interact in these. This includes transformation and mutagenicity tests, and systems to measure enzyme activities and DNA binding. It has become clear that the chemopreventive agents can be discriminated upon their mechanism of action, but also that many of the agents belong to more than one category.[19] The agents are naturally occurring or synthetic and can be divided into several classes based on their chemical structure.[19] They will be discussed here with respect to their mechanism of action. Three major groups can be distinguished:

- agents that block the activity of a carcinogen;
- antioxidants; and
- antiproliferative or antiprogression agents.

Carcinogen-blocking agents

This type of agent is found to be active in the initiation and promotion phase of carcinogenesis. An example of carcinogen-blocking activity is the inhibition of uptake, which may for instance be achieved by the use of chelating agents. To the group of carcinogen-blocking agents also belong those capable of inhibiting the formation or the activation of a carcinogen. Well-known examples are the inhibiting effects that vitamins C and E have on the formation of *N*-nitroso compounds and nitrosamines, respectively.[11]

The interaction with DNA is another target for chemopreventive agents. A drug that receives attention at this moment is oltipraz. This drug has been found to inhibit the formation of aflatoxin–DNA adducts[30] and is active in many animal models, including the hamster-MNU-lung cancer model.[35]

Antioxidants

Antioxidant activity is the scavenging of reactive electrophiles or oxygen radicals (e.g. singlet oxygen, peroxyl and hydroxyl radicals). Potentially, all these electrophiles and radicals can act in the initiation, promotion and progression phase of carcinogenesis. Radicals give DNA strand breaks which can lead to chromosomal instability in the form of deletions and rearrangements. The most important drugs with antioxidant activity are: *N*-acetylcysteine, β-carotene and vitamin E, neutralizing hydroxyl radicals, singlet oxygen and peroxyl radicals, respectively. *N*-Acetylcysteine is found to be active in the hamster-MNU-lung cancer model.[35]

The application of antioxidants is not without danger. Under aerobic conditions high levels of *N*-acetylcysteine[6] or β-carotene[14] can have an adverse, pro-oxidant effect. These findings together with the negative results with β-carotene in a large chemoprevention trial[36] has led to a more critical attitude to the use of antioxidants in cancer chemoprevention.[38]

Agents with antiproliferation and antiprogression activities

Once a tumor cell is beyond the process of promotion it starts to proliferate in an uncontrolled manner and progresses to a more malignant phenotype characterized by invasion and metastasis. A large variety of drugs have the potential to interfere in the processes of signal transduction, apoptosis, angiogenesis or metastasis. An example of a drug that is active in signal transduction is tamoxifen; it prevents the binding of estrogen to nuclear receptors. Large clinical trials are going on testing the activity of tamoxifen on the development of breast cancer. In addition, retinoids (vitamin A and natural and synthetic analogs) are also important agents in this group. They have an array of mechanisms of action of which the most important are signal transduction, terminal differentiation and intercellular communication.[19] Retinoids have shown to have activity in HNSCC, not only in preclinical,[9,33] but also in clinical studies.[21]

Clinical trials

General characteristics

A chemoprevention trial is characterized by a long duration, as the end point of a trial is the development of cancer and/or survival. Another consequence is that drug administration has a chronic character, being often a daily intake for more than a year. An important issue is the level of toxicity that can be tolerated. It has to be realized that individuals will be treated who will not develop a tumor at all. As a general rule it can be stated that a higher level of toxicity can be tolerated when the risk for cancer increases. The chronic character of the trials and the fact that side effects may occur can have consequences for compliance. This can be monitored by asking the patients to bring their empty pill boxes to the follow-up visit. Moreover, it is possible to measure the drug or metabolites in the urine of plasma. Another complicating factor is that patients can violate the treatment protocol by taking additional chemopreventive agents. Most of them, especially the vitamins and antioxidants, can be bought in most countries without prescription.

Two major types of chemoprevention trials can be performed. The primary prevention trials address a general population or a population with a higher risk, such as long-term smokers. Secondary chemoprevention trials apply to patients with precancerous lesions or patients at very high risk for a second primary tumor. The cancer risk is much higher in secondary prevention trials and therefore a higher level of toxic side effects is acceptable in the study population.

It is clear that chemoprevention trials require long-term follow-up and large subject populations. One of the most important goals of prevention is to identify morphologic, genetic and biochemical markers that can accurately detect early changes associated with a phase of carcinogenesis that precedes the final end point, cancer.[18] This task of characterization and validation of the markers should be an integral part in all chemopreventive research. Markers should be used to identify the individuals who have the highest cancer risk and to monitor and predict the outcome of intervention. With validated markers, trials will be performed in a shorter time, at reduced costs and fewer patients will be overtreated. The ideal marker would fulfil the following criteria:

- to define and monitor in a quantitative fashion an individual's risk for cancer development; and
- to monitor the impact of a prevention strategy.

For a list of markers that may be of importance for HNSCC we refer to a recent review.[28]

Another area that could be explored is assessing cancer risk based on host factors. Although smoking is the major risk factor in HNSCC, inherent host factors play an important role as well. *In vitro* cytogenetic analyses of sensitivities to genotoxicity are gaining approval for use in the assessment of cancer risk. A mutagen sensitivity assay developed by Hsu *et al.* quantifies the number of bleomycin-induced chromatid breaks in cultured lymphocytes.[16] A recent multicenter analysis of 667 individuals showed that mutagen-sensitive smokers had a much higher risk for HNSCC than mutagen-insensitive smokers with odds ratios of 44.7 and 11.5, respectively.[7]

In the clinical development of a new chemopreventive agent various types of trials can be discriminated. Based on preclinical studies, new chemopreventive agents can be selected.[20] Subsequently, a phase I trial is performed on healthy normal subjects. Single-dose pharmacokinetics and acute toxicity are determined and, in addition, a repeated daily dose schedule over a period of more than a month is tested and combined with pharmacokinetics and chronic toxicity.

A phase II trial is performed to evaluate the relationship between dose and intermediate markers as an end point. All phase II trials are performed in subjects at high risk for cancer. In case a marker has not been identified first, a dose–response chronic dosing study is indicated with candidate markers (a phase IIa trial). The ultimate phase IIb trial should be a randomized, blinded and placebo-controlled trial and must be performed at one or more dose levels in order to select a dose level that is safe and effective in biomarker modulation.

Phase III studies would be randomized, blinded, placebo-controlled clinical trials with cancer incidence as the end point and with the aim to validate the intermediate end points.

Carcinomas of the upper aerodigestive tract are the best studied system for chemoprevention. This is related to the relatively high frequency of this type of tumor and the fact that high-risk groups are available. Secondary prevention trials have been performed in patients with leukoplakia and patients who have been cured for their first tumor and are now at risk for a second malignancy. It is also an attractive tumor type in the sense that biomarker studies have a promising outlook. Tissue samples are relatively easy to obtain and molecular markers have been identified that may reflect the multistep carcinogenic process of HNSCC.[5,28]

Completed trials

Many clinical chemoprevention studies have been performed in patients with oral leukoplakia. Several drugs, including retinyl palmitate, β-carotene and vitamin E, are able to induce a response.[10] Regression of this premalignant lesion is commonly taken as the endpoint but, strictly speaking, the occurrence of a carcinoma would be a better endpoint. One chemoprevention trial has been performed on a patient group with a premalignant lesion of the larynx.[17] The authors report a 75% response rate as a result of treatment with retinyl palmitate.

For patients who have been curatively treated for an early stage HNSCC, the risk of dying from a second primary tumor is greater than the risk of recurrence. Second primary tumors develop in this group in 15–35% of individuals. With the first tumor in the larynx there is a relatively high chance that the second tumor will develop in the lungs.[8] In 1990 the first results of a chemoprevention trial in HNSCC were reported.[15] 103 patients,

Table 58.1 Ongoing clinical chemoprevention trials of second primary tumors following an initial tumor in the respiratory or upper digestive tract

Organization/Code/Principal investigator	*Type of trial*	*Treatment*	*Initial tumor*
EUROSCAN, EORTC 24871 and 08871/ N de Vries, Amsterdam, The Netherlands†	Phase III, randomized	*N*-acetylcysteine; retinyl palmitate; both agents; nothing	Larynx and oral cavity (early stage) and non-small cell lung (early stage)
CRCH-9302, NCI-H96-0002/ L Le Marchand, Hawaii, USA	Randomized	Intensive nutrition intervention; non-intensive nutrition intervention	HNSCC (early stage) and lung (early stage)
EST-C-0590, NCI-P92-0026, MAYO-887451/H A Pinto, Stanford, USA	Phase III, randomized, double blind	Low-dose isotretinoin; placebo	HNSCC (early stage)
UMCC-9212, NCI-T92-0121C/ B A Conley, Baltimore, USA*	Phase I*	Low-dose tretinoin, once daily; low-dose tretinoin, 3 × daily; high-dose tretinoin, once daily; high-dose tretinoin, 3 × daily	HNSCC (all stages)
RTOG-9115, NCI-C92\1-0002, MDA-CCOP, DM-90094, NCI-P91-0024, CLB-9499/W K Hong, Houston, USA	Single arm	Low-dose isotretinoin	HNSCC (early stage)
Institute National de cancer de Canada/ I Bairati, Quebec, Canada	Randomized, double blind	β-Carotene; α-tocopherol	HNSCC
NCI-R01-CA64567/S T Mayne, New Haven, USA	Randomized	β-Carotene; placebo	HNSCC (early stage)

Except for the study indicated by *, all studies refer to patients who have been curatively treated for HNSCC or lung cancer.
*This study intends to establish the optimal dose, pharmacokinetics, biomarkers and response (chemotherapeutic and chemopreventive).
†The results of the Euroscan trial have recently been analysed; no protective effect of treatment could be observed.

who were free of disease following local therapy with surgery and/or radiotherapy for HNSCC, were randomized to receive isotretinoin or a placebo for 12 months. At the time of publication, at a median follow-up of 32 months, there was no difference in the number of patients who had recurrence of the initial tumor but there was a statistically significant difference with respect to the occurrence of a second primary tumor. Two patients in the treatment group and 12 patients in the placebo group had developed secondary tumors. An update was presented at a median follow-up time of 54.4 months.[1] At the time the difference in secondary tumors between the two groups was less, but still significant. A major complication of the trial was that 32% of the patients did not finish the total course of the treatment due to toxicity or non-compliance.

Bolla *et al.* have studied the effect of etretinate on the development of secondary tumors following HNSCC.[4] When compared to the trial of Hong *et al.*[15], this trial had more patients and included only patients who were initially treated for early stage disease. The analysis was performed after a mean follow-up period of 65 months and did not show a difference between the synthetic retinoid and the placebo group.[3]

At present a number of trials is ongoing focusing on the prevention of secondary cancer following HNSCC (Table 58.1). With the exception of the Baltimore trial all trials have the occurrence of secondary tumors as the endpoint. Two trials focus on the effect of treatment with a low dose of isotretinoin, based on the expectation to cause less toxic side effects. The Euroscan trial is the largest of the series; it started in 1988 and has accrued 2700 patients and a recent analysis showed that treatment had no effect on the occurrence of second primary cancer (Dr N. de Vries, personal communication). As can be seen from Table 58.1, some of the studies are phase III trials; the schedules and doses are based on clinical experience. To our knowledge phase II trials, with the intention to detect marker modulation at the safest dose possible (see above), have not been performed.

Results of other chemoprevention trials relevant for HNSCC

The effect of vitamin A (retinyl palmitate) was tested on 307 patients that had been curatively treated by surgery for stage I lung cancer.[29] After a median follow-up of 46 months the number of patients with either recurrence or new primary tumors was 37% in the treated arm and 48% in the untreated control arm. A small, but significant difference in favor of treatment was observed with respect to the occurrence of second primary tumors.

Two large-scale primary chemoprevention trials in heavy smokers have come up with negative results. The α-tocopherol, β-carotene cancer (ATBC) prevention study group reported on the effect of daily α-tocopherol (50 mg), β-carotene (20 mg), both, or a placebo and this was studied in 29 133 Finnish smokers.[36] Unexpectedly, an 18% higher lung cancer rate was found in the β-carotene arm versus the placebo arm. The β-carotene and retinol efficacy trial (CARET) investigated the effect of chemoprevention on 18 314 US smokers, ex-smokers or asbestos workers.[27] The results of this trial pointed in the same direction: a 28% higher lung cancer risk in the subjects that were supplemented with β-carotene (30 mg/day). Another large-scale trial studied 22 071 male physicians, of whom 11% were smokers and 39% former smokers. Here no effect of β-carotene (50 mg on alternate days) on lung cancer was found.[13]

The outcome of the ATBC and CARET trials showed a harmful effect of a supplementation with β-carotene in smokers; this is in contrast to what was expected from animal and epidemiologic studies. There are a few studies that may shed some light on the adverse effect of β-carotene. Although β-carotene is known for its antioxidant properties, theoretically, the effect of β-carotene can be pro-oxidant, especially with a high oxygen tension, as is found in the lung.[38] *In vitro*, a pro-oxidant effect for *N*-acetylcysteine, vitamin C and other antioxidants, has been found.[6] Ingestion of large amounts of β-carotene seems to cause a decreased uptake of other natural occurring carotenoids, so this could lower the uptake of compounds with greater potential to prevent oxidative stress.[26] Another detrimental effect has been reported in the hamster cheek pouch model, showing that the administration of β-carotene led to a higher vascularization in malignant tissue.[32] Altogether, these data have led to the conclusion that the pharmacologic use of supplemental β-carotene for the prevention of lung cancer, particularly in smokers, can no longer be recommended.[23]

Future perspectives

The concept of chemoprevention is attractive and deserves further attention. As for larynx cancer, there are two patient groups that may profit from chemoprevention in the near future: patients with a premalignant lesion in the larynx and patients that have been curatively treated for larynx cancer and who are at high risk to develop a second primary tumor in the lungs or the upper digestive tract. A positive and two negative results (no effect) have been reported on the chemoprevention of second primary tumors following HNSCC. Results will soon become available from more trials (see Table 58.1).

Important drawbacks of the presently performed chemoprevention trials are the long duration and the need for a large study group. To make rapid progress in clinical chemoprevention it is essential to identify markers and select proper agents. These agents should be capable of altering cancer cell biology in ways that can be measured by the markers. This means that candidate markers should be tested in carefully designed phase II trials. A drug dose should be chosen that is safe and induces marker modulation. Eventually this integral approach should lead to carefully designed phase III trials with an early outcome as the key characteristic.

The basis of future chemoprevention research is the cooperation between laboratory and clinical researchers; only then will it become a successful treatment strategy.

References

1. Benner SE, Pajak TF, Lippman SM *et al.* Prevention of second primary tumors with isotretinoin in patients with squamous cell carcinoma of the head and neck: long-term follow-up. *J Natl Cancer Inst* 1994; **86**: 140–1.
2. Berenblum I. The modifying influence of dichloroethyl sulfide on the induction of tumours in mice by tar. *J Pathol Bacteriol* 1929; **32**: 1096–8.
3. Bolla M, Laplanche A, Lefur R *et al.* Prevention of second primary tumours with a second generation retinoid in squamous cell carcinoma of oral cavity and oropharynx: long term follow-up. *Eur J Cancer* 1996; **32A**: 375–6.
4. Bolla M, Lefur R, Ton Van J *et al.* Prevention of second primary tumours with etretinate in squamous cell carcinoma of the oral cavity and oropharynx. Results of a multicentric double-blind randomised study. *Eur J Cancer* 1994; **30A**: 767–72.
5. Califano J, van der Riet P, Westra W *et al.* Genetic progression model for head and neck cancer: implications for field cancerization. *Cancer Res* 1994; **56**: 2488–92.
6. Cloos J, Gille JJP, Steen I *et al.* Influence of the antioxidant *N*-acetylcysteine and its metabolites on damage induced by bleomycin in PM2 bacteriophage DNA. *Carcinogenesis* 1996; **17**: 327–31.
7. Cloos J, Spitz MR, Schantz SP *et al.* Genetic susceptibility to head and neck squamous cell carcinoma. *J Natl Cancer Inst* 1996; **88**: 530–5.
8. de Vries N. The magnitude of the problem. In: de Vries N, Gluckman JL, eds. *Multiple primary tumors in the head and neck.* Stuttgart; Thieme Verlag, 1990: 1–25.
9. Gijare PS, Rao KV, Bhide SV. Modulatory effects of snuff, retinoic acid and beta-carotene on DMBA-induced hamster cheek pouch carcinogenesis in relation to keratin expression. *Nutr Cancer* 1990; **14**: 253–9.
10. Gonzalez PM, Benner SE. Clinical studies in head and neck cancer chemoprevention. *Cancer Metast Rev* 1996; **15**: 113–18.
11. Hartman PE, Schankel DM. Antimutagens and anticarcinogens: a survey of putative interceptor molecules. *Environ Mol Mutagen* 1990; **15**: 145–82.
12. Heller B, Kluftinger AM, Davis NL, Quenville NF. A modified method of carcinogenesis induction in the DMBA hamster cheek pouch model of squamous neoplasia. *Am J Surg* 1996; **172**: 678–80.

13. Hennekens CH, Buring JE, Manson JE *et al.* Lack of effect of long-term supplementation with beta carotene on the incidence of malignant neoplasms and cardiovascular disease. *N Engl J Med* 1996; **334**: 1145–9.
14. Herbert V. The antioxidant supplement myth. *Am J Nutr* 1994; **60**: 157–8.
15. Hong WK, Lippman SM, Itri LM *et al.* Prevention of second primary tumors with isotretinoin in squamous cell carcinoma of the head and neck. *N Engl J Med* 1990; **323**: 795–801.
16. Hsu TC, Cherry L M, Samaan NA. Differential mutagen susceptibility in cultured lymphocytes of normal individuals and cancer patients. *Cancer Genet Cytogenet* 1985; **17**: 307–13.
17. Issing WJ, Struck R, Naumann A. Long-term follow-up of larynx leukoplakia under treatment with retinyl palmitate. *Head Neck Surg* 1996; **18**: 560–5.
18. Kelloff GJ, Malone WF, Boone CW, Steele VE, Doody LA. Intermediate biomarkers of precancer and their application in chemoprevention. *J Cell Biochem* 1992; **S16G**: 15–21.
19. Kelloff GJ, Boone CW, Steele VE *et al.* Mechanistic considerations in chemopreventive drug development. *J Cell Biochem* 1994; **S20**: 1–24.
20. Kelloff GJ, Johnson JR, Crowell JA *et al.* Guidance for development of chemopreventive agents. *J Cell Biochem* 1994; **S20**: 25–31.
21. Khuri FR, Lippman SM, Spitz MR, Lotan R, Hong WK. Molecular epidemiology and retinoid chemoprevention of head and neck cancer. *J Natl Cancer Inst* 1997; **89**: 199–211.
22. La Vecchia C, Franceschi S, Levi F, Lucchini F, Negri E. Diet and human oral carcinoma in Europe. *Oral Oncol Eur J Cancer* 1993; **29B**: 17–22.
23. Mayne ST. Beta-carotene, carotenoids, and disease prevention in humans. *FASEB J* 1996; **10**: 690–701.
24. Nomura AMY, Ziegler RG, Stemmermann GN, Chyou PH, Craft NE. Serum micronutrients and upper aerodigestive tract cancer. *Cancer Epidemiol Biomarkers Prev* 1997; **6**: 407–12.
25. Notani PN, Jayant K. Role of diet in upper aerodigestive tract cancer. *Nutr Cancer* 1987; **10**: 103–13.
26. Olsen J. Absorption, transport and metabolism of carotenoids in humans. *Pure Appl Chem* 1994; **66**: 1101–16.
27. Omnenn GS, Goodman GE, Thornquist MD *et al.* Effects of a combination of beta carotene and vitamin A on lung cancer and cardiovascular disease. *N Engl J Med* 1996; **334**: 1150–5.
28. Papadimitrakopoulou VA, Shin DM, Hong WK. Molecular and cellular biomarkers for field cancerization and multistep process in head and neck tumorigenesis. *Cancer Metastasis Rev* 1996; **15**: 53–76.
29. Pastorino U, Infante M, Maioli M *et al.* Adjuvant treatment of stage I lung cancer with high-dose vitamin A. *J Clin Oncol* 1993; **11**: 1216–22.
30. Roebuck BD, Liu YL, Rogers AE, Groopman JD, Kensler TW. Protection against aflatoxin B1-induced hepatocarcinogenesis in F344 rats by 5-(2-pyrazinyl)-4-methyl-1,2-dithiole-3-thione (oltipraz): predictive role for short-term molecular dosimetry. *Cancer Res* 1991; **51**: 5501–6.
31. Schwartz JL, Shklar G. Glutathione inhibits experimental oral carcinogenesis, p53 expression, and angiogenesis. *Nutr Cancer* 1996; **26**: 229–36.
32. Schwartz JL, Shklar G. Retinoid and carotenoid angiogenesis: a possible explanation for enhanced oral carcinogenesis. *Nutr Cancer* 1997; **27**: 192–9.
33. Shklar G, Schwartz J, Grau D, Trickler DP, Wallace KD. Inhibition of hamster buccal pouch carcinogenesis by 13-cis-retinoid acid. *Oral Surg Oral Med Oral Pathol* 1980; **50**: 45–52.
34. Sporn MB, Newton DL. Chemoprevention of cancer with retinoids. *Fed Proc* 1979; **38**: 2528–34.
35. Steele VE, Moon RC, Lubet RA *et al.* Preclinical efficacy evaluation of potential chemopreventive agents in animal carcinogenesis models: methods and results from the NCI Chemoprevention Drug Development Program. *J Cell Biochem* 1994; **S20**: 32–54.
36. The Alpha-Tocopherol Beta Carotene Cancer Prevention Study Group. The effect of vitamin E and beta carotene on the incidence of lung cancer and other cancers in male smokers. *N Engl J Med* 1994; **330**: 1029–35.
37. van den Brandt PA, Goldbohm RA, van 't Veer P *et al.* A prospective cohort study on selenium status and the risk of lung cancer. *Cancer Res* 1993; **53**: 4860–5.
38. Woodall AA, Jack CI, Jackson MJ. Caution with β-carotene supplements. *Lancet* 1996; **347**: 967–70.
39. Zheng W. Risk factors for oral and pharyngeal cancer in Shanghai, with emphasis on diet. *Cancer Epidemiol Biomarkers Prev* 1992; **1**: 441–8.
40. Zheng W, Blot WJ, Diamond EL *et al.* Serum micronutrients and the subsequent risk of oral and pharyngeal cancer. *Cancer Res* 1993; **53**: 795–8.

Voice rehabilitation after total laryngectomy

Ranny van Weissenbruch

The eradication of the intrinsic human characteristic of voice and verbal communication is generally considered to be the most disabling consequence of laryngectomy. Not surprisingly, the earliest efforts to introduce total laryngectomy as a treatment method for advanced laryngeal cancer were already accompanied by innovative artificial larynges or prostheses. However, treatment of this disease has often been complicated by reluctance to drastically alter the quality of life. With time, considerable progress has been made to salvage the laryngeal framework with radiation therapy and conservation laryngectomy procedures.

History of surgical voice restoration

In 1873, Gussenbauer devised an artificial larynx, which provided communication from the tracheostoma to the pharyngostoma for the first successfully laryngectomized patient by Th. Billroth.[42] Aspiration was prevented by a trapdoor flap while expired air was directed to the pharynx through a tracheal cannula, which consisted of a metal reed for sound production. As reported, 3 weeks after surgery the patient developed an intelligible though monotonous voice.

In 1894, Gluck and Sorensen were the pioneers of the primary closure of the pharynx following laryngectomy.[24a] This abolished the troublesome pharyngostoma, but at the same time eliminated the prosthetic tracheo-esophageal shunt for voice production. After pharyngeal closure, voice restoration methods were primarily directed towards external artificial larynges or intrinsic methods of voice production.

In 1932, Guttman described a procedure by which a fistula between the trachea and esophagus was created under surgical control with a diathermic needle.[43,44] By occluding the tracheostoma, this fistula allowed shunting of expired air from the airway to the digestive tract, where it elicited sound. This procedure allowed fast but temporarily vocal rehabilitation, because of spontaneous closure of the fistula. In 1952, Briani introduced a surgical technique for creating a pharyngocutaneous fistula connected to the tracheostoma by means of external acrylic and polyethylene devices.[18,19] After initially using an anterior neck flap, a simple puncture technique was described to create this fistula.

In order to prevent leakage or stenosis of the fistula, several modified surgical techniques were developed. Conley used a tubed esophageal mucosa or reversed autogenous vein grafts for esophagocutaneous fistulization at the level superior to the tracheostoma or the posterosuperior tracheal wall.[23–25] In 1965, Asai modified this approach with a three-stage method to establish an internal cervical 'dermal tube'.[8,9] A superiorly placed tracheostoma created at the time of laryngectomy was followed with secondary construction of a superior pharyngostoma in the midline hypopharynx. Upon manual closure of the tracheostoma, expiratory airflow could be diverted through this vertical shunt into the pharynx. Despite several modifications, its use was limited by aspiration, shunt disruption, strictures and troubles of hair growth in the fistula tract.

In 1969, Staffieri introduced the 'neoglottis phonatoria' using a tracheohypopharyngeal shunt with satisfactory functional speech results.[95,99,101,103,104,108] Following narrow field laryngectomy the cricoid ring, thyroid perichondrium, hyoid bone and epiglottic remnant were joined in a single-stage procedure to create a slit-like fistula in the anterior pharyngoesophageal wall and the proximal tracheal end. Satisfactory results were obtained with this type of shunt speech.[99] However, this procedure encountered a relatively high percentage of aspiration, shunt stenosis and recurrent carcinoma.[62,95,98,99]

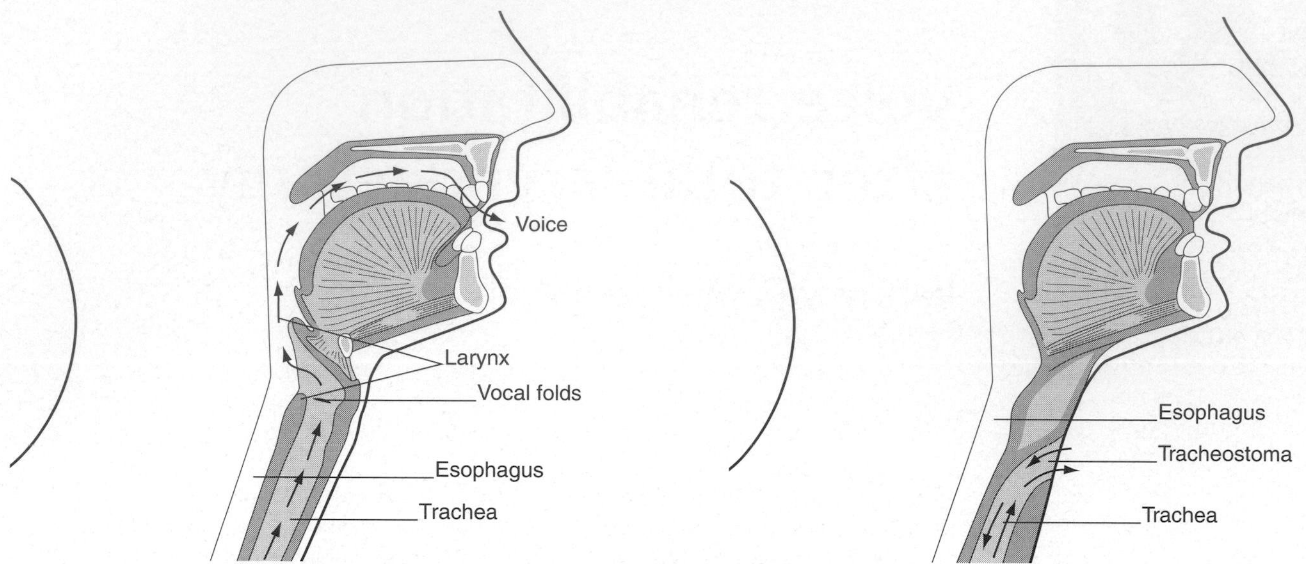

Figure 59.1 *Preoperative status. Laryngeal phonation is produced by passing exhaled air over the vocal cords, resulting in vibrations which are modified in the oral cavity.*

Figure 59.2 *Postoperative status. After laryngectomy the trachea is proximally attached to a permanent stoma. Respiration is carried on through the tracheostoma.*

Surgical voice restoration with tracheoesophageal shunt methods results in good voice quality when compared with other methods of substitute voice production. Aspiration through the shunt and stenosis of the fistula have been known as the most important drawbacks.[113]

Several techniques have been developed to prevent aspiration. The neoglottis procedure was introduced in 1972.[6,7] A primitive valved glottis was created after narrow field laryngectomy by preserving the cricoid ring, thyroid perichondrium, hyoid bone and suprahyoid epiglottic stump. Unlike some, good speech results were obtained with this procedure; it was accompanied by high percentages of complications.

Amatsu used two esophageal muscle flaps, a tracheal mucosal flap, and a tracheoesophageal side-to-side anastomosis in an attempt to gain control over the valve mechanism of the shunt.[1–3] Montgomery and Lavelle tried to regulate the opening of the tracheopharyngeal shunt with a myoplasty, using the sternocleidomastoid muscle.[70] Herrmann and Zenner created a valve with homogenous cartilage to close the shunt during swallowing.[50] Despite these efforts acceptable voice without aspiration was not always achieved. The high rate of failure of shunt and neoglottis procedures, along with an unacceptable rate of local tumor recurrence, stimulated new interest in laryngeal substitutes.

In 1972, Mozolewski was the first to introduce a prosthetic device which effectively prevented stenosis as well as aspiration.[73] By insertion of a valve prosthesis, the shunt became a 'protected' tracheoesophageal fistula.

In 1979, Blom and Singer further revolutionized this field with their description of endoscopic insertion of a tracheoesophageal one-way duckbill valve following total laryngectomy.[11] This stimulated new interest in prosthetic voice rehabilitation, including the introduction of various types of shunt valved prostheses.

Methods of voice rehabilitation

The result of a laryngectomy is not limited to the loss of the larynx and its vocal folds; the lower respiratory tract is separated from the vocal tract as well as from the upper digestive tract (Figs 59.1 and 59.2). Breathing is performed through the created tracheostoma and there is no connection between the oral cavity and the airways. After laryngectomy the laryngectomee has to develop a new sound source and a new energy source in order to acquire a substitute voice. In a way, both the sound and energy source should be connected to the vocal tract and oral cavity.

Today, the three most common methods of communication used by laryngectomees are the artificial electric larynx, esophageal speech, and tracheoesophageal speech.[101]

The artificial larynges

The function of an artificial larynx is to replace the voice source, and not to replace the natural larynx. These internally or externally applicable mechanical vibration sources have been developed to set the air in the vocal tract in vibration. The energy sources for these vibrators are either powered by air pressure (pneumatic larynges), or they are electrically (battery) powered (electric larynges).

The pneumatic larynges are driven by pulmonary air channeled across a reed vibrator and coupled to the permanent tracheostoma. The different devices are available in neck-type and mouth-type models. In the mouth-type devices, exhaled air carries the sound produced by the reed within the external tubing to the mouth. The advantages of a pneumatic larynx are the proper coordination of phonation by respiration and the unchanged dynamics of speech without mechanical or electronic noises. The manual use, necessary access to the tracheostoma with external tubings, and visual distractions during usage are considered major drawbacks of this method.

The principle of the electric larynx consists of vibrations generated by an electromagnetic mechanism. The devices can be divided into types that can be used transcervically, and mouth types. The oral devices (e.g. Cooper-Rand Electric Speech Aid) directs the battery-powered sound into the oral cavity via a small tube placed in the mouth. Immediately after surgery the oral devices may be advantageous, because the patient can use it without interfering with neck healing or causing discomfort.

The Servox Inton® and the Western Electric® AT&T electrolarynges are examples of widely known neck-held devices. The hand-held sound sources are placed against the neck to direct sound through the skin into the vocal tract. More recent types have variable pitch and loudness adjustments. In case of edematous swollen necks postoperatively and in necks with thick scar tissue formation, positioning of the devices against the neck is difficult. Some electric larynges feature an intraoral connector to permit the use of the device immediately after surgery. Another disadvantage is the hand-held feature, which may draw special attention to the disability. This could partially be compensated by using a neck strap. However, a more significant drawback of the use of electric artificial larynges is the production of monotonous and mechanical sounds.[113]

Esophageal speech

The intrinsic forms of alaryngeal speech make use of the anatomic structures which remain after the laryngectomy procedure.[64,113]

Esophageal speech is considered to be the best intrinsic form of alaryngeal speech.[113] Acquiring esophageal speech successfully after laryngectomy ranges from 20% to 83%.[40,54,64,87,115] To produce sound in esophageal speech, an energy source and a sound source are needed (Fig 59.3).

An air reservoir in the upper part of the esophagus is used as the energy source of esophageal voice production. The small air reservoir available for esophageal speech will limit the esophageal speaker's ability to produce long utterances on a single charge of air. However, this limited air supply need not be a significant limitation to good sound production. To produce sound in esophageal speech, air must first be transferred into the esophagus. However, the injection technique can be considered as the most efficient method to fill this esophageal reservoir.

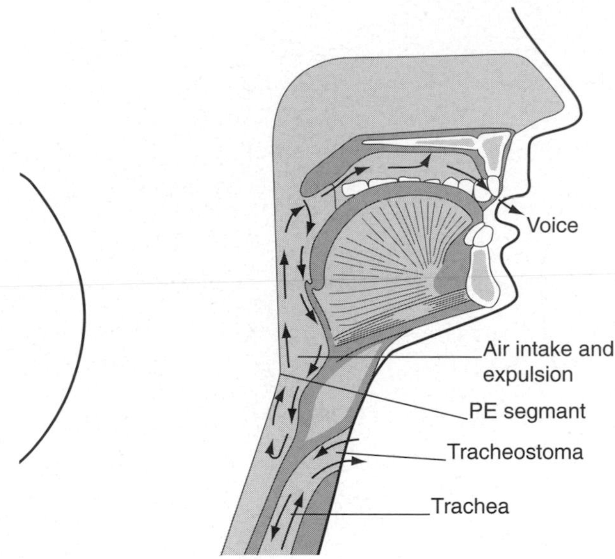

Figure 59.3 *Esophageal speech arises from vibrations of the pharyngoesophageal segment during eructation of injected esophageal air.*

When the injection method is used, the patient uses movements of the floor of the mouth to increase oral and pharyngeal pressure which causes the pharyngoesophageal (PE) segment to open and allows air into the esophagus.[64,113] The oropharyngeal cavity is enclosed by the lips and the velopharyngeal closing mechanism. The entrapped air can be sufficiently pressurized to overcome the resistance of the PE segment.

Air injection can be accomplished in two ways. The consonant injection or plosive injection method makes use of pressure buildup in the production of voiceless plosive consonants (/p/, /t/, /k/). The air is injected into the esophagus before the consonant is produced.[26,111] Another method of injecting air into the esophagus is known as the glossal press, glossopharyngeal press, or the tongue pump injection method.[113]

The actual sound source of esophageal speech has been a topic of intensive discussion. A structure within the PE segment, called the pseudoglottis, is generally considered to be the activator of esophageal sound production.

The pseudoglottis is located at a level between the fourth and sixth cervical vertebrae. It is also identical with the entrance of the esophagus.[28,30,79,82–84,109] The term pharyngoesophageal segment is used to describe the region where the pseudoglottis is located within the surroundings of the esophageal entrance. The shape and length of the PE segment varies depending on the exact surgical procedure. The pseudoglottis may be regarded as a sphincter muscle.[15,39,64,117] The location and shape of the pseudoglottis may be of influence on the quality of the esophageal voice production.[10,26,29,32,63,64,82–84] Massively shaped pseudoglottides are associated with poor esophageal voice.[64]

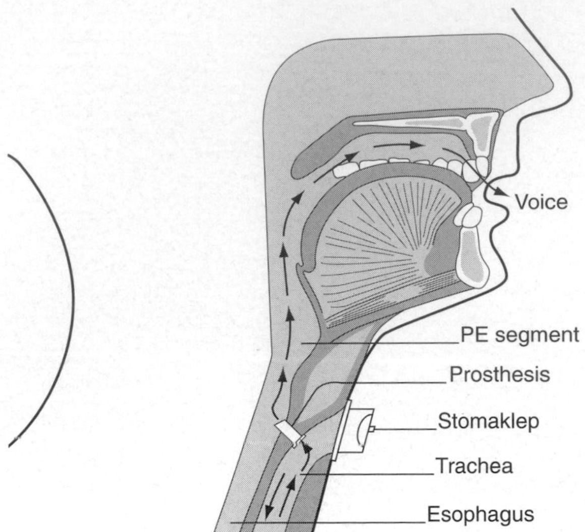

Figure 59.4 *Tracheoesophageal speech is produced by directing exhaled air from the trachea through the prosthesis into the esophagus where vibrations are produced. During phonation the stoma is closed manually or by using a tracheostoma valve.*

Tracheoesophageal speech

After a total laryngectomy no laryngeal structures are left for reconstruction of a neoglottis. The extrinsic forms of alaryngeal speech rely on procedures involving creation of an internal shunt with or without a voice prosthesis.

Most of the surgical methods used to restore speech after laryngectomy have consisted of internal and external tracheopharyngeal or tracheoesophageal shunt techniques. With these techniques voice rehabilitation is attempted with a connecting canal between the respiratory tract and the digestive tract (Fig 59.4).

Upon closure of the tracheostoma, expired air will be transported through the shunt to the digestive tract. The sound source depends on the type of technique used. In low tracheopharyngeal shunts and tracheoesophageal shunts, sound is produced in the PE segment by the pseudoglottis. This is the similar sound producing structure used in esophageal speech. High tracheopharyngeal shunts have their anastomosis located above the pseudoglottis. The sound produced with these shunts is not comparable with esophageal speech.

Various operative techniques and often complicated devices have been designed to cope with problems associated with these shunt methods, but they remained unsuccessful. The problems of leakage of saliva or food with subsequent aspiration, and spontaneous closure of the shunt necessitating revision surgery are considered major drawbacks of the procedure, which limited the use of these methods.

The development of valve prostheses that are introduced in the internal shunt have not only eliminated most of these surgical related complications, but prevented stenosis of the shunt as well.[47,64,74]

Table 59.1 Different types of tracheoesophageal voice prostheses

Algaba voice prosthesis
Bivona voice prostheses
Duckbill
Low-resistance
Ultra-low-resistance
Bivona-Colorado prosthesis
Blom-Singer voice prostheses
Duckbill
Low-pressure
Indwelling low-pressure
Bonelli valve
Groningen voice prostheses
Standard button
Low-resistance
Ultra-low-resistance
Henley-Cohn voice prosthesis
Herrmann ESKA voice prosthesis
Nijdam voice prosthesis
Panje voice button
Provox voice prosthesis
Type 1
Type 2
Staffieri voice prosthesis
Supratracheal semi-permanent valve prosthesis (Mozolewski)
Traissac voice prosthesis
Voicemaster

The first real tracheoesophageal valve prosthesis was introduced by Mozolewski in 1972.[73] Renewed interest for surgical voice rehabilitation was obtained after the introduction of the 'duckbill' voice prosthesis by Blom and Singer in 1979.[11] This valved prosthesis could be inserted by a simple endoscopic tracheoesophageal puncture technique. It was constructed of a medical biocompatible grade silicone polymer, resistant against chemical influences.

Since than many different silicone-made prostheses have been developed (see Table 59.1). The non-self-retaining prostheses (Bivona, Blom-Singer Duckbill and low-pressure devices, Herrmann) are designed for secondary placement some time following laryngectomy. The patient should be able to remove and replace the device for maintenance. The disadvantages of these non-self-retaining devices are the attachment of the prosthesis to the skin with glue, regular removal for maintenance, reinsertion problems with spontaneous closure of the fistula, irritation of the tracheoesophageal shunt, extrusion of the prosthesis and shunt migration.[74] The self-retaining prostheses (Blom-Singer indwelling, Groningen, Nijdam, Provox, Traissac) need daily maintenance without removal. During voice production these prostheses are self-cleaning. This type of prosthesis is ideal for the laryngectomee who is unable to perform daily removal

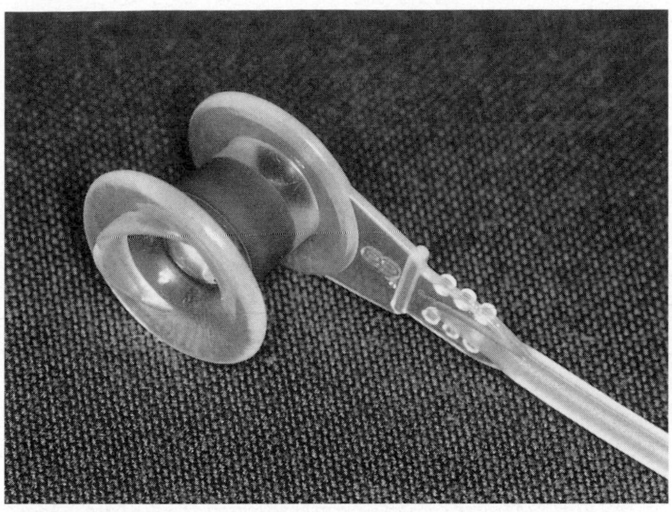

Figure 59.5 *Provox type 2 voice prosthesis. The valve is seated at the esophageal flange of the prosthesis. At the tracheal site a string is attached for secured anterograde insertion or retrograde insertion through the pharynx.*

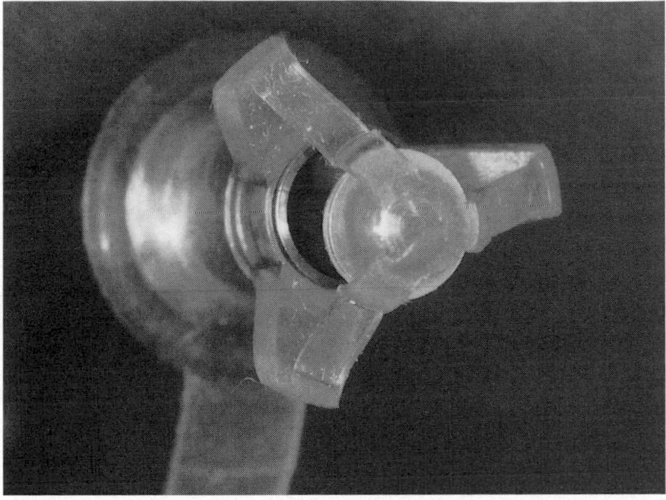

Figure 59.6 *Voicemaster voice prosthesis. Leakage through this prosthesis is prevented by using a retractable ball valve.*

and reinsertion of the prosthesis. They can be placed during laryngectomy, or as a secondary procedure after laryngectomy. Replacement of the prosthesis is performed by a clinician or physician, often as an outpatient procedure. For the introduction and replacement of indwelling prostheses, a flexible guidewire with a connector for attachment of the introduction string of the new prosthesis is used. After retrograde introduction of the guidewire through the esophagus and pharynx, the new prosthesis can be inserted transorally. The introduction and replacement of indwelling prostheses can be facilitated by using anterograde insertion techniques, which are available for the Provox 2 and Voicemaster voice prostheses (Figs 59.5 and 59.6). Just a few complications are reported with the standard procedures which are often limited to dislodgment of the prosthesis, aspiration, external leakage, hypertrophy and granulation of the shunt.[74]

During shunt esophageal speech the intratracheal air pressure is dependent on the tonicity of the esophagus and the PE segment, and on the airway resistance of the prosthesis used. The early developed prostheses (Duckbill, Groningen button, Herrmann, Traissac) are considered to be high-resistance prostheses. The newer ones (Blom-Singer low-pressure, ultra low-resistance Groningen, Provox 2, Voicemaster) are made of low-pressure valve designs or are even valveless (Nijdam prosthesis). The low-pressure prostheses should allow easier passage of air through the shaft, due to improved aerodynamic properties of the valve. By altering the size of the inner diameter of the shaft and by modifying the valve design, the prostheses can improve the efficiency of shunt esophageal speech. However, the size of the diameter of the prosthesis is limited as larger prostheses may interfere with wall strength and give rise to shunt insufficiency.[51]

High success rates (50–95%) of speech rehabilitation have been reported consistently by laryngectomees using several types of voice prostheses.[33,56,64,67,68,94,115] A high percentage of patients is able to produce tracheo-esophageal shunt speech almost immediately following puncture. The success rate of speech rehabilitation in patients with a secondary puncture appears to be lower compared to primarily punctured patients.[64,115]

The device life is determined by the normal wear and tear of the silicone rubber, and by colonization and deterioration of the silicone surface by a mixed biofilm containing fungi, bacteria and food residua (Fig 59.7). This may

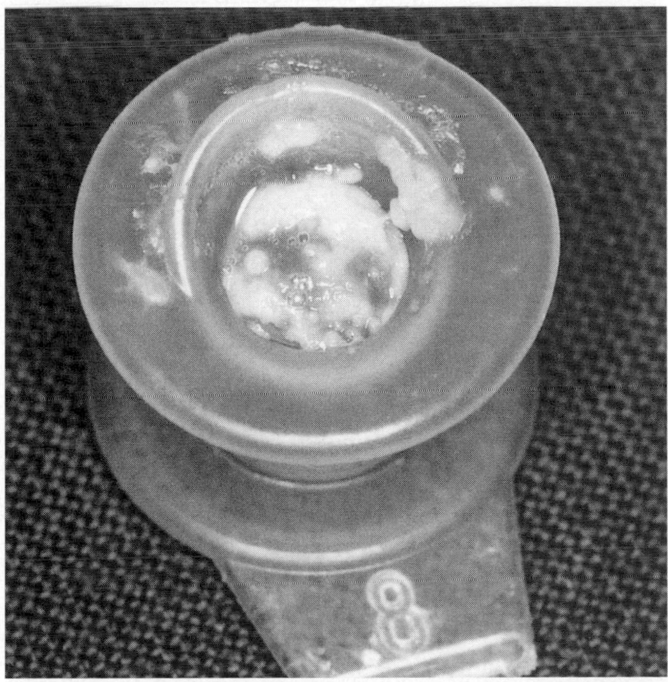

Figure 59.7 *Deposits at the esophageal flange of a dysfunctional Provox voice prosthesis.*

lead to stiffening of the valve with secondary leakage of pharyngeal contents into the trachea, and an increased airflow resistance of the valve.[47,51,74] A prolonged device life may be expected after surface-coating techniques to prevent fungal and bacterial contamination.

The properties of an ideal tracheoesophageal shunt prosthesis are:

- possible insertions during and following total laryngectomy;
- self-cleaning;
- maintenance free;
- low flow resistance; and
- unlimited device life.[100]

General principles of surgical voice rehabilitation

Preoperative speech evaluation

Good candidates for tracheoesophageal puncture should be motivated and mentally stable patients.[78] Understanding of the anatomy and function of the prosthesis, as well as manual dexterity and visual acuity, are necessary factors in order to guarantee maintenance and care for the stoma and prosthesis. However, patient selection criteria may vary according to whether rehabilitation is a primary or a secondary procedure.

Active and passive air insufflation tests with or without video fluoroscopy should be routinely undertaken to find out if the patient will be able to produce tracheoesophageal speech following total laryngectomy. Additional tests via multiple level manometry may be necessary.[114] This allows the examiner to assess the presence or lack of the vibrating pharyngoesophageal segment. Patients should also have good to moderate pulmonary ventilation and a sufficient cough reflex. Patients with low pulmonary flow rates may have difficulty with the speech fistula.[16]

Patients who undergo pharyngeal reconstruction with a skin flap or visceral transposition may effectively use tracheoesophageal phonation.[16,89,101] In these cases the prognosis for esophageal speech acquisition and effective artificial larynx use is relative poor.[101]

After total laryngectomy a complex of speech options becomes possible. The esophageal speech and artificial larynx speech options have already been discussed. All methods have one major communication goal: to accomplish patient satisfaction in meeting his or her communication needs.

Surgical techniques

Treatment for laryngeal malignancies is inextricably linked to quality of life after diagnosis. Fundamental concern revolves around voice production, whereas secondary consideration of the maintenance of good deglutition is of prime importance. The decision for primary or secondary tracheoesophageal puncture rests with the surgeon and the patient.

Tracheoesophageal puncture at the time of laryngectomy: the primary procedure

The technique of total laryngectomy should be carefully assessed in order to obtain good tracheoesophageal speech.

The tracheostoma must be of adequate size to accomplish sufficient closure with a finger. Tendency for stenosis of the stoma should also be prevented. The pharyngeal vocal tract must have efficient aerodynamic properties to enable good airflow. A right muscular tonus of the pharyngeal wall is necessary to generate a good pitch.[89]

The procedure of total laryngectomy is performed after intubation and creation of a tracheostomy. After resection of the larynx with or without a hemithyroidectomy from the surrounding neck structures, the specimen is taken out after making a horizontal incision at the first tracheal ring. The U-shaped incision length is dependent on the length of the neck and the required elevation of the superior skin flap to expose the hyoid. The tracheostoma is created by suturing the skin to the upper tracheal ring.[35]

The tracheoesophageal puncture is placed through the back wall of the trachea from the cervical esophagus. In the methods described for the Groningen and Provox prostheses, a pharynx protector is used and placed inside the open pharynx wound and positioned just cranially of the tracheostoma. A trocar or sharp pointed wire is used for puncturing the tracheoesophageal wall. The cutting device is placed in the midline of the trachea and between 1 and 1.5 cm below the cut edge of the posterior tracheal wall. If the tracheoesophageal wall has been separated to or below this level, a primary puncture should not be performed to avoid possible abscess formation.

After puncturing the wall, the mandrin of the trocar is removed, and a flexible or metal guidewire is introduced. After the tip of the wire is visible in the pharynx opening, the string of a prosthesis of the proper size is attached to it. By pulling the guidewire with the prosthesis backward, the prosthesis will be inserted into the tracheoesophageal shunt. The tracheal flange should be brought into position to accomplish accurate fitting of the prosthesis. The introduction string of the prosthesis is then cut off.

Hypopharyngeal closure is achieved by approximating the mucosal edges in a Y fashion, allowing a low-tension closure adapted to the defect. Running or interrupted sutures are used for mucosal closure. This is followed by submucosal and muscular sutures. The muscular closure may pull the eventually myotomized edges apart. Very tight closure of this layer is not recommended. To prevent false routes a nasogastric tube is introduced before mucosal closure.

Skin closure is performed after unilateral dissection of pharyngeal plexus branches, and introduction of wound drains for vacuum suction. A cuffed Shiley® cannula is introduced into the tracheostoma for 24–48 hours. Prosthetic voice rehabilitation may start 10–12 days postoperatively, as soon as the nasogastric tube has been removed.[75,89]

Secondary voice restoration

A number of factors are considered in selecting patients for secondary endoscopic voice restoration following laryngectomy. Patients who are not successful in obtaining satisfactory esophageal or artificial laryngeal speech are candidates for secondary prosthetic voice restoration.

A barium pharyngoesophagogram is indicated before the puncture to evaluate the size and mobility of the PE segment, and if there is a history of significant deglutition problems, stricture, or pharyngoesophageal reconstruction. The factors described at the primary puncture section are also judged.

The tracheostoma is evaluated with regard to location and diameter. The minimal stomal diameter to accommodate a voice prosthesis without obstructing respiration is 1.5 cm. The small stoma is managed by dilatation with silicone vents or surgical revision. Stoma vents may also be used in combination with the voice prosthesis.[35]

The secondary puncture is best performed under general anesthesia when the procedure requires rigid esophagoscopy,[21,31,46,93] although secondary puncture techniques are described for local or topical anesthesia.[41,102] A rigid esophagoscope is introduced into the hypopharynx, and advanced towards the tracheostoma while the midline of the neck is palpated with a hand. The tip of the esophagoscope is rotated 180°, to direct the open side of the instrument upwards. After removing the intubation tube from the trachea, a trocar or sharp, pointed wire is used again to puncture the tracheoesophageal wall. A metal or flexible guiding wire is advanced upwards through the esophagoscope into the mouth, after removal of the mandrin. After attaching the prosthesis to the wire, it is pulled back and inserted into the created tracheoesophageal shunt. Voice rehabilitation may start almost immediately after this procedure.[53,67,68,89]

Pharyngeal constrictor myotomy

A pharyngeal constrictor myotomy may be a very important single step to facilitate tracheoesophageal puncture speech, as well as esophageal speech. In general, constrictor myotomy is created at the time of laryngectomy, especially if the muscles are not repositioned in the closure.[35]

Hypertonicity of the PE segment and constrictor spasm are considered to be major causes of failing shunt esophageal speech. A tight PE segment will prevent the passage of air, whereas relaxation will facilitate air expulsion and subsequent phonation.[64] Pharyngoesophageal myotomies were originally performed as a secondary procedure to improve voice rehabilitation after laryngectomy. A primary myotomy is recommended for prevention of spasms and hypertonicity of the PE segment. A primary myotomy is preferred to a second-stage operation, because after extensive neck surgery and radiation this may be a difficult procedure. During total laryngectomy, it is easily performed. Patients often refuse to undergo a second operation. Myotomies or pharyngeal plexus neurectomy of the PE segment have been advocated to treat or prevent this hypertonic PE segment.[63,64,94,96]

When too much musculature has been dissected, a hypotonic state of the PE segment may be caused, which results in a breathy quality of the shunt esophageal speech. Modified procedures have been reported to prevent these problems.[64] The present technique is performed in the posterior midline from the level of the tongue base to the puncture site. All the musculature is incised to the depth of the submucosal vasculature.

To prevent embarrassment of vertical vasculature, straight myotomy incisions should be made.[35] The mucosa should be carefully examined for mucosal lacerations after performing the myotomy.

A pharyngeal constrictor myotomy is advocated even if the tracheoesophageal puncture has been delayed to a secondary procedure.[35]

Pharyngeal plexus neurectomy

During tracheoesophageal speech a critical tension in the muscular wall of the pharynx must exist to permit airflow for speech production. Hypertonicity or spasm of the PE segment will trap air, forcing it into the stomach with resultant distension. In the majority of cases, a unilateral myotomy of the cricopharyngeus muscle and inferior pharyngeal constrictor muscle is successful in preventing elevated tensions in the PE segment during phonation.[35,96] The resultant tonicity of the PE segment will affect the pitch in alaryngeal phonation.

A unilateral neurectomy of the pharyngeal plexus may have the advantage over a myotomy in that it is less anatomically destructive.[96] In addition, the vascular supply to the pharyngeal wall is preserved. A neurolytic procedure may result in a finer adjustment of the pharyngeal wall tensions. One of the disadvantages of a myotomy procedure may be a hypotonic state of the PE segment. A weak or absent PE segment will develop lower pitches. Vocal intensity and pitch can be improved by applying external pressure to the pharynx.

The pharyngeal plexus neurectomy can be performed simultaneously with total laryngectomy.[96] After separating the constrictor pharyngeal muscles from the laryngeal specimen, the posterolateral pharyngeal wall is stretched by grasping the edges of the pharyngostomy. At the level of the middle pharyngeal constrictor muscle, the pharynx and carotid artery are separated in the prevertebral space. The plexus fibers emanate from the vagus nerve and are frequently identified at the level of the superior thyroid artery. After checking the plexus by electrical stimulation, the identified branches are divided and the edges are separated by electrocautery. In the secondary setting the identification of the pharyngeal branches is more difficult

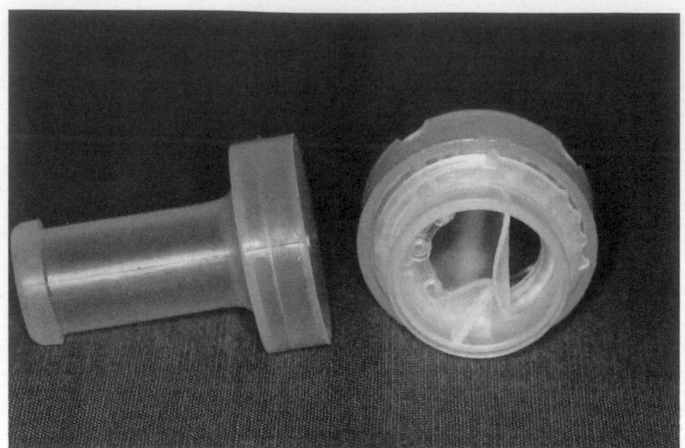

Figure 59.8 *A Blom-Singer adjustable tracheostoma valve which can be attached to a disposable plastic housing or tracheostoma button.*

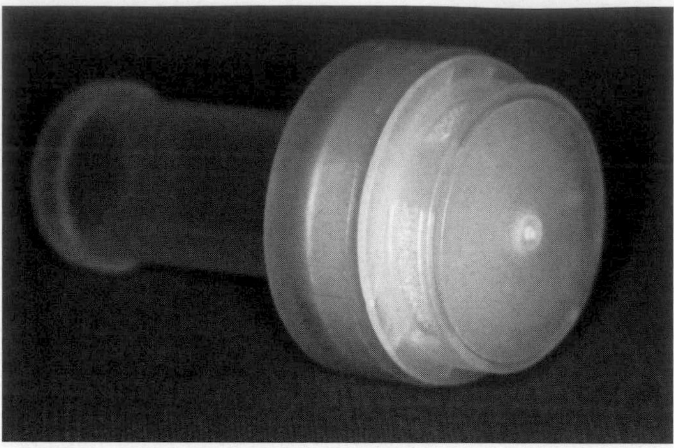

Figure 59.9 *A heat and moisture exchanger (Provox Stomafilter) can be used for digital stoma occlusion combined with a Barton-Mayo Tracheostoma Button.*

or impossible because of scarring and previous dissection in this area. In secondary cases, the use of botulinum A neurotoxin intramuscularly can be considerd as a suitable alternative for a surgical procedure.[53a]

Pharyngeal plexus neurectomy is another way to improve alaryngeal speech acquisition and quality.[12]

Tracheostoma valves

During tracheoesophageal speech with a voice prosthesis the patient is committed to manual occlusion of the airway. These limitations were recognized and tracheal valves were developed that close the trachea for phonation, but remain open during respiration. This allows tracheoesophageal speech without digital occlusion of the tracheostoma. During shunt phonation a thin diaphragm responds to the increase in air pressure by closing. These tracheostoma valves should enable a better social and professional reintegration of the laryngectomee.

The employment of a flexible valve housing or collar (Blom-Singer tracheostoma valve, Provox stomafilter) must be sealed for attachment to the peristomal skin (Figs 59.8 and 59.9).[2,3,13,97] This is done with the use of double-faced tape and/or liquid adhesives. A valve part can easily be inserted in the housing and can be quickly removed. In combination with a heat and moisture exchanger, the ease of prosthetic vocal rehabilitation can also be improved by reducing dryness, mucous secretions and coughing. A significant disadvantage of this type of tracheostoma valve is insufficient durability of the adhesive seal attachment.[2,3,13,112]

The ESKA-Herrmann tracheostoma valve has been developed to eliminate the above-mentioned sealing problems.[49] The tracheostoma valve consists of a cannula part with three different silicone outer flanges to retain the device in the stoma. A similar concept is provided by the Barton-Mayo tube, which consists of a customized tracheal cannula for a tight stomal occlusion. Fluent speech can be achieved with this valve when it is properly fitted and a functional voice prosthesis is inserted. This tracheostoma valve may interfere with the intensity of voice.

The application and use of tracheostoma valves are described as disappointing, due to application problems. Patients must be selected and fitted appropriately with a valve. Before the valve is attempted, the patients should be able to speak effectively using digital stoma occlusion. Sneezing and coughing are difficult to manage. In cases of significant respiratory problems, excessive mucous discharge, or secretions, the use of tracheostoma valves may be problematic.

Postoperative speech evaluation

The quality of tracheoesophageal speech can be assessed by using questionnaires, videofluoroscopy, videotaped interviews, and head and neck examinations. The appearance of the reconstructed pharyngoesophageal segment can be examined by videofluoroscopy during swallowing, esophageal phonation, and phonation during air insufflation. The esophageal segment must be examined dynamically.[101]

Voice production by means of a voice prosthesis resembles normal laryngeal voice production. Pulmonary air is used as the energy source. The pseudoglottis is known as the alternative sound source. Voice rehabilitation may start 10–12 days after primary puncture.

The laryngectomee should learn how to achieve a good breath and voice coordination. This can be achieved by optimal occlusion of the stoma, a good upright and relaxed body position, and abdominal breathing pattern without forced expiration.[88]

The majority of patients benefit from a brief program of speech therapy provided simultaneously with daily instructions in prosthesis management. Patients are instructed to use a continuous pulmonary airflow to speak fluently and

Table 59.2 Analysis of alaryngeal speech (Groningen criteria, 1988)

I Specific judgment			
A Phonatory skills	**Good (a)**	**Moderate (b)**	**Poor (c)**
Fluency (syllables per intake of air)	>18 (>4*)	10–18 (2–4*)	<10 (<2*)
Maximal phonation time (s)	>9 (>2*)	4–9 (0.5–2*)	<4 (<0.5*)
Dynamic range (dB)	>24 (>15*)	16–14 (6–14*)	<16 (<6*)
Maximal SPL [30 cm dB (A)]	mean 78 dB (>70 dB*), normal range 65–95 dB		
Availability of the voice	Immediate	Interval >4 s	No response
Articulation	Normal	Decreased intelligibility	Insufficient
Voice modulation (pitch)	Sufficient	Limited	Monotonous
Speech rate	Normal	Variable	Too high/low
B Additional factors			
Stoma noise	–	+	++
Audibility of inspiration	–	+	++
Redundant movements	–	+	++
C General judgment			
Voice quality	++	+	±
Intelligibility	++	+	±
II Final judgment	< 4 b scores in categories A & B	< 2 c scores in categories A & B	2 c in A or B, or > 2 c

Semiquantitative criteria used to assess alaryngeal speech. For each criteria group (A, B, C) a three-point scale was used: good, moderate, and poor. As the vocal performance of shunt esophageal speech differs from injection esophageal speech, separate criteria were applied to assess both speech modes.
*Criteria for injection esophageal speech.

with natural phrasing. By varying expiratory pressure and flow they can influence duration, stress and intonation of their communication pattern. Articulation therapy should be directed toward consonant voicing, speech intelligibility, and specific phoneme difficulties in case of anatomic alterations by surgery in the mouth or oropharynx.

Unsatisfactory voice production may be caused by several problems. Articulation problems are often due to a dysfunction of the tongue, soft palate, jaw or lips.

In cases of pharyngoesophageal spasm, voice production will be poor. The injection of air into the esophagus is usually sufficient, but regurgitation gives an uncoordinated, strained and strangled voice. With a stricture the patient will not be able to inject sufficient air into the esophagus for phonation to occur. This may be solved with the already described myotomy and or neurectomy procedures of this segment. In the case of hypotonicity of the pharyngoesophageal segment, the pharynx and esophagus dilate on swallowing, and the voice is weak and whispery. This can be corrected by digital pressure on the pharynx externally.[35] In addition, prosthesis-related problems should be checked in cases of no voice or poor voice. Insufficient stoma closure and excessive mucous production may also interfere with tracheoesophageal voice. The laryngectomee should learn how to effectively clean his self-retaining device daily with a specially developed brush or cotton swab.

A temporary decrease of shunt esophageal voice production may occur during radiotherapy due to swelling and rigidity of the pharyngeal wall. Nonetheless, speech therapy should continue, and the laryngectomee must be reassured that the voice quality will improve after the radiotherapy sessions.

The evaluation of tracheoesophageal voice production is standardized to conform to the criteria discussed at the Third International Congress on Voice Prosthesis (Groningen, 1988) (see Table 59.2).[14] The phonatory skills of voice production are judged on the following criteria: fluency (quantity of syllables per intake of air), maximum phonation time, dynamic range, availability of the voice, articulation, voice modulation and speech rate. The fluency of speech, measured by the number of syllables produced on one breath, is suggested to determine the quality of perception of tracheoesophageal voice.[14,64] Additional factors such as stoma noise, audibility of inspiration and redundant movements of the head and neck are also evaluated. Vocal quality and intelligibility are to be judged subjectively during the entire examination. The voice should be relaxed and pleasantly and easily understood.[14]

Speech therapy should both consist of injection esophageal speech and tracheoesophageal speech. Tracheoesophageal speech can be acquired faster than the original esophageal voice. Patients with tracheoesophageal voice are also able to acquire the injection esophageal

Table 59.3 Tracheoesophageal speech results

Study	*Results*
Singer and Blom[93]	90%
Wetmore *et al.*[118]	71%
Annyas *et al.*[5]	86%
Hall *et al.*[45]	57%
Wetmore *et al.*[119]	64%
Perry *et al.*[77]	73%
Stiernberg *et al.*[106]	65%
Lavertu *et al.*[61]	85%
Maniglia *et al.*[66]	85%
Recher *et al.*[80]	64%
Hilgers and Balm[52]	92%
Kerr *et al.*[59]	54%
Van Weissenbruch and Albers[115]	95%
Izdebski *et al.*[55]	92%
Kao *et al.*[57]	93%

voice easier.[115] The long-term results of tracheoesophageal speech as reported in literature are summarized in Table 59.3. Eventually the laryngectomee may choose which form of communication is preferable.

Voice failure and complications

The esophageal voice rehabilitation method is generally regarded as the most desirable method of non-prosthetic post-laryngectomy voice acquisition. In the literature, large differences are reported in the number of patients who successfully acquired esophageal voice. The percentage of laryngectomees that failed to achieve satisfactory esophageal voice, ranges from 14% to 76%.[54,87] Besides the differences in research design of the different studies, the causes of the lack of abilities and facilities of the laryngectomee should be taken into account.[34]

The PE segment, functioning as the sound source, can be associated with major physiologic problems causing a dysfunction of the air intake, air expulsion and vibratory movements of the pseudoglottis. The condition of this voice mechanism is dependent on factors related to air intake, i.e. flexibility of the neoglottis,[105] dysfunction of closure of the mouth,[64] tongue strength and movements,[76] velopharyngeal dysfunction, denture problems,[43] and factors related to air expulsion. Problems concerning the expulsion of air which interfere with the acquisition of esophageal voice occur less frequently than associated with the intake of air.[64] Incompetence of the distal esophageal sphincter has been suggested to interfere with the acquisition of esophageal voice.[38,120] Lack of coordination of the diaphragmatic ascent and relaxation of the PE segment may be associated with problems of air expulsion.[85,86]

Factors related to radiotherapy may have a negative influence on the acquisition of esophageal voice, as a result of the loss of elasticity of the PE segment and of the walls of the esophageal reservoir. Patients undergoing radiation therapy may experience a slower rate of progress. However, studies comparing the acquisition of esophageal speech between speakers who received radiotherapy postoperatively with non-irradiated esophageal speakers, are controversial.[20,40,64,81,87]

Anatomic factors may interfere with the acquisition of esophageal voice.[10,26,27,32,48,91] The described abnormalities are scar tissue formation, strictures, pouches and diverticulas located in or above the level of the PE segment.

Surgery-related factors involve the extent of the procedure on the PE segment. The shape and length of the PE segment varies depending on the extent of the carcinoma and the surgical requirements for removal of the larynx with or without other structures in the neck. A longer time interval between the time of surgery and the onset of speech therapy is also associated with a negative influence on esophageal voice acquisition.

Age- and gender-related factors have shown a controversial influence on the acquisition of esophageal voice.[17,20,22,32,58,60,91,110]

Auditory factors such as impaired hearing may negatively influence the acquisition of esophageal voice.[32,69,107] Auditory rehabilitation is suggested for laryngectomees with a hearing impairment.[64]

Surgical removal of the larynx may have serious emotional consequences for the laryngectomee. This can be accompanied by insufficient psychologic adjustments, which are necessary to cope with the traumatizing effect of this surgical procedure.

Factors such as a higher intelligence, a higher educational level, a favorable self-image, a good body image, a high achievement level, less depression and lower levels of anxiety are also related to a good esophageal speech development.[64]

The most important factors, which will have a major influence on the acquisition of esophageal voice, are the available teaching time and the moment at which speech therapy may be started. Speech therapy should start as early as possible after the laryngectomy, to achieve the best rehabilitation results.[36,37,58,71,72,90]

A training program for esophageal speech rehabilitation is supposed to be managed by a well-trained and motivated speech therapist. There should be sufficient teaching time available and a guaranteed continuation of the voice rehabilitation program.[64]

As described in previous sections, tracheoesophageal speech has many advantages above other methods of voice rehabilitation. As foreign bodies, voice prostheses for vocal rehabilitation of the laryngectomee may also be accompanied by frequent minor or severe complications.

Primary voice fistulas created at the time of laryngectomy were prone to more severe complications, i.e. infections. Fistula creation required a longer course of treatment in this group, compared to secondary created fistulas. The secondary procedures were often associated with complications such as esophageal perforation, peristomal cellulitis or cervical osteomyelitis.[116] By modifying the techniques of performing these punctures the complication rate has declined drastically.[53,67,68]

Proper fit of the prosthesis is necessary for good quality tracheoesophageal speech and to prevent complications. The length of the device and the angle of the prosthesis entering the posterior wall of the trachea into the esophagus are important factors. A long shaft of the prosthesis may injure the posterior pharyngeal wall. When excessive digital pressure is applied in occlusion of the stoma, the stoma may be pushed to the posterior esophageal wall. This may of course cause obstruction of the airflow through the prosthesis.

Development of a biofilm consisting of a mixed oropharyngeal microflora, may cause dysfunction of the one-way valve mechanism of the tracheoesophageal voice prosthesis. A dysfunctional valve is marked by leakage of esophageal contents through the prosthesis and increased phonatory efforts to produce sound. Average device life depends on the type of voice prosthesis and the ever-changing chemical, mechanical and microbiological factors in the upper digestive tract. In some patients, device life is extremely low and will result in a continuing series of device replacements. This group of patients can profit from the use of antifungal drugs, which can be applied topically. Application of amphotericin B lozenges or a slow-release system containing miconazole can significantly increase the device life of indwelling prostheses.[64,116] Other described complications[4] encountered with voice prostheses are summarized in Table 59.4.

Many of the above-mentioned problems can be solved by simple measures such as conservative antibiotic treatment, prosthetic replacement procedures, or surgical revisions.

Table 59.4 Complications with voice prostheses

Local	*Regional*
Candida colonization	Spasm or hypertonicity of PE segment
Leakage through the prosthesis	Hypotonicity of PE segment
Increased airflow resistance	Esophageal stenosis or stricture
Granulation tissue formation	Pulmonary aspiration
Local inflammation and infection	Pneumothorax
Migration of the fistula tract	Peristomal or cervical cellulitis
False tract	Subcutaneous emphysema
Dislocation of the prosthesis	Stomal stenosis
Closure of the fistula tract	Esophageal abscess
Leakage around the prosthesis	Vertebral osteomyelitis
Hypertrophic scarring	Mediastinitis

Conclusions

Tumors of the larynx are not only significant because they present treatment dilemmas but also because most treatment modalities have a profound impact on the life of a patient.

The loss of the larynx requires social adjustment secondary to changes in respiration, speech and deglutition. The primary goal of laryngectomy rehabilitation is to efficiently restore these dynamic functions after accomplishing radical tumor extirpation.[35] Achieving this goal depends significantly on the patient's adaptation to the loss of normal speech.

The most common methods of alaryngeal communication that may be used are the artificial larynx, esophageal speech and tracheoesophageal speech.

The disadvantages of the hand-held electrolarynx are the monotonous mechanical sounding voice, maintenance and care, and the fact that the user should always carry it with him or her. In comparison, esophageal speech has the advantage of hands-free voice production. Traditionally, esophageal speech has been considered the method of choice for vocal rehabilitation after total laryngectomy. However, approximately 50% of the patients using esophageal speech fail to acquire functional communication.[101] Among those who do, therapy time is considerable and the resultant speech proficiency is variable. Characteristically, the quality of acquired esophageal voice is limited with respect to intensity, pitch, and rate.[35]

Tracheoesophageal phonation produces higher success rates of useful voice, but requires an operative procedure and patient compliance. The fistula techniques, which allow tracheoesophageal speech, have been complicated with a high failure rate due to aspiration, local infection, stenosis, and migration of the tract. In 1979, Singer and Blom revolutionized the speech restoration field with their description of an endoscopic technique in which a tracheoesophageal one-way silicone valve was placed in a tracheoesophageal fistula after total laryngectomy. Increased amplitude levels of tracheoesophageal voice production are possible because the pulmonary system generates and sustains greater esophageal pressures. The characteristics of tracheoesophageal speech are more similar to normal laryngeal speech because of the powerful advantage of pulmonary supported airflow. Esophageal speakers have a reduced maximum phonation time due to their limited esophageal volume (80 ml). The finding that tracheoesophageal speech production is acoustically more similar to laryngeal speech encouraged several researchers to develop a more ideal prosthesis for vocal rehabilitation. Compared to the original developed prostheses, the self-retaining prostheses ensure easier maintenance and care for the prosthesis by the patient. This could be the reason for less reported complications concerning the fistula tract. Primary placement of the prosthesis at the time of laryngectomy leads to higher success rates without increased postoperative complications. In addition, primary introduction of the prosthesis at the time of laryngectomy made stenting of the created fistula unnecessary, which resulted in a reduction of postoperative wound healing. The replacement of the self-retaining (indwelling) prostheses can be performed as a simple outpatient procedure. This can be further enhanced by the introduction of front loader systems (Blom-Singer Gel Cap Insertion System, Provox 2, Voicemaster).

Preoperative evaluation of the candidates for surgical voice rehabilitation has proved to increase the success rate of tracheoesophageal speech. Factors such as visual acuity, manual dexterity, sufficient pulmonary reserve and coughing reflexes, and the muscular tonus of the cricopharyngeal segment appear to be important parameters for patient selection. However, the anatomic changes that follow surgical tumor resection will obviously determine which option for communication is adaptable.

With the development of self-retaining low-resistance prostheses, a reduction of airflow resistance has been achieved. These prostheses are considered comfortable because less effort is needed to produce adequate speech. However, not every laryngectomee may profit from the benefits of low-pressure devices. The tonicity of the PE segment seems to play a major role in the airflow resistance during tracheoesophageal speech.

The mean device life of the different prostheses ranges from a few weeks to 2 or more years. Deterioration of the prostheses may lead to increased airflow resistance and leakage of fluids through the device. Device life may be influenced by microbial (yeast) colonization of the silicone material, which leads to irreversible damage of the valve mechanism. Early failure of the voice prostheses can be prevented by using antifungal drugs (e.g. amphotericin B) lozenges in patients who tend to have rapid shunt valve deterioration.[65]

The complications encountered with the self-retaining low-resistance prostheses are not significant and mainly consist of hypertrophic scarring, granulation formation and minor leakage around the device. Usually, these problems can easily be overcome with limited measures.

The ideal voice prosthesis with self-retaining, self-cleaning and low-pressure properties combined with an unlimited device life, has yet to be developed. As device life seems to be limited in most cases, improved techniques should be advocated that reduce the sometimes inconvenient methods for replacement of indwelling prostheses.

Considering the quality of life, primary prosthetic voice rehabilitation seems to be an adequate method of alaryngeal communication following laryngectomy.

References

1. Amatsu M. A one stage surgical technique for postlaryngectomy voice rehabilitation. *Laryngoscope* 1980; **90:** 1378–86.
2. Amatsu M. Amatsu's technique using the Blom-Singer tracheostoma valve. In: Herrmann IF, ed. *Speech Restoration via Voice Prostheses.* Berlin: Springer-Verlag, 1986: 177–81.
3. Amatsu M, Makino K, Kinishi M, Tani M, Kokubu M. Primary tracheoesophageal shunt operation for postlaryngectomy speech with sphincter mechanism. *Ann Otol Rhinol Laryngol* 1986; **95:** 373–6.
4. Andrews JC, Mickel RA, Hanson DG, Monahan GP, Ward PH. Major complications following tracheoesophageal puncture for voice rehabilitation. *Laryngoscope* 1987; **97:** 562–7.
5. Annyas AA, Nijdam HF, Escajadillo JR, Mahieu HF, Leever H. Groningen prosthesis for voice rehabilitation after laryngectomy. *Clin Otolaryngol* 1984; **9:** 51–4.
6. Arslan M. Reconstructive laryngectomy. Report on the first 35 cases. *Ann Otol* 1972; **81:** 479–87.
7. Arslan M, Serafini I. Restoration of laryngeal function after total laryngectomy. Report on the first 25 cases. *Laryngoscope* 1972; **82:** 1349–60.
8. Asai R. Asai's new voice production method: substitution for voice and speech. In: Ono Y, ed. *Proceedings of the VIIIth International Congress of Otorhinolaryngology.* Amsterdam: Excerpta Medica, 1965: 730.
9. Asai R. Laryngoplasty after total laryngectomy. *Arch Otolaryngol* 1972; **95:** 114–19.
10. Bentzen N, Guld A, Rasmussen H. X-ray video tape studies of laryngectomized patients. *J Laryngol Otol* 1976; **90:** 655–66.
11. Blom ED, Singer MI. Surgical-prosthetic approaches for postlaryngectomy voice restoration. In: Keith RL, Darley FL, eds. *Laryngectomee Rehabilitation.* Houston: College-Hill Press, 1979: 251–76.
12. Blom ED, Pauloski BR, Hamaker RC. Functional outcome after surgery for prevention of pharyngospasms in tracheoesophageal speakers. Part I: speech characteristics. *Laryngoscope* 1995; **105:** 1093–103.
13. Blom ED, Singer MI, Hamaker RC. Tracheostoma valve for postlaryngectomy voice rehabilitation. *Ann Otol Rhinol Laryngol* 1982; **91:** 576–8.
14. Bors EFM. Indwelling voice prostheses for voice restoration after total laryngectomy: criteria for evaluation of speech with a voice-button. In: *Teaching Course on Indwelling Voice Prostheses for Voice Restoration after Total Laryngectomy.* Amsterdam: The Netherlands Cancer Institute, 1991: 50–7.
15. Brankel O. Formung und gestalt der pseudoglottis laryngektomierter im stroboskopischen rontgenbild. *Folia Phoniatr (Basel)* 1957; **9:** 18–31.
16. Brendebach J, Schmidt M, Brugger E. Lung function tests in laryngectomized patients. In: Herrmann IF, ed. *Speech Restoration via Voice Prostheses.* Berlin: Springer-Verlag, 1986: 130–4.
17. Breuninger H. Zur Rehabilitation nach Laryngektomie. *Laryngorhinootologie* 1982; **61:** 267–71.
18. Briani AA. Riabilitazione fonetica di laringectomizzati a mezzo della corrente aerea espiratoria polmonare. *Arch Ital Otolaringol* 1952; **63:** 469–75.
19. Briani AA. Il recupero sociale dei laringecomizzati attraverso un metodo personale operatorio. *Med Soc* 1958; **8:** 265–9.
20. Brouwer B, Snow GB, van Dam FS. Experiences of patients who undergo laryngectomy. *Clin Otolaryngol* 1079; **4:** 109–18.

21. Brown DH, Evans PH. A simplified method of tracheoesophageal puncture for speech restoration. *Laryngoscope* 1992; **102:** 579–80.
22. Brusis T, Schöning A. Wie gut ist die oesophagusstimme? *Laryngorhinootologie* 1984; **63:** 585–8.
23. Conley JJ. Vocal rehabilitation by autogenous vein graft. *Ann Otol* 1959; **68:** 990–5.
24. Conley JJ. Surgical techniques for the vocal rehabilitation of the postlaryngectomized patient. *Trans Am Acad Ophthalmol Otolaryngol* 1969; **73:** 288–99.
24a. Conley JJ, Vonfraenkel PH. Historical aspects of head and neck surgery. *Ann Otol* 1956; **65:** 643–53.
25. Conley JJ, De Amesti F, Pierce MK. A new surgical technique for the vocal rehabilitation of the laryngectomized patient. *Ann Otol* 1958; **67:** 655–64.
26. Damsté PH. *Oesophageal speech after laryngectomy.* Thesis. Groningen: Gebr. Hoitsema, 1958.
27. Damsté PH. Methods of restoring the voice after laryngectomy. *Laryngoscope* 1975; **85:** 649–55.
28. Damsté PH. Some obstacles in learning oesophageal speech. In: Keith RL, Darley FL, eds. *Laryngectomee Rehabilitation.* Houston: College-Hill Press, 1979: 49–62.
29. Damsté PH, Lerman JW. Configuration of the neoglottis: an x-ray study. *Folia Phoniatr (Basel)* 1969; **21:** 347–58.
30. Decroix G, Libersa CI, Lattard R. Bases anatomique et physiologiques de la reeducation vocale des laryngectomises. *J Fr Otorhinolaryngol* 1958; **7:** 549–73.
31. Deeb ZE, Arenstein MH, Lerner DN. A new simple technique for tracheoesophageal puncture. *Laryngoscope* 1992; **102:** 837–8.
32. Diedrich WM, Youngstrom KA. *Alaryngeal Speech.* Springfield: CC Thomas, 1966.
33. Donegan JO, Gluckman JL, Singh J. Limitations of the Blom-Singer technique for voice restoration. *Ann Otol* 1981; **90:** 495–7.
34. Duguay M. Special problems of the alaryngeal speaker. In: Keith RL, Darley FL, eds. *Laryngectomee Rehabilitation.* Houston: College-Hill Press, 1979: 423–44.
35. Duguay MJ, Feudo P Jr. The process of postlaryngectomy rehabilitation. In: Fried MP, ed. *The Larynx. A Multidisciplinary Approach.* Boston: Little, Brown, 1988: 603–13.
36. Edels Y. Pseudo-voice: its theory and practice. In: Edels Y, ed. *Laryngectomy, Diagnosis to Rehabilitation.* London: Croom Helm, 1983: 107–41.
37. Fontaine A, Mitchell J. Oesophageal voice: a factor of readiness. *J Laryngol Otol* 1960; **74:** 870–6.
38. Frith CK, Buffalo MD, Montague JC Jr. Reported dietary effects on esophageal voice production. *Folia Phoniatr (Basel)* 1985; **37:** 238–45.
39. Fumeaux J. Structure de la pseudoglotte des laryngectomises étudiée par radiocinématographie. *Rev Laryngol Otol Rhinol (Bord)* 1961; **82:** 241–6.
40. Gates GA, Ryan W, Cooper JC Jr *et al.* Current status of laryngectomee rehabilitation: I. Results of therapy. *Am J Otolaryngol* 1982; **3:** 1–7.
41. Gross M, Hess M. A new method for tracheoesophageal puncture under topical anaesthesia. *Laryngoscope* 1994; **104:** 233–4.
42. Gussenbauer C. Ueber die erste durch Th. Billroth am menschen ausgeführte kehlkopf-extirpation und die anwendung eines künstlichen kehlkopfes. *Arch Klin Chir* 1874; **17:** 343–56.
43. Guttman MR. Rehabilitation of voice in laryngectomized patients. *Arch Otolaryngol* 1932; **15:** 478–9.
44. Guttman MR. Tracheohypopharyngeal fistulization (a new procedure for speech production in the laryngectomized patient). *Trans Am Laryngol Rhinol Otolol Soc* 1935; **41:** 219–26.
45. Hall JG, Dahl T, Arnesen AR. Speech protheses, failures, problems and success. In: Myers EN, ed. *New Dimensions in Otorhinolaryngology, Head and Neck Surgery.* Vol. I. Amsterdam: Elsevier, 1985: 418–21.
46. Heatley DG, Anderson AG Jr. Tracheoesophageal puncture for speech rehabilitation after laryngectomy. *Laryngoscope* 1992; **102:** 581–2.
47. Herrmann IF. Introduction to speech restoration. In: Herrmann IF, ed. *Speech Restoration via Voice Prostheses.* Berlin: Springer-Verlag, 1986: 3–4.
48. Herrmann IF. Glottoplasty with functional pharynx surgery and tracheostomaplasty. In: Herrmann IF, ed. *Speech Restoration via Voice Prostheses.* Berlin: Springer-Verlag, 1986: 116–24.
49. Herrmann IF, Koss W. Experience with the ESKA-Herrmann tracheostoma valve. In: Herrmann IF, ed. *Speech Restoration via Voice Prostheses.* Berlin: Springer-Verlag, 1986: 184–6.
50. Herrmann IF, Zenner HP. Erfahrungen mit der Blom-Singer prothese nach Blom-Singer punktion und nach funktiongestorter Neoglottis Phonatoria. *HNO* 1984; **32:** 286–93.
51. Herrmann IF, Poschet G, Zohren J. Wear and tear on the silicon of valve prostheses in the upper digestive tract. A study using electron microscope scanning. In: Herrmann IF, ed. *Speech Restoration via Voice Prostheses.* Berlin: Springer-Verlag, 1986: 69–73.
52. Hilgers FJM, Balm AJM. Long-term results of vocal rehabilitation after total laryngectomy with the low-resistance, indwelling Provox voice prosthesis system. *Clin Otolaryngol* 1993; **18:** 517–23.
53. Hilgers FJM, Schouwenburg PF. A new low-resistance self-retaining prosthesis (Provox) for voice rehabilitation after total laryngectomy. *Laryngoscope* 1990; **100:** 1202–7.
53a. Hoffman HT, McCulloch TM. Botulinum neurotoxin for tracheoesophageal voice failure. In: Blom ED, Singer MI, Hamaker RC, eds. *Tracheoesophageal voice restoration following total laryngectomy.* San Diego: Singular Publishing Group, 1998: 83–7.
54. Hunt RB. Rehabilitation of the laryngectomee. *Laryngoscope* 1964; **74:** 382–95.
55. Izdebski K, Reed CG, Ross JC, Hilsinger RL Jr. Problems with tracheoesophageal fistula voice restoration in totally laryngectomized patients. A review of 95 cases. *Arch Otolaryngol Head Neck Surg* 1994; **120:** 840–5.
56. Johns ME, Cantrell RW. Voice restoration of the total laryngectomy patient: the Blom-Singer technique. *Otolaryngol Head Neck Surg* 1991; **89:** 82–6.
57. Kao WW, Mohr RM, Kimmel CA, Getch C, Silverman C. The outcome and techniques of primary and secondary tracheoesophageal puncture. *Arch Otolaryngol Head Neck Surg* 1994; **120:** 301–7.

58. Kelly DR, Adamovich BLB, Roberts TA Jr. Detailed investigation of alaryngeal speech to elucidate etiology of variation in quality. *Otolaryngol Head Neck Surg* 1981; **89:** 613–23.
59. Kerr AI, Denholm S, Sanderson RJ, Anderson SJ. Blom-Singer prosthesis: an 11 year experience of primary and secondary procedures. *Clin Otolaryngol* 1993; **18:** 184–7.
60. Kitzing P, Toremalm NG. The situation of the laryngectomized patient. *Acta Otolaryngol Suppl (Stockh)* 1969; **263:** 119–23.
61. Lavertu P, Scott SE, Finnegan EM, Levine HL, Tucker HM, Wood BG. Secondary tracheoesophageal puncture for voice rehabilitation after laryngectomy. *Arch Otolaryngol Head Neck Surg* 1989; **115:** 350–5.
62. Leipzig B, Griffiths CM, Shea JP. Neoglottic reconstruction following total laryngectomy. The Galveston experience. *Ann Otol* 1980; **89:** 204–8.
63. Mahieu HF. Laryngectomee voice rehabilitation using the Groningen button voice prosthesis. *Rev Laryngol Otol Rhinol* 1987; **108:** 113–19.
64. Mahieu HF. *Voice and speech rehabilitation following laryngectomy.* Thesis. Groningen: Groningen University Press, 1988.
65. Mahieu HF, van Saene HKF, Rosingh HJ, Shutte HK. Aantasting van siliconrubber stemprothese door *Candida*-vegetaties. *Ned Tijdschr Geneeskd* 1986; **130:** 891.
66. Maniglia AJ, Lundy DS, Casiano RC, Swim SC. Speech restoration and complications of primary versus secondary tracheoesophageal puncture following total laryngectomy. *Laryngoscope* 1989; **99:** 489–91.
67. Manni JJ, van den Broek P, de Groot MAH. Voice rehabilitation after laryngectomy with the Groningen voice prosthesis: experiences made in Nijmegen. In: Herrmann IF, ed. *Speech Restoration via Voice Prostheses.* Berlin: Springer Verlag, 1986: 33–6.
68. Manni JJ, van den Broek P, de Groot MAH, Berends E. Voice rehabilitation after laryngectomy with the Groningen prosthesis. *J Otolaryngol* 1984; **13:** 333–6.
69. Martin DE, Hoops HR. The relationship between esophageal speech proficiency and selected measures of auditory function. *J Speech Hear Res* 1974; **17:** 80–5.
70. Montgomery WW, Lavelle WG. A technique for improving esophageal and tracheopharyngeal speech. *Ann Otol* 1974; **83:** 452–61.
71. Moolenaar-Bijl AJ. The importance of certain consonants in oesophageal voice after laryngectomy. *Ann Otol* 1953; **62:** 979–89.
72. Moolenaar-Bijl AJ. Het spreken zonder strottehoofd. *Logoped Foniatr* 1979; **51:** 50–68.
73. Mozolewski E. Surgical rehabilitation of voice and speech after laryngectomy. *Otolaryngol Pol* 1972; **26:** 653–61.
74. Nijdam HF. Indwelling voice prostheses for voice restoration after total laryngectomy: the development of an indwelling voice prosthesis. In: *Teaching Course on Indwelling Voice Prostheses for Voice Restoration after Total Laryngectomy.* Amsterdam: The Netherlands Cancer Institute, 1991: 8–10.
75. Nijdam HF, Annyas AA, Schutte HK, Leever H. A new prosthesis for voice rehabilitation after laryngectomy. *Arch Otorhinolaryngol* 1982; **237:** 27–33.
76. Noll JD, Torgeson JK. A cinefluorographic observation of the tongue in esophageal speakers. *Folia Phoniatr (Basel)* 1967; **19:** 343–50.
77. Perry A, Cheesman AD, McIvor J, Chalton R. A British experience of surgical voice restoration techniques as a secondary procedure following total laryngectomy. *J Laryngol Otol* 1987; **101:** 155–63.
78. Pfrang H. Social and psycho-social aspects of vocal rehabilitation in laryngectomized patients preliminary results. In: Herrmann IF, ed. *Speech Restoration via Voice Prostheses.* Berlin: Springer-Verlag, 1986: 165–9.
79. Precechtel A. Contribution a la discussion de conférences concernant la voice oesophagienne au XXe Congress de Societé Francais de Phoniatrie. *J Fr Otorhinolaryngol* 1961; **10:** 69–73.
80. Recher G, Pesavento G, Cristoferi V, Ferlito A. Italian experience of voice restoration after laryngectomy with tracheoesophageal puncture. *Ann Otol Rhinol Laryngol* 1991; **100:** 206–10.
81. Richardson JL. Surgical and radiological effects upon the development of speech after total laryngectomy. *Ann Otol Rhinol Laryngol* 1981; **90:** 294–7.
82. Robe EY, Moore P, Andrews AH Jr, Holinger PH. A study of the role of certain factors in the development of speech after laryngectomy: type of operation. *Laryngoscope* 1956; **66:** 173–86.
83. Robe EY, Moore P, Andrews AH Jr, Holinger PH. A study of the role of certain factors in the development of speech after laryngectomy: site of pseudoglottis. *Laryngoscope* 1956; **66:** 382–401.
84. Robe EY, Moore P, Andrews AH Jr, Holinger PH. A study of the role of certain factors in the development of speech after laryngectomy: coordination of speech with respiration. *Laryngoscope* 1956; **66:** 481–99.
85. Samuel P, Adams FG. The effect of oesophageal speech on dyspeptic symptoms. *J Laryngol Otol* 1976; **90:** 1099–103.
86. Samuel P, Adams FG. The role of oesophageal and diaphragmatic movements in alaryngeal speech. *J Laryngol Otol* 1976; **90:** 1105–11.
87. Schaefer SD, Johns DF. Attaining functional esophageal speech. *Arch Otolaryngol* 1982; **108:** 647–9.
88. Scholtens BEGM. Indwelling voice prostheses for voice restoration after total laryngectomy: speech therapy. In: *Teaching Course on Indwelling Voice Prostheses for Voice Restoration after Total Laryngectomy.* Amsterdam: The Netherlands Cancer Institute, 1991: 42–9.
89. Schouwenburg PF. Indwelling voice prostheses for voice restoration after total laryngectomy: technical aspects of laryngectomy and primary and secondary TE puncture. In: *Teaching Course on Indwelling Voice Prostheses for Voice Restoration after Total Laryngectomy.* Amsterdam: The Netherlands Cancer Institute, 1991: 28–33.
90. Shames GH, Font J, Matthews J. Factors related to speech proficiency of the laryngectomized. *J Speech Hear Dis* 1963; **28:** 273–87.
91. Simpson IC, Smith JCS, Gordon MT. Laryngectomy: the influence of muscle reconstruction on the mechanism of oesophageal voice production. *J Laryngol Otol* 1972; **86:** 961–90.

92. Singer MI. Tracheoesophageal speech: vocal rehabilitation after total laryngectomy. *Laryngoscope* 1983; **93:** 1454–65.
93. Singer MI, Blom ED. An endoscopic technique for restoration of voice after laryngectomy. *Ann Otol* 1980; **89:** 529–33.
94. Singer MI, Blom ED, Hamaker RC. Further experience with voice restoration after total laryngectomy. *Ann Otol* 1981; **90:** 498–502.
95. Singer MI, Blom ED, Hamaker RC. Voice rehabilitation after total laryngectomy. *J Otolaryngol* 1983; **12:** 329–34.
96. Singer MI, Blom ED, Hamaker RC. Pharyngeal plexus neurectomy for alaryngeal speech rehabilitation. *Laryngoscope* 1986; **96:** 50–4.
97. Singh W. New tracheostoma flap valve for surgical speech reconstruction. In: Myers EN, ed. *New Dimensions in Otorhinolaryngology, Head and Neck Surgery.* Vol II. Amsterdam: Elsevier, 1985: 480–3.
98. Sisson GA, Goldman ME. Pseudoglottis procedure: update and secondary reconstruction techniques. *Laryngoscope* 1980; **90:** 1120–9.
99. Sisson GA, Bytell DE, Becker SP, McConnel FN, Singer MI. Total laryngectomy and reconstruction of a pseudoglottis: problems and complications. *Laryngoscope* 1978; **88:** 639–50.
100. Smith JK, Rise EN, Gralnek DE. Speech recovery in laryngectomized patients. *Laryngoscope* 1966; **76:** 1540–6.
101. Snyderman NL. Surgical vocal rehabilitation. In: Paparella MM, Schumrick DA, Gluckman JL, Meyerhoff WL, eds. *Otolaryngology.* Vol. III. Philadelphia: Saunders, 1991: 2371–8.
102. Spofford B, Jafek B, Barcz D. An improved method for creating tracheoesophageal fistulas for Blom-Singer or Panje voice prostheses. *Laryngoscope* 1984; **94:** 257–8.
103. Staffieri M. Laringectomia totale con ricostruzione di 'glottide fonatoria'. *N Arch Ital Otol Rinol Laringol* 1973; **1:** 181–8.
104. Staffieri M, Procacini A, Steiner W, Staffieri A. Chirurgische rehabilitation der stimme nach laryngectomie. *Laryngorhinootologie* 1978; **57:** 477–88.
105. Stetson RH. Esophageal speech for any laryngectomized person. *Arch Otolaryngol* 1937; **26:** 132–42.
106. Stiernberg CM, Bailey BJ, Calhoun KH, Perez DG. Primary tracheoesophageal fistula procedure for voice restoration: the University of Texas Medical Branch experience. *Laryngoscope* 1987; **97:** 820–4.
107. Svane-Knudsen V. The substitute voice of the laryngectomized patient. *Acta Otolaryngol (Stockh)* 1960; **52:** 85–93.
108. Tanabe M, Honjo I, Isshiki N. Neoglottic reconstruction following total laryngectomy. *Arch Otolaryngol* 1985; **111:** 39–42.
109. Taptapova SL. Methode d'enseignement de la voix oesophagienne. *Rev Laryngol Otol Rhinol (Bord)* 1979; **100:** 189–99.
110. Van den Berg JW. Myoelastic-aerodynamic theory of voice production. *J Speech Hear Res* 1958; **1:** 227–44.
111. Van den Berg JW, Moolenaar-Bijl AJ, Damsté PH. Oesophageal speech. *Folia Phoniatr (Basel)* 1958; **10:** 65–84.
112. Van den Hoogen FJA, Meeuwis C, Oudes MJ, Janssen P, Manni JJ. The Blom-Singer tracheostoma valve as a valuable addition in the rehabilitation of the laryngectomized patient. *Eur Arch Otorhinolaryngol* 1996; **253:** 126–9.
113. Van Geel RC. *Pitch inflection in electrolaryngeal speech.* Thesis. Utrecht: University of Utrecht, 1983.
114. Van Weissenbruch R. *Voice restoration after total laryngectomy.* Thesis. Groningen: University of Groningen, 1996.
115. Van Weissenbruch R, Albers FWJ. Voice rehabilitation after total laryngectomy using the Provox voice prosthesis. *Clin Otolaryngol* 1993; **18:** 359–64.
116. Van Weissenbruch R, Bouckaert S, Remon JP, Nelis HJ, Aerts R, Albers FWJ. Chemoprophylaxis of fungal deterioration of the Provox silicone tracheoesophageal prosthesis in postlaryngectomy patients. *Ann Otol Rhinol Laryngol* 1997; **106:** 329–37.
117. Vrticka K, Svoboda M. A clinical and X-ray study of 100 laryngectomized speakers. *Folia Phoniatr (Basel)* 1961; **13:** 174–86.
118. Wetmore SJ, Johns ME, Baker SR. The Singer-Blom voice restoration procedure. *Arch Otolaryngol* 1981; **107:** 674–6.
119. Wetmore SJ, Krueger K, Wesson K, Blessing ML. Long-term results of the Blom-Singer speech rehabilitation procedure. *Arch Otolaryngol* 1985; **111:** 106–9.
120. Wolfe RD, Olson JE, Goldenberg DB. Rehabilitation of the laryngectomee: the role of the distal esophageal sphincter. *Laryngoscope* 1971; **81:** 1971–8.

Secondary neoplasms of the larynx

Adel K El-Naggar

Metastasis is distant colonies arising from the dissemination of circulating primary tumor cells. Although this catastrophic event is typically a manifestation of late-stage widespread disease, it may rarely present as a localized synchronous or metachronous lesion. It is the latter form that may occasionally give rise to diagnostic and clinical management difficulties. In contrast to other anatomic locations, the larynx is an uncommon site for metastasis because of its terminal lymphovasculature and possibly to locoregional homing factors. Laryngeal metastasis is generally associated with poor prognosis.

Incidence

The reported incidence of laryngeal metastasis in comprehensive reviews of this subject ranged from 0.09% to 0.4% of all neoplasms at this location. Approximately 3–4% of these lesions are detected prior to primary tumor identification. The rate of localized metastasis, however, is difficult to estimate but it is suspected to be extremely low and most probably is limited to a few case reports. Nevertheless, the true incidence of such occurrence is relatively higher in studies of autopsy series.[2,11,12,17,18,24,56]

Laryngeal locations

The majority of reported laryngeal metastases have been localized to the supra- and subglottic regions because of their relatively abundant vascular and lymphatic supply.[19] In most instances the metastasis involves the submucosa but it may also involve ossified laryngeal cartilage due to the enhanced vascularization.[26]

Origin of primary tumor

Virtually any malignant neoplasm originating below the neck may metastasize to the larynx.[2] The frequency of laryngeal metastasis from common primary malignancies varied greatly. The most common primary tumors are melanoma, renal cell carcinoma, gastrointestinal, breast and pulmonary carcinomas. Less frequent tumors are from head and neck, bone and soft tissue and germ cell origin (see Tables 60.1 and 60.2).

Pathogenetic mechanisms

Metastasis is the most significant adverse sign of cancer. The underlying factors causing cancer cells to dispatch and form secondary nodules at distant sites are complicated and partially understood. It is believed that tumor cells with metastatic potential possess unique features that are restricted to only a few cells of primary tumors. Understanding the local and systematic factors involved

Table 60.1 Distribution of laryngeal metastasis by diagnosis

Histological type	*No. cases*	*Percentage*
Carcinomas	94	60.6
Melanomas	48	30.9
Sarcomas	7	4.5
Other	6	3.8
Total	155	100.0

Table 60.2 Incidence of laryngeal metastasis by primary site

Primary tumor	*No. cases*	*Percentage*
Skin (melanoma)	46	29.6
Kidney (RCC)	40	25.8
Gastrointestinal tract	17	10.9
Lung and trachea	15	9.6
Breast	14	9.0
Prostate	7	4.5
Head and neck	6	3.8
Bone	4	4.6
Testis	2	1.3
Trunk	2	1.3
Endocrine glands	1	0.6
Ovary	1	0.6
Total	155	100.0

RCC = renal cell carcinoma.

in the metastatic process, therefore, may impact on future management of cancer patients. Current theories underlying laryngeal metastasis are as follows.

Mechanical

Based on the anatomic location and the vascular distribution of the larynx, three different routes for circulating primary tumor cells to reach the larynx have been suggested:[2,11,12,17–19,24,56]

- through the terminal tributaries of the superior thyroid artery as it arises from the external carotid. This occurs as a consequence of the passage through low-pressure systemic circulation of the vena cava, right cardiopulmonary route, left heart, aorta to the external carotid artery;
- via the vertebral venous plexus from the infraclavicular region by a retrograde spread caused by alteration in the pelvic pressure; or
- through the free communication between lymphatic and the vascular systems in the subglottic region.

Biological (homing)

Early metastasis is a non-random, highly organized and organ-selective process that involves interaction between several heterologous molecules for successful secondary growth formation. The propensity of certain primary tumors to preferentially disseminate to a particular site in early stage of this process suggests that a paracrine interaction between metastatic cells and the metastatic site may take place.[26,33,34,47,58,64,65,70]

For metastasis to succeed, malignant cells must detach from neighboring cells or connective tissue, permeate into vascular spaces, circulate and evade host immune defenses, penetrate basement membrane and extravasate to form new growth at the metastatic site. At the new site, metastatic deposits generate neovascularization (angiogenesis) (Fig 60.1) for successful growth and survival.

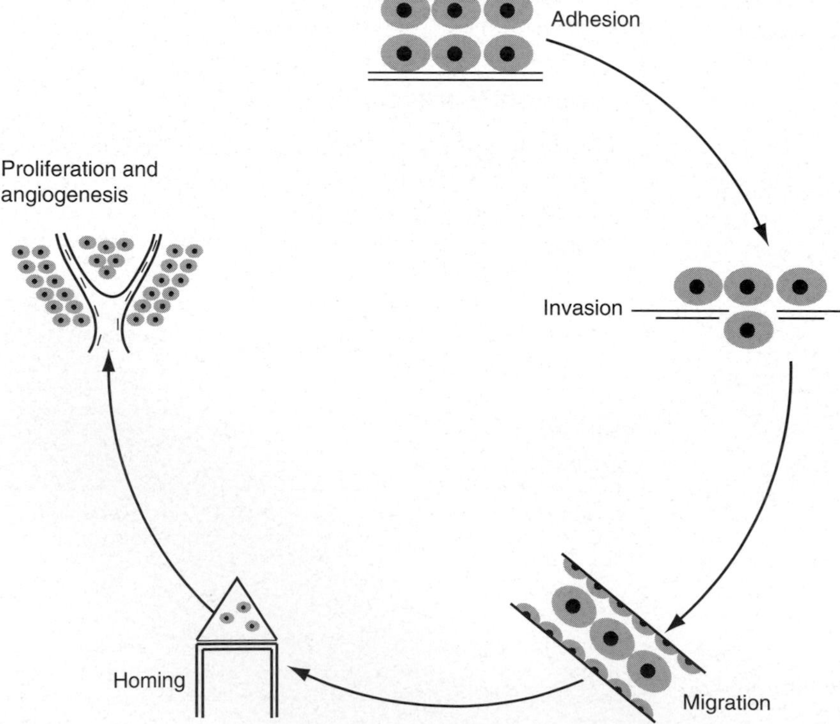

Figure 60.1 *Metastatic cascade to the larynx. (Reproduced with permission from Ohlms LA, McGill T, Healy GB. Malignant laryngeal tumors in children.* Ann Otol Rhinol Laryngol *1994;* ***103****: 686–92.)*

Recently, several organ-derived growth promoting and inhibiting factors have been found to play a critical role in metastasis. The interaction between these molecules in the sequential phases of the metastatic cascade has been the subject of intense investigations. Current understanding of this phenomenon indicates that an equilibrium between several growth-stimulating and inhibitory factors plays a central role in the ultimate success of the metastatic process.

Angiogenesis

The development of new vasculature is critical to the continued growth of both primary tumors and metastatic deposits of less than 2.0 mm in size. Neovascularization at the primary site facilitates cells to metastasize and sustain survival and growth at the secondary site. Tumor angiogenesis is regulated by angiogenic promoting and inhibitory factors released by tumor cells and the surrounding stroma.[39] The balancing interaction between these factors influences the neovascularization status in primary and secondary tumors. Among the well known angiogenic stimulators are fibroblast growth factors (α and β), epidermal growth factor, vascular endothelial growth factor (VEGF), interleukin-1 and 6, transforming growth factor α and β, tumor necrosis factor α, perlecan, and platelet-derived endothelial growth factor. Putative angiogenic inhibitors include angiostatin, interferon α and β, thrombospondin and heparinase. The mechanism(s) regulating these antagonistic factors is currently unknown. However, understanding this process is essential for the development of novel therapy of metastatic deposits. In this context, it has been shown that with reduced angiostatin level, a cleavage product of plasminogen found in non-vascularized tumor after excision of the primary tumor leads to reduced growth of metastatic lesions. These findings underscore the potential utilization of a similar approach in the treatment of cancer metastasis.[22,39,69]

Clinical presentation

The sign and symptoms of laryngeal metastasis are typically similar to those of primary tumors at the site.[3,27,44,46,68] Hoarseness, stridor, dyspnea and cough are the most common symptoms. Metastatic renal cell carcinomas in particular are more prone to present with hemoptysis. Symptomatic metastasis is especially important in solitary submucosal laryngeal lesions of unknown primary. Recognition of this setting is important in early diagnosis and management of these instances.[6,20,38,49,53] The endoscopic appearance of metastatic laryngeal lesions may not differ from those of primary lesions, except that ulceration favors primary rather than secondary lesions. Laryngeal metastasis may be nonsymptomatic and masked by the widespread disseminated disease or incidentally discovered at autopsy.[24,41,52,56]

Diagnosis

Clinical

In the absence of known primary tumors, the possibility of laryngeal primary should remain a consideration.[3] The finding of non-ulcerated mucosal surface of a single laryngeal nodule favors a secondary tumor. The ultimate diagnosis, however, should be based on biopsy examination. In lesions involving primarily cartilage, CT-guided biopsy may be used as an alternative to the traditional method.

Pathologic

Histologic examination

Except for metastatic squamous carcinoma to the larynx, metastasis can readily be identified by the histologic examination.[3] For localized metastatic laryngeal lesions of clear cell type, the differentiation between primary clear cell carcinoma poses a differential diagnostic dilemma.[15] The presence of rich intralesional vascularity and high lipid content favors metastatic renal cell carcinoma.[15,32,40,42,54,67] Similarly, the differentiation between primary melanoma and restricted metastasis may rest on the past history of the melanoma and the presence of junctional activity.[7,21,23,29,43] Primary mucosal melanoma, mesenchymal and minor salivary gland tumors of the larynx are extremely rare.[5,7,15,16,20,21,23,25,29,32,37,40,42,43,54,59,60,62,63,67]

Immunohistochemical staining

The use of the battery of immunohistochemical markers is pivotal to the final diagnosis of certain rare primary and metastatic lesions. The most useful include keratin, smooth muscle actin, desmin, S-100, HMB-45, PSA, CA125 and surfactant (PE-10) antibodies. The use of these antibodies individually or in combination along with the hematoxylin and eosin stained slide evaluation resolves the vast majority of nonsquamous lesions occurring at the site.

Electron microscopy

Except for occasional cases where histologic examination and immunostaining failed to establish the histogenesis, electron microscopic examination is rarely utilized.

Differential diagnosis

Any primary subclavicular tumor may metastasize to the site.[8,9,28,30,31,35,36,48,51,55,57] The differential diagnosis of secondary laryngeal nodules, especially of the solitary form from primary neoplasms, is a challenging task. Combined clinical, histopathologic and immunohistochemical information leads to the definitive diagnosis in most of these instances. Primary neuroendocrine tumors, paraganglioma, clear cell carcinoma of minor salivary gland and melanoma are rare but may lead to diagnostic difficulties[3,5] and mandate careful workup to exclude metastasis. Occasionally primary laryngeal carcinoid may manifest histomorphologic and immunostaining features that closely resemble metastatic medullary thyroid carcinoma.[13,61,66] Some of these patients have undergone unnecessary thyroidectomy, especially in cases presented with neck node metastasis. Careful clinical and laboratory examination of the thyroid and awareness of this situation is emphasized.

Management

The management of patients with laryngeal metastasis depends largely on the extent of the disease, the overall clinical status and the locoregional symptomatology. The treatment, therefore, should be tailored to the individual patient based on the knowledge of the biological behavior of the primary tumor, the physical characteristics of the laryngeal lesion, the patient's general condition and the outcome of the metastatic workup.[1,4,14,18,45,50]

In general, curative surgery should be restricted to localized symptomatic metastasis. Superficial and polypoid growth can be managed by endoscopic polypectomy or resection. Nonpolypoid and invasive lesions may require partial or total laryngectomy. Although radiation with and without chemotherapy is of unknown benefit for these lesions, small biologically sensitive metastases may respond to such treatment. Successful surgical management of localized seminoma, melanoma and small cell carcinomas has been reported. Palliative treatment to relieve local symptoms, especially airway obstruction, may be attempted and may include laser endoscopic resection.

Outcome

Most patients with laryngeal metastasis succumb to their disease, but occasional long-term survival has been reported. In the latter instances, a solitary metastasis from a relatively less aggressive primary has been reported. Laryngeal metastasis in children is extremely rare[52] but direct laryngoscopy and carbon dioxide laser can be performed.

Current and future experimental approaches

New modalities that may block the metastatic cascade and reduce angiogenesis may play an important role in the future management of these lesions. The application of anti-cytokines, anti-adhesion molecular and antisense nucleotides may block dislodgment, circulation and implantation of metastatic tumors. Similarly, anti-angiogenic reagents may interfere with tumor growth and survival at the metastatic site.[10] The use of vector-mediated gene therapy may also be useful in the future management of selected patients.

References

1. Abemayor E, Cochran AJ, Calcaterra TC. Metastatic cancer to the larynx: diagnosis and management. *Cancer* 1983; **52:** 1944–8.
2. Batsakis JG, Luna MA, Byers RM. Metastases to the larynx. *Head Neck Surg* 1985; **7:** 458–60.
3. Batsakis JG, Luna MA, El-Naggar AK. Non-squamous carcinoma of the larynx. *Ann Otol Rhinol Laryngol* 1992; **101:** 1024–6.
4. Bergstedt M, Herberts G. Hypernephrome metastasis in the larynx: radical extirpation before diagnosis of primary tumour. *Acta Otolaryngol (Stockh)* 1962; **54:** 95–8.
5. Blatchford SJ, Koopmann CF Jr, Coulthard SW. Mucosal melanoma of the head and neck. *Laryngoscope* 1986; **96:** 929–34.
6. Cavicchi O, Farneti G, Occhiuzzi L, Sorrenti G. Laryngeal metastasis from colonic adenocarcinoma. *J Laryngol Otol* 1990; **104:** 730–2.
7. Chamberlain D. Malignant melanoma metastatic to the larynx. *Arch Otolaryngol* 1996; **83:** 231–2.
8. Coakley JF, Ranson DL. Metastasis to the larynx from a prostatic carcinoma: a case report. *J Laryngol Otol* 1984; **98:** 839–42.
9. Cullen JR. Ovarian carcinoma metastatic to the larynx. *J Laryngol Otol* 1990; **104:** 48–9.
10. Effert PJ, Gastl G, Strohmeyer T. Current and future strategies to block tumor angiogenesis, invasion and metastasis. *World J Urol* 1996; **14:** 131–40.
11. Ellis M, Winston P. Secondary carcinoma of the larynx. *J Laryngol Otol* 1957; **71:** 16–24.
12. El-Naggar AK. Secondary neoplasms. In: Ferlito A, ed. *Surgical Pathology of Laryngeal Neoplasms.* London: Chapman & Hall, 1996: 456–74.
13. El-Naggar AK, Batsakis JG, Sellin RV. Medullary carcinoma of the thyroid presenting as tumor of the pharynx and larynx. *J Laryngol Otol* 1991; **105:** 683–6.
14. Eschwège F, Cachin Y, Micheau C. Treatment of adenocarcinoma of the larynx. *Can J Otolaryngol* 1975; **4:** 291–2.
15. Eversole LR. On the differential diagnosis of clear cell tumours of the head and neck. *Eur J Cancer B Oral Oncol* 1993; **29B:** 173–9.
16. Faaborg-Anderson K. Melanoma malignum laryngis. *Acta Otolaryngol (Stockh)* 1953; **43:** 539–41.
17. Ferlito A. Secondary neoplasms. In: Ferlito A, ed. *Neoplasms of the Larynx.* Edinburgh: Churchill Livingstone, 1993: 349–60.
18. Ferlito A, Caruso G. Secondary malignant melanoma of the larynx. Report of two cases and review of 79 laryngeal secondary cases. *ORL J Otorhinolaryngol Relat Spec* 1984; **46:** 117–33.
19. Ferlito A, Caruso G, Recher G. Secondary laryngeal tumors. Report of seven cases with review of the literature. *Arch Otolaryngol Head Neck Surg* 1988; **115:** 635–9.
20. Ferlito A, Pesavento G, Meli S, Recher G, Visoná A. Metastasis to the larynx revealing a renal cell carcinoma. *J Laryngol Otol* 1987; **101:** 843–50.
21. Fisher GE, Odess JS. Metastatic malignant melanoma of the larynx. *Arch Otolaryngol Head Neck Surg* 1951; **54:** 639–42.

22. Folkman J, Shing Y. Angiogenesis. *J Biol Chem* 1992; **267:** 10931–4.
23. Franzoni M. Melanomi metastatici della laringe. *Boll Mal Orecchio Gola Naso* 1951; **83:** 113–29.
24. Freeland AP, van Nostrand AWP, Jahn AR. Metastases of the larynx. *J Otolaryngol* 1979; **8:** 448–56.
25. Gadomski SP, Zwellemberg D, Choi HY. Non-epidermoid carcinoma of the larynx: the Thomas Jefferson University experience. *Otolaryngol Head Neck Surg* 1986; **95:** 558–65.
26. Glanz H, Kleinsasser O. Metastasen im kehlkopf. *HNO* 1978; **26:** 163–7.
27. Greenberg RE, Richter RM, Cooper J, Kessler H, Krigel RI, Petersen RO. Hoarseness: a unique clinical presentation for renal cell carcinoma. *Urology* 1992; **40:** 159–61.
28. Grignon DJ, Ayala AG, Ro JY, Chong C. Carcinoma of prostate metastasizing to vocal cord. *Urology* 1990; **36:** 85–8.
29. Henderson LT, Robbins KT, Weitzner S. Upper aerodigestive tract metastases in disseminated malignant melanoma. *Arch Otolaryngol Head Neck Surg* 1986; **112:** 659–63.
30. Hessan H, Strauss M, Sharkey FE. Urogenital tract carcinoma metastatic to the head and neck. *Laryngoscope* 1986; **96:** 1352–6.
31. Hilger AW, Prichard AJ, Jones T. Adenocarcinoma of the larynx – a distant metastasis from a rectal primary. *J Laryngol Otol* 1998; **112:** 199–201.
32. Hittel JP, Born IA. Ungewöhnliche Metastasen-lokalisation eines Nierenkarzinoms. Ein Fallbericht mit Literaturübersicht. *Laryngorhinootologie* 1995; **74:** 642–4.
33. Klein EA, Ulchaker JC. Biology of metastasis and its clinical implications: renal-cell cancer. *World J Urol* 1996; **14:** 175–81.
34. Kohn EC, Liotta LA. Invasion and metastasis: new approaches to an old problem. *Oncology* 1993; 7: 47–62.
35. Kyríakos M, Berlin BD, DeSchryver Kecskemeti K. Oat cell carcinoma of the larynx. *Arch Otolaryngol* 1978; **104:** 168–76.
36. Levine HL, Applebaum EL. Metastatic adenocarcinoma to the larynx: report of a case. *Trans Am Acad Ophthalmol Otolaryngol* 1976; **82:** 536–41.
37. Loughead JR. Malignant melanoma of the larynx. *Ann Otol* 1952; **61:** 154–8.
38. Marlowe SD, Swartz JD, Koenigsberg R, Zwillenberg S, Marlowe FI, Looby C. Metastatic hypernephroma to the larynx: an unusual presentation. *Neuroradiology* 1993; **35:** 242–3.
39. Marmé D. Tumor angiogenesis: the pivotal role of vascular endothelial growth factor. *World J Urol* 1996; **14:** 166–74.
40. Maxwell JH. Metastatic hypernephroma of the larynx. *Mich Univ Hosp Bull* 1942; **8:** 29–30.
41. Mazzarella LA, Pina LH, Wolff D. Asymptomatic metastasis to the larynx. *Laryngoscope* 1996; **76:** 1547–54.
42. Miyamoto R, Helmus C. Hypernephroma metastatic to the head and neck. *Laryngoscope* 1973; **83:** 898–905.
43. Miyata T, Kishimoto S, Katto Y, Masuda T. Metastatic malignant melanoma involving the larynx and hypopharynx. Report of a case. *Larynx Jpn* 1989; **1:** 146–9.
44. Mochimatsu I, Tsukuda M, Furukawa S, Sawaki S. Tumors metastasizing to the head and neck: a report of seven cases. *J Laryngol Otol* 1993; **107:** 1171–3.
45. Morgan AH, Norris JW, Hicks JN. Palliative laser surgery for melanoma metastatic to the larynx: report of two cases. *Laryngoscope* 1985; **95:** 794–7.
46. Nicolai P, Puxeddu R, Cappiello J *et al.* Metastatic neoplasms to the larynx: report of three cases. *Laryngoscope* 1996; **106:** 851–5.
47. Nicolson GL. Cancer progression and growth: relationship of paracrine and autocrine growth mechanisms to organ preference of metastasis. *Exp Cell Res* 1993; **204:** 171–80.
48. Oeken J, Meister E, Behrendt W. Metastase eines Adenokarzinoms des Ovars in der subglottis. Eine laryngologische Rarität. *HNO* 1996; **44:** 27–31.
49. Ogata H, Ebihara S, Mukai K *et al.* Laryngeal metastasis from a pulmonary papillary adenocarcinoma: a case report. *Jpn J Clin Oncol* 1993; **23:** 199–203.
50. Ohlms LA, McGill T, Healy GB. Malignant laryngeal tumors in children: a 15-year experience with four patients. *Ann Otol Rhinol Laryngol* 1994; **103:** 686–92.
51. Oku T, Hasegawa M, Watanable I, Nasu M, Oaki N. Pancreatic cancer with metastasis to the larynx. *J Laryngol Otol* 1980; **94:** 1205–9.
52. Palacios EJ, Hanchey CC, White HJ. Renal cell carcinoma metastatic to the larynx: case report. *J Ark Med Soc* 1970; **66:** 484–5.
53. Park MH, Park YM. Vocal cord paralysis from prostatic carcinoma metastasizing to the larynx. *Head Neck* 1993; **15:** 455–8.
54. Petridis D, Filios D, Radopoulos D, Nikolaou A, Daniilidis I. Case report: laryngeal metastasis of a renal primary adenocarcinoma (Grawitz tumour). *Eur Arch Otorhinolaryngol* 1998; **255(Suppl 1):** S13 (Abstract).
55. Puxeddu R, Pelagatti CL, Ambu R. Colon adenocarcinoma metastatic to the larynx. *Eur Arch Otorhinolaryngol* 1997; **254:** 353–5.
56. Relic A, Brors D, Prescher A, Schick B. Metastasis to the larynx. *Eur Arch Otorhinolaryngol* 1998; **255(Suppl 1):** S46 (Abstract).
57. Ritchie WW, Messmer JM, Whitley DP, Gopelrund DR. Uterine carcinoma metastatic to the larynx. *Laryngoscope* 1985; **95:** 199–201.
58. Ruiz P, Gunthert U. The cellular basis of metastasis. *World J Urol* 1996; **14:** 141–50.
59. Selch MT, Fu Y-S, Anzai Y, Lufkin RB. Osteosarcoma metastatic to larynx. *Ann Otol Rhinol Laryngol* 1994; **103:** 160–3.
60. Shaheen OH. A case of metastatic amelanotic melanoma of the larynx. *J Laryngol Otol* 1960; **74:** 182–7.
61. Smets G, Warson G, Dehou M-F. Metastasizing neuroendocrine carcinoma of the larynx with calcitonin and somatostatin secretions and CEA production resembling medullary thyroid carcinoma. *Vichows Arch A Pathol Anat Histopathol* 1990; **416:** 539–43.
62. Snow GB, Esch EP, van der Slooten EA. Mucosal melanomas of the head and neck. *Head Neck Surg* 1978; **1:** 24–30.

63. Stankiewicz C, Mostowski L. Przerzut raka jasnokomorkowego nerki do krtani. *Otolaryngol Pol* 1979; **8:** 448–56.
64. Steeg PS, Lawrence JA. Mechanisms of tumor invasion and metastasis. *World J Urol* 1996; **14:** 124–30.
65. Steeg PS, Bevilacqua G, Kopper L *et al.* Evidence for a novel gene associated with low tumor metastatic potential. *J Natl Cancer Inst* 1988; **80:** 200–4.
66. Sweeny EC, McDonnell L, O'Brian C. Medullary carcinoma of the thyroid presenting as tumor of the pharynx and larynx. *Histopathology* 1981; **5:** 263–75.
67. Szmeja Z, Obrebowski A, Lukaszewski B. A case of metastasis of breast cancer to the larynx. *Otolaryngol Pol* 1986; **40:** 212–16.
68. Wanamaker JR, Kraus DH, Eliachar I, Lavertu P. Manifestations of metastatic breast carcinoma to the head and neck. *Head Neck* 1993; **15:** 257–62.
69. Weidner N. Tumor angiogenesis: review of current applications in tumor prognostication. *Semin Diagn Pathol* 1993; **10:** 302–13.
70. Zetter BR. The cellular basis of site-specific tumor metastasis. *N Engl J Med* 1990; **332:** 605–12.

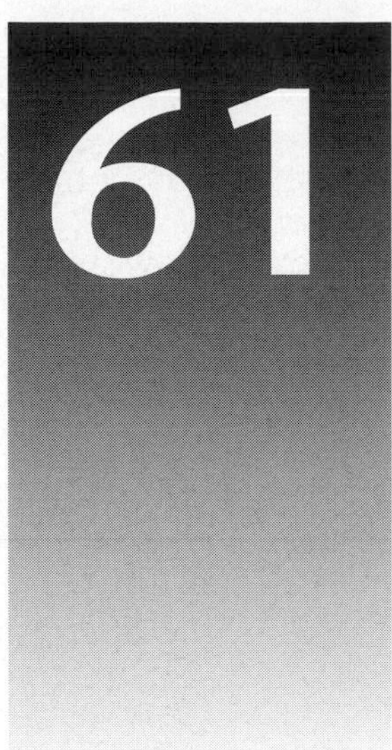

Neoplasms of the pediatric larynx

Laurie A Ohlms and Randal S Weber

Neoplasms of the pediatric larynx are relatively rare, with benign lesions occurring more commonly. The actual incidence of the various types of pediatric laryngeal tumor is difficult to estimate because such lesions occur infrequently. Since signs and symptoms of laryngeal tumors often mimic those of infectious or inflammatory disease, a high level of suspicion is necessary to rule out a neoplastic process.

Evaluation

Laryngeal tumors in children present with similar signs and symptoms, independent of histology. The infant usually develops stridor and airway obstruction; a hoarse cry and poor feeding may also be noted. In the older child, the first symptom may be voice change, with progressive airway obstruction as the lesion grows. Delay in diagnosis is not unusual as these findings commonly represent inflammatory disease such as croup in the young child. If symptoms do not respond to appropriate therapy, further evaluation is indicated. In the older child, especially the adolescent male, hoarseness may be attributed to pubertal voice change. Persistent voice changes in a child should always be investigated.

After recording a thorough history, a complete head and neck examination is performed. The neck is carefully palpated, noting any abnormal masses or adenopathy. Laryngoscopy is attempted in the office setting. An older, cooperative child may tolerate indirect, mirror examination. Flexible nasopharyngolaryngoscopy permits a more complete assessment, noting vocal cord motion and any unusual lesions. However, office laryngoscopy does not allow visualization of the subglottis or trachea and is often difficult in the young child. Formal direct laryngoscopy and bronchoscopy should be performed if the clinical situation warrants.

Radiographic studies supplement the physical examination. Anterior-posterior and lateral neck films, airway fluoroscopy and barium swallow can assess the tumor and rule out concomitant airway lesions. Computed tomography (CT) and magnetic resonance imaging (MRI) scans document tumor volume, local extension, and the presence of cartilage invasion. MRI is particularly useful for determining paraglottic and pre-epiglottic space invasion. These studies are also helpful in follow-up to document response to treatment.

Definitive diagnosis of a laryngeal tumor is based on endoscopic findings. Direct laryngoscopy and bronchoscopy under general anesthesia allow precise evaluation of the lesion and the surrounding tissues. Biopsy will establish the histology and guide treatment planning. A biopsy should be taken prior to laser excision of presumed papillomas to rule out coexisting malignancy. Follow-up endoscopy helps to assess treatment response and to rule out recurrent disease.

Treatment

Benign laryngeal neoplasms

Respiratory papillomas

Ninety-eight percent of pediatric airway tumors are benign; the most common benign lesions in children are squamous papillomas (also known as respiratory papillomas).[27] Often associated with human papilloma virus types 6 and 11, juvenile onset papillomas are benign, yet relentless, lesions that tend to recur after treatment.[25] Papillomas typically involve the true vocal cords (Fig 61.1), as well as the supraglottis and subglottis. Distal tracheal spread has been associated with tracheotomy (and disruption of the tracheal mucosa) and more aggressive disease.

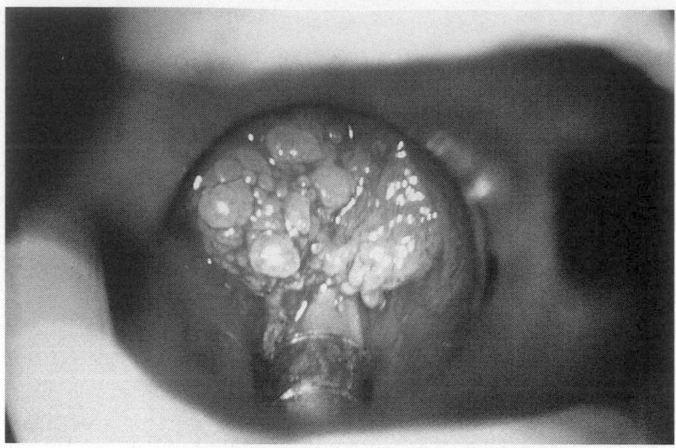

Figure 61.1 *Respiratory papillomas involving the larynx.*

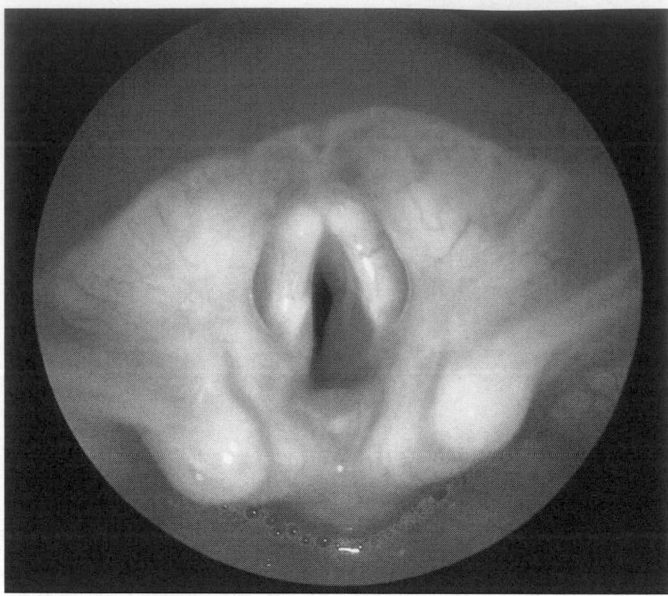

Figure 61.2 *Subglottic hemangioma.*

A definitive cure for respiratory papillomas is not available. The current goal of therapy is to maintain a stable airway while preserving as much normal tissue as possible. The most commonly used therapy for papillomas is laser vaporization with the carbon dioxide (CO_2) or potassium titanyl phosphate (KTP) laser. The lesions frequently recur, necessitating multiple endoscopic procedures.

Many adjuvant therapies have been suggested. Several studies have evaluated the use of interferon, an antiviral agent.[7–9,13] When used along with laser excision, interferon may initially slow papilloma growth in some patients. However, prolonged interferon use may actually be associated with accelerated papilloma growth.[9] Interferon does not cause a lasting remission; once the drug is discontinued, papilloma growth often recurs.

Recently, photodynamic therapy has been suggested as an alternative treatment. A photosensitizer (often a purified form of a hematoporphyrin derivative) is selectively absorbed and retained in the hyperplastic, neoplastic tissue (the papillomas). The treated tissue is then activated by light at a specific wavelength and cells that have concentrated the photosensitizer are destroyed.[21] Light sources include the argon pumped dye laser and the gold vapor laser. Although not yet widely used for the treatment of papillomas, initial results are encouraging.[1]

Subglottic hemangioma

The subglottic hemangioma, a less common benign neoplasm, forms as a result of endothelial proliferation. The lesion is usually not present at birth, but grows rapidly in the first few weeks of life. The child presents with biphasic stridor and increasing respiratory distress, usually at around 8–10 weeks of age. Fifty percent of patients with subglottic hemangiomas will have a cutaneous hemangioma as well.[24] Endoscopy reveals a smooth, pink, compressible mass, usually in the subglottis (Fig 61.2).

The natural history of subglottic hemangiomas is proliferation until about 1 year of age, followed by spontaneous involution over the next several years. The goal of treatment is to maintain a stable airway, preserving normal function and anatomy, until involution occurs. Tracheotomy can maintain the airway, but is associated with increased morbidity in infants. The isolated subglottic hemangioma is frequently amenable to laser excision using the CO_2 or KTP laser.[24] Several laser procedures may be necessary over several months. Open surgical excision of subglottic hemangiomas has been proposed, but can cause scarring in the airway.[28] Larger airway hemangiomas that extend beyond the larynx into the trachea or mediastinum may not be controlled by laser therapy. Interferon-α2A has been used successfully to treat these more extensive, life-threatening hemangiomas.[18]

Other benign laryngeal neoplasms in children include vascular malformations (venous and lymphatic) and neurogenic tumors (granular cell tumor, neurofibroma).[3,4,16] The goal of treatment remains the control of the lesion with preservation of laryngeal function, usually with surgical or laser excision.

Malignant laryngeal neoplasms

In the past, most pediatric laryngeal malignancies were squamous cell carcinomas, arising after radiation therapy of a benign condition such as papillomas or adenoid hypertrophy. Today malignant neoplasms are more often sarcomas, usually rhabdomyosarcoma.[5,14,27] Treatment of a malignant laryngeal tumor in a child depends upon the histology. Because these lesions are rare, decisions are often based on protocols for similar lesions at other sites.

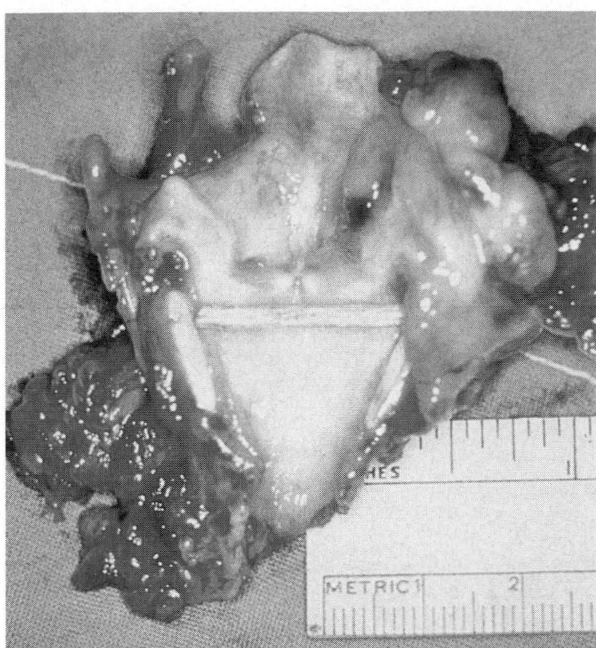

Figure 61.3 *Laryngeal rhabdomyosarcoma (laryngectomy specimen). (Reproduced with permission from Ohlms LA, McGill T, Healy GB. Malignant laryngeal tumors in children.* Ann Otol Rhinol Laryngol *1994;* ***103:*** *686–92.)*

The unique characteristics of the pediatric larynx may necessitate modification of established treatment protocols.

Rhabdomyosarcoma

Rhabdomyosarcoma is the most common soft tissue sarcoma in young children. In the head and neck, most tumors arise in the orbit (25%) or other parameningeal sites such as the nasopharynx, paranasal sinuses, temporal bone or infratemporal fossa. Laryngeal rhabdomyosarcoma is rare and usually presents as a localized, painless, enlarging mass (Fig 61.3).[10]

After diagnosis, a metastatic evaluation is performed, including skeletal survey, bone scan and bone marrow aspirate or biopsy. Metastasis can be via lymphatic and hematogenous spread. Staging is based on surgical–pathologic findings, including the amount of residual disease after resection.[12] Prognosis depends upon the extent of the tumor, histologic subtype and response to treatment.

Current treatment protocols include both chemotherapy and high-dose radiation therapy; surgery is usually reserved for diagnostic biopsy only or for easily accessible tumors that can be removed without creating a major functional or cosmetic defect.[10,27] Treatment of a pediatric laryngeal rhabdomyosarcoma raises unique concerns. Radiation of the developing larynx may result in a fibrotic, infantile larynx and is also associated with the potential risk of a second, radiation-induced malignancy.[17] Other options include hyperfractionation of the radiation therapy or no radiation in the child with a complete response after chemotherapy.

Squamous cell carcinoma

Squamous cell carcinoma of the larynx, although common in adults, is extremely rare in children.[5,6,19,20,22] Predisposing factors include prior laryngeal papillomatosis (with or without a history of radiation), tobacco and alcohol. There are reports of laryngeal carcinoma in children associated with human papilloma virus coinfection.[25]

These tumors are staged as in adults using the TNM classification system and treatment is based upon tumor stage. In the past, many pediatric patients were treated with a combination of surgery and radiation therapy, with poor survival rates. More recently, laryngeal preservation protocols have been used successfully in children with laryngeal carcinoma (Fig 61.4).[11,17,29] These protocols utilize induction chemotherapy and radiation therapy; surgery is reserved for patients with less than a 50% partial response to chemotherapy or for recurrent or residual disease after chemotherapy and radiation therapy.[15,23,26] Careful follow-up is essential to rule out recurrence in these patients.

Other laryngeal malignancies have been described in children, including lymphoma and primitive neuroectodermal tumor.[14,17] There are isolated case reports of adenocarcinoma and mucoepidermoid carcinoma arising from minor salivary glands in the larynx.[14] These glands are located in the supraglottic and subglottic larynx; the true vocal cords are devoid of minor salivary glands. Therefore, minor salivary gland tumors present with signs and symptoms of airway obstruction rather than voice changes. Metastasis to the larynx is rare at any age.[17] Again treatment is based upon current protocols for similar lesions at other sites.

Complications of treatment

Treatment of benign and malignant neoplasms can cause complications in the pediatric patient. Repeated laser excision of papillomas can create scarring of the vocal cords with subsequent voice change. Radiation therapy is associated with erythema, edema and desquamation in the acute phase; tracheotomy may be required for airway control. Radiation of the developing larynx may arrest growth; the larynx is not fully developed until puberty.[2] High-dose laryngeal radiation in a prepubescent child may result in an infantile larynx without useful voice, airway, or swallowing function.[17] Secondary tumors arising in the irradiated field (salivary glands, thyroid) are also a concern. In order to avoid radiation, partial laryngeal surgery is a definite consideration in the child with a malignant tumor. In some cases, however, surgical resection of a laryngeal tumor may necessitate total laryngectomy, creating serious psychosocial problems for the child and the family.

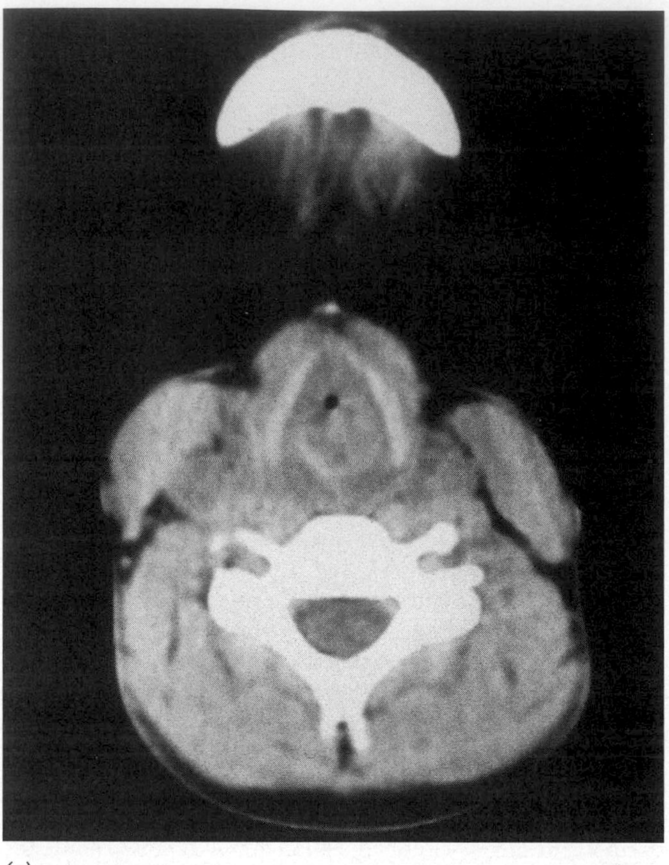

(a)

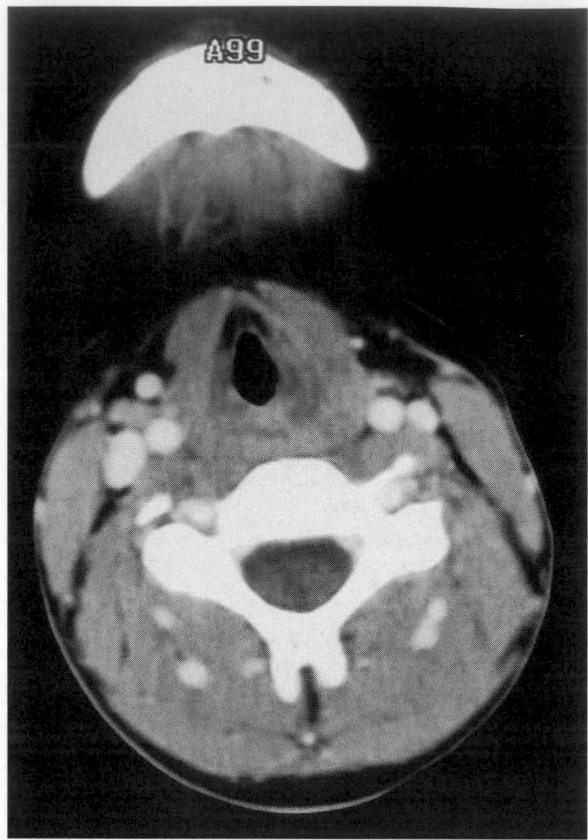

(b)

These risks emphasize the need for an individualized treatment plan for the child with a laryngeal tumor. Experience is limited with pediatric laryngeal malignancies; thus the risks and benefits must be considered as the treatment plan is designed. The plan must be flexible, allowing for modifications if the initial treatment response is incomplete.

Voice rehabilitation

Voice rehabilitation is important after treatment of laryngeal neoplasms. The child who has undergone multiple laser excisions of papillomas will likely benefit from speech therapy. When laryngectomy is necessary, the child will require an alternate method of communication. Children can learn to use esophageal speech effectively;[17] a voice prosthesis (tracheoesophageal puncture) is another option.

Conclusion

Laryngeal tumors in children are rare and a high index of suspicion is critical to make the diagnosis. Because experience with these tumors is limited, a careful individualized treatment approach to each child is crucial to control the tumor and preserve normal function whenever possible.

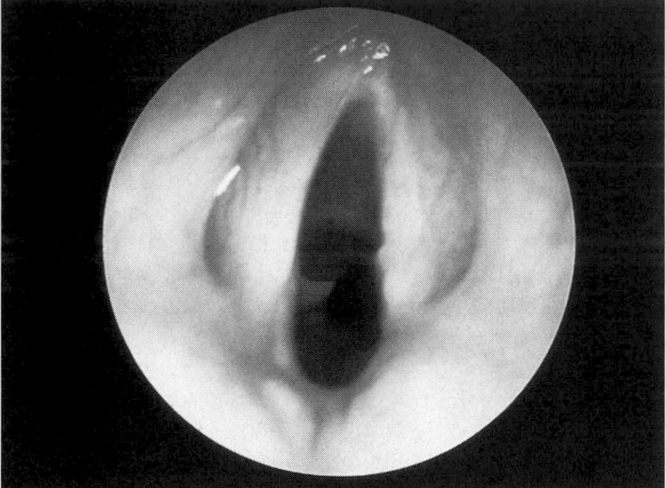

(c)

Figure 61.4 *(a) Pretreatment CT scan of an adolescent male with laryngeal squamous cell carcinoma. (b) Post-treatment CT scan. (c) Post-treatment endoscopic view of the larynx. (Reproduced with permission from Ohlms LA, McGill T, Healy GB. Malignant laryngeal tumors in children.* Ann Otol Rhinol Laryngol *1994;* ***103:*** *686–92.)*

References

1. Abramson AL, Shikowitz MJ, Mullooly VM, Steinberg BM, Amella CA, Rothstein HR. Clinical effects of photodynamic therapy in recurrent laryngeal papillomas. *Arch Otolaryngol Head Neck Surg* 1992; **118:** 25–9.
2. Benjamin B. Congenital disorders of the larynx. In: Cummings CW, Fredrickson JM, Harker LA, Krause CJ, Schuller DE, eds. *Otolaryngology – Head and Neck Surgery*, 2nd edn. St Louis: Mosby, 1993: 1831–53.
3. Conley SF, Milbrath MM, Beste DJ. Pediatric laryngeal granular cell tumor. *J Otolaryngol* 1992; **21:** 450–3.
4. Ejnell H, Jarund M, Bailey M, Lindeman P. Airway obstruction in children due to plexiform neurofibroma of the larynx. *J Laryngol Otol* 1996; **110:** 1065–8.
5. Ferlito A, Rinaldo A, Marioni G. Laryngeal malignant neoplasms in children and adolescents. *Int J Pediatr Otorhinolaryngol* 1999; **49:** 1–14.
6. Gindhart TD, Johnston WH, Chism SE, Dedo HH. Carcinoma of the larynx in childhood. *Cancer* 1980; **46:** 1683–7.
7. Goepfert H, Sessions RB, Gutterman JV, Cangir A, Dichtel WJ, Sulek M. Leukocyte interferon in patients with juvenile laryngeal papillomatosis. *Ann Otol* 1982; **91:** 431–6.
8. Haglund S, Lundquist P, Cantell K, Strander H. Interferon therapy in juvenile laryngeal papillomatosis. *Arch Otolaryngol* 1981; **107:** 327–32.
9. Healy GB, Gelber RD, Trowbridge AL, Grundfast KM, Ruben RJ, Price KN. Treatment of recurrent respiratory papillomatosis with human leukocyte interferon. Results of a multicenter randomized clinical trial. *N Engl J Med* 1988; **319:** 401–7.
10. Kato MA, Flamant F, Terrier-Lacombe MJ *et al.* Rhabdomyosarcoma of the larynx in children: a series of five patients treated in the Institut Gustave Roussy (Villejuif, France). *Med Pediatr Oncol* 1991; **19:** 110–14.
11. Laurian N, Sadov R, Strauss M, Kessler E. Laryngeal carcinoma in childhood. Report of a case and review of the literature. *Laryngoscope* 1984; **94:** 684–7.
12. Maurer HM. The Intergroup Rhabdomyosarcoma Study (NIH): objectives and clinical staging classification. *J Pediatr Surg* 1975; **10:** 977–8.
13. McCabe BF, Clark KF. Interferon and laryngeal papillomatosis: the Iowa experience. *Ann Otol Rhinol Laryngol* 1983; **92:** 2–7.
14. McGuirt WF, Little JP. Laryngeal cancer in children and adolescents. *Otolaryngol Clin North Am* 1997; **30:** 207–14.
15. Merlano M, Vitale V, Rosso R *et al.* Treatment of advanced squamous-cell carcinoma of the head and neck with alternating chemotherapy and radiotherapy. *N Engl J Med* 1992; **327:** 1115–21.
16. Ohlms LA, Forsen J, Burrows PE. Venous malformation of the pediatric airway. *Int J Pediatr Otorhinolaryngol* 1996; **37:** 99–114.
17. Ohlms LA, McGill TJ, Healy GB. Malignant laryngeal tumors in children: a 15-year experience with four patients. *Ann Otol Rhinol Laryngol* 1994; **103:** 686–92.
18. Ohlms LA, Jones DT, McGill TJ, Healy GB. Interferon alfa-2A therapy for airway hemangiomas. *Ann Otol Rhinol Laryngol* 1994; **103:** 1–8.
19. Ossoff RH, Tucker GF, Norris CM. Carcinoma of the larynx in an 11-year-old boy with late cervical metastasis: report of a case with a ten-year follow-up. *Otolaryngol Head Neck Surg* 1980; **88:** 142–5.
20. Pandey R, Choudhury C. Case report of cancer of the larynx in an adolescent. *J Laryngol Otol* 1968; **82:** 469–71.
21. Pransky SM, Kang DR. Tumors of the larynx, trachea, and bronchi. In: Bluestone CD, Stool SE, Kenna MA, eds. *Pediatric Otolaryngology*, 3rd edn. Philadelphia: Saunders, 1996: 1402–14.
22. Seth RRS, Yadav YC, Kala DM. Epidermoid carcinoma of the laryngopharynx in a young girl. *J Laryngol Otol* 1978; **92:** 925–6.
23. Shirinian MH, Weber RS, Lippman SM *et al.* Laryngeal preservation by induction chemotherapy plus radiotherapy in locally advanced head and neck cancer: the M.D. Anderson Cancer Center experience. *Head Neck* 1994; **16:** 39–44.
24. Sie KC, McGill TJ, Healy GB. Subglottic hemangioma: ten years' experience with the carbon dioxide laser. *Ann Otol Rhinol Laryngol* 1994; **103:** 167–72.
25. Simon M, Kahn T, Schneider A, Pirsig W. Laryngeal carcinoma in a 12-year-old child. Association with human papillomavirus 18 and 33. *Arch Otolaryngol Head Neck Surg* 1994; **120:** 277–82.
26. The Department of Veterans Affairs Laryngeal Study Group. Induction chemotherapy plus radiation in patients with advanced laryngeal cancer. *N Engl J Med* 1991; **324:** 1685–90.
27. Ward RF, Healy GB. Neoplasia of the pediatric larynx. In: Fried MP, ed. *The Larynx: A Multidisciplinary Approach*, 2nd edn. St Louis: Mosby, 1996: 171–7.
28. Wiatrak BJ, Reilly JS, Seid AB, Pransky SM, Castillo JV. Open surgical excision of subglottic hemangioma in children. *Int J Pediatr Otorhinolaryngol* 1996; **34:** 191–206.
29. Zalzal GH, Cotton RT, Bove K. Carcinoma of the larynx in a child. *Int J Pediatr Otorhinolaryngol* 1987; **13:** 219–25.

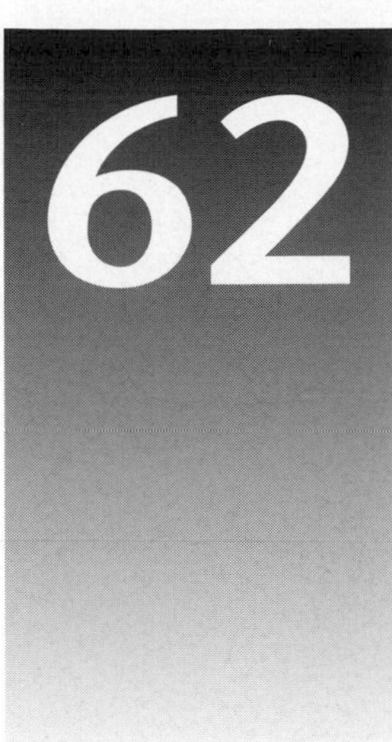

Pregnancy and cancer of the larynx

Alfio Ferlito and Jan Olofsson

Cancer of the larynx is a relatively rare disease, but it is the most common head and neck cancer (excluding the skin) in most countries. It is primarily a disease affecting adults, with a peak incidence in the sixth and seventh decades; less than 1% of laryngeal cancers occur under the age of 30 years. It has a higher incidence among blacks than among whites and a distinct male predominance, though recent data show that the male-to-female ratio is tending to change.[7,12,21] More than 20% of laryngeal cancers now occur in women[7,21] and there is evidence that changes in women's smoking and drinking habits in recent years would be responsible for this trend. Differences in the use of known cancer-promoting agents (such as alcohol and tobacco), hormonal effects and sociocultural influences probably have a role in gender differences in cancer of the larynx. The majority of men develop glottic cancers, whereas women in some countries are more likely to develop supraglottic cancer.[32,37] The ratio of glottic to supraglottic tumors in women is 0.56:1.[37]

Hematologic malignancies, cancers of the breast and of the female genital tract, thyroid cancer, and hepatocellular cancer may occasionally be encountered in association with pregnancy. Experience of laryngeal cancer in pregnancy is very rare, inasmuch as this tumor does not usually affect women, especially when they are young, so the pregnant woman does not belong to the age or sex groups with a high incidence of laryngeal cancer. There have been no studies correlating pregnancy with cancer of the larynx due to the rarity of the association.[9] The larynx is a secondary sex organ and the demonstration of estrogen, androgen and progesterone receptors in laryngeal tumors is well documented in the literature,[3,5,6,14,17,18,25,30,31,33–36,38,39,41,42] but any association of laryngeal cancer with pregnancy remains unclear and clinical experience of cases of laryngeal cancer during pregnancy remains very limited due to the small number of cases reported.

The first report of cancer of the larynx in pregnancy came in 1956 from Lehnhardt,[23] who described a case occurring in a 40-year-old woman in Germany. The tumor involved the false cord and was treated with hemilaryngectomy and radiation therapy. The patient was alive after 10 months. In 1957, Eckel[13] reported a case, again in Germany, of a woman with laryngeal papillomatosis since the age of 18 that degenerated into cancer during the first months of her second pregnancy. The therapeutic modality adopted was total laryngectomy followed by radiation therapy. In 1970, Chumakov and Paramonova[10] described a case in Russia of laryngeal carcinoma in a 27-year-old pregnant woman who received radiation therapy as primary treatment. At 2 years, the results appeared to be satisfactory for both mother and child. Later, in 1973, Brophy[8] reported another case occurring in a 24-year-old white woman of Anglo-Saxon extraction in which the cancer persisted after radiation therapy and the patient, a non-smoker, underwent hemilaryngectomy during the mid-trimester of pregnancy. In 1980, Ferlito and Nicolai[15] described a laryngeal cancer in a 26-year-old Italian female, whose disease had not been detected in time despite hoarseness from the mid-trimester. Total laryngectomy and radical neck dissection were performed after the delivery. No metastases were found in the lymph nodes. Voice restoration using a Blom-Singer prosthesis, producing an intelligible voice, was performed 9 years after the diagnosis. The patient is alive and well after 17 years and 7 months. In 1986, Mikaelian *et al.*[27] reported a case of epithelial-myoepithelial carcinoma involving the subglottic region in a 30-year-old woman treated by laryngofissure with excision of the tumor during the pregnancy and radiation therapy after the delivery. In 1994, Albrechtsen *et al.*[1] reported a case in Norway in a 23-year-old,

Table 62.1 Reported cases of laryngeal cancer in pregnancy

Author(s)	*Year*	*Age (years)*	*Gestation time*	*Previous pregnancy*	*Presentation*	*Site*	*Histology*	*Meta-stasis*	*Treatment*	*Follow-up*
Lehnhardt[23]	1956	40	4 mo	3 (2 abortions)	Hoarseness	Right false cord	Squamous carcinoma	None	Hemilaryngectomy, radiation therapy	NED 10 mo
Eckel[13]	1957	20	4 wk	1	Hoarseness, dyspnea	Right vocal cord	Squamous carcinoma	None	Total laryngectomy, radiation therapy during the pregnancy	NED 3 yr
Chumakov and Paramonova[10]	1970	27	7 mo		Hoarseness	Middle third of the right vocal cord	Squamous carcinoma	None	Radiation therapy during the pregnancy	NED 2 yr
Brophy[8]	1973	24		1	Hoarseness	Right vocal cord	Squamous carcinoma	None	Radiation therapy before diagnosis of pregnancy, intralaryngeal right cordectomy at first, hemi-laryngectomy during the pregnancy	NED 1 yr 4 mo
Ferlito and Nicolai[15]	1980	26	4 mo		Hoarseness	Right false and true vocal cords	Squamous carcinoma	None	Total laryngectomy and right radical neck dissection after the delivery	NED 17 yr 7 mo*
Mikaelian *et al.*[27]	1986	30	28 wk		Progressive shortness of breath, hoarseness	Right subglottic region, cricoid to the first true ring, inferior surface of the right true vocal cord	Epithelial-myoepithelial carcinoma	None	Laryngofissure with excision of the tumor during the pregnancy, radiation therapy after the delivery	NED 2 yr
Albrechtsen *et al.*[1]	1994	23	5 mo	2 (1 abortion)	Progressive shortness of breath, hoarseness, dyspnea during the delivery	Pyriform sinus	Squamous carcinoma	None	Laryngopharyngectomy and left radical neck dissection after the delivery, reconstruction with a pectoralis major myocutaneous flap and postoperative radiotherapy	NED 13 yr*
Matschke *et al.*[24]†	1994	33	28 wk	2 abortions	Painful swelling of the left neck, hoarseness	Left vocal cord, ventricle, left pyriform sinus	Squamous carcinoma	Lymph nodes, bones, soft tissues of the neck	Total laryngectomy and left radical neck dissection during the pregnancy, radiation therapy and chemo-therapy after the delivery	Died 2 yr (carotid hemor-rhage)
Pytel *et al.*[29]	1995	33	10 wk		Intermittent difficulty in swallowing	Both false vocal cords, laryngeal surface of the epiglottis	Squamous carcinoma	None	Supraglottic horizontal laryngectomy	NED 3 yr
Ferlito††		28	8 wk	1 spontaneous abortion	Hoarseness, cough with initial dyspnea	Left true vocal cord	Squamous carcinoma	None	Total laryngectomy, hemithyroidectomy, bilateral functional neck dissection after the delivery	NED 4 yr 1 mo

NED, no evidence of disease.
*Additional information obtained subsequent to original report.
†This case has been already published by Panagiotopoulos *et al.*[28]
††Unpublished case.

non-smoking woman whose pyriform sinus squamous cell carcinoma was diagnosed a few days after the delivery. The therapeutic modality adopted was laryngopharyngectomy and left radical neck dissection, reconstruction with a pectoralis major musculocutaneous flap and postoperative radiotherapy. The patient later received a Provox speech valve and a Bivona stomal valve and had a good voice. There was no evidence of recurrence after 10 years. Another case was reported in 1994 in the German literature of a 33-year-old pregnant woman with a large squamous cell carcinoma of the left vocal cord that had spread into the left pyriform sinus and infiltrated the soft tissues of the thyroid cartilage. The tumor was treated by total laryngectomy and left radical neck dissection during the pregnancy, plus radiation therapy and chemotherapy after the delivery. Bone metastases were present and there was a large recurrence in the soft tissue of the neck. The patient died 2 years after the diagnosis due to carotid hemorrhage.[24] In 1995, Pytel *et al.*[29] reported a case observed in Hungary in a 33-year-old patient, with supraglottic laryngeal cancer detected in the first trimester of her twin pregnancy following *in vitro* fertilization after a 10-year nulliparous period of married life. A supraglottic laryngectomy was performed during the pregnancy and she subsequently delivered a pair of premature twins, a boy and a girl, by cesarean section. Three years after surgery, the mother and twins were in good health. Another pregnant woman with cancer of the larynx observed in Italy involved a 28-year-old female treated by total laryngectomy, hemithyroidectomy, and bilateral functional neck dissection after the delivery. Voice restoration using the Blom-Singer prosthesis was done and the patient acquired an intelligible voice. She was alive and well 4 years and 1 month after surgery (unpublished case). The clinicopathological data on the patients with cancer of the larynx associated with pregnancy are summarized in Table 62.1.[1,8,10,13,15,23,24,27–29]

In a chapter entitled 'Cancer of the larynx in unusual hosts' in the book *Cancer of the Larynx*, Bryce[9] mentioned two patients with cancer of the larynx in pregnancy observed at the Princess Margaret Hospital, Toronto. In one, a tubal pregnancy was terminated and the cancer was treated using radiotherapy. In the second, the pregnancy was terminated and the patient received radiotherapy. In both cases, the therapy was successful and the voice was saved. In 1992, Werner *et al.*[43] reported the first case of the coexistence of laryngeal paraganglioma and pregnancy in a 30-year-old woman, though the association of extralaryngeal paraganglioma and pregnancy is well documented in the literature.[20,40] The case reported by Werner *et al.*[43] is not included in the table because the biologic behavior of this lesion in the larynx is generally benign.[4,16] In 1992, a case considered as the first report of a maternal death from laryngeal papillomatosis during pregnancy was reported by Helmrich *et al.*[19]

The treatment of laryngeal cancer is controversial and adding the variable of pregnancy further complicates the choice of appropriate treatment. The organogenesis period (lasting from day 10–14 to the eighth week) is the most sensitive to any kind of teratogenic insult. Teratogenicity may be caused by radiation, chemotherapy and general anesthesia, but the anesthesia-related teratogenic risks are almost nonexistent by comparison with the risks relating to radiation and chemotherapy. Typical anesthetic agents readily reach the fetus but are not known to be teratogenic in humans.

General anesthesia during pregnancy is complicated for various reasons (increased blood volume, increased heart rate and cardiac output, supine positional hypotension, decreased pulmonary functional residual capacity, elevated diaphragm, etc.). Pregnancy is not an absolute contraindication for surgery during the first trimester, however, providing specific precautions are taken concerning the general anesthesia (monitoring the mother's period of apnea and hemodynamic parameters, preventing any inhalation of vomit, and keeping a check on fetal heart rate as of the 16th week of gestation) and the postoperative period (monitoring uterine activity).

As concerns the type of anesthesia to use, a classic neuroleptic anesthesia is always suitable in the first trimester. Sodium thiopental is administered as a short-term hypnotic drug, followed by nitrogen protoxide to maintain the hypnotic state. For analgesic purposes, fentanyl can be used – which is associated with haloperidol for sedation. Succinylcholine is used initially to relax the muscles and thus facilitate intubation. Pancuronium, or any other curarizing preparation, is administered throughout the operation. None of the above-mentioned drugs has revealed any teratogenic effects,[2,11,22,26] apart from nitrogen protoxide, which has only proved teratogenic in animal models after prolonged exposure (24–48 hours) and at very high doses. Minimal doses of inhalation anesthetic and short exposure times cannot induce to teratogenic effects.

Surgical treatment could also be carried out during the second trimester, when there is no longer any risk of teratogenesis, but prior to the third trimester, when premature labor secondary to general anesthesia becomes a major hazard.

Alternatively, radiotherapy may be administered while shielding the patient's abdomen and the fetus from the radiation. This treatment has proved an effective therapeutic modality, but the risk of radiation therapy in young patients must be borne in mind. Radiotherapy can induce the occurrence of a new neoplasm at the site of radiation or in neighboring structures.

Chemotherapy should be avoided because of its harmful effects on organogenesis during the first trimester.

As in the nonpregnant patient, either surgery or radiotherapy may be appropriate. All our patients treated with surgery are alive and well. Close cooperation is required between the laryngologist, radiotherapist, obstetrician and anesthesiologist to select the most valid treatment.

Almost all the patients with pregnancy-associated cancer had negative lymph nodes; in fact, only one presented local and distant metastases (to the bones) and died after 2 years. There is no significant difference in the actual survival between pregnant and nonpregnant patients with laryngeal tumors of equivalent stage and the same phenotype.

References

1. Albrechtsen S, Julseth E, Olofsson J, Dalaker K. Outcome of pregnancy and childbirth following laryngectomy. *Acta Obstet Gynecol Scand* 1994; **73:** 83–4.
2. Aldridge LM, Tunstall ME. Nitrous oxide and the fetus. A review and the results of a retrospective study of 175 cases of anaesthesia for insertion of Shirodkar suture. *Br J Anaesth* 1986; **58:** 1348–56.
3. Altissimi G, Simoncelli C, Angelini A. Recettori ormonali nel cancro della laringe. *Acta Otorhinolaryngol Ital* 1988; **8:** 423–35.
4. Barnes L. Paraganglioma of the larynx. A critical review of the literature. *ORL J Otorhinolaryngol Relat Spec* 1991; **53:** 220–34.
5. Beckford NS, Rood SR, Schaid D, Schanbacher B. Androgen stimulation and laryngeal development. *Ann Otol Rhinol Laryngol* 1985; **94:** 634–40.
6. Berg NJ, Colvard DS, Neel HB III, Weiland LH, Spelsberg TC. Progesterone receptors in carcinomas of the upper aerodigestive tract. *Otolaryngol Head Neck Surg* 1989; **101:** 527–36.
7. Boring CC, Squires TS, Heath CW. Cancer statistics for African-Americans. *CA Cancer J Clin* 1992; **42:** 7–17.
8. Brophy JW. Squamous cell carcinoma of the larynx in pregnancy. *Arch Otolaryngol* 1973; **97:** 480–1.
9. Bryce DP. Cancer of the larynx in unusual hosts. In: Ferlito A, ed. *Cancer of the Larynx*. Boca Raton: CRC Press, 1985: 26–32.
10. Chumakov FI, Paramonova EA. Cancer of the larynx in a pregnant woman. *Vestn Otorhinolaryngol* 1970; **32:** 113–14.
11. Cohen EN, McGreenfield G, Brown BW, Wu ML. Occupational disease in dentistry and chronic exposure to trace anesthetic gases. *J Am Dent Assoc* 1980; **101:** 21–31.
12. DeRienzo DP, Greenberg SD, Fraire AE. Carcinoma of the larynx. Changing incidence in women. *Arch Otolaryngol Head Neck Surg* 1991; **117:** 681–4.
13. Eckel W. Kehlkopfpapillome und deren carcinomatöse Entartung, entstanden jeweils während der Schwangerschaft. Ein Beitrag zur Kasuistik des Kehlkopfcarcinoms der Frau. *HNO* 1957; **6:** 197–200.
14. Ferguson BJ, Hudson WR, McCarty KS Jr. Sex steroid receptors distribution in the human larynx and laryngeal carcinoma. *Arch Otolaryngol Head Neck Surg* 1987; **113:** 1311–15.
15. Ferlito A, Nicolai P. Laryngeal cancer in pregnancy. *Acta Otorhinolaryngol Belg* 1980; **34:** 706–9.
16. Ferlito A, Barnes L, Wenig BM. Identification, classification, treatment, and prognosis of laryngeal paraganglioma. Review of the literature and eight new cases. *Ann Otol Rhinol Laryngol* 1994; **103:** 525–36.
17. Grenman R, Virolainen E, Shapira A, Carey T. *In vitro* effects of tamoxifen on UM-SCC head and neck cancer cell lines: correlation with the estrogen and progesterone receptor content. *Int J Cancer* 1987; **39:** 77–81.
18. Haidoutova R, Melamed M, Dimitrova S, Kyossovska R. Investigations of serum testosterone levels in patients with laryngeal cancers. *Arch Otorhinolaryngol* 1985; **241:** 213–17.
19. Helmrich G. Stubbs TM, Stoerker J. Fetal maternal laryngeal papillomatosis in pregnancy. A case report. *Am J Obstet Gynecol* 1992; **166:** 524–5.
20. Kleiner GJ, Greston WM, Yang PT, Levy JL, Newman AD. Paraganglioma complicating pregnancy and the puerperium. *Obstet Gynecol* 1982; **59:** 2S-6S.
21. Kokoska MS, Piccirillo JF, Haughey BH. Gender differences in cancer of the larynx. *Ann Otol Rhinol Laryngol* 1995; **104:** 419–24.
22. Konieczko KM, Chapple JC, Nunn JF. Fetotoxic potential of general anaesthesia in relation to pregnancy. *Br J Anaesth* 1987; **59:** 449–54.
23. Lehnhardt E. Kehlkopfkrebs bei Frauen. Zugleich ein kasuistischer Beitrag über Kehlkopfkrebs in der Schwangerschaft. *Laryngorhinootologie* 1956; **35:** 732–7.
24. Matschke RG, Gräber T, Panagiotopoulos A. Ein Kehlkopfkarzinom in der Schwangerschaft. *HNO* 1994; **42:** 505–8.
25. Mattox DE, Von Hoff DD, McGuire WL. Androgen receptors and antiandrogen therapy for laryngeal carcinoma. *Arch Otolaryngol* 1984; **110:** 721–4.
26. Mazze RI, Wilson AI, Rice SA, Baden IM. Reproduction and fetal development in rats exposed to nitrous oxide. *Teratology* 1984; **30:** 259–65.
27. Mikaelian DO, Contrucci RB, Batsakis JG. Epithelial-myoepithelial carcinoma of the subglottic region: a case presentation and review of the literature. *Otolaryngol Head Neck Surg* 1986; **95:** 104–6.
28. Panagiotopoulos A, Matschke R, Faber P. Schwangerschaft und Larynxkarzinom. *Geburtshilfe Frauenheilkd* 1993; **53:** 64–5.
29. Pytel J, Gerlinger I, Arany A. Twin pregnancy following in vitro fertilisation coinciding with laryngeal cancer. *ORL J Otorhinolaryngol Relat Spec* 1995; **57:** 232–4.
30. Reiner Z, Cvrtila D, Petric V. Cytoplasmic steroid receptors in cancer of the larynx. *Arch Otorhinolaryngol* 1988; **245:** 47–9.
31. Resta L, Fiorella R, Marsigliante S *et al.* Stato recettoriale del carcinoma laringeo: studio dei recettori per estrogeni, progesterone, androgeni e glucocorticoidi. *Acta Otorhinolaryngol Ital* 1994; **14:** 385–92.
32. Robbins KT. Prognostic and therapeutic implications of gender and menopausal status in laryngeal cancer. *J Otolaryngol* 1988; **17:** 81–5.
33. Robbins KT, Vu TP, Diaz A, Varki NM. Growth effects of tamoxifen and estradiol on laryngeal carcinoma cell lines. *Arch Otolaryngol Head Neck Surg* 1994; **120:** 1261–6.
34. Saez S, Sakai F. Androgen receptors in human pharyngo-laryngeal mucosa and pharyngo-laryngeal epithelioma. *J Steroid Biochem* 1976; **7:** 919–21.
35. Scambia G, Benedetti Panici P, Battaglia F *et al.* Receptors for epidermal growth factor and steroid hormones in primary laryngeal tumors. *Cancer* 1991; **67:** 1347–51.
36. Schuller DE, Abou-Issa H, Parrish R. Estrogen and proges-

terone receptors in head and neck cancer. *Arch Otolaryngol* 1984; **110:** 725–7.
37. Stephenson WT, Barnes DE, Holmes FF, Norris CW. Gender influences subsite of origin of laryngeal carcinoma. *Arch Otolaryngol Head Neck Surg* 1991; **117:** 774–8.
38. Tuohimaa PT, Kallio S, Heinijoki J *et al.* Androgen receptors in laryngeal carcinoma. *Acta Otolaryngol (Stockh)* 1981; **91:** 149–54.
39. Vecerina-Volic S, Romic-Stojkovic R, Krajina Z, Gamulin S. Androgen receptors in normal and neoplastic laryngeal tissue. *Arch Otolaryngol Head Neck Surg* 1987; **113:** 411–13.
40. Verstraeten PR, de Boer R. Pregnancy and functional paraganglioma. *Eur J Obstet Gynecol Reprod Biol* 1987; **26:** 157–64.
41. Virolainen E, Vanharanta R, Carey TE. Steroid hormone receptors in human squamous carcinoma cell lines. *Int J Cancer* 1984; **33:** 19–25.
42. Virolainen E, Tuohimaa P, Aitasalo K, Kyttä J, Vanharanta-Hiltunen R. Steroid hormone receptors in laryngeal carcinoma. *Otolaryngol Head Neck Surg* 1986; **94:** 512–16.
43. Werner JA, Hansmann M-L, Lippert BM, Rudert H. Laryngeal paraganglioma and pregnancy. *ORL J Otorhinolaryngol Relat Spec* 1992; **54:** 163–7.

Paraneoplastic syndromes in patients with laryngeal and hypopharyngeal cancers*

Alfio Ferlito and Alessandra Rinaldo

Cancer patients may present different signs and symptoms that are generally determined locally, regionally and remotely by the location and size of the neoplastic lesion. In a minority of patients, the signs and symptoms are due to the presence of an evident or occult cancer, but are not directly related to the primary mass or its metastases, appearing rather to be associated with the tumor on the basis of other, as yet ill-understood mechanisms. These conditions are usually referred to as paraneoplastic syndromes and their location does not coincide with the site of the tumor.

Small cell lung cancer is the most frequent cause of paraneoplastic syndromes and a wide array of conditions are associated with this oncotype, though they may occur in almost all types of malignant neoplasm involving various organs.

The association of paraneoplastic syndromes with tumors of the larynx and hypopharynx has occasionally been reported. They are also called paraneoplastic conditions, paraneoplastic effects, nonmetastatic syndromes, paraneoplastic phenomena, paraneoplastic disturbances, or remote effects, and they may precede the clinical manifestations of a tumor (persistent or recurrent tumor) or of asymptomatic metastases and their appearance may thus be the first sign of a malignancy in a minority of cancer patients. Paraneoplastic syndromes have been identified with increasing frequency because of a greater clinician awareness and the identification of specific autoantibodies for some syndromes – neurologic syndromes in particular.

Paraneoplastic syndromes associated with laryngeal and hypopharyngeal cancer can be divided into four main groups:

- paraneoplastic cutaneous or dermatologic syndromes;
- paraneoplastic endocrine syndromes;
- paraneoplastic hematologic syndromes; and
- paraneoplastic neurologic syndromes.

Different oncotypes, such as squamous cell carcinoma, typical carcinoid, atypical carcinoid, and small cell neuroendocrine carcinoma, have been associated with paraneoplastic syndromes in patients with cancer of the larynx and hypopharynx.

Dermatologic syndromes

Dermatologic syndromes include a very long list of cutaneous lesions. Acanthosis nigricans, Bazex's syndrome, Bowen's disease, bullous pemphigoid, dermatomyositis, pruritus, Sweet's syndrome, yellow nail syndrome, and tylosis have been observed in patients with laryngeal and hypopharyngeal cancer.

Acanthosis nigricans

Acanthosis nigricans is the most frequent paraneoplastic lesion of the skin. It is a cutaneous paraneoplastic syndrome characterized by the presence of symmetric, light or dark brown areas of hyperpigmentation with orthokeratosis, hyperkeratosis, exaggerated skin markings, and warty lesions, particularly involving the intertriginous and flexural areas, especially the axilla, posterior neck, anogenital region, umbilicus and areola. However, widespread involvement of the hands, feet and mucosal membranes has also been seen. The most frequent association is with abdominal cancers, and particularly gastric

*This chapter has been recently published and has been reproduced with the permission of the Editor of the *Annals of Otology, Rhinology and Laryngology*.

carcinomas, but the process has also been described in association with squamous cell carcinoma of the hypopharynx.[48,59]

Bazex's syndrome

Bazex's syndrome (also termed Bazex's acrokeratosis paraneoplastica, acrokeratosis paraneoplastica, acrokeratosis Bazex) was described in 1965,[7] as a paraneoplastic process associated with a carcinoma of the pyriform sinus, but it had already been reported by Gougerot and Rupp in 1922[29] in association with a squamous cell carcinoma of the tongue. The initial reports came mainly from the European literature, and from French authors in particular, but the lesion is now reported with increasing frequency all over the world.[11]

This paraneoplastic dermatosis has been seen mainly in white men over the age of 40 years and only a few cases have been documented in black men and women.[1,5,6,26,31,45,65,68]

Clinically, it is characterized by erythematous squamous cutaneous plaques that spread centripetally – a psoriasiform cutaneous eruption – with a predilection for the extremities (ears, nose, fingers, toes) and, less frequently, the elbows, knees, and trunk, when the neoplastic mass is detected with difficulty or persists untreated, and nail dystrophy. Sometimes, even vesicles, bullae and scabs have been described, particularly on the fingers, hands, and feet. The distribution of the cutaneous manifestations is generally symmetric.

According to Bazex and Griffiths,[6] the skin lesions develop in three stages.[11,41,62] The first stage begins with a psoriasiform eruption confined to the fingers and toes, the bridge of the nose, and the helix of the ear. Nail plate destruction can occur. In the second stage, the eruption becomes more extensive: the palms of the hands and soles of the feet become erythematous and scaly, with a characteristic violaceous color. The erythema and scaling spread to involve the cheeks and the external ear is affected. The third stage is characterized by involvement of the back of the hands, the elbows, knees, arms, thighs, legs, scalp and trunk. The lesions are erythematous to violaceous, with a fine adherent scale.

Histologically, these lesions are nonspecific. The most common histologic features are orthokeratosis with parakeratotic foci, an irregularly acanthotic epidermis with an intact basal cell layer, and a predominantly perivascular lymphocytic infiltrate in the upper dermis. Less commonly reported histologic changes in the epidermis include psoriasiform acanthosis, focal dyskeratosis, vacuolar degeneration of the prickle cells and focal liquefaction of the basal cells with an infiltrate at the dermoepidermal interface.[79]

To date, a total number of 113 cases of Bazex's syndrome have been reported in association with malignancies[8,11,20,35,36,41,50,52,67,76] and nearly half of the tumors were located in the oral cavity, pharynx, and larynx.[67] In the past, this dermatosis was erroneously defined as a process associated with supradiaphragmatic malignancies. It occurs more commonly, however, in patients with a primary squamous cell carcinoma of the head and neck metastasizing to the cervical lymph nodes,[11] especially with a cancer of the oral cavity, pharynx, and larynx, with lung and esophageal cancers, and with squamous cell carcinomas of unknown primary site with cervical nodal involvement. However, this process has been related to malignancies occurring in the bronchus, thymus, prostate, uterus, stomach, liver, bladder, and vulva. This dermatologic condition is associated with various oncotypes (squamous cell carcinoma, adenocarcinoma, anaplastic carcinoma, neuroendocrine carcinomas, transitional cell carcinoma, myeloma, etc.).[41]

Bazex's acrokeratosis is the most frequent paraneoplastic syndrome associated with cancer of the larynx and hypopharynx and it is well documented in the literature.[7,8,10,11,18,27,41,44,50,52,67] Exceptionally, an association of different paraneoplastic cutaneous syndromes (Bazex's syndrome, hyperpigmentation, acquired ichthyosis and pruritus) has been reported in a patient with laryngeal cancer.[8]

The syndrome often appears before the initial symptoms or diagnosis of the cancer. In a review of 93 patients with Bazex's syndrome, 63% revealed this syndrome an average of 11 months (range 1–72) before any clinical manifestation of the tumor.[11]

How this cutaneous syndrome develops in response to an underlying malignancy is unknown. Possible mechanisms include a cross-reactivity between skin antigens and the tumor, or the secretion of growth factors by the tumor.[11]

The differential diagnosis of these skin lesions includes psoriasis, dermatitis, pityriasis rubra pilaris, Reiter's syndrome, tinea, hereditary palmoplantar keratoderma, chronic arsenic ingestion, secondary syphilis, porphyria cutanea tarda, bullous pemphigoid, and acquired epidermolysis bullosa.[41,52]

In 91% (64/70) of the patients reported with this syndrome, the cutaneous lesions improved significantly after treatment of the underlying malignancy. In general, the cutaneous lesions are resistant to a variety of topical treatments.[11] The recognition of this cutaneous paraneoplastic syndrome may lead to the diagnosis and treatment of the underlying cancer.[47,76] This condition responds to the removal of the primary cancer[35] and may respond to etretinate (Tigason®),[78] systemic retinoids[43] and corticosteroids.[45] A trial of octreotide, a long-acting synthetic somatostatin analog, would be reasonable as a palliative measure in inoperable cases.[35]

Bowen's disease

Bowen's disease appears clinically as an asymptomatic, persistent, progressive, non-elevated, often red, scaly, or crusted skin plaque caused by an intraepithelial neoplasm, and it has sometimes been reported to have an internal malignancy. It may occasionally be associated with laryngeal cancer.[14] The designation of Bowen's disease as a paraneoplastic cutaneous syndrome has been questioned, however.[14]

Bullous pemphigoid

Bullous pemphigoid is a fairly common subepidermal blistering disease and has been reported in association with many tumors, including carcinoma of the larynx.[37] The association of bullous pemphigoid with malignancies still remains controversial, nonetheless.

Dermatomyositis

Dermatomyositis is an inflammatory disease affecting the skin and skeletal muscle, causing widespread degenerative and inflammatory changes. The disease is characterized clinically by progressive proximal, symmetrical muscle weakness and skin lesions. Its cause is unknown. Approximately 15–20% of cases are associated with underlying malignancies, most commonly carcinomas of the lung, breast, stomach, ovary and kidney. In elderly patients in particular, it has also been reported in association with laryngeal carcinoma.[12,33]

Pruritus

Pruritus is rare in patients with a laryngeal malignancy. In a letter to the editor, Rantuccio[64] described one patient with 'idiopathic' pruritus who subsequently developed cancer of the larynx. Paraneoplastic pruritus has been reported in patients with hematologic malignancies, particularly Hodgkin's lymphoma, and with solid tumors.[19,40,61,64] Only generalized pruritus (not localized pruritus) may be an uncommon symptom of malignancy.

Sweet's syndrome

Sweet's syndrome (acute febrile neutrophilic dermatosis) was originally described by Robert Douglas Sweet, a British dermatologist, in 1964.[70] It may occur as a cutaneous paraneoplastic syndrome. It has been associated mainly with hematologic disorders such as leukemia (acute myelogenous leukemia in particular) and with solid tumors.[16] The female sex is more often involved, and a recent upper respiratory tract infection and elevated erythrocyte sedimentation rate are reportedly frequent findings. The clinical characteristics included pyrexia, neutrophilia, anemia, painful erythematous cutaneous plaques, and nodules, mainly localized on the upper extremities, face and neck. This condition has been reported in association with solid tumors of the breast and of the genitourinary and gastrointestinal organs. The absence of fever or neutrophilia does not rule out the possibility of Sweet's syndrome in patients with solid tumors.[17] Microscopically, the cutaneous lesions are characterized by a dense neutrophilic infiltrate primarily involving the superficial dermis. Exceptionally, Sweet's syndrome may occur in association with a squamous cell carcinoma of the pyriform sinus.[17] A complete malignancy workup is indicated in patients after the onset of Sweet's syndrome skin lesions, because an unsuspected primary or recurrent cancer may be detected. Approximately 10–20% of patients reported with Sweet's syndrome had an associated neoplasm.[17]

Corticosteroid therapy is the treatment of choice. All the manifestations of Sweet's syndrome improved dramatically with corticosteroid therapy, regardless of the response of the associated neoplasm to tumor-directed therapy.[15,16] Potassium iodide or colchicine have also proved effective therapeutic alternatives.

Yellow nail syndrome

Yellow nail syndrome has been reported in a patient with laryngeal carcinoma, and this disorder regressed after excision of the cancer.[32] The syndrome is characterized by a yellow or greenish discoloration of the nails preceded and accompanied by stunted growth and is associated with lymphedema (usually confined to the ankles but sometimes involving other areas) and occasionally also with bronchiectasis and sinusitis.

Tylosis

Tylosis (palmaris et plantaris) is characterized by hyperkeratosis of the palms and soles; it is often associated with esophageal cancer, and more rarely, with laryngeal cancer.[34] This hereditary disorder is assumed to be paraneoplastic.

Paraneoplastic endocrine syndromes

Paraneoplastic endocrine syndromes are caused by the production of polypeptide hormones and are usually associated with lung cancer, medullary carcinoma of the thyroid, breast cancer, carcinoids, etc. Endocrine syndromes are very rarely associated with malignant laryngeal neoplasms.

Carcinoid syndrome

Carcinoid syndrome (carcinoidosis or argentaffinosis), as its name suggests, is most commonly associated with metastatic carcinoid tumors involving various organs (lung, stomach, colon, ovary, etc.). This syndrome occurs very rarely in patients with small cell lung cancer. The four main clinical components of this syndrome are skin flushing, usually localized in the face and upper trunk, episodic watery diarrhea, manifestations of carcinoid heart disease, and wheezing. Less common changes include dermatitis and episodes of depression. Few patients display all the symptoms.

The majority of typical and atypical carcinoids of the larynx reported in the literature have been nonfunctional[23] and therefore did not lead to clinical syndromes,

Table 63.1 Paraneoplastic syndromes associated with laryngeal neuroendocrine carcinomas

Author(s)	*Year*	*Syndrome*	*No. cases*	*Type of tumor*	*Follow-up*
Trotoux *et al.*[73]	1979	SIADH	1	SCNC	DOD
Medina *et al.*[46]	1984	Eaton–Lambert	1	SCNC	DOD
Bishop *et al.*[9]	1985	ACTH	1	SCNC	DOD
Baugh *et al.*[4]	1987	Carcinoid	1	AC	DOD
Takeuchi *et al.*[71]	1989	SIADH	1	SCNC	DOD
Wenig and Gnepp[77]	1989	Carcinoid	1	TC	NED*
Myers and Kessimian[56]	1995	SIADH	1	SCNC	DOD
Overholt *et al.*[60]	1995	Carcinoid	1	AC	DOD

ACTH, adrenocorticotropic hormone; AC, atypical carcinoid; DOD, dead of disease; NED, no evidence of disease; SCNC, small cell neuroendocrine carcinoma; SIADH, syndrome of inappropriate antidiuretic hormone; TC, typical carcinoid.
*Personal communication, 1997.

such as carcinoid syndrome, adrenocorticotropic hormone (ACTH) syndrome, etc. Three cases of laryngeal carcinoid tumors (one typical and two atypical) associated with a carcinoid syndrome have been reported, however.[4,60,77] One case, of typical carcinoid tumor, was identified from the files of the Department of Otolaryngic Pathology, Armed Forces Institute of Pathology, Washington, DC. Based on the diagnosis of a malignant tumor, a total laryngectomy was performed. The patient remained disease-free for 3 years, then noted a lump in his left neck that proved to be a metastasis from the primary laryngeal neoplasm. A left-sided radical dissection was performed, revealing multiple lymph node involvement. Six months later, the patient presented to his physician complaining of fever, malaise and right-sided upper quadrant abdominal pain. A computed tomography scan of the abdomen revealed multiple liver nodules that were submitted to biopsy and proved morphologically identical to the laryngeal neoplasm. This patient developed carcinoid syndrome following the liver metastases. Urinalysis revealed a 5-hydroxy indolacetic acid (5-HIAA) level increased to 195 mg/24 h (1–5 mg/24 h is normal), which decreased following therapy with streptozotocin and 5-fluorouracil. The patient was much improved after treatment and was alive and well at last follow-up[77] (and personal communication, 1997).

The second case was a supraglottic atypical carcinoid. Twenty-six months after therapy, the patient was admitted with abdominal cramps, distension, alternating diarrhea and constipation, and a generalized warm feeling. Urinary vanillylmandelic acid and 5-HIAA levels were normal. Multiple liver metastases and a retroperitoneal mass were found. The patient died 41 months after surgical treatment.[4]

The third case involved a 57-year-old man with an atypical carcinoid of the aryepiglottic fold. The patient presented with sore throat, flushing, diarrhea and hypertension consistent with a carcinoid syndrome. The patient underwent supraglottic laryngectomy and modified radical neck dissection and remained well for 1 year. However, he developed recurrent local disease with evidence of distant metastases to the small bowel, mesentery and skin. An attempt to control the disease with chemotherapy was unsuccessful, and the patient died after 26 months.[60]

Of the eight patients reported with various paraneoplastic syndromes (carcinoid syndrome, Schwartz–Bartter syndrome, Eaton–Lambert syndrome, ACTH syndrome) in association with neuroendocrine carcinomas of the larynx (typical carcinoid, atypical carcinoid, small cell neuroendocrine carcinoma), seven died (see Table 63.1).[4,9,46,56,60,71,73,77]

ACTH syndrome

Ectopic ACTH syndrome in association with a squamous cell carcinoma of the larynx was reported by Imura *et al.* in 1975.[38] The authors described a Japanese patient, a 66-year-old man, who underwent surgical excision of the larynx for squamous cell carcinoma. One year later, he developed hyperadrenocorticism, and postmortem examination revealed metastases to the liver and other organs. Bioassayable and immunoassayable ACTH, as well as bioassayable melanocyte-stimulating hormone, were detected in the metastatic tumor tissue.[38]

In 1985, Bishop *et al.*[9] reported the first case of laryngeal small cell neuroendocrine carcinoma associated with ectopic ACTH syndrome. The cell cytoplasm was immunoreactive for ACTH, gastrin-releasing polypeptide, neuron-specific enolase, β-endorphin, calcitonin, and keratin, by indirect immunoperoxidase techniques.

Ectopic production of ACTH by tumors does not always result in classical Cushing's syndrome,[38] which was absent in the two mentioned reported cases.[9,38]

Schwartz–Bartter syndrome

Schwartz–Bartter syndrome (syndrome of inappropriate secretion of antidiuretic hormone – SIADH) was first described by Schwartz *et al.* in 1957.[69] It is characterized by excessive blood levels or actions of vasopressin associated with hyponatremia without edema. The inability to excrete a dilute urine implies a subsequent retention of ingested fluids, with expansion of the extracellular fluid volume without edema. Hyponatremia is due both to sodium dilution in a larger extracellular fluid volume, and to its higher urinary excretion caused by its decreased reabsorption in the proximal renal tubular tract because of the increased extracellular fluid volume.

This condition is the most frequently detected paraneoplastic syndrome in patients with small cell lung cancer,[75] but it has been associated with many different types of tumors, including pancreatic carcinoma, duodenal carcinoma, prostatic carcinoma, bladder carcinoma, mesothelioma, lymphoma, Hodgkin's disease, acute myelogenous leukemia, thymoma and adrenocortical carcinoma.

In the head and neck region, in particular, SIADH is a well-recognized form of paraneoplastic syndrome that may accompany malignancies. In a recent review of the literature, Ferlito *et al.*[24] collected 70 cases of this syndrome associated with cancers of the head and neck. The most common site of occurrence was the oral cavity, with 29 cases detected; the larynx was involved in 13 patients, and the hypopharynx in seven. The most frequent histologic tumor type was squamous cell carcinoma[39,51,66,72,80] and three cases were small cell neuroendocrine carcinoma.[56,71,73] The SIADH may precede the presentation of the cancer by several weeks or months.

The first two cases of this syndrome associated with squamous cell carcinoma of the larynx were described in 1976 by Moses *et al.*[51] Other cases associated with squamous cell carcinoma were subsequently reported by various authors.[39,66,72,80]

In 1979, Trotoux *et al.*[73] described the first case of small cell neuroendocrine carcinoma of the subglottic region associated with SIADH. The patient presented with initial headache, confusion and temporospatial disorientation, hyperreflexia, hyponatremia, hypochloremia, serum hypo-osmolarity, reduced hematocrit, negative free water clearance, and high plasma levels of antidiuretic hormone. The diagnosis of the subglottic tumor was only reached 3 months later.

In 1989, Takeuchi *et al.*[71] reported a case of small cell neuroendocrine carcinoma of the larynx in a 53-year-old man. The tumor was associated with SIADH, and hyponatremia persisted until the patient's death, despite the administration of salt. Postmortem examination revealed no central nervous system lesions or lung diseases.

In 1995, Myers and Kessimian[56] described a patient with small cell neuroendocrine carcinoma of the larynx who had clinical complications of SIADH. The diagnosis of this endocrine syndrome was confirmed by the finding of serum hyponatremia and hypo-osmolarity, urine hypo-osmolarity, and an increased urinary sodium concentration. Careful patient evaluation identified only the laryngeal neoplasm as the cause of SIADH and excluded any other potential causes (pulmonary neoplastic or non-neoplastic diseases, central nervous system lesions, drugs).

Hypercalcemia

Hypercalcemia is the most common metabolic complication of malignancy[54] and often presents in the terminal stage of neoplastic disease. It has been associated with many neoplasms, including carcinomas (especially of the head and neck, esophagus, lung, kidney and ovary), sarcomas and hematopoietic malignancies.[55,63] Bone metastasis is an uncommon cause.[2] Many cancers produce hypercalcemia by an ill-understood hormonal mechanism. Nonmetastatic hypercalcemia is not uncommon in patients with laryngeal malignancies.[2] Clinical signs of mild hypercalcemia include dehydration, anorexia, nausea, vomiting, constipation, ileus, fatigue and confusion. Severe hypercalcemia is considered a medical emergency.[49] Hypercalcemia complicating malignant disease is a poor prognostic sign and correlates with advanced disease, but it is important to distinguish this from hypercalcemia due to other causes, i.e. sarcoidosis, primary hyperparathyroidism, or thiazide therapy.

Treatment of malignancy-induced hypercalcemia is primarily directed toward controlling the underlying cancer.[49]

Paraneoplastic hematologic syndromes

Paraneoplastic hematologic syndromes may occur in many neoplasms, but have only occasionally been observed in association with laryngeal cancer.

Trousseau's syndrome

Trousseau's syndrome (thrombophlebitis migrans, migratory thrombophlebitis, disseminated intravascular coagulation or thromboembolism) was first reported, in 1865, by Armand Trousseau,[74] who described a high incidence of venous thrombosis in a series of patients with gastric carcinoma. Historically, Trousseau's syndrome has been associated with pancreatic carcinoma, but it has also been reported in association with stomach, breast, lung, colon and ovarian carcinoma.[22] The prevalence of this syndrome with head and neck cancers is less than 1%, and it has only occasionally been observed in laryngeal carcinoma.[58]

This process is characterized by disseminated intravascular coagulation and is detected by laboratory tests (elevated levels of fibrin, thrombocytosis, hyperfibrinogenemia).

An unexplained thromboembolism may indicate the presence of a malignancy before any signs or symptoms of the tumor itself become apparent.[57]

Paraneoplastic neurologic syndromes

Paraneoplastic neurologic syndromes occur frequently in cancer patients, but have been described only occasionally in association with laryngeal cancers.

Cerebellar degeneration

Cerebellar degeneration, or cerebellar cortex degeneration, is a relatively common paraneoplastic effect of

Table 63.2 Paraneoplastic syndromes occurring in patients with laryngeal and hypopharyngeal cancers

Syndrome	*Author(s)*	*Type of tumor*
Cutaneous syndromes		
Acanthosis nigricans*	Miller and Davis[48]	SCC
	Oppolzer *et al.*[59]	SCC
Bazex's syndrome*	Bazex *et al.*[7]	SCC
	Bolognia *et al.*[11]	SCC
	Laccourreye *et al.*[41]	SCC
	Mounsey and Brown[52]	SCC
	Bazex *et al.*[8]	SCC
	Sarkar *et al.*[67]	SCC
	Miquel *et al.*[50]	SCC
	Legros *et al.*[44]	SCC
	Gaillard *et al.*[27]	SCC
	Blanchet *et al.*[10]	SCC
	Colomb *et al.*[18]	SCC
Bowen's disease	Cohen[14]	SCC
Bullous pemphigoid	Hodge *et al.*[37]	SCC
Dermatomyositis*	Bonnetblanc *et al.*[12]	SCC
Pruritus*	Rantuccio[64]	SCC
Sweet's syndrome*	Cohen *et al.*[17]	SCC
Yellow nail syndrome	Guin and Elleman[32]	SCC
Tylosis	Haines[34]	SCC
Endocrine syndromes		
Carcinoid syndrome*	Baugh *et al.*[4]	AC
	Wenig and Gnepp[77]	TC
	Overholt *et al.*[60]	AC
ACTH syndrome*	Bishop *et al.*[9]	SCNC
	Imura *et al.*[38]	SCC
Schwartz–Bartter syndrome*	Trotoux *et al.*[73]	SCNC
	Takeuchi *et al.*[71]	SCNC
	Myers and Kessimian[56]	SCNC
	Moses *et al.*[51]	SCC
	Zohar *et al.*[80]	SCC
	Talmi *et al.*[72]	SCC
	Roth *et al.*[66]	SCC
	Kandylis *et al.*[39]	SCC
Hypercalcemia*	Angel *et al.*[2]	SCC
Hematologic syndromes		
Trousseau's syndrome*	Nikšic and Balogh[58]	SCC
Neurologic syndromes		
Cerebellar degeneration*	Garcin and Lapresle[28]	SCC
	Müller *et al.*[53]	SCC
Eaton–Lambert myasthenic syndrome*	Medina *et al.*[46]	SCNC
	Fontanel *et al.*[25]	SCC

AC, atypical carcinoid; ACTH, adrenocorticotropic hormone; SCC, squamous cell carcinoma; SCNC, squamous cell neuroendocrine carcinoma; TC, typical carcinoid.
*True paraneoplastic syndrome.

small cell lung cancer, but it also occurs with other types of lung cancer, as well as with tumors arising elsewhere (ovary and breast cancer). It has also been occasionally reported in association with laryngeal cancer.[28,53] It is characterized by subacute symptoms of diffuse cerebellar dysfunction: vertigo, dysarthria, intention tremor, and progressive limb and truncal ataxia. Ocular disturbances, nystagmus, ocular dysmetria, and opsoclonus are also common. This syndrome may be caused by immunologic cross-reactions, and anti-neural antibodies are found in about half the patients. The most specific autoantibody is the anti-Purkinje cell antibody, found in women with gynecologic tumors.[3] Paraneoplastic syndromes usually occur before the malignancy is diagnosed, and the best described are those associated with specific antibodies.[13]

Eaton–Lambert myasthenic syndrome

Eaton–Lambert myasthenic syndrome was reported in abstract form by Lambert *et al.* in 1956[42] and again in more detail by Eaton and Lambert in 1957,[21] though the same condition had been reported by Gray and Halton in 1948.[30] It is usually seen in association with lung cancer, but may also be associated with laryngeal cancer. Fontanel *et al.*[25] described a case of this syndrome in a 58-year-old man that led to the detection of a squamous cell carcinoma of the larynx.

In 1984, Medina *et al.*[46] reported a case of primary small cell neuroendocrine carcinoma of the larynx associated with clinical and electromyographic evidence of the myasthenic syndrome. The upper extremities may become involved. Ocular and bulbar involvement is rare and, when present, less severe than in the case of myasthenia gravis. Deep tendon reflexes are hypoactive or absent, but sensory function is preserved. Unlike myasthenia gravis, muscle strength improves with exercise. Electromyography is essential in the diagnosis of this syndrome, and electromyographic findings differ from those observed in patients with myasthenia gravis. The electrophysiologic diagnosis of Eaton–Lambert syndrome relies on the observation of a progressive increase in the amplitude – by 200% or more – of the compound muscle action potential evoked by repetitive supramaximal nerve stimulation.

Diagnostically useful serum and cerebrospinal fluid autoantibodies have recently been identified in several neurologic paraneoplastic syndromes, including cerebellar degeneration and Eaton-Lambert myasthenic syndrome.

Table 63.2 summarizes the paraneoplastic syndromes reportedly occurring in patients with cancer of the larynx and hypopharynx.[2,4,7–12,14,17,18,25,27,28,32,34,37–39,41,44,46,48,50–53,56,58–60,64,66,67,71–73,77,80]

References

1. Amblard P, Reymond JL, Jerome P, Detante J. Double syndrome paranéoplasique dermatomyosite et acrokératose de Bazex. *Rev Med Alpes Fr* 1979; **8**: 39.
2. Angel MF, Stewart A, Pensak ML, Pillsbury HRC, Sasaki CT. Mechanisms of hypercalcemia in patients with head and neck cancer. *Head Neck Surg* 1982; **5**: 125–9.
3. Baloh RW. Paraneoplastic cerebellar disorders. *Otolaryngol Head Neck Surg* 1995; **112**: 125–7.
4. Baugh RF, Wolf GT, Lloyd RV, McClatchey KD, Evans DA. Carcinoid (neuroendocrine carcinoma) of the larynx. *Ann Otol Rhinol Laryngol* 1987; **96**: 315–21.
5. Baxter DL Jr, Kallgren DL, Leone KC. Acrokeratosis paraneoplastica of Bazex: report of a case in a young black woman. *Cutis* 1992; **49**: 265–8.
6. Bazex A, Griffiths A. Acrokeratosis paraneoplastica – a new cutaneous marker of malignancy. *Br J Dermatol* 1980; **102**: 301–6.
7. Bazex A, Salvador R, Dupré A, Christol B. Syndrome paranéoplasique à type d'hyperkératose des extrémités. Guérison après le traitement de l'épithélioma laryngé. *Bull Soc Fr Dermatol Syphil* 1965; **72**: 182.
8. Bazex J, El Sayed F, Sans B, Marguery MC, Samalens G. Acrokératose paranéoplasique de Bazex associée a une ichtyose acquise, des troubles de la pigmentation et un prurit: révélation tardive d'un néoplasme laryngé. *Ann Dermatol Venereol* 1992; **119**: 483–5.
9. Bishop JW, Osamura RY, Tsutsumi Y. Multiple hormone production in an oat cell carcinoma of the larynx. *Acta Pathol Jpn* 1985; **35**: 915–23.
10. Blanchet F, Leroy D, Deschamps P. Acrokératose paranéoplasique de Bazex. A propos de 8 cas. *J Fr Otorhinolaryngol* 1980; **29**: 165–72.
11. Bolognia JL, Brewer YP, Cooper DL. Bazex syndrome (acrokeratosis paraneoplastica). An analytic review. *Medicine (Baltimore)* 1991; **70**: 269–80.
12. Bonnetblanc JM, Bernard P, Fayol J. Dermatomyositis and malignancy: a multicenter cooperative study. *Dermatologica* 1990; **180**: 212–16.
13. Cher LM, Hochberg FH, Teruya J *et al.* Therapy for paraneoplastic neurologic syndromes in six patients with protein A column immunoadsorption. *Cancer* 1995; **75**: 1678–83.
14. Cohen PR. Bowen's disease. *Am Fam Physician* 1991; **44**: 1325–9.
15. Cohen PR, Kurzrock R. Treatment of Sweet's syndrome [letter]. *Am J Med* 1990; **89**: 396.
16. Cohen PR, Talpaz M, Kurzrock R. Malignancy-associated Sweet's syndrome: review of the world literature. *J Clin Oncol* 1988; **6**: 1887–97.
17. Cohen PR, Holder WR, Tucker SB, Kono S, Kurzrock R. Sweet syndrome in patients with solid tumors. *Cancer* 1993; **72**: 2723–31.
18. Colomb D, Reboul MC, Mauduit G, Forestier JY. Forme diffuse d'acrokératose paranéoplasique de Bazex révélatrice d'une récidive et de métastases d'un cancer de l'épiglotte antérieurement traité. *Ann Dermatol Venereol* 1981; **108**: 885–8.
19. Cormia FE. Pruritus, an uncommon but important symptom of systemic carcinoma. *Arch Dermatol* 1965; **92**: 36–9.
20. Douglas WS, Bilsland DJ, Howatson R. Acrokeratosis paraneoplastica of Bazex. A case in the UK. *Clin Exp Dermatol* 1991; **16**: 297–9.
21. Eaton LM, Lambert EH. Electromyography and electric stimulation of nerves in diseases of motor unit: observation on the myasthenic syndrome associated with malignant tumors. *JAMA* 1957; **183**: 183–99.
22. Evans TRJ, Mansi JL, Bevan DH. Trousseau's syndrome in association with ovarian carcinoma. *Cancer* 1996; **77**: 2544–9.
23. Ferlito A, Friedmann I. Review of neuroendocrine carcinomas of the larynx. *Ann Otol Rhinol Laryngol* 1989; **98**: 780–90.
24. Ferlito A, Rinaldo A, Devaney KO. Syndrome of inappropriate antidiuretic hormone secretion associated with head and neck cancers: review of the literature. *Ann Otol Rhinol Laryngol* 1997; **106**: 878–83.
25. Fontanel J-P, Betheuil MJ, Sénéchal G, Haguenau M. Un cas de syndrome de Lambert-Eaton secondaire à un épithélioma laryngé. *Ann Otolaryngol Chir Cervicofac* 1973; **90**: 314–17.

26. Gago S, Jimenez M, Montes B, Molina L. Síndrome de Bazex o dermatosis psoriasiforme acromélica. *Actas Dermosifiliogr* 1975; **66:** 321–4.
27. Gaillard J, Haguenauer JP, Dubreuil C, Romanet P. Acrokératose de Bazex, syndrome paranéoplasique révélateur d'une métastase d'un cancer de la vallécule guéri localement à trois ans. *J Fr Otorhinolaryngol* 1978; **27:** 353–7.
28. Garcin R, Lapresle J. Sur un cas d'atrophie cérébelleuse corticale subaigue en relation avec un épithélioma du larynx. *Arch Pathol* 1956; **62:** 399–402.
29. Gougerot, Rupp. Dermatose érythémato-squameuse avec hyperkératose palmo-plantaire, porectasies digitales et cancer de la langue latent. Contribution à l'étude des dermatoses monitrices de cancer. *Paris Med* 1922; **43:** 234–7.
30. Gray TC, Halton J. Idiosyncracy to d-tubocurarine chloride. *Br Med J* 1948; **1:** 784–6.
31. Grimwood RE, Lekan C. Acrokeratosis paraneoplastica with esophageal squamous cell carcinoma. *J Am Acad Dermatol* 1987; **17:** 685–6.
32. Guin JD, Elleman JH. Yellow nail syndrome. Possible association with malignancy. *Arch Dermatol* 1979; **115:** 734–5.
33. Hagedorn M, Hauf GF, Thomas C. *Paraneoplasien, Tumorsyntropien und Tumorsyndrome der Haut.* Wien: Springer, 1978.
34. Haines D. Primary carcinoma duplex associated with tylosis. *J R Nav Med Serv* 1967; **53:** 75–8.
35. Halpern SM, O'Donnell LJD, Makunura CN. Acrokeratosis paraneoplastica of Bazex in association with a metastatic neuroendocrine tumour. *J R Soc Med* 1995; **88:** 353P–4P.
36. Handfield-Jones SE, Matthews CNA, Ellis JP, Das KB, McGibbon DH. Acrokeratosis paraneoplastica of Bazex. *J R Soc Med* 1992; **85:** 548–50.
37. Hodge L, Marsden RA, Black MM, Bhogal B, Corbett MF. Bullous pemphigoid: the frequency of mucosal involvement and concurrent malignancy related to indirect immunofluorescence findings. *Br J Dermatol* 1981; **105:** 65–9.
38. Imura H, Matsukura S, Yamamoto H *et al.* Studies on ectopic ACTH-producing tumors. II. Clinical and biochemical features of 30 cases. *Cancer* 1975; **35:** 1430–7.
39. Kandylis KV, Vasilomanolakis M, Efremides AD. Syndrome of inappropriate antidiuretic hormone secretion in pyriform sinus squamous cell carcinoma. *Am J Med* 1986; **81:** 946. [Letter to the Editor]
40. Kantor GR, Lookingbill DP. Generalized pruritus and systemic disease. *J Am Acad Dermatol* 1983; **9:** 375–82.
41. Laccourreye O, Laccourreye L, Jouffre V, Brasnu D. Bazex's acrokeratosis paraneoplastica. *Ann Otol Rhinol Laryngol* 1996; **105:** 487–9.
42. Lambert E, Eaton L, Rooke E. Defect of neuromuscular conduction associated with malignant neoplasm. *Am J Physiol* 1956; **187:** 612. [Abstract]
43. Le T, Pierard GE. Etude clinique et histologique de l'effet d'un rétinoïde aromatique Ro 10-9359 sur un syndrome apparenté à l'acrokératose paranéoplasique de Bazex. *Dermatologica* 1982; **165:** 559–67.
44. Legros M, Kalis B, Brunetaud P, Longuebray A. Cancer pharyngo-laryngé et acrokératose de Bazex. *Ann Otolaryngol Chir Cervicofac* 1977; **94:** 47–52.
45. Martin RW, Cornitius TG, Naylor MF, Neldner KH. Bazex's syndrome in a woman with pulmonary adenocarcinoma. *Arch Dermatol* 1989; **125:** 847–8.
46. Medina JE, Moran M, Goepfert H. Oat cell carcinoma of the larynx and Eaton–Lambert syndrome. *Arch Otolaryngol* 1984; **110:** 123–6.
47. Milewski Ch, Wieland W. Paraneoplastische Akrokeratose: M. Bazex Eine tumorspezifische Dermatose bei Plattenepithelkarzinomen im Kopf-Halsbereich. *HNO* 1988; **36:** 158–60.
48. Miller TR, Davis J. Acanthosis nigricans occurring in association with squamous carcinoma of the hypopharynx. *NY State J Med* 1954; **54:** 2333–6.
49. Minotti AM, Kountakis SE, Stiernberg CM. Paraneoplastic syndromes in patients with head and neck cancer. *Am J Otolaryngol* 1994; **15:** 336–43.
50. Miquel FJ, Zapater E, Vilata JJ, Gil MP, Garin L. Paraneoplastic acral hyperkeratosis: Initial sign of laryngeal neoplasia. *Otolaryngol Head Neck Surg* 1997; **117** (Suppl): S239–42.
51. Moses AM, Miller M, Streeten DHP. Pathophysiologic and pharmacologic alterations in the release and action of ADH. *Metabolism* 1976; **25:** 697–721.
52. Mounsey R, Brown DH. Bazex syndrome. *Otolaryngol Head Neck Surg* 1992; **107:** 475–7.
53. Müller E, Spanke O, Lehmann I. Neurogene Störungen bei extrazerebralen Malignomen. *Med Klin* 1969; **64:** 1470–5.
54. Mundy GR. Ectopic production of calciotropic peptides. *Endocrinol Metab Clin North Am* 1991; **20:** 473–87.
55. Mundy GR, Ibbotson KJ, D'Souza SM, Simpson EL, Jacobs JW, Martin TJ. The hypercalcemia of cancer: clinical implications and pathogenic mechanisms. *N Engl J Med* 1984; **310:** 1718–27.
56. Myers TJ, Kessimian N. Small cell carcinoma of the larynx and ectopic antidiuretic hormone secretion. *Otolaryngol Head Neck Surg* 1995; **113:** 301–4.
57. Naschitz JE, Yeshurun D, Eldar S, Lev LM. Diagnosis of cancer-associated vascular disorders. *Cancer* 1996; **77:** 1759–67.
58. Nikšic M, Balogh M. Über Gerinnungsstörungen bei Kehlkopf- und Rachen-Malignomen. *Laryngorhinootologie* 1976; **55:** 414–19.
59. Oppolzer G, Schwarz T, Zechner G, Gschnait F. Acanthosis nigricans in squamous cell carcinoma of the larynx. *Z Hautkr* 1986; **61:** 1229–37.
60. Overholt SM, Donovan DT, Schwartz MR, Laucirica R, Green LK, Alford BR. Neuroendocrine neoplasms of the larynx. *Laryngoscope* 1995; **105:** 789–94.
61. Paul R, Paul R, Jansen CT. Itch and malignancy prognosis in generalized pruritus: a 6-year follow-up of 125 patients. *J Am Acad Dermatol* 1987; **16:** 1179–82.
62. Pecora AL, Landsman L, Imgrund SP, Lambert WC. Acrokeratosis paraneoplastica (Bazex's syndrome). Report of a case and review of the literature. *Arch Dermatol* 1983; **119:** 820–6.
63. Plimpton CH, Gellhorn A. Hypercalcemia in malignant

disease without evidence of bone destruction. *Am J Med* 1956; **21:** 750–9.
64. Rantuccio F. Incidence of malignancy in patients with generalized pruritus. *J Am Acad Dermatol* 1989; **21:** 1317. [Letter]
65. Richard M, Giroux J-M. Acrokeratosis paraneoplastica (Bazex's syndrome). *J Am Acad Dermatol* 1987; **16:** 178–83.
66. Roth Y, Lightman SL, Kronenberg J. Hyponatremia associated with laryngeal squamous cell carcinoma. *Eur Arch Otorhinolaryngol* 1994; **251:** 183–5.
67. Sarkar B, Knecht R, Sarkar C, Weidauer H. Bazex syndrome (acrokeratosis paraneoplastica). *Eur Arch Otorhinolaryngol* 1998; **255:** 205–10.
68. Scarpa C, Nini G, Pasqua MC, Franchi A, Frati C. Singolare osservazione di eritroacrocheratosi paraneoplastica. *G Ital Dermatol* 1971; **112:** 17–25.
69. Schwartz WB, Warren B, Curelop S, Bartter FC. A syndrome of renal sodium loss and hyponatremia probably resulting from inappropriate secretion of antidiuretic hormone. *Am J Med* 1957; **23:** 529–42.
70. Sweet RD. An acute febrile neutrophilic dermatosis. *Br J Dermatol* 1964; **76:** 349–56.
71. Takeuchi K, Nishii S, Jin CS, Ukai K, Sakakura Y. Anaplastic small cell carcinoma of the larynx. *Auris Nasus Larynx* 1989; **16:** 127–32.
72. Talmi YP, Hoffman HT, McCabe BF. Syndrome of inappropriate secretion of arginine vasopressin in patients with cancer of the head and neck. *Ann Otol Rhinol Laryngol* 1992; **101:** 946–9.
73. Trotoux J, Glickmanas M, Sterkers O, Trousset M, Pinel J. Syndrome de Schwartz–Bartter: révélateur d'un cancer laryngé sousglottique à petites cellules. *Ann Otolaryngol Chir Cervicofac* 1979; **96:** 349–58.
74. Trousseau A. Phlegmasia alba dolens. *Clinique Medicale de l'Hôtel-Dieu de Paris*, Vol. 3. London: New Sydenham Society, 1865; **3:** 695–727.
75. van Oosterhout AGM, van de Pol M, ten Velde GPM, Twijnstra A. Neurologic disorders in 203 consecutive patients with small cell lung cancer. Results of a longitudinal study. *Cancer* 1996; **77:** 1434–41.
76. Wareing MJ, Vaughan-Jones SA, McGibbon DH. Acrokeratosis paraneoplastica: Bazex syndrome. *J Laryngol Otol* 1996; **110:** 899–900.
77. Wenig BM, Gnepp DR. The spectrum of neuroendocrine carcinomas of the larynx. *Semin Diagn Pathol* 1989; **6:** 329–50.
78. Wishart JM. Bazex paraneoplastic acrokeratosis: a case report and response to Tigason. *Br J Dermatol* 1986; **115:** 595–9.
79. Witkowski JA, Parish LC. Bazex's syndrome. Paraneoplastic acrokeratosis. *JAMA* 1982; **248:** 2883–4.
80. Zohar Y, Talmi YP, Finkelstein Y, Nobel M, Gafter U. The syndrome of inappropriate antidiuretic hormone secretion in cancer of the head and neck. *Ann Otol Rhinol Laryngol* 1991; **100:** 341–4.

Human laryngeal transplantation – reality grounded in research

Marshall Strome

In 1954, the first successful solid organ transplant was performed at the Peter Bent Brigham Hospital in Boston. In the four ensuing decades, organ transplantation has extended life for patients with varied non-neoplastic diseases affecting vital visceral organs. Despite general acceptance, transplantation following ablative surgery for malignancy remains limited because of an increased risk of recurrence and/or metastases, secondary to protracted systemic immunosuppression. Further, the known increased incidence of new primary tumors as well as other significant acknowledged adverse effects of requisite immunomodulatory measures has until now limited transplantation to organs considered vital.

The larynx has been classically considered to be nonvital because survival following resection is acknowledged. However, beyond survival, functional losses and social stigmata following laryngectomy make the designation of nonvital circumspect. A reduction of risk should make laryngeal transplantation a treatment option for patients requiring laryngectomy. Further, aphonic patients following multiple reconstructive efforts for laryngeal trauma are transplantation candidates today in light of current research data generated under my aegis.

A recent commentary in *The Lancet* stated that on January 4, 1998 Marshall Strome of the Cleveland Clinic performed the first real human laryngeal transplantation.[1] It further inferred that no matter what the eventual outcome, it was a historic event that altered forever concepts concerning transplantation. Clearly, replacing kind with kind was achieved. In a 12-hour procedure a total larynx, 70% of the pharynx, five tracheal rings, the total thyroid and parathyroids were transplanted. The donor was an otherwise healthy, middle-aged male. The recipient was a healthy 40-year-old male whose laryngotracheal complex, crushed in a motorcycle accident, was clearly not reconstructable with even the most advanced surgical techniques. Following multiple procedures at another institution, he had used an electrolarynx for 19 years. He sought a laryngeal transplant and after exhaustive hematologic testing, radiographic imaging, and a thorough psychiatric evaluation, he was deemed a suitable candidate. We rode on the shoulders of giants – Billroth, Boles,[2] Ogura,[5] Silver[6] – fulfilling their dreams and our own, hopefully providing one man with long-term voicing and in general betterment for society. Further, this accomplishment was more significant in that it was one of an infinitesimally small number of transplanted organs that was successfully transferred the first time. The details and management are beyond the scope of this rendering; however, it is clear that our procedure differed significantly from the procedure performed by Kluyskens in 1970.[3] His transplant was subtotal, preserving recipient perichondrium to revascularize the donor organ. Ours was total, composite and had bilateral microvascular arterial and venous anastomoses. Further, sensory and motor neuronal units were reestablished.

Did this patient have the right of choice even if fully informed? Did we have the right to transplant a nonvital organ into an otherwise healthy male? Can we, should we, take otherwise healthy individuals and make them medically dependent for life? Is it justified to subject otherwise healthy individuals to hypertension, convulsions, renal failure, hyperlipidemia, malignancy and lymphoma? I submit the decision rests not with the ethicists and naysayers, but with the informed individual patient. We do not walk in their shoes. We don't have diminished smell, an altered body habitus, a voice imprint clearly and identifiably beyond the norm, nor do we blow air through a neck opening during intimacy. Our oath and obligation is to help heal and support, if not cure.

Approximately a decade ago a program project was initiated to evaluate the potential for transplanting a human larynx. Ethical considerations were among the first issues addressed.[9] The inherent dilemma to be confronted by otolaryngologists and society is acceptable risk versus potential benefit. A prerequisite for ethical analysis is an understanding of purpose. Laryngeal transplantation should be able to attain serviceable speech, swallowing and cosmesis with limited aspiration. For this, the recipient accepts certain risks, cancer recurrence or arising *de novo*, graft rejection, and the morbidity of chronic immunosuppression. Objectively reviewing the incidence of transplantation-associated malignancy, it is clearly related to the dose and type of immunosuppressant. In fact, most notably Pittsburgh's liver transplant program has performed transplants in patients with primary hepatic malignancy with a low incidence of recurrence.

A second issue is patient acceptance of total laryngectomy. I have had patients choose death to the procedure in the face of malignancy. In an effort to quantify patient attitudes towards laryngectomy, McNeil interviewed 37 healthy firefighters and executives.[4] Queried as to whether they would choose radiation or laryngectomy for advanced laryngeal cancer given a 20% increase in survival for laryngectomy, 20% chose radiation therapy rather than lose normal voicing. It appears that there is a population willing to assume risk for an individually perceived quantum leap in quality of life.

Our research effort has been to consider varied immunomodulators used sequentially and synchronously in low doses to control rejection, decrease morbidity, limit mortality and thereby potentially improve life's quality for those choosing organ transplantation. The sentinel contribution of my laboratory was to develop a rat model of a vascularized laryngeal allograft.[7] The salient features of this model include a vascular pedicle based on a carotid artery to superior thyroid artery inflow and superior thyroid artery to external jugular vein arteriovenous shunt for outflow. There is no recipient airway intrusion, the allograft being placed in tandem with the recipient larynx. Laryngeal innervation using this model was not our intent, but such was successfully accomplished by the Vanderbilt group using the recurrent laryngeal nerves in our model.

If developing the rat model represented my sentinel contribution, defining a reproducible rejection pattern was a close second.[11] By so doing, all therapeutic modalities tested had a histologic reference base against which their efficacy could be judged. In brief, laryngeal allografts reject in a definable sequence. Using a gradation of 0–5, these changes can be standardized. Zero represents normal anatomy. Stage 1 has some limited edema in the lamina propria and limited polymorphonuclear cell infiltration. Stage 2 includes some lymphocyte presence and identifiable change in minor salivary glands, e.g. dilated acini, distortion of the lobular architecture and loss of specialized granular cytoplasm. In this grouping, the respiratory lining is intact, yet may have some leukocyte infiltration. In stage 3 there was significant atrophy of the minor salivary gland acini, focal squamous metaplasia of the formerly respiratory epithelium, and an increased presence of inflammatory cells in the lamina propria. With stage 4, irregularly thickened allograft mucosa has the surface completely replaced by squamous metaplasia. There is reactive intimal proliferation and focal thrombi of medium- to large-size blood vessels as well as a paucity of minor salivary glands. In stage 5 there was little recognizable mucosa or cartilage, the latter being destroyed and replaced by sensitized lymphocytes. Recanalizing thrombi, reactive endothelial cell proliferation and thickening and duplication of the layers of the vascular wall are all in evidence. Of course, the above represent a continuum. However, stages 1 and 2 are early in the rejection milieu corresponding loosely to days 1–5. Stage 3 occurs at days 5–7, stage 4 at days 7–10, and stage 5 at days 10–14. These histologic parameters were the standard used in assessing monitoring biopsies in our human transplant recipient. With no yet standardized hematologic or functional determinants for human larynx transplantation, interval biopsies will continue to be requisite for monitoring ongoing processes and accordingly immunosuppressive regimens.

Cyclosporin A (CSA) made solid organ transplantation feasible, modulating both the cellular and humoral responses by down-regulating the IL-2 receptor and as such a reduction in IL-2 production. Further, it spares CD8 T-cells. Our published data has established that when used alone, daily doses of CSA as low as 7.5 mg/kg can eliminate histologic evidence of rejection.[10] The latter information was also used in determining the dose of cyclosporin in our patient.

Glucocorticoids, such as methylprednisolone, at increased dose levels suppress inflammatory and immunologic responsivity. In excess, they inhibit T-cell function and synthesis of interleukins, lymphokines and prostaglandins, among other responses. Importantly, this class of steroids does not permanently affect the immune system. Using our animal model, we showed that methylprednisolone can lower the cyclosporin dose required to prevent rejection of the transplanted larynx. This information, again, was directly transferable to the human experience.

It was essential to establish the ischemic time interval within which viability would be assured upon transfer. In this animal study, heparinized saline was compared to the Wisconsin solution.[8] Each cold solution was used to completely flush the isolated organ immediately upon harvest. The animals flushed with iced heparinized saline tolerated only a 3-hour ischemic interval, whereas, the University of Wisconsin's solution extended the viable ischemic time to 20 hours. It is postulated that the addition of impermeants in the University of Wisconsin's solution effectively prevents cell swelling and interstitial edema, extending viability. Currently, our first flush is lactated Ringer's until the return is clear. Then, the Wisconsin solution is administered. The latter sequence was used in the human donor at harvest with a total ischemic time of 10 hours.

Initially described for liver rescue following impending rejection with standard modalities, FK-506 (tacrolimus) seemed promising should a similar circumstance arise with human laryngeal transplantation. Mechanistically inhibiting cytotoxic T-cell generation and IL-2 production, its efficacy was obtainable at doses significantly lower than those of CSA. Not a classic nephrotoxin, it does affect renal function. Moderate hyperkalemia associated with FK-506 administration can cause decreased glomerulofiltration. Hypertension, troublesome with CSA, is less so with FK-506. Interestingly, although 1 mg/kg/day and 3 mg/kg/day given for 14 days extended survival of both cardiac and skin allografts in one study, these doses did little in our study and those of others. However, at 1.2 mg/kg/day, efficacy was established in our laboratory. Should the situation arise, it is apparent that FK-506 could be used as a rescue agent in the human experience.

Rapamycin (sirolimus) also has potential as a rescue agent. It reportedly has an even greater immunosuppression potential than FK-506. In addition, it has acknowledged activity against CDF-1 mammary tumor, colon-38 tumor, and ependymoblastoma, e.g. an immunosuppressant with antitumor activity. Unfortunately, as tested by my group for animal laryngeal transplantation, rapamycin was not effective. Based on our earlier study, the IM route of administration was chosen. A few other studies have reported success with this route and dose sequence; however, most studies reporting success with rapamycin used an intraperitoneal delivery. When time permits, intraperitoneal delivery will be evaluated and if successful, a second trial would be initiated. Rapamycin, relative to the growth of a squamous cell carcinoma line should be investigated. The implications of the latter are obvious.

Pushing the envelope to ultimately enable transplantation in the presence of malignancy in my opinion will require the sequencing of immunomodulators. For example, CTLA-4Ig has a greater affinity for B7 than its natural ligand, thereby limiting T-cell activity. As yet unpublished data in our laboratory suggest efficacy if administered only on days 2–9. Used in concert and sequence with other immunomodulators, independent dose requirements can be decreased. Currently under active investigation are donor irradiation *in vitro*, donor specific transfusion, and a number of specific monoclonal antibodies.

A decade ago, it was my belief that human laryngeal transplantation was achievable. Having now accomplished that, the technique can be improved, extending the procedure to many. It is my current belief that in the next decade precision molecular scalpels will become available, targeting selective areas of our complex immune system, making transplantation from a specific donor feasible whilst leaving all other immunologic functions intact. Ongoing unpublished research in our laboratory has shown that the use of short-duration immunomodulators in concert with traditional immunosuppressants can significantly reduce the requisite dose of the latter. The goal of transplanting larynges for malignancy is within our grasp.

References

1. Birchall MA. Human laryngeal allograft: shift of emphasis in transplantation. *Lancet* 1998; **351**: 539–40.
2. Boles R. Surgical reimplantation of the larynx in dogs: a progress report. *Laryngoscope* 1966; **76**: 1057–64.
3. Kluyskens P, Ringoir S. Follow-up of a human larynx transplantation. *Laryngoscope* 1970; **80**: 1244–50.
4. McNeil B, Weichselbaum R, Pauker S. Speech and survival. *N Engl J Med* 1981; **305**: 982–7.
5. Ogura JH, Kawasaki M, Takenouchi S, Yagi M. Replantation and transplantation of the canine larynx. *Laryngoscope* 1966; **75**: 295–311.
6. Silver GE, Liebert PS, Som ML. Autologous transplantation of the canine larynx. *Arch Otolaryngol* 1967; **86**: 95–102.
7. Strome M, Wu J, Strome S, Brodsky G. A comparison of preservation techniques in a vascularized rat laryngeal transplant model. *Laryngoscope* 1994; **104**: 666–8.
8. Strome M, Strome S, Darrell J, Wu J, Brodsky G. The effects of cyclosporin A on transplanted rat allografts. *Laryngoscope* 1993; **103**: 394–8.
9. Strome S, Strome M. Laryngeal transplantation: ethical considerations. *Am J Otolaryngol* 1992; **13**: 75–7.
10. Strome S, Brodsky G, Darrell J, Wu J, Strome M. Histopathologic correlates of acute laryngeal allograft rejection in a rat model. *Ann Otol Rhinol Laryngol* 1992; **101**: 156–60.
11. Strome S, Sloman-Moll E, Samonte B, Wu J, Strome M. A rate model for a vascularized laryngeal allograft. *Ann Otol Rhinol Laryngol* 1992; **101**: 950–3.

Psychologic aspects of laryngeal cancer and its treatment

Lawrence W DeSanto

The emotional impact of the diagnosis and treatment of any cancer is a life crisis. Because of the functions of the larynx a patient who has laryngeal cancer will obviously experience intense stress and anxiety.[2] He or she must confront the possibility of death, the fear of mutilation, and the functional changes to breathing, eating and talking. A patient also must endure the impact of the disease and its treatment on life's activities and relationships. Head and neck professionals are concerned about the functional aspects of laryngeal cancer and its treatment. Our efforts are focused on survival while preserving function. We, or at least the author, have not deliberated much about the impact of treatment on the patient's life. In other professions such as speech pathology and psychology, more attention has been given to these aspects of a patient's treatment. Perhaps the concerns of the professionals and those of the patients are not always the same.

Case report

A 44-year-old married communications executive with two teenage daughters was seen after referral. His past history included alcohol-related problems. He became hoarse in October 1996. After a few weeks of antibiotics therapy he was examined by a laryngologist, had a biopsy, and was advised that he had an early cancer of the vocal cord. He was shown photographs of the cancer taken at the time of biopsy. He was told that it was at the front of the right vocal cord and that the vocal cord moved normally. The laryngologist discussed treatment options, including radiation and an open operation. The patient was told that his voice would be altered permanently with the operation but that there was a 10% better chance of success with the operation than with radiation. He then visited a radiation specialist, who reviewed the records and examined the patient with a fiberoptic instrument. The radiation option was discussed. The radiation specialist disagreed with the recommendations of the laryngologist, stating that the success with radiation was equal to that of the operation. The radiation doctor said the voice would be better after radiation, and the chance of getting well was cited at about 90%. The patient was confused and he consulted his family physician who said that he did not know much about laryngeal cancer, suggesting that the patient see an oncologist. The patient continued to work and fit his medical appointments into his schedule. Each appointment required half a day. From the date of the biopsy to the oncology appointment 3 weeks had passed. The oncologist reviewed the record but did not examine the patient. The oncologist then told the patient that some promising research suggested that chemotherapy given before radiation shrunk the tumor and improved the radiation results. The oncologist emphasized that this research was being done in regional cancer centers but that the same program could be used at home. Despite the patient's confusion regarding the three different opinions, he thought the concept of shrinking the tumor and then 'killing' it with the radiation made sense.

The patient agreed to the experimental program and received three weekly courses of chemotherapy. There was a 1 week delay while he waited to have a magnetic resonance imaging (MRI) scan which was ordered by the oncologist. Each chemotherapy session required that he stay home from work. He was hospitalized for 4 days to treat dehydration and nausea. After a month's wait the radiation treatments began. Before the treatments were started the radiation specialist examined the larynx with a fiberoptic instrument and noted that the vocal cord moved and the tumor 'seemed smaller'. The radiation treatments took 6 weeks; during this time the patient worked most days, but on some days he came home early because of fatigue.

The patient's voice improved, and by early February 1997 it was nearly normal. In mid-April his voice changed again. He returned to the laryngologist who had done the initial biopsy. This physician had reports from the radiation specialist and the oncologist.

The laryngologist examined his larynx and said there was something 'up in the front' and recommended antibiotic and steroid therapy. The medications were taken for 10 days but the patient's voice remained the same. He returned to the laryngologist who recommended another biopsy. A biopsy, performed on a Friday, was done as an outpatient with the patient under anesthesia. The pathology report, which was delayed until Tuesday, revealed squamous cell carcinoma. Another MRI scan was ordered and it was obtained a week later. It was compared with the first scan and no obvious change was noted. The laryngologist recommended that the patient have his larynx removed. The patient said he would rather die than lose his larynx. A second opinion was recommended, and I was asked to see the patient. I met with him the next Monday. Ten days had passed since the biopsy. I saw a mobile vocal cord and evidence of a recent biopsy on the right side at or very near the anterior commissure. The patient told me that a laryngectomy was not an option. With a mobile vocal cord and no documentation that it was ever fixed, I agreed to attempt a partial operation. I was reluctant for two reasons. First I had never examined the patient before; however, I did have complete records and knew the laryngologist. Second, although the patient's voice was severely altered, my findings did not explain the voice change. I rationalized that the voice was altered because of the previous treatment and the recent biopsy; an operation was thus scheduled. Permission to proceed to a total laryngectomy was denied. During the operation the larynx was opened to the right of the midline vertically. The now obvious cancer was limited to the left side but went up to the anterior commissure – about 10 mm of tumor extending subglottically nearly to the cricothyroid membrane. A vertical hemilaryngectomy, including a portion of the anterior cricoid, was done. Multiple frozen sections at the margins were all free of tumor. There was no evidence of thyroid cartilage invasion. There was a very obvious Delphian lymph node; biopsy of the node was positive for squamous cancer. Because of the Delphian node, an unplanned left neck dissection, a left hemithyroidectomy and a left paratracheal node dissection also were performed. A tracheotomy was sited. Convalescence was complicated by extensive subcutaneous emphysema, but the patient left the hospital in 6 days. The final pathology report noted two positive cervical lymph nodes and two positive paratracheal lymph nodes. The tracheotomy was removed in 14 days. The patient returned to work in 3 weeks.

Throughout this sequence the patient was stoic, but his wife was visibly disturbed and required almost daily reassurance. She continued to work as a schoolteacher but used many days of her family leave to provide transportation for the patient. Regular follow-up visits were uneventful until June 1997, when some stridor and exertional dyspnea were noted. Fiberoptic examinations showed a narrowed airway, consistent with the operation, but no obvious growths. A tracheotomy was suggested but refused. Steroid and antibiotic therapy was given and the situation improved. After use of the medications was stopped, the stridor returned, there was an emergency room visit, replacement of the tracheotomy, and a direct laryngoscopy. No tumor was found and biopsy results were negative for cancer. In early July the patient had sudden onset of swelling in the right side of the neck. The neck skin was erythematous and the patient was febrile. A large drain was placed and antibiotic therapy was started. The right-sided swelling subsided gradually and a subtle fullness remained in the lower left side of the neck. I examined the patient with mirrors and fiberoptic scopes multiple times but found nothing suggesting tumor. A few weeks later, after the inflammatory response was gone, needle biopsies of the lower left side of the neck were done and were positive for cancer. More chemotherapy was given but it was unsuccessful and a laryngectomy and a second left neck dissection were planned. There is doubt that the neck mass is surgically resectable. A few days ago I saw the patient in the lobby of the clinic. I did not recognize him. He was thin, grey, old and ill-appearing. His wife was distraught and angry.

The physician's perspective is different from the patient's

Our patients interact with us in our environment. We work in clinics and hospitals and are comfortable in those venues. Earlier in my career I thought that a patient's encounter with cancer was merely an unpleasant interlude in an otherwise meaningful life. The patients come to us, we fix their problems, and they go back to what they did before. Only after asking many patients about what disease and its treatment did to their and their spouses' lives did I realize that what we do to and for patients can have negative effects on their lives forever. They may not die, but their lives are never the same.

Our patient found that his disease and its treatment gradually consumed his entire physical and emotional life. He was disappointed at every turn of his illness. He was told things that later were found to be untrue. He lost time from work and finally had to leave work. His home life evolved into turmoil as the illness and treatment consumed every minute and all the emotional energy of the family. His wife was bewildered, and his children were frightened. He was taking pain medication that dulled his senses. He was never at peace with his future because its prospect kept changing. He lost weight, he aged visibly, and sexual interaction with his spouse stopped. He lived with his disease for 24 hours every day.

Much of the time his physicians were unaware of what was happening to the patient outside the clinic. We were involved with his disease for minutes a week. We worried about him occasionally; he worried constantly. Obviously, what we see is different from what the patient lives.

In the case described the time to definitive operation was more than a delay. There were delays with appointments, long days waiting for reports, and a continuous sequence of heartbreaking disappointments. There was a big difference between what was anticipated from the physician's statements and what actually happened.

'Anxiety', 'depression' and 'altered quality of life' are the words we use to describe a patient's situation. The human experience is not well depicted by these words.

The spouse's perspective

The partner or spouse of a patient with cancer has another view of events. In our patient's case, the spouse saw her partner change over a period of months from the fiercely independent leader of the family to a dependent, old-appearing man. Her life was disrupted, her career was threatened, and her security system was diminished. She was angry at a system that seemed to do nothing but bad things to her husband without helping him. She was distressed by the continuous series of unmet expectations and what to her seemed like deception.

Background

There is a comprehensive literature on the impact of illness and its treatment on patients' adaptability (coping), socialization, depression, and even sexuality.[2,6–9,13,14]

A common theme is that communications with family and friends deteriorate, particularly after a total laryngectomy. In the older literature, there is a sense that patients with cancer of the larynx, even after laryngectomy, continue to have a quality of life that is better than that of patients with other head and neck cancers. The basis for 'better' is unclear because normative data for comparison are scarce. Most of the impressions about life after treatment of larynx cancer were advanced when treatment programs were rather straightforward. The poorest quality of life is said to occur after treatment for laryngopharyngeal cancer. The inference is that hospitalization is generally longer, combination therapy is used more often, and there are functional changes in swallowing and speech.

Krouse *et al.*[8] noted that about 88% of patients with larynx cancer returned to work, although not all of the patients studied had a total laryngectomy. Harwood and Raawlinson[6] noted that, of patients treated surgically after radiation failure, only 44% returned to work whereas most of those who were treated with radiation, if they did not die, returned to work. In a group of patients treated with partial and total laryngectomy Schuller *et al.*[15] found that 43% either left the workforce or changed their jobs. Despite the forced vocational changes, 88% of the patients were satisfied with their postoperative vocal function. Gates[5] reported that his patients experienced a loss of self-esteem and confidence as well as job loss. Natvig[12] observed that loss of voice is a problem in less than half (40%) of patients, but loss of smell and taste were serious concerns. Natvig also noted the obvious: well-adjusted people do better than those who are more vulnerable. Personality traits and precancer life adjustment predicted mastery of problems and adaptation better than any other situational or social factor, such as income or marital status.[11]

The patient's experiences during treatment are important variables for subsequent adjustment. The patients who do the best (all other variables considered) are those who:

- are counseled preoperatively;
- have a brief hospital stay;
- are satisfied that they have a support system regardless of whether it is needed;
- have their expectations and needs met by the medical profession; and
- have expectations that were the same as the results.

In the case report described the level of complexity was high and there was a long sequence of treatment with disappointments all along the way. In earlier times, treatment was simple. Patients had a laryngectomy, a partial laryngectomy, or radiation quickly after biopsy. Now treatment schemes are complex, such as chemotherapy linked with radiation and operations for salvage. Scans, subsequent biopsies and long waits between phases cause uncertainty. A recent study of coping found several important relationships between complexity of treatment and coping after treatment. Dropkin,[4] an oncology nurse, studied 117 patients for their coping success after treatment. Forty-four of these patients had salvage surgery after radiation or chemotherapy or both. Several important independent variables were related to the treatment sequence. Preoperative chemotherapy, which was related statistically to radiation, significantly reduced the postoperative coping effectiveness. The anticipation of a disfiguring operation was a negative variable. The greater the number of postoperative complications the less effective was subsequent coping ability. I assumed that preoperative radiation or chemotherapy contributes to postoperative complications such as wound infections, fistulas and long hospitalization. In fact, these treatment variables were independent of complications that contributed to length of stay and subsequent coping dysfunction. In other words, the longer the treatment sequence, the longer the hospital stay, the greater the subsequent coping difficulty, even if there were no complications. Lengthy preoperative treatment seriously taxes a patient ability to cope with subsequent operation and later life.

There is evidence that patients and spouses see life issues differently than do health care providers. Mohide *et al.*[10] asked 20 professionals and 20 patients who had a laryngectomy to rate areas of life that seemed most important to adjustment after operation. Patients commented that lifestyle changes and the physical consequences of laryngectomy, such as the stoma and its associated problems, were the most important. The professionals emphasized voice, risk of recurrence, self-image and self-esteem concerns as more important. Such studies emphasize the highly subjective nature of the cancer experience. In the absence of data on preferences, caution is required about professional assumptions about impact of disease and its treatment on quality of life. This is particularly so now when organ preservation schemes with chemotherapy and radiation, when successful, are assumed to enhance a patient's quality of life. There are no data to support such a conclusion.

It is easy to assume that the most important quality-of-life issue is loss of voice. Unfortunately, discussion is hampered by a deficient understanding of what is meant by 'quality of life'. My personal view is that quality of life is much more than just voice quality. It is also more than a permanent stoma. Quality of life is composed of many things: a beautiful sunset, an amenable and loving spouse, admiring and accomplished children, healthy and proximate grandchildren, satisfying work, political and economic security, a grooved golf swing and a descending handicap, time for reflection, spirituality, and many others. Quality of life is certainly not enhanced by waiting for reports, taking chemotherapy, changing dressings or having food go down the wrong way or not going down at all.

One way of looking at the quality of life question is to try to understand the impact of a disease and its treatment on the various roles we have in life. Some of life's roles are those of worker, partner in relationships (such as spouse), and participant in activities including socializing with family and friends. Other aspects of life that are affected by illness are economic and psychologic status.

Our questionnaires

Using two questionnaires, the PAIS (Psychosocial Adjustment to Illness Scale)[1] and an institutionally designed questionnaire (Mayo Clinic Post Laryngectomy Questionnaire), we attempted to learn from patients and spouses the impact that operation for laryngeal cancer had on various areas of their lives. The PAIS questionnaire addresses quality of life. The test consists of 46 questions with four possible responses.

For example, the question 'Has your illness interfered with your ability to do your job?' can be answered:

- no problem;
- some problems, only minor ones;
- some serious problems; or
- illness has totally prevented me from doing my job.

The sequence of possible answers was periodically reversed to counter the possibility of invalid responses. The questions were grouped into seven areas of life experiences (domains):

- health attitudes;
- work or school;
- relationships with spouse;
- sexuality;
- family relationships other than spouse;
- hobbies and activities; and
- psychologic.

The instrument was given to both patients and their spouses or partners at different times. The partner was asked how the patient's illness affected the partner's life. The PAIS questionnaire is not specifically designed for patients with larynx cancer. There is no normal comparison group, that is, the impact of illness cannot be compared with people who are not ill.

The PAIS scores were referenced to a group of other patients with cancer, including breast and lung cancer. The survey group included 111 patients who had a laryngectomy and their partners, 38 patients who had near-total laryngectomy and their partners, and 55 patients who had partial laryngectomy and their partners. These patients were compared with 113 patients with other kinds of cancer. The inventory was scored by domain, and an overall T score and a T score for each domain were generated. A T score of 50 is average for each domain, that is, a patient who had laryngeal cancer surgery with a T score of 50 adjusted no better nor worse than the comparison group of patients. A score of 40 or 60 is 1 standard deviation from the mean. Scores between 40 and 50 reflect psychosocial adjustment superior to the comparison group. The lower the score the better the adjustment. Scores between 50 and 60 reflect adjustment in that domain that is less favorable than that of the comparison group. The higher the score the poorer the adjustment. The group of questions within the domain generated an overall view of adjustment.[3]

The Mayo Clinic Post Laryngectomy Questionnaire focused more on demographics and functional data such as speech, swallowing and general health. The questions in this instrument about adjustment are more direct. The patient should have no ambiguity about the purpose of the question. The patients were self-selected and entrance to the survey was sequential. There were no exclusions, except patients who were dead obviously could not participate. Patients were queried 1–2 years after treatment.

Findings

Overall adjustment

Figure 65.1 compares the domain T scores for the three surgical treatment groups, total, near-total and partial laryngectomy.[3] The extremes of the ranges of T scores varied nearly 2 standard deviations in both directions from a neutral score of 50. Only the patients with partial laryngectomy scored more favorably than the comparison cancer group in all domains. Both the patients with total and those with near-total laryngectomy indicated less satisfactory adjustment in all domains, except for the

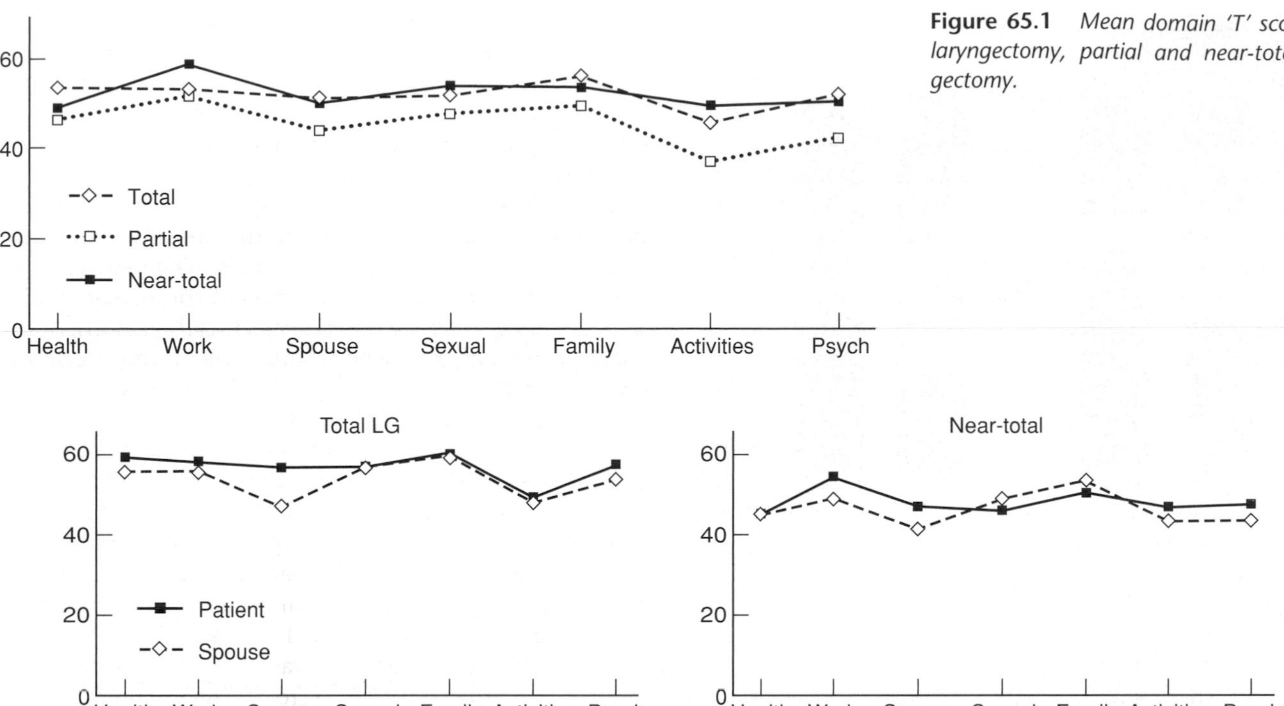

Figure 65.1 *Mean domain 'T' score: total laryngectomy, partial and near-total laryngectomy.*

Figure 65.2 *Patient and spouse domain 'T' scores.*

'activities' domain in the patients with the total laryngectomy. The only domain that was statistically different was the work domain. The patients with total laryngectomy had a score of 53 and those in the near-total group had a composite score of 59. The scores mean that, as a group, the patients with near-total laryngectomy experienced greater difficulty with work than those in the total laryngectomy group. These scores indicate that, as a group, patients with total or near-total laryngectomy have less satisfactory psychosocial adjustment than patients with other and often more serious forms of cancer in terms of prognosis. Patients with partial laryngectomy adjusted better than the comparison patients.

We observed that the psychosocial adjustment in all domains was not much different between the patients with total laryngectomy who had to learn to talk again and patients with near-total laryngectomy who had a built-in speaking fistula. There are no data to explain this finding. One would expect that the patients who could talk without a lot of training would do better. Several conjectures can be made. The first is that the stoma has the biggest impact on adjustment. I believe this to be true. We have always put a strong emphasis on voice quality, but the patients with partial laryngectomy adjusted as a group much better than the total and near-total laryngectomy groups, even with altered voices. A second conjecture is that we promised more than we delivered to the patients with near-total laryngectomy. We stressed that they would be able to talk and eat but we did not dwell enough on the stoma. Expectations were different from the final effect.

Patient and partner adjustment to illness

Figure 65.2 compares patients with permanent stomas and their partner adjustment to illness. The partner scores nearly paralleled the patient scores. A husband's illness affects his spouse's life just as it does his.

Work

A person's occupation during the working years is important for defining self and for acquiring and maintaining self-esteem. For some people, their work is their life. An altered, mechanical, or absent voice with or without a permanent stoma has an impact on a person's work. To what degree is uncertain. In regard to the ability to work, among the 111 patients who had total laryngectomy, we were told that 40% of them had no problems with work. Nearly 20% were either unable to work or had serious difficulty working (Fig 65.3). These percentages were nearly the same as those of patients who had partial laryngectomies (where speech is retained and no permanent stoma is required). After partial laryngectomy, 40% of patients had no trouble with work, about 10% could not work, and the remainder reported minor difficulty with work. In the patients we surveyed who had the near-total operation (voice is retained but a permanent stoma is required), about 15% could not work, about 15% had what they thought were serious problems at work, and the rest (about 70%) reported only minor problems. These findings indicate that work issues are age-related. Patients who must work can continue to work and many of those who can quit working will retire.

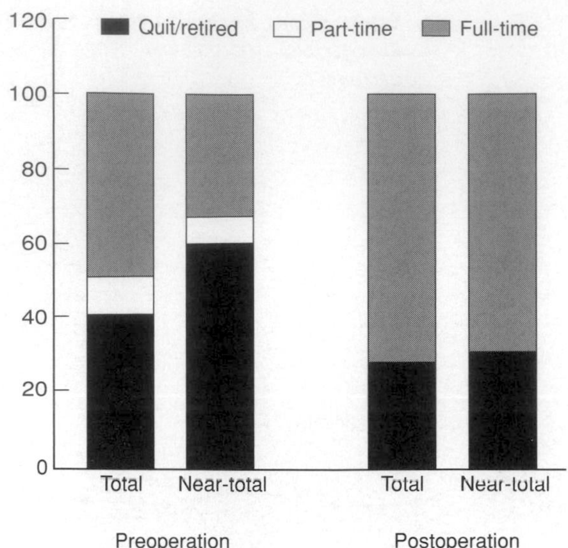

Figure 65.3 *Pre- and postoperation work status.*

We also asked the patients about the economic impact of their operation. About 10% of patients with stomas (total and near-total operation) experienced significant economic consequences from their operation. No patient with a partial operation (no stoma) but with voice alteration noted a severe economic impact of the operation. About 25% of the patients with partial operation noted some negative economic impact after operation. The work issues vary a great deal from one society and economy to another. Social systems and support for physically handicapped persons vary from place to place. In the USA, middle class patients who want to or must work will return to work.

Spousal relationships

Domestic relationships were another area of inquiry. Of patients who had total laryngectomy, more than 90% reported good or at least fair overall relationships with

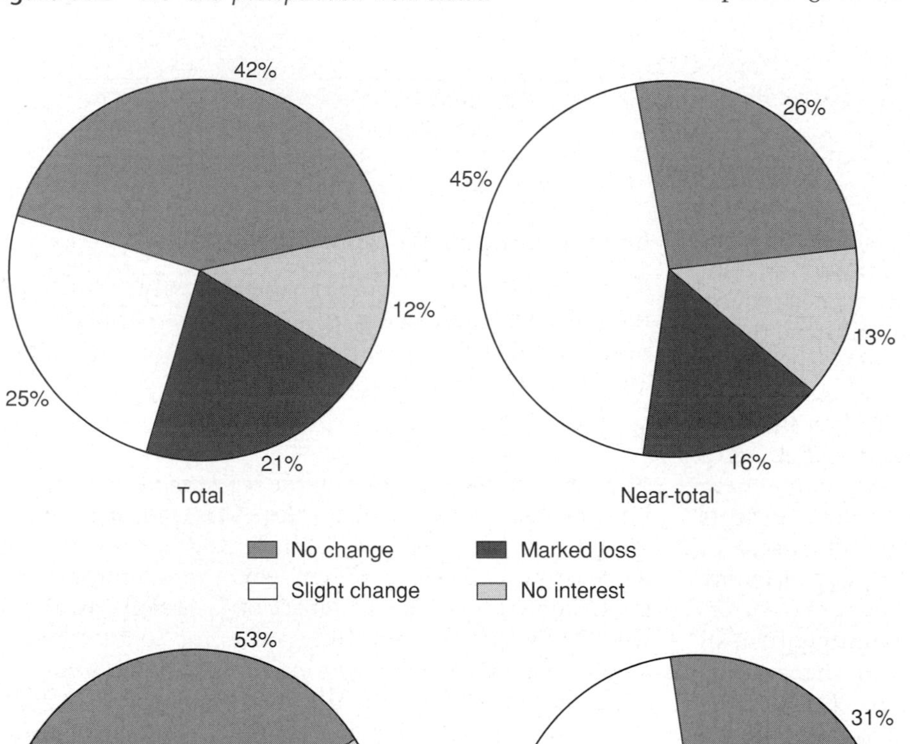

Figure 65.4 *'Have you experienced less sexual interest since surgery?*

Figure 65.5 *'Has your ability to perform sexually changed since surgery?*

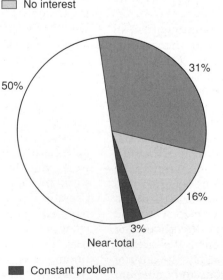

their partner after operation. These percentages were not very different from those reported by patients with less than total operations. One aspect of the domestic relationship that changed in patients with stomas was in sexual activity and sexual performance, which decreased significantly. Whereas 60% of patients with total laryngectomy reported little or no change in sexual activity, 40% had a large decrease or no sexual activity at all. The same percentage of patients with a near-total operation reported a significant decrease in sexual activity. Sexual performance in those who continued to have a sexual dimension to their lives was cited as a problem (Figs 65.4 and 65.5). Twenty percent of patients without stomas noted less sexual performance capability. These findings are consistent with other observations in the literature. Many couples find no change in their sexuality, but others are troubled by the stoma or fear suffocation. We realize that these patients tend to be older but they still have an interest in sex. Most laryngectomy rehabilitation programs ignore human sexuality and focus on speech, but the sexual dimension should be a part of counseling.

Conclusions

A broad view of what patients experience after treatment is evolving. Attention is beginning to be given to the treatment process. Treatment variables such as duration, length of hospitalization, associated morbidity, and speed of convalescence all seem to be important to the patient's ultimate quality of life. Treatment programs that extend for months, have multiple phases, and are physically, financially, and emotionally debilitating must offer a clear survival advantage to be justified. As more studies are done it seems clear that illness and its treatment affects patients' lives forever. Survival after consuming treatment is often a hollow victory.

The first measure of success of treatment of cancer of the larynx is survival. The provision for a lung-powered voice is another goal, as is voice quality. A review of the literature provides no consensus (nor can there be) on whether survival (life) or voice is the preeminent consideration. Some who treat larynx cancer feel that life is more important than voice, others argue that life without a quality voice may not be worth living. Elaborate treatment schemes exist to preserve both life and voice.

The cancer experience is psychologically demanding. Adjustment after treatment is influenced by many variables. Some of them, which the patients bring to their treatment, are age, gender, general health, support systems, economic situation, and coping experience. Other variables are those that the treatment personnel can control. We determine expectations. We are responsible for length of treatment. We can control, to some extent, length of hospitalization and morbidity. We should be able to prevent some complications. Decisions we make, such as using or withholding multimodality programs, influence the duration of treatment, pain and suffering, physical and emotional degradation, complication rates and the length of hospital stay. Treatment programs that continue for months and consume much of a patient's life and programs that have multiple phases and are financially, physically and spiritually debilitating must be justified by an increase in survival. We cannot assume that voice quality is all there is to quality of life. The more negative experiences that patients have, the poorer they will adjust. There will be some lasting impact on their subsequent life. As treatment schemes become more complicated with worthy goals of increasing survival and saving functional larynges, the more we diminish our patients' potential for a high-quality adjustment. An awareness that quality of life is more than avoiding death is a hard message for physicians to learn.

Note: The patient reported at the beginning died of uncontrolled local disease 1 year after his cancer was diagnosed.

References

1. Derogatis LR. The psychosocial adjustment to illness scale (PAIS). *J Psychosom Res* 1986; **30:** 77–91.
2. Derogatis LR, Morrow GR, Fetting J *et al.* The prevalence of psychiatric disorders among cancer patients. *JAMA* 1983; **249:** 751–7.
3. DeSanto LW, Olsen KA, Perry WC, Rohe DE, Keith RL. Quality of life after surgical treatment of cancer of the larynx. *Ann Otol Rhinol Laryngol* 1995; **104:** 763–9.
4. Dropkin MJ. Coping with disfigurement/dysfunction and length of hospital stay after head and neck surgery. *ORL Head Neck Nurs* 1997; **15:** 22–6.
5. Gates GA. Current status of laryngectomy rehabilitation. In: Chretien PB, Johns ME, Shedd DB, Strong EW, Ward PH, eds. *Head and Neck Cancer.* Vol. 1. Philadelphia: BC Decker, 1985: 6–13.
6. Harwood AR, Raawlinson E. The quality of life of patients following treatment for laryngeal cancer. *Int J Radiat Oncol Biol Phys* 1983; **9:** 335–8.
7. Hilgers FJ, Ackerstaff AH, Aaronson NK, Schouwenburg PF, Van Zandwijk N. Physical and psychosocial consequences of total laryngectomy. *Clin Otolaryngol* 1990; **15:** 421–5.
8. Krouse JH, Krouse HJ, Fabian RL. Adaptation to surgery for head and neck cancer. *Laryngoscope* 1989; **99:** 789–94.
9. Metcalfe MC, Fischman SH. Factors affecting the sexuality of patients with head and neck cancer. *Oncol Nurs Forum* 1985; **12:** 21–5.
10. Mohide EA, Archibald SD, Tew M, Young JE, Haines T. Postlaryngectomy quality-of-life dimensions identified by patients and health care professionals. *Am J Surg* 1992; **164:** 619–22.
11. Natvig K. Laryngectomees in Norway. Study No 4. Social, occupational, and personal factors related to vocational rehabilitation. *J Otolaryngol* 1983; **12:** 370–6.
12. Natvig K. Laryngectomees in Norway. Study No 5. Problems of everyday life. *J Otolaryngol* 1984; **13:** 15–22.
13. Olson ML, Shedd DP. Disability and rehabilitation in head and neck cancer patients after treatment. *Head Neck Surg* 1978; **1:** 52–8.

14. Pruyn JF, de Jong PC, Bosman LJ *et al*. Psychosocial aspects of head and neck cancer. A review of the literature. *Clin Otolaryngol* 1986; **11**: 469–74.

15. Schuller DE, Trudeau M, Bistline J, La Face K. Evaluation of voice by patients and close relatives following different laryngeal cancer treatments. *J Surg Oncol* 1990; **44**: 10–14.

Index